7/23/0

To John Seals,

Many happy days of neuroimaging to a fine pediatric neurologist – neuroimager. You have made our seminars very enjoyable – keep coming.

Jack Greenberg M.D.

NEUROIMAGING

NEUROIMAGING

A Companion to ADAMS and VICTOR'S PRINCIPLES OF NEUROLOGY

Second Edition

EDITOR

Jack O. Greenberg, M.D.

Clinical Professor of Neurology
Medical College of Pennsylvania–Hahnemann
Philadelphia, Pennsylvania
Clinical Professor of Neurology
University of South Florida
Tampa, Florida

McGraw-Hill
Health Professions Division

New York St. Louis San Francisco Auckland Bogotá Caracas Lisbon London Madrid
Mexico City Milan Montreal New Delhi San Juan Singapore Sydney Tokyo Toronto

McGraw-Hill
*A Division of The **McGraw-Hill** Companies*

NEUROIMAGING
A Companion to Adams and Victor's Principles of Neurology

1234567890 QPKQPK 99

ISBN 0-07-134615-5

This book was set in Times Roman by The PRD Group, Inc.
The editors were Joseph A. Hefta and Lester A. Sheinis.
The production supervisor was Richard C. Ruzycka.
The text and cover designer was José R. Fonfrias.
The indexer was Alexandra Nickerson.
Quebecor Printing/Kingsport was printer and binder.

This book is printed on acid-free paper.

Cataloging-in-Publication Data is on file for this title at the Library of Congress.

For Gillian Hope Shenkman

CONTRIBUTORS

Abass Alavi, M.D. [10]*
Professor of Radiology, Neurology, and Psychiatry
Chief, Division of Nuclear Medicine
Hospital of the University of Pennsylvania
Philadelphia, Pennsylvania

Luiz Alberto Bacheschi, M.D. [13]
Associate Professor of Neurology
Department of Neurology
School of Medicine
University of São Paolo
São Paolo, Brazil

Rob Ashforth, M.D. [1]
Assistant Clinical Professor
Department of Radiology
University Hospital
Edmonton, Alberta, Canada

Antonio Alci Barone, M.D. [13]

Joseph R. Berger, M.D. [14]
Department of Neurology
University of Kentucky College of Medicine
Lexington, Kentucky

Stefan Bluml, Ph.D. [24]
Huntingdon Medical Research Institute
Pasadena, California

Kelly N. Botteron, M.D. [9]
Departments of Psychiatry and Radiology
Washington University School of Medicine
St. Louis, Missouri

Orest B. Boyko, M.D. [9]
Department of Neuroradiology
Temple University
Philadelphia, Pennsylvania
Ambler, Pennsylvania

* The numbers in brackets following the contributors' names indicate the chapters written or co-written by the contributors.

Joan C. Breen, M.D. [15]
Department of Neurology
Tufts University
Boston, Massachusetts

Louis R. Caplan, M.D. [15]
Neurology Department
Beth Israel Deaconess Hospital
Boston, Massachusetts

Michael E. Charness, M.D. [18]
Department of Neurology (Neuroscience)
Harvard Medical Center
Brigham and Women's Hospital
Boston, Massachusetts
West Roxbury VA Medical Center
West Roxbury, Massachusetts

John B. Chawluk, M.D. [10]
Good Samaritan Regional Medical Center
Pottsville, Pennsylvania

L. Dana DeWitt, M.D. [15]
Department of Neurology
Tufts University
Boston, Massachusetts

M. Judith Donovan Post, M.D. [14]
Professor of Radiology
Department of Radiology
University of Miami School of Medicine
Miami, Florida

Carl Ellenberger, Jr., M.D.
Medical Director
Lebanon Magnetic Imaging
Lebanon, Pennsylvania

Franz Fazekas, M.D. [16]
Professor of Neurology
Department of Neurology
Karl-Franzens University
Graz, Austria

Gary S. Figiel, M.D. [9]
Wesley Woods Geriatric Hospital
and Psychiatric Center
Atlanta, Georgia

Marc Fisher, M.D. [20]
Department of Neurology
Medical Center of Central Massachusetts
University of Massachusetts Medical School
Worcester, Massachusetts

David Friedman, M.D. [4]
Associate Professor of Radiology
Division of Neuroradiology
Thomas Jefferson University Hospital
Philadelphia, Pennsylvania

Jack O. Greenberg, M.D. [12]
Clinical Professor of Neurology
Medical College of Pennsylvania–Hahnemann
Clinical Professor of Neurology
University of South Florida
Tampa, Florida

Camilo R. Gomez, M.D. [25]
University of Alabama at Birmingham
Birmingham, Alabama

David J. Hewitt, M.D. [3]
Neurology Section
Emory University
Atlanta, Georgia

Lawrence Jacobs, M.D. [17]
Professor of Neurology
Buffalo General Hospital
Buffalo, New York

Peter Kapeller, M.D. [16]

Suzan Khoromi, M.D. [11]
Department of Neurology
University of South Florida
College of Medicine
Tampa, Florida

K. Ranga Rama Krishnan, M.D. [9]
Associate Professor of Psychiatry
Head, Division of Biological Psychiatry
Director, Affective Disorders Program
Duke University Medical Center
Durham, North Carolina

Robert M. Levy, M.D., Ph.D.
Associate Professor of Neurosurgery
Northwestern University of Medicine
Chicago, Illinois

Álvardo C. de Almeida Magalhães, M.D. [13]
Associate Professor of Radiology
School of Medicine
University of São Paolo
São Paolo, Brazil

W. R. Wayne Martin, M.D., F.R.C.P.C. [1]
H. M. Toupin Professor of Neurological Sciences
Department of Medicine (Neurology)
University of Alberta
Edmonton, Alberta, Canada

Joseph C. Masdeu, M.D. [2, 21]
Professor and Chairman of Neurology
New York Medical College
New York, New York

Michael K. Matthews, Jr., M.D., Ph.D. [8]
Bala Cynwyd, Pennsylvania

Eduard Michel, M.D., Ph.D. [19]
Department of Neuroradiology
University of Minnesota
Minneapolis, Minnesota

Maromi Nei, M.D. [7]
Fellow in Neurology
Jefferson Medical College
Jefferson Comprehensive Epilepsy Center
Philadelphia, Pennsylvania

Julie Pickholtz, M.D. [8]
Department of Psychiatry
Division of Neuropsychology
Hahnemann School of Medicine
Philadelphia, Pennsylvania

Ilydio Polachini, Jr., M.D. [12, 23]
Director of Neuroimaging
Kalamazoo Neurologic Institute
Kalamazoo, Michigan

Leon D. Prockop, M.D. [11]
Professor and Chairman
Department of Neurology
University of South Florida
College of Medicine
Tampa, Florida

Disya Ratanakorn, M.D. [22]

Laura Vitale Romo, M.D. [6]
Neuroradiologist
Department of Radiology
Massachusetts Eye and Ear Infirmary
Boston, Massachusetts

Brian D. Ross, M.D. [24]
Huntington Medical Research Institute
Pasadena, California

Todd D. Rozen, M.D. [4]
Jefferson Headache Center
Philadelphia, Pennsylvania

Wolf Schaebitz, M.D. [20]
University of Heidelberg Neurology Clinic
Heidelberg, Germany

Holly Shue, M.D. [8]
Head, Division of Biological Psychiatry
Duke University Medical Center
Durham, North Carolina

Stephen D. Silberstein, M.D. [4]
Professor of Neurology
Director, Jefferson Headache Center
Thomas Jefferson University Hospital
Philadelphia, Pennsylvania

Jack H. Simon, M.D. [17]
Associate Professor
Department of Radiology
University of Colorado Health Sciences Center
Denver, Colorado

Barry Snow, M.D. [1]
Department of Neurosciences
Auckland Hospital
Auckland, New Zealand

Michael R. Sperling, M.D. [7]
Associate Professor of Neurology
Director, Epilepsy Center
Jefferson Medical College
Philadelphia, Pennsylvania

Charles H. Tegeler, M.D. [22]
Associate Professor
Department of Neurology
Director of Neurosonology Laboratories
Bowman-Gray School of Medicine
Wake Forest University Medical Center
Winston-Salem, North Carolina

Chip Truwit, M.D. [19]
Department of Neuroradiology
University of Minnesota
Minneapolis, Minnesota

Steven J. Warach, M.D., Ph.D. [18]
Department of Neurology
Harvard Medical School
Beth Israel Hospital
Boston, Massachusetts

Alfred L. Weber, M.D. [6]
Chief of Radiology
Massachusetts Eye and Ear Infirmary
Boston, Massachusetts

Marco A. Zenteno, M.D. [25]
Professor of Radiology
Director, Neuroendovascular Therapy Service
Instituto Nacional de Neurologia
y Neurocirugia
Mexico City, Mexico

PREFACE

As with any worthwhile revision, this new edition of *Neuroimaging* features many exciting changes. Some of the original chapters have additional contributors. Two chapters have been completely revised by individuals considered to be real leaders in their fields, Steve Silberstein in "Headache" and Chip Truwit in "Pediatric Neuroimaging." Three new chapters are also included. Ilydio Polachini, who has been a pioneer in the field of magnetic resonance angiography, has written a stimulating chapter in this area, in addition to helping me revise our chapter on brain tumors. Camilo Gomez has been a bright light for neurologists in the exciting field of interventional neuroimaging and shares his experiences in this area. Finally, a text on magnetic resonance imaging is not complete without spectroscopy. Brian Ross, who has really been an innovator in this field, elucidates this area most completely.

To the skilled neurodiagnostician the manifestations of nervous system activity are readily apparent. The malfunctioning nervous system lends itself to clinical interpretation better than any other organ system. Thus, the single "best test" in the diagnosis of neurologic disorders remains the neurologic history and examination performed by someone trained in such skills.

For almost a century these fundamental techniques have led to a "differential" diagnosis of the cause of symptoms, but in many cases, the exact nature of the suspected lesion was not revealed until its exposure at the operating table or in the autopsy room. By midcentury, the arteriogram and pneumoencephalogram were developed to guide the surgeon, but these invasive, painful, and risky procedures usually provided only hints of the size, location, and relationship of lesions to normal structures. In the early 1970s, new imaging techniques began to reveal, in living patients, unprecedented information about brain structure and disease. Computed tomography (CT) scanning was a quantum leap in detecting pathology that causes morphologic change. Even more exciting is the ongoing development of magnetic resonance imaging (MRI); MRI provides almost a "live autopsy" for the clinician. Not only can we obtain images with superb morphologic accuracy and detail, but we have begun to "see" biochemical and pathophysiologic processes. MRI is now the mainstay of imaging diagnosis of many neurologic diseases. Signal characteristics, as well as morphologic changes, have become a basis for sound clinical, pathologic, and biochemical correlations. Happily, MRI and CT pose little risk to the patient, but their expense requires that they be used selectively and efficiently. The latter task remains the role of the astute clinician, who must also interpret the meaning of the many findings of these exquisitely sensitive techniques and decide upon their relevance to the patient's current symptoms and lifetime well-being.

Conventional MRI is only one part of this new adventure for the clinician. Functional MRI may surpass other diagnostic techniques in revealing pathophysiology as well as pathology of brain disorders. Carotid ultrasound, color flow imaging, and transcranial Doppler are informative, cost-efficient, safe modalities utilized in the workup of patients with vascular lesions of the brain. In addition, MR spectroscopy, flow imaging techniques, MR angiography (MRA), single photon emission tomography (SPECT), and positron emission tomography (PET) are also important to the neurodiagnostician. They are covered generally and specifically in several chapters of this book.

The leading textbook of neurology for many years has been Adams and Victor's *Principles of Neurology.* In 1997, the sixth edition was a welcomed update. This classic book presents the clinical phenomena resulting from physiologic and pathologic changes in the nervous system, in conformity with the Oslerian method.

When approached by McGraw-Hill to be the editor of an imaging companion to Adams and Victor's *Principles of Neurology,* I welcomed the opportunity. Neuroimaging has evolved so rapidly that a separate companion to this text would provide readers with the additional information necessary in this important area. Another reason for accepting this task was that I knew the people who could do it. Contributors to this volume are all highly experienced in their fields. Eight of them are radiologists who are imaging full-time, as are several of the authors who are neurologists. Still others are neurologists and psychiatrists who are specialists in fields where they utilize imaging with expertise. As Dr. Adams and Dr. Victor stated, "The sequence of symptoms to syndrome to disease recapitulates the rational process by which the neurologist makes a diagnosis." It is felt that having *clinicians* write about the use of imaging in their various areas of expertise would aid the reader in this exercise.

We have tried to follow the outline of Dr. Adams and Dr. Victor's book as closely as possible. Our book differs from all other textbooks of imaging in that it is correlated with a standard textbook of neurology. It is hoped that practitioners and residents in neurology, neurosurgery, psychiatry, and radiology and all students of the nervous system will find this to be a true companion to what is considered a neurologic classic.

JACK O. GREENBERG, M.D.

ACKNOWLEDGMENTS

I am particularly grateful to my past teachers in neurology and neuroimaging, from whom I have had inspiration and excellent teaching. This includes the late Dr. William Oldendorf, who inspired me to go into the field of neurology and, later, neuroimaging. The late Dr. John Sullivan of Boston and Dr. Hugh Garland of Leeds, England, were both master neurologic clinicians who guided me through my early neurologic training. I am indebted to Dr. Murray Solomon and Dr. William Bradley, both neuroradiologists, who taught me magnetic resonance imaging and continue as leaders in this field.

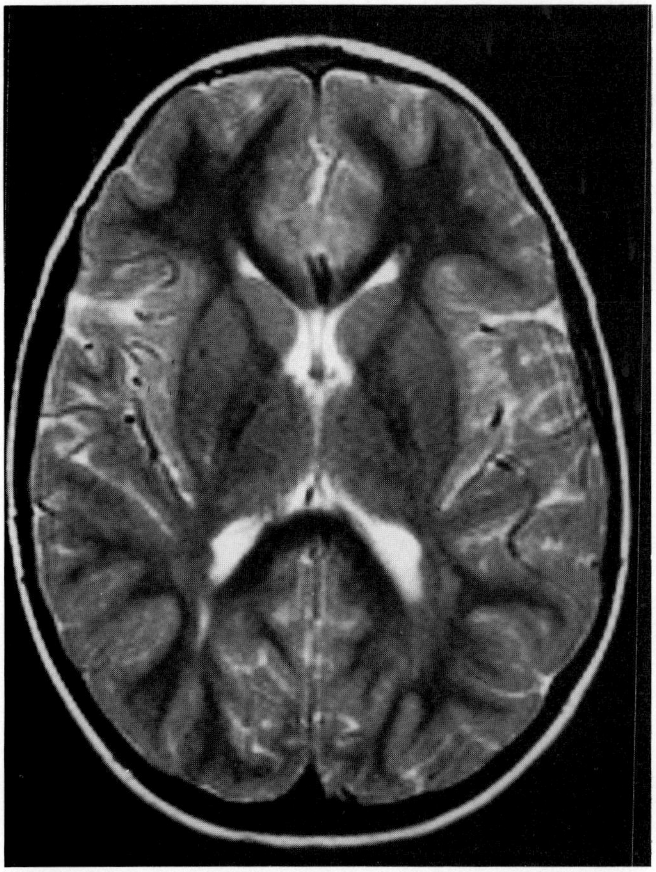

Figure 1-2
Normal transverse T2-weighted MRI. The globus pallidus has lower signal than does the putamen because of the accumulation of iron in the globus pallidus.

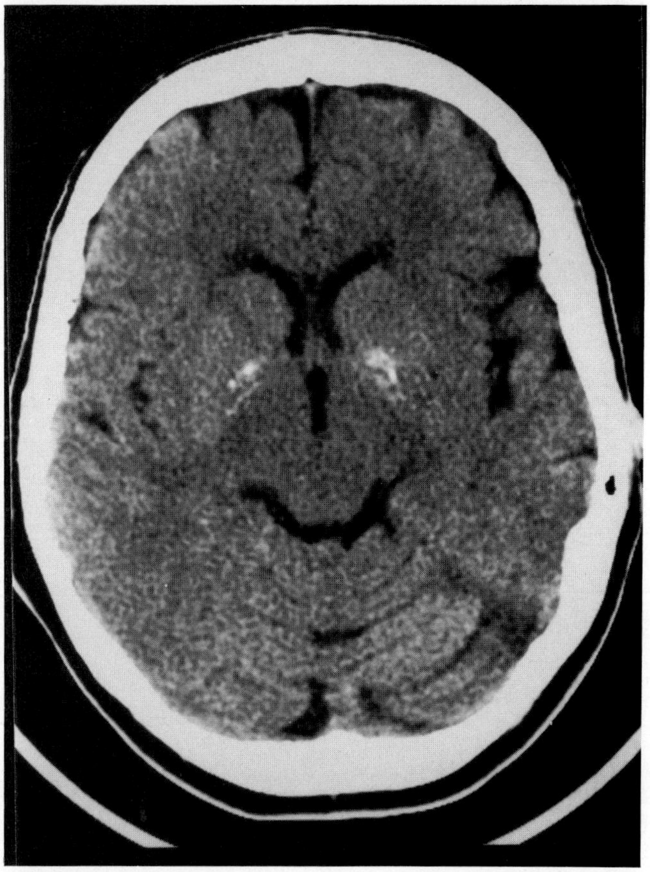

Figure 1-3
Normal transverse CT image. Note physiologic calcification in the globus pallidus bilaterally.

common cause of this is Fahr disease (familial idiopathic cerebral calcification), which can present with various movement disorders, seizures, dementia, ataxia, and pyramidal tract signs. This disorder has an unknown etiology and tends to be slowly progressive.

In contrast to CT, calcified areas may be difficult to identify with MRI. Because of the lack of mobile hydrogen atoms, calcific deposits appear on MRI as foci of diminished signal intensity on T1-weighted, T2-weighted, and proton-density pulse sequences. When calcification is the only abnormality seen with CT, it often goes undetected on MRI.[4]

The functional anatomy of the striatum is well demonstrated with PET studies of cerebral metabolism and blood flow. Like all interneuronal synaptic connections, the connections in the striatum are highly active metabolically. As a result, the head of the caudate nucleus and the putamen are easily seen on high-resolution images of regional glucose and oxygen metabolism (Fig. 1-4). Because regional cerebral metabolism tends to be coupled with regional cerebral blood flow, the striatum is also readily seen on images of regional perfusion. The resolution of current PET systems does not permit the direct identification of the globus pallidus or smaller basal ganglia structures such as the subthalamic nucleus and the substantia nigra. The functional anatomy of the dopaminergic system is readily seen with ligands that bind to presynaptic nigrostriatal terminals (Fig. 1-5A) or D2 dopamine receptors (Fig. 1-5B).

Table 1-1
Causes of symmetrical calcification of the basal ganglia

Physiologic
Hypoparathyroidism (including pseudohypoparathyroidism)
Hyperparathyroidism (?)
Familial idiopathic cerebral calcification (Fahr syndrome)
Birth anoxia
Carbon monoxide intoxication
Lead poisoning
Tuberous sclerosis
Cockayne syndrome
Postinfectious (cytomegalic inclusion disease, measles, varicella, toxoplasmosis)
Acquired immune deficiency syndrome
Radiation therapy
Methotrexate therapy
Kearns-Sayre syndrome and other mitochondrial diseases
Down syndrome

From Ref. 80.

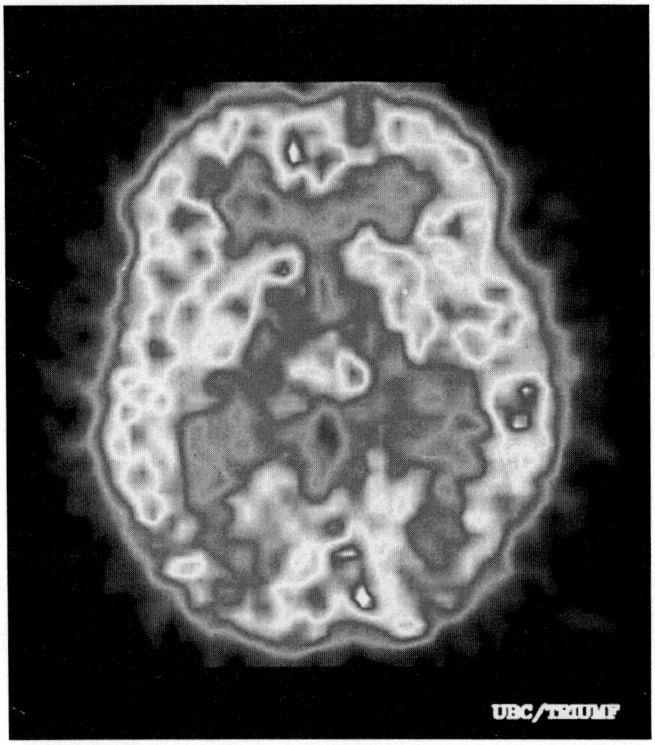

Figure 1-4 (Plate 1)
Normal PET scan of glucose metabolism. Note the high metabolic rate in cortex and deep gray matter structures. White matter has a low metabolic rate and cannot be separated from the ventricle at this resolution.

DISORDERS CHARACTERIZED BY HYPOKINESIA AND BRADYKINESIA

These disorders are characterized clinically by a poverty of movement (hypokinesia or akinesia), slowness of movement (bradykinesia), and increased tone (rigidity); this explains the use of the term *akinetic-rigid syndrome.* Although the presence of these clinical manifestations implies impaired function of the basal ganglia, structural abnormalities are only rarely demonstrated with CT or MRI. In an akinetic-rigid patient with purely unilateral signs and symptoms, neuroimaging may demonstrate pathologic changes in the basal ganglia on the contralateral side.

Parkinson Disease

The most common cause of the akinetic-rigid syndrome is Parkinson disease (PD). The diagnosis of PD is based on the characteristic clinical syndrome: varying combinations of resting tremor, rigidity, and bradykinesia or hypokinesia. PD is characterized neuropathologically by a loss of dopaminergic nigrostriatal neurons from the pars compacta of the substantia nigra. This cell loss leads to a dramatic depletion in dopamine concentration in the striatum, particularly the putamen. Structural imaging may be of value in a patient with an unusual

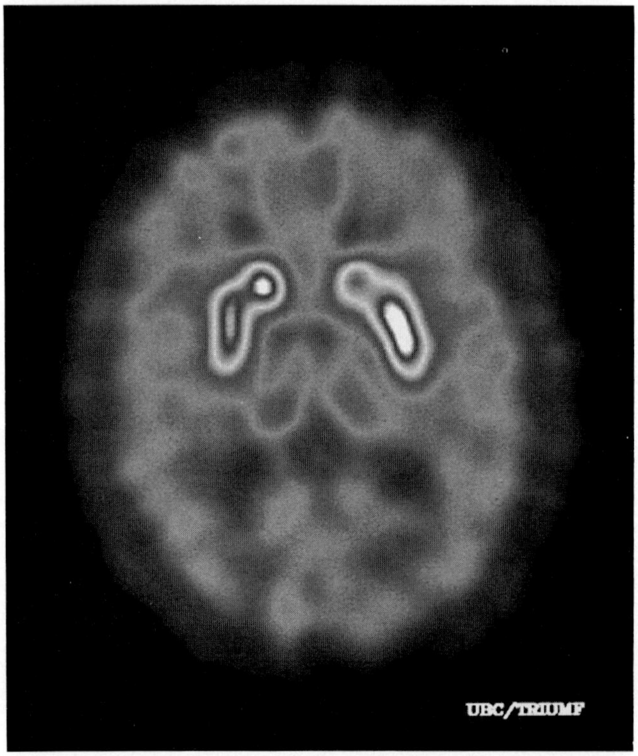

A

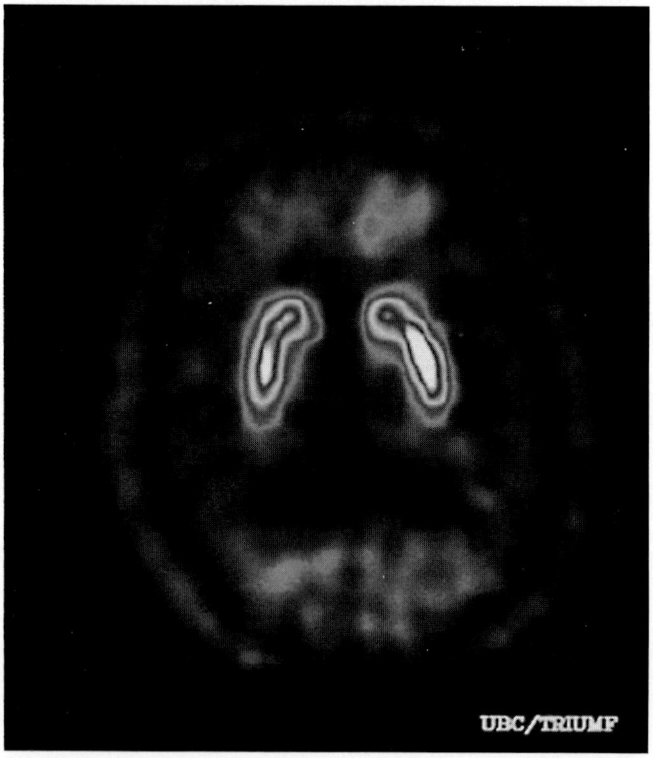

B

Figure 1-5 (Plates 2 and 3)
PET images of the normal dopaminergic system. **(A)** *Fluorodopa uptake showing normally functioning presynaptic neuronal endings in the caudate and putamen.* **(B)** *Raclopride uptake showing normal accumulation of this D2 receptor binding ligand, implying normally functioning D2 receptors.*

degree of asymmetry in clinical manifestations to rule out a contralateral structural lesion, but in most patients these techniques have not revealed significant abnormalities and have not played a major role in diagnosis.

High-field-strength MRI systems produce a detailed image of the midbrain, and the substantia nigra is readily visualized by virtue of its high iron content and the T2* effect. Some investigators have reported midbrain abnormalities in PD patients in the form of narrowing or smudging of the high signal region that separates the substantia nigra from the red nucleus.[1,2] The demonstration of these changes may ultimately be of diagnostic (or prognostic) value, but current systems are not sufficiently sensitive for routine clinical application. Although nigral changes in PD are readily detected in population studies, technical factors such as slice thickness, image averaging, and positioning make it difficult to define these abnormalities with certainty in individual patients.

The absence of major abnormalities with structural imaging techniques is consistent with the absence of gross neuropathologic changes in PD. In view of the prominent neurochemical findings, one would anticipate significant changes in basal ganglia function with appropriate methods of functional imaging. Abnormalities of cerebral metabolism and blood flow have been demonstrated with PET in the basal ganglia of patients with predominantly unilateral PD.[5] These studies suggest abnormal pallidal function opposite the most severely affected limbs. The presence of consistent abnormalities in patients with bilateral parkinsonism is less clear. In general, PET studies of cerebral metabolism are of little clinical utility in confirming a diagnosis of PD, although they may reveal cortical or striatal changes that suggest an alternative diagnosis (see below).

The pathology of PD affects primarily the nigrostriatal pathway. Hence, any PET tracer whose uptake is dependent on normal nigrostriatal function would be expected to show abnormalities in PD. Indeed, uptake of the levodopa analog 6-fluorodopa, which requires decarboxylation and intravesicular trapping within functionally intact nigrostriatal nerve endings, is decreased markedly in PD patients.[5,6] The depletion is most marked in the posterior striatum, consistent with postmortem neurochemical studies that indicate that the dopamine depletion is most marked in the putamen [Fig. 1-6A (Plate 4)]. While 6-fluorodopa remains the standard tracer for PET imaging of the presynaptic dopaminergic system, new tracers add valuable extra information. After decarboxylation of levodopa, dopamine is stored in vesicles in the presynaptic nerve terminals. Dihydrotetrabenazine binds to these vesicles, providing a measure of the relative density of the nerve terminals.[7] The advantage of this tracer is that it may not be subject to regulatory changes, as may be the case with fluoro-

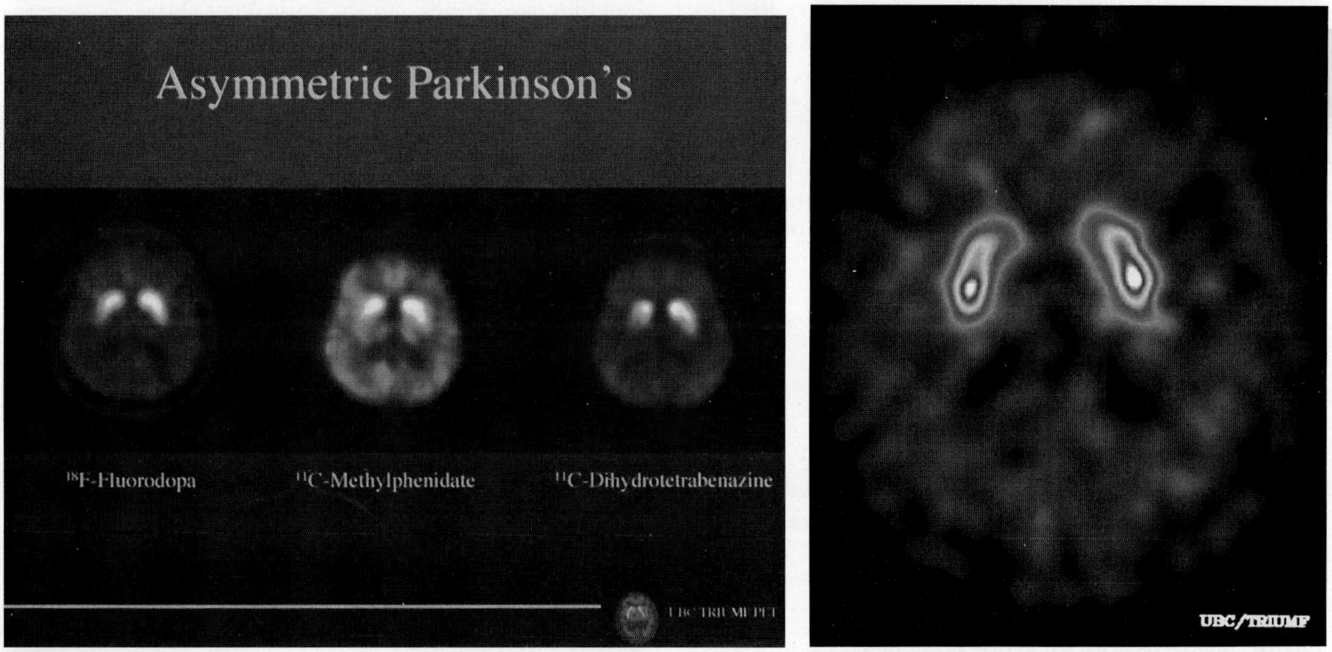

A B

Figure 1-6 (Plates 4 and 5)
PET images in Parkinson disease. **(A)** *Asymmetrical Parkinson disease with decreased tracer uptake in the left posterior striatum. The fluorodopa image indicates reduced decarboxylation of fluorodopa, the methylphenidate image the density of presynaptic dopamine reuptake sites, and the dihydrotetrabenazine image the density of dopamine-containing vesicles in dopaminergic nerve terminals (compare with Fig. 1-5A).* **(B)** *Raclopride binding showing increased uptake in the posterior striatal region (compare with Fig. 1-5B).*

dopa. After release into the dopaminergic synapse, dopamine is taken up by the presynaptic terminal. The dopamine reuptake site may be imaged with PET by using methylphenidate or various cocaine analogs.[8–10] Similar studies can be performed with single photon emission computed tomography (SPECT) and appropriately labeled cocaine analogs.[11] These techniques appear to be sensitive to changes in early PD and ultimately may prove to be clinically useful in the investigation of patients with mild symptoms in whom the diagnosis is uncertain. The distribution of striatal dopaminergic function may discriminate PD from other forms of parkinsonism, especially progressive supranuclear palsy, in which there seems to be a more generalized loss of striatal dopaminergic function (see below).

It may be possible to assess neural transplant function in PD with fluorodopa-PET. After adrenal medullary tissue transplantation into the striatum of patients with PD, a procedure that has demonstrated little clinical efficacy, fluorodopa uptake does not increase.[12] In contrast, after fetal mesencephalic tissue implantation, there has been clinical improvement associated with increased fluorodopa uptake.[13]

In untreated PD, there is an increase in specific binding of the dopamine D2 antagonist raclopride, indicating an upregulation of D2 receptors (Fig. 1-6C).[14] Treated patients probably have normal D2 receptor numbers, whereas advanced PD patients who have motor fluctuations may have reduced raclopride binding. The demonstration of increased D2 antagonist binding with PET or SPECT in an untreated patient with mild parkinsonism provides supportive evidence for a diagnosis of idiopathic PD.

Although PD traditionally has been considered a disorder of motor function, many investigators have described cognitive changes in a significant number of patients. Studies of glucose metabolism with PET have shown diffuse cortical hypometabolism in all patients with PD but more marked hypometabolism affecting parietotemporal cortex in patients with PD and dementia.[15] Similar changes in regional cerebral perfusion have been demonstrated with SPECT.[16] This focal decrease in metabolism and blood flow is similar to the cortical changes seen in Alzheimer disease and may indicate some commonality between these two disorders or perhaps the coexistence of two age-related disease processes.

Other Neurodegenerative Causes of Parkinsonism

Progressive Supranuclear Palsy

Progressive supranuclear palsy (PSP) is characterized pathologically by neurofibrillary tangles distributed through the brainstem. The substantia nigra is involved, and these patients usually present with parkinsonism. In addition, the striatum is affected, and perhaps for this reason these patients often respond poorly to levodopa. Involvement of other midbrain pathways is responsible for the characteristic gaze palsy of PSP. Fluorodopa-PET shows reduced striatal uptake affecting the whole striatum (in contrast to the reduction in PD, which is maximal in the putamen).[17] In addition to the motor signs, in PSP there is claimed to be a distinctive pattern of dementia, suggesting impairment of frontal lobe function. Imaging of cerebral glucose metabolism with PET demonstrates cortical changes consistent with this pattern of dementia, with a depression in the frontal cortex metabolic rate (Fig. 1-7).[18,19] These cortical changes are significantly different from those of PD and Alzheimer disease.

Structural imaging in PSP reveals atrophy of the midbrain with a dilated cerebral aqueduct and enlarged perimesencephalic cisterns (Fig. 1-8).[20] An increased signal in periaqueductal regions is seen occasionally, coincident with the neuropathologic finding of gliosis in this region. Some patients presenting with PSP may have vascular disease rather than an idiopathic neurodegenerative disorder. As many as 33 percent of patients with a clinical presentation of PSP (versus 13 percent of patients with PD) have had multiple cerebral infarcts reported on CT or MRI.[21]

Multiple System Atrophy

Multiple system atrophy (MSA) is a general term that includes conditions whose pathology shows degeneration of neurons in the pons, cerebellum, olivae, substan-

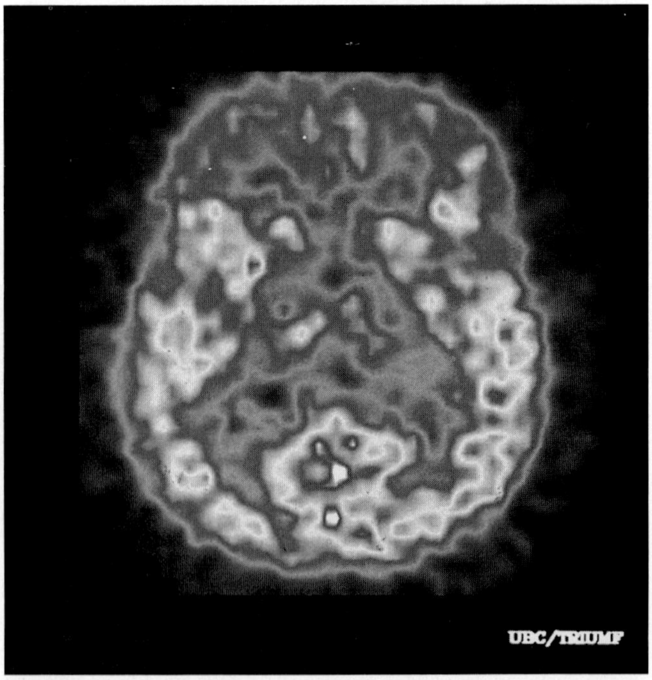

Figure 1-7 (Plate 6)
PET scan from a patient with progressive supranuclear palsy showing decreased glucose metabolism in frontal cortex.

caudate and putamen, with resultant striatal atrophy. As early as 1936, pneumoencephalography was used to demonstrate focal caudate atrophy in advanced HD. The diagnosis, however, has remained primarily clinical, based on a positive family history and the characteristic neurologic and/or psychiatric manifestations.

Structural imaging in HD shows nonspecific changes of caudate atrophy in the intermediate and more advanced stages of the disease. Various indexes have been developed with CT for quantifying the caudate changes.[40] In general, these indexes have referenced the distance between the medial surfaces of the caudate heads (bicaudate diameter) to other structures, such as the width of the outer table of the skull (at the same level as the bicaudate diameter) or the frontal horns (also at the same level). There are substantial differences in these indexes between normal subjects and patients with advanced HD. Caudate atrophy is more readily demonstrated with MRI because of its superior spatial resolution and the ability to perform direct coronal imaging (Fig. 1-13A). Putamen volume reduction on MRI appears to exceed caudate changes in mild disease.[41] In early HD, however, before the development of significant striatal atrophy, routine imaging with CT and MRI is usually normal. These techniques are therefore of little value in a mildly affected patient with suspected disease or an asymptomatic individual who is at risk for HD by virtue of having an affected parent. There is some evidence, however, that quantitation of basal ganglia volume with MRI may be of added benefit, including a recent report that measurable basal ganglia atrophy may precede the development of symptomatic HD.[42]

Other abnormalities on MRI have been reported. These abnormalities include increased signal intensity in both caudate and putamen on T2-weighted images in the rigid form of HD[43] and, with high-field-strength magnets, decreased signal in the globus pallidus and striatum (Fig. 1-13B and C).[2,44] Cortical atrophy has been reported on CT, usually beginning in frontal regions and progressing posteriorly with disease progression.[45] Cognitive change has been shown to correlate with the degree of cortical atrophy.

The ability to measure regional cerebral metabolism with PET represents a major advance in the ability to demonstrate striatal changes in HD.[40] A characteristic decrease in striatal metabolism precedes the development of atrophy (Fig. 1-13D).[46–48] PET therefore can demonstrate clear changes in HD while CT and MRI still appear normal. The demonstration of striatal hypometabolism with PET correlates more closely with the presence of symptomatic HD than does the demonstration of striatal hypoperfusion with SPECT.[49] Striatal hypometabolism is not specific for HD, however. It is also seen in neuroacanthocytosis,[50] benign hereditary chorea,[51] Lesch-Nyhan syndrome,[52] and striatonigral degeneration.[25] Clinical information is required to adequately interpret the presence of the striatal metabolic changes seen with PET. Nevertheless, in appropriately selected patients, that is, those with a positive family history with early symptoms consistent with HD and minimal caudate atrophy, impaired striatal metabolism provides clinically useful supportive evidence for a diagnosis of HD. Similarly, since only the rare symptomatic patient will have preserved striatal metabolism, a normal PET scan in a patient with definite neurologic signs makes a diagnosis of HD very unlikely. PET also shows cortical changes in symptomatic HD with hypometabolism that is most marked in frontal cortex.[53,54]

Some investigators have reported the presence of striatal hypometabolism in individuals at risk for HD before the development of objective neurologic abnormalities.[55,56] There is some evidence, however, of a close temporal relationship between the development of clinical symptomatology and the appearance of impaired striatal metabolism. Individuals are not likely to have striatal changes preceding neurologic features for a prolonged period.

Other Causes of Generalized Chorea

Neuroacanthocytosis is a slowly progressive familial disorder that is characterized by abnormal involuntary movements, including chorea, dystonia, and tics; parkinsonism; peripheral neuropathy; and a peripheral smear containing acanthocytes. The findings on neuroimaging are similar to those of HD. Caudate atrophy is present on CT or MRI; increased signal from the striatum has been reported with MRI.[57,58] PET scans show striatal glucose hypometabolism, decreased fluorodopa uptake in the posterior striatum (similar to that seen in PD), and a loss of dopamine D2 receptors from the striatum.[50,59]

Benign hereditary chorea is an autosomal dominant disorder that is characterized by chorea with an early onset and little or no progression. In contrast to HD, there is no significant mental deterioration. PET scans often show reduced caudate metabolism similar to that seen in HD.[51]

Any metabolic or toxic disorder that affects the basal ganglia can be associated with chorea, but in most of these disorders structural and functional imaging remains unaffected. In chorea associated with *systemic lupus erythematosus,* for example, striatal glucose metabolism remains normal.[60]

Dystonia

Dystonia is characterized by slower, more sustained movements, often of a twisting nature, usually resulting in an abnormal posture of the affected body part. The term *dystonia* has come to describe an objective neurologic sign that may be present in a variety of basal ganglia disorders as well as a disease process that may be considered either primary (idiopathic) or secondary dystonia.

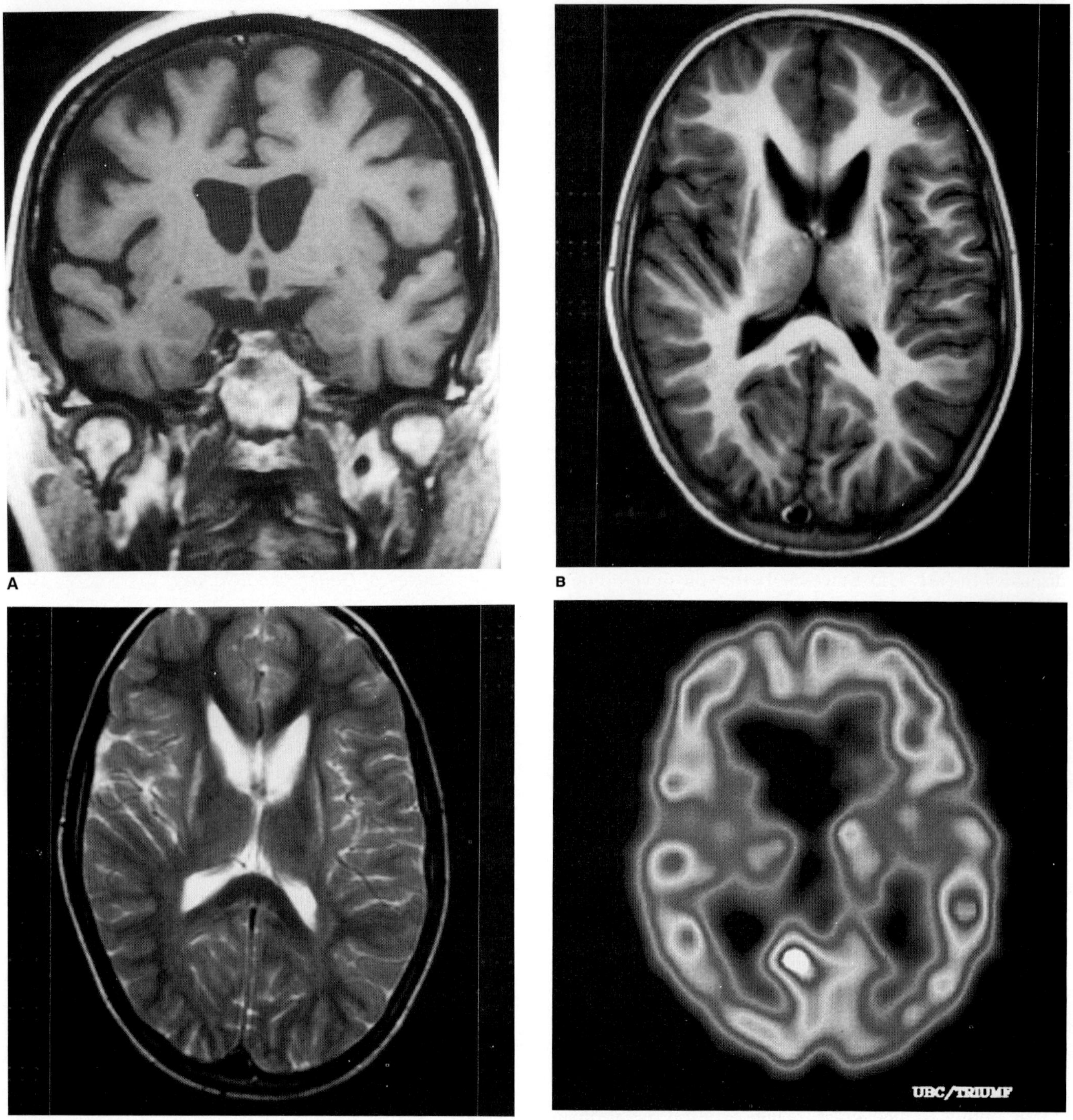

A B C D (Plate 8)

Figure 1-13
Huntington disease. **(A)** *Coronal MRI showing marked atrophy of the head of the caudate nucleus, associated with ventricular enlargement.* **(B and C)** *Transverse MRI from a patient with juvenile-onset Huntington disease. Note decreased signal in the putamen on the T1-weighted image* **(B),** coinciding with increased signal on the T2-weighted image **(C).** **(D)** *PET image of glucose metabolism. Note decreased metabolism in the caudate and putamen.*

Primary Dystonia

The idiopathic form of the disorder does not have a known neuropathologic correlate and is not associated with structural changes on CT or MRI. Although impaired basal ganglia function is assumed, PET studies generally have been unimpressive and inconsistent.

Secondary Dystonia

Dystonia may be secondary to numerous different metabolic disorders, many of which are inherited. An ever-increasing series of CT and MRI reports have implicated abnormalities in the region of the basal ganglia in many of these conditions. The changes seen with these structural imaging techniques, however, are seldom specific in regard to the precise etiology of the disorder. At present, the major role of neuroimaging in the investigation of generalized dystonia is in the depiction of structural lesions. The literature is replete with reports of various forms of dystonia occurring in association with focal lesions on MRI or CT. The presence of these lesions in a dystonic patient suggests the presence of secondary dystonia, but not all patients with the secondary form have lesions that are visible on CT or MRI. Even when lesions are visible, additional investigations usually are required to determine the nature of the underlying disease process.

The most frequently seen structural change associated with generalized dystonia is bilateral striatal necrosis (Table 1-2). *Subacute necrotizing encephalopathy* (Leigh disease) is associated with infantile onset, dystonia (as well as other neurologic signs), and bilateral symmetrical hypodensities in the putamen and caudate as well as the hypothalamus and areas adjacent to the fourth ventricle (Fig. 1-14A and B).[61] A similar CT-MRI appearance has been associated with a progressive generalized dystonia occurring in older patients (Fig. 1-15A and B), sometimes associated with an optic neuropathy, and may be secondary to a *mitochondrial encephalopathy*.[62]

Wilson disease is a very important diagnostic consideration in all patients who present with dystonia in childhood, adolescence, or young adulthood. This autosomal recessive disorder of copper metabolism is associated with two different clinical presentations. In one form dystonia is the prominent neurologic feature, whereas in the other form parkinsonism with tremor, rigidity, and bradykinesia is dominant. On CT or MRI, striatal lesions may be seen in more advanced patients, primarily affecting the putamen (Fig. 1-16A and B). On long TR images, a combination of high signal and low signal changes may be seen in the striatum, with the former presumed to be secondary to gliosis, edema, and/or necrosis and the latter probably being due to accumulation of copper or another paramagnetic substance.[63] Extensive striatal damage may be evident in patients with severe dystonia more than it is in patients with parkinsonism. Midbrain atrophy is commonly seen. T2-weighted midbrain images reveal a characteristic "face of the giant panda" sign that consists of high signal intensity in the tegmentum except for the red nucleus, preservation of signal intensity of the lateral portion of the pars reticulata of the substantia nigra, and hypointensity of the superior colliculus.[64] PET scans have shown decreased glucose metabolism in frontal and parietal cortex and white matter and in caudate and lenticular nuclei.[65] In Wilson disease patients the greatest focal hypometabolism is in the lenticular nucleus. Striatal fluorodopa uptake is also decreased in some patients, particularly in the putamen, indicating a nigrostriatal dopaminergic defect.[66]

Hallervorden-Spatz disease (HSD) is an autosomal recessive disorder, often with prominent dystonia but also with other neurologic abnormalities, including men-

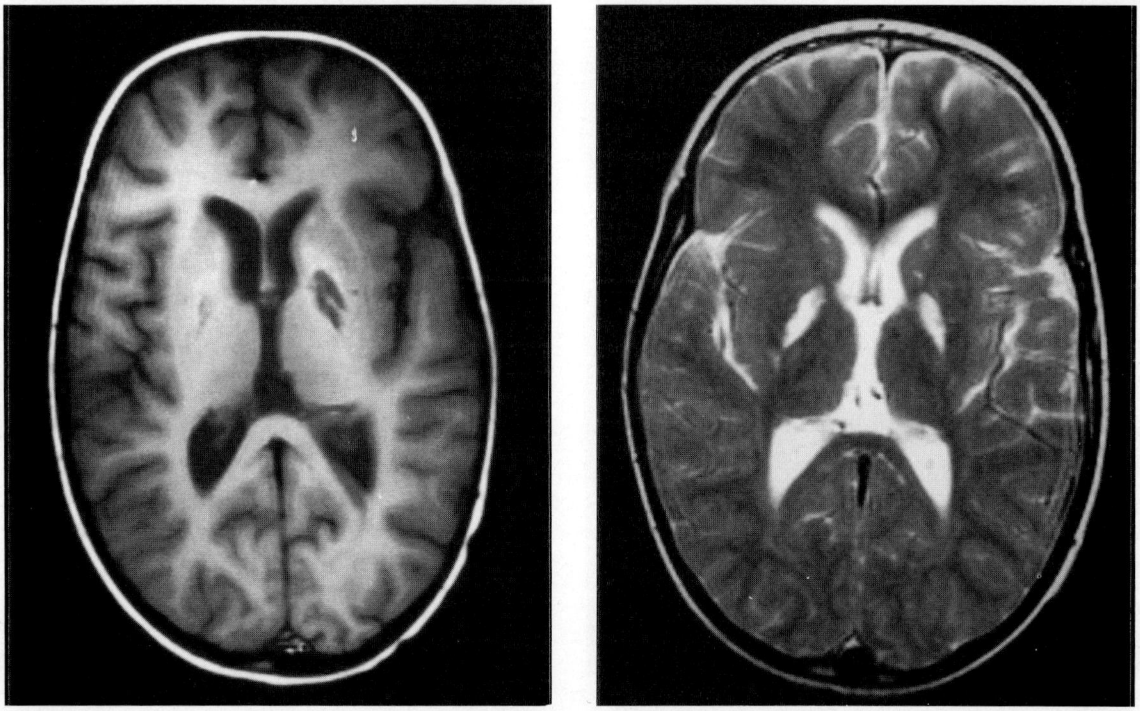

A **B**

Figure 1-14
Transverse MRIs from a 7-year-old child with Leigh disease. Note decreased signal in the globus pallidus on the T1-weighted image **(A)** *and increased signal on the T2-weighted image* **(B).**

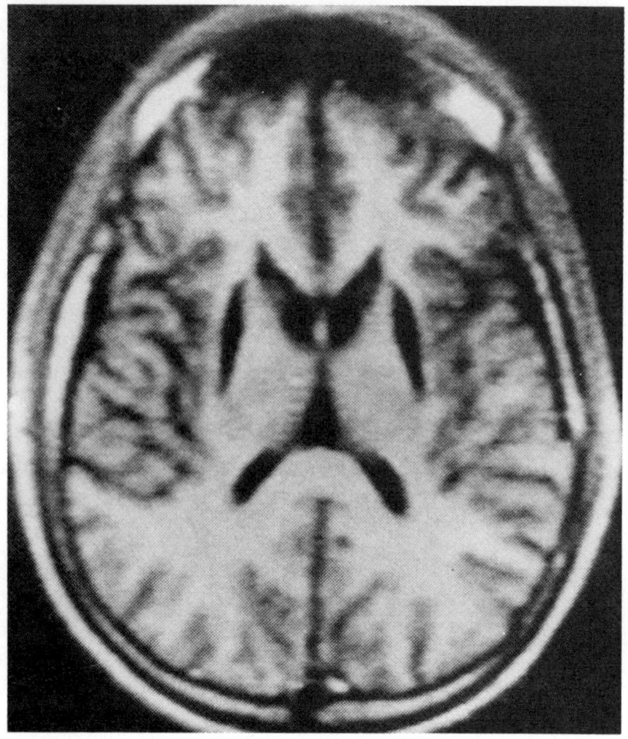

A B

Figure 1-15
MRIs from an adult with dystonia of unknown etiology showing bilateral lucencies in the putamen on transverse **(A)** *and coronal* **(B)** *scans. (Used with permission from Ref. 84.)*

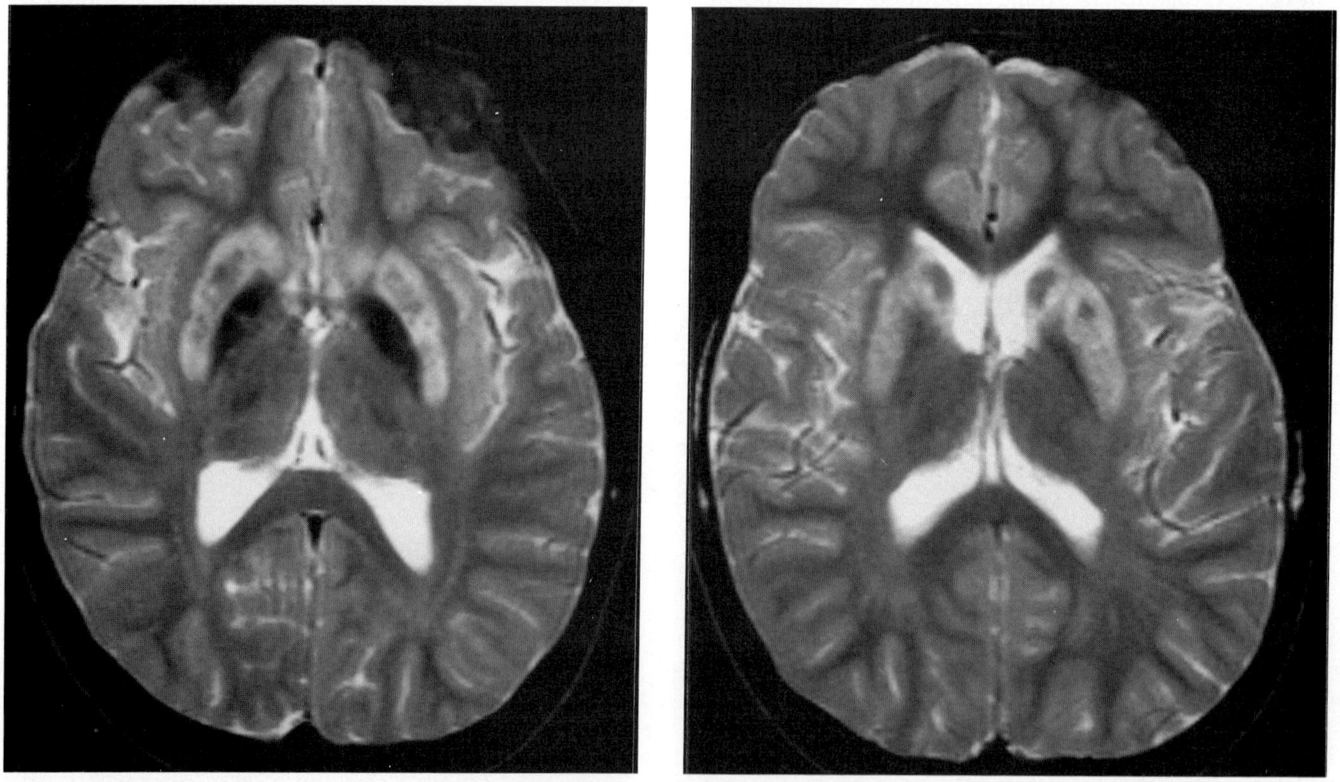

A B

Figure 1-16
Transverse T2-weighted MRIs from two adjacent levels in a patient with Wilson disease. Note the decreased signal in the globus pallidus associated with heterogeneous signal increase in the caudate and putamen.

tal retardation, seizures, parkinsonism, spasticity, ataxia, and optic atrophy. It was difficult to diagnose on a clinical basis in the past. CT findings are nonspecific, showing primarily caudate atrophy, although increased density in the globus pallidus secondary to increased iron content also has been reported.[67] In contrast, MRI can show a very distinctive picture that is highly suggestive of this disorder in the appropriate clinical setting. There is pronounced low signal in the pallidum (caused by iron accumulation), particularly prominent on gradient echo images, with a small central high signal area, the "eye of the tiger" sign (Fig. 1-17).[68]

Unilateral Hyperkinetic Disorders

These syndromes are usually described according to the clinical characteristics of the involuntary movements. Therefore, terms such as *hemiballismus, hemichorea,* and *hemidystonia* refer to the symptomatology rather than to a specific disease process. The presence of one of these unilateral syndromes strongly suggests a structural abnormality in the region of the basal ganglia contralateral to the involuntary movement. Investigations therefore should be directed toward the demonstration of the responsible anatomic lesion.

Hemiballismus refers to a unilateral, often disabling disorder that is characterized by violent, flinging movements of the arm and leg. These symptoms are known to result from a focal lesion of the contralateral subthalamic nucleus, although they also may occur in conjunction with lesions in the caudate, putamen, globus pallidus, precentral gyrus, or thalamic nuclei.[69] Hemiballismus occurs most commonly as a result of a vascular lesion but also has been described with tumors, infection, head trauma, and demyelination and as a result of stereotactic surgery for PD. MRI is more sensitive than CT for small lesions and has been reported to show evidence of lacunar infarction in the lateral subthalamic nucleus in patients with hemiballismus and normal CT scans.[70] Hemiballismus occurring in Sydenham chorea has been reported to be associated with high signal changes on T2-weighted images in the contralateral striatum, pallidum, perirubral area, and substantia nigra.[71]

Hemidystonia is characterized by slower, more sustained dystonic movements and postures. Hemidystonia must be distinguished clinically from the more common syndromes of focal dystonia. In hemidystonia both upper and lower limbs are involved, whereas in focal dystonia only a single muscle group is affected. In contrast to the hemidystonias, the focal dystonias are rarely associated with structural damage. Lesions involving striatopallidothalamic pathways, or pathways between the thalamus and the premotor cortex, are the most commonly described lesions in hemidystonic patients.[72,73] Striatopallidal lesions may more likely be associated with dystonia itself, while thalamic lesions can be associated with the combination of dystonia and myoclonus.[74] A vascular etiology is probably the most common. The

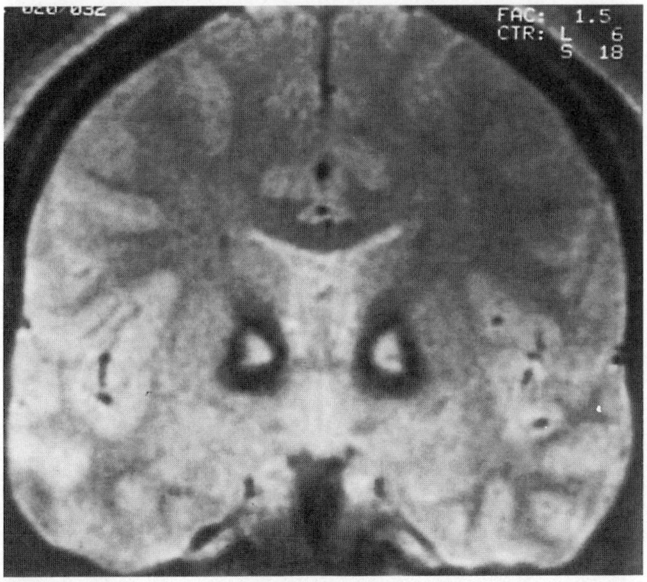

A

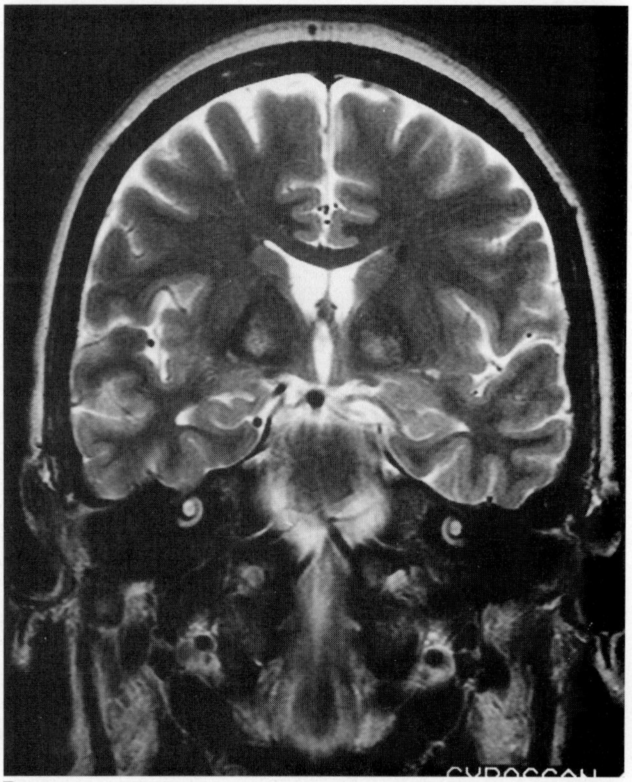

B

Figure 1-17
(A) *Gradient echo coronal image in a patient with Hallervorden-Spatz disease. Note the "eye of the tiger" sign with pronounced bilateral pallidal hypointensity peripherally and hyperintensity centrally. (Used with permission from Ref. 82.)* **(B)** *"Eye of the tiger" sign obtained with a turbo spin echo sequence. Note the less pronounced pallidal hypointensity compared with the gradient echo image in* **A**.

ability of MRI to perform direct coronal imaging is particularly useful in determining the precise anatomic localization of these lesions (Fig. 1-18A and B).

CEREBELLAR DISORDERS

The cerebellum is concerned primarily with the regulation of muscle tone, the coordination of skilled voluntary movement, and the control of posture and gait. The presenting complaints of patients with cerebellar disease depend more on the location within the cerebellum and the rate of progression of the lesion than on the pathology.

Until the development of MRI, the ability to image the cerebellar structure was somewhat limited because of the susceptibility of CT to artifacts related to the bony structure of the posterior fossa. Nevertheless, CT has been useful in demonstrating mass lesions and infarcts within the cerebellum and showing cerebellar atrophy, especially severe atrophy (Fig. 1-19A). Idiopathic (physiologic) calcification in the dentate nucleus is seen occasionally, although not as commonly as in the globus pallidus. MRI has provided a major advantage by virtue of its ability to view brain tissue without degradation from adjacent bone and to image orthogonal planes directly (Fig. 1-19B). This allows, for example, the demonstration of cerebellar atrophy on a sagittal section through the midline. On T2-weighted images, areas of low signal often are evident in the region of the dentate, suggesting the accumulation of iron. This iron is not present at birth but appears at about 5 to 10 years of age, a few years later than it appears in the globus pallidus, substantia nigra, and red nucleus.

The following CT criteria have been established for the presence of cerebellar atrophy: visualization of four or more vermian sulci on a single section, two or more cerebellar hemispheric sulci, a fourth ventricular index greater than 0.178, and a fourth ventricular diameter greater than 19 mm.[75] The use of these multiple objective measures decreases the likelihood of errors in determining the presence of atrophy that may result from variable gantry positions and transverse section levels.

Cerebellar atrophy is a nonspecific finding and can result from numerous acquired disorders. *Paraneoplastic cerebellar degeneration,* occurring as a nonmetastatic

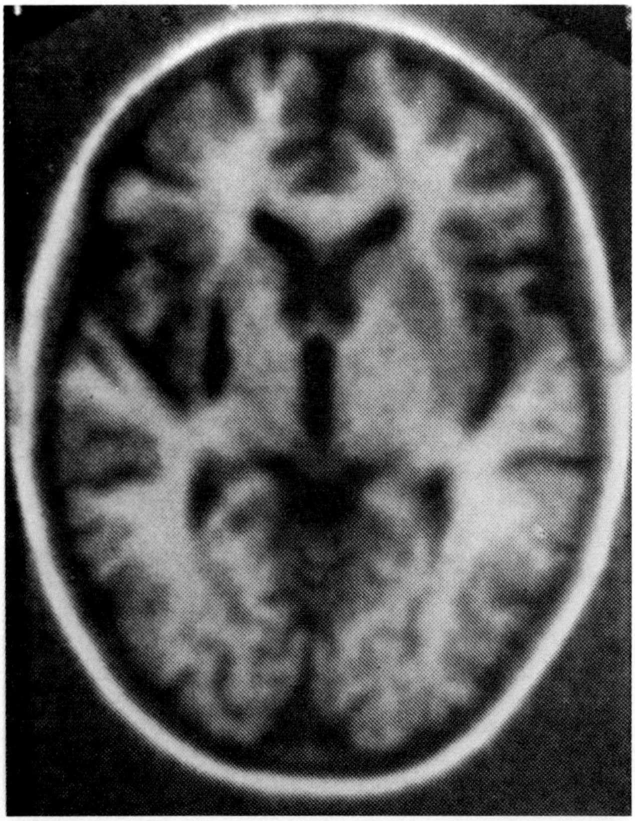

A

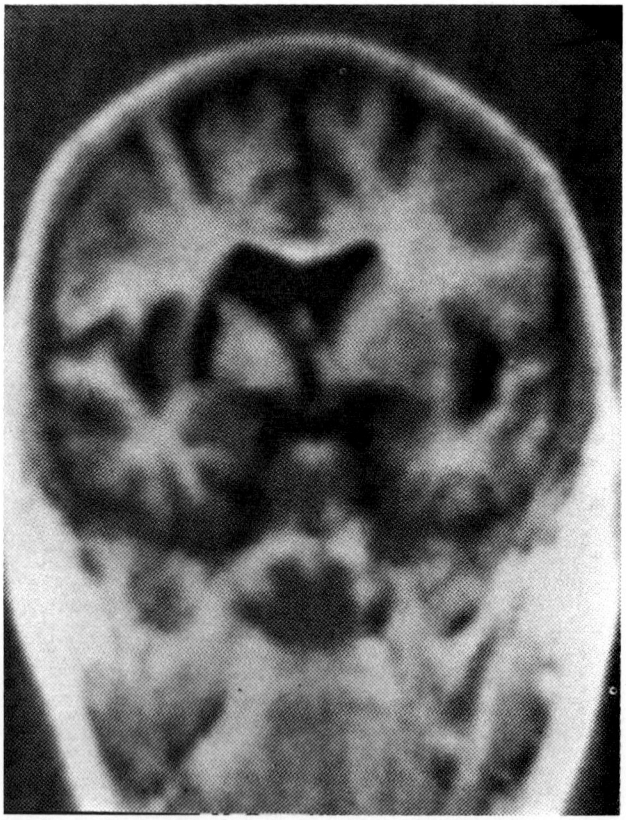

B

Figure 1-18

Transverse **(A)** *and coronal* **(B)** *MRIs from a patient with left-sided hemidystonia that developed after an infarct almost completely restricted to the right putamen. (Used with permission from Ref. 85.)*

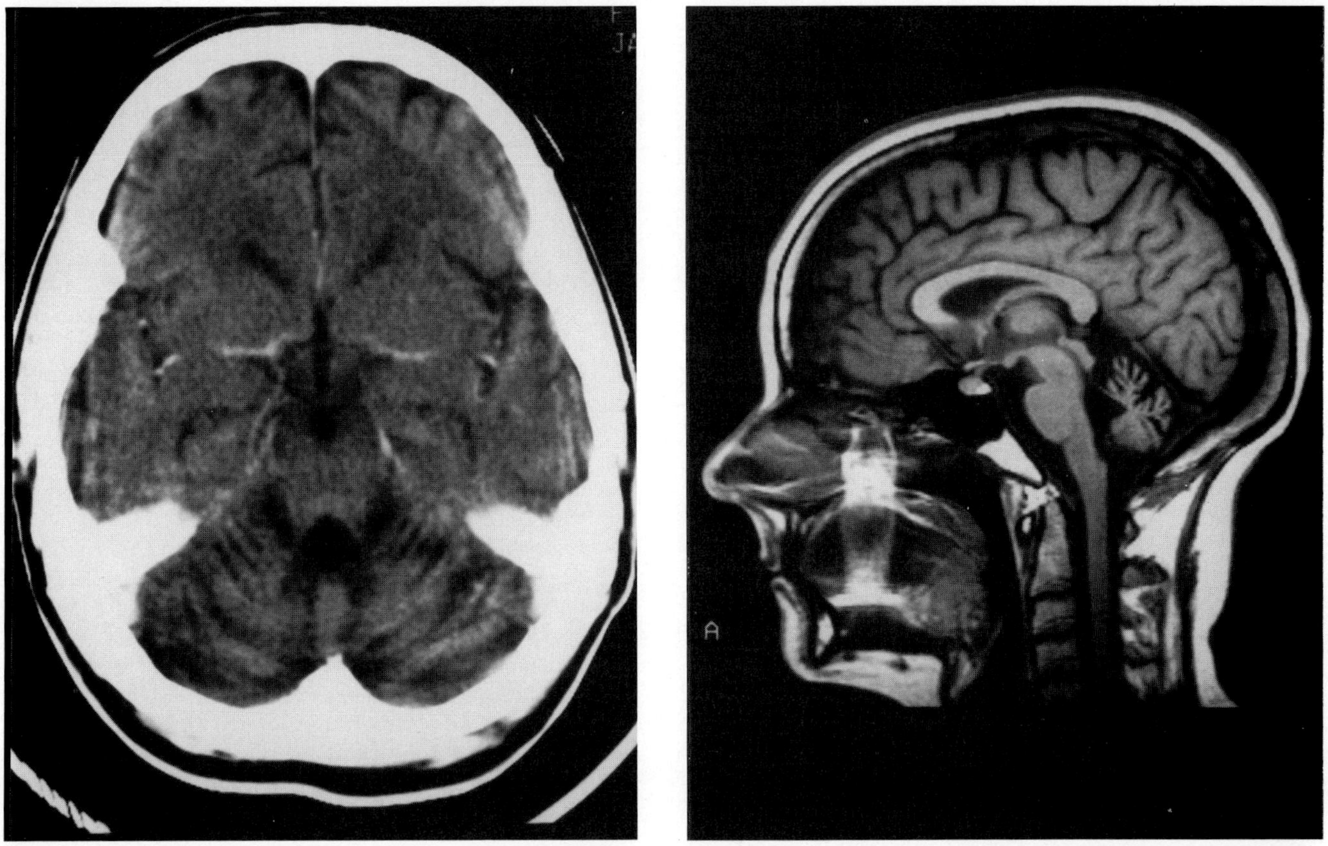

A B

Figure 1-19
Cerebellar atrophy. **(A)** *Transverse CT scan showing enlarged fourth ventricle and widening of hemispheral sulci.* **(B)** *Sagittal T1-weighted MRI showing marked widening of sulci over the superior vermis (compare with Fig. 1-1D).*

complication of malignancy, often is associated with atrophy on CT or MRI.[76] Structural imaging is particularly important in this setting to exclude metastatic disease, which is a much more common cause of cerebellar dysfunction in patients with cancer. *Alcoholism* and *thiamine deficiency* can be associated with signs and symptoms of cerebellar dysfunction and with prominent atrophy, primarily affecting the anterior lobe of the cerebellum.[77] Multiple toxic causes exist, such as chronic phenytoin toxicity, high-dose cytosine arabinoside, and chronic toluene exposure.

The degenerative cerebellar and spinocerebellar disorders are a complex group and are classified primarily on a clinical basis. *Friedreich ataxia* is probably the most common specific disorder in this group. The diagnostic features include progressive limb and gait ataxia starting before age 25, autosomal recessive inheritance, absent tendon reflexes in the lower limbs, and an axonal sensory neuropathy. The major pathology involves the peripheral nerves and spinal cord, with the cerebellum being largely spared. Structural imaging is not diagnostic but may reveal mild cerebellar atrophy. The absence or mild nature of the cerebellar atrophy in Friedreich ataxia on CT or MRI is a feature that helps differentiate it from the primary cerebellar degenerations.[78] In contrast to other degenerative disorders associated with ataxia, in Friedreich ataxia PET scans demonstrate widespread cerebral and cerebellar hypermetabolism in ambulatory patients with metabolic rates close to normal control levels in patients who are no longer ambulatory.[79] The *late-onset cerebellar ataxias,* often labeled as olivopontocerebellar atrophy by some authors, have numerous subtypes. Many of these ataxias are idiopathic, although some are inherited, usually in an autosomal dominant fashion. Structural imaging often reveals nonspecific cerebellar and brainstem atrophy that can be severe but does not appear to be useful for clinical classification. In similar patients classified as having OPCA by Gilman and associates, PET studies of cerebral metabolism have shown a marked reduction in cerebellar and brainstem glucose utilization that precede the development of cerebellar atrophy on CT.[27] The demonstration of cerebellar metabolic and structural changes in patients suspected of having cerebellar degeneration provides information that helps support this diagnosis.

REFERENCES

1. Olanow CW: Magnetic resonance imaging in parkinsonism, in Cedarbaum JM, Gancher ST (eds): *Neurol Clin* 10:405–420, 1992.
2. Rutledge JN, Hilal SK, Silver AJ, et al: Study of movement disorders and brain iron by MR. *AJNR* 8:397–411, 1987.
3. Puvanendran K, Low CH, Boey HK, Tank KP: Basal ganglia calcification on computer tomographic scan: A clinical and radiological correlation. *Acta Neurol Scand* 66:309–315, 1982.
4. Holland BA, Kucharcyzk W, Brant-Zawadzki M, et al: MR imaging of calcified intracranial lesions. *Radiology* 157:353–356, 1985.
5. Martin WRW: Parkinson's disease: Positron emission tomographic studies. *Semin Neurol* 9:351–356, 1989.
6. Leenders KL, Palmer AJ, Quinn N, et al: Brain dopamine metabolism in patients with Parkinson's disease measured with positron emission tomography. *J Neurol Neurosurg Psychiatry* 49:853–860, 1986.
7. Frey KA, Koeppe RA, Kilbourn MR, et al: Presynaptic monoaminergic vesicles in Parkinson's disease and normal aging. *Ann Neurol* 40:873–884, 1996.
8. Guttman M, Burkholder J, Kish SJ, et al: [^{11}C]RTI-32 PET studies of the dopamine transporter in early dopa-naive Parkinson's disease: Implications for the symptomatic threshold. *Neurology* 48:1578–1583, 1997.
9. Rinne JO, Laihinen A, Nagren K, et al: PET examination of the monoamine transporter with [^{11}C]β-CIT and [^{11}C]β-CFT in early Parkinson's disease. *Synapse* 21:97–103, 1995.
10. Volkow ND, Pappas N, Schlyer DJ, et al: A new PET ligand for the dopamine transporter: Studies in the human brain. *J Nucl Med* 36:2162–2168, 1995.
11. Marek KL, Seibyl JP, Zoghbi SS, et al: [^{123}I]β-CIT/SPECT imaging demonstrates bilateral loss of dopamine transporters in hemi-Parkinson's disease. *Neurology* 46:231–237, 1996.
12. Guttman M, Burns RS, Martin WRW, et al: PET studies of parkinsonian patients treated with autologous adrenal transplants. *Can J Neurol Sci* 16:305–309, 1989.
13. Lindvall O, Brundin P, Widner H, et al: Grafts of fetal dopamine neurons survive and improve motor function in Parkinson's disease. *Science* 247:574–577, 1990.
14. Brooks DJ, Ibanez V, Sawle GV, et al: Striatal D_2 receptor status in patients with Parkinson's disease, striatonigral degeneration and progressive supranuclear palsy, measured with ^{11}C-raclopride and positron emission tomography. *Ann Neurol* 31:184–192, 1992.
15. Peppard RF, Martin WRW, Carr GD, et al: Cerebral glucose metabolism in Parkinson's disease with and without dementia. *Arch Neurol* 49:1262–1267, 1992.
16. Spampinato U, Habert MO, Mas JL, et al: (^{99m}Tc)-HM-PAO SPECT and cognitive impairment in Parkinson's disease: A comparison with dementia of the Alzheimer type. *J Neurol Neurosurg Psychiatry* 54:787–792, 1991.
17. Brooks DJ, Ibanez V, Sawle GV, et al: Differing patterns of striatal [18F]-dopa uptake in Parkinson's disease, multiple system atrophy, and progressive supranuclear palsy. *Ann Neurol* 28:547–555, 1990.
18. D'Antona R, Baron JC, Samson Y, et al: Subcortical dementia: Frontal cortex hypometabolism detected by positron tomography in patients with progressive supranuclear palsy. *Brain* 108:785–799, 1985.
19. Foster NL, Gilman S, Berent S, et al: Cerebral hypometabolism in progressive supranuclear palsy studied with positron emission tomography. *Ann Neurol* 24:399–406, 1988.
20. Savoiardo M, Strada L, Girotti F, et al: MR imaging in progressive supranuclear palsy and Shy-Drager syndrome. *J Comput Assist Tomogr* 13:555–560, 1989.
21. Dubinsky RM, Jankovic J: Progressive supranuclear palsy and a multi-infarct state. *Neurology* 37:570–576, 1987.
22. Huang YP, Plaitakis A: Morphological changes of olivopontocerebellar atrophy in computed tomography and comments on its pathogenesis, in Duvoisin RC, Plaitakis A (eds): *The Olivopontocerebellar Atrophies.* New York, Raven Press, 1984, pp 39–85.
23. Brown R, Polinsky RJ, Di Chiro G, et al: MRI in autonomic failure. *J Neurol Neurosurg Psychiatry* 50:913–914, 1987.
24. Lang AE, Curran T, Provias J, Bergeron C: Striatonigral degeneration: Iron deposition in putamen correlates with the slit-like void signal of magnetic resonance imaging. *Can J Neurol Sci* 21:311–318, 1994.
25. Eidelberg D, Takikawa S, Moeller JR, et al: Striatal hypometabolism distinguishes striatonigral degeneration from Parkinson's disease. *Ann Neurol* 33:518–527, 1993.
26. DeVolder AG, Francart J, Laterre C, et al: Decreased glucose utilization in the striatum and frontal lobe in probable striatonigral degeneration. *Ann Neurol* 26:239–247, 1989.
27. Gilman S, Markel DS, Koeppe RA, et al: Cerebellar and brainstem hypometabolism in olivopontocerebellar atrophy studied with positron emission tomography. *Ann Neurol* 23:223–230, 1988.
28. Savoiardo M, Strada L, Girotti F, et al: Olivopontocerebellar atrophy: MR diagnosis and relationship to multisystem atrophy. *Radiology* 174:693–696, 1990.
29. Sawle GV, Brooks DJ, Marsden CD, Frackowiak RSJ: Corticobasal degeneration. *Brain* 114:541–556, 1991.
30. Eidelberg D, Dhawan V, Moeller JR, et al: The metabolic landscape of cortico-basal ganglionic degeneration: Regional asymmetries studied with positron emission tomography. *J Neurol Neurosurg Psychiatry* 54:856–862, 1991.
31. Hauser RA, Olanow CW, Gold M, et al: Magnetic resonance imaging of corticobasal degeneration. *J Neuroimaging* 6:222–226, 1996.
32. Sciarra D, Sprofkin B: Symptoms and signs referable to the basal ganglia in brain tumor. *Arch Neurol Psychiatry* 69:450–461, 1953.
33. Van Eck JH: Parkinsonism as a misleading brain tumor syndrome. *Psychiatr Neurol Neurochir* 64:109–123, 1961.
34. Nicholson AN, Turner EA: Parkinsonism produced by parasagittal meningiomas. *J Neurosurg* 21:104–113, 1964.
35. Jankovic J, Newmark M, Peter P: Parkinsonism and acquired hydrocephalus. *Mov Disord* 1:59–64, 1986.
36. Glatt S, Fine S, Kaplan J: Parkinsonism as a presentation of subdural hematoma. *Neurology* 33(suppl 2):61, 1983.
37. Zijlmans JCM, Thijssen HOM, Vogels OJM, et al: MRI in patients with suspected vascular parkinsonism. *Neurology* 45:2183–2188, 1995.
38. Muenter MD, Whisnant JP: Basal ganglia calcification, hypoparathyroidism, and extrapyramidal motor manifestations. *Neurology* 18:1075–1083, 1968.

39. Davis PL: The magnetic resonance imaging appearances of basal ganglia lesions in carbon monoxide poisoning. *Magn Reson Imaging* 4:489–490, 1986.
40. Mazziotta JC: Huntington's disease: Studies with structural imaging techniques and positron emission tomography. *Semin Neurol* 9:360–369, 1989.
41. Harris GJ, Pearlson GD, Peyser CE, et al: Putamen volume reduction on magnetic resonance imaging exceeds caudate changes in mild Huntington's disease. *Ann Neurol* 31:69–75, 1992.
42. Aylward EH, Codori A-M, Barta PE, et al: Basal ganglia volume and proximity to onset in presymptomatic Huntington disease. *Arch Neurol* 53:1293–1296, 1996.
43. Savoiardo M, Strada L, Oliva D, et al: Abnormal MRI signal in the rigid form of Huntington's disease. *J Neurol Neurosurg Psychiatry* 54:888–891, 1991.
44. Kozachuk W, Salagna V, Conomy J, Smith A: MRI (magnetic resonance imaging) in Huntington's disease. *Neurology (Cleve)* 36(suppl 1):310, 1986.
45. Sax DS, O'Donnell B, Butters N, et al: CT, neurologic and neuropsychological correlates of Huntington's disease. *Int J Neurosci* 18:21–36, 1983.
46. Kuhl DE, Phelps ME, Markham CH, et al: Cerebral metabolism and atrophy in Huntington's disease determined by 18-FDG and computed tomographic scan. *Ann Neurol* 12:425–434, 1982.
47. Hayden MR, Martin WRW, Stoessl AJ, et al: Positron emission tomography in the early diagnosis of Huntington's disease. *Neurology* 36:888–894, 1986.
48. Young AB, Penney JB, Starosta-Rubinstein S, et al: PET scan investigations of Huntington's disease: Cerebral metabolic correlates of neurologic features and functional decline. *Ann Neurol* 20:296–303, 1986.
49. Martin WRW, Hoskinson M, Kremer B, et al: Functional caudate imaging in symptomatic Huntington's disease: PET vs SPECT. *J Neuroimaging* 5:227–232, 1995.
50. Dubinsky RM, Hallett M, Levey R, Di Chiro G: Regional brain glucose metabolism in neuroacanthocytosis. *Neurology* 39:1253–1255, 1989.
51. Suchowersky O, Hayden MR, Martin WRW, et al: Cerebral metabolism of glucose in benign hereditary chorea. *Mov Disord* 1:33–44, 1986.
52. Palella TD, Hichwa RD, Ehrenkaufer RL, et al: 18-F-fluorodeoxyglucose PET scanning in HPRT deficiency. *Am J Hum Genet* 37:A70, 1981.
53. Martin WRW, Clark C, Ammann W, et al: Cortical glucose metabolism in Huntington's disease. *Neurology* 42:223–229, 1992.
54. Kuwert T, Lange HW, Langen K-J, et al: Cortical and subcortical glucose consumption measured by PET in patients with Huntington's disease. *Brain* 113:1405–1423, 1990.
55. Hayden MR, Hewitt BSC, Stoessl AJ, et al: The combined use of positron emission tomography and DNA polymorphisms for preclinical detection of Huntington's disease. *Neurology* 37:1441–1447, 1987.
56. Mazziotta JC, Phelps ME, Pahl JJ, et al: Reduced cerebral glucose metabolism in asymptomatic subjects at risk for Huntington's disease. *N Engl J Med* 316:357–362, 1987.
57. Hardie RJ, Pullon HWH, Harding AE, et al: Neuroacanthocytosis: A clinical, haematological, and pathological study of 19 cases. *Brain* 114:13–50, 1991.
58. Serra S, Xerra A, Scribano E, et al: Computed tomography in amyotrophic chorea-acanthocytosis. *Neuroradiology* 29:480–482, 1987.
59. Brooks DJ, Ibanez V, Playford ED, et al: Presynaptic and postsynaptic striatal dopaminergic function in neuroacanthocytosis: A positron emission tomographic study. *Ann Neurol* 30:166–171, 1991.
60. Guttman M, Lang AE, Garnett ES, et al: Regional cerebral glucose metabolism in SLE chorea: Further evidence that striatal hypometabolism is not a correlate of chorea. *Mov Disord* 2:201–211, 1987.
61. Davis PC, Hoffman JC Jr, Braun IF, et al: MR of Leigh's disease (subacute necrotizing encephalomyelopathy). *AJNR* 8:71–75, 1987.
62. Novotny EJ, Singh G, Wallace DC, et al: Leber's disease and dystonia: A mitochondrial disease. *Neurology* 36:1053–1060, 1986.
63. De Haan J, Grossman RI, Civitello L, et al: High-field magnetic resonance imaging of Wilson's disease. *J Comput Assist Tomogr* 11:132–135, 1987.
64. Hitoshi S, Iwata M, Yoshikawa K: Mid-brain pathology of Wilson's disease: MRI analysis of three cases. *J Neurol Neurosurg Psychiatry* 54:624–626, 1991.
65. Hawkins RA, Mazziotta JC, Phelps ME: Wilson's disease studied with FDG and positron emission tomography. *Neurology* 37:1707–1711, 1987.
66. Snow BJ, Bhatt M, Martin WRW, et al: The nigrostriatal dopaminergic pathway in Wilson's disease studied with positron emission tomography. *J Neurol Neurosurg Psychiatry* 54:12–17, 1991.
67. Tennison MB, Bouldin TW, Whaley MD: Mineralization of the basal ganglia detected by CT in Hallervorden-Spatz syndrome. *Neurology* 38:154–155, 1988.
68. Sethi KD, Adams RJ, Loring DW, El Gamm T: Hallervorden-Spatz syndrome: Clinical and magnetic resonance imaging correlations. *Ann Neurol* 24:692–694, 1988.
69. Buruma OJS, Lakke JPWF: Ballismus, in Vincken PJ, Bruyn GW, Klawans HL (eds): *Handbook of Clinical Neurology,* vol. 49: *Extrapyramidal Disorders.* Amsterdam, Elsevier, 1986, pp 369–380.
70. Biller J, Graff-Radford NR, Smoker WRK, et al: MR imaging in "lacunar" hemiballismus. *J Comput Assist Tomogr* 10:793–797, 1986.
71. Konagaya M, Konagaya Y: MRI in hemiballism due to Sydenham's chorea. *J Neurol Neurosurg Psychiatry* 55:238–239, 1992.
72. Marsden CD, Obeso JA, Zarranz JJ, Lang AE: The anatomical basis of symptomatic hemidystonia. *Brain* 108:463–483, 1985.
73. Pettigrew LC, Jankovic J. Hemidystonia: A report of 22 patients and a review of the literature. *J Neurol Neurosurg Psychiatry* 48:650–657, 1985.
74. Lehericy S, Vidailhet M, Dormont D, et al: Striatopallidal and thalamic dystonia: A magnetic resonance imaging anatomoclinical study. *Arch Neurol* 53:241–250, 1996.
75. Claus D, Aschoff JC: Evaluation of infrantentorial atrophy by computed tomography. *J Neurol Neurosurg Psychiatry* 45:979–983, 1982.
76. Hammack J, Kotanides H, Rosenblum MK, Posner JB: Paraneoplastic cerebellar degeneration: II. Clinical and immunologic findings in 21 patients with Hodgkin's disease. *Neurology* 42:1938–1943, 1992.

77. Hillbom M, Muuronen A, Holm L, Hindmarsh T: The clinical versus radiological diagnosis of alcoholic cerebellar degeneration. *J Neurol Sci* 73:45–53, 1986.
78. Ramos A, Quintana F, Diez C, et al: CT findings in spinocerebellar degneration. *AJNR* 8:635–640, 1987.
79. Gilman S, Junck L, Markel DS, et al: Cerebral glucose hypermetabolism in Friedreich's ataxia detected with positron emission tomography. *Ann Neurol* 28:750–757, 1990.
80. Riley DE, Lang AE: Movement disorders, in Bradley WG, Daroff RB, Fenichel GM, Marsden CD (eds): *Neurology in Clinical Practice.* Boston, Butterworth-Heinemann, 1991, chap 76.
81. Marsden CD, Lang AE, Quinn NP, et al: Familial dystonia and visual failure with striatal CT lucencies. *J Neurol Neurosurg Psychiatry* 49:500–509, 1986.
82. Braffman BH, Trojanowski JQ, Atlas SW: The aging brain and neurodegenerative disorders, in Atlas SW (ed): *Magnetic Resonance Imaging of the Brain and Spine.* New York, Raven Press, 1991, pp 567–624.
83. Gilman S: Olivopontocerebellar atrophy, in Martin WRW (ed): *Functional Imaging in Movement Disorders.* Boca Raton, CRC Press, 1990, pp 157–176.
84. Fross RD, Martin WRW, Li D, et al: Lesions of the putamen: Their relevance to dystonia. *Neurology* 37:1125–1129, 1987.
85. Burton K, Farrell K, Li D, Calne DB: Lesions of the putamen and dystonia: CT and magnetic resonance imaging. *Neurology* 34:962–965, 1984.

CHAPTER 2

DISORDERS OF STANCE AND GAIT

Joseph C. Masdeu

INTRODUCTION: CLINICAL BACKGROUND

From a clinical standpoint, the emphasis of this chapter is not on the imaging of neurologic disorders that secondarily result in ambulation difficulties, such as stroke that causes hemiplegia, but on disorders that primarily affect the ability to stand or walk, often without overt weakness. Many of these disorders elude even the most sophisticated neuroimaging procedures. To this category belong idiopathic gait disorders in elderly individuals. Some diseases, such as Parkinson disease, cause only nonspecific changes in the available imaging modalities or share changes with other degenerative brain disorders when investigated with positron emission tomography (PET) and single photon emission computed tomography (SPECT). A few cause characteristic imaging patterns etiologically or, more often, topographically.

Stance, equilibrium, and balance refer to the ability to maintain or the act of maintaining erect posture. Gait and ambulation pressupose the ability to stand, although the neural mechanisms underlying these two motor functions are far from identical. Surprisingly, some patients experience more difficulty standing than walking, for instance, those with orthostatic tremor.[1] Disorders of stance and gait can be the presenting syndrome of many different pathologies along the neuroaxis. Clinical localization before the use of neuroimaging is essential if neuroimaging procedures are to be applied in a focused and economical manner that will minimize the likelihood of false-positive findings.

Stance and gait disorders are particularly common in the elderly population. The Duke study of normal aging estimated that gait disturbances affect 15 percent of the elderly, constituting the most common neurologic impairment in this age group.[2] Among the elderly, falls are the leading source of injury-related deaths.[3] In the United States about 9500 deaths among people age 65 years or older are attributed each year to a falling episode. Falling is also a major cause of morbidity among older people. Eighty-four percent of the approximately 200,000 hip fractures that occur yearly affect people older than age 65 years. Most of these cases are related to a fall. Hip fracture is the most common injury leading to hospitalization.[4] In the last few years several imaging patterns, including white matter changes,[5–8] lacunar disease,[5,9] and hydrocephalus,[10,11] have been found to correlate with impaired ambulation in this age group. Still, in many patients conventional imaging with computed tomography (CT) and magnetic resonance imaging (MRI) is normal for age.[9] Among 18 patients with "primary progressive freezing gait," Achiron and associates reported deep lacunae in 3 patients and normal studies, with some atrophy, in 15.[9]

This chapter will cover only those pathologic processes which most often present with disorders of stance and gait and in which imaging can be of some help. A more extensive review of the imaging patterns in some of the specific etiologies, for instance, vascular disorders and hydrocephalus, can be found in other chapters in this book. The functional mechanisms of many of these disorders, such as cerebellar or vestibular ataxia, have been known for a long time and will not be discussed here. However, the anatomic underpinnings of some of the newly described clinicopathologic syndromes, such as thalamic or mesencephalic astasia, will be discussed in some detail.[12] The description of these disorders will follow a topographic pattern, covering first the supratentorial compartment, then the posterior fossa, and finally the spinal cord.

SUPRATENTORIAL LESIONS

Since the advent of CT and, particularly, MRI the ubiquitous changes observed in the white matter of older individuals have fascinated both clinicians and radiologists. The clinical significance of these changes has not been fully elucidated, but the best data point to gait and balance impairment as the main clinical correlate of white matter disease in the elderly. Lacunar events, which are easily imaged with CT or MRI in the chronic stage although they are elusive acutely, are often responsible for the sudden onset of impaired balance and gait in an older individual, particularly when the lesion affects structures that play a key role in ambulation, such as the thalami, basal ganglia, and projection fibers from the paracentral lobule. Other supratentorial disorders that course with early gait and balance changes, such as primary lateral sclerosis, are much more rare (Fig. 2-1).

White Matter Disease

White matter changes in the elderly and their relation to impaired equilibrium and gait will be described first.

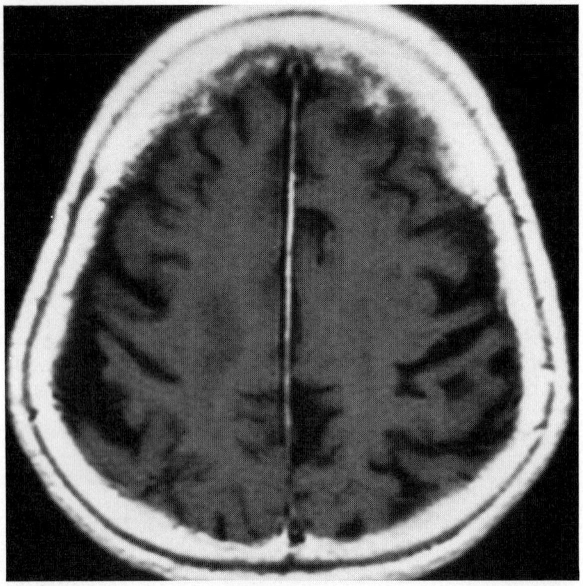

A

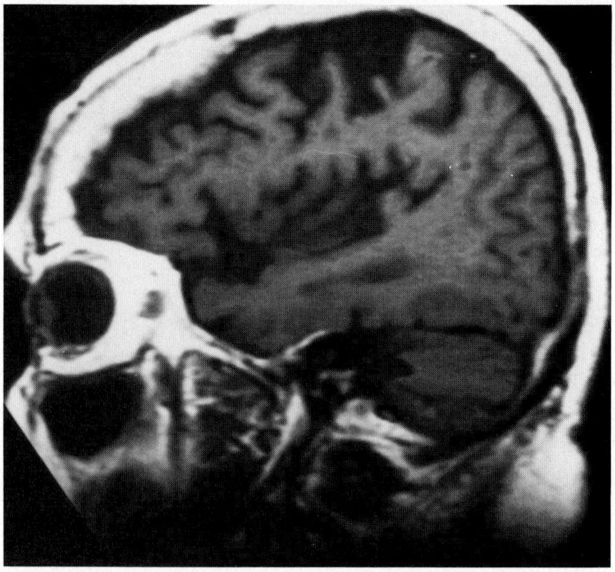

B

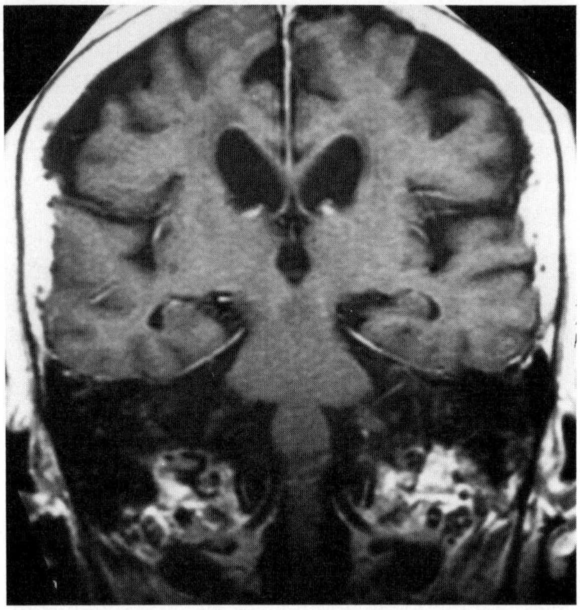

C

Figure 2-1

Primary lateral sclerosis. MRI and SPECT of an 85-year-old woman with primary lateral sclerosis. After a slowly progressive course beginning with gait impairment, the patient had a severe spastic quadriplegia and dysarthria. Note the widening of the rolandic, precentral, and postcentral sulci on axial **(A)**, *sagittal* **(B)**, *and coronal* **(C)** *MRI. Coronal sections show preservation of the temporal lobes. SPECT* **(D)** *shows markedly decreased perfusion of the paracentral regions and some decrease in the prefrontal cortex but normal perfusion of the association cortex of the parietal and temporal lobes.*

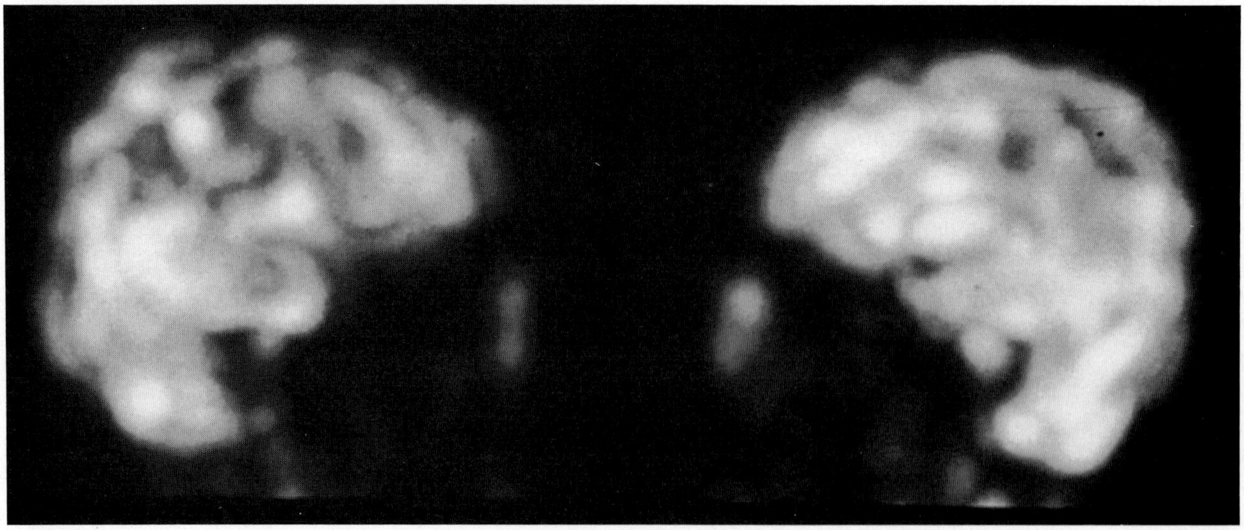

D (Plate 9)

A number of other disorders that are identifiable on CT or MRI will be discussed in the second part of this section.

White Matter Disease of the Elderly

White matter changes on CT or MRI are very common in older people. On MRI, some degree of white matter change is present in about 30 percent of subjects over age 65.[13] Since these changes are unusual before age 50, it is clear that they are somehow related to the aging process.[14,15] On CT, the density of the centrum semiovale has been reported to decrease with age.[16] The prevalence and severity of white matter changes have been found to increase with age.[13,14,16–20] White matter hypodensity in the elderly, which is subtle on CT, has striking visual characteristics when imaged by MRI.[17,21–23] Areas of the periventricular white matter that are hypodense on CT appear markedly hyperintense on T2-weighted images and hypointense on T1-weighted images.[24] (Fig. 2-2). However, high-intensity areas on T2-weighted MRI often are not detected on CT. On T2-weighted MRI it may be difficult to differentiate areas of increased water content caused by dilation of perivascular spaces with normal aging or transependymal cerebrospinal fluid (CSF) absorption from areas of tissue damage because both have increased intensity values.[23,25,26] For this reason, it seems preferable to make the diagnosis of significant white matter changes only when the abnormalities are visible on T1-weighted images. However, there are no data available on the functional significance of white matter changes on only T2-weighted images versus changes on both T2-weighted and T1-weighted images.

Because the histology underlying these changes remains elusive, Hachinski and associates proposed the descriptive term *leuko-araiosis* for the CT findings.[27] Several authors have reported normal histology, but vascular or ischemic disease has been present in cases with pronounced changes on MRI or CT.[24,28–33] Amyloid angiopathy has been incriminated in the genesis of white matter disease in some elderly individuals.[34,35] In addition to white matter changes, amyloid angiopathy results in subcortical hemorrhages (Fig. 2-3). Pronounced white matter changes on T1-weighted MRI and CT most often correspond to ischemic changes similar to the findings in subcortical arteriosclerotic encephalopathy (SAE) or Binswanger disease.[24,28–33,36] Cerebrovascular disease and hypertension are common correlates of subcortical arteriosclerotic encephalopathy.[21,37]

Although several reports have addressed the possible correlation of CT-MRI white matter changes with the presence of dementia,[14,21,22,37–42] few have commented on gait disturbances.[43] Disorders of gait were pronounced among 41 well-documented cases of progressive arteriopathic white matter disease described with histology since 1978 (males = 23, females = 18, mean age at onset 60 ± 9.7 years, mean length of illness 5.8 ± 4.2 years).[14,33–35,44–47] Impairment of ambulation preceded cognitive impairment in 43 percent of these patients, whereas dementia developed before gait impairment in only 17 percent; in 20 percent they evolved simultaneously, and in 20 percent insufficient data precluded the timing of gait abnormality versus dementia. Two of the patients in whom dementia occurred first had amyloid angiopathy and senile changes in the cortex.[34] A large proportion of patients with abnormal white matter on CT or MRI have gait abnormalities.[24,48,49] Comparing demented elderly subjects with controls for dementia, George and coworkers[20] and Hendrie and coworkers[50] failed to find a significant correlation between white matter disease and dementia, but white matter disease seemed to correlate with gait impairment. Periventricular white matter changes were present in the cases of "lower body parkinsonism" described in elderly subjects by Thompson and Marsden[43] and FitzGerald and Jankovic.[51] In a controlled study of elderly persons prone to falling, Masdeu and coworkers found that impaired gait and balance correlated with the presence of white matter disease on CT.[52] This finding was corroborated by MRI studies.[6,7]

Leukoencephalopathies

In younger age groups, disease of the white matter may manifest itself as impaired gait early in the course of a disease. Congenital disorders include enzymatic defects resulting from disorders of the lysosome, mitochondria, peroxisome, or nucleus as well as disorders of amino acid metabolism and several diseases without a known metabolic defect (Fig. 2-4).[10,53,54] Some familial leukoencephalopathies, such as cerebral autosomal dominant arteriopathy with subcortical infarcts and leukoencephalopathy (CADASIL), manifest in adulthood.[55,56] CT and MRI show abnormal white matter that is hypodense on CT, hyperintense on T2-weighted MRI, and hypointense on T1-weighted MRI (Fig. 2-5). Imaging changes are often present in presymptomatic individuals.[56] CADASIL has been mapped to a mutation of the Notch 3 gene on chromosome 19.[57,58] A periodic acid–Schiff (PAS)-positive granular material is deposited in the media of the arterioles of the brain and other organs, including skin.[59] When positive, a skin biopsy is helpful, but there have been genetically proven cases with negative skin biopsy.[60] Other vascular familial leukoencephalopathies include familial amyloid angiopathy and disorders that are less well characterized.[35,61–63]

Less common among the acquired white matter disorders are multiple sclerosis, other noninfectious inflammatory disorders, AIDS encephalopathy[64,65] (Fig. 2-6), progressive multifocal leukoencephalopathy (Fig. 2-7), subacute sclerosing panencephalitis, radiation leukoencephalopathy, and toxicity by chemotherapeutic agents, including methotrexate and cytarabine (Ara-C).[66]

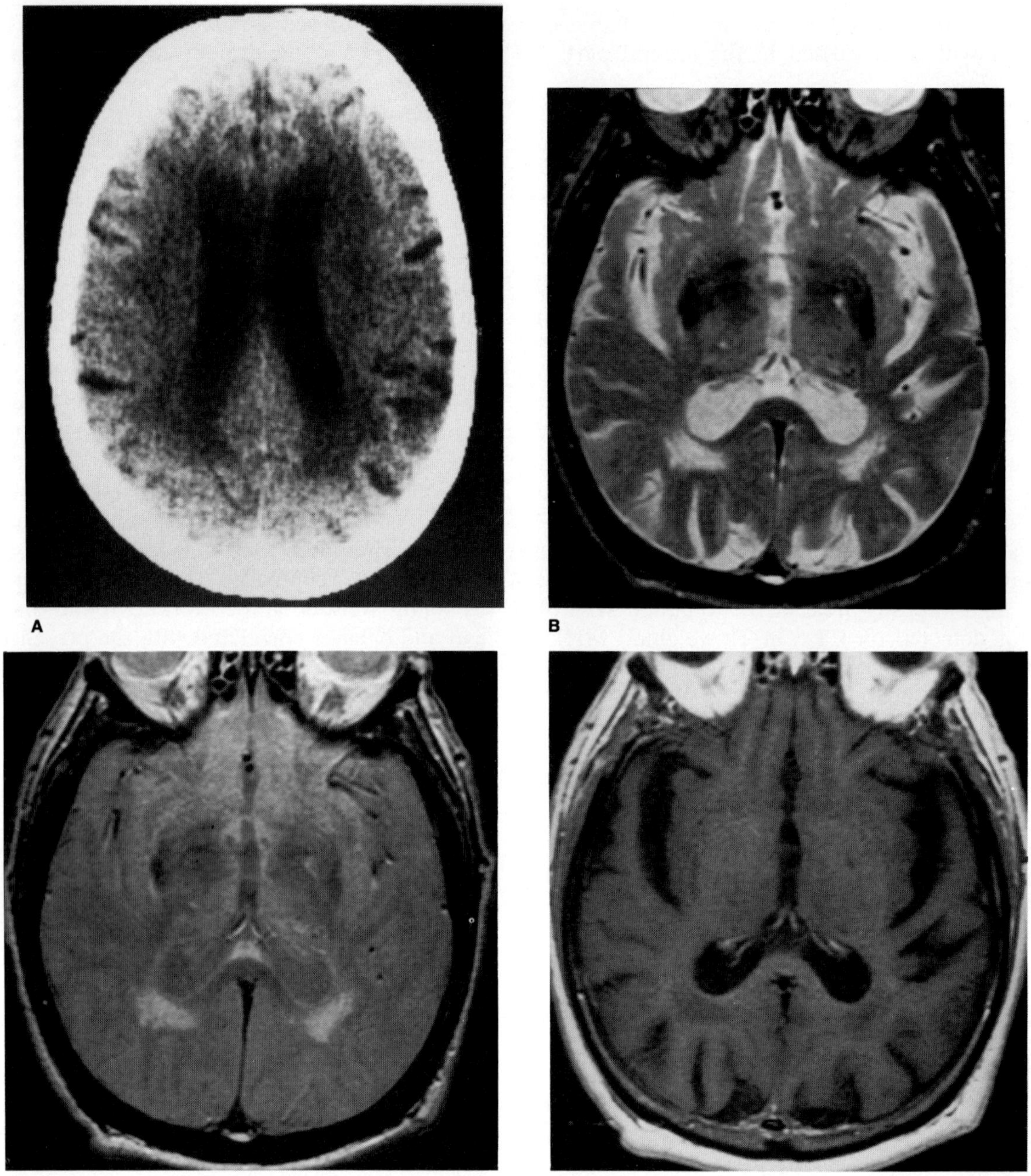

Figure 2-2
White matter changes in the elderly, CT and MRI of a normotensive 79-year-old woman with normal mentation but a slow, hesitating gait and a propensity to fall. Areas of low density on CT **(A)***, particularly in the periatrial white matter, appear to be of high intensity on T2-weighted MRI* **(B)** *and proton-density MRI* **(C)** *and low intensity on T1-weighted MRI* **(D)***.*

Acute Vascular Disease

Vascular disease is the most common clinically identifiable neurologic cause of gait impairment.[67,68] Ischemic brain disease tends to follow one of three patterns that are discernible by clinical evaluation and with the help of neuroimaging procedures: (1) cortical infarcts, most often related to embolic disease, (2) subcortical disease, often in the form of widespread lacunae and white matter changes, most often related to arteriolar disease, and (3) a mixture of the two patterns, often related to atheromatous disease of the major vessels. The second and third types of cerebrovascular disease tend to cause gait and balance impairment early in the course of the disease, as was mentioned above. Subcortical infarcts that are strategically located may impair equilibrium and gait with little or no limb weakness on isometric testing. These lesions tend to affect structures that play

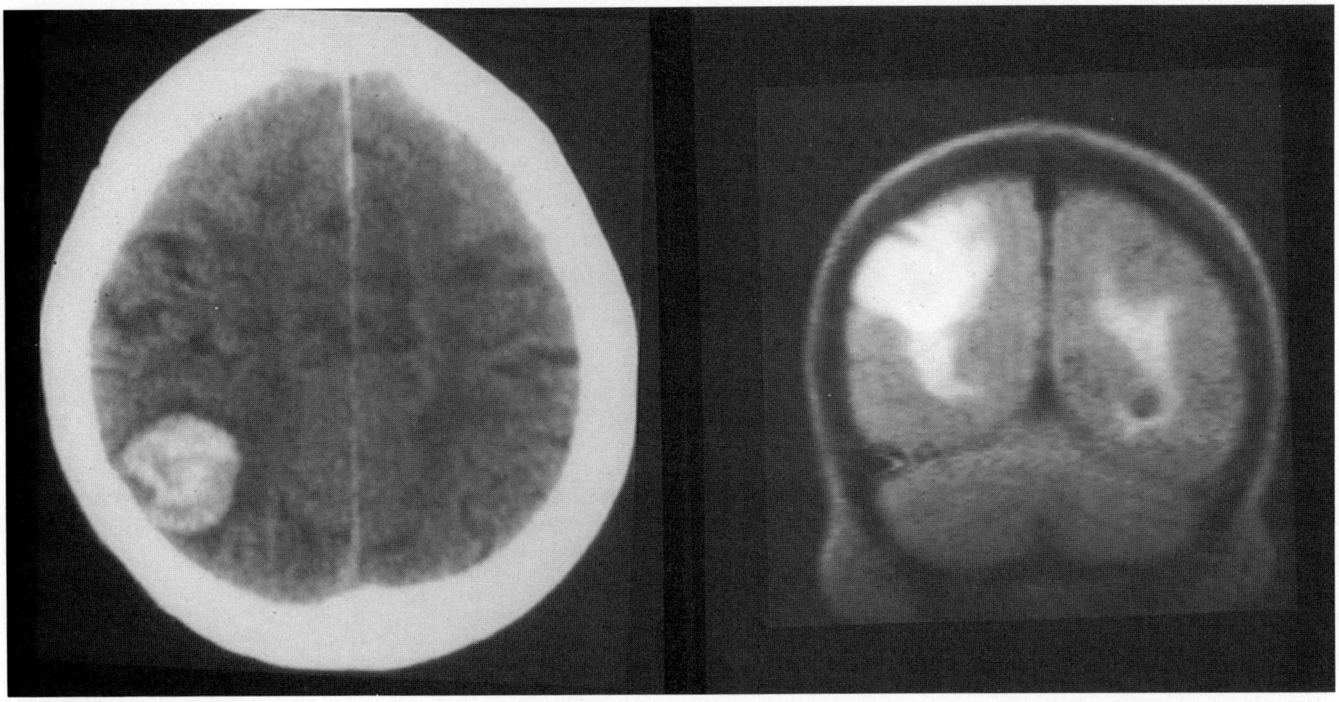

Figure 2-3
Amyloid angiopathy. CT of a 79-year-old woman showing a recent hemorrhage in the right supramarginal gyrus (left). On T2-weighted MRI, the lesion appears bright because of the high methemoglobin content, and the abnormal white matter is hyperintense on both hemispheres (right).

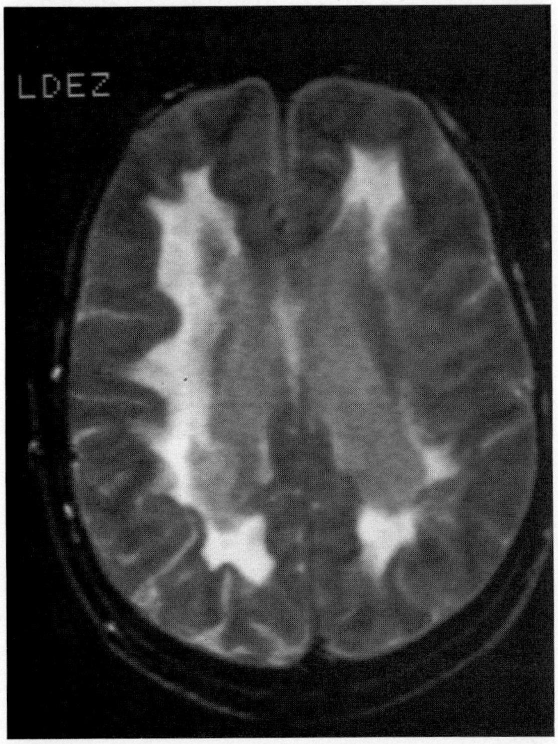

Figure 2-4
Congenital leukoencephalopathy. Proton-density MRI of a 43-year-old man with a 25-year history of progressive spastic quadriparesis and dysarthria but no dementia. The disorder presented as difficulty running. Note the marked involvement of the white matter with some preservation of the U fibers.

a critical role in gait and balance mechanisms, including the cortico/basal-ganglionic/thalamo/cortical loop (Fig. 2-8). Although acute stroke tends to be associated with overt neurologic findings, gait impairment may be neglected as a neurologic finding despite being the result of small, "silent" lacunar strokes.[69] In a cohort of clinically asymptomatic patients studied during the Asymptomatic Carotid Artery Stenosis trial, Brott and coworkers documented lacunar strokes with CT in 11 percent of the patients.[70] These patients were more likely to have gait impairment.

The disturbances caused by cerebellar or vestibular lesions are well known. Recently, striking abnormalities of gait and balance were described with lesions in the thalamus, the basal ganglia, and, the infratentorial compartment in the pedunculopontine region.

Thalamic Astasia

Inability to stand or walk despite minimal weakness has been recorded in patients with thalamic infarction[71,72] and hemorrhage.[73,74] It also has been reported in patients with lesions in the internal capsule or corona radiata who have the syndrome of unilateral ataxia and crural paresis (ataxic hemiparesis).[75–78] Masdeu and Gorelick described 15 patients with thalamic lesions (13 of a vascular nature) that caused a syndrome of "thalamic astasia."[79] Alert, with normal or nearly normal strength on isometric muscle testing and a variable degree of sensory

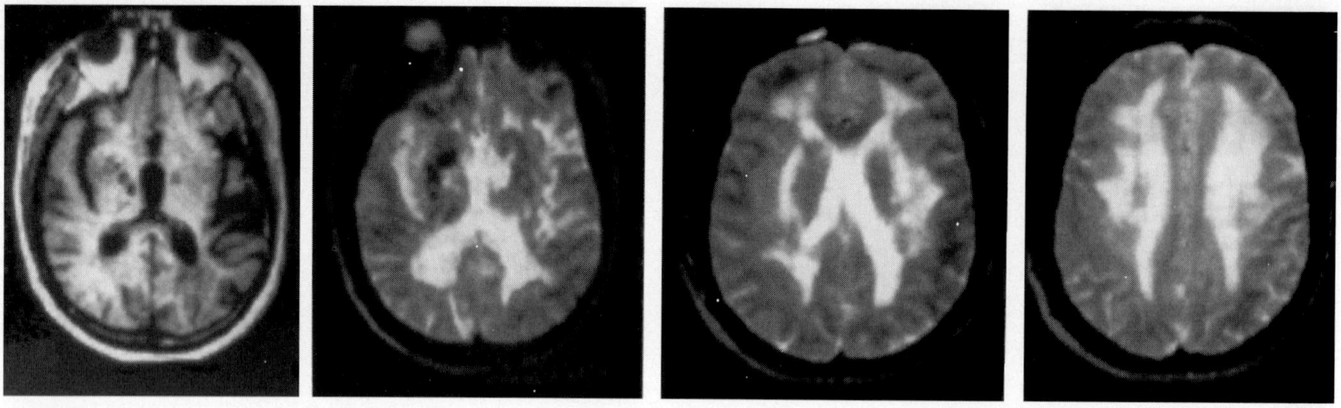

Figure 2-5

Cerebral autosomal dominant arteriopathy with subcortical infarcts and leukoencephalopathy (CADASIL). **(A and B)** *T1-weighted and T2-weighted MRIs of a 40-year-old who had sustained several strokes, leaving him with a quadriparesis. CADASIL was confirmed by brain biopsy and genetic typing.* **(C and D)** *T2-weighted MRIs of an asymptomatic 40-year-old relative of the first patient at 50 percent genetic risk of having CADASIL. (From Sabbadini G, Francia A, Calandriello L, et al: Cerebral autosomal dominant arteriopathy with subcortical infarcts and leukoencephalopathy (CADASIL): Clinical, neuroimaging, pathological and genetic study of a large Italian family.* Brain *118:207–215, 1995, with permission.)*

loss, these patients could not stand, and seven of them could not sit up unassisted. They fell backward or toward the side contralateral to the lesion. They appeared to have a deficit of overlearned motor activity of an axial and postural nature. In the 13 vascular cases, the deficit improved in a few days or weeks (Fig. 2-9). However, these patients had a tendency to sustain falls during the rehabilitation period. The lesions were clustered mainly in the superior portion of the ventrolateral nucleus of the thalamus, and in some cases the suprathalamic white matter was affected (Fig. 2-10).

The propensity of thalamic lesions to cause balance and gait impairment is easily understood if one reviews thalamic connectivity. The ventrolateral nucleus of the

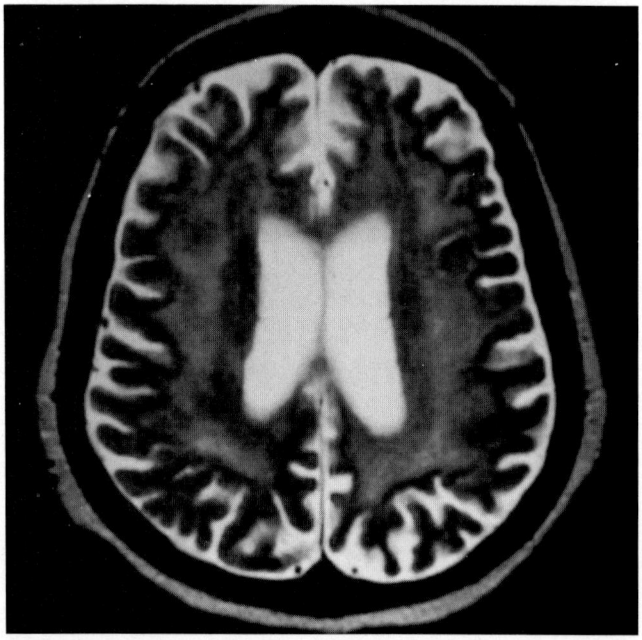

Figure 2-6

Human immunodeficiency virus (HIV) encephalopathy. T2-weighted MRI of a 43-year-old woman with a 7-year history of HIV infection and a 3-month history of progressive gait impairment. Improvement followed therapy with zidovudine. Note the diffuse hyperintensity of the hemispheric white matter.

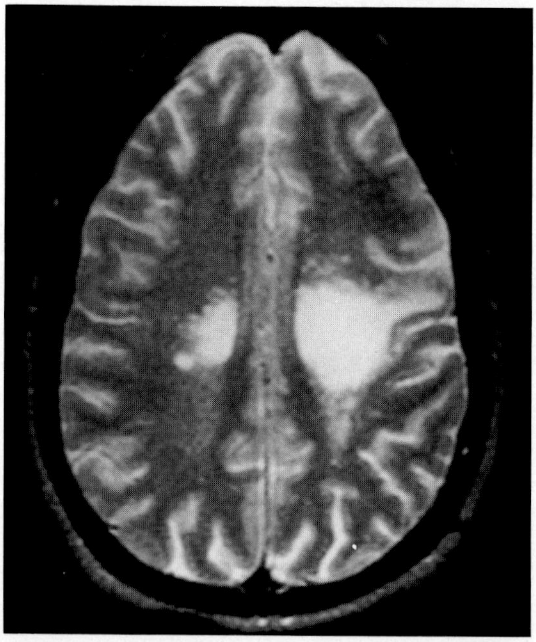

Figure 2-7

Progressive multifocal leukoencephalopathy (PML). T2-weighted MRI of a 32-year-old woman with a 6-week history of progressive gait impairment. PML genome was recovered from the CSF and the infection was confirmed at autopsy. Note the areas of hyperintensity involving the paracentral white matter bilaterally.

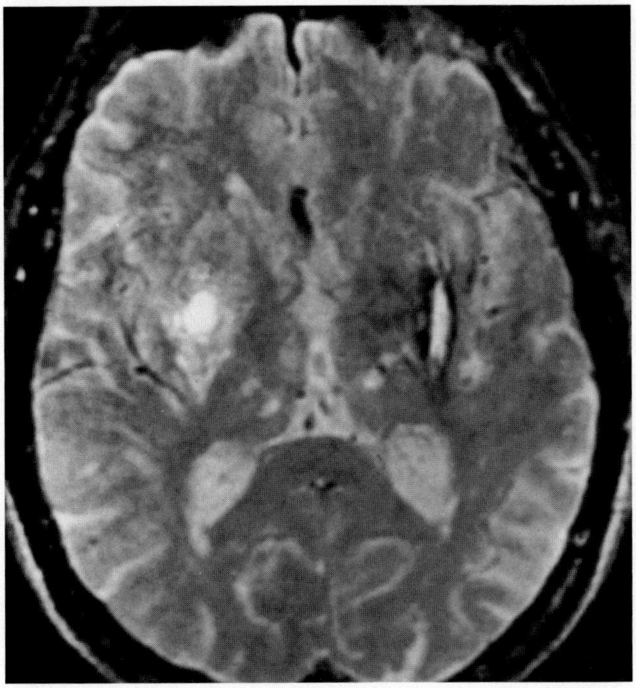

Figure 2-8
Lacunar disease. MRI of a 73-year-old male chronic hypertensive with a transient episode of mild left-sided weakness but progressive gait impairment. In addition to multiple thalamic lacunae and a larger infarct in the right lenticular nucleus, there is an organizing hematoma in the left external capsular region.

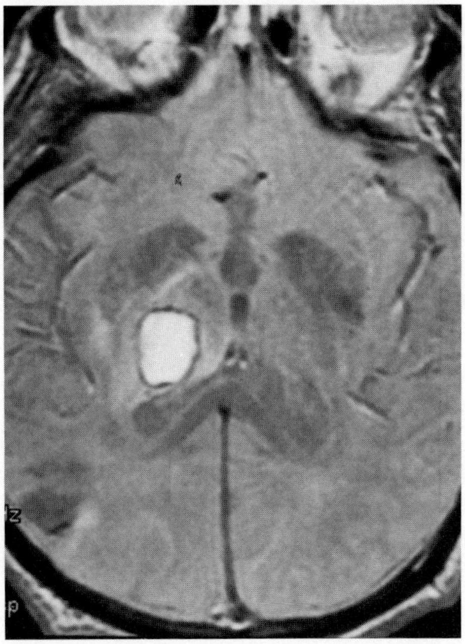

Figure 2-9
Thalamic hematoma. MRI of an 86-year-old man with a transient mild left hemiparesis but inability to walk for 8 weeks despite recovery of isometric strength. A right thalamic hematoma involves the ventrolateral and ventral posterior nuclei as well as the pulvinar.

thalamus consists of two portions.[80,81] The smaller anterior portion (VLa) receives projections from the medial globus pallidus via the thalamic fasciculus and projects to area 6 of the frontal cortex, including the supplementary motor area. The larger posterior portion (VLp) receives cerebellar, spinothalamic, and vestibular afferents and projects in a somatotopic fashion to area 4 of the precentral gyrus.[80] Laterosuperior neurons project to the medial portion of the precentral gyrus, where the trunk and leg are represented. Fibers destined for the leg region course in the posterior limb of the internal capsule and then ascend in the more medial portion of the corona radiata, near the wall of the lateral ventricle. Impairment of gait in the elderly with periventricular white matter disease may be related to involvement of this pathway.[52] Through the fastigial projection, VLp

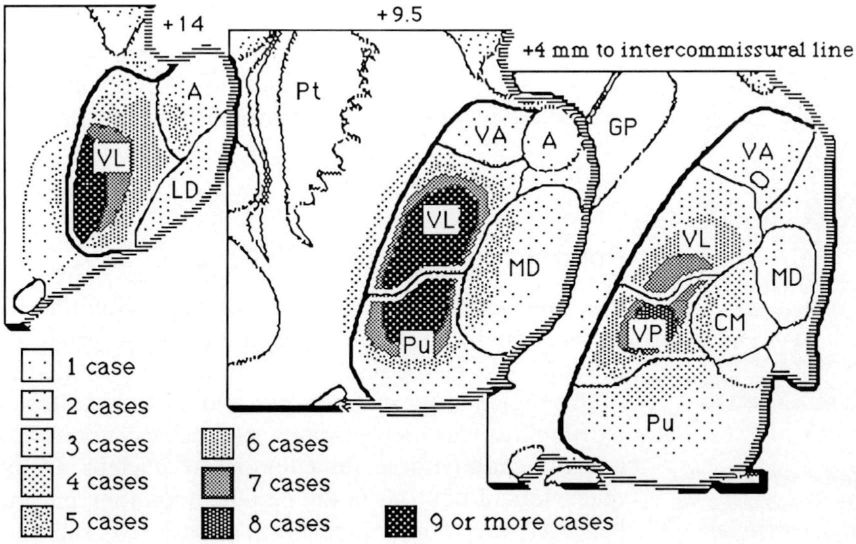

Figure 2-10
Thalamic astasia. Horizontal sections of the thalamus showing the regional frequency distribution of lesions in the patients with thalamic astasia reported by Masdeu and Gorelick.[79] Note that anterior is on top, posterior at the bottom, medial to the right, and lateral to the left. The most rostral section is at the left, and the most caudal is at the right.

receives information from the vestibulocerebellum.[82] Bilateral representation of this projection may be one of the factors explaining the transient nature of balance impairment when only one side is affected. Bilateral involvement of these structures by lacunar disease or disease of the white matter may result in permanent impairment of gait and balance.

Capsular and Basal Ganglia Lesions

A tendency to fall despite good strength was recorded by Groothuis and associates.[83] in a patient with a small medial capsular hemorrhage involving the most lateral portion of the ventrolateral nucleus of the thalamus and by Labadie and coworkers in patients with acute lesions in the basal ganglia.[84] Multiple bilateral lacunae involving the basal ganglia can be accompanied by gait impairment (Fig. 2-8).

Hydrocephalus

Hydrocephalus is a well-recognized and treatable cause of gait impairment, particularly among older people.[68,85,86] Not as common as was suspected when it first was reported,[87] this entity nevertheless should be recognized when present because shunting is helpful.[88] The ventricles are dilated, and the callosocaudal angle is blunted (Fig. 2-11). Ventricular dilation includes the third and fourth ventricles. The subarachnoid space may be obliterated, but this finding is not always present, particularly in the elderly population. In patients with shunt-responsive hydrocephalus, white matter lesions on MRI are uncommon and their presence correlates negatively with a good outcome after shunting.[89,90] Other helpful clinical and imaging findings were defined by Graff-Radford and coworkers[88] on the basis of a good outcome from shunting (Table 2-1). Because the imaging of hydrocephalus is reviewed in detail in Chap. 11, it is mentioned here only in connection with gait impairment.

Table 2-1
Predictors of good outcome after shunting in hydrocephalus of the elderly ("normal-pressure" hydrocephalus)

1. Gait impaired first or at same time as cognition
2. Patient demented less than 2 years
3. No history of alcohol abuse
4. History of subarachnoid hemorrhage, meningitis, brain surgery, head injury
5. Head circumference < 59 cm (men) or < 57 cm (women)
6. No aphasia
7. Improvement after draining 30–50 mL
8. Flow void in sylvian aqueduct on MRI
9. Lowered frontoparietal perfusion ratio on SPECT

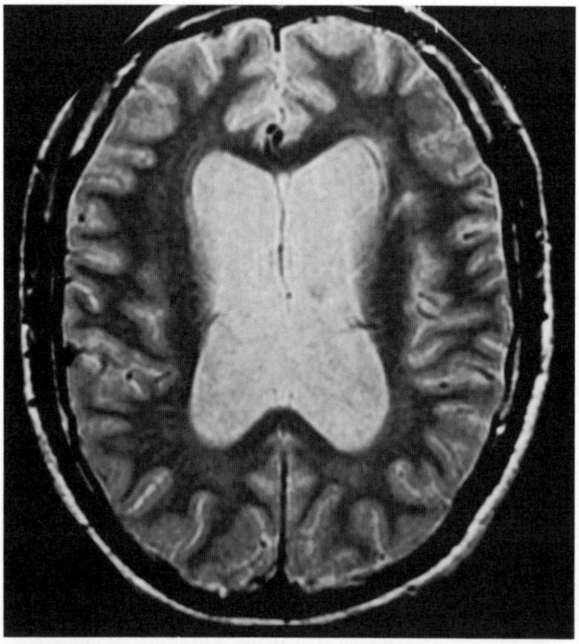

Figure 2-11
Hydrocephalus. MRI of a 58-year-old man with gait impairment that had progressed over 3 years after moderate head trauma. Note the ventricular dilation and the rounding of the callosocaudal angle.

Bilateral Subdural Hematomas

Chronic subdural hematomas cause generally mild hemiparesis and aphasic or apractic syndromes. When bilateral, they may present predominantly as gait failure, particularly in elderly individuals.[91] These lesions are prominent on MRI on both T1- and T2-weighted images.

INFRATENTORIAL LESIONS

Infratentorial lesions often cause impairment of balance and gait. Two major classical syndromes are cerebellar ataxia and vestibular dysequilibrium. Less often reported are dysequilibrium syndromes arising from midbrain or high pontine lesions in the area of the mesencephalic locomotor region.

Pontomesencephalic Gait Failure

The laterodorsal region of the midbrain contains the mesencephalic locomotor region, which plays an important role in locomotion in animals.[92] Stimulation of this region in the cat induces rapid walking, followed by running. This area contains the nucleus cuneiformis and the cholinergic pedunculopontine nucleus. In humans, loss of neurons in the pedunculopontine nucleus has been found in patients with progressive supranu-

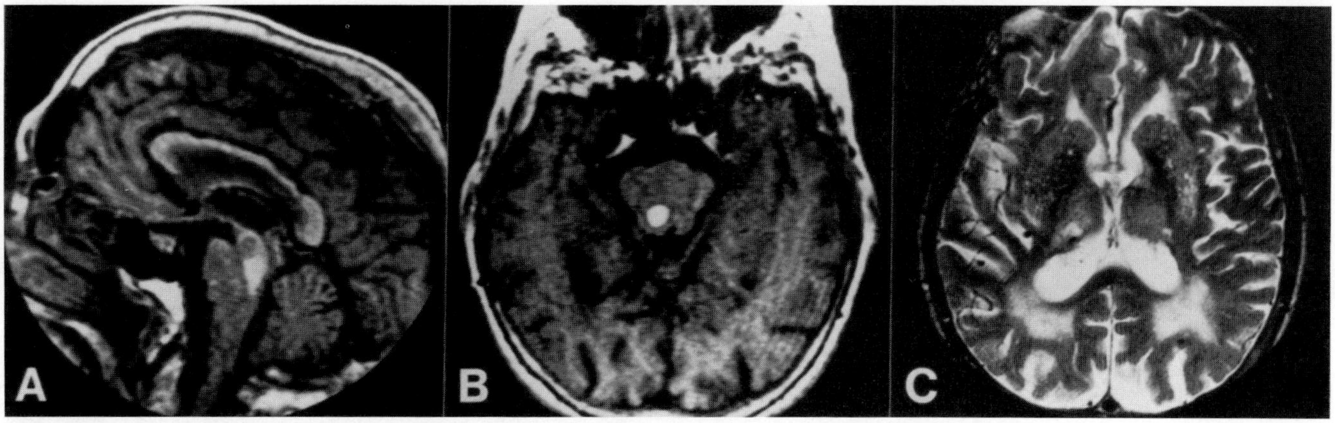

Figure 2-12
Pedunculopontine gait failure. MRI of an 83-year-old woman with gait failure after a hemorrhage in the locomotor mesencephalic region. The lesion is shown in the sagittal **(A)** *and coronal* **(B)** *planes. In addition, periventricular white matter changes and small thalamic lacunae were present in this chronically hypertensive individual* **(C)**.

clear palsy and Parkinson disease but not in patients with Alzheimer disease, perhaps implying a role of this nucleus in ambulatory mechanisms. The patient whose MRI is shown in Fig. 2-12 had the acute onset of inability to walk without hemiparesis or sensory loss. She was able to draw a circle with either leg when sitting down but could not generate regular stepping movements with her feet. Holding on to a walker and stooping forward, she could walk with short, shuffling, irregular steps. Her base of ambulation was only minimally wide. Regular stepping was not initiated either in attempted walking or in response to loss of balance. The steps were of irregular amplitude and direction, sometimes directed laterally. The left foot seemed to step less readily than did the right. Often there would be two steps with one foot while the other foot remained motionless. There was no cadence or rhythmicity to this patient's gait. The deficit of gait observed in this patient bears a striking resemblance to the gait failure experienced by many elderly individuals, which in most cases does not have a clear anatomic correlate.[93] They lack the ability to generate spontaneous, rhythmic stepping movements. Imaging studies may show hemorrhagic or ischemic lesions in these patients.[94,95]

The connectivity of the pedunculopontine region suggests an important role in motor behavior for this area. It receives projections from the deep cerebellar nuclei,[96] substantia nigra[97] and globus pallidus[98] as well as from the nucleus locus coeruleus and the raphe nuclei[99] and projects to the substantia nigra, globus pallidus, subthalamic nucleus, ventrolateral nucleus of the thalamus, and motor cortex[100] as well as to pontomedullary reticular nuclei that are known to influence the pattern generators in the spinal cord.[99,101] In addition to the effects of electric stimulation mentioned above, the results of injection in this area of putative neurotransmitters suggest a role for the pedunculopontine area in locomotion. Spontaneous locomotion, which occurs in the precollicular-premammillary transected cat, can be blocked by the injection of γ-aminobutyric acid (GABA). In contrast, when increasing amounts of GABA antagonists or substance P are given, the step cycle frequency can be increased from a walk to a trot to a gallop.[99] Lesions of the pedunculopontine nucleus lead to a reduction of locomotor activity in experimental animals.[102]

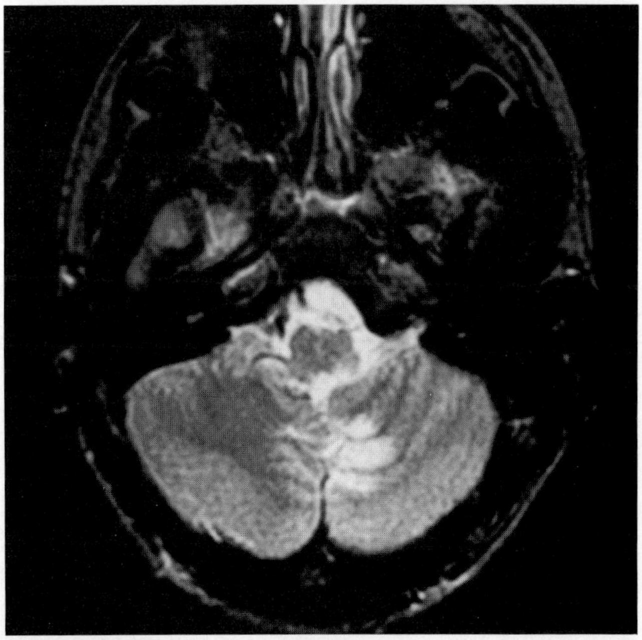

Figure 2-13
Wallenberg syndrome. MRI of a 31-year-old man with a left lateral medullary infarction after spontaneous dissection of the left vertebral artery. The cerebellar tonsil is also affected.

Vestibular Lesions

Lesions of the vestibular region may present with unilateral or bilateral findings. Unilateral findings are not uncommon in vascular disorders such as Wallenberg syndrome (Fig. 2-13), with multiple sclerosis, and with neoplasms of the cerebellopontine angle. These patients tend to fall to the side of the lesion. Bilateral findings are present in Wernicke encephalopathy of vitamin B_1 deficiency. On MRI, changes have been documented in the periventricular gray matter, consisting of reversible high intensity on T2-weighted images and transient gadolinium enhancement.[103,104]

Cerebellar Lesions

Cerebellar lesions, particularly those affecting the flocculonodular lobe, or vestibulocerebellum, can present with acute or progressive impairment of balance and gait (Fig. 2-14). Although patients with cerebellar lesions most often tend to fall to the side of the lesion, some patients with lesions in the tonsilar area develop increased tone (and increased reflexes) in the ipsilateral side and fall to the contralateral side. This was the case with the 64-year-old whose CT is shown in Fig. 2-15.

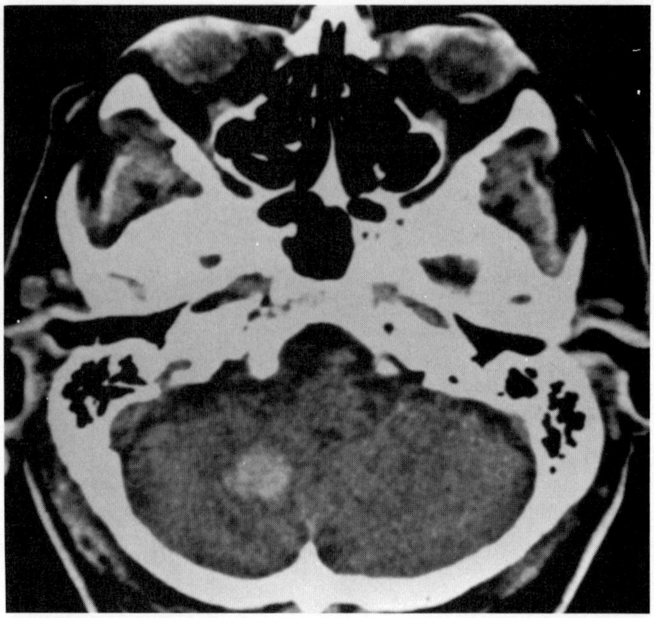

Figure 2-15
Cerebellar hematoma. CT of a 64-year-old man with sudden onset of inability to walk and a tendency to fall to the left side. A hemorrhage involves the right supratonsilar region.

MYELOPATHY

When advanced, spinal cord lesions give rise to unmistakable corticospinal tract findings. However, the initial manifestations of a myelopathy are often gait and balance impairment. In young patients the complaint may be difficulty running. The most common findings among patients with spinal cord lesions are cervical spondylosis in the elderly and multiple sclerosis in young individuals.

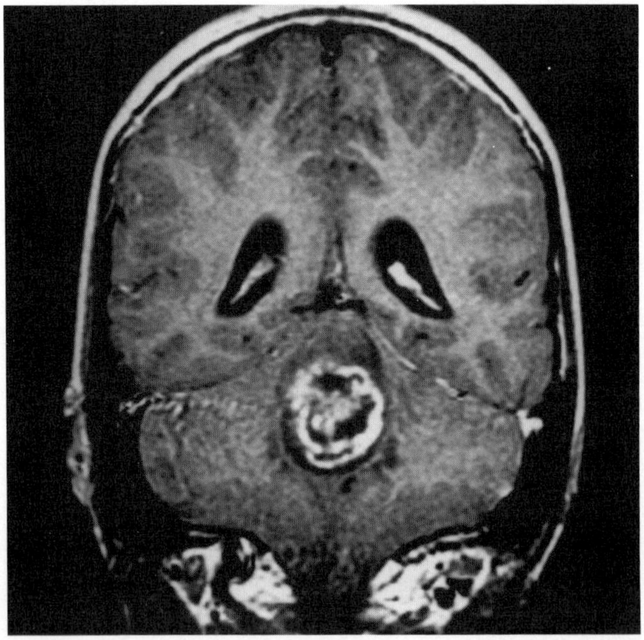

Figure 2-14
Cerebellar astrocytoma. Gadolinium-enhanced MRI of a 14-year-old boy with progressive difficulty running.

Cervical Spondylosis

Cervical spondylosis is generally severe before it causes impairment of gait. The changes in ambulation often are accompanied by radicular findings such as pain and reflex changes. If the lesion is central and mild, the patient may experience only subtle changes in locomotion. In some of these mild cases the clinical role of the degenerative changes visualized on MRI is often difficult to define.[105] The patient whose MRI is shown in Fig. 2-16 noticed a tendency to trip over high stairs and not clear the curb with her toes while walking in the street. Bony osteophytes are responsible for narrowing of the canal and questionable compression of the cervical cord. No change in signal intensity is demonstrated in the cord itself. More advanced disease (Fig. 2-17) gave rise to a quadriparesis with a spastic-ataxic gait. On T2-weighted images the spinal cord appears hyperintense below the area of maximal compression. Identification of cervical myelopathy is important because this entity can be treated.[106–110] After surgery, decreased cord compression and lessening of the increased T2 signal on MRI may predict clinical

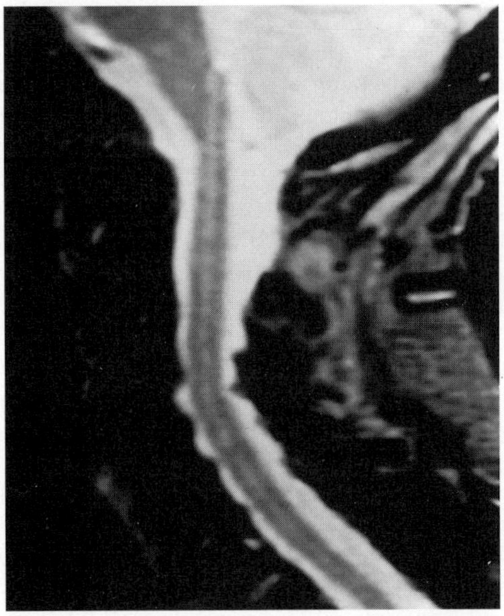

Figure 2-16

Cervical spondylosis. MRI of a 75-year-old woman with mild gait impairment and a left-sided inverted radial reflex. Although there is narrowing of the subarachnoid space because of degenerative disc disease, the signal intensity of the spinal cord is normal.

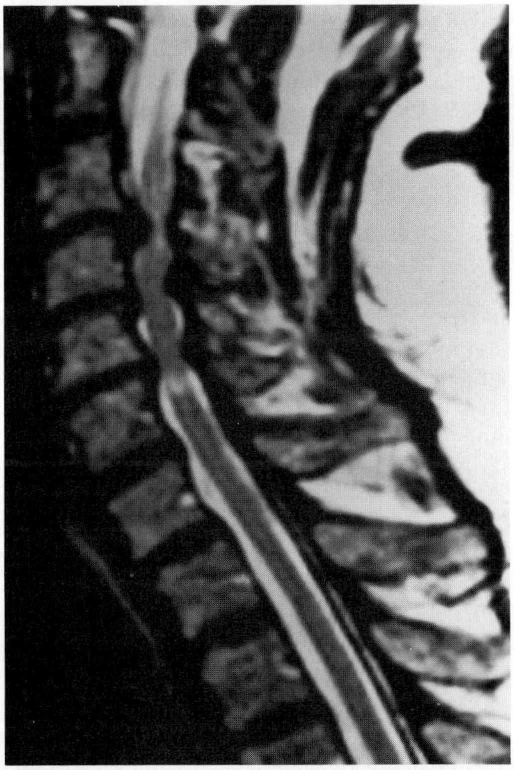

Figure 2-17

Cervical spondylosis with cervical myelopathy. MRI of a 67-year-old woman with a progressive quadriparesis and a spastic gait. The spinal cord is compressed at the C3–4–5 levels. Increased signal intensity in the substance of the cord indicates the presence of a myelopathy.

recovery.[111,112] In a series of 102 patients, Statham and coworkers showed that MRI was sufficient for the imaging evaluation of cervical myelopathy and that myelography did not change management.[113] MRI is very helpful in the evaluation of progression of clinical findings in patients who previously were treated surgically.[114]

Multiple Sclerosis

Gait or balance impairment may be the only manifestation of multiple sclerosis involving the spinal cord or some of the higher levels of the neuraxis discussed above. Because of the frequency with which multiple sclerosis becomes symptomatic when it affects the spinal cord and its propensity to cause gait disturbances, this disorder is mentioned here.[115] In addition to the impairment of gait or balance, many of these patients experience sensory changes. The patient whose MRI is shown in Fig. 2-18 presented with sensory ataxia and numbness below the level of C4. These lesions appear bright on T2-weighted images and may have some mass effect (Fig. 2-18). T1-weighted images may show hypointensity but are often negative unless gadolinium is administered. Enhancement is common with acute lesions. Although the rate of negative studies is not known, approximately 15 percent of these patients may have a negative MRI on the first presentation. Multiple sclerosis may be associated with cervical spondylosis, in which case both conditions should be treated.[116]

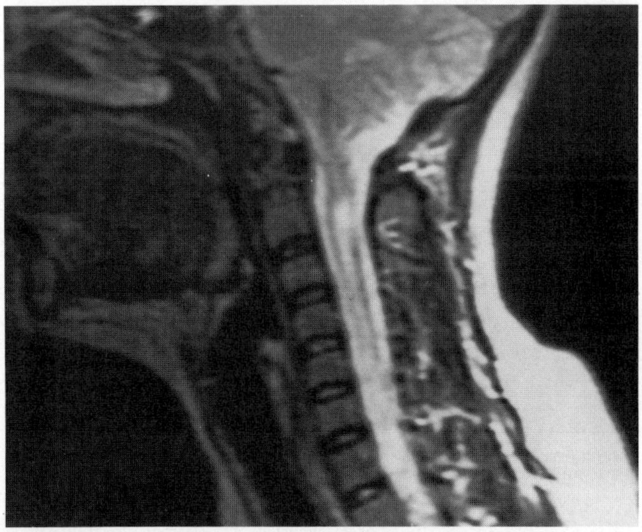

Figure 2-18

Multiple sclerosis. MRI of a 38-year-old woman with sensory ataxia and numbness below the level of C4. The lesion appears bright on this T2-weighted image and has some mass effect.

REFERENCES

1. Britton TC, Thompson PD, van der Kamp W, et al: Primary orthostatic tremor: Further observations in six cases. *J Neurol* 239:209–217, 1992.
2. Newman G, Dovenmuehle R, Busse E: Alterations in neurologic status with age. *J Am Geriatr Soc* 8:915–917, 1960.
3. Baker S, Harvey A: Fall injuries in the elderly, in Radebaugh T, Hadley E, Suzman R (eds) *Falls in the Elderly: Biologic and Behavioral Aspects.* Clinics in Geriatric Medicine, vol 1. Philadelphia, Saunders, 1985, pp 501–512.
4. Haupt B, Graves E: Detailed diagnoses and surgical procedures for patients discharged from short-stay hospitals, 1979, in DHHS Pub. (PHS) 82-1274-1 U.S. Washington, D.C., Department of Health and Human Services, 1982.
5. Zhang WW, Ma KC, Andersen O, et al: The microvascular changes in cases of hereditary multi-infarct disease of the brain. *Acta Neuropathol Berl* 87:317–324, 1994.
6. Hennerici MG, Oster M, Cohen S, et al: Are gait disturbances and white matter degeneration early indicators of vascular dementia? *Dementia* 5:197–202, 1994.
7. Baloh RW, Yue Q, Socotch TM, Jacobson KM: White matter lesions and disequilibrium in older people: I. Case-control comparison. *Arch Neurol* 52:970–974, 1995.
8. Baloh RW, Vinters HV: White matter lesions and disequilibrium in older people: II. Clinicopathologic correlation. *Arch Neurol* 2:975–981, 1995.
9. Achiron A, Ziv I, Goren M, et al: Primary progressive freezing gait. *Mov Disord* 8:293–297, 1993.
10. Blaser SI, Clarke JT, Becker LE: Neuroradiology of lysosomal disorders. *Neuroimaging Clin North Am* 4:283–298, 1994.
11. Malm J, Kristensen B, Karlsson T, et al: The predictive value of cerebrospinal fluid dynamic tests in patients with the idiopathic adult hydrocephalus syndrome. *Arch Neurol* 52:783–789, 1995.
12. Masdeu JC: Cerebrovascular disorders, in Masdeu JC, Sudarsky L, Wolfson L (eds): *Gait Disorders of Aging,* vol 22. Philadelphia, Lippincott & Raven, 1997, pp 221–243.
13. Fazekas F, Niederkorn K, Schmidt R, et al: White matter signal abnormalities in normal individuals: Correlation with carotid ultrasonography, cerebral blood flow measurements, and cerebrovascular risk factors. *Stroke* 19:1285–1288, 1988.
14. Goto K, Ishii N, Fukasawa H: Diffuse white-matter disease in the geriatric population: A clinical, neuropathological, and CT study. *Radiology* 141:687–695, 1981.
15. Meyer JS, Kawamura J, Terayama Y: White matter lesions in the elderly. *J Neurol Sci* 110:1–7, 1992.
16. Zatz L, Jernigan T, Ahumada AJ: White matter changes in cerebral computed tomography related to aging. *J Comput Assist Tomogr* 6:19–23, 1982.
17. Gerard G, Weisberg I: MRI periventricular lesions in adults. *Neurology* 36:998–1001, 1986.
18. McQuinn B, O'Leary D: CT periventricular lucencies: Association with systemic disease states and with subacute arteriosclerotic encephalopathy (SAE, "Binswanger's disease"). *Stroke* 17:135, 1986.
19. Pullicino P, Eskin T, Ketonen L: Prevalence of Binswanger's disease. *Lancet* 1:939, 1983.
20. George A, de Leon M, Gentes C, et al: Leukoencephalopathy in normal and pathologic aging: CT of brain lucencies. *AJNR* 7:561–566, 1986.
21. Awad I, Spetzler R, Hodak J, et al: Incidental subcortical lesions identified on magnetic resonance imaging in the elderly: I. Correlation with age and cerebrovascular risk factors. *Stroke* 17:1084–1089, 1986.
22. Brant-Zawadzki M, Fein G, Van Dyke C, et al: MR imaging of the aging brain: Patchy white-matter lesions and dementia. *AJNR* 6:675–682, 1985.
23. Zimmerman R, Fleming C, Lee B, et al: Periventricular hyperintensity as seen by magnetic resonance: Prevalence and significance. *AJR* 146:443–450, 1986.
24. Kinkel W, Jacobs L, Polachini I, et al: Subcortical arteriosclerotic encephalopathy (Binswanger's disease): Computed tomographic, nuclear magnetic resonance, and clinical correlations. *Arch Neurol* 42:951–959, 1985.
25. Awad I, Johnson P, Spetzler R, Hodak J: Incidental subcortical lesions identified on magnetic resonance imaging in the elderly: II. Postmortem pathological correlations. *Stroke* 17:1090–1097, 1986.
26. Kirkpatric J, Hayman L: White-matter lesions on MR imaging of clinically healthy brains of elderly subjects: Possible pathologic basis. *Radiology* 162:509–511, 1987.
27. Hachinski V, Potter P, Merskey H: Leuko-araiosis. *Arch Neurol* 44:21–23, 1987.
28. Braffman B, Zimmerman R, Trojanowski J, et al: Pathologic correlation with gross and histopathology: II. Hyperintense white-matter foci in the elderly. *AJNR* 9:629–636, 1988.
29. Johnson K, Davis K, Buonanno F, et al: Comparison of magnetic resonance and roentgen ray computed tomography in dementia. *Arch Neurol* 44:1075–1080, 1987.
30. Lotz P, Ballinger W, Quisling R: Subcortical arteriosclerotic encephalopathy: CT spectrum and pathologic correlation. *AJR* 147:1209–1214, 1986.
31. Marshall V, Bradley W, Marshall C, et al: Deep white matter infarction: Correlation of MR imaging and histopathologic findings. *Radiology* 167:517–522, 1988.
32. Rezek D, Morris J, Fulling K, Gado M: Periventricular white matter lucencies in senile dementia of the Alzheimer type and in normal aging. *Neurology* 37:1365–1368, 1987.
33. Rosenberg G, Kornfeld M, Stovring J, Bicknell J: Subcortical arteriosclerotic encephalopathy (Binswanger): Computerized tomography. *Neurology* 29:1102–1106, 1979.
34. Dubas F, Gray F, Roullet E, Escourolle R: Leucoencephalopathies artériopathiques (17 cas anatomo-cliniques). *Rev Neurol (Paris)* 141:93–108, 1985.
35. Gray F, Dubas F, Roullet E, Escourolle R: Leukoencephalopathy in diffuse hemorrhagic cerebral amyloid angiopathy. *Ann Neurol* 18:54–59, 1985.
36. Yamanouchi H: Loss of white matter oligodendrocytes and astrocytes in progressive subcortical vascular encephalopathy of Binswanger type. *Acta Neurol Scand* 83:301–305, 1991.
37. van Swieten JC, Geyskes GG, Derix MM, et al: Hypertension in the elderly is associated with white matter

lesions and cognitive decline. *Ann Neurol* 30:825–830, 1991.
38. Almkvist O, Wahlund LO, Andersson-Lundman G, et al: White-matter hyperintensity and neuropsychological functions in dementia and healthy aging. *Arch Neurol* 49:626–632, 1992.
39. Mirsen TR, Lee DH, Wong CJ, et al: Clinical correlates of white-matter changes on magnetic resonance imaging scans of the brain. *Arch Neurol* 48:1015–1021, 1991.
40. Rao S, Mittenberg W, Bernardin L, et al: Neuropsychological test findings in subjects with leukoaraiosis. *Arch Neurol* 46:40–44, 1989.
41. Valentine A, Moseley I, Kendall B: White matter abnormality in cerebral atrophy: Clinicoradiological correlations. *J Neurol Neurosurg Psychiatry* 43:139–142, 1980.
42. Zeumer H, Hacke W, Kolmann H, Ringelstein E: Subcortical arteriosclerotic encephalopathy (Binswanger disease). *Exp Brain Res* 5(suppl 5):272–276, 1982.
43. Thompson P, Marsden C: Gait disorder of subcortical arteriosclerotic encephalopathy: Binswanger's disease. *Mov Disord* 2:1–8, 1987.
44. Caplan L, Schoene W: Clinical features of subcortical arteriosclerotic encephalopathy (Binswanger disease). *Neurology* 28:1206–1215, 1978.
45. Dupuis M, Brucher J, Gonsette R: Obsevation anatomoclinique d'une encéphalopathie sous-corticale artérioscléreuse ("maladie de Binswanger") avec hypodensité de la substance blanche au scanner cérébral. *Acta Neurol Belg* 84:131–140, 1984.
46. Huang K, Wu L, Luo Y: Binswanger's disease: Progressive subcortical encephalopathy or multi-infarct dementia? *Can J Neurol Sci* 2:88–94, 1985.
47. Janota I: Dementia, deep white matter damage and hypertension: "Binswanger's disease." *Psychol Med* 11:39–48, 1981.
48. Loizou L, Kendall B, Marshall J: Subcortical arteriosclerotic encephalopathy: A clinical and radiological investigation. *J Neurol Neurosurg Psychiatry* 44:294–304, 1981.
49. Steingart A, Hachinski V, Lau C: Cognitive and neurologic findings in subjects with diffuse white matter lucencies on computed tomographic scan (leuko-araiosis). *Arch Neurol* 44:32–35, 1987.
50. Hendrie H, Farlow M, Austrom M, et al: Foci of increased T2 signal intensity on brain MR scans of healthy elderly subjects. *AJNR* 10:703–707, 1989.
51. FitzGerald P, Jankovic J: Lower body parkinsonism: Evidence for vascular etiology: *Mov Disord* 4:249–260, 1987.
52. Masdeu J, Wolfson L, Lantos G, et al: White matter disease in the elderly prone to falling. *Arch Neurol* 46:1292–1296, 1989.
53. McCombe PA, McLaughlin DB, Chalk JB, et al: Spasticity and white matter abnormalities in adult phenylketonuria. *J Neurol Neurosurg Psychiatry* 55:359–361, 1992.
54. van der Knaap M, Valk J, de Neeling N, Nauta J: Pattern recognition in magnetic resonance imaging of white matter disorders in children and young adults. *Neuroradiology* 33:478–493, 1991.
55. Sabbadini G, Francia A, Calandriello L, et al: Cerebral autosomal dominant arteriopathy with subcortical infarcts and leukoencephalopathy (CADASIL): Clinical, neuroimaging, pathological and genetic study of a large Italian family. *Brain* 118:207–215, 1995.
56. Chabriat H, Vahedi K, Iba-Zizen MT, et al: Clinical spectrum of CADASIL: A study of 7 families: Cerebral autosomal dominant arteriopathy with subcortical infarcts and leukoencephalopathy [see comments]. *Lancet* 346:934–939, 1995.
57. Ducros A, Nagy T, Alamowitch S, et al: Cerebral autosomal dominant arteriopathy with subcortical infarcts and leukoencephalopathy, genetic homogeneity, and mapping of the locus within a 2-cM interval. *Am J Hum Genet* 58:171–181, 1996.
58. Joutel A, Vahedi K, Corpechot C, et al: Strong clustering and stereotyped nature of Notch3 mutations in CADASIL patients [see comments]. *Lancet* 350:1511–1515, 1997.
59. Ruchoux MM, Maurage CA: CADASIL: Cerebral autosomal dominant arteriopathy with subcortical infarcts and leukoencephalopathy. *J Neuropathol Exp Neurol* 56:947–964, 1997.
60. Rubio A, Rifkin D, Powers JM, et al: Phenotypic variability of CADASIL and novel morphologic findings. *Acta Neuropathol (Berl)* 94:247–254, 1997.
61. Gutierrez-Molina M, Caminero Rodriguez A, Martinez Garcia C, et al: Small arterial granular degeneration in familial Binswanger's syndrome. *Acta Neuropathol (Berl)* 87:98–105, 1997.
62. Jen J, Cohen AH, Yue Q, et al: Hereditary endotheliopathy with retinopathy, and stroke (HERNS). *Neurology* 49:1322–1330, 1997.
63. Quattrocolo G, Leombruni S, Vaula G, et al: Autosomal dominant late-onset leukoencephalopathy: Clinical report of a new Italian family. *Eur Neurol* 37:53–61, 1997.
64. Bornstein RA, Chakeres D, Brogan M, et al: Magnetic resonance imaging of white matter lesions in HIV infection. *J Neuropsychiatry Clin Neurosci* 4:174–178, 1992.
65. Broderick DF, Wippold FII, Clifford DB, et al: White matter lesions and cerebral atrophy on MR images in patients with and without AIDS dementia complex. *AJR* 161:177–181, 1993.
66. Patel AG, Rao R: Transient Ara-C leukoencephalopathy: MR findings. *J Comput Assist Tomogr* 20:161–162, 1996.
67. Fuh JL, Lin KN, Wang SJ, et al: Neurologic diseases presenting with gait impairment in the elderly. *J Geriatr Psychiatry Neurol* 7:89–92, 1994.
68. Sudarsky L, Ronthal M: Gait disorders among elderly patients. *Arch Neurol* 40:740–743, 1983.
69. Boon A, Lodder J, Heuts-van-Raak L, Kessels F: Silent brain infarcts in 755 consecutive patients with a first-ever supratentorial ischemic stroke: Relationship with index-stroke subtype, vascular risk factors, and mortality. *Stroke* 25:2384–2390, 1994.
70. Brott T, Tomsick T, Feinberg W, et al: Baseline silent cerebral infarction in the Asymptomatic Carotid Atherosclerosis Study. *Stroke* 25:1122–1129, 1994.
71. Cambier J, Elghozi D, Strube E: Lésions du thalamus droit avec syndrome de l'hémisphère mineur: Discussion du concept de négligence thalamique. *Rev Neurol (Paris)* 136:105–116, 1980.
72. Laplane D, Escourolle R, Degos J, et al: La négligence motrice d'origine thalamique: A propos de deux cas. *Rev Neurol (Paris)* 138:201–211, 1982.
73. Jenkyn L, Alberti A, Peters J: Language dysfunction,

somasthetic hemi-inattention, and thalamic hemorrhage in the dominant hemisphere. *Neurology (NY)* 31:1202, 1981.
74. Verma A, Maheshwari M: Hypesthetic-ataxic-hemiparesis in thalamic hemorrhage. *Stroke* 17:49–51, 1986.
75. Fisher C, Cole M: Homolateral ataxia and crural paresis: A vascular syndrome. *J Neurol Neurosurg Psychiatry* 28:48–55, 1965.
76. Huang C, Lui F: Ataxic-hemiparesis, localization and clinical features. *Stroke* 15:363–366, 1984.
77. Iragui V, McCutchen C: Capsular ataxic hemiparesis. *Arch Neurol* 39:528–529, 1982.
78. Sage J, Lepore F: Ataxic hemiparesis from lesions of the corona radiata. *Arch Neurol* 40:449–450, 1983.
79. Masdeu J, Gorelick P: Thalamic astasia: Inability to stand after unilateral thalamic lesions. *Ann Neurol* 23:596–603, 1988.
80. Jones E: *The Thalamus.* New York, Plenum Press, 1985.
81. Van Buren J, Borke R: Variations and connections of the human thalamus. Berlin, New York, Springer-Verlag, 1972.
82. Asanuma C, Thach W, Jones E: Distribution of cerebellar terminations and their relation to other afferent terminations in the thalamic ventral lateral region of the monkey. *Brain Res Rev* 5:237–265, 1983.
83. Groothuis D, Duncan G, Fisher C: The human thalamocortical sensory path in the internal capsule: Evidence from a small capsular hemorrhage causing a pure sensory stroke. *Ann Neurol* 2:328–333, 1977.
84. Labadie E, Awerbuch G, Hamilton R, Rapcsak S: Falling and postural deficits due to acute unilateral basal ganglia lesions. *Arch Neurol* 261:492–496, 1989.
85. Fisher C: Hydrocephalus as a cause of disturbances of gait in the elderly. *Neurology* 32:1358–1363, 1982.
86. Koller W, Wilson R, Glatt S, et al: Senile gait: Correlation with computed tomographic scans. *Ann Neurol* 13:343–344, 1983.
87. Adams R, Fisher C, Hakim S, et al: Symptomatic occult hydrocephalus with "normal" cerebrospinal fluid pressure. *N Engl J Med* 273:117–126, 1965.
88. Graff-Radford N, Godersky J, Jones M: Variables predicting outcome in symptomatic hydrocephalus in the elderly. *Neurology* 39:1601–1604, 1989.
89. Krauss JK, Droste DW, Vach W, et al: Cerebrospinal fluid shunting in idiopathic normal-pressure hydrocephalus of the elderly: Effect of periventricular and deep white matter lesions. *Neurosurgery* 39:292–299, 1996.
90. Kristensen B, Malm J, Fagerland M, et al: Regional cerebral blood flow, white matter abnormalities, and cerebrospinal fluid hydrodynamics in patients with idiopathic adult hydrocephalus syndrome. *J Neurol Neurosurg Psychiatry* 60:282–288, 1996.
91. Goto I, Kuroiwa Y, Kitamura K: The triad of neurological manifestations in bilateral chronic subdural hematoma and normal pressure hydrocephalus. *J Neurosurg Sci* 30:123–128, 1986.
92. Garcia-Rill E: The pedunculopontine nucleus. *Prog Neurobiol* 36:363–389, 1991.
93. Nutt J, Marsden C, Thompson P: Human walking and higher-level gait disorders, particularly in the elderly. *Neurology* 43:268–279, 1993.
94. Felice K, Keilson G, Schwartz W: "Rubral" gait ataxia. *Neurology* 40:1004–1005, 1990.
95. Sand J, Biller J, Corbett J, et al: Partial dorsal mesencephalic hemorrhages: Report of three cases. *Neurology* 36:529–533, 1986.
96. Hazrati LN, Parent A: Projection from the deep cerebellar nuclei to the pedunculopontine nucleus in the squirrel monkey. *Brain Res* 585:267–271, 1992.
97. Granata AR, Kitai ST: Inhibitory substantia nigra inputs to the pedunculopontine neurons. *Exp Brain Res* 86:459–466, 1991.
98. Moriizumi T, Hattori T: Separate neuronal populations of the rat globus pallidus projecting to the subthalamic nucleus, auditory cortex and pedunculopontine tegmental area. *Neuroscience* 46:701–710, 1992.
99. Skinner R, Garcia-Rill E: Brainstem modulation of rhythmic functions and behaviors, in Klemm W, Vertes R (eds): *Brainstem Mechanisms and Behavior.* New York, Wiley, 1990, pp 465–496.
100. Nakano K, Hasegawa Y, Tokushige A, et al: Topographical projections from the thalamus, subthalamic nucleus and pedunculopontine tegmental nucleus to the striatum in the Japanese monkey, Macaca fuscata. *Brain Res* 537:54–68, 1990.
101. Grofova I, Keane S: Descending brainstem projections of the pedunculopontine tegmental nucleus in the rat. *Anat Embryol (Berl)* 184:275–290, 1991.
102. Mogenson G, Wu M, Brudzynski S: The role of pedunculopontine nucleus in locomotor activity. *Neurosci Abstr* 16:753, 1990.
103. Gallucci M, Bozzao A, Splendiani A, et al: Wernicke encephalopathy: MR findings in five patients. *AJNR* 11:887–892, 1990.
104. Schroth G, Wichmann W, Valavanis A: Blood-brain-barrier disruption in acute Wernicke encephalopathy: MR findings. *J Comput Assist Tomogr* 15:1059–1061, 1991.
105. Rowland LP: Surgical treatment of cervical spondylotic myelopathy: Time for a controlled trial. *Neurology* 42:5–13, 1992.
106. Arnold H, Feldmann U, Missler U: Chronic spondylogenic cervical myelopathy: A critical evaluation of surgical treatment after early and long-term follow-up. *Neurosurg Rev* 16:105–109, 1993.
107. Dillin W, Uppal GS: Analysis of medications used in the treatment of cervical disk degeneration. *Orthop Clin North Am* 23:421–433, 1992.
108. Klara PM, Foley K: Surgical treatment of osteophytes and calcified discs of the cervical spine. *Neurosurg Clin North Am* 4:53–60, 1993.
109. Maurer PK, Ellenbogen RG, Ecklund J, et al: Cervical spondylotic myelopathy: Treatment with posterior decompression and Luque rectangle bone fusion. *Neurosurgery* 28:680–683, 1991.
110. Tan JC, Nordin M: Role of physical therapy in the treatment of cervical disk disease. *Orthop Clin North Am* 23:435–449, 1992.
111. Harada A, Mimatsu K: Postoperative changes in the spinal cord in cervical myelopathy demonstrated by magnetic resonance imaging. *Spine* 17:1275–1280, 1992.
112. Matsuda Y, Miyazaki K, Tada K, et al: Increased MR

signal intensity due to cervical myelopathy: Analysis of 29 surgical cases. *J Neurosurg* 74:887–892, 1991.

113. Statham PF, Hadley DM, Macpherson P, et al: MRI in the management of suspected cervical spondylotic myelopathy. *J Neurol Neurosurg Psychiatry* 54:484–489, 1991.
114. Goto S, Mochizuki M, Watanabe T, et al: Long-term follow-up study of anterior surgery for cervical spondylotic myelopathy with special reference to the magnetic resonance imaging findings in 52 cases. *Clin Orthop* 291:142–153, 1991.
115. Poser CM: MRI of spinal cord in multiple sclerosis [letter]. *Lancet* 341:1025, 1993.
116. Burgerman R, Rigamonti D, Randle JM, et al: The association of cervical spondylosis and multiple sclerosis. *Surg Neurol* 38:265–270, 1992.

SECTION TWO

PAIN, HEADACHE

CHAPTER 3

NEUROIMAGING OF PAIN

David J. Hewitt

INTRODUCTION

Pain is one of the most common symptoms that bring a patient to seek neurologic consultation, and the assessment often leads to the selection of an imaging study. Radiologic techniques, including plain radiography, radionuclide scans, computed tomography (CT), and magnetic resonance imaging (MRI), are commonly employed to confirm the diagnosis, direct further workup, or guide treatment. More controversial techniques include thermography and discography. There are also other neuroradiologic techniques, such as positron emission tomography (PET), single photon emission computed tomography (SPECT), and MR neuronography, which are used in special clinical circumstances or in clinical neurologic research.

Normal radiologic study results in the setting of a clinical impression of a serious pathologic condition should not deter the clinician from pursuing the diagnosis. The symptom of pain frequently precedes the identification of a pathologic process by radiographic techniques that are usually employed or that are currently available.

The patient who complains of pain in the absence of radiographic evidence of a pathologic condition is often considered a malingerer or worse. But not all pain leads to structural changes that can be visualized by the imaging techniques now available. Posttraumatic myofascial or muscular pain is an example; plain radiography and MRIs of the spine may be negative, but appropriate therapy can lead to an improvement in symptoms and a return to normal function. Similarly, an abnormal radiographic finding in an asymptomatic patient or in a symptomatic patient that does not explain the complaint of pain should not lead the clinician to clinical therapies that are not indicated or necessary. Many studies have demonstrated the presence of radiographic abnormalities in asymptomatic patients. Abnormalities such as disc protrusions have been discovered in asymptomatic individuals by plain radiography, myelogram, and CT.[1] Disc protrusions, spinal cord impingement, and spinal cord compression have also been documented on MRI in asymptomatic individuals.[2] In a study focusing on the thoracic spine using MRI, 73 percent of 90 asymptomatic individuals had positive anatomic findings at one or more levels, including disc herniation (37 percent), bulging discs (53 percent), anular tears (58 percent), deformations of the spinal cord (29 percent), and Scheuermann end-plate irregularities or kyphosis (38 percent).[3]

The first step in deciding on the appropriate radiologic study is a careful clinical evaluation of the patient. The physician should be aware of the indications for a particular study, understand how to interpret subsequent findings, personally review the studies with the neuroradiologist as appropriate, and develop a plan to direct therapeutic interventions accordingly. The patient should not endure any test unless the results will help to clarify the diagnosis or lead to a therapeutic intervention. Recent studies suggest, from a review of utilization of medical services, that there is both an overutilization and an underutilization of diagnostic and therapeutic services.[4] A good clinical evaluation and knowledge of the indications for the selection of a diagnostic intervention help in utilizing these services more effectively.

Accurate diagnosis depends on a logical approach to the clinical evaluation. Neuroanatomy and pathophysiology should be correlated with a detailed and relevant history. The neurologic history usually supplies 80 percent of the total diagnostic information, more than the neurologic examination or other investigations.

Critical to the assessment of the patient with pain is the establishment of a trusting relationship with the physician. A pain complaint is a symptom, not a diagnosis, and pain perception is not only a function of the amount of physical injury sustained by the patient but also a complex state determined by multiple factors. It is important to remember that the diagnosis of a specific pain syndrome and a complete understanding of the psychologic state of the patient is not always made on the initial evaluation. It may take several weeks to define the nature of the pain because of the lack of radiologic or pathologic verification. It may take a similar period to fully comprehend the psychologic makeup of the individual patient. Numerous examples in the assessment of patients with pain and neurologic illness illustrate the limitation of diagnostic procedures. For example, it is not uncommon for patients with tumor infiltration of the brachial plexus from lung or breast cancer to have pain for several weeks or months prior to the onset of objective radiologic and neurologic findings.

A comprehensive evaluation starts with a careful history; includes a detailed medical, neurologic, and psychologic evaluation; requires the development of a series of diagnosis-related hypotheses; and necessitates ordering the appropriate diagnostic studies. A careful history of the pain complaint includes the patient's description of the site of pain, its quality, exacerbating and alleviating factors, its temporal pattern, the precise time of onset, associated symptoms and signs, and interference with activities of daily living—all critical in helping establish the pain diagnosis. At the same time, a careful assessment of the patient's psychologic state and response to previous and current analgesic therapies can help to further define the problem. Multiple pain complaints are common and need to be ordered in terms of priority and classified.

During the initial assessment, it is critical to evaluate the psychologic state of the patient by trying to clarify the patient's level of anxiety and depression. It is useful to know whether the patient has had a previous history of psychiatric illness or past history or family history of acute or chronic pain. Information on how the patient has handled previous painful events may provide insight into whether the patient has a history of chronic illness behavior. A personal family history of alcohol or drug dependence may explain why the patient may be fearful of taking or refuse to take certain analgesic drugs, such as opioids. It is also useful to have the patient elaborate on the meaning of the pain, and, in patients with cancer, the meaning of pain often implies the possibility of recurrent tumor; in patients with rheumatoid arthritis, the recurrence of pain often implies acute exacerbation of their chronic disease. There is now sufficient evidence to demonstrate that persistent chronic pain interferes with a patient's quality of life and that a number of psychologic factors can often play a significant role in accounting for the differences in pain experienced in patients with neurologic illness.

At times, it is not possible to obtain detailed information about the patient's pain, psychologic state, and complex medical and neurologic history. Moreover, it may be necessary to verify the history with a family member who may provide information that the patient is unable or unwilling to provide. Similarly, with a patient who is a poor historian, the family member may be able to provide essential information that may alter the diagnostic approach. At all times, attempts should be made to compile a careful history and define the medical, neurologic, and psychologic profile of the pain complaint.

During the neurologic examination, finding changes in motor or sensory function can help provide the necessary data to substantiate the history and support or refute a working hypothesis. Knowledge of referral patterns (Fig. 3-1) of pain can often direct the neuroradiologic studies.[5] Through the physical and neurologic examination, the sites of pain can be inspected visually, and assessment of associated physical and neurologic signs can be pursued. For example, with hydronephrosis, the pain may be referred to the low back, mimicking spine disease (Fig. 3-2). Similarly, abdominal masses

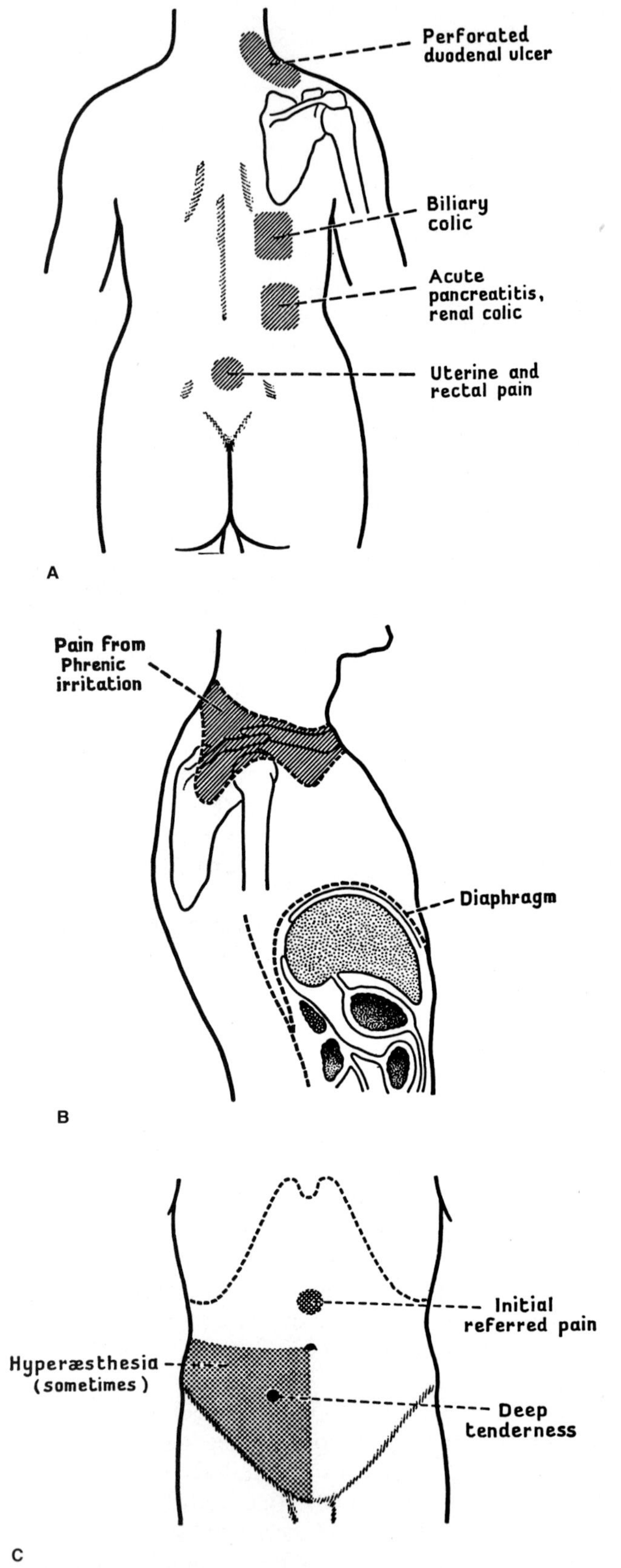

Figure 3-1
Demonstration of patterns of referred pain: **(A)** *referral from visceral sites to cutaneous sites on the back and front of the body,* **(B)** *pattern of referral of diaphragmatic irritation,* **(C)** *hyperesthesia as referred pain from appendicitis.*[5]

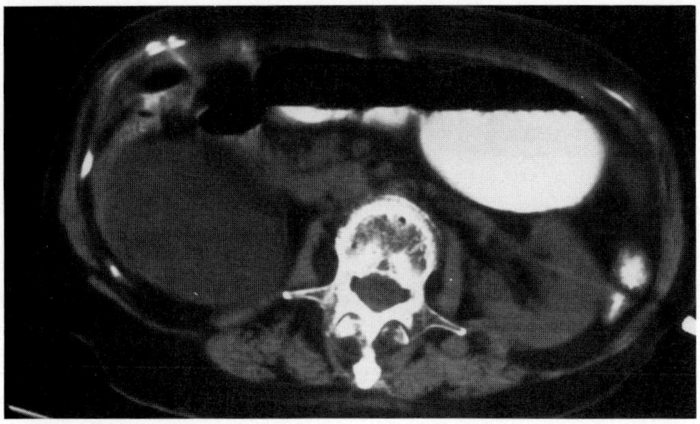

Figure 3-2
CT scan showing hydronephrosis from metastatic disease causing flank and back pain.

that cause distortion of tissues can cause nociceptive visceral pain to be referred to the back (Fig. 3-3).

Defining the degree of motor or sensory changes can help determine the specific site in the nervous system that may be involved. Similarly, the presence of sensory loss, allodynia, and hyperesthesia can further define the nature of the sensory problem.

As stated, diagnostic studies can confirm the clinical diagnosis and define the site and extent of the neuroanatomic area involved.

The next step in the assessment of the pain complaint is to decide on and then order and personally review the appropriate diagnostic studies. The importance of personally reviewing the appropriate diagnostic studies cannot be stressed enough, and this is not always easy. The demands on a physician's time may make it impractical to personally review all films, but relying on a radiologist's report may lead to a missed or wrong diagnosis. For example, in a worker's compensation case, a radiologist failed to report the presence of arachnoiditis that was present 6 weeks after a man fell off a roof and then developed back pain, leg pain, and impotence. The radiologist did not have an appropriate history and was only looking for disc disease. The most common diagnostic studies for the evaluation of patients with pain and neurologic illness include plain radiographs, bone scans, CT scans, and MRI scans. In the following section, the utility of the various modalities for determining the cause of various syndromes and diseases is discussed.

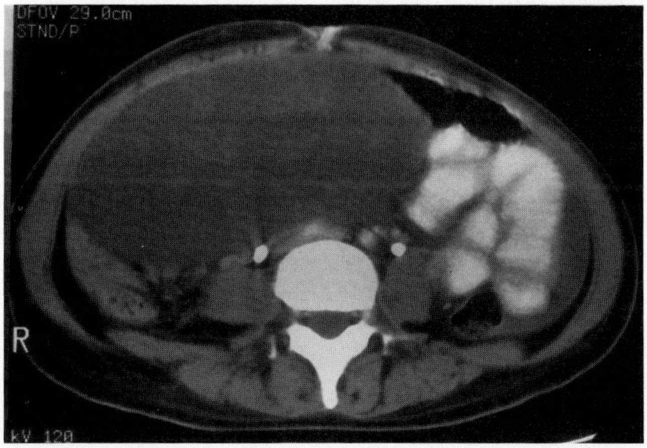

Figure 3-3
Intra-abdominal mass presenting as back and left leg pain in a 30-year-old Asian woman. She developed severe low back pain in the setting of increasing abdominal girth, decreased appetite, and increased fatigue. She was diagnosed with gastric adenocarcinoma on endoscopic biopsy. Her abdominal CT identifies a 14 × 10 × 13 cm well-encapsulated mass with both a solid and a cystic component. A moderate amount of ascites fluid and diffuse infiltration of the omentum with peritoneal seeding are also seen.

RADIOGRAPHY

Plain radiography is the most common screening test for demonstrating bony abnormalities and assessing the structural integrity of bone. For example, in determining the stability of the spine following trauma, flexion and extension films of the cervical spine are routinely obtained. Plain radiographs are most helpful in detecting degenerative and congenital diseases, primary and metastatic tumors, metabolic bone disease, and fractures of vertebral bodies. Osteophytes in the neural foramina in the cervical, thoracic, and lumbar spine are screened using plain radiographs. Plain radiographs of the spine are often used to screen patients before myelography, CT, or MRI in order to identify segmental anomalies at the thoracolumbar and lumbosacral junctions. They are also helpful in determining the location and extent of lesions so that CT and MRI studies can be tailored to concentrate on specific areas. Although characteristic bony changes can lead to a specific diagnosis (e.g., the classical changes of osteomyelitis of the spine), plain films are often normal or demonstrate nonspecific changes. Plain films are the least sensitive of the available techniques used to assess patients with neurologic disease (e.g., patients with pain in the base of the skull or in specific vertebral bodies, such as C2, C7, or T1), and the sacrum. If the results are negative, the degree of overlap of bone shadows makes this diagnostic procedure an inadequate test to fully assess neurologic complaints arising from these areas.

BONE SCAN

This technique represents a useful screening test for evaluating skeletal pain. Radiopharmaceuticals labeled with technitium 99m are used to localize areas of increased blood flow and increased bone turnover, which are associated with high rates of osteoblastic activity. Abnormalities in a bone scan can occur at any one of three phases of transit: flow, soft tissues, and bone uptake. Radionuclide bone imaging is more sensitive than plain radiographs demonstrating abnormalities up to 3 months prior to changes in plain radiographs.[6] Thirty percent of patients with known malignant disease with pain and normal radiographs demonstrate metastatic lesions on bone scan. Although this radiographic technique is more sensitive, it is not specific and does not differentiate among trauma, osteonecrosis, infection, and inflammation or osteoarthritis. It provides confirmatory information of changes in bone, but other diagnostic procedures, such as CT and MRI, are often necessary to clearly define the cause of the pain. Since the bone scan assesses increased osteoblastic activity, it misses osteolytic lesions. In patients with aggressive cancer, the osteolytic process may be occuring faster than the osteoblastic activity. Therefore, a negative bone scan in a patient who complains of bone pain requires further diagnostic investigation with plain radiography, CT, or MRI.

COMPUTED TOMOGRAPHY

Computed tomography provides a two-dimensional view of anatomic sites and is most useful in assessing changes in bone and soft tissues contiguous with neural structures. Because nerves are radiopaque, changes in local soft tissue and bone are used to suggest secondary compression or infiltration of nerve structures. The CT scan is most useful in assessing visceral pain and referred pain, as well as defining anatomic changes associated with brachial and lumbosacral plexopathies. It can detect bony abnormalities earlier than both plain radiographs and bone scans, but it appears that MRI is even more sensitive than CT. CT is useful in assessing vertebral body and disc disease. The use of fine sagittal and coronal cuts, bone windows, and reconstructed images further extends the indications for this procedure. The addition of an intravenous contrast medium can demonstrate vascular tumors of the spinal cord and meninges as well as differentiate recurrent herniation of lumbar intervertebral discs from postsurgical scarring. Images are usually obtained in the axial plane. Multiplanar reformation of data can be performed in any plane, but the results lack the spatial resolution of the original images.

QUANTITATIVE CT

Quantitative CT (QCT) has become a valuable technique (see below) in the measurement of bone mineral density in assessing patients with bone pain from osteoporosis. It does not require the injection of a nuclide and provides a quantitative image measuring trabecular, cortical, or integral bone centrally or peripherally. It provides precise three-dimensional anatomic localization, distinguishes cancellous from cortical bone, and can exclude extraosseous minerals from measurement, making QCT superior to other techniques that measure bone density.[7,8]

THREE-DIMENSIONAL CT

Three-dimensional CT utilizes recent advances in software and multiplanar CT imaging. It reformats the transaxial two-dimensional CT data into simulated three-dimensional images, creating with simulated lighting and shading the illusion of three dimensions on a two-dimensional screen or hard copy. This technique is most useful in assessing musculoskeletal trauma, especially acetabular fractures, and spinal, facial, and neck trauma to better define the neuroanatomy of the base of skull and plan the operative approach.[9,10]

CT MYELOGRAPHY

The technique of CT myelography detects intradural mass lesions of the spine. It can help clarify equivocal myelographic and MRI findings.

Postmyelogram CT can help delineate subtle nerve root displacement due to posterolateral herniation of the intervertebral discs and associated osteophytes. It is also useful in demonstrating cysts and hydromyelia of the spinal cord. Avulsion of nerve roots can also be detected by this technique. The procedure has become a second-line diagnostic test after gadolinium-enhanced MRI but remains a useful approach, as mentioned.

MYELOGRAPHY

Although once the gold standard for assessing anatomic abnormalities of the spinal cord, myelography has been replaced by MRI, CT, and CT myelography. Myelography is useful in studying the patency of the cerebrospinal space in patients who have undergone spinal stabilization procedures and in whom orthopedic hardware produces extensive artifact. Similarly, in patients who refuse MRI scanning because of phobia, it remains an important diagnostic test.

MAGNETIC RESONANCE IMAGING

Magnetic resonance imaging is superior to CT for evaluation of the spine, giving far better resolution of the spinal cord, subarachnoid space, and vertebral anatomy and their relationships. Intervertebral discs are well visualized, and MRI demonstrates the state of hydration of the nucleus pulposus and the condition of the annulus, including rupture of the annulus.[11–13] The addition of gadolinium defines spinal cord tumors and inflammatory processes of the meninges and differentiates recurrent disc herniation from postoperative scar tissue. Sagittal imaging of the spine can help detect multiple anomalies of the spine. While MRI of the abdomen, chest, and pelvis to assess plexopathies is useful, its superiority to detailed CT with fine cuts and three-dimensional reconstructions has not been fully demonstrated.[14,15] Some surgeons prefer to have information from both MRI and CT myelography when planning spine surgery.

THERMOGRAPHY

Infrared thermography records the emission of infrared energy from the surface of the body and has been used to evaluate the cutaneous vascular changes that occur with nerve root irritation and compression, peripheral nerve injury, reflex sympathetic dystrophy, occlusive disease of cranial vessels and mechanisms associated with headaches, and spinal cord abnormality and has been used in distinguishing neuropathic from nonphysiologic pain syndromes. It is generally believed to represent skin surface temperatures, essentially reflecting cutaneous blood flow regulated by the autonomic nervous system and other factors. Its use has generated a heated debate in the evaluation of neurologic disability. At this time, the test is considered to have limited value in evaluation of neurologic dysfunction or deficit,[13] and it should be used only in conjunction with established neurodiagnostic evaluative procedures.[16] This is a technique that continues to be used and has recently been shown to be of no value in the evaluation of low back pain.[17]

DISCOGRAPHY

Discography is the injection of a contrast medium into the center of the nucleus pulposus of a disc under fluoroscopic guidance. The volume of contrast, the force of the injection, the morphologic characteristics of the contrast accumulation, and, most important, whether the injection reproduces the patient's pain symptoms, are used to decide whether the disc is causing the patient's symptoms.[12,13] Discography has been used to look for disc disease when no evidence has been found on CT or MRI. The decision to operate on a patient with no focal disc protrusion or extrusion apparent on CT or MRI imaging but solely on the reproduction of pain is controversial, since the mechanism of such pain reproduction is not completely understood; tears in the anulus fibrosus with subsequent extension of the nucleus pulposus peripherally and later reparative processes is thought to be the likely cause of the pain. Reparative processes can be detected on T2-weighted spin-echo and on gadolinium-enhanced T1-weighted images on MRI. The prevalence of asymptomatic concentric and radial anular tears is quite high and probably an incidental finding in the aging process.

In addition, the safety of discography has even been debated, but a large review of cases, 269 disc injections, demonstrated a complication rate of 1.49 or 2.48 percent per case.[18] Another study showed significant complications from diagnostic discography procedures occurring in less than 0.6 percent of patients and 0.16 percent of the cervical disc injections.[19]

Discography is a hotly debated area. Prospective, controlled clinical trials are needed.[23] The North American Spine Society Diagnostic and Therapeutic Committee has issued a position statement on discography.[24]

Discography remains controversial. A study of posterior high-intensity zones on T2-weighted MRI studies versus discography demonstrates[25] that the high-intensity zone is a reliable marker of painful outer anular disruption.

TECHNIQUES USED PRINCIPALLY IN RESEARCH TO ASSESS PAIN

Single photon emission computed tomography uses radionuclides, such as technetium 99m and iodine 123, that emit a single photon with nuclear decay to measure regional organ function by reconstructing cross-sectional images. Nuclides cross the blood-brain barrier, distribute within the brain in proportion to regional blood flow, and remain fixed for sufficient time to permit cross-sectional imaging; SPECT has been used as a tool to study acute cerebral infarction, in the diagnosis of Alzheimer disease, and in finding an epileptic focus that might lead to surgical resection. Studies with SPECT can also yield important information about bony abnormalities, better defining the changes in overlapping osseous structures that are found on planar scintigraphy, since it can produce increased image contrast and improved spatial resolution.[20,21] Its use in the assessment of bone pain is currently under study. SPECT is often considered a less costly and more easily available version of PET, yielding important information about brain metabolism, since blood flow is a reflection of metabolism. SPECT may also have a role in identifying patients with back pain who might benefit from facet joint injection.

Positron emission tomography has been used predominantly as a research tool in the assessment of patients with pain. It has demonstrated focal changes in blood flow and glucose metabolism in both the thalamus and bilateral cingulate regions in patients studied in experimental pain paradigms, and it has been used to study patients following central brain stimulation, thalamic hemorrhage, and high cervical cordotomy.[22,26,27]

Magnetic resonance neurography is a new technique that permits visualization of nerves in cross section. In traditional MRI, nerves do not stand out from surrounding tissues. This new technique uses traditional MRI and a custom-built phased array frequency coil system. A fast spin-echo sequence is used with fat suppression and spatial radiofrequency pulses for vessel suppression. Individual fascicles can be clearly visualized by this experimental technique.[28] By using planes parallel or transverse to the long axis of the nerve and standard or phased-array coils, perineural masses can be distinguished from intraneural masses, and areas of nerve discontinuation after trauma can be located.[28]

Gadolimum has also been added to this technique for the evaluation of tumors.[30] Cervical radiculopathy has been evaluated using base-arrayed coils. The T2-weighted and fast short tau inversion recovery images demonstrated markedly increased signals in the proximal portion of the spinal nerves.[31]

PUBLIC POLICY

While the belief persists that imaging studies are overutilized, good studies assessing clinical efficacy are lacking. Boos et al[34] reviewed the literature and found that evaluations occur mostly at a technical efficacy level, with fewer evaluations of diagnostic accuracy, and that studies of diagnostic and therapeutic impact, patient outcome, and cost-benefit analysis were sparse. Prospective studies are badly needed in this area.

Retrospective studies are often fraught with the authors' biases.[35] Prospective studies are needed to determine the predictive value of these modalities based on an initial assessment of prior probability. Specifically what data from the history, physical examination, and neurologic examination went into the decision to order a particular study?

The diagnosis of clinical efficacy cannot be based solely on the number of normal versus abnormal images obtained, but must also be based on the subsequent cost of not performing an imaging study (e.g., missing a tumor or recommending physical therapies that may be contraindicated and may cause harm. For example, how many negative CTs should be allowed for the evaluation of severe headache presenting to an emergency department.[36] There are a number of factors that are used by the clinician to determine whether an imaging study should be performed in addition to those mentioned above: fear of missing serious pathology, fear of malpractice, the presence of litigation or workers' compensation. There is also the expectation on the part of the patient that an imaging study should be performed. Studies should also seek to evaluate the role of disability versus the role of pain. Activities of daily living and the chronicity of the complaint should be considered, since chronicity of neck pain correlates with the number of levels of intervertebral disc degeneration.[37]

Patients' characteristics have been studied to determine utilization of specific imaging modalities. Patients who received MRI had higher socioeconomic status, greater utilization of health care resources, more functional impairment, sciatica, and signs and symptoms consistent with nerve root compromise.

A number of clinical factors and the physician's specialty are major correlates of the use of imaging studies.[40] Patients getting radiography had pain that began more than 2 weeks before the index visit, had no previous episodes of low back pain, and had seen a chiropractor, orthopedic surgeon, or solo practitioner. The use of CT and MRI was associated with white race, neurologic deficit at baseline, sciatica, poor functional states at baseline, and small group practice size.

Investigations utilizing MRI have demonstrated that morphologic changes correspond to clinical outcome and that clinical improvement preceded MRI changes in half of patients.

Studies to determine the reasons behind current utilization practices are badly needed. Changing practice habits regarding utilization of imaging for the evaluation of pain can be very difficult. In one study, primary care physicians were given practice guidelines on the appropriate use of imaging studies for the evaluation of low back pain. They were compared to a control group that was not given these guidelines. There was no decrease in the utilization rates or in the variability of use rates of spine x-rays, CT, and MRI of the lumbar spine.[38]

One good clinical outcomes study assessed the predictive value of clinical findings combined with a quantitative measure of disc versus canal areas in patients with sciatica.[39] Outcomes judged satisfaction, activity, and medications intake and reported pain at follow-up. For the nonoperative group, the shorter duration of sciatica, no litigation, and young age were the most important predictors of a good outcome. The only good MRI parameter associated with a good outcome was a small ratio of disc hemirarea to remaining canal hemiarea. In surgical patients, a positive outcome was associated with a larger anteroposterior disc length, as were larger ratios of disc area to canal area. Poor outcomes in surgical patients were associated with concurrent medical illness, worker's compensation, and female gender.

USE OF NEURODIAGNOSTIC PROCEDURES

Examples of the use of these diagnostic procedures in various painful neurologic syndromes are described in the following sections. The most important decision the neurologist must make is choosing the most sensitive and specific study to define the clinical symptoms. These imaging studies not only provide diagnostic information but can also be used to direct treatment, for example, to determine the direction for needle biopsy, define radiation ports, and evaluate the results of therapy.

Low Back Pain

Low back pain is one of the most common complaints that bring a patient to a neurologist, and up to 80 percent of adults at some time in their lives will suffer from it. Clinical criteria have been proposed to limit the use of lumbosacral spine roentgenograms in patients with acute low back pain. Acute low back pain is most frequently self-limited (the majority getting better within 6 weeks) and due to benign, unspecific causes, such as lumbosacral strain or sprain.[22] Serious causes of acute low back pain are rare; herniated discs are found in less than 2 percent of patients, cancer in 6 in 1000, and osteomyelitis in 1 in 100,000.[29] Disc herniations resolve with conservative therapy alone, and only 5 to 10 percent of patients have pain that lasts more than 6 weeks. Criteria that select for radiographic evaluation patients at risk for vertebral tumor, acute fracture, osteomyelitis, and herniated disc include (1) age over 50 years, (2) significant trauma, (3) neuromotor defects, (4) weight loss, (5) history of cancer, (6) treatment with corticosteroids, (7) abuse of alcohol or illicit drugs, (8) fever, (9) failure to improve with conservative therapy, (10) suspicion of ankylosing spondylitis, and (11) patients seeking compensation for back pain.[45] Other criteria recommend immediate testing of patients with unrelenting pain at rest, an evolving neurologic deficit, or known cancer. Otherwise, spinal roentgenograms are considered unnecessary in the acute phase.

Congenital Abnormalities

The onset of acute back or neck pain requires immediate evaluation, often revealing suspected or unsuspected pathologic conditions Figure 3-4 shows congenital spondylolisthesis that was discovered in a 19-year-old woman who was in a motor vehicle accident.[33] She had pain and tenderness along the trapezius muscle on the right side with some discomfort at extremes of range of motion. Plain radiographs show a 2-mm anterior displacement of the C6 vertebral body relative to the C7 body. Flexion and extension films show no abnormal motion. A lucency in the posterior elements seen on oblique views was suggestive of a defect in the pars interarticularis region. A follow-up CT scan (Fig. 3-5) demonstrated bilateral well-corticated bony clefts involving the pars interarticularis regions of the C6 vertebra. Anomalous-appearing facet articulations were noted bilaterally at the C5–C6 and C6–C7 levels. A well-defined midline bony cleft involving the C6 spinous process was seen as well. There was no evidence of fracture. The combination of plain radiography and CT defined the pathophysiology of her symptoms.

Traumatic Disorders

Radiographic Evaluation

The evaluation of acute back or neck pain associated with trauma to the spine is commonly started with plain radiographs to determine areas of fracture and dislocation and to focus further evaluation with CT or MRI scans.[8,9,41] Flexion and extension radiographs of the cervical spine are taken following trauma to the neck in order to detect instability due to ligamentous injury

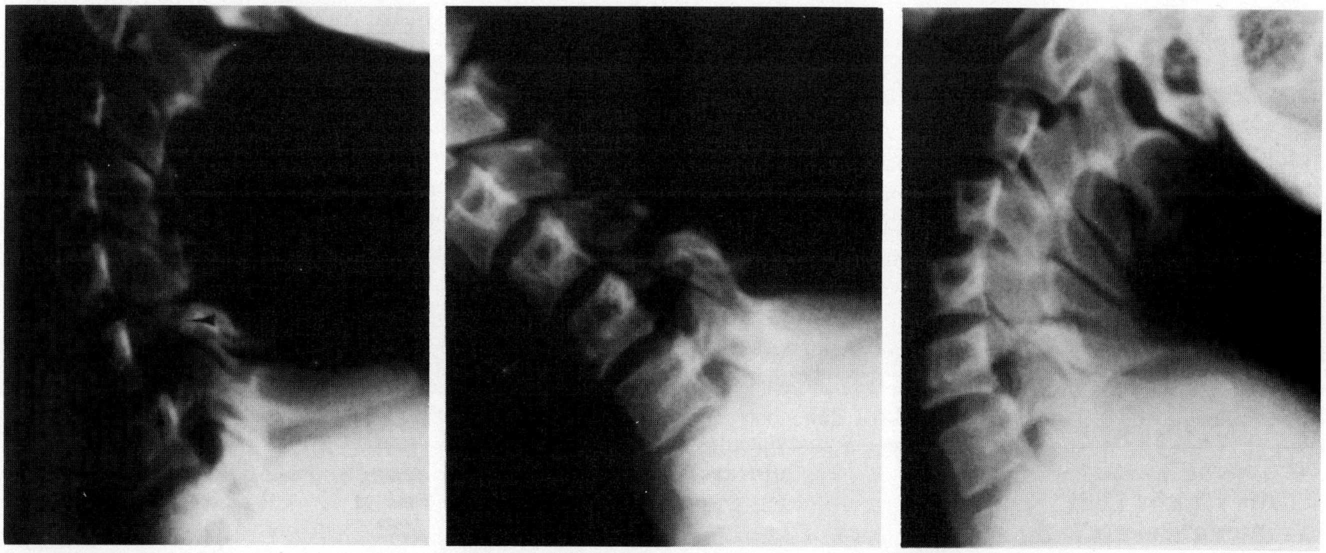

A B C

Figure 3-4
Congenital spondylolisthesis. Plain radiographs in neutral, flexion, and extension demonstrate a 2-mm subluxation of the C6 body anteriorly on C7. No abnormal motion was seen on flexion and extension films.[33]

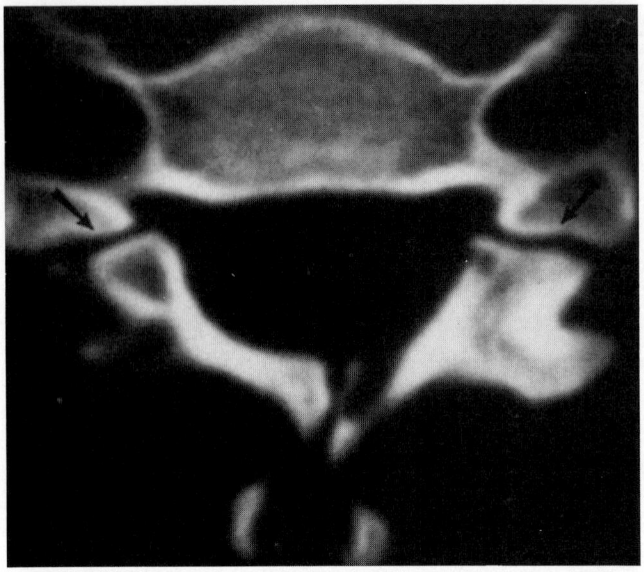
A

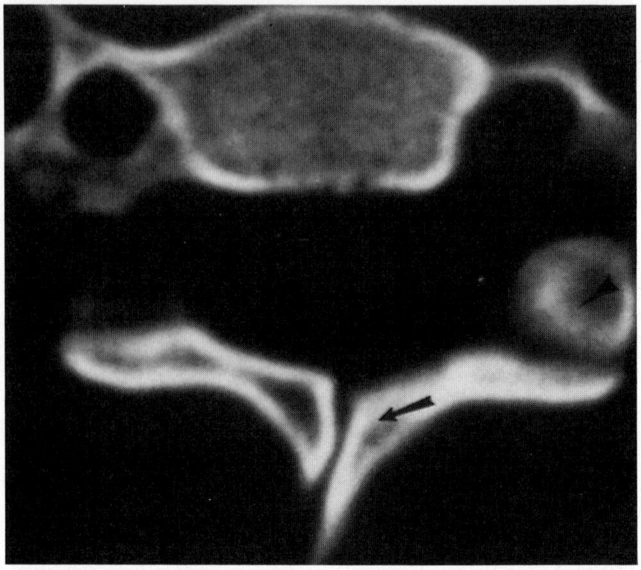
B

Figure 3-5
(A) *Axial CT of C6 vertebral body shows well-corticated bony clefts in the pars interarticularis regions bilaterally (arrows).* **(B)** *At a slightly inferior level, anomalous facet joints are present bilaterally at C6–C7 (arrowhead). There is a midline cleft involving the C6 spinous process.*[33]

after midposition views with a collar have demonstrated normal alignment and an intact odontoid process. Studies utilizing CT can demonstrate fractures of the neural arch and articular facets, transverse fractures of the vertebral body, and posttraumatic disc herniations that may lead to cord or nerve root compression. Hematomyelia and epidural hematoma are best evaluated by MRI. Negative plain x-rays in the setting of severe pain should force the use of MRI or CT using bone windows with fine cuts.

Vertebral Body Fracture

Figure 3-6 demonstrates on plain x-ray a fracture of the vertebral body of T11 in a patient who developed a flaccid paraplegia secondary to a transection of the spinal cord when she was injured in a motor vehicle accident. She underwent a five-level spinal fusion from L1 to L3 without improvement in her back pain. The patient had severe osteoporosis with disabling back pain, bilateral lower extremity pain, and rectal pain. On examination, she had a complete sensory level to T10 on the right and to T12 on the left and had complete loss of bowel and bladder function. Figure 3-6B demonstrates further collapse and subluxation in the same patient 10 years after the surgery.

Degenerative Disease of the Spine

Disc Disease

In the evaluation of low back pain associated with degenerative disc disease, plain radiographs can detect disc space narrowing; flexion and extension views can demonstrate instability at the intervertebral articulation. Both CT and MRI can be used in the evaluation of disc protrusion. However, MRI can provide information about the integrity of the disc, since a degenerating disc, owing to chemical changes, can be discerned on MRI prior to change in the disc contour. The water content of the nucleus pulposus and the inner anular fibers leads to the high signal intensity on T2-weighted images. The proteoglycans in the nucleus break down, and gradual dessication of the disc occurs with age. Studies with MRI can delineate small radial tears in the annulus on T2-weighted images. Herniation leads to degeneration of the disc and a subsequent decrease in signal intensity. Degenerative changes may also be found in adjacent vertebral body endplates and can be detected by both CT and MRI, although MRI is more sensitive in staging the severity of the degenerative changes. In addition, MRI is more accurate than CT myelography in differentiating a sequestered disc fragment (hyperintense on T2-weighted images) from other forms of disc herniation.[42,43]

Since MRI is the best method of demonstrating degeneration or prolapse of the disc, it should be considered the procedure of choice in assessing patients with degenerative disc disease. Views are taken in the sagittal and oblique axial planes through the intervertebral discs using T1- or T2-weighted spin-echo sequences or gradient-echo techniques; disc prolapse with annular defect is often observed. Spinal cord or cauda equina compression or spinal stenosis may also be detected. In addition, MRI has demonstrated some very important clinical findings regarding the natural history of disc

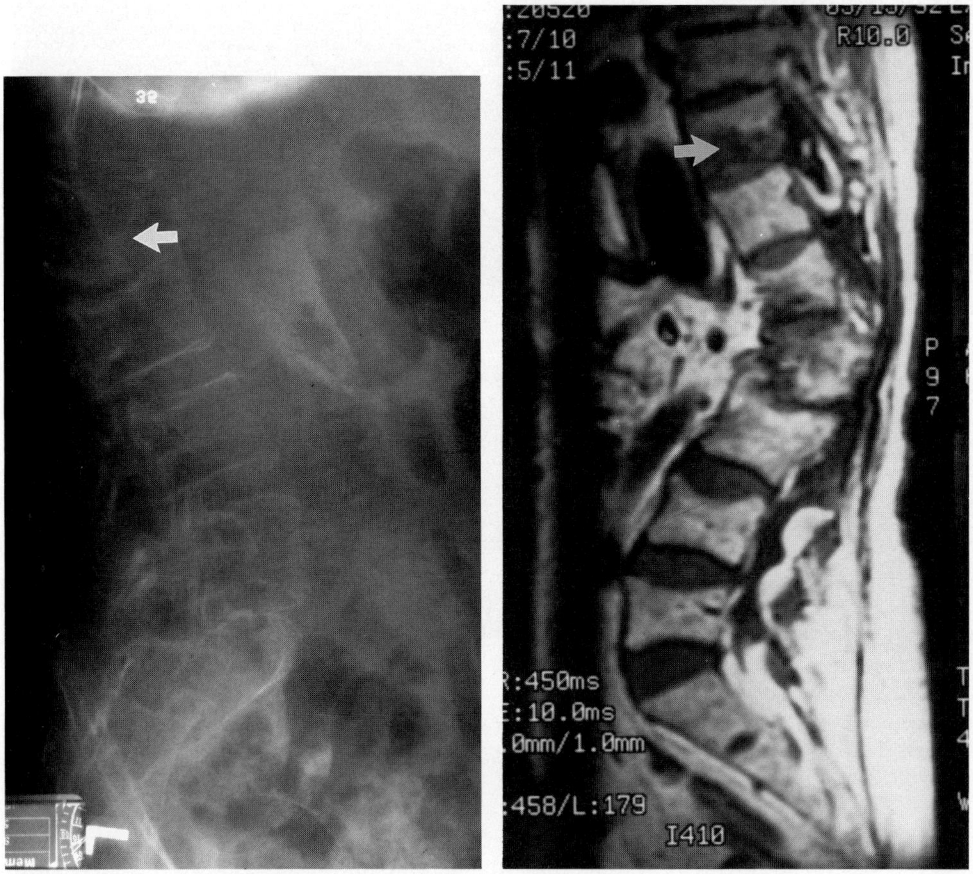

A B

Figure 3-6
L2 vertebral body fracture. ***(A)*** *Radiograph demonstrates vertebral body fracture with significant osteoporosis involving all vertebral bodies.* ***(B)*** *Sagittal MRI view of T11 fracture in the same patient 10 years later, shows further collapse and subluxation of L1–L2 secondary to osteoporosis.*

herniation.[49] In a prospective evaluation of cervical herniation with radicular-type symptoms and objective neurologic findings, 12 of 13 patients demonstrated a regression of the cervical disc herniation and an improvement in their symptoms.

An important neurodiagnostic consideration is the evaluation of whiplash injuries. Whiplash includes a symptom complex of neck pain and/or occipital headache. Studies using MRI are able to assess various types of soft tissue injuries. Dynamic imaging, use of flexion/extension views, high-resolution static MRI, and dynamic MRI should help improve the correlation between imaging and the patient's pain.[51]

Examples of the usefulness of MRI in assessing disc disease are presented below.

Cervical Disc Disease

A 45-year-old woman developed the gradual onset of pain radiating up the lateral aspect of her right arm into her biceps and neck. She also described paresthesias up and down her arm and a spasm of her biceps muscle. There was no weakness or sensory change, but she did have slightly decreased biceps and brachioradialis reflexes. The MRI showed a herniated disc at C5–C6 with distortion of the nerve roots as they exit the spinal canal (Fig. 3-7).

Lumbar Disc Disease

The patient is a 45-year-old woman who complains of low back pain that radiates into her legs bilaterally. On sagittal cuts (Fig. 3-8), the L3–L4, and L4–L5 disc herniations can be readily seen on MRI. On axial images, the L3–L4 disc has a lateral herniation and the L4–L5 lesion is a central herniation. The symmetric nature of the pain concurs with the radiologic findings of a centrally placed disc with compression of the L5 and S1 nerve roots bilaterally.

Facet Arthrosis

Facet arthrosis is a significant cause of back pain due to degeneration. It is best delineated by CT to detect early erosions, cystic changes, hyperostosis, and fat capsular calcification. Studies using MRI (Fig. 3-9) can resolve facet hypertrophy, osteophytic spurring, cartilage narrowing, joint effusion, and capsular hypertrophy.[43,44] Plain radiography can be a helpful screening technique. In the evaluation and treatment of back pain, a CT-guided facet block can be diagnostic and therapeutic.

Spinal Stenosis

Spinal stenosis can be the result of hyperostotic spurring of the vertebral body endplates, uncinate processes, and

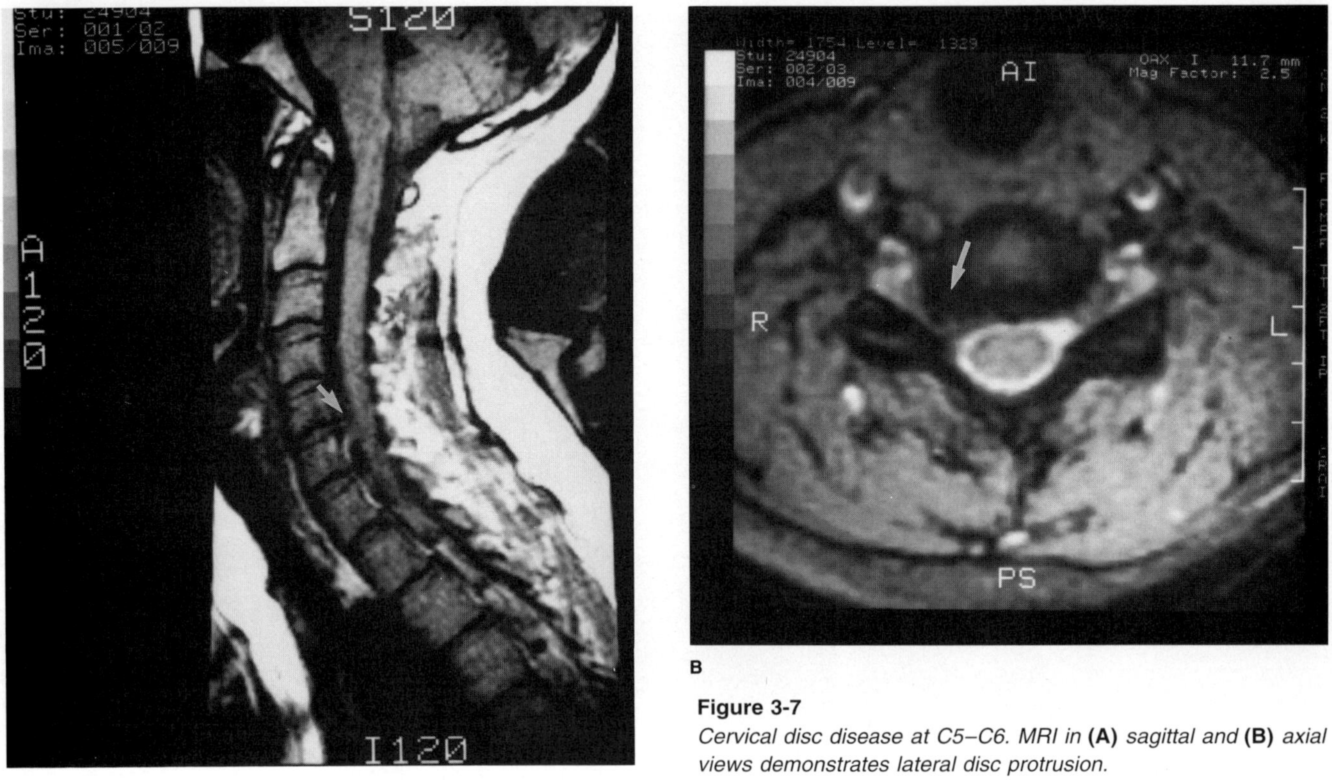

A

B

Figure 3-7
Cervical disc disease at C5–C6. MRI in **(A)** *sagittal and* **(B)** *axial views demonstrates lateral disc protrusion.*

facet joints, along with hypertrophy of the ligamentum flava and anterior facet capsules. Congenitally stenotic canals are most common in the lumbar region and are characterized by a triangular, or trefoil, morphology, with short pedicles and medially bowing laminae. While CT can differentiate between disc herniations and spondylotic spurs, MRI is better at delineating the effect of the spondylotic changes on the neural elements in the central and intervertebral canal. A developmentally narrowed central canal coupled with degenerative spondylitic changes can lead to the myelopathic symptoms of spinal stenosis. Modic et al[11] prospectively examined 60 patients with clinical suspicion of lumbar disc herniation and/or central stenosis with MRI, CT, and/or myelography and compared their findings with findings on surgery. Surgical findings of stenosis concurred with the MRI findings in 82.6 percent, CT findings in 83 percent, and myelographic findings in 71.8 percent of patients. In addition, MRI is more helpful than CT in exploring the differential diagnosis of cervical myelopathy, including spinal cord tumors, intra- and extradural masses, metastatic disease, and demyelinating processes.

Central Lumbar Stenosis

The patient is a 71-year-old man with central lumbar stenosis and back and leg pain markedly exacerbated by walking. Figure 3-10 demonstrates a combination of disc bulge (solid arrows), facet hypertrophy (open arrow), and thickening of the ligamentum flavum (arrowheads) that is causing circumferential constriction of the canal. Myelography showed a complete block at this level.[45]

Foraminal Stenosis

The patient is a 48-year-old man with left arm pain secondary to foraminal stenosis at C5–C6, seen in Fig. 3-11. Hypertrophy of the uncinate process (arrowhead) and/or facet joint (arrow) leads to foraminal stenosis. As seen here, the left intervertebral foramen is moderately narrowed.[45]

Osteoporosis of the Spine

Osteoporosis of the spine is more common in the elderly and presents as a significant acute and chronic pain problem. Plain radiographs do not reliably detect early changes in bone density, and they are not helpful as predictors for risk of fracture. Plain radiographs have a characteristic striated appearance that results from horizontal trabecular loss and primary trabecular reinforcement (Fig. 3-6A). Typically, there is an increase in lucency of the trabecular part of the vertebral body with preservation of cortical outline and an increase in endplate opaqueness that produces a "picture framing" or "empty box" appearance. Schmorl's nodes are areas where preserved intervertebral disc protrudes into adjacent and weakened vertebral bodies, giving a characteristic appearance. Various studies are now available that

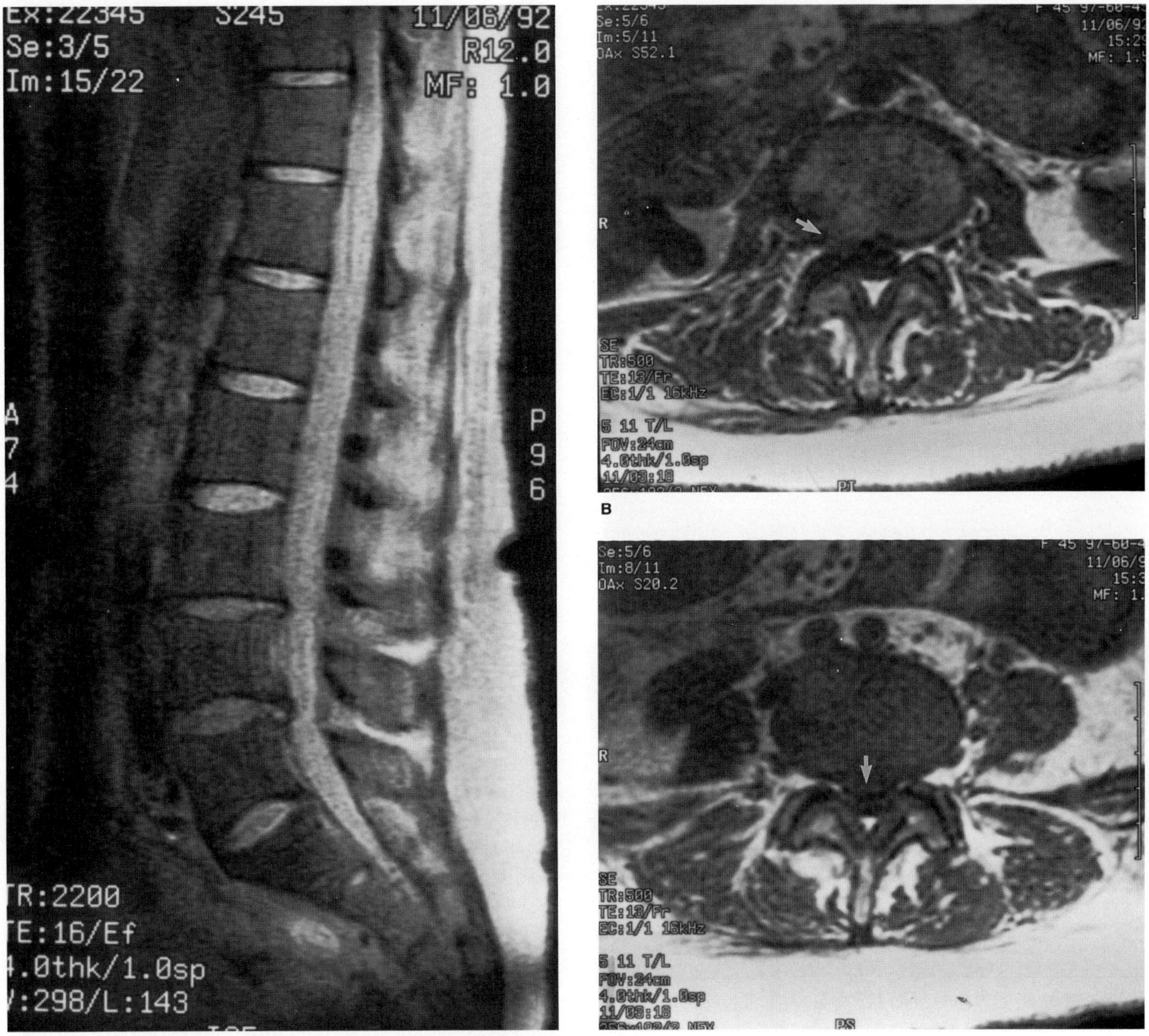

A B C

Figure 3-8

MRI of lumbar disc herniation. **(A)** *Sagittal image demonstrates disc herniation at L3–L4 and L4–L5.* **(B)** *Axial image shows L3–L4 lateral disc herniation and* **(C)** *L4–L5 midline disc herniation.*

are very precise at measuring bone density, including rectilinear scanning, high-speed dual-energy x-ray absorptiometry, and QTC, which is the diagnostic procedure of choice for assessing bone density. It is the most sensitive method of monitoring changes in trabecular bone in response to osteoporotic therapy and serially in patients with metabolic bone disease.[7,8] In addition, QTC is superior in predicting relative risk of definitive vertebral body fracture. Decrease in bone mass is directly correlated with increased risk of fracture, and the use of these accurate techniques of measuring bone mineral density is important in implementing preventive measures and, most important, in preventing vertebral body collapse and severe pain. Since estrogen therapy has been shown to prevent both bone loss and fracture, the results of densitometry can clarify whether such therapy needs to be instituted.

Vertebral body collapse and/or fracture from osteoporosis can be demonstrated on plain radiographs. In elderly patients, particularly patients with a history of cancer, the differential diagnosis of vertebral body collapse from osteoporosis versus tumor infiltration can be difficult and may even require bone biopsy (Fig. 3-16A). The characteristic preservation of the endplates and diffuse changes in bone density on CT scan support the diagnosis of osteoporosis. With MRI

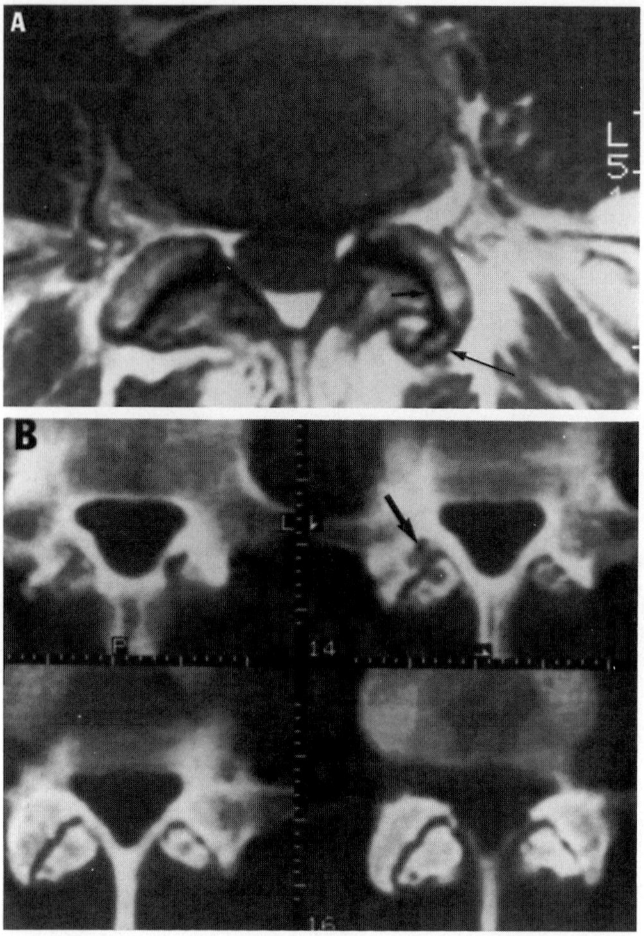

Figure 3-9
Facet arthrosis. MRI shows **(A)** *axial proton-density-weighted images revealing degeneration of the left facet joint, as identified by narrowing of the articular cartilage (short arrow) and osteophytic spurring of the dorsal surface (long arrow) of the left superior articular process. The multiplanar reformatted CT evaluation of the lumbar spine* **(B)** *provides excellent delineation of the subchondral cystic changes (black arrow) involving the facet joints.*[44]

gadolinium enhancement may occur and is often used as a sign to suggest possible tumor infiltration of bone. CT scanning with fine cuts and bone windows through the vertebral body can sometimes detect punched-out lesions within the body suggestive of tumor. If a radiologic diagnosis cannot be made, the patient should be considered for bone biopsy to provide a definitive cause of the collapse.

Arachnoiditis

The patient who presents with arachnoiditis may have characteristic symptoms of a root compression or irritation but may present with neuropathic pain syndrome, which is unfamiliar to many clinicians, often prompting the misdiagnosis of psychiatric disease. This is unfortunate, since patients frequently have debilitating pain. Symptoms include spasm of leg muscles, cramps, radicular pain, and even chills.[52] In one series of 68 cases, patients presented with multiple nerve root involvement, producing back pain, leg pain, sphincter disturbances, and motor, sensory, and reflex changes in two-thirds of cases.[53] Symptoms are frequently bilateral. A series of 100 patients describes low back and leg pain that increased with activity and straight leg pains, tenderness of the sciatic notch, decreased trunk range of motion, and muscle spasm.[53]

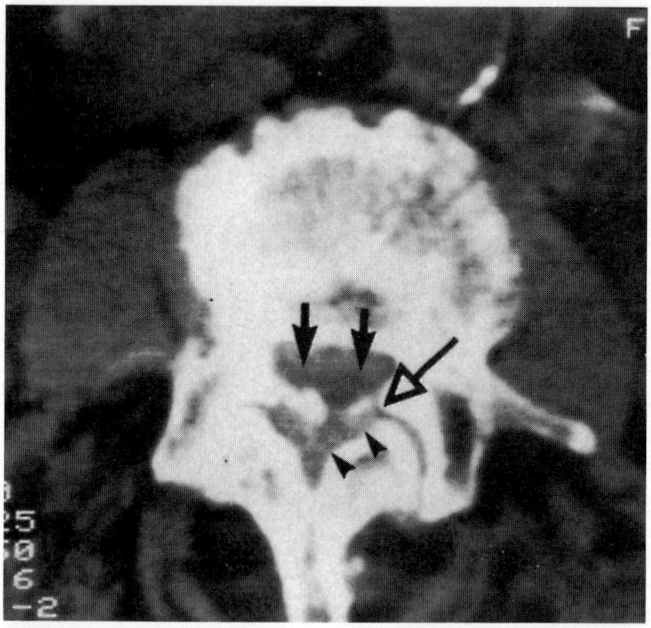

Figure 3-10
Spinal stenosis. Disc bulge (solid arrows), facet hypertrophy (open arrow), and thickening of ligamentum flavum are revealed.[45]

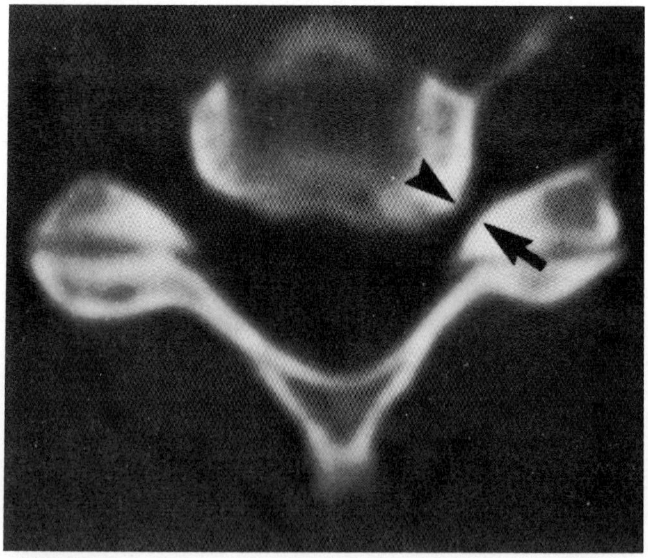

Figure 3-11
Foraminal stenosis. Hypertrophy of uncinate process (arrowhead) and facet joint (arrow) are shown.[45]

One author has described the symptoms as "bizarre—and commonly dismissed as neurotic or functional."[54,55]

Some of the more unusual symptoms describe burning in the sacral area, gripping, clawing pain in the calves and ankles, severe pain radiating down the legs in a nondermatomal distribution, paresthesias in the insteps and feet and burning at the medial area of the knees. Patients may have significant hyperalgesia and allodynia, and some describe the pain as a toothache-type pain of the legs.

Arachnoiditis presents most commonly with nonspecific back pain but may present with radiculopathy or myelopathy. Myelography (Fig. 3-12A) in the past was used to confirm the diagnosis, demonstrating a "formless" or "sleeveless" appearance.[48] The nerve root sheaths do not fill out, owing to adhesion of nerve roots peripherally. Myelography may also show filling defects, differentially filling compartments or even blockage of the thecal sac.[48] Postmyelographic CT shows either peripheral clumping, causing an empty sac appearance, or central clumping of the roots. Figure 3-12B shows a postmyelographic CT scan with asymmetric clumping of nerve roots within the thecal sac posterior to the L4 vertebral body. Magnetic resonance imaging has replaced myelography in making this diagnosis. The MRI appearance of arachnoiditis (Fig. 3-13) may show three different patterns:[65] centrally clumped roots in the thecal sac, best seen on T2-weighted images; peripheral adhesion of roots to the thecal sac similar to the empty sac pattern demonstrated on myelography; and increased soft tissue signal intensity within the thecal sac below the conus medullaris, which makes the differentiation between cerebrospinal fluid (CSF) and nerve roots difficult. The latter pattern looks similar to a subarachnoid block, producing an irregular distal subarachnoid space, as seen on CT myelography.

Other Common Sites of Pain

Magnetic resonance imaging has become the study of choice for evaluation of pain in a number of structures and parts of the body, including the evaluation of heel pain.[56,57] Magnetic resonance imaging of the hip can be useful, but, when compared to arthroscopy, chondral softening, fibrillation, and partial-thickness defects less than 1 cm in diameter were less consistently detected with MRI, and osteochondral loose bodies and labral tears were not well demonstrated.[58]

Shoulder pathology is often evaluated using MRI. It provides an accurate method of evaluation of rotator cuff pathology.[59]

Magnetic resonance imaging has a diagnostic accuracy of 97 percent in patients undergoing arthroscopy, is a cost-effective technique of avoiding unnecessary surgery, and improves patients' outcomes by improving surgical decision making regarding knee surgery.[60]

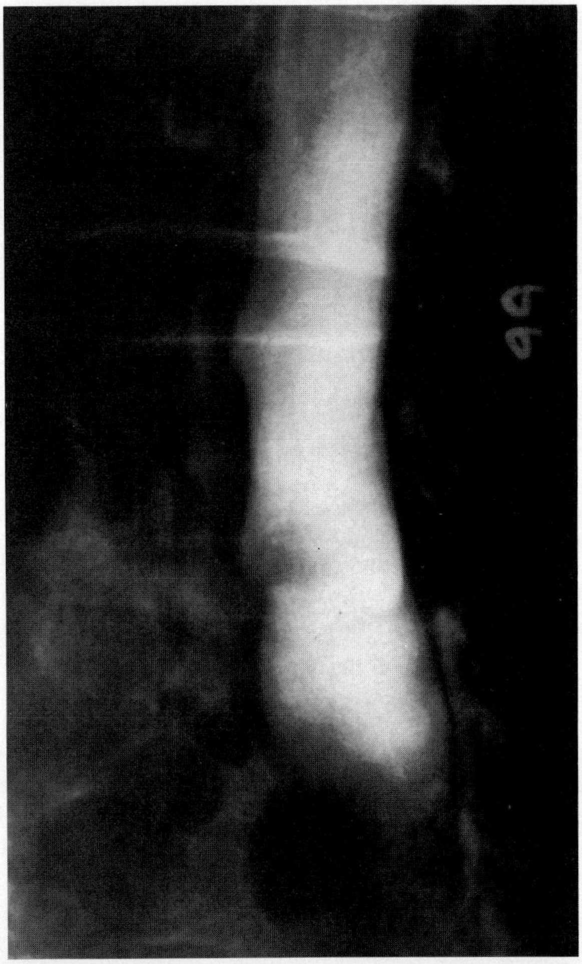

A

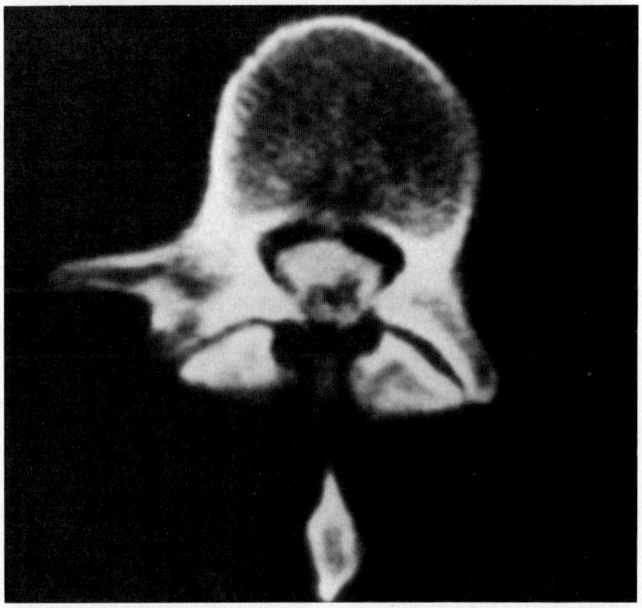

B

Figure 3-12
(A) *Myelographic pattern of arachnoiditis. A featureless thecal sac is seen without a nerve sheath filling or delineation of the roots within the contrast column.* **(B)** *Postmyelogram CT shows asymmetrical clumping of nerve roots in the thecal sac posterior to the L4 vertebral body.*[48]

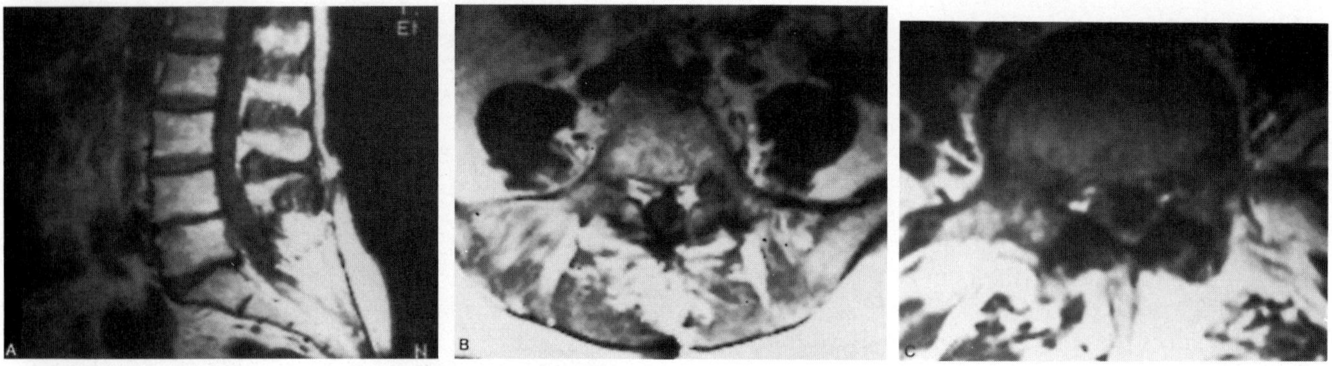

Figure 3-13
Three common MRI patterns of arachnoiditis. **(A)** *Thickened nerve roots are present within the thecal sac.* **(B)** *Peripheral and* **(C)** *lateral placement of nerve roots is shown in thecal sac.*[50]

For the evaluation of avascular necrosis (AVN), MRI is the modality of choice for diagnosis, monitoring therapy, and assessing risk of AVN. MRI provides a more specific diagnosis and gives information about lesion size and location.[61]

In addition, MRI has become an important tool in the evaluation of pelvic pain. Chronic pelvic pain often requires a multidimensional approach to treatment and frequently requires use of pelvic ultrasound and MRI, with laparoscopy providing the final diagnosis.[62] MRI has been shown to be better at preoperative screening of suspected ovarian masses than ultrasound.[63]

Groin pain can frequently be difficult to diagnose. Findings on MRI can include broadened and irregular symphysis with low T1- and high T2-weighted signal localized in the pubic ramus superior to the symphysis.[64] Muscle pain is often a difficult diagnosis to confirm. The use of MRI has demonstrated increased T2-weighted images in torn and overused muscles.[65]

Magnetic resonance imaging is more sensitive (95 percent) and superior to quantitative sacroiliac (SI) scintigraphy (48 percent) or conventional radiography (19 percent) for the detection and confirmation of active sacroiliitis. In addition, MRI had a higher specificity (100 percent) than did scintigraphy (97 percent) or plain radiography (47 percent) for the assessment of inflammatory signs.[66]

Metastatic Disease to Spine

Metastatic disease to the spine is the most common cause of pain in patients with cancer. Breast, prostate, and lung are the most common tumors that metastasize to bone. Bone metastases from breast cancer and multiple myeloma are most commonly osteolytic, whereas osteosclerotic changes occur most commonly with prostate cancer. A 30- to 50-percent change in bone mass is necessary before being detected on plain radiographs. Bone scans are most sensitive, requiring only a 5- to 10-percent change. Bone pain results from periosteal involvement and injury to pain-sensitive fibers. It is interesting to note that bone scans do not always correlate with the patient's pain complaint. Two examples of this phenomenon are seen in Fig. 3-14A and B. Both scans are in men with metastatic prostate cancer. The patient in Fig. 3-14A reported bone pain. Figure 3-14B shows a markedly abnormal scan in a patient who had this study for staging purposes only and who reported no pain. Bone scans can often be falsely negative. This is seen in purely osteolytic metastatic disease, as occurs in multiple myeloma. Such false-negative scans have been reported to occur in lung cancer and malignant melanoma. Bone scans are commonly negative in sites of previous radiation therapy.

Epidural spinal cord compression is a common associated finding in patients with metastatic vertebral body disease. Back pain is the first symptom in 95 percent of such patients. Prompt evaluation and treatment markedly improve outcome. The degree of neurologic impairment on presentation is an important prognostic factor. Ambulation is retained by approximately 75 percent of ambulatory patients, 30 to 50 percent of paretic patients, but can only be regained in 10 percent of paraplegic patients. Gadolinium-enhanced MRI is the diagnostic procedure of choice to facilitate a treatment approach and assess prognosis.

Changes in plain radiographs in patients with back pain and normal neurologic examination findings can help to direct an emergent need for an MRI.[72] Eighty-seven percent of patients with greater than 50 percent collapse of the vertebral body have epidural disease, as do 31 percent with pedicle erosion without major vertebral body collapse and 7 percent of patients with tumor limited to the vertebral body without collapse.[73] In patients with multiple vertebral metastases, 10 percent have asymptomatic spinal cord compression.[74] Epidural spinal cord compression can also occur without bony metastatic disease, resulting from paraspinal tumors that grow through the neural foramina. This condition is most common in lymphoma but is well

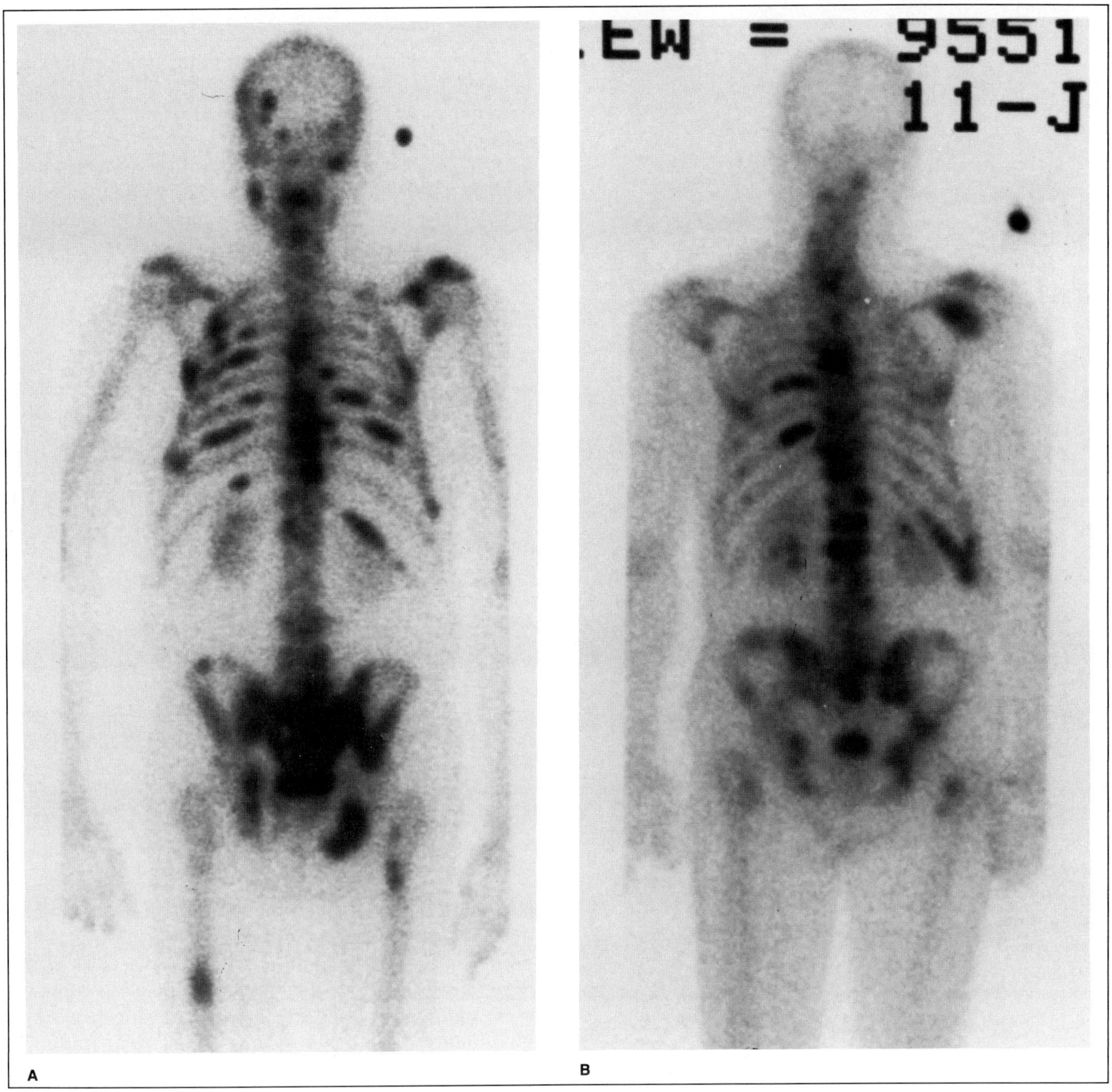

Figure 3-14
(A) *A 64-year-old man with prostate cancer and diffuse multifocal pain involving his ribs, back, and pelvis.*
(B) *Bone scan done for staging purposes in an asymptomatic 70-year-old man with prostate cancer.*

described in patients with breast and lung cancer. Leptomeningeal disease often presents with back pain and radicular symptoms, and gadolinium-enhanced MRI is the radiologic procedure of choice. Double-dose gadolinium may further increase the diagnostic accuracy of MRI.

Destruction of Pedicle

Plain radiography demonstrates the destruction of a pedicle that corresponds with an area of back pain in a patient with a known history of cancer. The subsequent myelogram (Fig. 3-15) demonstrates both the absence of a pedicle and the presence of a complete block. In patients with back pain and a normal findings on neurologic examination, destruction of the pedicle alone is associated with epidural disease in 12 to 20 percent of patients and is a radiologic change that requires further assessment with CT, MRI, or myelography.

Metastatic Thyroid Carcinoma to Lumbar Spine

A 45-year-old woman developed low back pain that increased in a crescendo pattern over the course of a

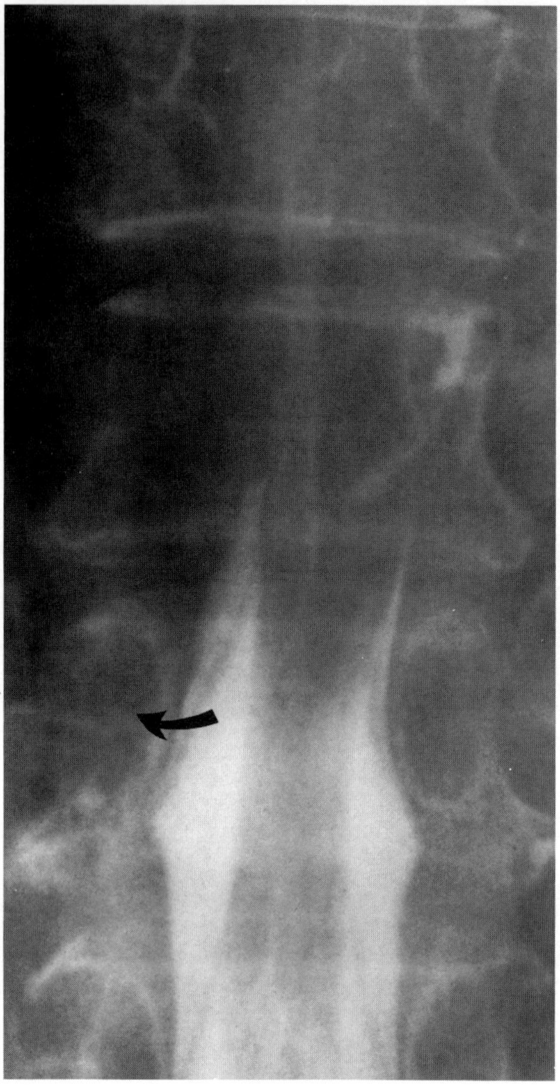

Figure 3-15
Myelographic evidence of cord compression with complete block. The patient was a 54-year-old woman with metastatic colon cancer and severe midback pain. The myelogram demonstrates a complete block to flow at T9. Note the absence of the left pedicle of T9.

week and a half. The pain radiated down the lateral aspect of both legs to her ankles. It was made worse by the Valsalva maneuver and by lying flat; she had taken to sleeping in a recliner. She had increased her use of analgesics. Many of these features are characteristic of epidural disease and make a more benign process less likely. The crescendo pattern, for instance, is not consistent with a benign process. Back pain from more benign processes, such as disc disease, is usually made better by lying flat. On the plain film (Fig. 3-16A), there is a destruction of both the vertebral body and the pedicle of L5–S1 and a collapse of the L5 vertebral body. On CT, an axial image (Fig. 3-16B) shows a pathologic burst-type destruction of the vertebral body. Open biopsy demonstrated metastatic thyroid cancer.

Metastatic Breast Cancer to Thoracic Spine

A 52-year-old woman with metastatic breast cancer developed midback pain. She was paretic in her lower extremities, with increased tone. Her reflexes were increased, and both plantar reflexes were extensor. She had a sensory level to T4. Studies utilizing MRI in both sagittal and axial planes (Fig. 3-17A, B) demonstrated a T4 metastasis that had extruded its contents into the epidural space, producing bony compression.

Metastatic Lung Cancer to Thoracic Spine

A 56-year-old woman with metastatic adenocarcinoma of the lung developed severe pain that radiated across her back and down into both of her legs. The pain also radiated up her back. She had been constipated for the past 5 days and had difficulty completely emptying her bladder. The MRI demonstrates replacement of the T11 vertebral body by tumor, with compression of the cord at that level (Fig. 3-18).

Cord Compression due to Local Invasion

Epidural disease can arise from bony metastases to the spine, leading to collapse of a vertebral body, or by direct tumor growth through a neuroforamina, as seen in Fig. 3-19. The CT scan demonstrates a lung tumor invading through a neuroforamina and causing cord compression.

Radiation-Induced Osteoporosis

Radiation therapy to the spine is not without complications. Although the most serious complication of radiation therapy to the spine is injury to the cord in the form of radiation myelitis, this has become less common as optimum dosing and fractionation have been worked out. Figure 3-20 demonstrates a collapsed vertebral body with posterior subluxation that occurred in a 47-year-old woman radiated 16 years previously. The hyperintense changes in the adjacent vertebra are seen following radiation therapy. A 2-year follow-up showed no change in this area on MRI.

Tumor Involving the Cauda Equina

A 35-year-old woman developed pain in her right buttock in the fourth month of pregnancy that radiated into her right medial thigh and sometimes into the lateral aspect of her right leg. She also complained of paresthesias involving her right leg that were worse in the morning. The MRI shows an intradural tumor that becomes hyperintense on T2 and enhances with gadolinium (Fig. 3-21). The mass extends from L2 to between

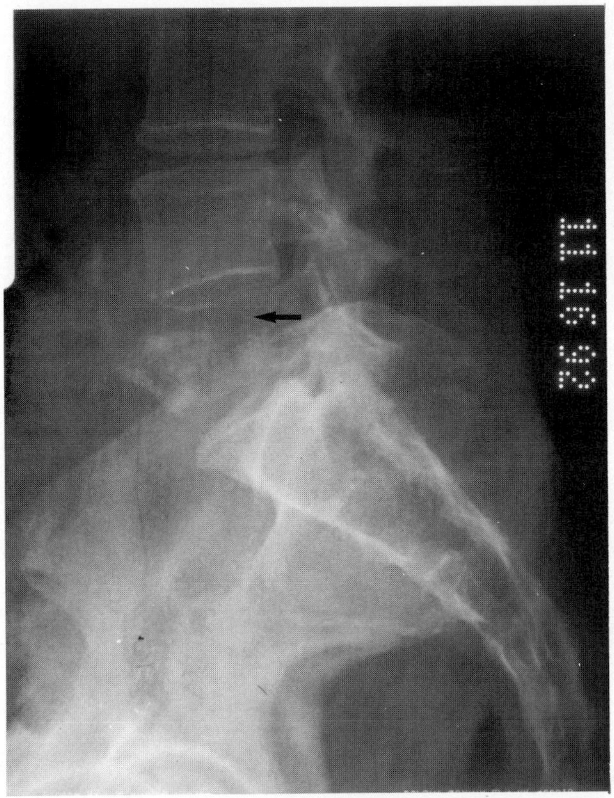

A

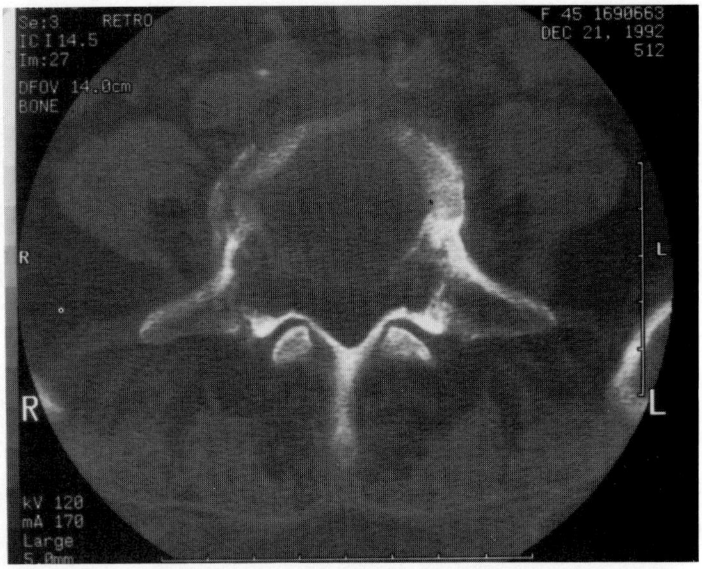

B

Figure 3-16
(A) *Radiograph of compression of L5 vertebral body from metastatic thyroid osteolytic lesion.* **(B)** *CT of complete block with burst fracture of L5 vertebral body.*

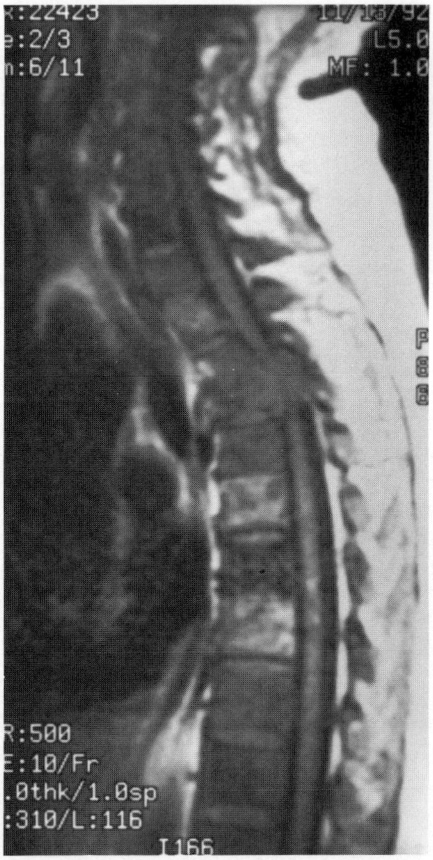

A

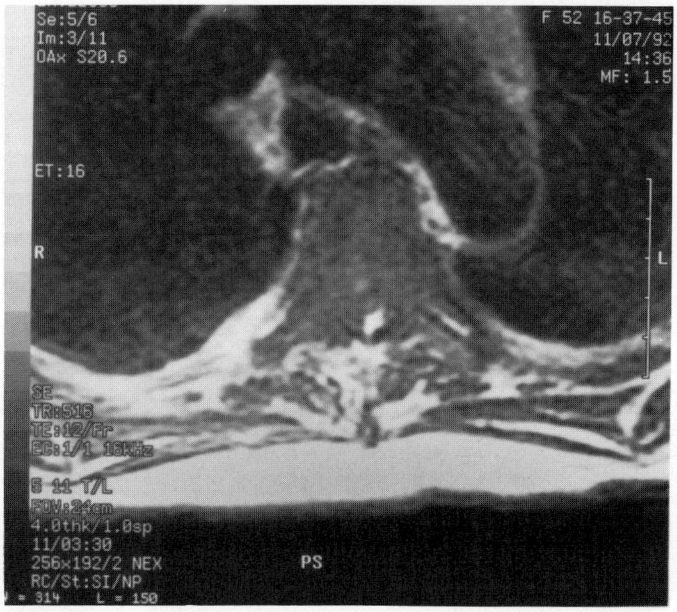

B

Figure 3-17
MRI of metastatic breast lesion to T4 vertebral body causing back pain and epidural disease with cord compression. **(A)** *Sagittal and* **(B)** *axial images show high-grade block.*

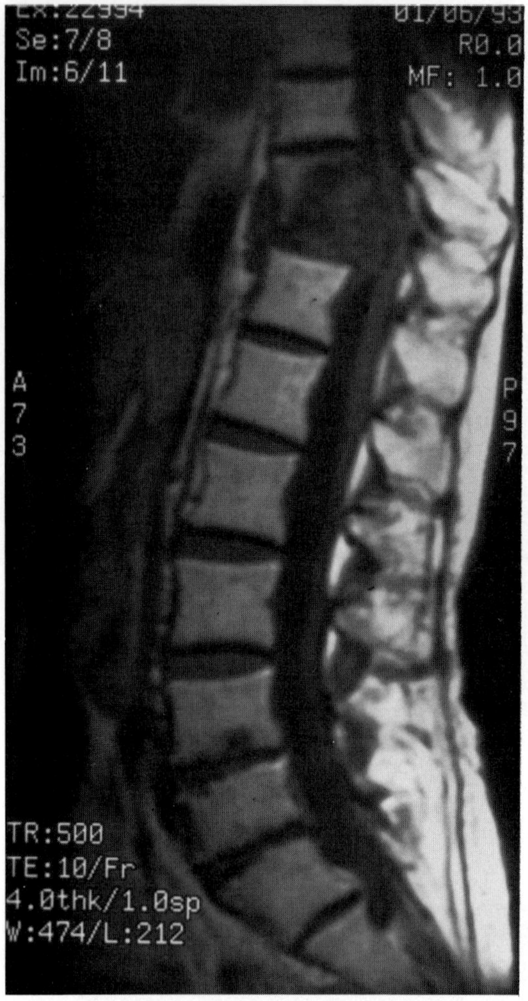

A

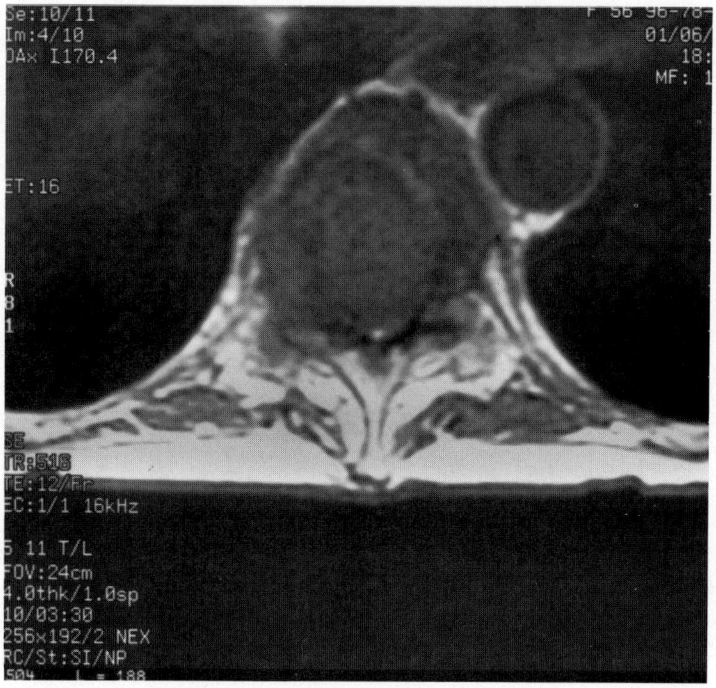

B

Figure 3-18
MRI in sagittal and axial views showing T9 and T10 subluxation and cord compression.

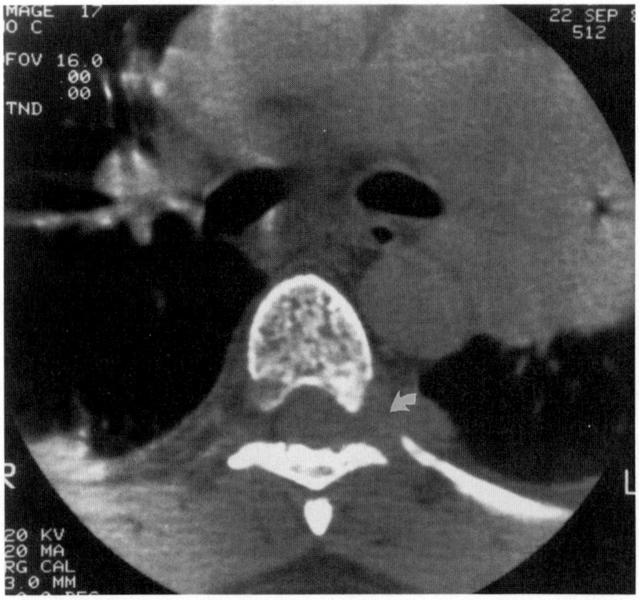

Figure 3-19
CT of lung tumor growing through vertebral foramina and causing epidural disease with spinal cord compression.

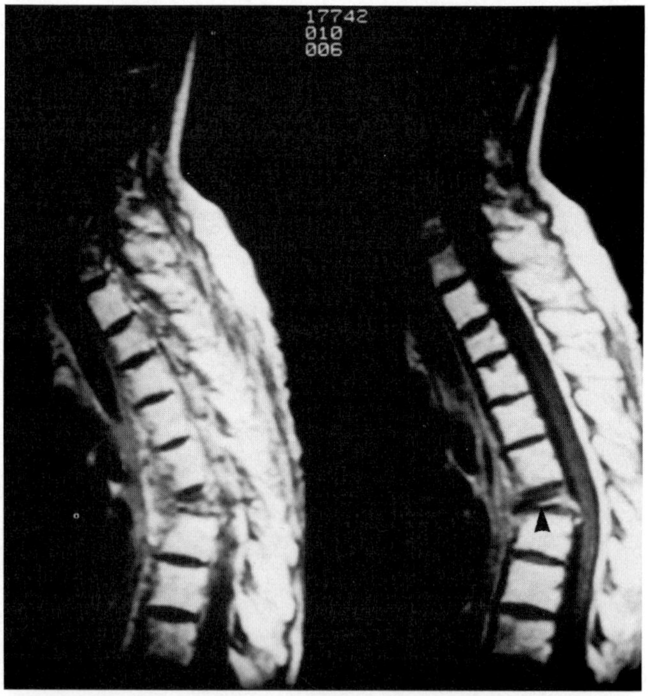

Figure 3-20
Radiation-induced osteoporosis. MRI demonstrates collapse of T9 vertebral body. Note the bone signal intensity on T1 images. Radiation therapy decreases the fat content within bone, causing increased signal intensity in the adjacent vertebrae.

L3 and L4. Involvement of the nerve roots explains the sensory symptoms that the patient described. The patient underwent a lumbar laminectomy and excision of a schwannoma.

Leptomeningeal Disease of the Cauda Equina

A 26-year-old woman with widely metastatic breast cancer, including metastasis to brain as well as significant involvement of multiple bones, complained of pain in the pelvic area and base of the spine that was made worse with sitting and walking. She developed a numbness in her lower extremities and difficulty with urination. The MRI (Fig. 3-22) demonstrates leptomeningeal disease with clumping of the cauda equina. This area is hyperintense on T2 and enhances after administration of gadolinium.

Multiple Myeloma

A 56-year-old woman with an IgAK-spike multiple myeloma has severe back and abdominal pain. She has widely disseminated disease. There are multiple levels of metastatic disease (Fig. 3-23) throughout the spine, with tumor replacing multiple vertebral bodies. In addition to replacement of the L1 vertebra by tumor, there is also compression of the thecal sac at that level.

Plasmacytoma

A 40-year-old woman complained of disabling sciatic pain for 3 months. Although presenting multiple times to her HMO for care, she was given nonsteroidal anti-inflammatory drugs, and bed rest was recommended. She had significant pain that she described as radiating

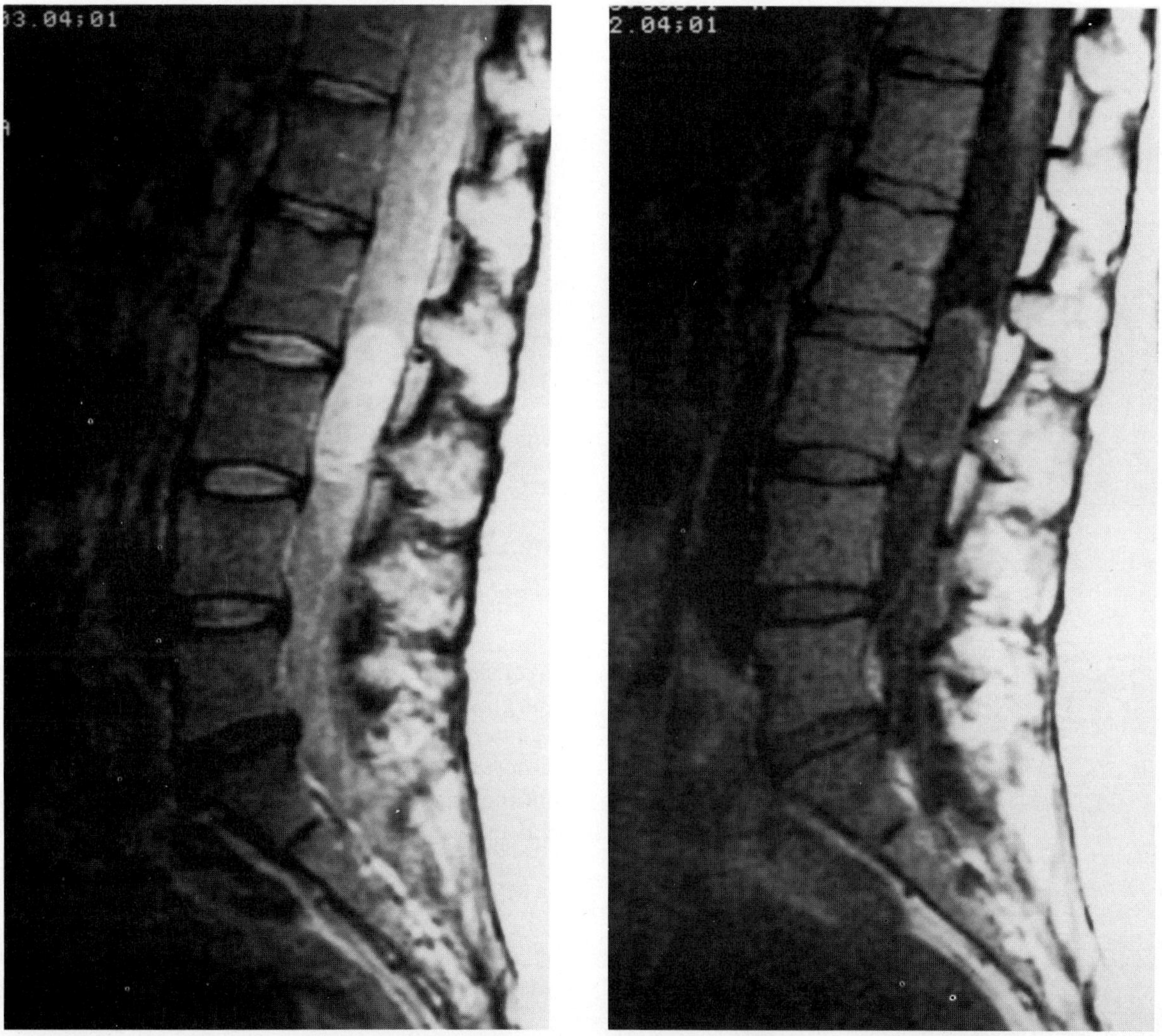

A **B**

Figure 3-21
(A) *MRI of intradural schwannoma of the cauda equina on T2.* **(B)** *Gadolinium-enhanced scans showing hyperintensity in the periphery of the lesion.*

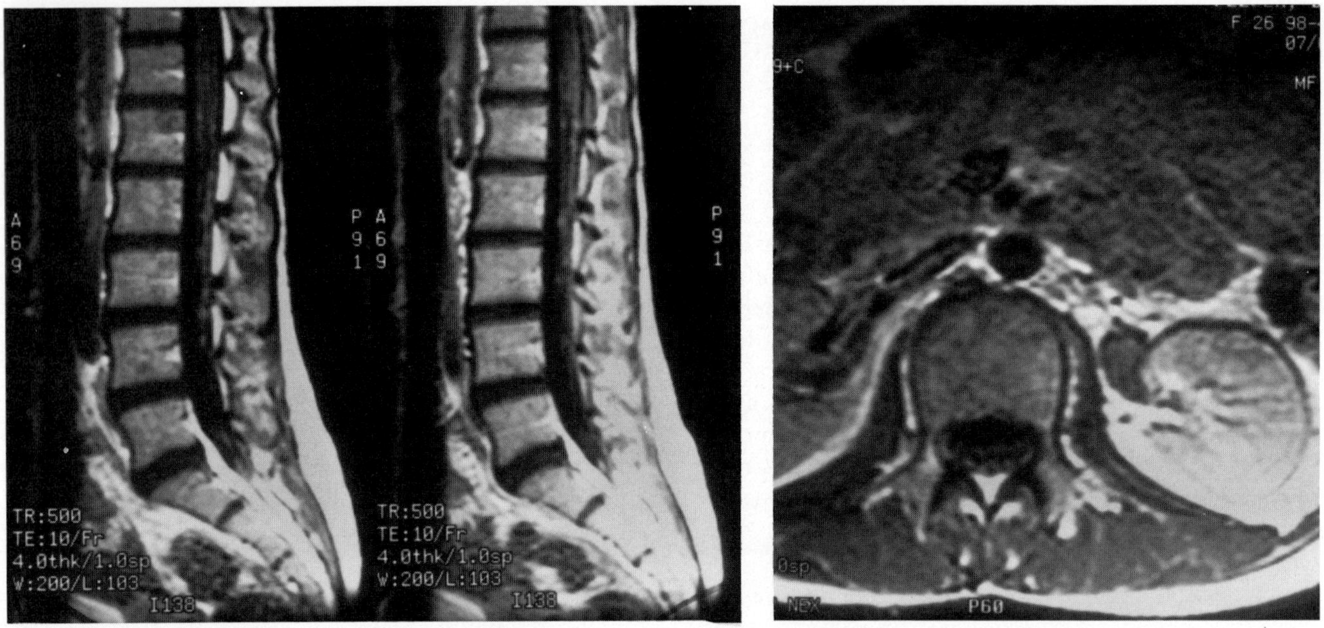

A B

Figure 3-22

Leptomeningeal disease involving the cauda equina in a 26-year-old woman with widely metastatic breast cancer and bilateral buttock pain. Beading of the nerve roots is seen on sagittal **(A)** *and axial* **(B)** *postgadolinium scans.*

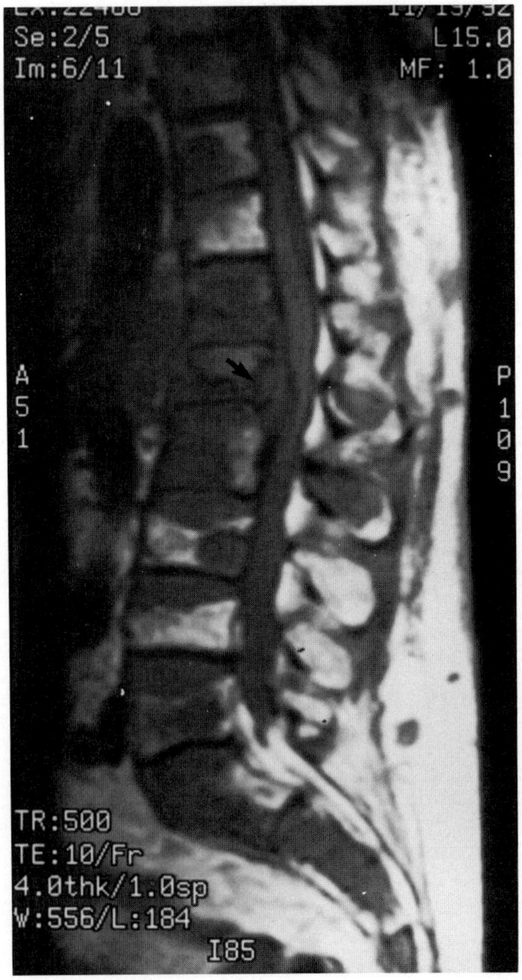

Figure 3-23

Multiple myeloma. MRI demonstrates significant multilevel vertebral body disease, with minimal involvement of multiple spinous processes, including epidural disease at L1.

down the posterior aspect of her right leg. The week prior to admission, she presented to her HMO with constipation. Medication was given, and she was able to move her bowels. She also complained of increased difficulty emptying her bladder. The patient was severely anemic when she presented to the emergency room. The mass seen in Fig. 3-24 was diagnosed as plasmacytoma by needle biopsy, and the patient was diagnosed with multiple myeloma.

Infectious Processes

Vertebral Osteomyelitis

Plain films demonstrate characteristic changes in osteomyelitis and include loss of definition of the endplate margins, narrowing of intervertebral disc height, an associated soft tissue swelling, and, in severe cases, destruction of the vertebral body. These are often late findings not occurring for 2 to 8 weeks.[75,76] A CT scan will demonstrate soft tissue swelling with obliteration of the fat planes around the vertebral body and fragmentation or erosive changes in the vertebral endplates. When disc space infection is suspected, MRI is the study of choice. When MRI fails to pick up a suspected osteomyelitis, radionuclide imaging can be helpful.[76] The MRI

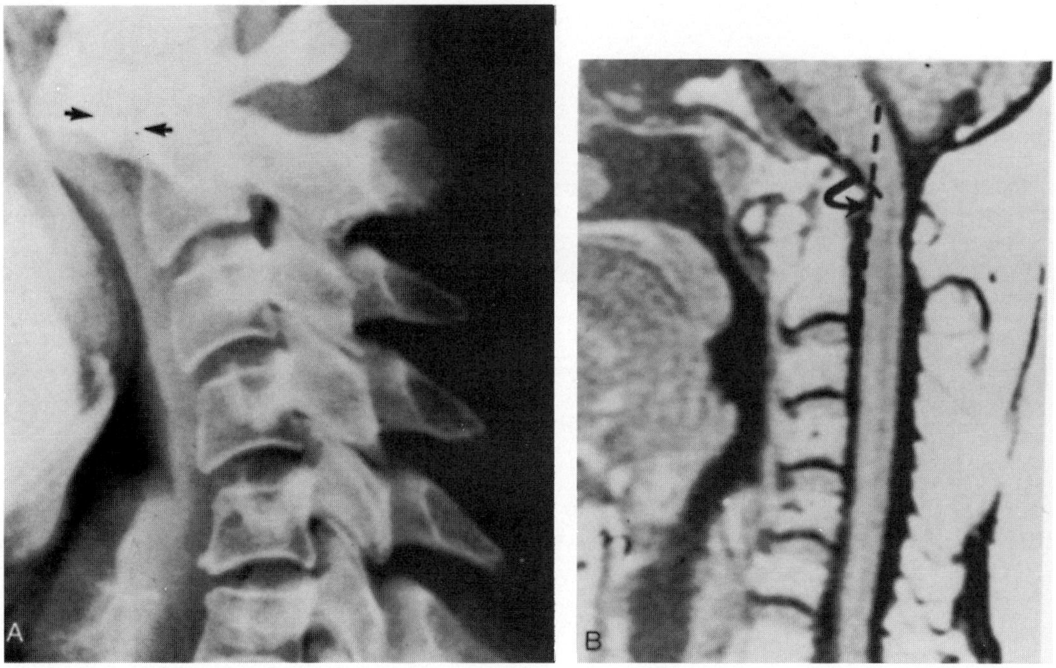

Figure 3-30

Rheumatoid arthritis. There is anterior subluxation of C1 on C2. **(A)** *Lateral radiograph in flexion shows 1 cm of anterior subluxation (arrow). At C5–C6, there is an anterior osteophyte with C5–C6 disc narrowing.* **(B)** *The MRI in flexion confirms the degree of deformity but also documents compression of the cervicomedullary junction. The cervicomedullary angle (arrow) is drawn (dashed lines).*[81]

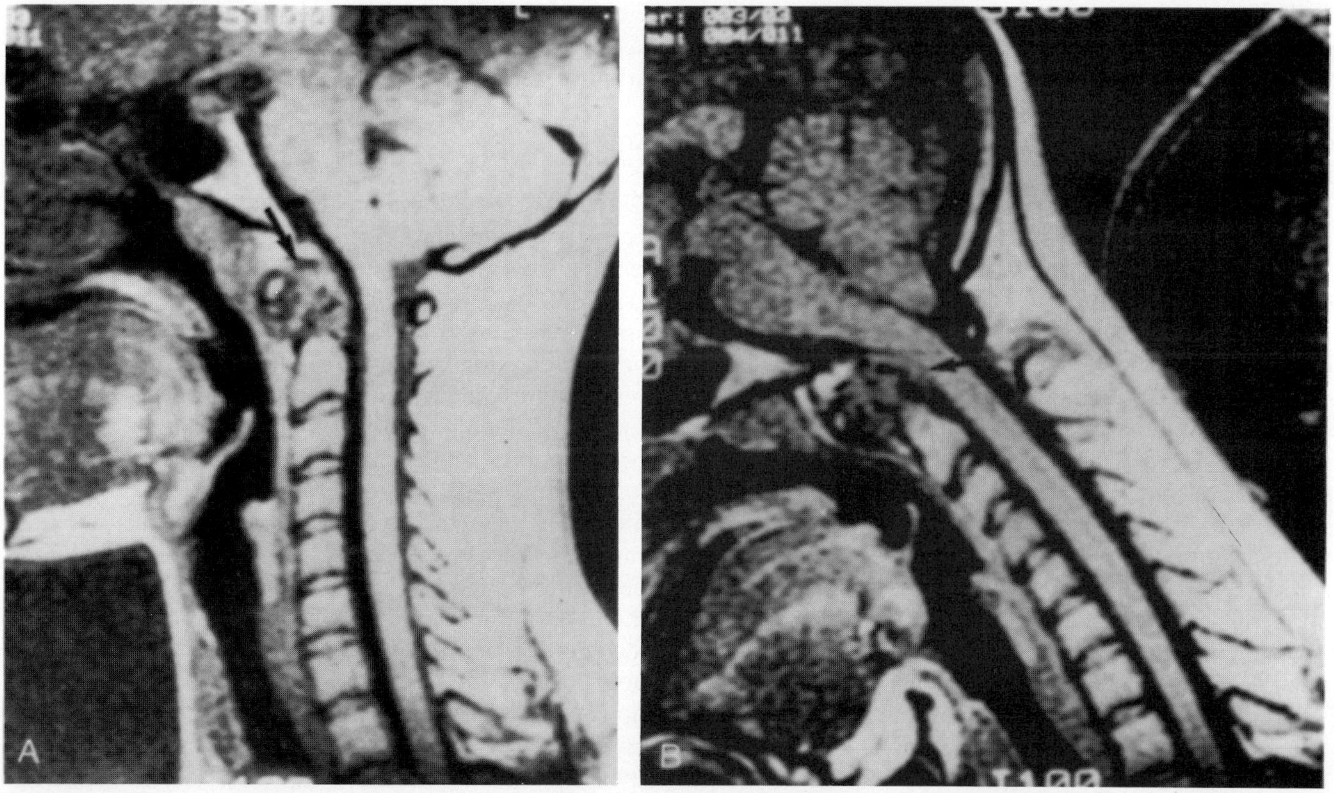

Figure 3-31

MRI demonstrating pannus-producing spinal cord compression. **(A)** *In extension, the soft tissue mass of intermediate signal intensity (arrows) is replacing the odontoid process, filling C1–C2 space, but is not causing compression on the thecal sac.* **(B)** *In flexion, compression of thecal sac occurs (arrow).*[81]

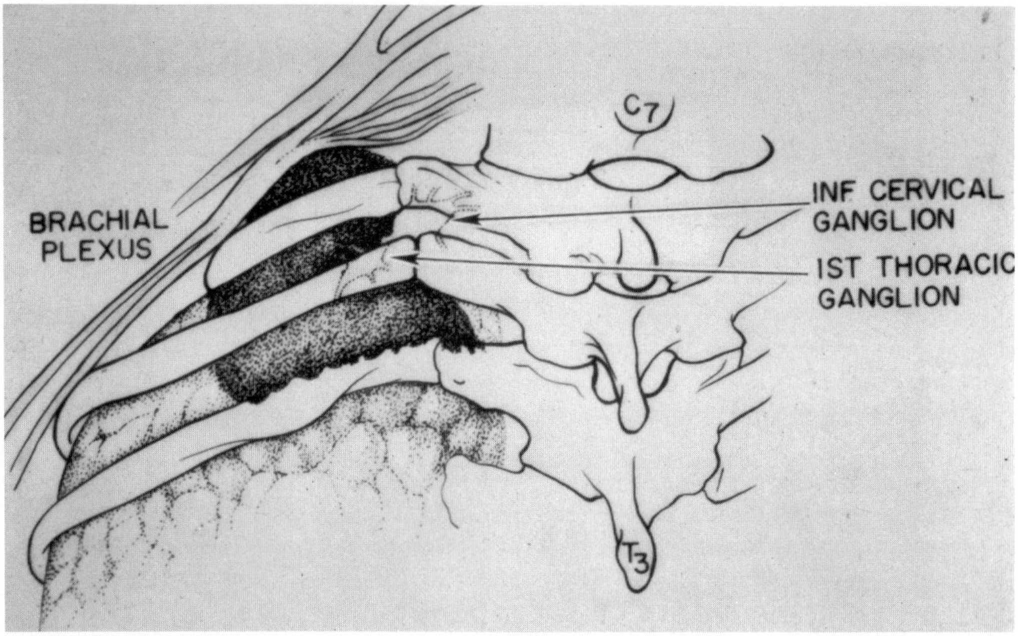

Figure 3-32
Pancoast tumor schematic shows compression of the brachial plexus, inferior cervical ganglion, and first thoracic ganglion from tumor growing from the superior sulcus of the lung.[84]

larly vulnerable to injury; traction injuries can occur when the head and neck and shoulder and arm are forced in opposite directions, as occurs in motorcycle accidents and during surgery. Malignant disease can affect the brachial plexus in Pancoast syndrome (superior pulmonary sulcus tumor) by extension of the tumor from the apex of the lung into the brachial plexus (Fig. 3-32).[84] The most common cause of malignant brachial plexopathy occurs from tumor infiltration of the brachial plexus by breast and, less commonly, lung cancer. Radiation injury to the plexus as well as radiation-induced second primaries may be difficult to distinguish radiologically. Table 3-1 summarizes the various brachial plexus syndromes that can occur in patients with breast cancer.[73] Thoracic outlet syndrome can also compromise the brachial plexus.[86] Compression of the brachial plexus by hypertrophied muscles or due to congenital or developmental abnormalities can be detected radiographically.

While MRI has significant advantages over CT myelography in the evaluation of the brachial plexus, traumatic injuries may be more accurately evaluated using CT myelography, as found when intraoperative intradural findings were assessed. An 85-percent accuracy was determined for CT myelography versus 52 percent for MRI when compared to intradural exploration during hemilaminectomy.[67]

Magnetic resonance imaging is the imaging modality of choice in the evaluation of the brachial plexus,[70] with T1-weighted axial and oblique coronal images supplemented by T2-weighted or short TI inversion recovery (STIR) images and can diagnose nerve root avulsion, neuromas, tumor and radiation fibrosis.

Three-dimensional MRI myelography can show the majority of traumatic lesions that involve the proximal portion of the brachial plexus and had 89-percent sensitivity, 95-percent specificity, and 92-percent diagnostic accuracy in the evaluation of nerve root integrity.[68] The development of signs and symptoms of brachial plexopathy in a patient with a history of cancer and radiation to the area of the brachial plexus can suggest either disease recurrence or a radiation-induced brachial neuropathy. One study found that fibrosis may appear on either high or low signal intensity on T2-weighted images.[69] In one case, fibrosis enhanced 21 years after radiation therapy.

Tumor Infiltration of the Brachial Plexus

Computed tomography, MRI, and myelography have been used to investigate malignant invasion of the brachial plexus. Plain radiographs, such as chest radiographs, are sometimes helpful if there is an associated apical or paraspinal mass, but CT and MRI provide better definition of the plexus (Fig. 3-33).

Computed tomography can demonstrate bony and soft tissue definition in two planes, and multiplanar reconstructions in coronal, sagittal, and orthogonal planes help to further evaluate the brachial plexus; this technique has been demonstrated to be useful in breast cancer.[15] Since a CT study includes both sides of the body, the symptomatic plexus may be compared with the asymptomatic one, rendering a valuable diagnostic technique. The use of narrow-section (4-mm) CT with bolus intravenous enhancement facilitates examination of the base of the neck and axilla. Thicker slices miss subtle anatomic changes, particularly changes associated with fibrosis in the upper axilla. Vascular enhancement allows for identification of vascular structures that relate to the plexus. In 28 of 42 patients with neurologic symptoms affecting the arm or hand, CT changes were seen in 96 percent.[83] In the use of postoper-

Table 3-1
Clinical features of brachial plexus syndromes in patients with breast cancer

Clinical feature	*Tumor infiltration*	*Radiation fibrosis*	*Reversible radiation injury*	*Acute ischemic brachial plexopathy*
Incidence of pain	89%	18%	40%	Painless
Location of pain	Shoulder, upper arm, elbow, radiating to fourth and fifth fingers	Shoulder, wrist, hand	Hand, forearm	Hand, forearm
Nature of pain	Dull aching in shoulder; lancinating pain in elbow and ulnar aspect of hand; occasional dysesthesias, burning, or freezing sensations	Aching pain in shoulder; paresthesias in C5, C6 distribution in hand	Aching pain in shoulder; paresthesias in hand and forearm	Paresthesias in hand and forearm
Severity of pain	Moderate to severe (severe in 98% of patients)	Mild to moderate; severe in 35% of patients	Mild	
Course	Progressive neurologic dysfunction; atrophy and weakness with C7–T1 distribution; persistent pain; Horner syndrome	Progressive weakness with C5, C6 distribution; stabilizing pain with appearance of weakness	Transient weakness and atrophy affecting C6–C7, T1; complete resolution of motor findings	Acute nonprogressive weakness and sensory changes
CT scan findings	Circumscribed mass; diffuse infiltration of tissue planes	Diffuse infiltration of tissue planes	Normal	Normal; angiography shows subclavian artery segmental obstruction
MRI findings	High signal intensity in circumscribed mass on T2-weighted images may enhance with gadolinium	Diffuse low signal intensity on T2-weighted images; no change with gadolinium	No available data	Normal
EMG findings	Segmental slowing; no myokymia	Myokymia	Segmental slowing; no myokymia	Segmental slowing; no myokymia

Source: Adami et al.[47]

ative CT scans in 19 patients with breast cancer and suspected local or regional recurrence, CT correctly identified the recurrence in all 15 biopsy-proven cases.[15] It is interesting to note that, in 2 cases, suspicious areas on the CT scans proved to be residual pectoralis muscle. In a study of patients with known tumor involving the brachial plexus, the CT scan was abnormal in 89 percent of patients. Paravertebral extension and tumor erosion of bone are frequently demonstrated despite normal plain radiographs and bone scans. Bone scans to detect bony changes and screen for vertebral body tumor were found not to be helpful and were falsely negative, especially in patients who had received prior radiation therapy. Computed tomography studies of the brachial plexus (Figs. 3-34, 3-35, and 3-36) can demonstrate paravertebral extension of soft tissue masses, vertebral body and rib erosion, and epidural extension.[83] In patients with a normal CT scan but significant plexopathy, surgical exploration through a posterior scapular approach may be necessary to define the tumor pathology.

Magnetic resonance imaging is replacing CT as the radiologic technique of choice for evaluating the brachial plexus because it provides multiplanar views that better delineate soft tissue structures, such as nerves, from adjacent vessels and surrounding soft tissue. This ability to assess changes in soft tissue signal intensity allows tumor to be distinguished from radiation fibrosis and radiation necrosis of bone. Unlike CT, contrast enhancement is not a necessity with MRI in evaluating soft tissue structures. Multiple views are obtained; sagittal views assess the cervical and upper thoracic spinal cord, axial views can define a paraspinal mass, and coronal views evaluate the peripheral components of the brachial plexus. T2-weighted images are useful because fibrosis is associated with low signal intensity and tumor is characterized by high signal intensity. In addition, MRI can be used to define radiation ports, particularly in patients with epidural extension of tumor. Nerves can be followed from the ventral rami through the brachial plexus to the peripheral nerve branches.[82] Com-

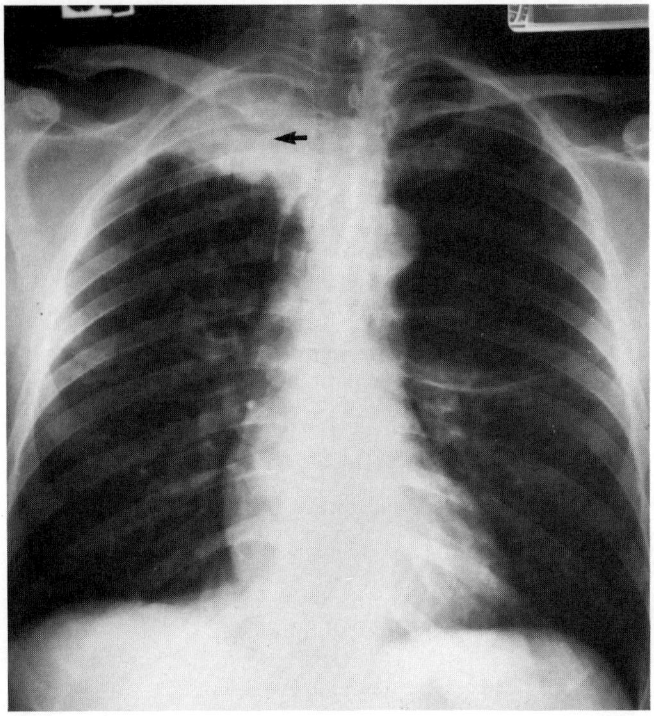

A

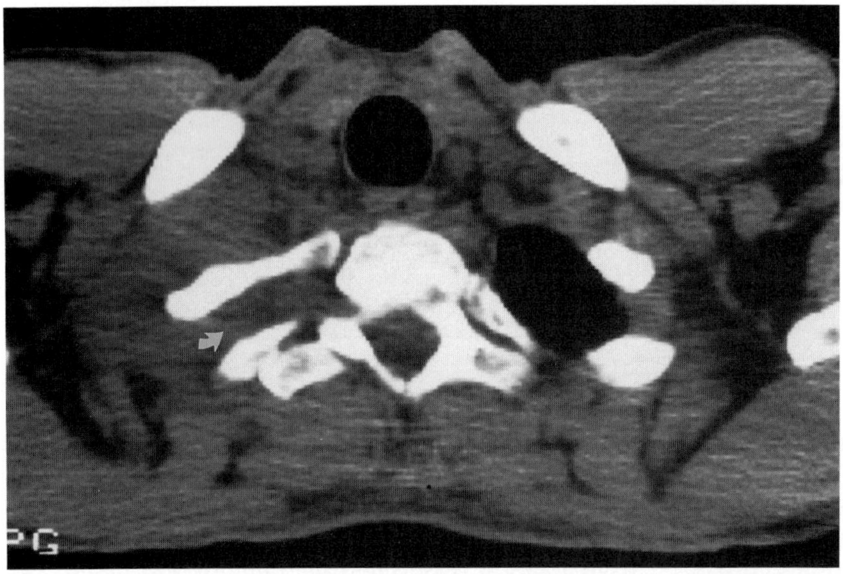

B

Figure 3-33
Pancoast tumor. This 63-year-old man had an apical tumor of the right lung involving the brachial plexus. **(A)** *A soft tissue mass is seen arising from the apical surface of the lung.* **(B)** *CT scan demonstrates soft tissue invasion of the brachial plexus and extension into the intervertebral foramen.*

puted tomography has significant limitations, including restriction to the axial plane, streak artifacts from the shoulders, and difficulty in distinguishing soft tissue structures.

Thoracic Outlet Syndrome

A 25-year-old man (Fig. 3-37) presented with a 5-year history of pain along the medial aspect of the right arm and forearm and the fourth and fifth fingers; playing rugby or driving his car made the pain worse. Plain radiographs and CT scan showed the entire first rib involved by a mass, with swelling of the cortical bone. Excision of the medial two-thirds of the clavicle through a supraclavicular approach demonstrated expansion of the first rib, which, on pathologic testing, showed fibrous dysplasia.[86]

Painful Lesions of the Lumbosacral Plexus

The lumbosacral plexus can be affected by malignant invasion, primary tumors, postradiation syndrome, retroperitoneal hemorrhage, psoas abscess, diabetic radiculoplexopathy, nondiabetic lumbosacral plexopa-

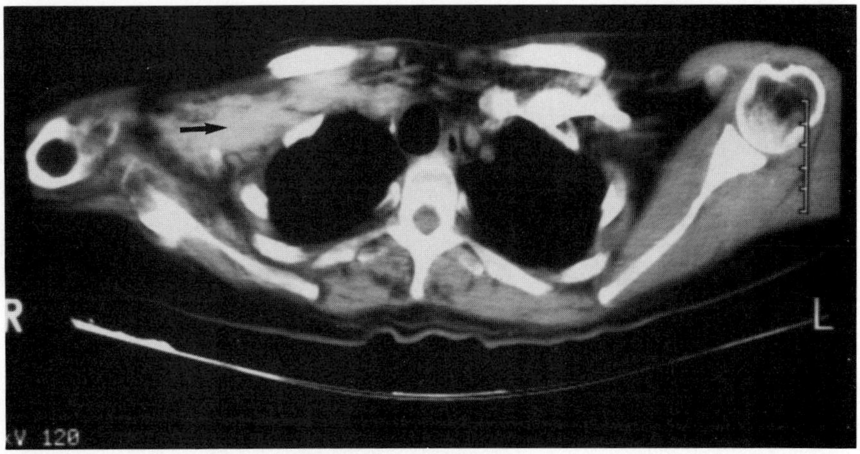

Figure 3-34
CT scan shows diffuse infiltration of soft tissues with loss of normal tissue planes in a patient without a history of previous radiation therapy. Exploration revealed diffusely infiltrating tumor.

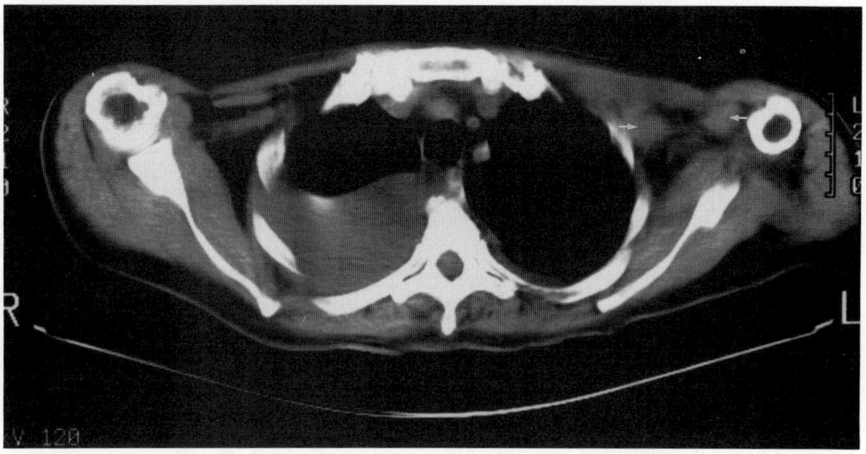

Figure 3-35
CT scan shows discrete mass lesions (arrows) involving the left brachial plexus in a 70-year-old woman with breast cancer who developed severe pain that radiated down the ulnar aspect of the left arm into her hand.

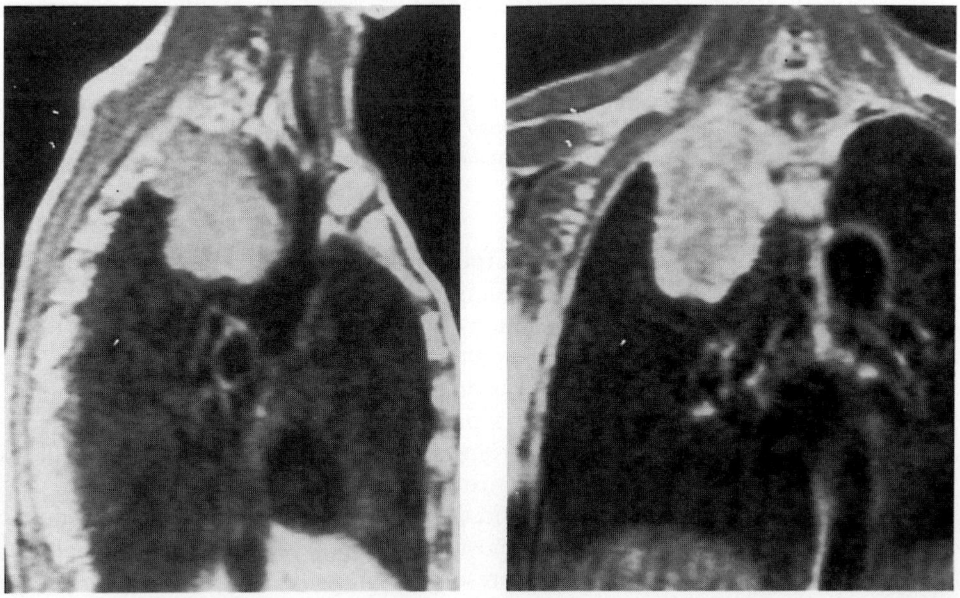

A B

Figure 3-36
(A) *MRI in sagittal section shows tumor extending to the posterior chest wall.* **(B)** *Coronal MRI shows extension of tumor into the vertebral body.*

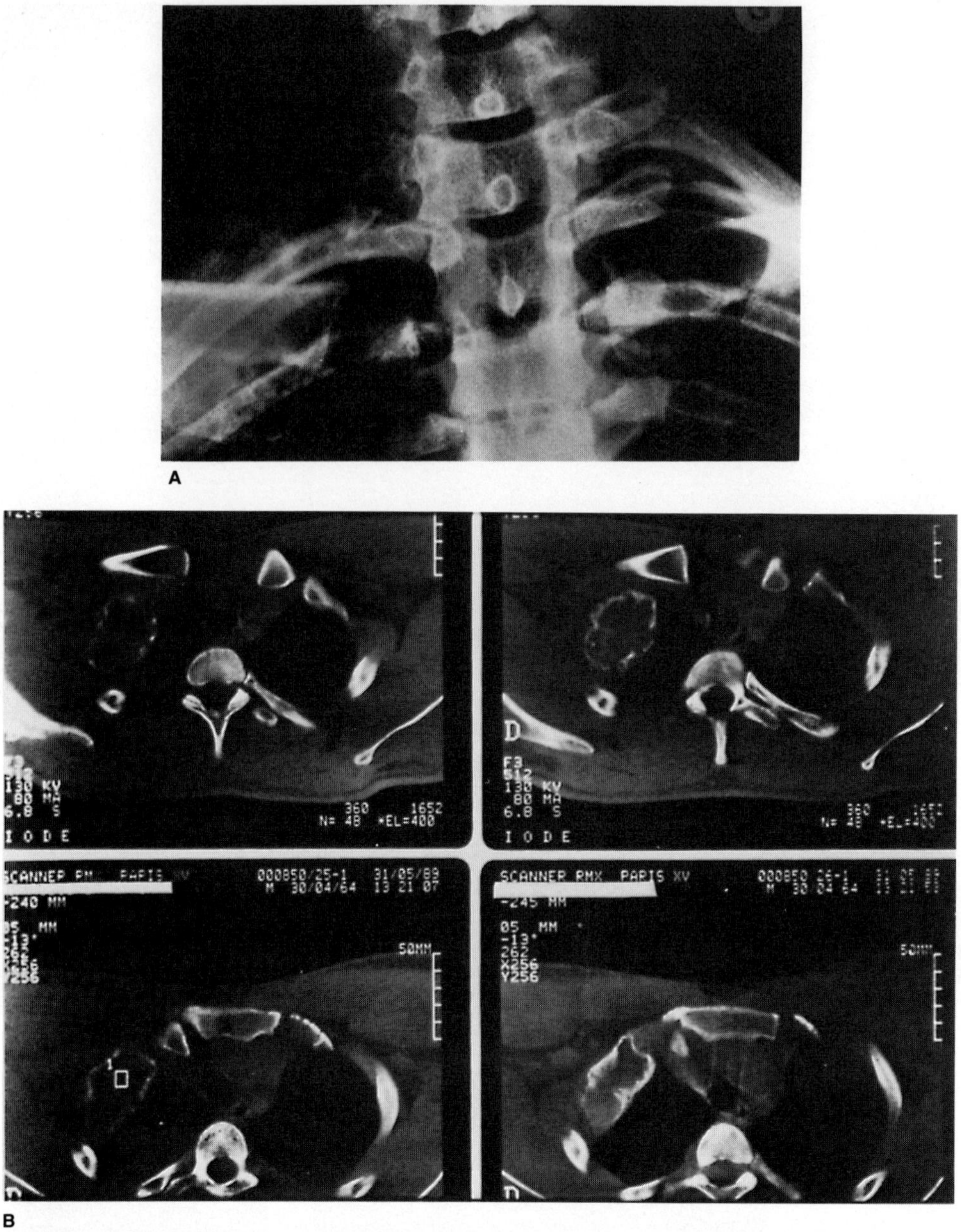

Figure 3-37
Thoracic outline syndrome. **(A)** *Radiograph shows hypertrophic right rib, expanded by a large and hypodense tumor.* **(B)** *CT scan shows tumor involving the whole rib, cortical bone swelling, and no calcification or extension into the adjacent tissues.*[86]

thy, injections, ischemia, trauma, and herpesvirus infection. The lumbosacral trunk can be compromised by trauma, including fractures and dislocation of the pelvis, sacrum, and sacroiliac joints; compression during childbirth and benign pelvic masses; and invasion from sacral metastatic tumor. Symptoms include low back or pelvic pain that often radiates into the leg. Clinical features include neurologic abnormalities that extend beyond the distribution of a single nerve or individual peripheral nerve. In cancer patients with lumbosacral plexus involvement, pain is the most common presenting symptom, followed weeks to months later by numbness, paresthesias, and weakness. Pain may be local, radicular, or referred. Mild weakness, sensory signs, and reflex asymmetry occur initially and are followed by focal paralysis of muscle groups.[87,88]

Imaging of the Lumbosacral Plexus

Plain radiographs of the sacrum and lumbar spine often demonstrate bony disease. A retroperitoneal mass involving the psoas muscle may obscure the psoas shadow on a plain x-ray. Bone scan can often help determine the presence of bone disease. Ultrasonography is often used in the investigation of abdominal and pelvic pathology to demonstrate a mass lesion. The CT scan is the

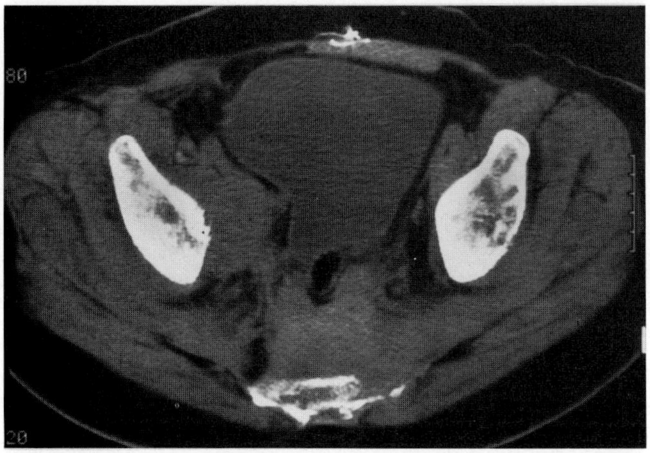

Figure 3-38
CT scan shows soft tissue infiltration, causing a lower sacral plexopathy. The patient was a 60-year-old man with bladder cancer who presented with pain radiating down the posterior aspect of both legs. A presacral mass is seen eroding the sacrum and extending to the right side of the pelvis.

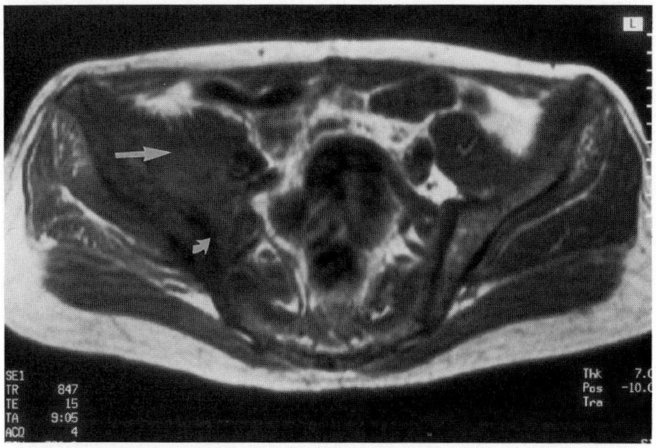

Figure 3-39
MRI shows a large tumor mass involving the right hemipelvis displacing psoas muscle and compressing the right sciatic nerve.

most common procedure used to demonstrate lesions of the lumbosacral plexus.[87,88] Figure 3-38 shows a 60-year-old man with cancer of the bladder who developed pain radiating down the posterior aspect of both legs. A CT scan of the pelvis showed a presacral mass eroding the sacrum and extending into the right side of the pelvic wall.

Studies utilizing CT myelography can demonstrate lesions affecting the cauda equina and nerve roots and distinguish these from extraspinal disorders involving spinal nerves and the lumbosacral plexus. Magnetic resonance imaging has this advantage as well and provides excellent delineation of particular soft tissue structures as well as bony involvement. Gradient-echo imaging can be used to help distinguish neural from vascular structures. Multiplanar examination aids in the assessment, with axial and oblique coronal planes distinguishing relevant structures more distinctly than does the sagittal plane. In a retrospective review of lumbosacral plexopathy, MRI was more sensitive than CT for diagnosing cancer-induced lumbosacral plexopathy.[71]

Figure 3-39 is of a 71-year-old man with transitional cell carcinoma who developed left leg pain that increased in severity, followed by leg weakness. An MRI of the pelvis demonstrated bony metastases to the right hemipelvis with pelvic extension and involvement of the right lumbosacral plexus.

Both CT and MRI can identify the specific lumbar nerve involved. Figure 3-40 shows a large hyperintense lesion in the left gluteal region compressing the sciatic nerve. Biopsy revealed a malignant fibroma. Figure 3-41 shows a lytic lesion in the left acetabulum and involving the pelvis. The patient complained of left leg and hip pain.

Figure 3-42 shows an MRI of a chloroma involving the sciatic nerve in a 9-year-old boy with acute nonlymphocytic leukemia who developed a tingling sensation over the lateral aspect and dorsum of his right foot that was followed by burning pain and a new pain behind his right knee. The foot pain was intermittent and worse at night. There was no back or buttock pain or pain with the Valsalva maneuver or movement. He consistently noticed paresthesia in the sole of his foot that was brought on with urination. He also developed weakness of dorsiflexion, plantar flexion, eversion, and inversion. There were diffuse wasting and distal weakness in all extremities and decrease in sensation in the L5 and S1 dermatomes on the right. Results of myelographic and all CSF studies were negative. Subsequently, the pain behind his knee worsened, and a swelling developed in the right popliteal fossa that was warm, erythematous,

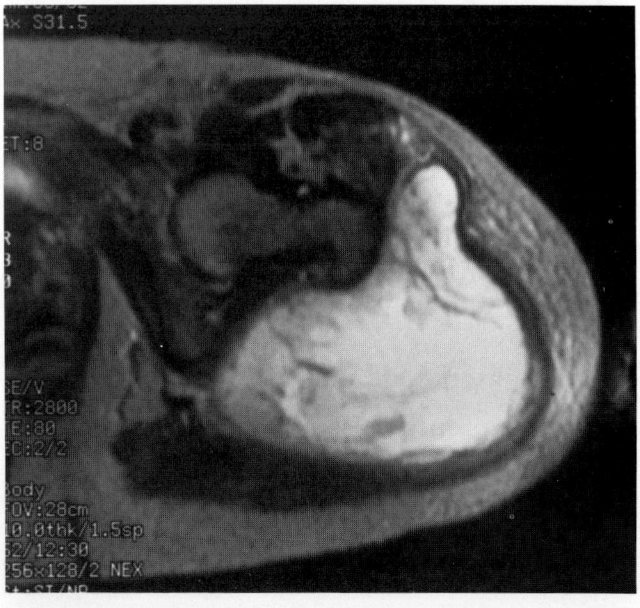

Figure 3-40
MRI shows a large hyperintense mass in the left gluteal region compressing the sciatic nerve.

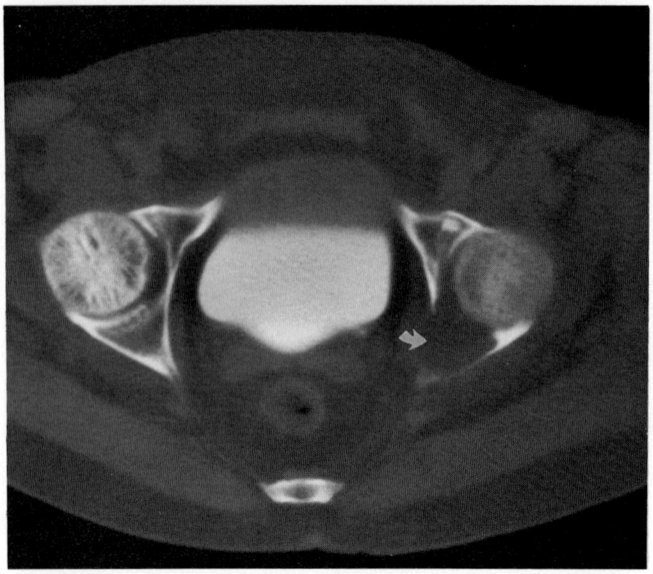

Figure 3-41
Lung tumor causing destructive lesion to the left acetabulum and invading the pelvis. The patient complained of left leg and hip pain.

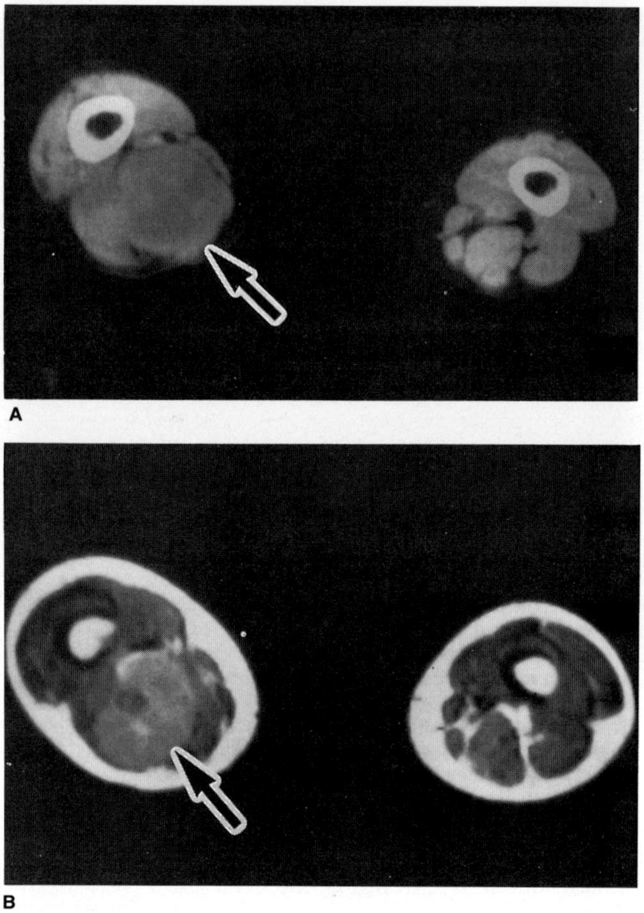

Figure 3-42
(A) *Contrast-enhanced CT scan of the leg shows a large, nonenhancing, inhomogeneous mass posterior to the femur and neurovascular bundle on the patient's right side (arrow).* **(B)** *A corresponding T1-weighted MRI scan of the leg shows a mass of higher signal intensity than the surrounding muscle (arrow). The subcutaneous fat and marrow appear as high intensity, and the bone appears dark.*[89]

and measured 8 by 12 cm. Studies with MRI and CT demonstrated a 5- by 13-cm mass, which was resected and, on pathologic study, was diagnosed as chloroma, a rare form of leukemic involvement of the peripheral nervous system (PNS) that usually occurs in the setting of epidural or leptomeningeal involvement.[89]

The ability to image a nerve in the axial plane and distinguish it clearly from other tissues, such as blood vessels, muscle, and fat, has recently been accomplished.[28] Figure 3-43 shows a magnetoneurographic image of a sciatic nerve in a 24-year-old man who underwent surgical repair of a stab wound, which occurred 7 months before, that had lacerated the tibial portion of his left sciatic nerve. Scarred segments of tibial nerve were resected until normal fascicular structures were encountered, leaving a gap of 5 cm. Fascicles of the tibial nerve were separated from each other for a distance of 3 to 4 mm and then sutured to autologous sural nerve cable grafts. Special pulse sequences and acquisition techniques were used for fat and vessel suppression to obtain this image of the nerve in both axial and longitudinal sections. This technique was so successful that individual fascicles were visualized.

Reflex Sympathetic Dystrophy

Reflex sympathetic dystrophy is a painful syndrome that results from an abnormal response of the sympathetic nervous system to trauma or minor injury. The pain is characteristically of a burning quality but can be knifelike or lancinating or even dull, throbbing, and aching in quality. It is accompanied by allodynia, hyperpathia, vasomotor and sudomotor disturbances, skeletal and muscle changes, and hypotonia. Slight changes in movement or emotional stress can exacerbate symptoms, and the pain is not relieved by rest. The pain does not conform to segmental or peripheral patterns of nerve injury, and the symptoms may spread proximally to include the entire limb or a quadrant of the body. In usually days to weeks, and less often months, following an injury there are local edema, muscle spasm, and tenderness, and the skin may become dry, warm, red, and later cyanotic and sweaty, with acceleration of hair and nail growth. The bone scan may show increased uptake in small joints, while plain x-rays show no changes. Later, skin may become cool, pale, gray, and often cyanotic and brawny. Hair growth becomes decreased or scant, nails become brittle and deeply grooved, joints become thickened, and muscle wasting develops, leading to a decrease in mobility. Osteoporosis becomes more evident, especially in the epiphyseal region. Even later, the skin may take on a smooth, glossy appearance, becoming drawn, pale, and cyanotic; skin temperature

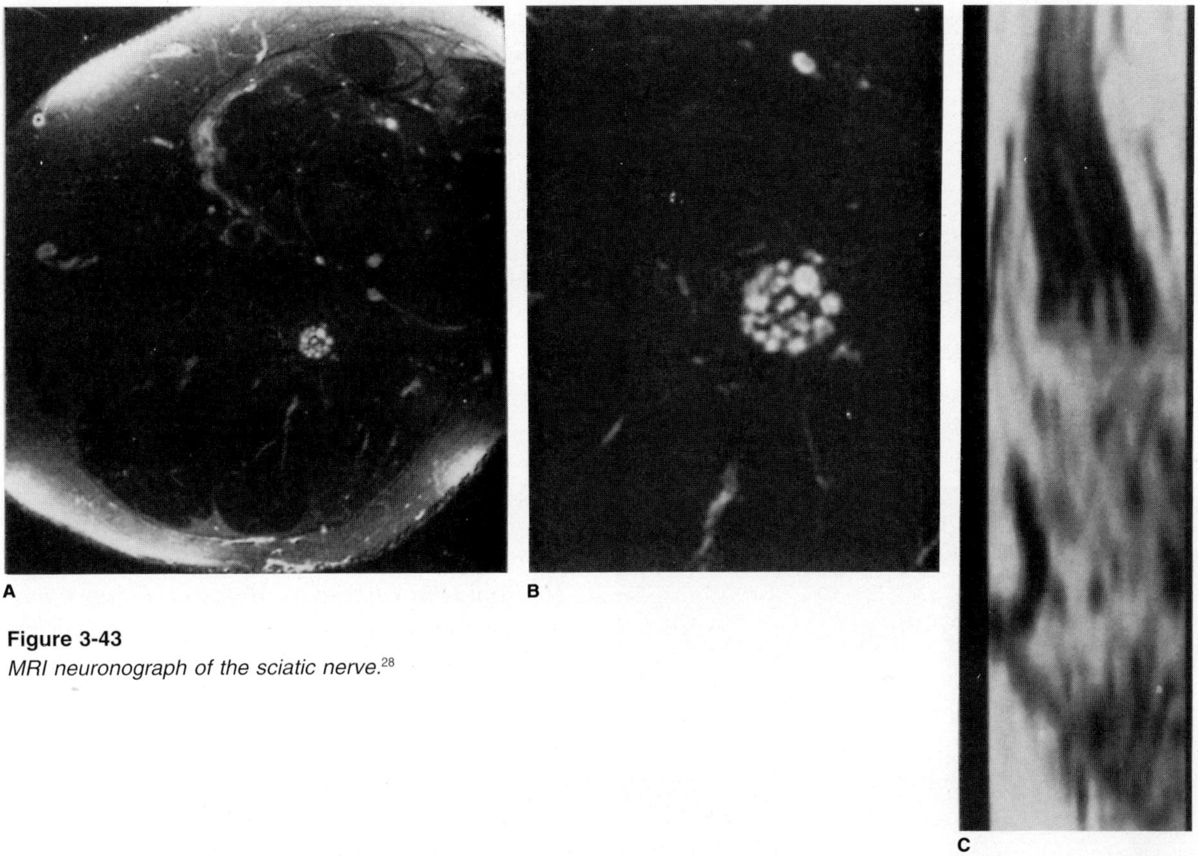

Figure 3-43
MRI neuronograph of the sciatic nerve.[28]

decreases in the affected area, and the nails become ridged and laterally arching; fat pads, hand muscles, and bones atrophy; and there may be ankylosing of the joints. Ultimately, fingers take on a thin and pointed appearance.

Reflex Sympathetic Dystrophy from Wrist Trauma

A 20-year-old woman had an accident at work in which she sustained a minor injury to her wrist. She developed pain and swelling in the hand and stopped using her hand because of the pain. Over the next 2 months her symptoms progressed, with edema involving her whole arm and flexion contractures involving her fingers. Figure 3-44 and Plates 10 and 11 show swelling of the hand and arm, smooth glossy skin, and tapering of the nails. Also seen is an x-ray of this patient's hands demonstrating the osteoarthropathy that is associated with this syndrome.

Central Nervous System Lesions Causing Pain

Central Cord Syndromes

Syringomyelic Syndrome The syringomyelic syndrome is due to syringomyelia, a central cavitation of the spinal cord of unknown cause. Other pathologic states can lead to a similar syndrome, including traumatic myelopathy, postradiation myelopathy, hematomyelia, intramedullary cord lesions, spinal arachnoiditis, infarction (myelomalacia), and, rarely, extramedullary tumors, cervical spondylosis, and cervical necrotizing myelitis. About 90 percent of cases of syringomyelia are associated with type I Chiari malformations. Pain of a burning, aching quality occurs in about 50 percent of patients with syringomyelia and is usually unilateral or more marked on one side.

Traumatic Syrinx A 27-year-old man (Fig. 3-45) had been left paraparetic after a motorcycle accident. He subsequently developed an intramedullary syrinx that required a shunt placement. He presented with severe right-sided headache that radiated down into the right side of his neck with a decrease in sensation in this area in the setting of a 4-month worsening numbness, tingling, and weakness over the right side of his body. He found it difficult to use his right hand to wheel himself around. His examination was significant for decrease in sensation over the right side of his face in a V1–V2 distribution. He had weakness in the right deltoid and in the muscles of the right hand; decrease in bulk in both lower extremities, with both proximal and distal weakness; and decreased sensation in his right upper and lower extremities to all primary modalities. The MRI showed a cervical syrinx cavity that extended into the medulla. After placement of a shunt into the syrinx, his headache and symptoms involving his right

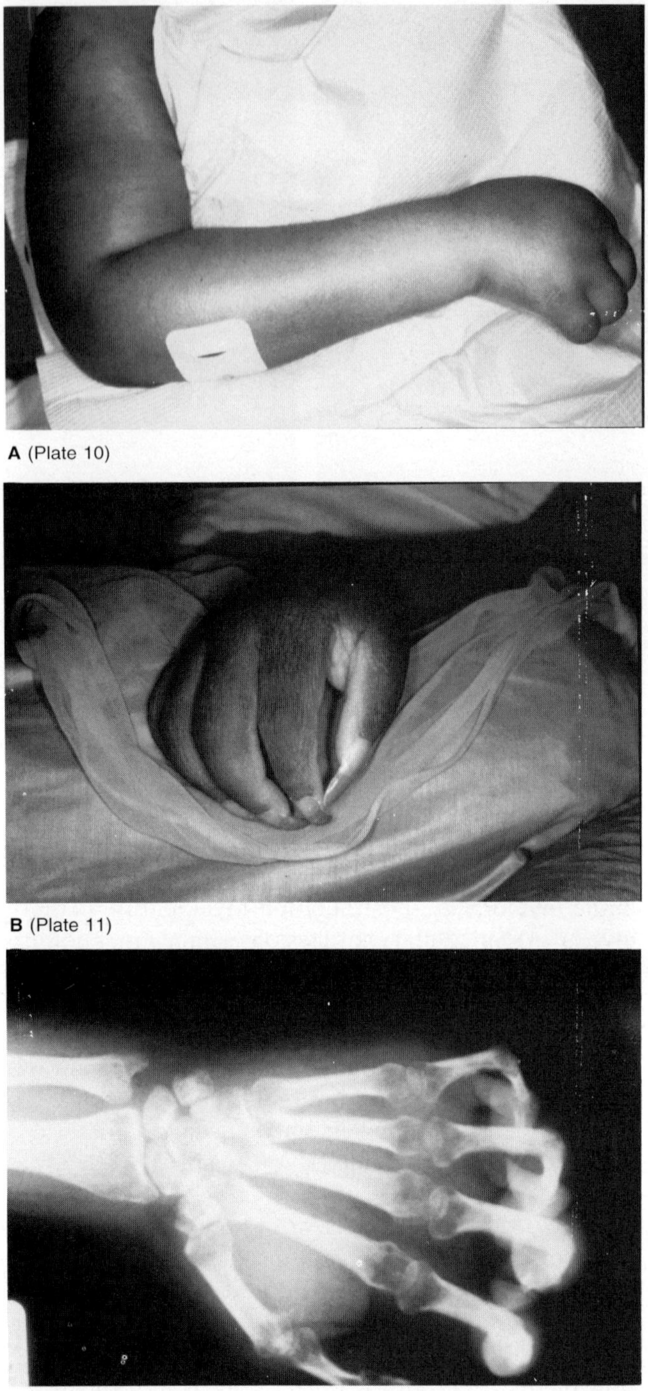

A (Plate 10)

B (Plate 11)

C

Figure 3-44
Photographs of characteristic soft tissue changes seen in reflex sympathetic dystrophy. **(A)** *Swelling of arm.* **(B)** *Pitting of nails and skin changes.* **(C)** *Radiograph showing characteristic changes of osteoporosis especially seen in joints.*

arm resolved. This case represents a more complicated form of a syringomyelic syndrome; the syrinx caused more than the suspended sensory loss characteristic of syringomyelia and affected the descending tract and nucleus of the trigeminal nerve in its course through both the medulla and the spinal cord.

Syrinx Causing Centrally Maintained Deafferentation Pain A 67-year-old woman was diagnosed in 1968 with a spinal lymphosarcoma. She was treated with surgery and radiation and did well until 1986, when she developed tingling and mild dysesthesias in her toes and increased difficulty with her gait. An MRI (Fig. 3-46) demonstrated a syrinx in the mid to lower thoracic spinal cord. She developed burning dysesthesia from the waist down, especially involving her feet and legs. She developed a squeezing and crushing sensation of her right leg. She had bilateral lower extremity edema and demonstrated vasomotor instability of her legs and feet. The MRI shows T7–T8 to L1 laminectomy with the cord posteriorly displaced. This is consistent with postoperative tethering. There is enlargement of the lower thoracic cord centrally, consistent with a syrinx that extends from T8 to T12 (Figs. 3-46 and 3-47).

Hydromyelia Caused by Metastatic Lung Cancer An 83-year-old woman with small cell lung cancer was admitted with excruciating pain that increased over a 2½-day course. The pain began in her upper thoracic spine and then radiated down her back and down into both her ankles. She also complained of constipation. The MRI (Fig. 3-48) showed a syrinx involving the spinal cord at the low cervical and high thoracic region. This lesion was due to an intramedullary metastatic tumor diagnosed by the demonstration of positive CSF cytologic test results for small cell lung cancer, which caused an associated hydromyelia. This area was hypointense on T1 and hyperintense on T2.

Vascular Malformations

Intramedullary Hemorrhage An 82-year-old man had a 6-year history of pain radiating up his right arm to his shoulder and neck. It was described as an aching dysesthesia, fluctuating in nature, associated with a sensitivity to heat and cold in an ulnar distribution. An MRI showed a hypointensity on both T1- and T2-weighted images at the C7 level that was consistent with a possible occult hemangioma of the cord. A year later he developed a symmetric-type pain in the left fourth and fifth fingers with a burning pain along the medial aspect of his left arm up to the elbow and swelling of the fifth digit and pain across his shoulders. The pain intensified over a 2-day period and abated with the development of acute paraparesis. An MRI showed hemorrhage in the lower cervical cord, and the right hand pain completely resolved. However, the pain returned in the right arm, along with hyperpathia, swelling, allodynia, deeply grooved fingernails, and vasomotor instability. The clinical diagnosis was a sympathetically maintained central pain syndrome. A subsequent MRI (Fig. 3-49) demonstrated myoedema of the midcervical and upper thoracic cord with evidence of residual chronic hemorrhage.

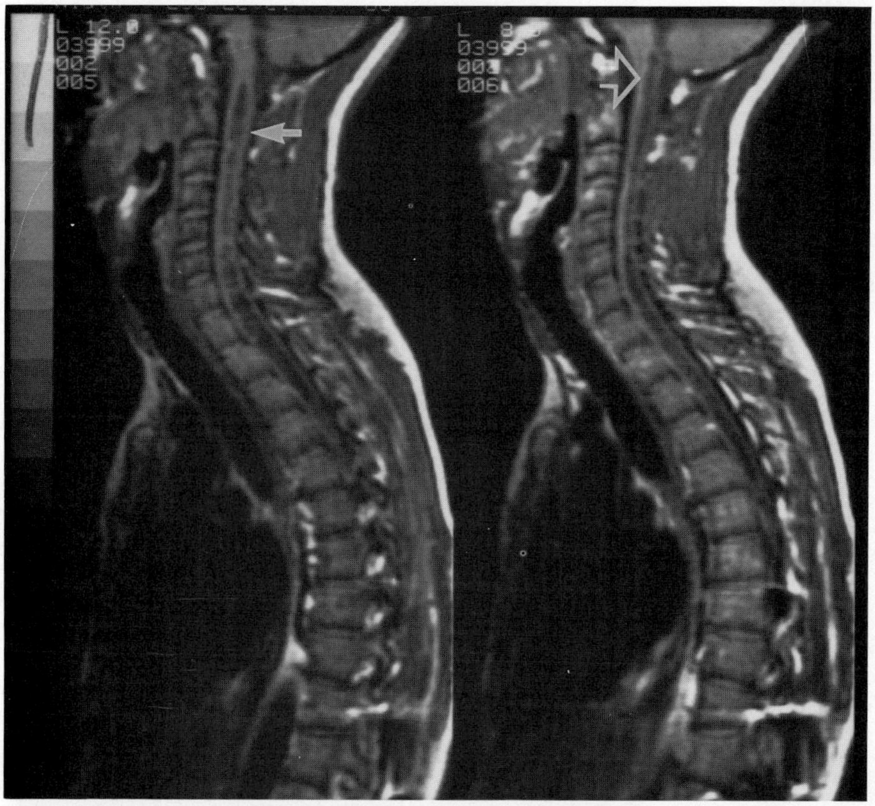

Figure 3-45
MRI shows T1 sagittal images of traumatic syrinx that extends up into the medulla.

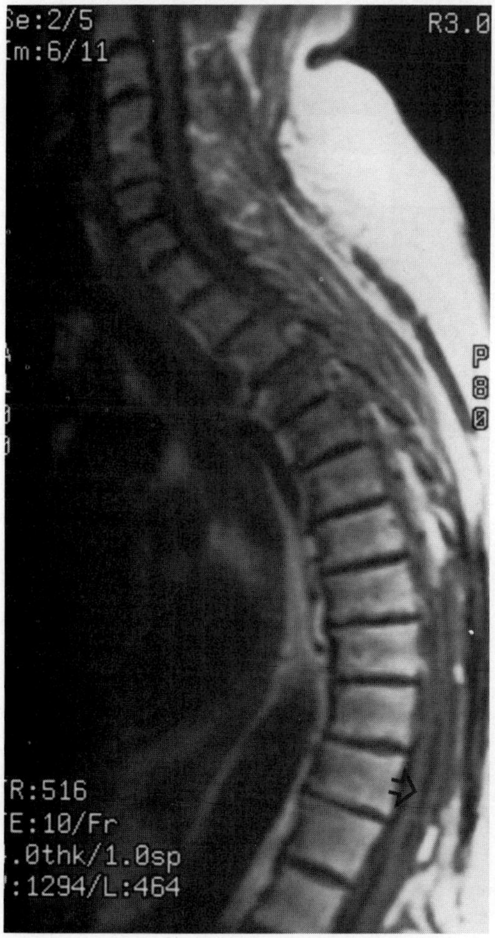

Figure 3-46
MRI of a patient with centrally maintained deafferentation pain. The enlargement of the lower thoracic cord with abnormal signal intensity centrally is consistent with a syrinx that extends from T8 to T12. The patient presented with this lesion 18 years after radiation therapy for lymphosarcoma. There is a T7–T8 to L1 laminectomy.

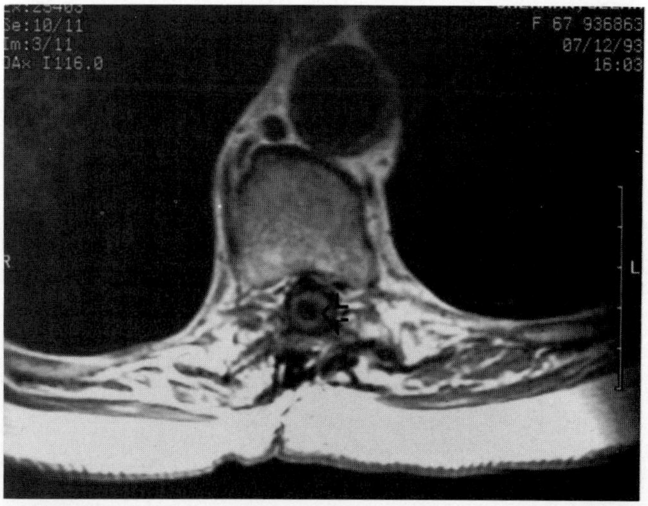

Figure 3-47
Axial MRI demonstrating a central hypodense region consistent with postradiation syrinx.

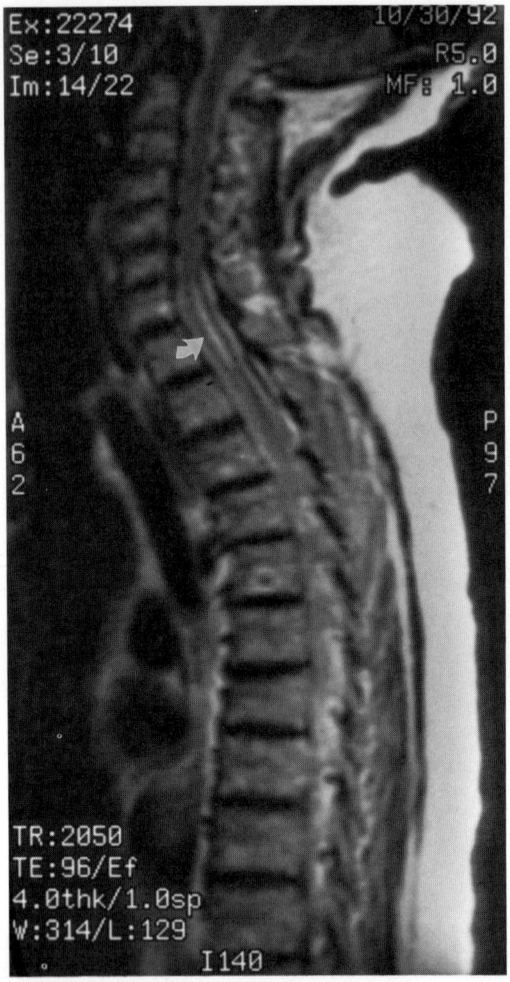

A

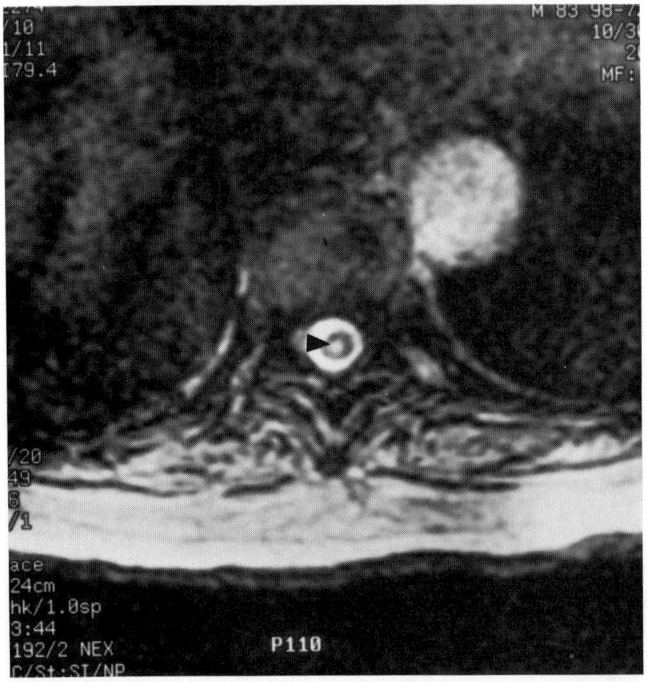

B

Figure 3-48

MRI showing syrinx **(A)** *associated with intramedullary metastasis from breast cancer.* **(B)** *Axial view shows hyperintensity on T2.*

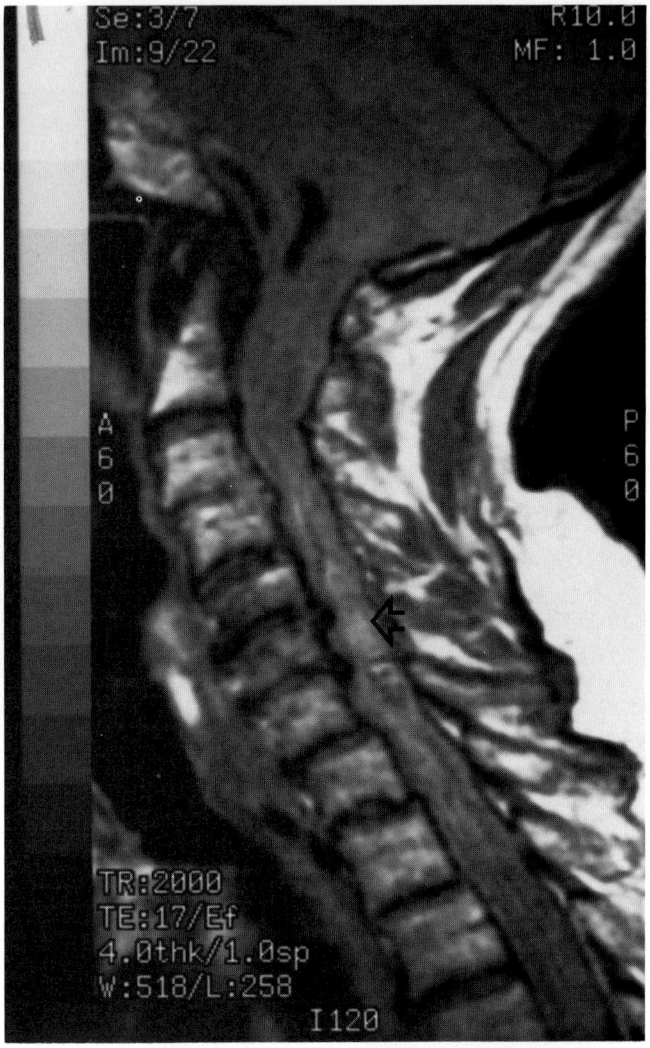

A

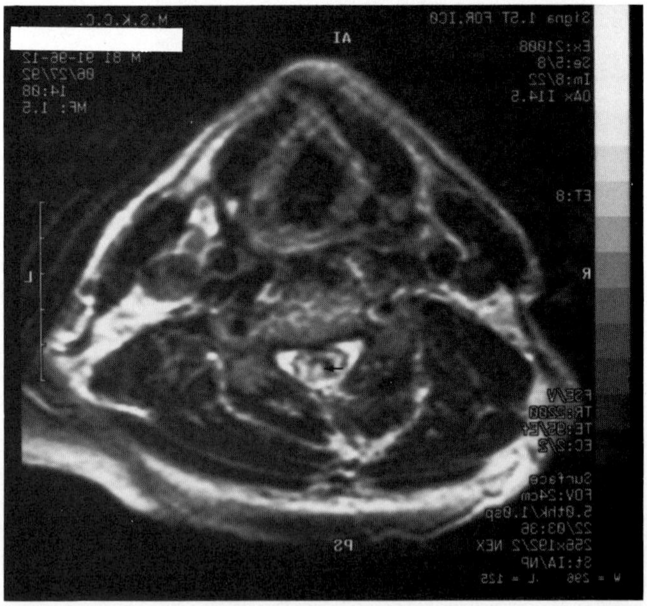

B

Figure 3-49

MRI showing area of chronic hemorrhage with myoedema in the cervical cord in sagittal and axial views.

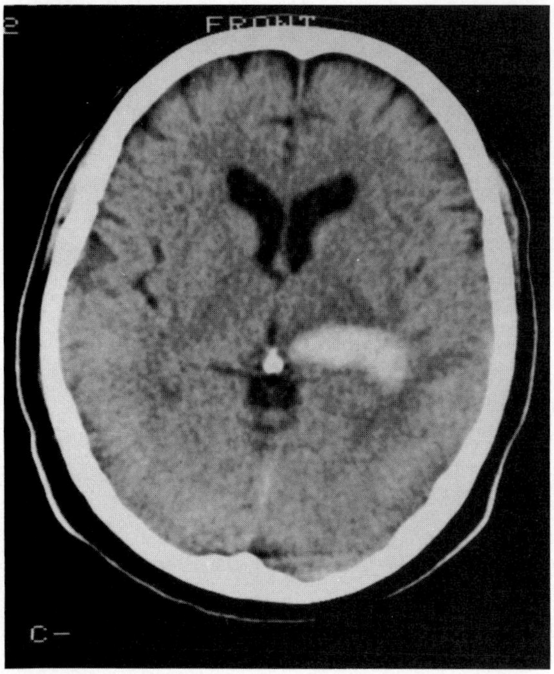

Figure 3-50
CT scan showing hemorrhagic lesion involving left thalamus.

Cerebral Causes of Pain

Central pain can occur with injury to the somatosensory pathways at any level of the central nervous system.[91] The pathophysiologic mechanism of such a lesion is controversial but may result from irritation of sensory fibers that terminate in the thalamic posterior nucleus or from disinhibition of normally inhibitory mechanisms that modulate nociceptive stimuli on their course along the neospinothalamic or paleospinothalamic pathways. Other mechanisms might be the loss of the filtering function of the thalamus for ascending input. At higher levels, lesions of the cortex or corticothalamic fibers might disrupt descending modulating input to the thalamus and lead to exaggerated thalamic responses.

Syndrome of Dejerine-Roussy The thalamic syndrome, or Dejerine-Roussy syndrome, results from a thalamic lesion and is associated with a contralateral dysesthesia, sensory loss, abnormal involuntary movements, and sometimes hemiparesis. It most commonly results from vascular lesions of the thalamus (Fig. 3-50). Recently, infectious agents have been shown to produce comparable lesions.[92]

Thalamic Lesion Due to Hemorrhagic Infarct A 58-year-old man developed acute right hemiplegia involving his right hand, trunk, and leg, and decreased sensation and a burning dysesthetic pain involving the right side of his body. A CT scan showed a hemorrhage involving his left thalamus. His symptoms improved, and he was left with a mild right hemiparesis and a slight ataxia of gait (Fig. 3-50).

Figure 3-51 shows a 45-year-old man with AIDS and a history of intravenous drug abuse who developed right-sided weakness. He had decreased sensation to pinprick on the right side of his body and poor tandem gait. A CT showed bilateral ring-enhancing lesions, and he was started on pyrimethamine and sulfadiazine for presumed *Toxoplasma* abscess. The right arm and leg weakness improved, and follow-up CT showed a clear radiographic response to therapy. Two months later he developed "pins and needles," deep aching pain, and hypersensitivity to touch in the right hand and arm. His symptoms worsened and progressed to involve his right thorax and right leg. He had decreased vibratory and temperature sensation on the right and developed mild choreaform movements of his right hand. The patient was treated with amitriptyline and did well. The patient died 5 months later, and autopsy showed a lesion in

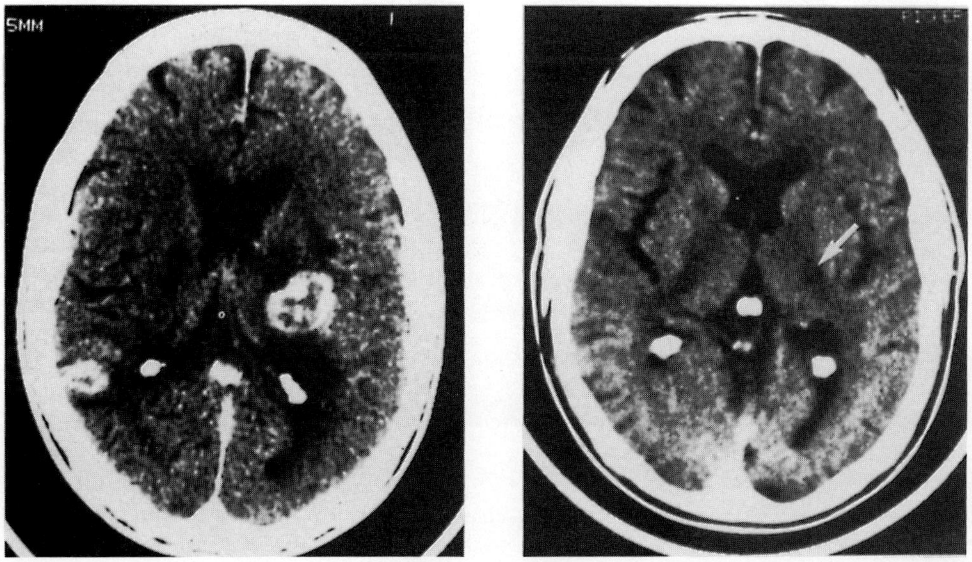

A B

Figure 3-51
Contrast-enhanced CT scan obtained at the time of diagnosis reveals **(A)** *ring-enhancing lesions.* **(B)** *Five months after treatment, a* Toxoplasma *abscess is revealed as a hypodense area in the left internal capsule (arrow).*[92]

the left internal capsule and the reticular nucleus of the thalamus.

Evaluation of Central Pain Syndrome with SPECT Single photon emission computed tomography has been used to study patients with thalamic pain, demonstrating changes in response to temperature and pressure stimuli on the affected side. The pathophysiology of these changes remains undefined.[90]

A 58-year-old man presented with weakness and numbness of the right hand, hypoesthesia to temperature and pinprick on the right side of the body, and slight aphasia.[93] A left thalamocapsular hyperdensity on CT scan (Fig. 3-52) was consistent with hematoma. Two months later he developed prolonged burning pain in his right hand when it was dipped into warm water. He also developed slow abnormal movements of the right hand. A SPECT study performed 15 min after the right hand was immersed in warm water showed a relative hyperactivity of the left thalamic area. No such asymmetry was noted when the left hand was similarly treated.

Verger-Dejerine Syndrome Spontaneous hemibody pain can also occur as the result of a lesion in the parietal lobe that results in a partial deafferentation of the lemniscal-thalamic-parietal pathway. A 69-year-old man (Fig. 3-53) presented with the acute onset of left hand weakness and decreased sensation to the left upper arm and the left side of his face.[81] A small right parietal subcortical hypodense lesion was found on CT scan that enhanced after injection of contrast material and thought to be consistent with an ischemic lacunar infarct. He developed a burning pain in his left hand brought on by light touch or pressure. One month later he developed spontaneous burning pain. He also developed hyperpathia of the left arm and face. A SPECT study was performed 15 min after the left hand was stimulated and demonstrated a relative right hyperactivity within the thalamic area. Stimulation of the painless right hand did not produce an asymmetry in thalamic activity, nor was an asymmetry found after the patient was successfully treated with 150 mg of amitriptyline daily.

Pain from Cranial Nerve Involvement Injury to cranial nerves by compression or by compromise of the blood supply to the nerve, resulting in ischemia, can be caused by both tumor and infection (Fig. 3-54). Destruction of soft tissue and bony structures also leads to cranial nerve injury and pain. Gadolinium-enhanced MRI provides more information than does CT in assessing the spread of tumor involving the base of the skull, demonstrating, in coronal and sagittal sections,

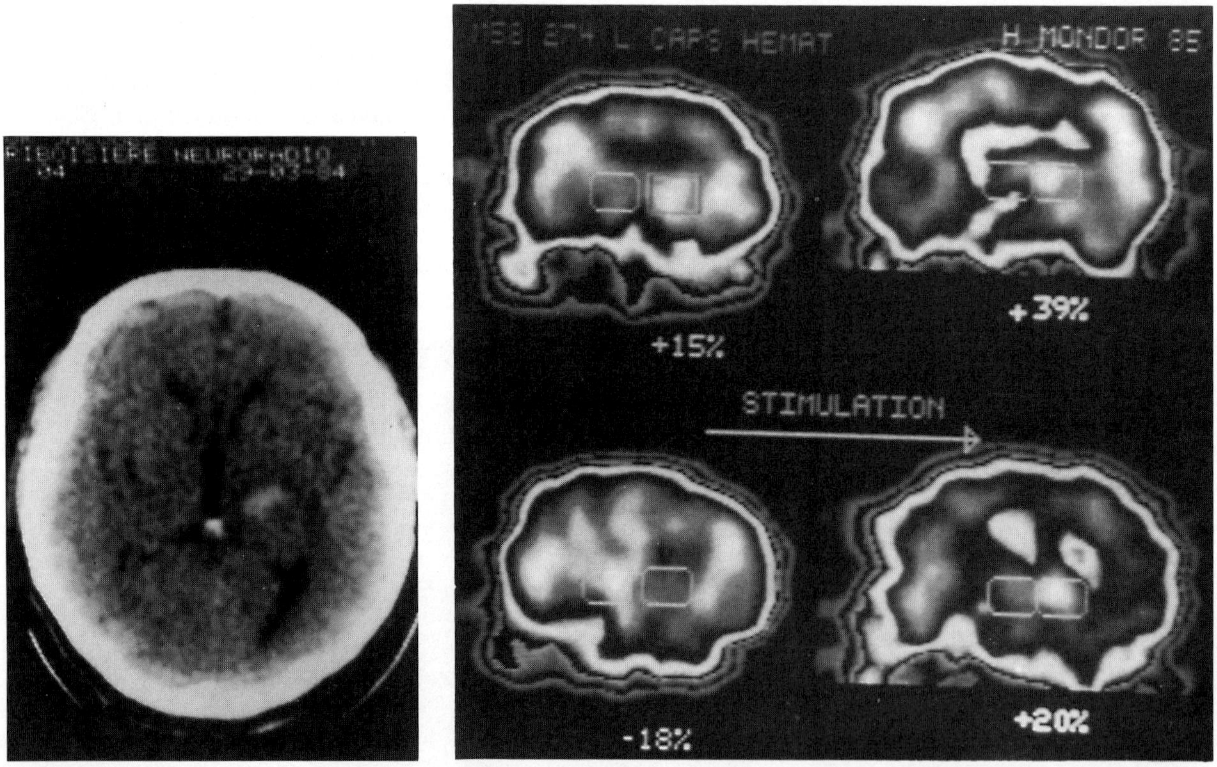

A B

Figure 3-52

(A) *CT scan shows left thalamic hematoma.* **(B)** *SPECT shows two consecutive coronal slices at the thalamic level. The slices on the left were obtained without stimulation of the painful right hand, while the slices on the right were obtained following 15-min stimulation of the right hand with warm water.*[93]

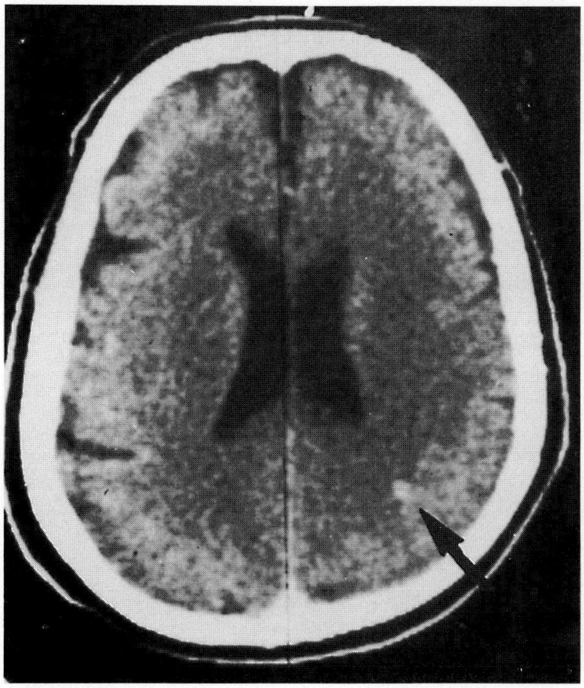

A

Figure 3-53

(A) *Contrast-enhanced CT scan showing a right parietal enhancing lesion adjacent to the cortical ribbon.* **(B)** *SPECT imaging. The four upper slices (one horizontal, one coronal, and three parasagittal, all at thalamic level) were obtained without any stimulation. The left-right difference of activity was within the control range (10 percent). The lower four slices were obtained 1 week earlier after 15 min of sensory tactile, smooth stimulation of the hyperpathic finger of the left hand. Each slice demonstrates a left-right difference ranging from 16 percent (coronal slide) to 26 percent (parasagittal slices) in favor of the right thalamic area.*[93]

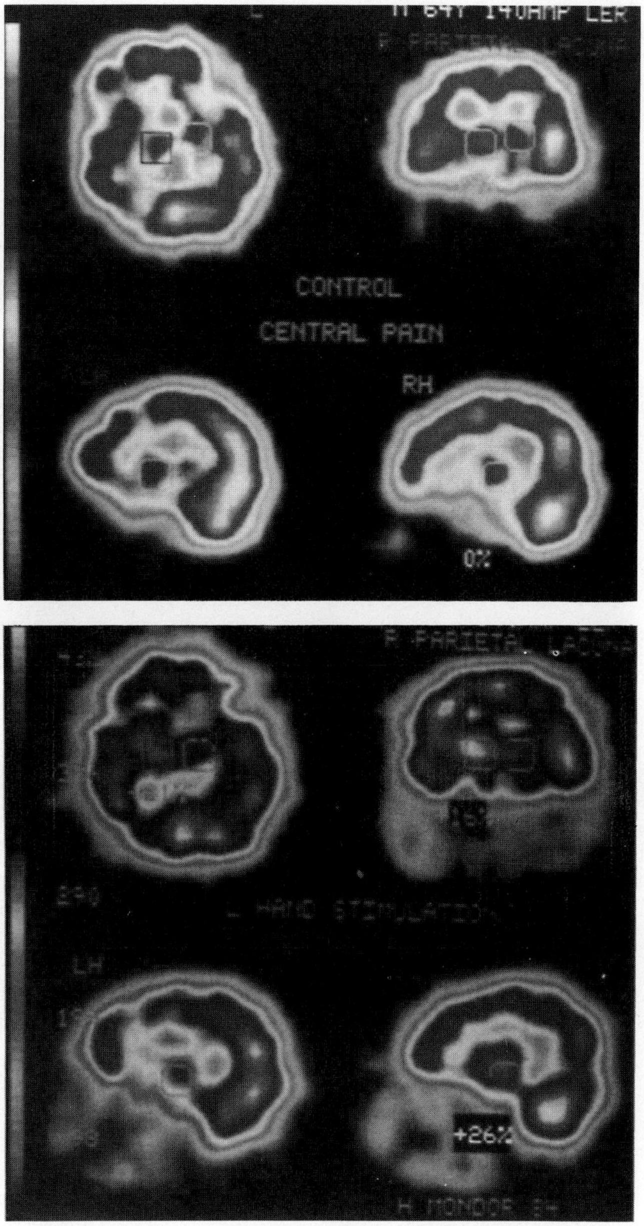

B

the involvement of the trigeminal nerve and its divisions. The presence of subtle bony changes is often better assessed by CT.

Ramsay Hunt Syndrome (Herpes Zoster Oticus) A 46-year-old man developed acute pain and fullness in his left ear and noted the presence of two fever blisters on his left auricle.[94] Facial paralysis, vertigo, and decreased hearing on the left developed 2 weeks later. On examination, the patient had a crusting blister lesion in the left external auditory canal; left lower motor neuron facial paralysis and mild loss of taste were present, as was decreased hearing on the left. The serum varicella zoster virus titer was 1:128. Results of CT with and without contrast material were normal. Magnetic resonance images with and without gadolinium were obtained using a head coil followed by 5-in surface coils on the top of both ears. There was abnormal enhancement of the horizontal and vertical segment of the left facial nerves as well as the cochlea, the vestibule, and the common crus of the semicircular canals. The blister lesion also enhanced (Fig. 3-54).

Trigeminal Neuroma A 27-year-old man was evaluated for a burning pain in the left jaw associated with paroxysmal sharp pain in the same region. Examination showed hypoesthesia and paresthesia of the left jaw and left corneal anesthesia. There was a trigger zone, and the other cranial nerves were normal.[95]

A CT study in axial and coronal planes showed an hourglass neuroma medial to the left petrous apex, extending to the middle cranial fossa and cerebellopontine angle. The lesion enhanced with contrast material and exerted mass effect on the left side of the pons. Studies

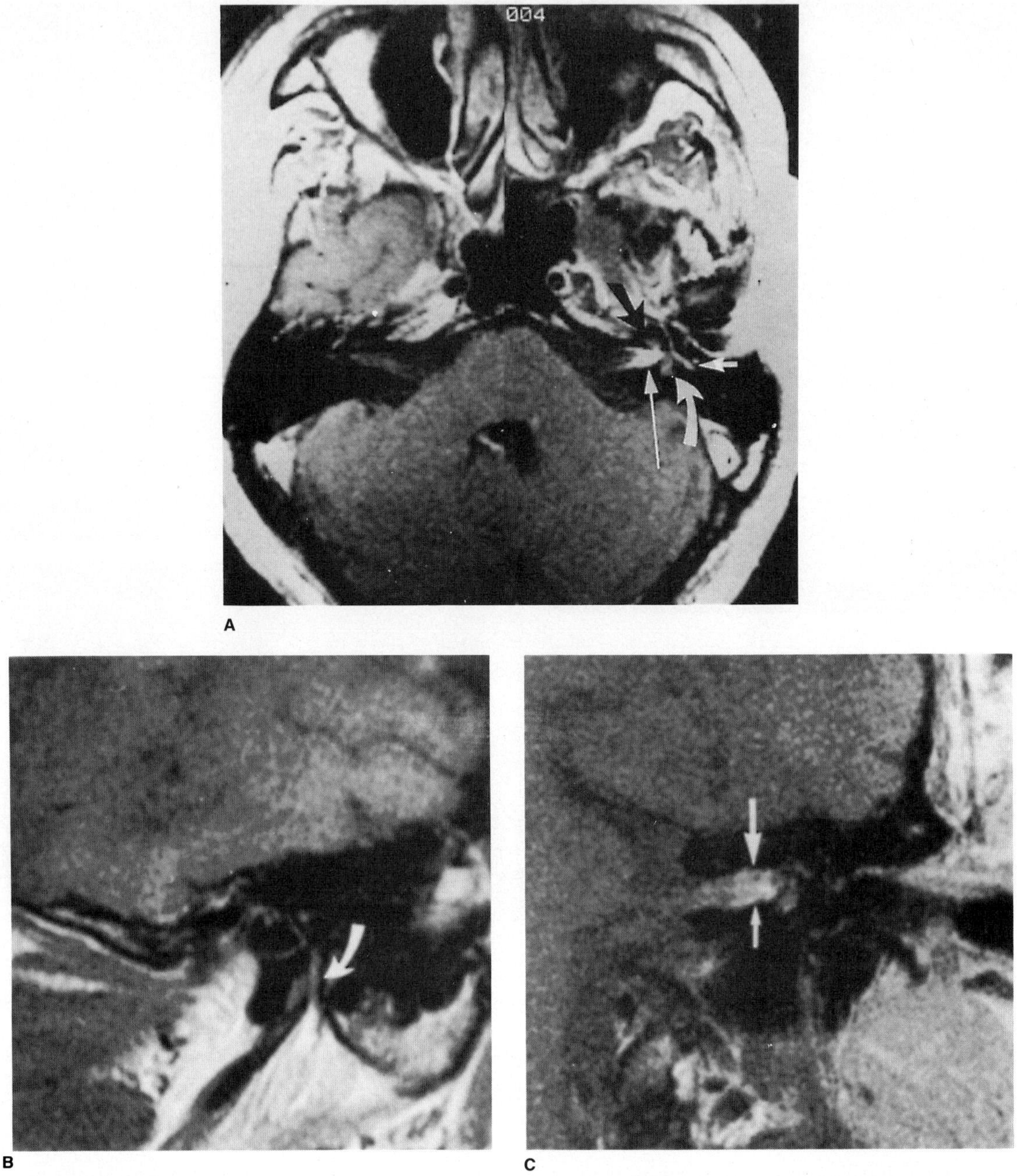

Figure 3-54
Ramsay Hunt syndrome. **(A)** *Postgadolinium T1-weighted images using a head coil shows enhancement in the left internal acoustic canal (long white arrow), the geniculate ganglion and the horizontal segment (short arrow) of the facial nerve, the cochlea (back arrow), and the vestibule and the common crus of the semicircular canals (curved white arrow).* **(B)** *Postgadolinium oblique sagittal T1-weighted image of the left facial nerve using a 5-in surface coil shows abnormal enhancement of the descending segment of the left facial nerve (arrow).* **(C)** *Postgadolinium oblique coronal T1-weighted image of the left internal acoustic canal with a 5-in surface coil demonstrates abnormal enhancement, apparently involving both the superior seventh (larger arrow) and inferior eighth (smaller arrow) nerves. Actual distinction of these two nerves is not possible in this image.*

using MRI (Fig. 3-55) with and without gadolinium were performed and, on coronal sections, showed a tumor in contact with the internal carotid artery and involvement of the left cavernous sinus. The tumor was isointense with gray matter on T1-weighted images, with a hyperintense component; it was mildly hyperintense and heterogeneous on T2-weighted images but strongly enhanced with contrast material, and a hypointense rim was noted on both sequences. Atrophy of the left pterygoid muscles was present.

Facial Pain and Weakness due to Tumor A 58-year-old woman had recently been diagnosed with gastric lymphoma when she developed a peripheral VII nerve palsy with severe facial pain. A CT scan demonstrated a soft tissue mass with bony destruction at the base of

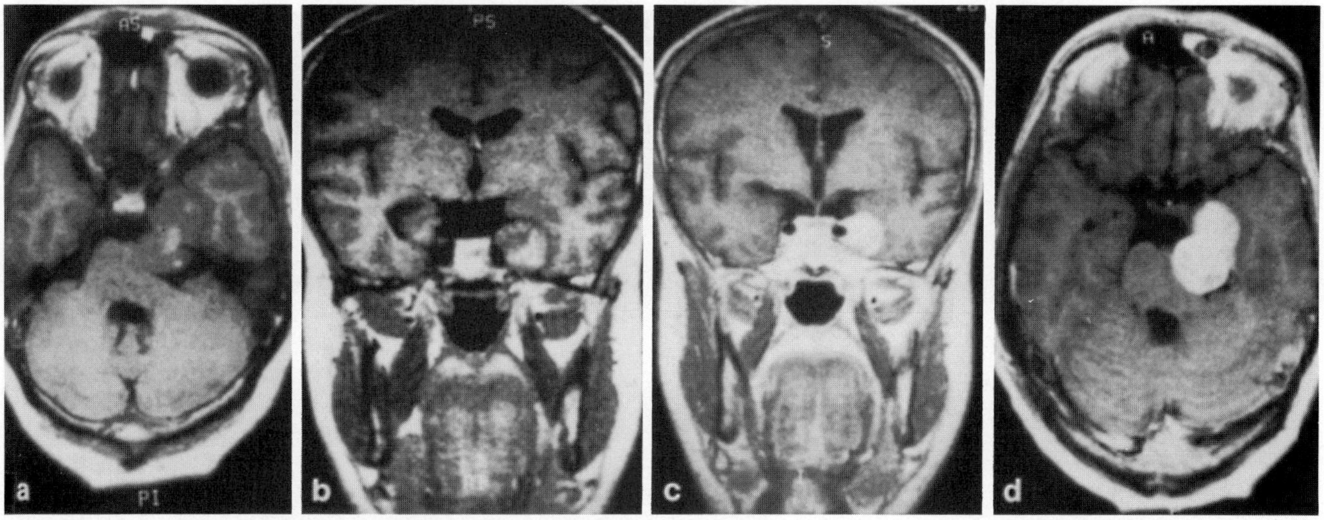

Figure 3-55
Trigeminal neuroma. MRI revealed left hourglass neuroma that is slightly hypointense with areas of high signal on an axial image **(A)** *with a hypointense rim on a coronal T1-weighted image* **(B).** *Note atrophy of the left pterygoid muscles. There was marked enhancement of the tumor, which involves the cavernous sinus and compresses the left side of the pons, on coronal* **(C)** *and axial* **(D)** *T1-weighted images after gadolinium.*

the skull (Fig. 3-56). The tumor had completely destroyed the facial canal and was compressing cranial nerve VII on its course through the facial canal.

Combining Imaging Modalities

Sometimes a number of imaging techniques must be used to fully characterize the extent and nature of a disease process. As discussed previously, it is very important to believe the patient's complaint of pain. When initial imaging studies fail to show the cause of the pain, physicians are often too quick to conclude that the patient does not have pain. However, it is important to understand the limitations of imaging studies. This is especially true when neurologic deficits are found.

Arterial Venous Malformation

A 16-year-old girl developed the gradual onset of a subacute spastic paraparesis. She had associated back pain. She was ultimately diagnosed with a juvenile onset

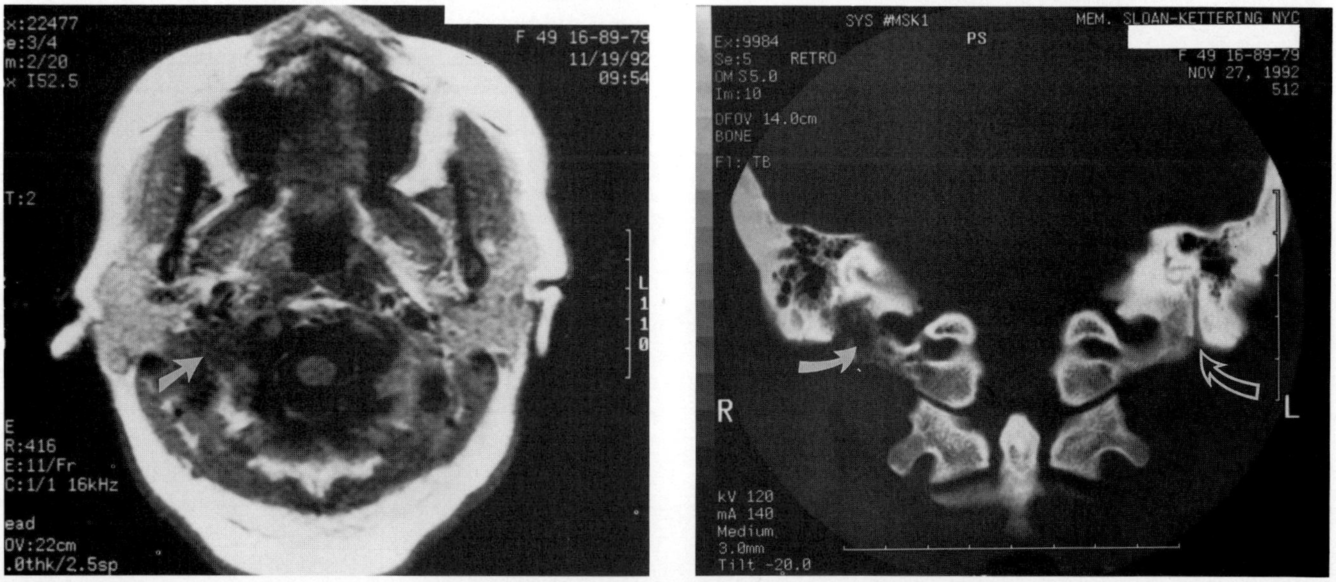

A B

Figure 3-56
CT shows **(A)** *axial and* **(B)** *coronal images of a hypointense lesion and bony destruction at the level of the stylomastoid foramen with destruction of the facial canal.*

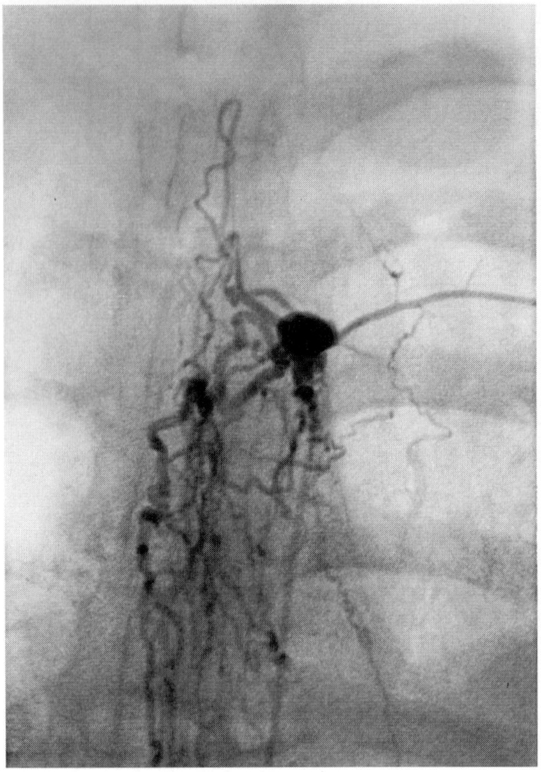

A

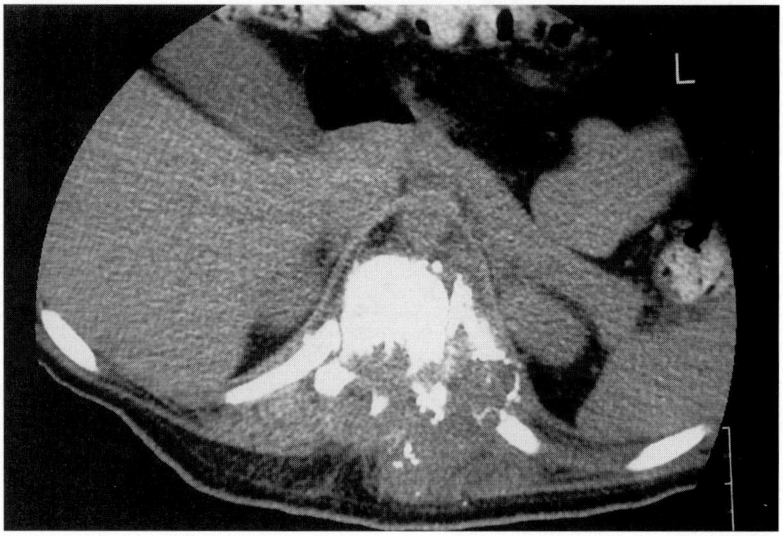

B

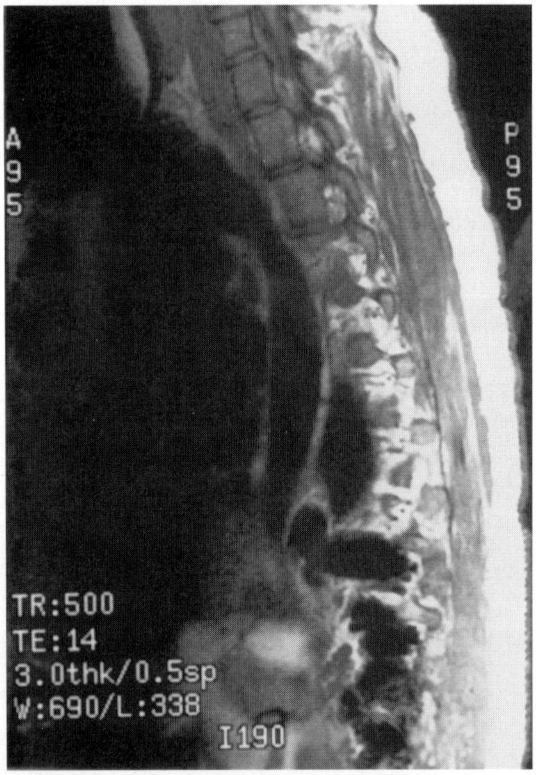

C

Figure 3-57

Angiogram demonstrates the extent of the AVM **(A).** *CT scan shows bone destruction of vertebral bodies due to AVM* **(B).** *MRI shows the relationship between the AVM and adjacent soft tissue structures* **(C).**

arterial venous malformation (AVM) at the T8 level (Fig. 3-57). The CT scan shows the significant bony destruction that has occurred with this vascular lesion. The angiogram has demonstrated the AVM and its dimensions. The MRI nicely demonstrates the relationship of the AVM to soft tissue structures and its extension outside the spinal canal.

Glioma

As mentioned previously, imaging studies may fail to demonstrate the source of pain for some time. A 60-year-old man developed a sharp pain in his left bicep that he described as being like a toothache and feeling as if the bone was broken. The work-up at that time centered on his cervical spine and was negative. One month later he developed some shooting pain in his left foot and ankle and heatlike pain in his leg. He described pain that surges into the left side of his body into his left arm, hip, and leg. Studies of his brain and cervical spine utilizing MRI were negative.

On examination, the patient had decreased sensation in V_2 and V_3 to pinprick, light touch, and temperature and decreased hearing on the left. Left pronator drift was present, and iliopsoas and dorsiflexion was $4^+/5$. Tone was increased in the left arm. He had an extensor plantar response on the left. He had decreased sensation to pinprick, light touch, and joint position sense on the left hemibody.

Figure 3-58 (Plate 12) is a SPECT scan showing an area of moderately increased uptake in the right temporoparietal region with slightly decreased uptake in the region of the left thalamus. Previous MRIs of the brain

Patient Name: JOHNSON WILLIAM
Patient Number: 559986
Study Name: TRANSVERSE-AC
Acquisition Date: 2/7/97, 12:00:00 AM

Emory University Hospital
Atlanta, GA

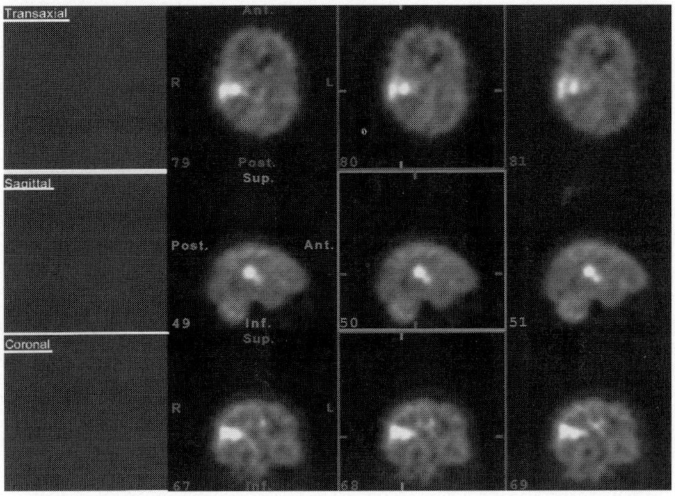

Figure 3-58 (Plate 12)
SPECT demonstrates thalamic and parietal increases in signal activity consistent with the presence of an infiltrating glioma in three views: axial, sagittal, and coronal.

were negative. A subsequent MRI showed a large area of abnormal signal intensity involving the right temporal lobe, extending into the right thalamus and the corpus callosum and into the left occipital lobe.

SUMMARY

Good clinical judgment is the most important element in the diagnostic and therapeutic process. This chapter has discussed the various imaging modalities that are commonly used and explored how they may be employed in the evaluation of pain syndromes. Appropriate management may not require further exploration by radiographic methods at all (e.g., most complaints of low back pain). Conservative therapy is often the best course to follow, reserving further evaluation when such methods fail. At other times, diagnosis by radiographic means demands a more urgent time course (e.g., back pain with leg weakness and loss of bowel and bladder function). The patient's best chance for avoiding both irreversible morbidity and inappropriate and useless diagnostic procedures is a clinician who understands the utility of and indications for the imaging modalities now available for the evaluation of patients in pain.

REFERENCES

1. Weisel SW, Tsourmas N, Feffer HL, et al: A study of computer-assisted tomography: I. The incidence of positive CAT scan in an asymptomatic group of patients. *Spine* 9:549–551, 1984.
2. Teresi LM, Lufkin RB, Reicher MA, et al: Asymptomatic degenerative disk disease and spondylosis of the cervical spine: MR imaging. *Radiology* 164:83–88, 1987.
3. Wood KB, Garvey TA, Gundry C: "Magnetic resonance imaging of the thoracic spine. Evaluation of asymptomatic individuals." *Am J Bone Joint Surg* 77:1631–1638, 1995.
4. Schroth WS, Schectman JM, Elinsky EG, Panagides JC: Utilization of medical services for the treatment of acute low back pain: Conformance with clinical guidelines. *J Gen Intern Med* 7:486–487, 1992.
5. Cope Z: *The Early Diagnosis of the Acute Abdomen,* 12th ed. London, Oxford, 1963.
6. Holder LE: Clinical radionuclide bone imaging. *Radiology* 176:607–614, 1990.
7. Lang P, Steiger P, Faulkner K, et al: Osteoporosis: Current techniques and recent developments in quantitative bone densitometry. *Radiol Clin North Am* 29:49–76, 1991.
8. Cann CE, Genant KH, Kolb FO, et al: Quantitative computed tomography for prediction of vertebral fracture risk. *Bone* 6:1–7, 1985.
9. Magid D, Fishman EK: Imaging of musculoskeletal trauma in three dimensions. *Radiol Clin North Am* 27: 945–956, 1989.
10. Mirvis SE: Applications of magnetic resonance imaging and three-dimensional computed tomography in emergency medicine. *Ann Emerg Med* 18(12):1315–1321, 1989.
11. Modic MT, Masaryk T, Bounphrey F, et al: Lumbar herniated disk disease and canal stenosis: Prospective evaluation by surface coil MR, CT and myelography. *Am J Roentgenology* 147: 757–765, 1986.
12. Ross JS, Perez-Reyes N, Masaryk TJ, et al: Tears in the annulus fibrosus: Assessment with Gd-DPTA-enhanced MR imaging. *Am J Neuroradiology* 10:1251–1254, 1989.

13. Kieffer SA, Stadlan EM, Mohandas A, et al: Discographic anatomical correlation of developmental changes with age in the intervertebral disc. *Acta Radiol Diagn (Stockh)* 9: 733–739, 1969.
14. Rapoport S, Blair DN, McCarthy SM, et al: Brachial plexus: Correlation of MR imaging with CT and pathologic findings. *Radiology* 167:161–165, 1988.
15. Fishman EK, Campbell JN, Kuhlman JE, et al: Multiplanar CT evaluation of brachial plexopathy in breast cancer. *J Comput Assist Tomogr* 15:790–795, 1991.
16. Report of American Academy of Neurology, Therapeutics and Technology Assessment Subcommittee. *Neurology* 40:523–525, 1990.
17. Leclaire R, Esdaile JM, et al: Diagnostic accuracy of technologies used in low back pain assessment: Thermography, triaxial dynamometry, spinoscopy and clinical examination. *Spine* 21:1325–1330, 1996.
18. Guyer RD, Ohnmeiss DD, et al: Complications of cervical discography: Findings in a large series. *J Spinal Disord* 10:95–101, 1997.
19. Zeidman SM, Thompson K, et al: Complications of cervical discography: Analysis of 4400 diagnostic disc injections. *Neurosurgery* 37:414–417, 1995.
20. Holman BL, Tumeh SS: Single-photon emission computed tomography (SPECT): Applications and potential. *JAMA* 263:561–564, 1990.
21. Weber DA: Options in camera technology for the bone scan: Role of SPECT. *Semin Nucl Med* 18:78–89, 1988.
22. Talbott JD, Marrett S, Evans AC, et al: Multiple representations of pain in human cerebral cortex. *Science* 251: 1355–1358, 1991.
23. Bogduk N, Modic MT: Lumbar discography. *Spine* 21: 402–404, 1996.
24. Guyer RD, Ohnmeiss DD: Lumbar discography: Position statement from the North American Spine Society Diagnostic and Therapeutic Committee. *Spine* 20:2048–2059, 1995.
25. Schellhas KP, Pollei SR, Gundry CR: Lumbar disc high-intensity zone: Correlation of magnetic resonance imaging and discography. *Spine* 21:79–86, 1996.
26. DiPiero V, Jones AKP, Iannotti F, et al: Chronic pain: A PET study of the central effects of percutaneous high cervical cordotomy. *Pain* 46:9–12, 1991.
27. Hoffman JM, Hanson MW, Coleman RE: Clinical positron emission tomography imaging. *Radiol Clin North Am* 31:939–959, 1993.
28. Filler AG, Howe FA, Hayes CE, et al: Magnetic resonance neurography. *Lancet* 341:659–661, 1993.
29. Currey HLF, Greenwood RM, Lloyd GG, et al: A perspective study of low back pain. *Rhematol Rehabil* 18:94–104, 1979.
30. Kuntz C IV, Blake L, Britz G: Magnetic resonance neurography of peripheral nerve lesions in the lower extremity. *Neurosurgery* 39:750–756, 1996.
31. Dailey AT, Tsuruda JS, Filler AG: Magnetic resonance neurography for cervical radiculopathy: A preliminary report. *Neurosurgery* 38:488–492, 1996.
32. Deyo RA, Diehl AK: Lumbar spine films in primary care: Current use and effects of selective ordering criteria. *J Gen Intern Med* 318:291–300, 1988.
33. Black KS, Gorey MT, Seidman B, et al: Congenital spondylolisthesis of the 6th cervical vertebra: CT findings. *J Comput Assist Tomogr* 15:335–337, 1991.
34. Boos N, Lander PH: Clinical efficacy of imaging modalities in the diagnosis of low back pain disorders. *Eur Spine J* 5:2–22, 1996.
35. Johnson MJ, Lucas GL: Value of cervical spine radiographs as a screening tool. *Clinical Orthop Rel Res* 340: 102–108, 1997.
36. Marik PE, Rakusin A, Sandhu SS: The impact of the accessibility of cranial CT scans on patient evaluation and management decisions. *J Intern Med* 241:237–243, 1997.
37. Marchiori DM, Henderson CN: A cross-sectional study correlating cervical radiographic degenerative findings to pain and disbability. *Spine* 21:2747–2751, 1996.
38. Freeborn DK, Shye D, Mulloly JP: Primary care physicians' use of lumbar spine imaging tests: Effects of guidelines and practice pattern feedback. *J Gen Intern Med* 12: 619–625, 1997.
39. Carragee EJ, Kim DH: A prospective analysis of magnetic resonance imaging findings in patients with sciatica and lumbar disc herniation: Correlation of outcomes with disc fragment and canal morphology. *Spine* 22:1650–1660, 1997.
40. Carey TS, Garrett J: Patterns of ordering diagnostic tests for patients with acute low back pain: The North Carolina Back Pain Project." *Ann Intern Med* 125:807–814, 1996.
41. Shaker L, Montanera W: Computed tomography versus magnetic resonance imaging and three dimensional applications. *Med Clin North Am* 75:1355–1366, 1991.
42. Masaryk TJ, Ross JS, Modic MT, et al: High resolution MR imaging of sequestered lumbar intervertebral disks. *Am J Roentgenol* 150:1155–1162, 1998.
43. Greiner N, Kressel HY, Schiebler ML, et al: Normal and degenerative posterior spinal structures: MR imaging. *Radiology* 170:489–493, 1989.
44. Saal JA (ed): *Physical Medicine and Rehabilitation: Neck and Back Pain. State of the Art Reviews.* Philadelphia, Hanley & Belfus, 1990.
45. Yoch DH: *Imaging of CNS Disease: A CT and MR Teaching File,* 2d ed. St. Louis, Mosby Year Book, 1991.
46. Adami S, Gatti D, Rossini M, et al: The radiologic assessment of osteoporosis. *Bone* 13:S33–S36, 1992.
47. Fogelman I, Ryan P: Measurement of bone mass. *Bone* 13:S23–S28, 1992.
48. Jorgensen J, Hansen PH, Steenskov V, et al: A clinical and radiological study of chronic lower spinal arachnoiditis. *Neuroradiology* 9:139–144, 1975.
49. Bush K, Chaudhuri R, Hiller S: The pathomorphologic changes that accompany the resolution of cervical radiculopathy: A prospective study with repeat magnetic resonance imaging. *Spine* 22:183–186, 1997.
50. Ross JS, Masaryk TJ, Modic MT, et al: MR imaging of lumbar arachnoiditis. *Am J Roentgenol* 8:885–892, 1987.
51. Van Geothem JW, Biltjes Ig, et al: Whiplash injuries: Is there a role for imaging? *Eur J Radiol* 22:30–37, 1996.
52. Auld AW: Chronic spinal arachnoiditis: A postoperative syndrome that may signal its onset. *Spine* 3:88–92, 1978.
53. Benner B, Ehni S: Spinal arachnoiditis: The postoperative variety in particular. *Spine* 3:40–41, 1975.
54. Burton CV: Lumbosacral arachnoiditis. *Spine* 1:24–30, 1978.
55. Bourne IHJ: Lumbo-sacral adhesive arachnoiditis: A review. *J R Soc Med* 83:262–265, 1990.

56. DiMarcangelo MT, Yu TC: Diagnostic imaging of heel pain and plantar fasciitis. *Clin Podiatr Med Surg* 14:281–301, 1997.
57. Stiskal M, Szolar DH, Stenzel I: Magnetic resonance imaging of Achilles tendon in patients with rheumatoid arthritis. *Investigat Radiol* 32:602–608, 1997.
58. Edwards DJ, Lomas D, Villar RN: Diagnosis of the painful hip by magnetic resonance imaging and arthroscopy. *Br J Bone Joint Surg* 77:374–376, 1995.
59. Imhoff AB, Hodler J: Correction of MR imaging, CT arthrography, and arthroscopy of the shoulder. *Bull Hosp Joint Dis* 54:146–152, 1996.
60. Trieshmann HW Jr, Mosure JC: The impact of magnetic resonance imaging of the knee on surgical decision making. *Arthroscopy* 12:550–555, 1996.
61. Bluemke DA, Zerhouni EA: MRI of avascular necrosis of bone. *Top Magn Reson Imaging* 8:231–246, 1996.
62. Duleba AJ, Keltz MD, Olive DL: Evaluation and management of chronic pelvic pain. *J Am Assoc Gynecol Laparoscopists* 3:205–227, 1996.
63. Medl M, Kulenkampff KJ, Stiskal M: Magnetic resonance imaging in the preoperative evaluation of suspected ovarian masses. *Anticancer Res* 15:1123–1125, 1995.
64. Ekberg O, Sjoberg S, Westlin N: Sports-related groin pain: Evaluation with MR imaging. *Eur Radiol* 6:52–55, 1996.
65. Rubin SJ, Feldman F, Staron RB: Magnetic resonance imaging of muscle injury. *Clin Imaging* 19:263–269, 1995.
66. Blum U, Buitrago-Tellez C, Mundinger A: Magnetic resonance imaging (MRI) for detection of active sacroiliitis: A prospective study comparing conventional radiography, scintigraphy, and contrast enhanced MRI. *J Rhematol* 23: 2107–2115, 1996.
67. Shapiro S: Long-term follow up of 57 patients undergoing automated percutaneous discectomy. *J Neurosurg* 83:31–33, 1995.
68. Gasparotti R, Ferraresi S Ginelli L: Three-dimensional MR myelography of traumatic injuries of the brachial plexus. *Am J Neuroradiol* 18:1733–1742, 1997.
69. Wouter van Es H, Engelen AM, Witkamp TD: Radiation-induced brachial plexopathy: MR imaging. *Skeletal Radiol* 26:284–288, 1997.
70. Panasci DJ, Holliday RA, Shpizner B: Advanced imaging techniques of the brachial plexus. *Hand Clin* 11:545–553, 1995.
71. Taylor BV, Kimmel DW, Krecke KN: Magnetic resonance imaging in cancer-related lumbosacral plexopathy. *Mayo Clin Proc* 72:823–829, 1997.
72. Portenoy RK, Galer BS, Salomon O, et al: Identification of epidural neoplasm: Radiography and bone scintigraphy in the symptomatic spine. *Cancer* 64:2207–2213, 1989.
73. Graus F, Krol G, Foley KM: Early diagnosis of spinal epidural metastases (SEM): Correlation with clinical and radiological findings (abstr). Abstract No. C-1047, Program/Proceedings American Society of Clinical Oncology 4:269, 1985.
74. Posner JB: Back pain and epidural spine cord compression. *Med Clin North Am* 71:185–205, 1987.
75. Waldvogel FA, Varsey H: Osteomyelitis: The past decade. *N Engl J Med* 303:360–370, 1980.
76. Smith AS, Blaser SI: Infectious and inflammatory processes of the spine. *Radiol Clin North Am* 29:809–827, 1991.
77. Hlavin ML, Kaminski HJ, Ross JS, et al: Spinal epidural abscess: A ten-year perspective. *Neurosurgery* 27:177–184, 1990.
78. Artinian MA, Leung AT, Tishler PV: Vertebral osteomyelitis, in Images in Clinical Medicine. *N Engl J Med* 329:399, 1993.
79. Swayne LC, Dorsky S, Caruana V, et al: Septic arthritis of a lumbar facet joint: Detection with bone SPECT imaging. *J Nucl Med* 30:1408–1411, 1989.
80. Weissman BN: Spondyloarthropathies. *Radiol Clin North Am* 25:1235–1262, 1987.
81. Westmark KD, Weissman BN: Complications of axial arthropathies. *Orthop Clin North Am* 21:423–435, 1990.
82. Blair DN, Rapoport S, Sostman HD, Blair OC: Normal brachial plexus imaging. *Radiology* 165:763–767, 1987.
83. Cascino TL, Kori S, Krol G, Foley KM: CT scanning of the brachial plexus in patients with cancer. *Neurology* 33:1553–1557, 1983.
84. Martini N: Pain associated with superior sulcus tumor and its management, in Arbit E (ed): *Management of Cancer-Related Pain.* New York, Futura Press, 1993, chap 25, pp 425–435.
85. Foley KM: Brachial plexopathy in patients with breast cancer, in Harris JR, Hellman S, Henderson IC, Kinne D (eds): *Breast Diseases.* Philadelphia, Lippincott, 1987, chap 23, pp 722–729.
86. Melliere D, Yahia EB, Etienne G, et al: Thoracic outlet syndrome caused by tumor of the first-rib. *J Vasc Surg* 2:236–240, 1991.
87. Jaeckle KA, Young DF, Foley KM: The natural history of lumbosacral plexopathy in cancer. *Neurology* 35:8–14, 1984.
88. Patchell RA, Posner JB: Neurologic complications of systemic cancer, in Nicholas A, Vick MD, Bigner DD (eds): *Neurologic Clinics Neuro-Oncology Now.* Philadelphia, Saunders, 1985, 3(4):729–750.
89. Stillman MJ, Christensen W, Payne R, Foley KM: Leukemic relapse presenting as sciatic nerve involvement by chloroma (granulocytic sarcoma). *Cancer* 62:2047–2050, 1988.
90. Bonica JJ: Causalgia and other reflex sympathetic dystrophies, in Bonica JJ (ed): *The Management of Pain.* Malverne, PA, Lea & Febiger, 1990, chap 11, pp 220–243.
91. Casey KL (ed): *Pain and Central Nervous System Disease: The Central Pain Syndromes.* New York, Raven Press, 1991.
92. Gonzales GR, Herskovitz S, Rosenblum M, Foley KM, et al: Central pain from cerebral abscess: Thalamic syndrome in AIDS patients with toxoplasmosis. *Neurology* 42(5):1107–1109, 1992.
93. Cesaro P, Mann MW, Moretti JL, et al: Central pain and thalamic hyperactivity: A single photon emission computerized tomography study. *Pain* 47:329–336, 1991.
94. Osumi A, Tie RD: MR findings in a patient with a Ramsay-Hunt syndrome. *J Comput Assist Tomogr* 6:991–993, 1990.
95. Berges C, Revel MP, Gaston A, et al: Trigeminal neuromas: Assessment of MRI and CT. *Neuroradiology* 34:179–183, 1992.

CHAPTER 4

NEUROIMAGING OF HEADACHE

Todd D. Rozen
Stephen D. Silberstein
David Friedman

INTRODUCTION

Headache is extraordinarily common, with a lifetime prevalence up to 90 percent.[1] Four percent of all doctor visits, or 10 million visits per year, are for a complaint of headache.[2] Migraine affects 18 million women and 5.6 million men in the United States.[3] Headache afflicts individuals in all socioeconomic classes and places a tremendous economic burden on society. The annual estimate of lost labor costs resulting from migraine is between $5 billion and $17 billion per year.[4]

In 1988 the International Headache Society (IHS) established operational diagnostic criteria for all headache disorders.[5] Primary headache syndromes (migraine, cluster, and tension-type headaches) are by definition not a symptom of an underlying medical condition, while secondary headache syndromes (headache associated with trauma, vascular disorders, infections, and mass lesions) are a symptom of another illness.

New developments in neuroimaging and neuropharmacology have advanced the diagnosis and treatment of headache. Many headache sufferers have had either a computed tomography (CT) or magnetic resonance imaging (MRI) scan of the brain during their lifetimes. Often the imaging procedure was done to reassure these patients that they did not have an underlying serious medical condition. Neuroimaging is expensive, and its role in patients who present with headache and have a normal neurologic examination is controversial. Physicians may feel pressured to image a patient because of fear of litigation, not because they think the study is medically indicated.

Before the introduction of CT in 1973, brain tissue could not be imaged. Skull x-rays could image bone, pneumoencephalograms could obtain the outline of brain tissue, and angiograms could identify the integrity of the cerebral vasculature, but the true intracranial contents of the brain appeared as shadows. CT and MRI have changed the way medicine is practiced. Structural abnormalities that can mimic primary headache disorders now can be diagnosed easily.

Headache is a subjective experience. Many recurrent stereotypic headache syndromes have been classified, but their causes remain basically unknown. Three distinct theories of migraine pathogenesis have been proposed. The vascular theory expounded by Wolff[6] suggests that the aura phase of migraine is secondary to vasoconstriction with transient ischemia to the cerebral cortex, while the pain phase is the result of reactive vasodilation causing the throbbing sensation that many migraineurs experience. The humoral hypothesis[7] suggests that neurochemicals (serotonin, nitric oxide) that circulate throughout the body can change acutely in concentration above or below a threshold and induce migraine. The most recent hypothesis involves the trigeminovascular system and neurogenic inflammation theory.[8] A headache trigger (e.g., stress, spreading depression) activates the trigeminal axons that surround intracranial vessels. The stimulated neurons release vasoactive peptides [substance P, neurokinin A, calcitonin gene-related peptide (CGRP)] that induce sterile neurogenic inflammation with resultant blood vessel dilation, plasma extravasation, and mast cell degranulation. In addition, the trigeminal axons send a signal centrally to brainstem structures and higher brain pain centers (thalamus, cortex). The trigeminovascular theory encompasses the vascular theory (vessel dilation) and the humoral theory (sumatriptan, a 5HT1D agonist, can abort neurogenic inflammation in animal models, suggesting serotonin involvement) and adds neurogenic centers that can initiate and modulate migraine attacks.

Neuroimaging has helped in the development of the theories of migraine pathogenesis. In 1941 Lashley plotted his own visual scotoma, which he calculated was due to a phenomenon that moved across his occipital cortex at a rate of 3 mm/min.[9] Leão[10] demonstrated spreading depression of cortical activity in experimental animals that moved at a rate of 3 mm/min. The cortical and brainstem neurologic dysfunction that manifests as the migraine aura appears to result from an event, associated with spreading oligemia, that moves across the cortex at a rate of 2 to 3 mm/min. Both single photon emission computed tomography (SPECT)[11] and positron emission tomography (PET)[12] imaging techniques have demonstrated spreading hypoperfusion in humans during migraine. The spreading oligemia did not respect vascular territories, placing in doubt focal vasospasm as the cause of the aura. SPECT data also showed that cerebral hypoperfusion does not reach ischemic thresholds, so that neuronal ischemia is an unlikely mechanism for aura initiation.[13] PET studies have identified a possible generator for both migraine (in the brainstem)[14] and cluster (in the hypothalamus).[15] Newer techniques such as functional MRI may allow "real-time" study of headache. Neuroimaging has expanded our knowledge of headache mechanisms and may result in improved treatment.

PRIMARY HEADACHES

Migraine

CT Evaluation in Migraine Patients

When CT technology was introduced, it was hoped that it could play a role in migraine diagnosis and help provide an understanding of the cause of migraine. CT is important in differentiating primary from secondary headache syndromes, especially in the acute setting, but is not helpful in diagnosing migraine. Most CT scans of migraineurs on state-of-the-art scanners are normal. Reported abnormalities have included cerebral atrophy, ventricular enlargement, and white matter lesions. Focal edema or ischemia may be found during an acute episode of complicated migraine. These CT changes usually resolve on subsequent imaging several weeks after the initial scan.[16] In 1976 Cala and Mastiglia[17] reported a high prevalence of CT abnormalities in 46 migraineurs age 17 to 35 years. Acute migraine attacks were imaged in 12 individuals, among whom 7 showed mild cerebral edema. Only 19.6 percent of the scans were normal. Cerebral atrophy was noted in 8 of 46 patients, but only in 2 patients was the atrophy considered significant. Hungersford and associates[18] found cerebral atrophy in 26.4 percent of 53 patients with a history of severe migraine whose average age was 42 years. Atrophy was felt to be related to the age of the patient and the frequency and severity of the migraine attacks and possibly represented chronic infarction. In 1983, duBoulay and Ruiz[19] reported that 58 percent of 53 migraineurs had cerebral atrophy on CT. However, Cuetter and Aita[20] looked at 435 CT scans of patients with migraine with aura, and all but 1 scan was normal. The high incidence of CT changes in migraineurs in early studies probably reflected artifact and a failure to recognize the range of normality on a new imaging technique.

MRI Evaluation in Migraine

MRI, which was introduced in 1984, provided new insights into the physical state of the brain. MRI is normal in most migraine patients. The most common abnormal finding (found in 6 to 40 percent of migraineurs) is punctate foci of white matter hyperintensity on T2-weighted images[21] (Fig. 4-1). The MRI literature is difficult to interpret, as disparate imaging parameters have been used in individual studies. Igarashi and colleagues[22]

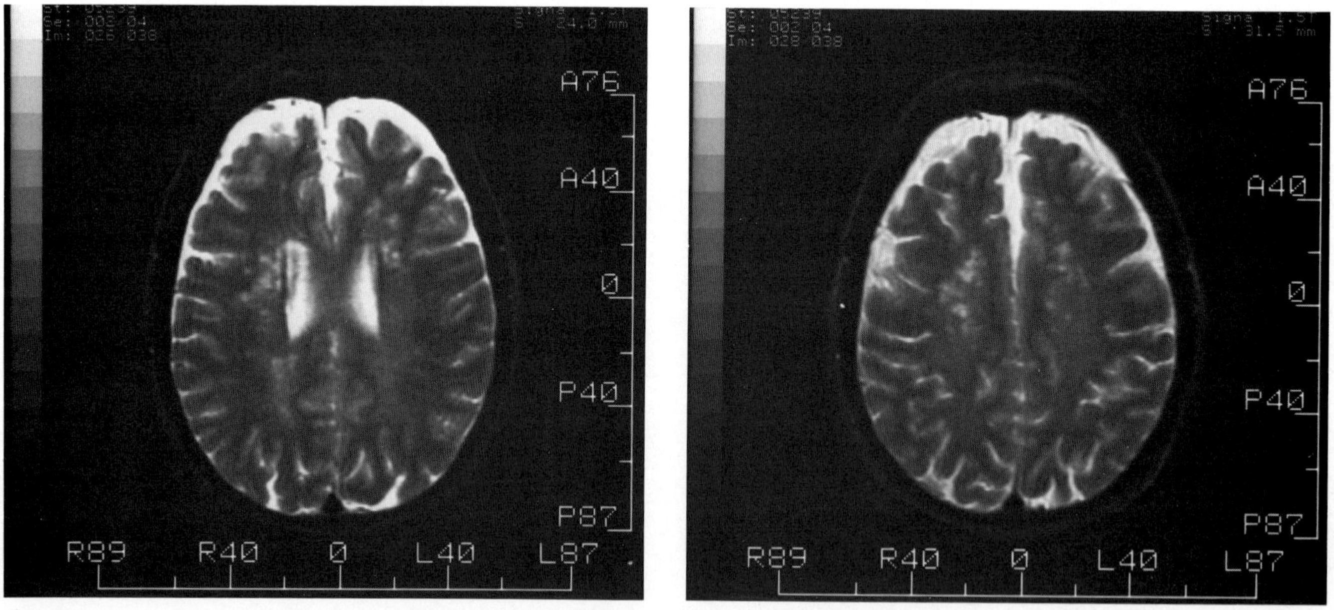

A B

Figure 4-1
A 35-year-old female with a history of migraine with aura since childhood. **(A)** *and* **(B)** *T2 WIs demonstrating areas of white matter hyperintensities.*

used MRI to study 91 patients with migraine and 98 age-matched controls, looking for the frequency of white matter lesions while controlling for risk factors that could lead to similar white matter changes (multiple sclerosis, diabetes mellitus, hypertension, hyperlipidemia, and polycythemia). All their MRI examinations were done interictally using T-1, T-2, and proton-density weighted imaging. Among the 91 IHS-classified migraine patients, 53 had migraine with aura, 33 had migraine without aura, and 5 had migraine with prolonged aura. Focal areas of high signal intensity on both T-2 and proton-density weighted images were identified in 39.6 percent of these patients. No significant differences were identified among the migraine subtypes. Among migraineurs under 40 years of age without risk factors for white matter changes, 29.4 percent showed focal white matter lesions, compared with 11.2 percent of age-matched controls. MRI abnormalities did not correlate with migraine frequency, duration, or intensity or past ergotamine use. White matter lesions increased with advancing age. In patients under age 40 years, high signal T2 lesions usually were located in the centrum semiovale and frontal white matter. In older migraineurs, lesions extended into the deep white matter at the level of the basal ganglia. The distribution of white matter lesions was not related to migraine subtype or side of head pain or aura. These results suggested that migraine alone may be associated with focal white matter lesions in an age-dependent manner.

Pavese and coworkers[21] imaged 129 migraine patients and excluded individuals older than age 45 years and those with cardiovascular risk factors (83 had migraine without aura, and 46 had migraine with aura); 19.3 percent of these patients had focal areas of hyperintensity on T2-weighted scans localized to the deep and subcortical white matter, largely the centrum semiovale. No periventricular lesions were noted. Changes on MRI imaging did not correlate with age, gender, migraine subtype, headache frequency or duration, and previous migraine therapy. Only 2 percent of age- and gender-matched controls had white matter changes.

Cooney and associates[23] found T2 white matter lesions (no location specified) in 16 percent of 185 patients with migraine. The changes on MRI correlated with increasing age and cardiovascular risk factors but not with migraine subtype or gender or the duration of migraine symptoms.

Most migraineurs never develop changes on MRI. White matter lesions in migraineurs are preferentially located to the centrum semiovale and frontal subcortical white matter in individuals less than 40 years of age and involve the deep white matter at the level of the basal ganglia in migraineurs over age 40. The lesions correlate with increasing age but not with migraine subtype or headache frequency or duration. The T2 lesions may not be specific or directly related to migraine. The same incidence of white matter lesions occurs in tension-type and migraine patients.[24]

The pathology of the white matter changes in migraine patients is not known. Lesions that are known to cause high signal on T2-weighted images include demyelination, infarction, and gliosis. A study looking at the histologic changes associated with white matter signal changes on MRI in 11 elderly patients identified periventricular lesions as areas of demyelination and deep white matter lesions as areas of ischemia.[25]

Lesions in older migraineurs involving deep white matter structures could be ischemic. Possible pathogenic mechanisms for the white matter changes in migraineurs include (1) hypoperfusion during the aura phase leading to ischemia, (2) multiple microemboli caused by increased platelet aggregation (present in migraine patients) leading to patchy white matter lesions,[22] (3) 5HT (serotonin) released from platelets during a migraine attack causing vasoconstriction of perforating cerebral arteries leading to ischemia,[26] and (4) abnormal cerebrovascular autoregulation, identified in migraineurs by transcranial Doppler,[27] leading to reduced cerebral perfusion and thus ischemia.

A subgroup of migraineurs may have a genetic predisposition for white matter lesions on MRI scans. Cerebral autosomal dominant arteriopathy with subcortical infarcts and leukoencephalopathy (CADASIL) is a familial genetic disease with migraine as a common symptom and severe white matter abnormalities on MRI as common stigmata[28] (see below). Chabriat and coworkers[29] described several members of a family with an autosomal dominant illness manifested by migraine attacks and a significant leukoencephalopathy on MRI but without other specific manifestations of CADASIL. There maybe a specific gene locus for migraine with white matter changes. Variable gene penetrance could result in CADASIL at one extreme and individuals with tiny T2 hyperintense white matter foci and migraine alone at the other extreme.

Magnetic Resonance Spectroscopy in Migraine

Most studies of magnetic resonance spectroscopy (MRS) in migraine have utilized phosphorous spectroscopy with ^{31}P, since this compound directly relates to energy metabolism. Adenosine triphosphate (ATP) and phosphocreatinine (Pcr) can be measured and intracellular magnesium concentrations can be calculated indirectly by utilizing the chemical shifts between phosphorylated compounds (Fig. 4-2). Welch and colleagues[30] used MRS to calculate intracellular brain pH in migraineurs. No significant difference was found in pH levels between normal controls and migraineurs (both with and without aura and between and during attacks), suggesting that tissue ischemia (and acidosis) does not occur during migraine attacks. This is consistent with

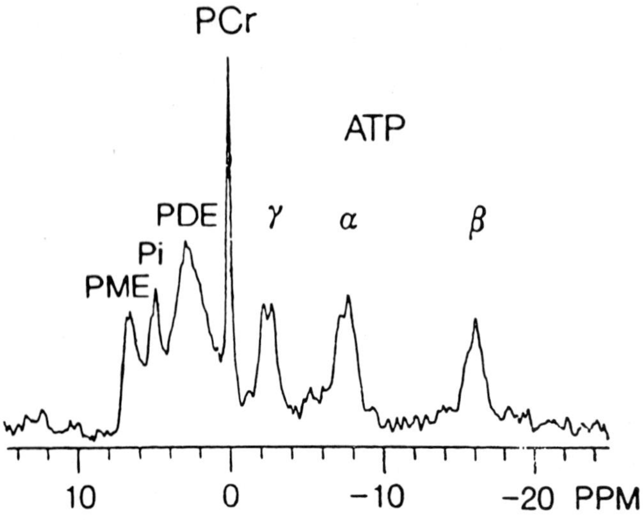

Figure 4-2
^{31}P Magnetic resonance spectrum from the occipital lobe of the brain. Phosphocreatinine (Pcr), phosphodiesters (PDE), phosphomonoesters (PME), and inorganic phosphate (Pi). (Reprinted from Montagna P: Magnetic resonance spectroscopy in migraine, Cephalalgia *15:323–327, 1995, by permission of the Scandinavian University Press.)*

SPECT evaluations.[13] Welch and associates,[31] using ^{31}P-MRS, found that phosphate metabolism is altered during a migraine attack with a loss of high-energy phosphates. Since ischemia was excluded in their previous study, this finding was most likely secondary to energy failure.

In 1989, Ramadan and coworkers,[32] using ^{31}P-MRS, found that during an attack migraineurs have lower calculated brain magnesium levels than do controls. Clinically, intravenous magnesium can abort migraine and cluster attacks.[33,34] This suggests that hypomagnesemia may be relevant in the pathogenesis of migraine and perhaps cluster headache.

Brain energy metabolism measured by ^{31}P-MRS has been shown to be abnormal in all migraine subtypes (with aura, without aura, and with prolonged aura) during and between migraine attacks.[35] The neurons and glia of migraineurs may have low energy reserves and thus less ability to tolerate the demands of increased energy expenditure than do those of normal individuals. When a migraineur is stressed (e.g., fasting, infection) and is unable to meet elevated energy demands, a metabolic crisis may ensue leading to a migraine attack.

Patients with mitochondrial cytopathies (migraine can be part of their clinical presentations) have metabolic deficiencies on MRS that are similar to those of migraineurs. In addition, MRS of muscle in migraineurs has demonstrated delayed phosphocreatinine recovery after exercise, which is a direct measure of mitochondrial function.[35] These findings suggest that in a subset of individuals, migraine is the result of mitochondrial dysfunction. Riboflavin, a mitochondrial respiratory chain cofactor, has been shown to be effective in migraine prophylaxis.[36]

Functional MRI in Migraine

Functional MRI (fMRI) can measure regional cerebral blood flow (rCBF), regional cerebral blood volume (rCBV), and tissue mean transit time. It can evaluate physiologic processes such as the mobility of water (diffusion), vascular hemodynamics (perfusion), brain activation (neuronal activity), and permeability of the blood-brain barrier. Echo planar imaging can acquire images in less than 100 ms, allowing the entire brain to be imaged within a few seconds.[37] Using fMRI, one could theoretically detect the ischemia that may occur with aura (trying to disprove previous SPECT investigations[13]), look for increasing rCBF that may indicate vasodilation during head pain, and possibly detect the presence (if it exists) of cortical spreading depression in humans, all in real time. Functional MRI also may be used to verify the presence of a possible migraine generator that has been demonstrated by PET investigations (see below).

Cutrer and coworkers[38] utilized perfusion- and diffusion-weighted fMRI in four patients with a spontaneous migraine aura. A reduction in rCBF and rCBV and an increase in mean tissue transit time occurred in the occipital gray matter contralateral to the visual hemifield experiencing the aura. This study confirmed hemodynamic changes identified in previous SPECT evaluations and suggested that the changes on SPECT are real and not a result of Compton scatter. Photons emitted by body tissues can be scattered by the electrons surrounding the atoms of the tissue (Compton scattering), and this can result in a degradation of SPECT images. It had been suggested that the spreading oligemia identified on SPECT was an artifact of Compton scatter.

Cao and associates,[39] using fMRI:BOLD (blood oxygen level–dependent T2 changes) in patients with visually induced migraine, showed an initial activation followed by a suppression of the BOLD effect, which moved across the cortex at a rate of 3 to 6 mm/min. This appeared to simulate the initial hyperperfusion and secondary hypoperfusion that occur with cortical spreading depression in animals. The BOLD propagation effect was noted in patients with and without aura, suggesting that spreading depression may induce migraine without aura. This investigation required artificial induction of headache, and so spontaneous spreading depression has not yet been visualized in humans.

Positron Emission Tomography in Migraine

PET can image the entire brain with 4- to 5-mm spatial resolution within a few seconds. This technique involves the detection of positron labeled tracers with image reconstruction utilizing CT.[40] It allows the measurement of the pathophysiologic changes that occur during a headache in almost real time.

In 1994 Woods and colleagues[12] reported the first PET scan of a patient with a spontaneous attack of migraine without aura. The subject, a participant in a visual activation study, was being scanned with 12 successive measurements of rCBF. After the sixth scan was completed, the patient developed an acute migraine episode. A bilateral decrease in rCBF spread across the cortex at a constant rate and spared the cerebellum, basal ganglia, and thalamus. Both middle cerebral artery (MCA) and posterior cerebral artery (PCA) territories were involved [Fig. 4-3 (Plate 13)]. The rCBF changes were transient, with substantial recovery at the time of the subsequent scan 12 to 15 min later. The maximum decrease in rCBF was 40 percent. The most intriguing finding from this study is that the rCBF changes occurred in a patient without aura, suggesting that spreading hypoperfusion exists in migraine both with and without aura.

PET studies also have suggested the possibility of a migraine generator in the brainstem. Weiller and associates[14] investigated nine patients with migraine without aura during spontaneous attacks. Three measurements of rCBF were undertaken: during the acute attack, after headache relief with subcutaneous sumatriptan injection, and during a headache-free interval 3 days to 4 months after the initial study. During the acute attack, elevated rCBF values were noted in medial brainstem structures contralateral to the side of the head pain. Increased rCBF levels also occurred in both visual and auditory association areas as well as in the inferior anterocaudal cingulate cortex [Fig. 4-4 (Plate 14)]. After alleviation of the head pain, nausea, and photophobia-phonophobia with sumatriptan, the cortical rCBF values returned to baseline levels, but rCBF was still increased in the brainstem. Brainstem areas affected by the rCBF changes included the periaqueductal gray region, the midbrain reticular formation, and the locus coeruleus. Brainstem activa-

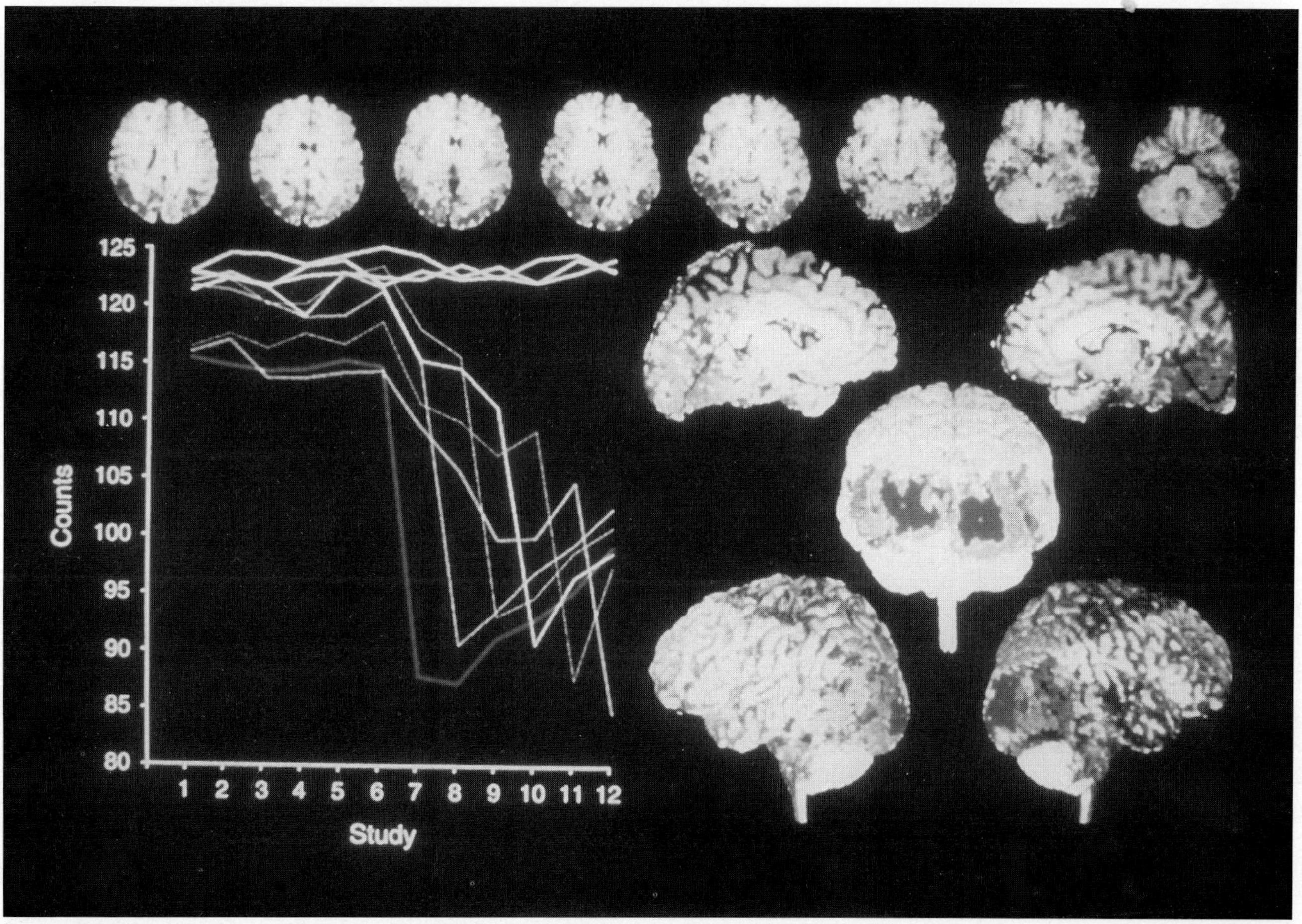

Figure 4-3 (Plate 13)
A 21-year-old woman who developed a spontaneous attack of migraine without aura while in a PET scanner. Figure demonstrates bilateral decreases in regional cerebral blood flow starting in the occipital region and spreading anteriorly with time. Areas in red were the first to show a reduction in regional blood flow. [Reprinted from Woods RP, Iacoboni M, Mazziotta JC: Brief report: Bilateral spreading cerebral hypoperfusion during spontaneous migraine headache, N Engl J Med *331(25):1689–1692, 1994, by permission of the Massachusetts Medical Society (Copyright 1994, Massachusetts Medical Society. All rights reserved.)]*

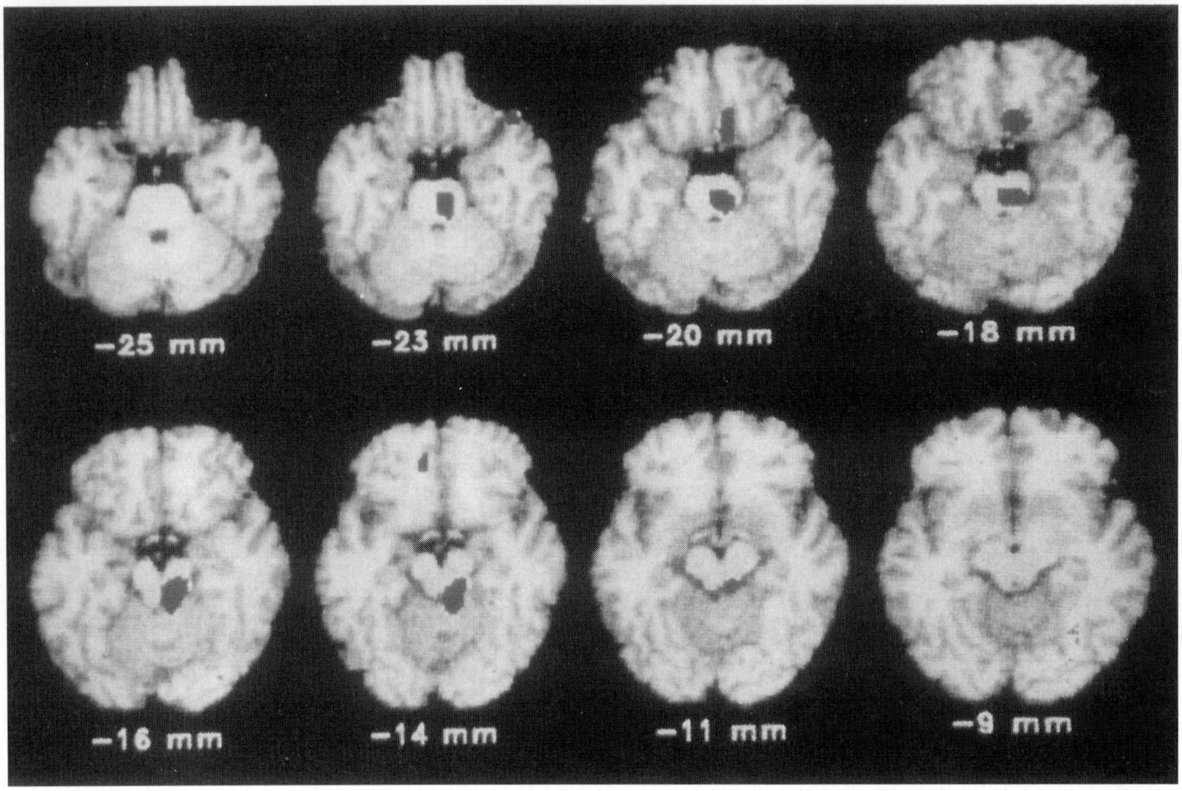

Figure 4-4 (Plate 14)
A PET scan study of nine patients with right-sided migraine without aura who were scanned within 6 h after the onset of headache. The activations during the attack are shown as statistical parametric maps that show the areas of significant increases in regional cerebral blood flow in red superimposed on an anatomic reference image derived from a T1-weighted MRI. The left side of each image is the right side of the brain. Significant increases in regional cerebral blood flow were noted in the brainstem slightly lateralized to the left in the periaqueductal gray matter and midbrain reticular formation, as well as the inferoanterocaudal cingulate gyrus. [Reprinted from Weiller C, May A, Limmroth V, et al: Brainstem activation in spontaneous human migraine attacks, Nature Med *1(7):658–660, 1995, by permission of* Nature Medicine.*]*

tion was absent at the 3-day to 4-month studies. The sustained increase in rCBF in the brainstem suggests the presence of a migraine generator. The persistent brainstem activation after sumatriptan symptomatic therapy may explain the high rate of headache recurrence in patients taking this 5HT1D/B agonist.

Role of Cerebral Angiography in Migraine

Reported cases of angiographic abnormalities in migraine patients are rare and include arterial narrowing, which may reflect vasospasm or arterial stenosis, and segmental stenosis and dilation, which may signify an underlying inflammation (Fig. 4-5).

Garnic and Schellinger[41] reported the angiographic findings in a patient with a history of migraine headache. The patient's four-vessel cerebral angiogram was originally normal, but during repeat catheterization of the right internal carotid artery the patient developed a typical migraine headache. Spasm of the anterior cerebral artery (ACA) and MCA and spasm around the catheter tip were found. These authors suggested that vasospasm may play a role in headache induction.

Schulman and Hershey[42] described a patient with status migrainosus and an angiographic picture of arterial segmental narrowing and dilation that suggested vessel inflammation. The patient had no evidence of systemic vasculitis and improved on steroids (Fig. 4-6).

Most migraineurs do not undergo cerebral angiography, and so the true state of cerebral blood vessels during and between migraine attacks is not known. If vasospasm occurs, it may reflect increased sympathetic outflow during a migraine attack. Vessel stenosis and dilation may reflect underlying isolated cerebral angitis but more likely are a reflection of neurogenic inflammation.[42]

Cerebral angiography is not part of the routine workup for headache. It should be requested only when an aneurysm, an arteriovenous malformation (AVM), or vasculitis is strongly suspected. In the setting of a stereotypic headache syndrome in a patient with a normal neurologic examination and normal CT or MRI, angiography adds very little useful diagnostic information and should not be undertaken. In past case reports migraineurs were falsely felt to have a higher complication rate with angiography than were nonmigraineurs. Shuaib and Hachinski[43] reviewed a series of 149 angiograms in migraine patients and did not find an increased

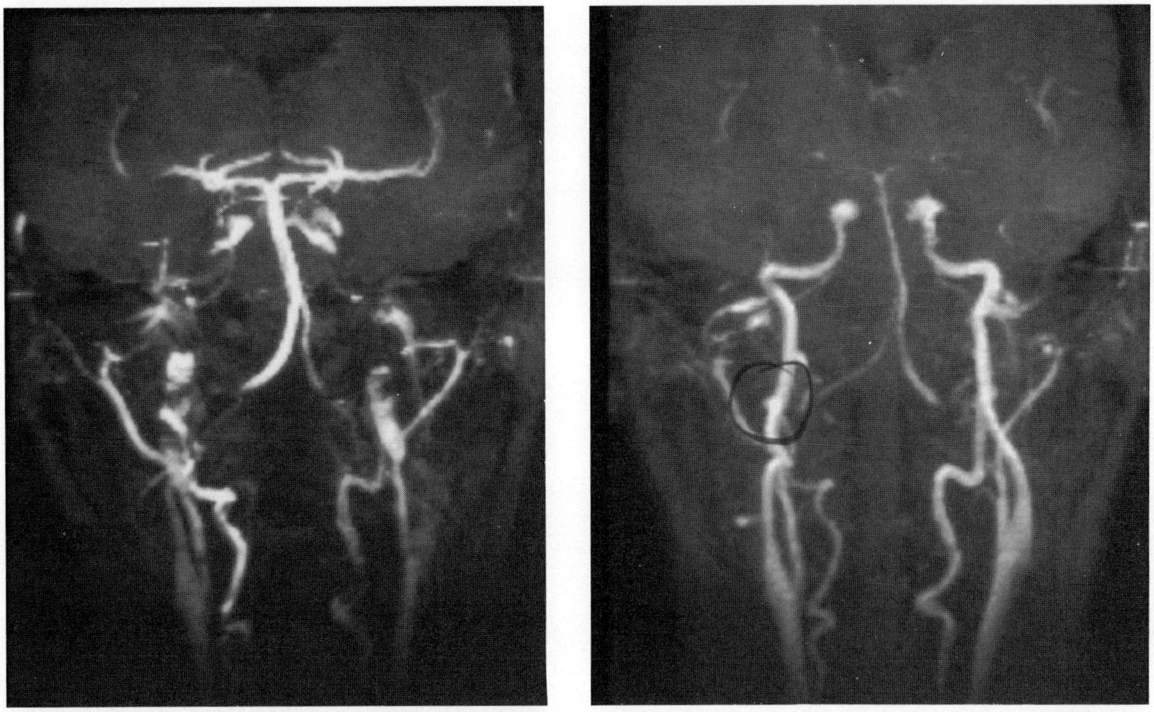

A C

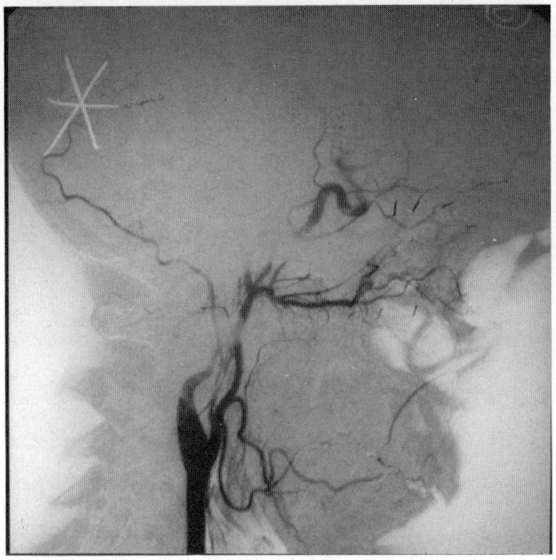

B

Figure 4-5

A 40-year-old female with a long history of "migraine headaches," increasing use of ergot medications, and the development of carotid bruits. **(A)** *MRA demonstrating marked decreased flow though both internal carotid arteries and the left vertebral artery.* **(B)** *Subtraction angiogram confirming high-grade stenosis of the internal carotid artery and demonstrating segmental stenosis of some intracranial vessels.* **(C)** *After withdrawal of ergots and use of calcium channel blocking medication, there is marked improvement in flow though the internal carotid arteries. A small aneurysm was seen in the right internal carotid artery. These findings were confirmed with repeat contrast angiography.*

risk of complications even during a migraine attack. Radiologists avoid performing angiograms in migraineurs because the procedure can precipitate a migraine attack. Low-osmolarity contrast is used in angiography of migraineurs in an attempt to reduce the induction of migraine headaches.

Cluster Headache

Cluster headache, which has been described since the seventeenth century, is a distinct headache syndrome with stereotypic signs and symptoms.[44] Features of cluster attacks include severe, strictly unilateral pain in an orbital or periorbital location that is of short duration (mean 45 minutes) and has a mean attack frequency of one to three episodes per day. Associated symptoms include ipsilateral nasal congestion or rhinorrhea, lacrimation, conjunctival injection, ptosis, and miosis (Horner syndrome). Cluster sufferers, unlike migraineurs, do not lie down during an attack but instead usually pace the floor. Cluster attacks often occur during times of relaxation or during rapid eye movement (REM) sleep. Attacks can be induced by alcohol or nitroglycerin during an active cluster period.

The pathogenesis of cluster headaches is unknown, but its periodicity and strong autonomic components suggest hypothalamic dysfunction. Moskowitz[45] inferred that the symptoms of cluster attacks represent sympa-

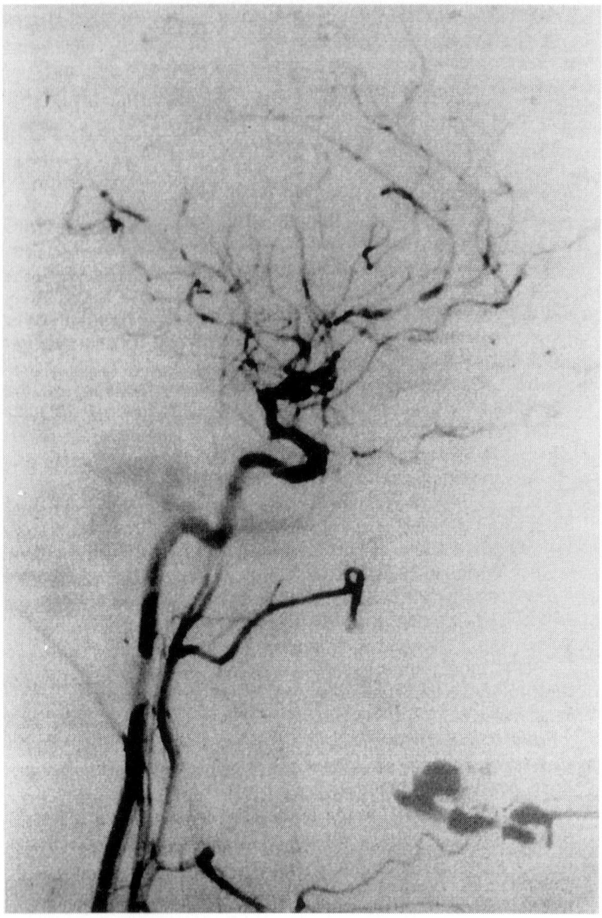

Figure 4-6
Cerebral angiogram from a 26-year-old woman in status migrainosus. Note the multiple areas of focal arterial stenosis and dilation. (Reprinted from Schulman EA, Hershey B: "An unusual angiographic picture in status migrainosus," Headache *31:396–398, 1991, by permission of* Headache.*)*

thetic failure (Horner syndrome), sympathetic activation (facial and forehead perspiration), and parasympathetic activation (rhinorrhea, lacrimation) that can be best localized to the superior pericarotid cavernous sinus plexus, where fibers from the ophthalmic and maxillary division of the trigeminal nerve, the sympathetic superior cervical ganglion, and the parasympathetic sphenopalatine ganglion come together.

Neuroimaging of cluster attacks has been very successful in identifying structural lesions that mimic cluster but until very recently has provided little information on the pathogenesis of cluster headaches. Russel and colleagues[46] studied 28 patients during a symptomatic cluster period and found no significant CT abnormalities. Sjaastad and Rinck[47] found no MRI abnormalities in 14 cluster patients during imaging the cavernous sinus and the base of the brain.

Ekbom and Greitz[48] reported angiographic abnormalities in 4 of 18 cluster patients, which included arterial narrowing (especially in the extradural part of the internal carotid artery) and dilation of the ipsilateral ophthalmic artery. Waldenlind and coworkers[49] studied two spontaneous cluster attacks in a 24-year-old male with magnetic resonance angiography (MRA). The ophthalmic artery ipsilateral to the cluster pain was significantly dilated during the event and normalized by 2 weeks after the attack (Fig. 4-7A and B). No changes were identified in the internal carotid artery or any other portion of the intracranial circulation.

Gallium SPECT scanning has been used in an attempt

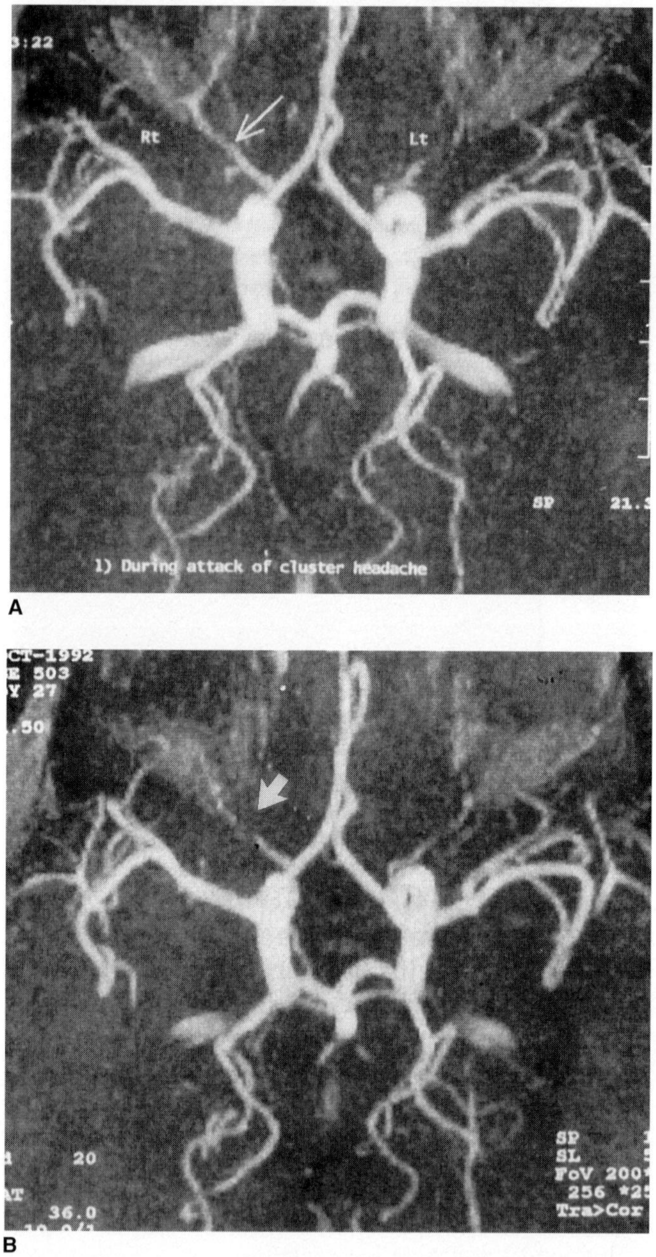

Figure 4-7
(A) *MRA of the circle of Willis during a spontaneous cluster attack. Note the dilation of the ophthalmic artery (arrow), which was ipsilateral to the symptomatic cluster side in this patient.* **(B)** *Same patient 2 weeks after clinical remission of episodic cluster headaches. Ophthalmic artery has resumed its normal caliber (arrow). (Reprinted from Waldenlind E, Ekbom K, Torhall J: MR-angiography during spontaneous attacks of cluster headache: A case report,* Headache *33:281–295, 1993, by permission of* Headache.*)*

to identify cavernous sinus pathology in cluster headaches. It has been speculated that cluster headache results from inflammation in the region of the cavernous sinus with involvement of local draining veins. Gawel and associates[50] found increased SPECT activity in the cavernous sinus of three of six cluster patients during an active cluster period, suggesting the presence of inflammation. Sianard-Gianko and colleagues[51] tried to verify this finding by using SPECT in 30 cluster patients and 7 migraineurs used as a control group. Unexpectedly, parasellar hyperactivity was noted in cluster patients both during attacks and in remission and was noted in most of the migraine patients. These authors concluded that increased parasellar activity on gallium SPECT is not specific for cluster and that this technique lacks reliability in identifying an inflammatory process in the region of the cavernous sinus.

Phosphorus MRS has identified altered brain energy metabolism in migraine patients, perhaps secondary to mitochondrial dysfunction.[35] Montagna and coworkers[52] performed ^{31}P MRS on 14 cluster patients and identified a defect in brain energy metabolism (a decrease in high-energy phosphates) during and after a cluster period. The changes mimicked what had been found previously in migraine patients, suggesting a similar biochemical-metabolic abnormality in both headache disorders and possible mitochondrial dysfunction in both migraine and cluster headache patients.

Hypothalamic involvement in cluster headache was initially suggested when lower levels of plasma testosterone were identified in male cluster headache patients during attacks compared with cluster free-periods.[53] Now a possible hypothalamic generator has been identified, using PET scanning techniques. May and associates[15] noted an isolated increase in hypothalamic rCBF ipsilateral to the side of cluster pain in nine study patients [Fig. 4-8 (Plate 15)].

Secondary causes of headache that can mimic cluster have been identified through the use of neuroimaging techniques (Fig. 4-9). Cavernous sinus lesions (aneurysm, vasculitis, meningioma), an invasive pituitary adenoma, a prolactinoma, an upper cervical meningioma, and lung metastases to the brain have all been reported to simulate cluster-like headaches.[54]

Neuroimaging of Uncommon Primary Headache Syndromes

Cadasil

Cerebral autosomal dominant arteriopathy with subcortical infarcts and leukoencephalopathy is a rare inherited neurodegenerative disorder that recently was mapped to chromosome 19q12.[28] It formally was called hereditary multi-infarct dementia.[28] The genetic defect involves the notch 3 gene, which codes for transmembrane receptor proteins.[55] The syndrome usually presents with migraine with aura in the third decade, stroke-like spells in the fourth decade, and subcortical dementia in the fifth decade. Affective disorders are an extremely common part of the syndrome. Death normally occurs by the sixth decade.[56] Neuroimaging has played a pivotal role in the study of CADASIL. MRI

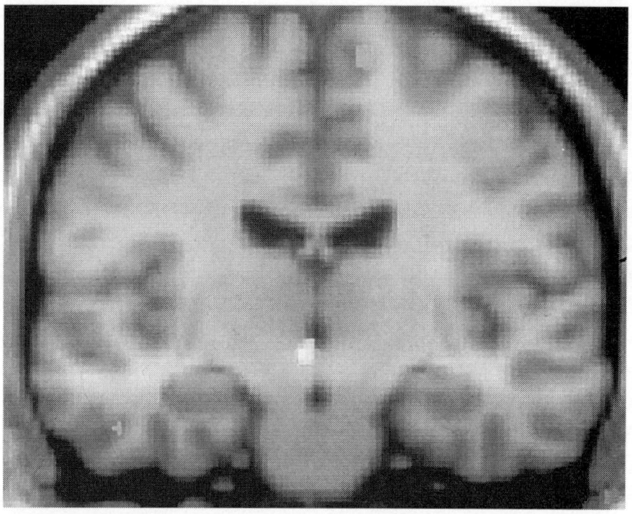

Figure 4-8 (Plate 15)
PET scan from a patient with a nitroglycerin-induced cluster headache. The activations during the attack are shown as statistical parametric maps that show the areas of significant increases; regional cerebral blood flow in color superimposed on an anatomic reference image derived from a T1-weighted MRI. The left side of the picture shows the left side of the brain. The area of greatest activation was ipsilateral to the painful cluster side and was localized to the hypothalamic gray matter. (Courtesy of P. J. Goadsby, M.D., The National Hospital for Neurology and Neurosurgery, London.)

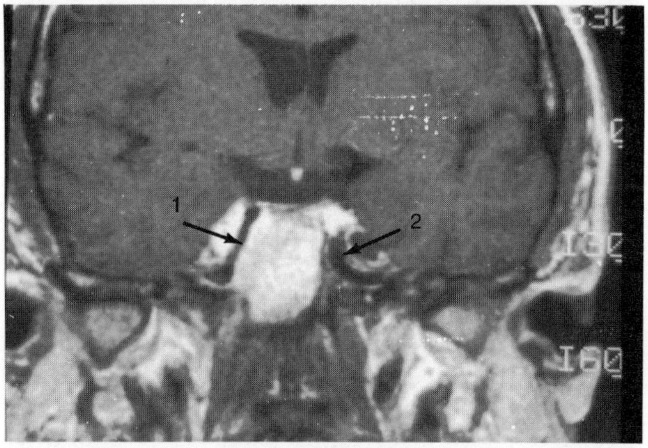

Figure 4-9
A 45-year-old white male with right periorbital headaches suggestive of cluster headaches. Coronal MRI scan after gadolinium demonstrating an enhancing soft tissue tumor in the region of the clivus eroding into the right inferior aspect of the sphenoid sinus and right cavernous sinus encasing the precavernous segment of the right internal carotid artery. The tumor extends superiorly to the sella turcica. Arrows: 1. Right internal carotid artery encased by tumor. 2. Left internal carotid artery. This tumor was found to be a thorotrast-induced tumor at the brain base.

findings are very suggestive of the diagnosis in the appropriate clinical setting.

Chabriat and associates[56] studied seven families with CADASIL and found that 50 percent of these subjects 30 to 40 years of age had an abnormal CT or MRI while only 25 percent had symptoms of the disease. In individuals who were asymptomatic, neuroimaging was diagnostic and not just an adjunctive procedure. Two main MRI abnormalities are observed in CADASIL: (1) extensive symmetrical white matter abnormalities involving both periventricular and lobar white matter with a preponderance in the anterior temporal regions, preference of the external capsule over the internal capsule, and an absence of cortical lesions and a sparing of the subcortical U fibers and (2) small, well-delineated deep lesions with decreased signal on T1-weighted images and increased signal on T2-weighted images, consistent with lacunar infarctions involving the basal ganglia and thalamus[28] (Fig. 4-10). Disorders that can potentially be confused with CADASIL on MRI include Biswanger disease, metachromatic leukodystrophy, subacute sclerosing panencephalitis, multiple sclerosis, and progressive multifocal leukoencephalopathy. Each disorder lacks the dominating history of migraine headache.

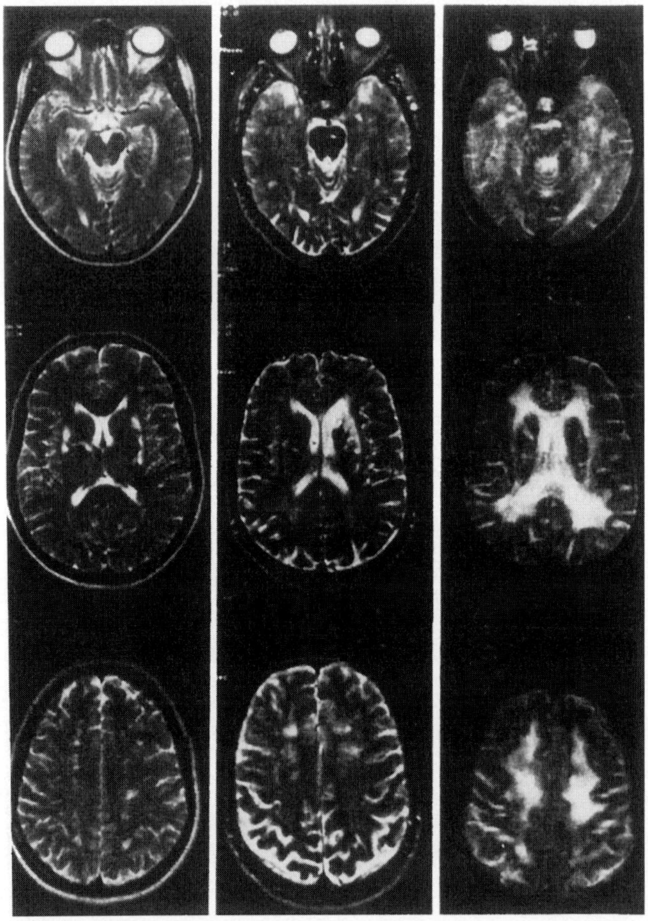

Figure 4-10
MRI images of three patients with CADASIL showing T2-weighted signal abnormalities in the white matter and basal ganglia of varying severity. (Reprinted from Chabriat H, Vahedi K, Joutel A, et al: Cerebral autosomal dominant arteriopathy with subcortical infarcts and leukoencephalopathy (CADASIL), The Neurologist *3:137–145, 1997, by permission of Williams & Wilkins.)*

Melas

Mitochondrial encephalomyopathy, with lactic acidosis, and stroke-like spells (MELAS) is a mitochondrial inherited disease in which 50 to 80 percent of sufferers have migraine.[57] In most individuals the onset of stroke, seizures, and lactic acidosis occurs before age 40. Headache (usually migraine), seizures, and gastrointestinal symptoms (nausea and vomiting) are the most common presenting symptoms. Initially most MELAS patients are neurologically intact, but they later develop focal neurologic abnormalities, usually a visual field deficit or hemiparesis. When the disease begins before age 20, about 30 percent of the patients die before age 30.[57]

Hirano and Pavlakis[57] reviewed 110 documented cases of MELAS. Infarcts occurred in 80 percent of imaged patients on CT examinations. All had hemispheric lesions, usually cortical in location. Only 5 of 56 patients had basal ganglia lesions. Almost half had cortical atrophy.

Common MRI findings in MELAS include ischemic signal changes involving the temporoparietal and occipital lobes (Fig. 4-11). In some individuals the MRI lesions disappear over time.[58] Matthews and associates[59] reported multifocal lesions of increased T2 signal localized to the cortex of the cerebrum, cerebellum, and adjacent subcortical white matter that may be a unique neuroimaging picture of MELAS.

SPECT studies in MELAS all showed decreased tracer accumulation [HMPAO, *N*-isopropyl-p-(^{123}I) iodoamphetamine] in areas of infarction.[60–65] Two patients had increased tracer levels 3 to 16 days before the appearance of infarcts on CT, suggesting that stroke results from metabolic dysfunction rather than from ischemia.

MRS has been done on only a small number of patients with MELAS. Mathews and associates[66] identified areas of increased lactate coinciding with T2 lesions on MRI during an attack with neurologic symptoms. Lactate elevation also was identified by MRS in a portion of brain with no T1 or T2 abnormalities on conventional imaging.[67]

Cerebral angiography was normal in 65 percent of studied patients with MELAS.[57] In two individuals, major arteries were affected: One showed occlusion of an extracranial internal carotid artery,[68] while the other demonstrated occlusion of a supraclinoid internal carotid artery similar to what is seen in moyamoya disease.[69]

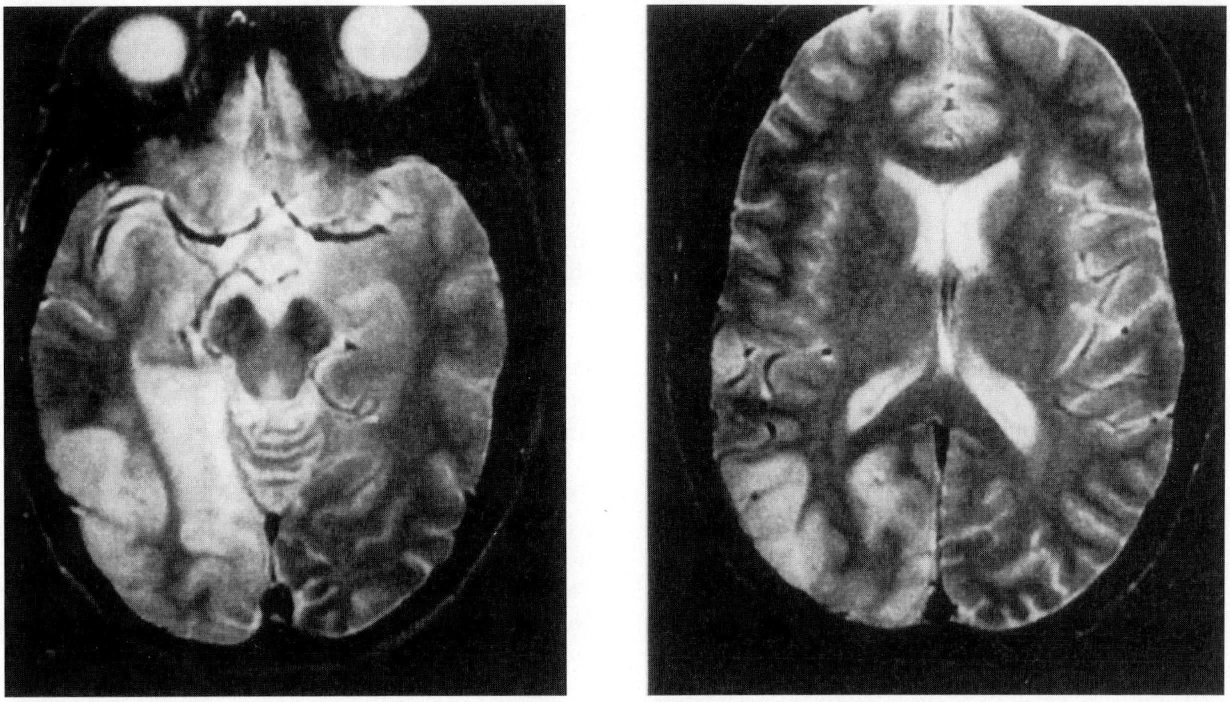

Figure 4-11
A 44-year-old woman with MELAS who presented with headache, nausea, and vomiting with a dense left homonymous hemianopia on examination. T2-weighted MRI showing signal hyperintensity in the right temporal and right occipital lobes confined to the cortical regions. These lesion resolved after 21 days on repeat scanning. (Reprinted from Clark JM, Marks MP, Adalsteinsson E, et al: MELAS: Clinical and pathologic correlations with MRI, xenon/CT, and MR spectroscopy, Neurology 46:223–227, 1996, by permission of Neurology.)

Exertional and Cough Headache

Cough headache is defined as head pain induced by coughing. It also may occur with sneezing, lifting, and straining. Exertional headache is a headache that is brought on specifically by physical exertion. Population-based studies suggest that there is a 1 percent prevalence of each of these two headache disorders.[70]

Benign cough headache is a rare disorder that has a male predominance and normally affects individuals over 40 years of age.[71] The pain begins immediately after coughing or other Valsalva maneuvers and is severe in intensity with an explosive quality.[72] The headache is usually bilateral and is not normally associated with concomitant nausea or vomiting. The presence of vomiting suggests an underlying organic pathology. Symptomatic (secondary) cough headache normally occurs in a younger population than does benign cough headache. Causes of secondary cough headache include posterior fossa meningiomas, craniospinal abnormalities (Chiari malformations, basilar impression, platybasia), brain tumors, and acoustic neuromas.[73–75] Unlike benign cough headaches, secondary cough headache normally does not respond to indomethacin therapy.

Benign exertional headache occurs in individuals younger than 40 years of age. It normally presents as bilateral throbbing head pain that lasts from 5 min to 24 h and is incited by physical exercise. The head pain is nonexplosive and occurs during protracted exertion or shortly after the completion of an activity. Symptomatic exertional headache is usually explosive in onset ("thunderclap"), severe, and bilateral. Underlying causes include tumors, sinusitis, and subarachnoid hemorrhage of any cause, especially a ruptured berry aneurysm.

Neuroimaging is mandatory in the evaluation of patients who present with cough headache and in selected cases of exertional headache, especially when the headache is of an explosive variety. Vomiting suggests an organic cause of the headache. MRI is the test of choice, as it provides excellent visualization of the posterior fossa and can define most intracranial mass lesions, vascular lesions, and craniospinal abnormalities.

SECONDARY HEADACHE SYNDROMES

Secondary headaches are a symptom of an underlying pathologic disorder. The causes include neoplasms, vascular malformations, toxic and/or metabolic abnormalities, infections, posttraumatic causes, and congenital malformations. Neuroimaging plays a pivotal role in diagnosing the organic conditions that produce these secondary headaches.

Brain Tumors

One of the greatest fears of patients with new-onset headache is that they have a brain tumor. Headaches are the presenting symptom in about 40 percent of brain tumor patients[76] (Fig. 4-12). Forsyth and Posner[77] reported on 111 patients with primary brain tumors or metastatic lesions. The classic "brain tumor headache" that is present on awakening, is severe in intensity, and is associated with nausea or vomiting was present in only 17 percent of their patients, six of whom had evidence of increased intracranial pressure. Most of the headaches produced by brain tumors fit the IHS criteria[5] for tension-type headache (77 percent), while 9 percent could be classified as migraine. A mixed headache syndrome that could not be classified easily by IHS criteria was noted in 14 percent of these patients. The typical brain tumor headache was a dull (usually bifrontal) ache that was worst ipsilateral to the tumor and could be aggravated by exertion. Nausea and vomiting also were common symptoms. Only 45 percent of the patients had headache as the worst symptom, and only 57 percent had neuroimaging because of their headaches. The most common site of head pain was frontal and usually was associated with supratentorial lesions or increased intracranial pressure. Unilateral headache was seen in 25 percent of these patients and was always ipsilateral to the lesion. Bilateral headache (78 percent) was associated with midline or bilateral tumors or increased intracranial pressure. The accompanying signs (vomiting, papilledema), rather than the headache itself, were more suggestive of the presence of a brain tumor.

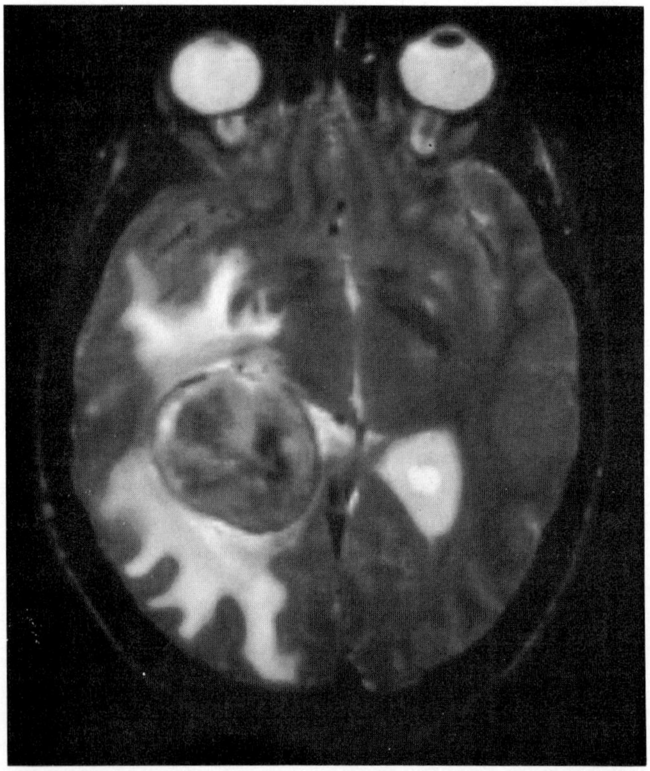

Figure 4-12
A 36-year-old patient with right hemicranial pain clinically suggestive of migraine. T2 W transverse image. This study demonstrates a large right intraventricular mass. White matter edema and a shift of midline structures to the left are visible. This mass was found to be an intraventricular meningioma.

The establishment of a brain tumor headache depended on several factors: the presence of increased intracranial pressure, the degree of midline shift (mean shift was 6.1 mm in patients with headache compared with 2.7 mm in those without head pain), tumor size (mean size, 18.3 cm^2 with headache and 9.3 cm^2 without), and a past history of headache. In this population 78 percent of the patients with a prior history of headache developed a brain tumor headache, while only 33 percent of individuals without a prior history of head pain developed tumor headache. The brain tumor headache was always more severe or more frequent than the patient's premorbid headache and was associated with changes in mental status, seizures, or motor symptoms. No specific headache subtype was more commonly associated with a brain tumor headache.[77]

Central Nervous System Infections

Headaches are an early symptom of central nervous system (CNS) infection, especially when they affect the meninges. The diagnosis is not difficult when fever, meningismus, and alterations in mental status are present, but these symptoms are not always obvious. Neuroimaging is mandatory before lumbar puncture if a brain abscess or another mass lesion is suspected on clinical examination. Contrast-enhanced CT or MRI can be used to diagnose intracranial abscesses (Fig. 4-13). Meningeal inflammation is seen almost exclusively after contrast administration.

Headaches in HIV-positive and AIDS patients are often secondary to CNS involvement by infectious agents (fungal, bacterial, tuberculosis) or lymphoma[78] (Fig. 4-14). Headache frequency in the HIV-infected population is between 11 and 55 percent, but headache is rare in recent seroconverters.[79] Lipton and coworkers[78] found that 82 percent of HIV-infected patients reporting to a metropolitan emergency room and AIDS clinic with a complaint of headache had underlying structural pathology, including neoplasms and opportunistic infections. MRI is the diagnostic test of choice in evaluating AIDS patients with headache, since it is more sensitive than CT for characterizing lymphomas, progressive multifocal leukoencephalopathy, and infectious processes.

Stroke

Headache occurs in 25 to 42 percent of patients with stroke[80] (Fig. 4-15). Headache can precede a stroke by hours to weeks in 10 to 43 percent of patients.[81] Headache characteristics are not helpful in distinguishing the underlying stroke type (embolic, thrombotic,

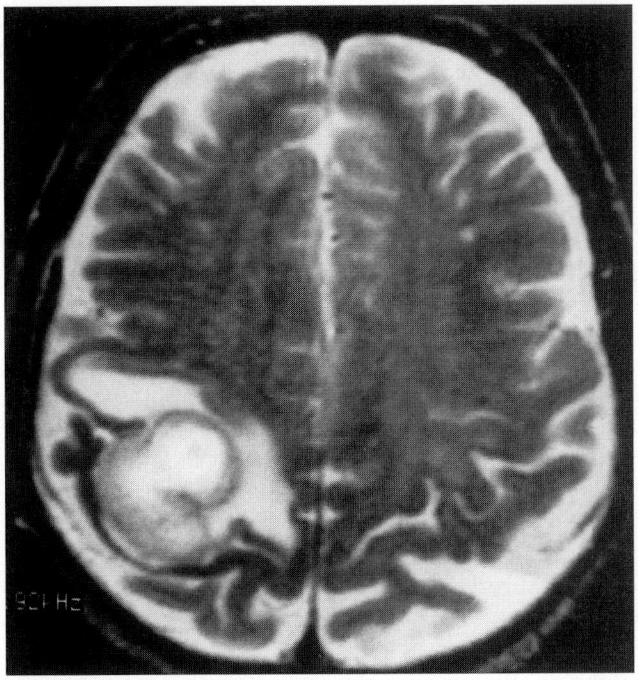

Figure 4-13
T2-weighted MRI shows large abscess with surrounding vasogenic edema.

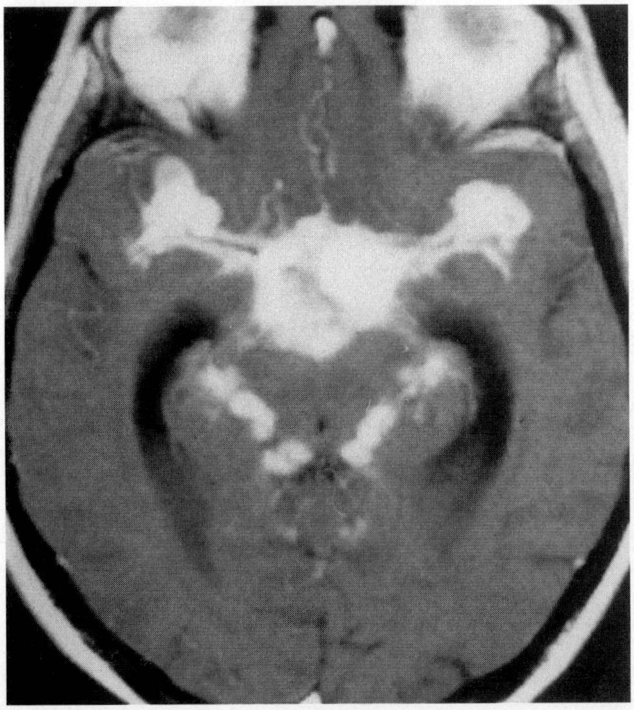

Figure 4-14
AIDS patient who presented with headache and fever and was found to have tuberculosis meningitis. Enhanced T1-weighted MRI shows intense, thick enhancement of basilar cisterns. The inflammatory process surrounds the middle cerebral arteries.

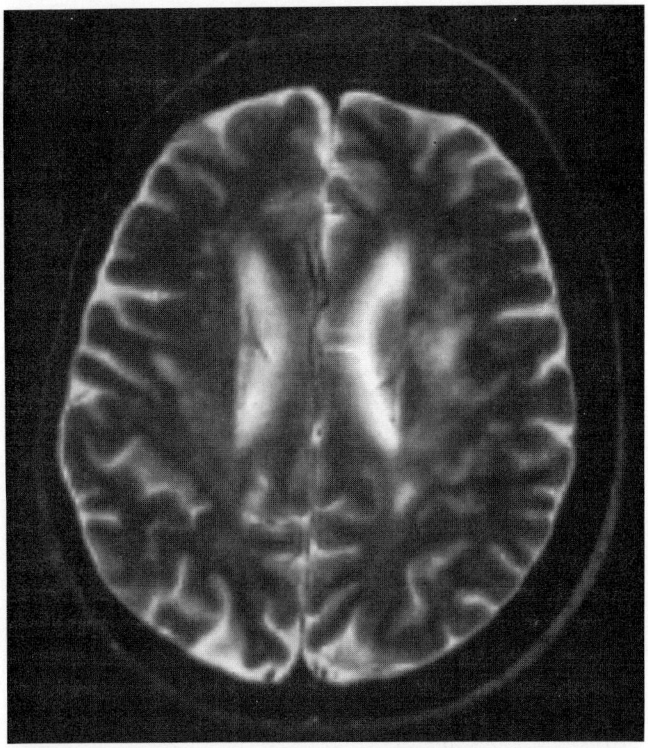

A

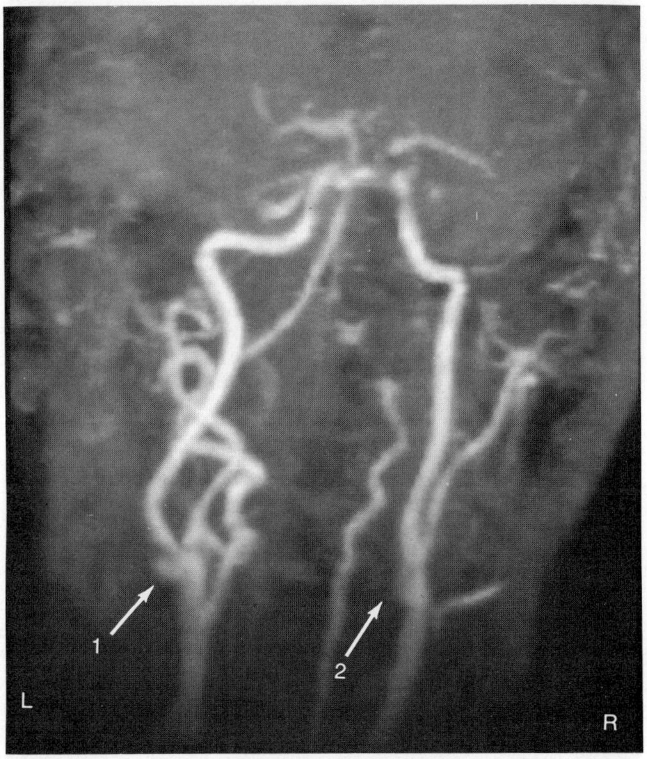

B

Figure 4-15
This 70-year-old patient developed sudden onset of left-sided headaches soon followed by right-sided weakness. T2 WI white matter hyperintensity in the left corona radiata consistent with an infarct in the left middle cerebral artery distribution. MRA: deeply ulcerated plaque in proximal left internal carotid artery causing approximately 50 percent stenosis (arrow 1) and a small plaque posterior right carotid bifurcation causing mild stenosis (arrow 2).

or hemorrhagic). Headache occurs 2 to 5 times more often with hemorrhagic infarction than with thrombic stroke.[80] Headache occurs in 3 to 23 percent of lacunar infarctions and 25 percent of transient ischemic attacks (TIAs).

Arboix and colleagues[80] evaluated headache in 240 patients with acute stroke. Headache occurred in 38 percent of their patients; 40.5 percent of those subjects had a history of headache. Only 23.5 percent of the nonheadache group after stroke had a previous headache history. Headache occurred in 58 percent of patients with hemorrhagic strokes, 41 percent of those with thrombotic strokes, 39 percent of those with cardioembolic strokes, and 26 percent of those with TIAs. Headache occurred in 56 percent of patients with cortical strokes compared with 26 percent of individuals with subcortical infarctions. Headaches were rare in patients with watershed infarctions and lacunar strokes. Headache was more common in patients with posterior circulation ischemic events, possibly because the vertebrobasilar circulation is more densely innervated than is the anterior circulation. Headache usually occurred ipsilateral to a stroke, but location was not a good indicator of the affected vessel.

Headache from stroke may be due to[80] (1) traction on pain-sensitive structures by large infarctions with possible activation of the trigeminovascular system, (2) dilation of pain-sensitive collateral vessels from arterial thrombosis, (3) release of neurochemicals from platelets that could produce pain sensitization and neurogenic inflammation, and (4) activation of spreading depression and then headache.

Intracranial Hematomas

Melo and associates[82] reported on 289 patients with intracerebral hemorrhage (ICH). Headache was present at the onset of ICH in 57 percent of these patients and was most common in those with cerebellar and lobar hematomas. Meningeal irritation secondary to subarachnoid blood was the best predictor for headache. The amount of blood needed to produce clinical signs of meningeal irritation can be lower than that needed for CT visualization. Midline shift and the volume of the hematoma were not strongly associated with the presence of headache.

Berry Aneurysms

Berry aneurysms can cause headaches both before and after rupture. Intracranial aneurysms are identified in 2 to 5 percent of autopsy cases, and the annual risk of aneurysmal rupture is approximately 2 percent[83] (Fig. 4-16). Aneurysms of the petrous internal carotid artery, which are usually posttraumatic, can produce localized or generalized headache with associated bruits, tinnitus, a seventh nerve palsy, and a pulsatile mass in the nasopharynx. Cavernous sinus aneurysms can produce pain in the ophthalmic and maxillary division of the trigeminal nerve and often are associated with palsies of cranial nerves III, IV, and VI. Ophthalmic artery aneurysms can present with retro-orbital pain associated with visual deficits in the affected eye. Third nerve palsies are associated with aneurysms of the posterior communicating artery, anterior choroidal artery, basilar tip, superior cerebellar artery, and proximal posterior cerebral artery. Unruptured MCA and ACA aneurysms typically are not associated with headache or other localizing signs. Vertebrobasilar aneurysms can be associated with headache, but the clinical symptoms rarely allow a diagnosis before rupture.[84] Headache related to unruptured aneurysms is usually size-related and thus probably is secondary to mass effect. Aneurysms known to present with headache (e.g., ophthalmic and cavernous sinus)

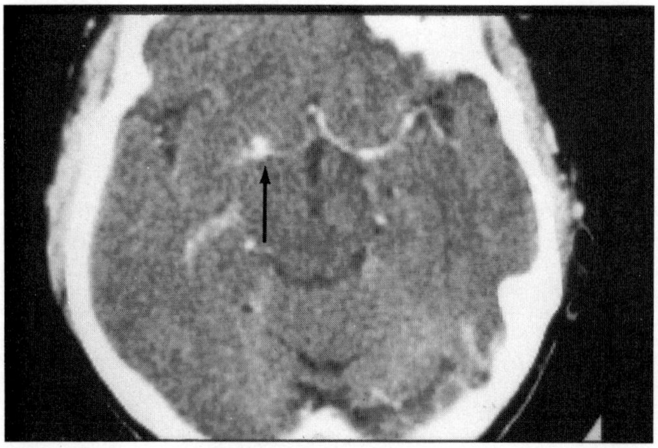

A

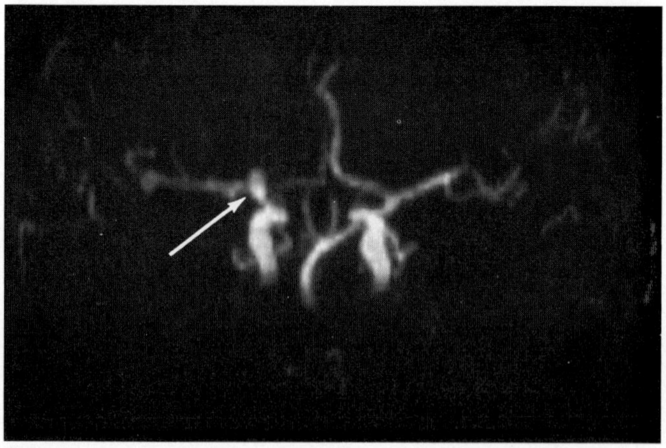

B

Figure 4-16

A 45-year-old female with right-sided headaches. **(A)** *CT scan after contrast demonstrating possible aneurysm in the right internal carotid artery (arrow).* **(B)** *4-mm berry aneurysm at the right internal carotid artery at the origin of the A1 and M1 segments.*

have a tendency not to rupture and to become quite large.

It is common for patients with ruptured aneurysms to report a past history of headache. About 30 percent of these patients complain of an isolated headache weeks to months before a subarachnoid hemorrhage (SAH). This sentinel headache may be secondary to a minor hemorrhage, aneurysmal enlargement, thrombosis of an aneurysm, or embolic strokes with the aneurysm as the clot source. Leblanc[85] found that 34 of 87 patients with SAH had had a previous sentinel bleed. Fifty percent had initially visited a physician before the onset of SAH, but in no case was the correct diagnosis of a sentinel bleed made. CT scanning was negative in 55 percent of the sentinel bleed group, but lumbar puncture, when performed, was always positive. Twenty-five of the 34 patients had a major hemorrhage within 1 to 28 days of the minor hemorrhage. Among the patients with internal carotid artery aneurysms, half presented with unilateral headache or periorbital pain at the time of the sentinel bleed. In a series of 422 patients with aneurysmal subarachnoid hemorrhage, Jakobsson and colleagues[86] found 84 patients with a history suggestive of a sentinel hemorrhage; 40.5 percent were examined by a physician, and an incorrect diagnosis was made in every case. In 75 percent of these patients the sentinel headache occurred within 2 weeks of the major SAH. Patients with a warning bleed had a poorer outcome than did those without a sentinel hemorrhage, emphasizing the need for accurate diagnosis by the physician at the time of the sentinel bleed.

Most intracranial aneurysms are diagnosed only after they rupture. The headache most commonly associated with aneurysmal rupture and resultant SAH has been deemed a "thunderclap headache."[87] The headache is typically of sudden onset (like a hand clap), is of severe intensity ("worst headache of my life"), and is associated with a change in the level of consciousness and with nausea and/or vomiting. This type of headache is readily recognized by physicians as a possible indicator of SAH, but the headache of aneurysmal rupture can be highly variable (Fig. 4-17). Walton and associates[88] looked at 192 cases of SAH and found that 10 percent of the patients had no headache, while 8 percent had an initial gradual headache that slowly worsened.

Patients presenting with a thunderclap headache should have an emergent CT scan without contrast to rule out SAH. If the CT is negative, a lumbar puncture should be performed to look for frank blood or xanthochromia. Some institutions have the capability of studying CSF with spectrophotometry, looking for oxyhemoglobin and bilirubin. Van Gijn and van Dongen[89] looked at 100 cases of SAH and found blood in the subarachnoid space on CT in 92 percent of the patients on day 0, while only 58 percent had blood on imaging on day 5. The ability to visualize an SAH on CT examination becomes increasingly difficult the longer the time since the initial hemorrhage; after 3 weeks SAH rarely can be detected.

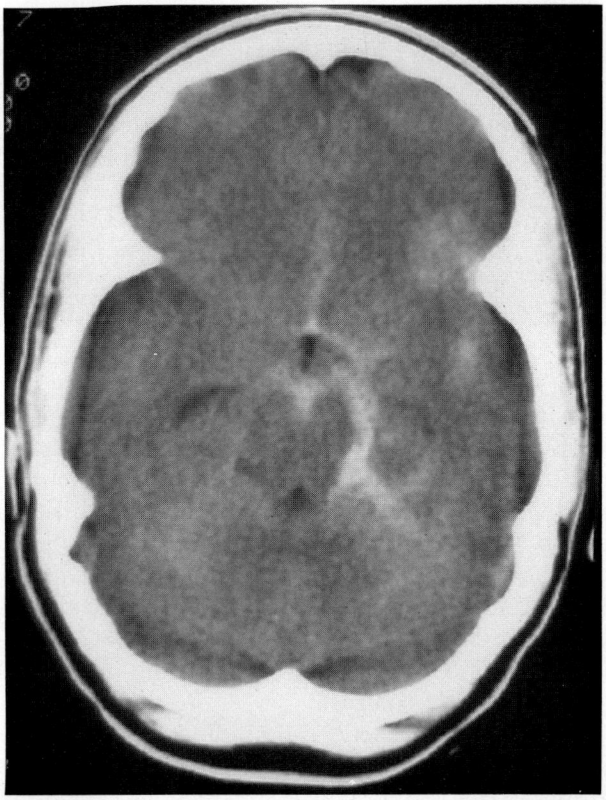

Figure 4-17
Sudden-onset occipital head pain. CT brain scan demonstrates abnormal increased density in the pontine cistern and ambient cistern, indicative of a recent subarachnoid hemorrhage.

There is still disagreement on the need for conventional cerebral angiography to rule out the presence of an unruptured aneurysm, in a patient with a thunderclap headache and a normal CT scan and normal cerebrospinal fluid (CSF) examination. Many clinicians would stop the workup at this point, especially if the studies were completed no more than 1 to 3 days after the ictus. Wijdicks and coworkers[90] reported on 71 patients who presented with acute severe headaches and had normal CT and lumbar puncture examinations and followed those patients for an average of 3.3 years. Headache recurred in 17 percent of the patients, and reevaluation at that time showed no evidence of SAH. Angiography was done on six patients, and all were normal. The study suggested that thunderclap headache without SAH on CT and CSF is a benign syndrome with no requirement for conventional cerebral angiography. However, in a retrospective study of 111 patients, Raps and collegues[91] did show that unruptured aneurysms can present as thunderclap headache in a small percentage of cases.

MRA is a valuable noninvasive tool for identifying intracranial aneurysms (Fig. 4-18). It has very high sensitivity for diagnosing aneurysms 3 mm or greater in size. Moreover, it is very uncommon for aneurysms less than

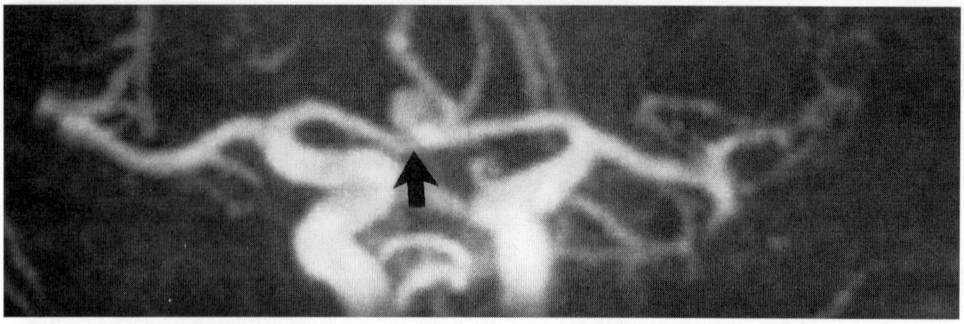

Figure 4-18
Coronal three-dimensional time of flight MRA revealing an anterior cerebral artery aneurysm (arrow).

3 mm in size to rupture. MRA is an excellent alternative to conventional angiography for excluding the presence of an unruptured aneurysm in patients with acute-onset thunderclap headache and normal CT and CSF examinations. MRA also can be utilized in the investigation of a patient with a remote history of thunderclap headache. More recently, CT angiography (CTA) has shown great promise in the diagnosis of intracranial aneurysms. However, CTA examination requires the intravenous administration of contrast.

Thunderclap headache also has been linked to cerebral venous sinus thrombosis,[92] pituitary apoplexy,[93] and carotid artery–vertebral artery dissections (Fig. 4-19A and B). MRI evaluation is necessary to characterize pituitary tumors and associated hemorrhage, as CT is less accurate. MRI and MR venography have become the techniques of choice in the diagnosis of intracranial venous thrombosis (Fig. 4-20).

Unruptured Arteriovenous Malformations

The association between arteriovenous malformations (AVMs) and headache is controversial. AVMs can be pial, dural, or mixed; dural AVMs typically are associated with headache. Distended vessels may impinge on innervated meninges, producing head pain. Monteiro and associates[94] reported recurrent headaches in 30 of 38 patients with AVMs and 10 of 13 patients with cavernous angiomas. Headache was the first symptom in 57 percent of the patients with vessel malformations. The AVM headaches fit the IHS criteria for migraine in 47 percent and those for tension-type headache in 31.4 percent. Head pain was on the side of the AVM in 88.8 percent of these patients. The "AVM migraine" is somewhat atypical, with a higher incidence of prolonged aura, no side shifting of pain, short duration of pain (less than 4 h), and a low prevalence of migraine

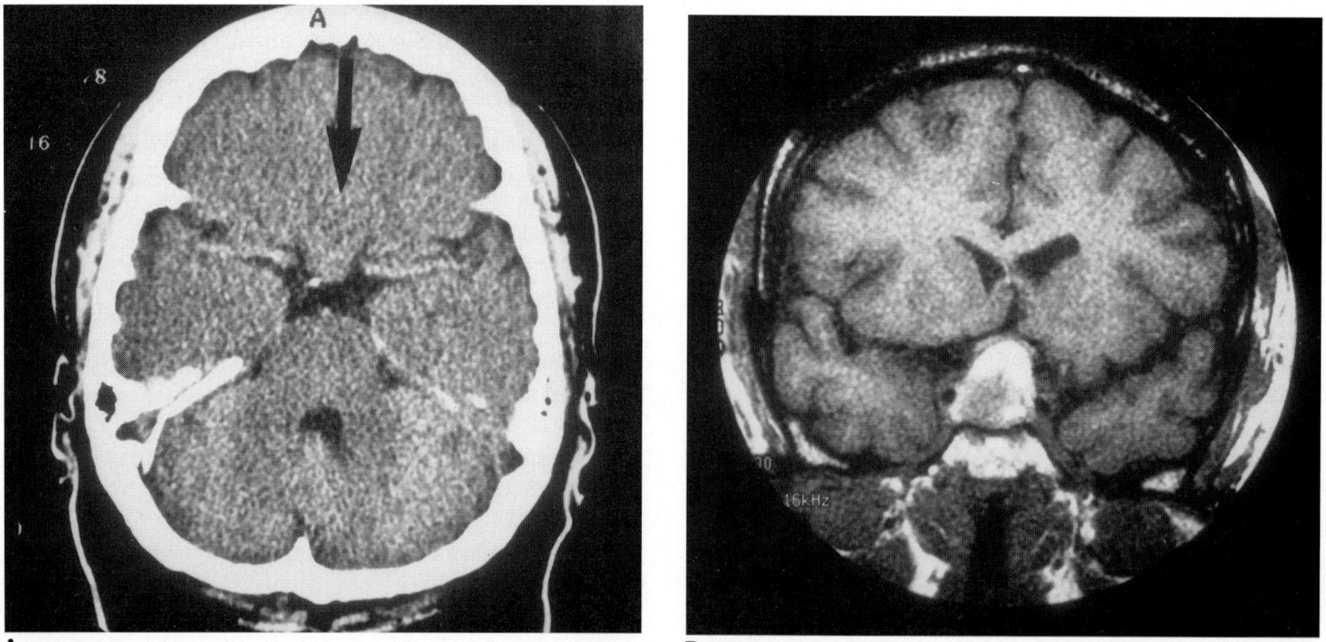

A B

Figure 4-19
A 50-year-old woman with thunderclap headache. **(A)** *CT scan demonstrating a distortion of the usual pentagonal shape of the suprasellar cistern by an isodense pituitary tumor.* **(B)** *Coronal T1-weighted MRI showing a pituitary mass with hyperintensities at the border suggesting a subacute hemorrhage. (Courtesy of D. W. Dodick and E. F. M. Wijdicks, Mayo Clinic and Mayo Foundation.)*

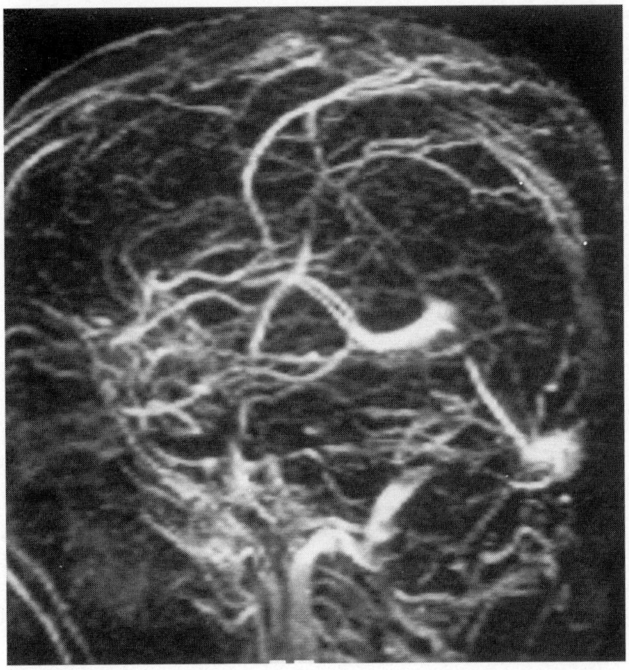

Figure 4-20
Sagittal two-dimensional MR venogram shows nonvisualization of the majority of the superior saggital sinus, indicating thrombosis.

in family members. AVMs also can present as short-lasting unilateral neuralgiform headache with conjunctival injection and tearing (SUNCT),[95] trigeminal neuralgia,[96] and chronic occipital neuralgia.[97]

Most AVMs can be identified on CT with contrast. MRI-MRA is more sensitive and can help therapeutically by providing a three-dimensional definition of the malformation. Most (80 percent) AVMs are supratentorial (Fig. 4-21). MRI is much less helpful in the characterization of dural AVMs.

Stereotactic radiosurgery (gamma knife) has become a supplement or alternative to microsurgery in the treatment of AVMs. There may be a headache associated with AVM treatment after the use of the gamma knife.[98] Rozen and Swanson[98] presented a case of a 62-year-old man with no prior history of headache who developed migraine 15 months after gamma knife surgery. The headache was associated with a rapid thrombosis of the AVM and a area of increased T2 signal around the AVM on MRI; there was no evidence of mass effect or shift. Other reports in the literature of headache after gamma knife have identified the same T2 signal changes. The nature of the T2 signal change is not known, but it may result from radiation-induced edema, demyelination, or gliosis. The true frequency of headaches after gamma knife is not known, but this type of headache may be a manifestation of local intracranial venous hypertension from an AVM undergoing thrombosis.

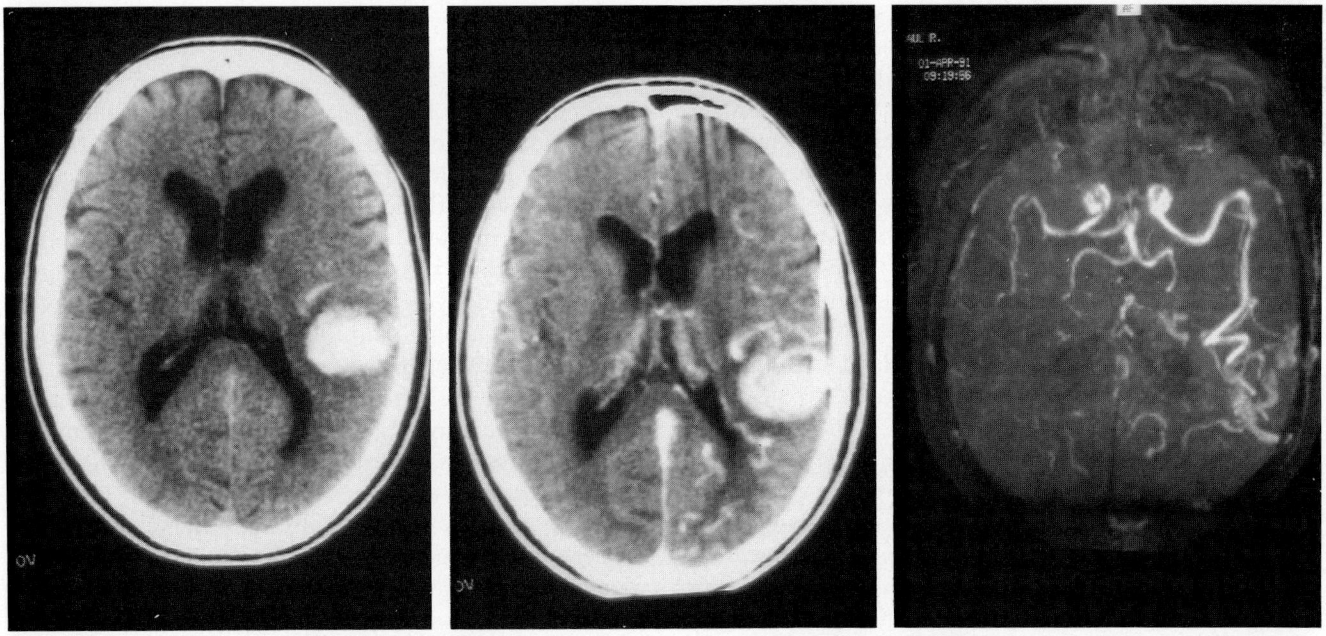

A B C

Figure 4-21
A 70-year-old male with a history of intermittent left hemispheral headaches with recent sudden exacerbation of left hemicranial pain. **(A)** *CT scan demonstrating left parietal intracerebral hematoma.* **(B)** *CT after contrast enhancement, again demonstrating the hematoma but revealing abnormal blood vessels in the region of the hematoma.* **(C)** *MRA demonstrating a left posterior parietal temporal AVM with the major feeding vessel from the left middle cerebral artery.*

Carotid Artery and Vertebral Artery Dissections

The most common site of arterial dissection in the cerebral circulation is the extracranial internal carotid artery (ICA), followed by the vertebral artery (VA).[99] The intracranial segment of the ICA rarely is involved, but extracranial vertebral dissection can extend intracranially. The true incidence of spontaneous ICA dissections is not known, since many are asymptomatic or misdiagnosed. In Rochester, Minn., the annual incidence of spontaneous ICA dissections was 2.6 per 100,000 persons.[100] VA dissections are about a third as common as ICA dissections. Dissection of cranial vessels is often spontaneous but also can occur secondary to major trauma (whiplash injury) or mild trauma such as coughing, sleeping in an abnormal position, and normal flexion and/or extension of the neck. Underlying connective tissue disorders such as Marfan syndrome, fibromuscular dysplasia, and Ehlers-Danlos syndrome can predispose an individual to arterial dissection. Migraine also may be a risk factor for cervical arterial dissection.[101] Most individuals who develop ICA or VA dissections are younger than 50 years of age.[99]

ICA dissections usually present with pain involving the face, neck, or head. Headache, the most common symptom of ICA dissection, occurs in 84 percent of these patients; this is followed in decreasing frequency by focal ischemic symptoms (61 percent), oculosympathetic paresis (Horner syndrome) (53 percent), neck pain (23 percent), and light-headedness (21 percent). Mokri and colleagues[102] found that stroke-like spells can occur minutes or up to 11 days after the onset of hemicrania. Bruits, either objective or subjective, are present in about 45 percent of these patients.[103] Less common symptoms include amaurosis fugax, scintillating scotomas, trigeminal nerve palsy, and dysgeusia. The headaches are usually one-sided and focal, most commonly involving the anterior head region in the orbit or periorbit. The head pain is usually nonthrobbing and constant and is the initial symptom in 47 percent of cases.[104] Headache onset is usually gradual but can be sudden (thunderclap) in 10 percent of patients. Facial pain occurs in about 30 percent of patients with ICA dissections.

The most common symptoms of VA dissection are neck pain and headache. Headache usually occurs at the base of the head (occipital area), often in association with neck pain. Focal ischemic symptoms in a vertebrobasilar distribution, frequently presenting as a lateral medullary infarction, can follow as early as 5 h but up to 2 weeks after the onset of headache.[99] Some patients have posterior circulation strokes or TIAs alone; others have headache or neck pain alone. Headache is the initial symptom in 33 percent of these patients, and unlike ICA dissections, orbital and facial pain is rare. VA dissections present as a thunderclap headache in 20 percent of cases; in this setting SAH has to be excluded. VA and ICA dissections can occur bilaterally, and the presence of dissections in both territories concomitantly is not rare.

The most common angiographic findings for both ICA and VA dissections include lumen stenosis (77 to 80 percent), pseudoaneurysm formation (14 to 39 percent), intimal flap (28 percent), and occlusion (11 to 17 percent). Other findings include attenuated flow in the affected intracranial territory and distal branch embolization.[102,105]

MRI and MRA have shown increasing usefulness in the diagnosis of ICA dissections. MRI-MRA is of only modest usefulness in VA dissections. Cross-sectional imaging of an artery on MRI can demonstrate the arterial lumen as well as a subintimal clot. The true lumen is represented as a dark flow void that is smaller than the normal diameter of the vessel, and the subintimal hematoma (methemoglobin) is of high signal on both T1-weighted and T2-weighted images and has a crescent or circular morphology.[99] MRI and MRA can visualize most pseudoaneurysms and lumenal stenoses caused by dissection. These techniques still can miss smaller pseudoaneurysms, mistake artifactual areas of attenuated flow-related enhancement for true stenoses, and not visualize intimal flaps. MRA and MRI may ultimately become the diagnostic procedures of choice for identifying extracranial head and neck dissections because they are noninvasive studies (Fig. 4-22). CTA also is showing great promise in the evaluation of dissection.

Colloid Cysts

Colloid cysts are the most common neuroepithelial tumors and have been documented to occur in patients 3 weeks to 72 years of age.[106] Young and Silberstein[107] recently reviewed the literature and found that headache occurs in 68 to 100 percent of patients with colloid cysts of the third ventricle and in many is the presenting complaint. The typical colloid cyst headache is a severe throbbing or aching pain that usually is precipitated by movement or a change in position. The headache can be aborted by the same maneuvers. In the initial course, the headache may begin and end abruptly, lasting minutes to days. As time progresses, the headache occurs more frequently and can be associated with vomiting, tinnitus, changes in heart rate, sixth nerve palsy, drop attacks, paresthesias, and light-headedness. Sudden death can occur.[108]

MRI is the diagnostic procedure of choice (Fig. 4-23). Colloid cysts usually are hyperdense on CT, but they may be isodense in up to 30 percent of cases. MRI is felt to be 100 percent sensitive and can rule out other causes of paroxysmal headaches, including pineal cysts, vascular malformations, and base of skull abnormalities (Chiari malformations, basilar impression).

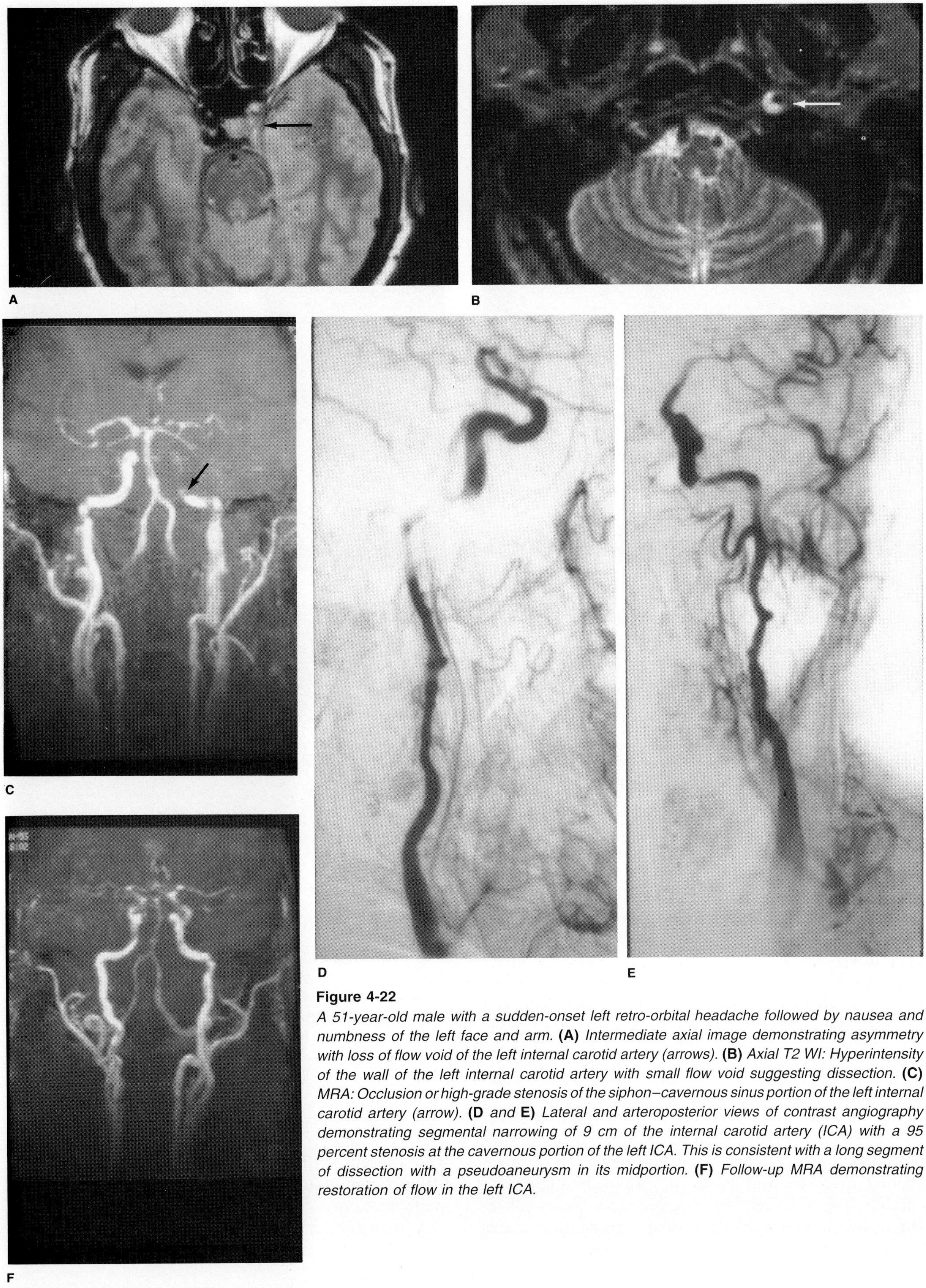

Figure 4-22
A 51-year-old male with a sudden-onset left retro-orbital headache followed by nausea and numbness of the left face and arm. **(A)** *Intermediate axial image demonstrating asymmetry with loss of flow void of the left internal carotid artery (arrows).* **(B)** *Axial T2 WI: Hyperintensity of the wall of the left internal carotid artery with small flow void suggesting dissection.* **(C)** *MRA: Occlusion or high-grade stenosis of the siphon–cavernous sinus portion of the left internal carotid artery (arrow).* **(D** *and* **E)** *Lateral and arteroposterior views of contrast angiography demonstrating segmental narrowing of 9 cm of the internal carotid artery (ICA) with a 95 percent stenosis at the cavernous portion of the left ICA. This is consistent with a long segment of dissection with a pseudoaneurysm in its midportion.* **(F)** *Follow-up MRA demonstrating restoration of flow in the left ICA.*

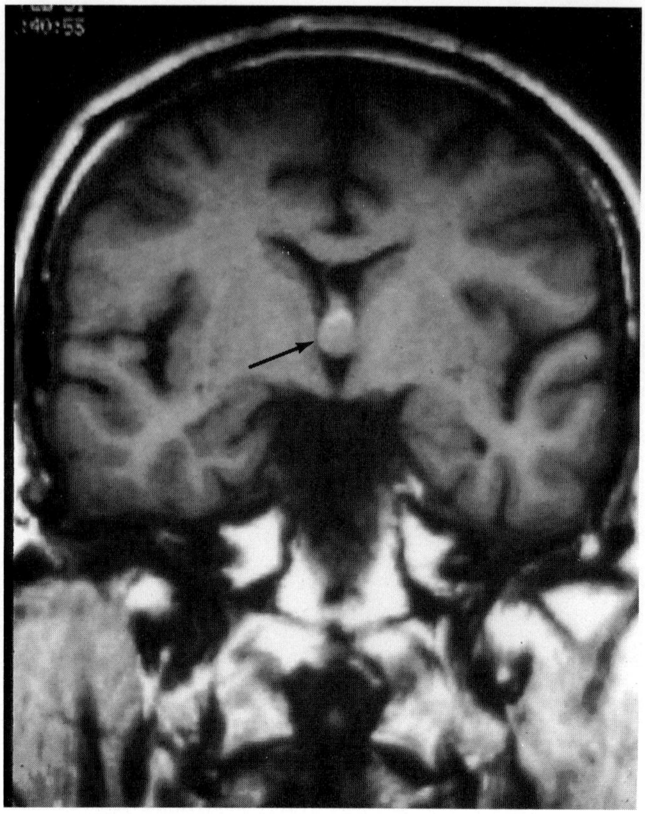

Figure 4-23
Chronic headaches. T1 W coronal image demonstrating a third ventricular cyst (arrow) with normal-size lateral ventricles.

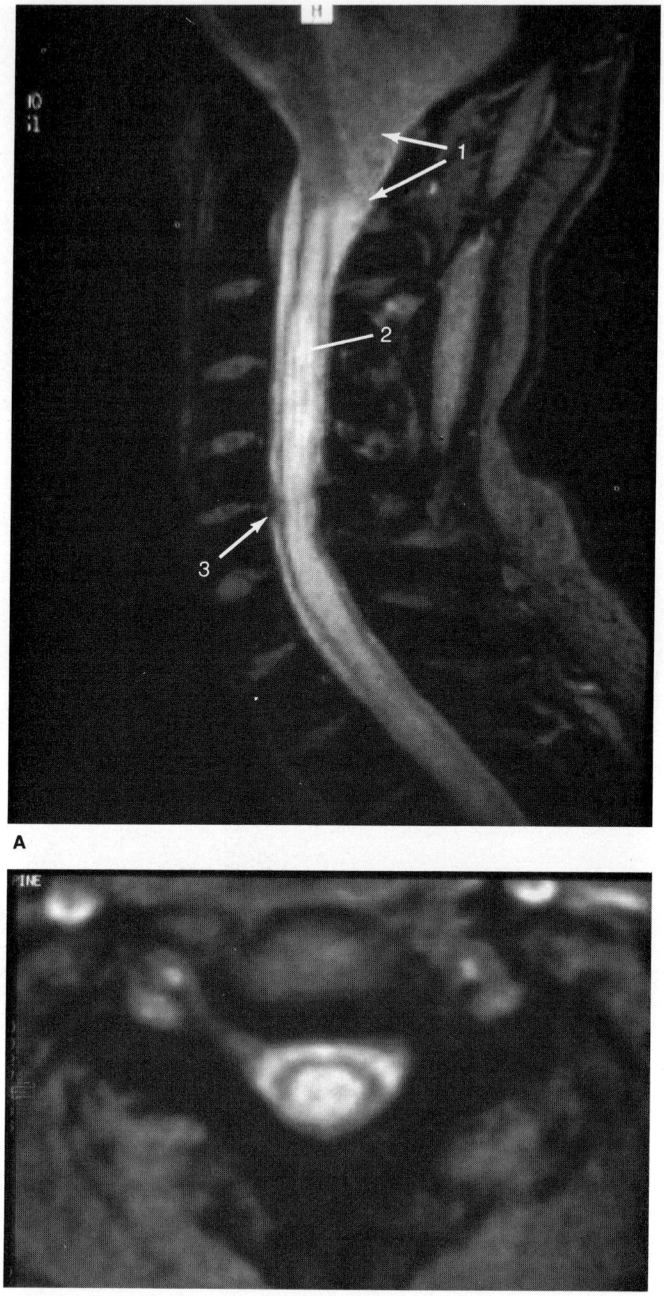

A

B

Figure 4-24
A 52-year-old patient with upper cervical, occipital, and temporal head pain. **(A)** *T2 WI demonstrating inferior displacement of the cerebellum into the upper spinal canal to the C2 level (arrow 1). A large central-fluid-filled spinal cord cavity is noted extending from the C2 level to the T10 level (arrow 2). A small herniated disc at the C5–C6 level (arrow 3).* **(B)** *T2 W axial image demonstrating the central-fluid-filled cavity within the spinal cord: type I Chiari malformation associated with syringomyelia.*

Chiari Malformations

Headache is a common presenting symptom of Chiari malformations. Chiari I malformation is associated with displacement of the cerebellar tonsils into the cervical spinal canal. Cerebellar ectopia less than 5 mm below the foramen magnum is common and generally is without clinical significance. In Chiari II malformations, there is caudal displacement of the brainstem and lower cerebellum; elongation of the fourth ventricle, which may descend below the foramen magnum; and associated myelomeningocele. Both Chiari I and Chiari II malformations are associated with hydromyelic cavities (Fig. 4-24).

In a recent review Ramadan[79] found that headache occurs in 15 to 75 percent of patients with Chiari I malformations. The typical headache is of short duration, is occipital or nuchal in location, and is aggravated or initiated by Valsalva maneuvers (symptomatic cough headache). The headache is likely to be due to distortion and stretching of craniocervical pain-sensitive structures.[79] Coughing, for example, produces increased intrathoracic pressure and secondary elevation of intracranial pressure; this leads to further herniation of already low-lying cerebellar tonsils and causes subsequent traction on pain-sensitive structures. Individuals who present with cough headache should have an MRI examination to rule out the presence of a Chiari malformation.

A recurrent, longer-lasting Chiari I malformation

headache that is not affected by Valsalva maneuvers has been described. This headache may have the characteristics of migraine, tension-type, or low- or high-CSF-pressure headaches. The pathogenesis of this headache subtype is unknown.

Posttraumatic Headaches

Headache is a common complaint after mild head injury, occurring in 30 to 80 percent of these patients.[109] Concussion or loss of consciousness is not a prerequisite for posttraumatic headache (PTH), but 79 to 90 percent of patients with the posttraumatic syndrome (PTS) have headache.[110,111] PTS consists of a collection of symptoms and signs occurring after head injury that normally begin within 24 to 48 h after the insult. In addition to headache, PTS patients complain of dizziness, vertigo, changes in mood, sleep disturbances, alteration of memory, and problems with concentration and alertness. The IHS[5] criteria for the diagnosis of acute PTH include onset of headache within 14 days of injury with or without loss of consciousness and alleviation of headache within 8 weeks. If the headache lasts beyond 8 weeks, it is considered chronic PTH. The IHS[5] does not specify headache type. In clinical practice, it is not unusual to see PTH develop months to years after trauma.

Most posttraumatic headaches often resemble tension-type headaches and are usually mild to moderate in intensity, with bilateral, generalized constant pain. In addition, new recurrent migraine-like headaches can occur after head trauma. Weiss and associates[112] described 35 patients with posttraumatic migraine, all of whom had had no prior history of headache. The migraine began instantaneously or several days after the insult and developed into a recurrent headache syndrome. The median age of onset of posttraumatic migraine appears to be higher than that of idiopathic migraine. Head injury also has been documented to cause cluster headache,[113] low-CSF-pressure-type headache, and idiopathic intracranial hypertension.[114]

Women have a higher risk for developing PTH (1.9×) compared with men.[115] The severity of the injury does not correlate with headache persistence. Yamaguchi[116] actually reported an inverse relationship between headache severity and trauma severity. Early headache onset, within 24 h of trauma, is associated with a higher incidence of headache at 6 weeks.[117]

Only a few studies have looked at the utility of neuroimaging in patients with PTS. Kelly and colleagues[118] found no specific MRI abnormalities in PTS patients. Levin and coworkers[119] identified MRI changes in 17 of 20 patients with mild to moderate head injury. The lesions were located at the gray-white junction or in the white matter and might have represented diffuse axonal injury. These lesions often decreased in size or resolved over time. Most of the resolution occurred within the first month after the injury; lesions present at 1 month were commonly present at 3 months. These lesions appear to correlate with a higher frequency of postinjury cognitive dysfunction. Young and Packard[109] suggested that the MRI changes in PTH patients may reflect diffuse axonal injury (DAI) secondary to the shearing forces inflicted on the brain at the time of head trauma. They went on to suggest that mild DAI may resolve over time, whereas severe DAI leads to permanent pathologic and radiographic changes. MRI is superior to CT in identifying diffuse axonal injury.

SPECT has been used to study head injury patients. In the acute setting, SPECT has demonstrated perfusion abnormalities; including focal areas of hypoperfusion (probably representing contusion) and diffuse occipital and temporal areas of hypoperfusion (probably representing diffuse axonal injury or multiple contusions). Masdeu and associates[120] identified SPECT abnormalities in 11 of 14 patients with normal CT scans. SPECT may be more sensitive than conventional MRI in showing residual injury weeks to months after head trauma. The Therapeutics and Technology Assessment Subcommittee of the American Academy of Neurology has not supported the routine use of SPECT in the evaluation of head injury patients and has recommended that this neuroimaging technique remain an investigational tool.[121]

PET also has been utilized as an investigational tool for the evaluation of head injury patients. Diffuse changes in cerebral glucose metabolism have been demonstrated after head trauma. Perfusion abnormalities also have been noted, and in some patients these areas have corresponded to changes found on neuropsychometric testing.[122]

Young and Packard[109] suggested that neuroimaging should be performed on all patients in the acute setting of head injury who present with evidence of mild behavioral changes, a Glasgow Coma Score less than 15, or equivocal findings on neurologic examination. In the emergency setting, a CT scan is adequate for diagnosing parenchymal or extra-axial hematomas that may warrant surgical intervention. MRI is more useful for identifying diffuse axonal injury and for prognostication. MRI is warranted when there is a discrepancy between the clinical status of a patient and the appearance of the CT scan.

If a patient presents days to weeks after head injury, CT or MRI should be performed (if it has not already been done) to exclude skull fractures, contusions, chronic subdural hematomas, posttraumatic hydrocephalus, and diffuse axonal injury (Fig. 4-25). If the patient presents with neck pain and/or radicular signs with abnormalities on neurologic examination, MRI of the cervical spine will help diagnose posttraumatic bone spurs, hematomas, or disc herniations. Evaluation for an occult carotid artery or VA dissection also may be clinically indicated.

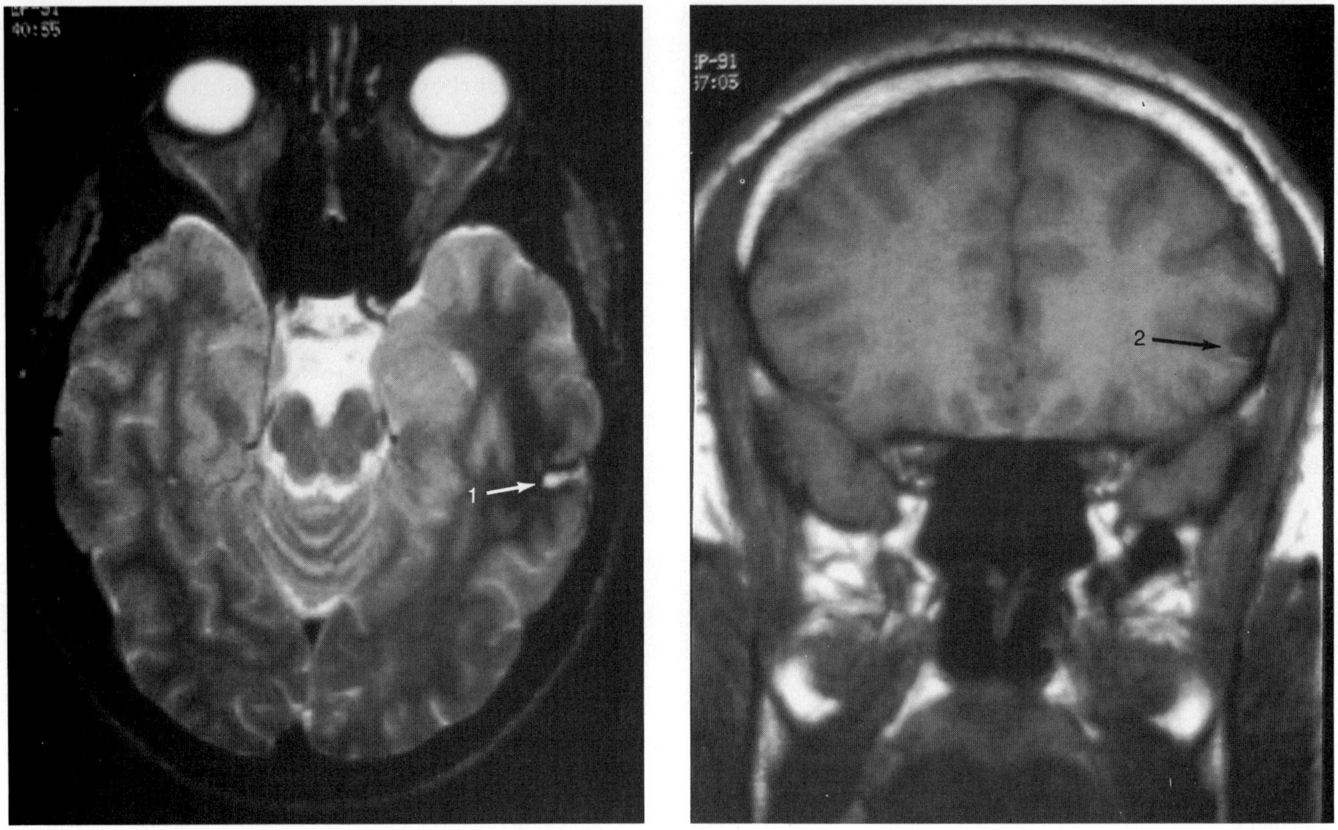

A B

Figure 4-25
A 28-year-old patient with persistent headaches 7 months after a severe head injury. **(A)** *T2 W axial image; left temporal contusion.* **(B)** *T1 W coronal image; left frontal contusion.*

Headaches Associated with Low Cerebrospinal Fluid Pressure

Low-CSF-pressure headache typically manifests as an orthostatic head pain. The headache begins a variable time after the patient has arisen from a recumbent position and is alleviated by returning to the supine position. Other exacerbating factors include coughing, straining, sneezing, and jugular venous compression. The headache is usually severe in intensity. It can be throbbing or dull in quality and either localized or diffuse in location. Associated symptoms include nausea, vomiting, light-headedness, vertigo, photophobia, tinnitus, visual blurring, and neck stiffness. The natural history of the disorder depends on the cause. The headache itself can last from days to years. The neurologic examination is usually normal except for an occasional sixth nerve palsy.

Low-CSF-pressure headaches are most commonly caused by lumbar puncture (LP). A post-LP headache probably results from an ongoing leakage of CSF from the site of the dural puncture. Intracranial hypotension occurs at a CSF pressure below 50 to 90 mmH_2O. Post-LP headaches occur in 10 to 30 percent of patients and are 2 times more common in women.[123] Headache onset can occur within minutes or up to 12 days after the procedure. Most of these headaches resolve spontaneously within 4 to 8 days.

Schaltenbrand[124] first developed the concept of a spontaneous low-CSF-pressure syndrome. Theories advanced for the cause of this syndrome include (1) decreased CSF production as a result of a reversible disturbance of the choroid plexus, (2) spontaneous CSF leakage from an arachnoid membrane rupture and (3) hyperabsorption of CSF. The most likely cause is CSF leakage through small occult meningeal tears. Physicians often can elicit a history of mild trauma that could have resulted in a CSF leak.

Brain MRI and routine CT scanning generally are not beneficial in defining the site of a CSF leak but have identified several pathologic consequences of the low-CSF-pressure syndrome. Murros and Fogelholm[125] described cranial CT findings in a patient with spontaneous intracranial hypotension. The patient's ventricles were slit-like, and there was concomitant effacement of basal cisterns. The CT abnormalities resolved after headache alleviation. Mokri and colleagues[126] were able to demonstrate diffuse pachymeningeal enhancement on brain MRI in patients with low-CSF-pressure headaches (Fig. 4-26A and B). This finding has been verified by other

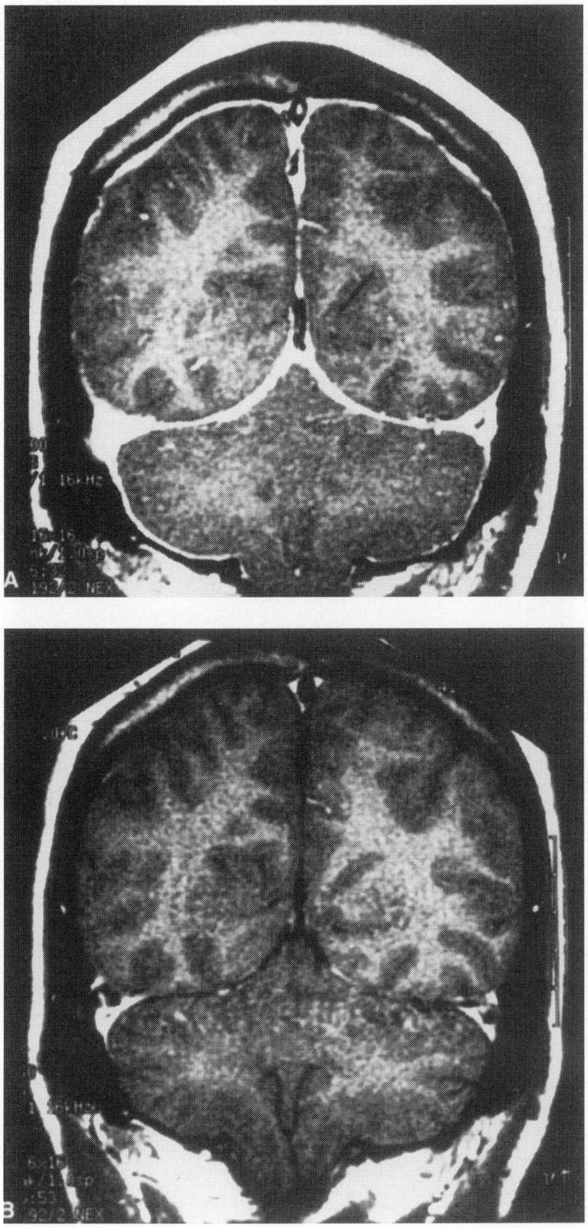

Figure 4-26
(A) *Coronal T1-weighted MRI with gadolinium exhibiting contiguous pachymeningeal enhancement involving the convexity, dura, falx, and tentorium in a patient with spontaneous intracranial hypotension.* **(B)** *Resolution of meningeal enhancement after surgical repair of a lumbar cerebrospinal fluid leak. [Reprinted from Lay CL, Campbell JK, Mokri B: Low cerebrospinal fluid pressure headache, in Goadsby PJ, Silberstein SD (eds): Blue Books of Practical Neurology, volume 17:* Headache. *Boston, Butterworth-Heinemann, 1997, pp 355–367, by permission from Butterworth-Heinemann.]*

investigators. The enhancement involves both the supratentorial compartment and the infratentorial compartment and does not involve the leptomeninges.[123] The MRI abnormality is believed to be secondary to vascular dilation in the pachymeninges, which is then identified as diffuse contrast enhancement. Some authors believe that the changes are secondary to inflammation.[127] An independent finding on MRI is a downward displacement of the brain with resultant cerebellar tonsilar herniation, flattening of the basis pontis, brainstem descent, and bowing of the optic chiasm over the pituitary gland.[128] The brain MRI changes resolve with treatment (Fig. 4-27A and B). Intracranial hypotension also may cause the formation of subdural hematomas or hygromas, presumably as a result of tearing of bridging veins

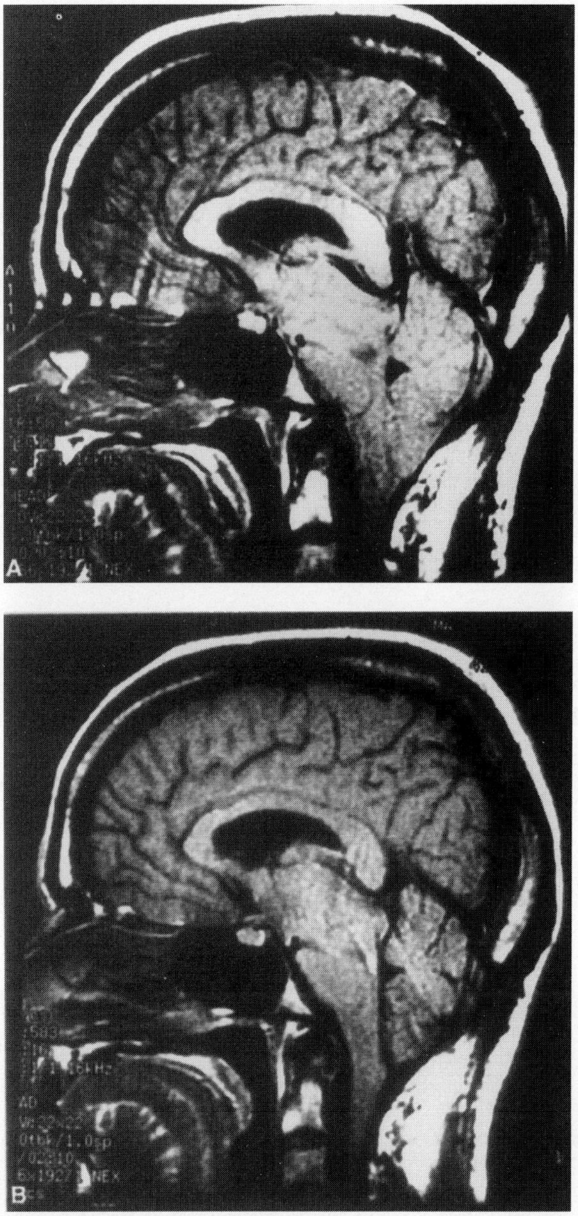

Figure 4-27
(A) *Patient with a lumbar cerebrospinal fluid leak. Saggital T1-weighted MRI showing descent of the brain and crowding of the posterior fossa structures.* **(B)** *Brain and posterior fossa return to normal appearance after surgical repair of CSF leak. [Reprinted from Lay CL, Campbell JK, Mokri B: Low cerebrospinal fluid pressure headache, in Goadsby PJ, Silberstein SD (eds): Blue Books of Practical Neurology, volume 17:* Headache. *Boston, Butterworth-Heinemann, 1997, pp 355–367, by permission from Butterworth-Heinemann.]*

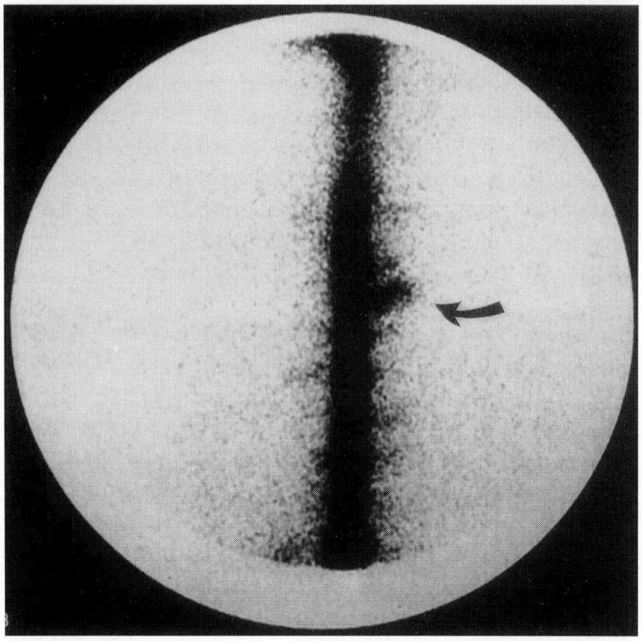

Figure 4-28

Radioisotope cisternography demonstrating extra-arachnoid leakage of isotope in the midthoracic region in a patient with a low cerebrospinal fluid pressure headache (arrow). [Reprinted from Lay CL, Campbell JK, Mokri B: Low cerebrospinal fluid pressure headache, in Goadsby PJ, Silberstein SD (eds): Blue Books of Practical Neurology, volume 17: Headache. *Boston, Butterworth-Heinemann, 1997, pp 355–367, by permission from Butterworth-Heinemann.]*

or arachnoid membranes as the brain descends away from the dura secondary to a reduction in CSF volume.[123]

In the absence of an obvious cause of a low-CSF-pressure headache, CSF analysis may be needed with accurate measurements of an opening pressure. In the presence of diffuse meningeal enhancement on MRI, a normal neurologic examination, and a typical history of low-CSF-pressure headache, some physicians might empirically treat a post-LP headache with an epidural blood patch. In most instances CSF analysis (total protein, cells, etc.) is normal. A moderate pleocytosis or elevated total protein can occur. Once the low pressure is documented, various studies can be utilized to identify a possible CSF leak. Radioisotope cisternography is an excellent imaging study to identify CSF leakage. A radioactive tracer (indium III-DTPA) is injected into the lumbosacral subarachnoid space, and a gamma camera then is used to follow the tracer in its course over the entire neuraxis. Extravasation of the radiotracer can then be imaged (Fig. 4-28). CT myelography and CT cisternography have a higher diagnostic yield than does radioisotope cisternography, although all these studies may fail to identify a CSF leak (Fig. 4-29).

Neuroimaging of Headaches in Children

Maytal and coworkers[129] did a retrospective chart review of children age 3 to 18 years who were evaluated for headache at a pediatric neurology clinic over a 2-year period. Most of the children were diagnosed with either migraine headache or tension-type headache. Among 133 records, 78 imaging studies were completed (45 MRIs, 27 CTs, and 6 with both), and no significant abnormalities were identified even though individuals were scanned for atypical headache and/or transient neurologic dysfunction during a headache. These authors concluded that neuroimaging is of limited value in the evaluation of pediatric headache unless there is clinical evidence of a mass lesion.

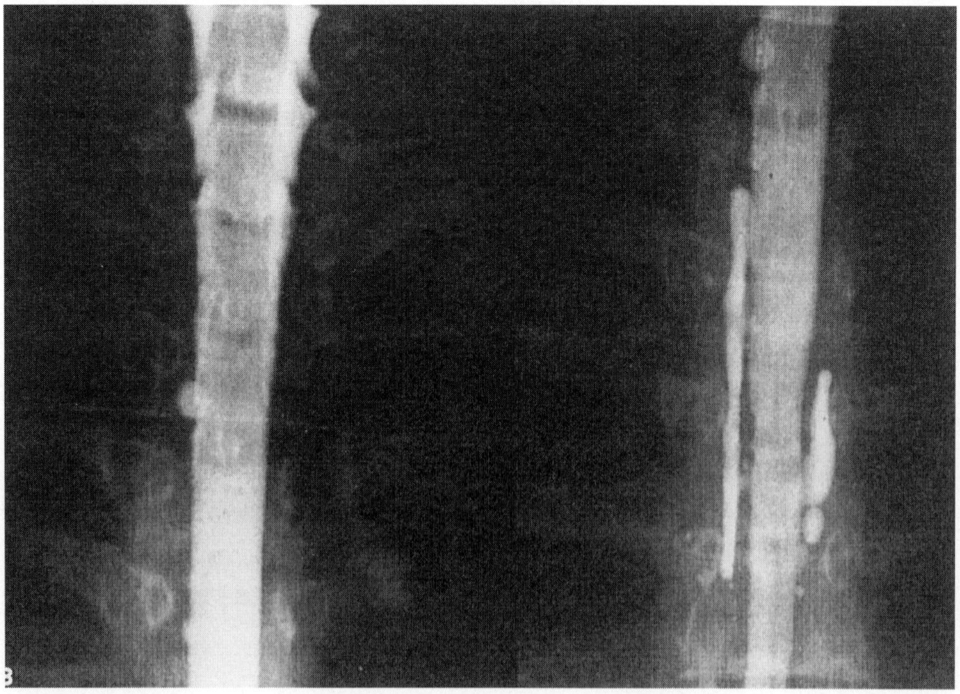

Figure 4-29

An oil-based pantopaque myelogram demonstrating extravasation of dye at T2 and an increasing subdural collection of dye through the ruptured root sleeve. [Reprinted from Lay CL, Campbell JK, Mokri B: Low cerebrospinal fluid pressure headache, in Goadsby PJ, Silberstein SD (eds): Blue Books of Practical Neurology, volume 17: Headache. *Boston, Butterworth-Heinemann, 1997, pp 355–367, by permission from Butterworth-Heinemann.]*

Wober-Bingol and colleagues[130] looked at 429 patients age 5 to 18 years who were diagnosed with tension-type headache or migraine headache. There were two study groups: one in which all patients had MRI scans and one in which only clinical examinations were completed. MRI was normal in 82.3 percent, while 17.7 percent had a structural abnormality such as a pineal cyst, asymmetry of the lateral ventricles, an arachnoid cyst, or cavum septum pellucidum. In all cases the lesions identified were not thought to be related to the headache. The authors concluded that MRI is not required for the evaluation of recurrent headache in children and adolescents with normal neurologic examinations.

Indications for Neuroimaging in Headache Patients

Evaluation of headache patients with neuroimaging techniques has changed with advancing technology. In 1978, Diamond and Dalessio[131] suggested that skull x-rays be performed at all initial evaluations of headache patients. In 1983, Sargent and Solbach[132] studied 193 migraineurs with isotope brain scans, CTs, electroencephalograms (EEGs), and skull x-rays and concluded that CT was the most effective screening test for headache and that the other diagnostic examinations could be eliminated from the workup. At the present time physicians usually choose either CT or MRI to image patients with headaches.

Since 1973, CT has been widely used in headache evaluation. In a single study all intracranial structures can be visualized, as well as the paranasal sinuses, calvarium, and skull base. In 1982, the National Institutes of Health consensus development conference on CT stated that "CT detection of intracranial lesions is now so well established that the suspicion of any intracranial mass lesion from history or neurologic examination constitutes a strong indication for the procedure."[133] Is isolated headache in a patient with a normal neurologic examination enough to raise suspicion of a mass lesion, and if so, should one consider CT or MRI?

Akpek and associates[134] reviewed 592 patients with headache and a normal neurologic examination who were studied with contrast-enhanced CT scans. No significant lesions were identified. These authors concluded that contrast-enhanced CT in patients with chronic headache and a normal neurologic examination is not useful. They estimated that the cost of finding intracranial pathology with this technique in a patient with a normal neurologic examination was $200,000.

Demaerel and colleagues[135] looked at 363 patients with chronic headache and normal neurologic examinations, each of whom had a contrast-and non-contrast-enhanced CT scan. Normal CT scans were found in 88.4 percent. Space-occupying lesions were noted in 3 percent, and the CT finding led to a specific treatment in 1.4 percent. The contrast-enhanced scan changed the diagnosis in only 3 percent of the patients. The authors concluded that an unenhanced CT is useful in the evaluation of all chronic headache patients, even those with a normal examination. The use of an unenhanced scan reduces costs and in most instances is sufficient to make the correct diagnosis. Contrast-enhanced CT or MRI is indicated if a suspicious lesion is noted on the noncontrast scan. CT scans play a pivotal role in the evaluation of secondary headache syndromes, especially in the emergency department. Cranial CT examinations in the evaluation of headache patients should include images from below the sphenoid sinus to the vertex of the head.

MRI is more sensitive than CT for identifying intracranial pathology, but at an increased cost. MRI can detect almost all lesions visualized by CT and also has a greater ability to assess intracranial vasculature utilizing MRA and pathophysiologic processes on fMRI. Kuhn and Shekar[136] reported a comparison evaluation of CT and MRI in migraine patients. They looked at 74 patients with migraine with aura. T2 lesions were identified in 26 percent of MRI scans, while no parenchymal changes were noted on CT. MRI was also more useful in identifying secondary causes of headache, including vascular malformations and carotid dissections. MRI is not as valuable as CT in the evaluation of acute SAH. Both imaging techniques have a place in headache evaluation, depending on a patient's history, presentation, and examination.

Which headache patients need to have neuroimaging? In 1994, the Quality Standards Subcommittee of the American Academy of Neurology (AAN) developed practice parameters looking specifically at the utility of neuroimaging in the evaluation of headache patients with normal neurologic examinations.[137] The study consisted of a MEDLINE search from 1974 to 1991 and an *Index Medicus* search to July 1993, reviewing CT and MRI usage in patients with headache and migraine. Only studies with more than 17 patients were utilized, and all patients had had normal neurologic exams. Seventeen studies eventually were analyzed. The investigations were divided into those with undefined headache (not defined in the article) and those with migraine. In the migraine patient population, 897 CTs or MRIs were completed. Three tumors and one AVM were found. The patient with the AVM also had a seizure disorder that greatly enhanced the suspicion of an intracranial lesion. The total yield of structural lesions was 0.4 percent. In the unspecified headache group, 1825 CTs or MRIs were completed. In this group, 6 AVMs, 21 tumors, 3 aneurysms, 5 subdural hematomas, and 8 cases of hydrocephalus were noted. The total yield of pathology was 2.4 percent. In regard to cost, if all 897 scans for migraine patients had been CTs, the estimated bill would have been $448,500, with a cost of $112,125 per positive lesion. In the unspecified headache group the cost per positive finding would have been $21,220.

In his review, which formed the basis of the AAN study, Dr. Benjamin Frishberg[138] related that health outcome from early detection of intracranial lesions in headache patients was difficult to assess. In many instances neuroimaging was utilized to defuse the fears of patients that they had a severe underlying neurologic condition. Fitzpatrick and Hopkins[139] looked at patient satisfaction after evaluation by a physician for headache. Among 109 patients, 60 percent had a fear of a serious illness and 40 percent, even after a normal neurologic exam, left the physician not feeling reassured. Some of these patients actually requested further neurologic testing.

The subcommittee's conclusion was that the routine use of neuroimaging is not warranted for adult patients with recurrent headache defined as migraine with or without aura who have no change in headache pattern, no history of seizures, and no focal neurologic signs or symptoms. If an atypical headache pattern evolves with neurologic dysfunction or seizures, imaging may be indicated. From the AAN study, insufficient evidence was available to define the role of CT and MRI in patients with headache syndromes other than migraine. In patients with chronic daily headache or posttraumatic headache, imaging probably is indicated.

Warning signs ("red flags") that warrant neuroimaging during headache evaluation include (1) the initial headache or "worst headache of my life," especially if the headache is of abrupt onset (thunderclap headache) or there is a change in the level of awareness, (2) headache that changes in quality, frequency, duration, or severity, (3) an abnormal neurologic examination, including the presence of orbital or cranial bruits or papilledema, (4) progressive or new persistent daily headache, (5) headache associated with seizures or abnormalities on EEG suggesting focal pathology, (6) headache associated with fever or nuchal rigidity before a lumbar puncture is performed, (7) new cough or exertional headache, and (8) migraineurs with atypical aura, stroke, or early-onset dementia (the latter may suggest CADASIL).

In spite of all the advances in neuroimaging techniques, there is still not a definitive diagnostic test for migraine and other primary headache syndromes. Neuroimaging may be the key to unlocking the secrets of headache pathogenesis.

REFERENCES

1. Rasmussen BK, Jensen R, Schroll M, Olesen J: Epidemiology of headache in a general population: A prevalence study. *J Clin Epidemiol* 44:1147–1157, 1991.
2. The National Ambulatory Medical Case Survey: 1977 Summary. United States, January–December 1977. *Vital Health Stat* [13] 13:1–107, 1980.
3. Lipton RB, Stewart WF: Migraine in the United States: A review of epidemiology and healthcare use. *Neurology* 43(suppl 3):S6–S10, 1993.
4. Stang PE, Osterhaus JT: Impact of migraine in the United States: Data from the National Health Interview Survey. *Headache* 33:29–35, 1993.
5. Headache Classification Committee of the International Headache Society: Classification and diagnostic criteria for headache disorders, cranial neuralgias, and facial pain. *Cephalalgia* 8(suppl 7):1–96, 1988.
6. Wolf HG: *Headache and Other Head Pain*. New York, Oxford University Press, 1963.
7. Bruyn GW: Whither migraine research? in Sandler M, Ferrari M, Harnett S (eds): *Migraine: Pharmacology and Genetics*. London, Chapman and Hall, 1996, pp 4–5.
8. Moskowitz MA: The trigeminovascular system, in Olesen J, Tfelt-Hansen P, Welch KMA (eds): *The Headaches*. New York, Raven Press, 1993, pp 97–104.
9. Lashley KS: Patterns of cerebral integration indicated by scotomas of migraine. *Arch Neurol Psychiatry* 46:331–339, 1941.
10. Leão AAP: Spreading depression of activity in cerebral cortex. *J Neurophysiol* 7:357–390, 1944.
11. Andersen AR, Friberg L, Skyloj-Olsen T, Olesen J: Delayed hyperemia following hypoperfusion in classic migraine: Single photon emission computed tomographic demonstration. *Arch Neurol* 45:154–159, 1988.
12. Woods RP, Iacaboni M, Mazziotta JC: Bilateral spreading cerebral hypoperfusion during spontaneous migraine headache. *N Engl J Med* 331:1689–1692, 1994.
13. Lauritzen M, Olesen J: Regional cerebral blood flow during migraine attacks by xenon-133 inhalation and emission tomography. *Brain* 107:447–461, 1984.
14. Weiller C, May A, Limmroth V, et al: Brainstem activation in spontaneous human migraine attacks. *Nature Med* 1:658–660, 1995.
15. May A, Bahra A, Buchel C, et al: Hypothalamic activation in cluster headache attacks. *Lancet* 352:275–278, 1998.
16. Selby G: Investigating migraine: When, why and how, in Blau JN (ed): *Migraine: Clinical and Research Aspects*. Baltimore, Johns Hopkins University Press, 1987, pp 83–84.
17. Cala LA, Mastiglia FL: Computerized axial tomography findings in patients with migrainous headaches. *Br Med J* 2:147–150, 1976.
18. Hungersford GD, du Boulay GH, Zilkha KJ: Computerized axial tomography in patients with severe migraine: A preliminary report. *J Neurol Neurosurg Psychiatry* 39:990–994, 1976.
19. duBoulay GH, Ruiz JS: CT changes associated with migraine. *AJNR* 4:472–473, 1983.
20. Cuetter AC, Aita JF: CT scanning in classic migraine. *Headache* 23:195, 1983.
21. Pavese N, Canapicchi R, Nuti A, et al: White matter MRI hyperintensities in a hundred and twenty-nine consecutive migraine patients. *Cephalalgia* 14:342–345, 1994.
22. Igarashi H, Fumihiko S, Kan S, et al: Magnetic resonance imaging of the brain in patients with migraine. *Cephalagia* 11:69–74, 1991.
23. Cooney BS, Grossman RI, Farber RE, et al: Frequency of magnetic resonance imaging abnormalities in patients with migraine. *Headache* 36:616–621, 1996.
24. DeBenedittis G, Lorenzetti A, Sina C, Bernasconi V: Magnetic resonance imaging in migraine and tension-type headache. *Headache* 35:264–268, 1995.
25. Fazekas F, Kleinert R, Offenbacher H, et al: Pathologic correlates of incidental MRI white matter signal hyperintensities. *Neurology* 43:1683–1687, 1993.

26. Lance JW, Anthony M, Gonski A: Serotonin, the carotid body and cranial vessels in migraine. *Arch Neurol* 16:553–558, 1967.
27. Harer C, vonKummer R: Cerebrovascular CO_2 reactivity in migraine assessment by transcranial doppler ultrasound. *J Neurol* 238:23–26, 1991.
28. Bousser MG, Tournier-Lasserve E: Summary of the proceedings of the first international workshop on CADASIL, Paris, May 19–21. *Stroke* 25:704–707, 1994.
29. Chabriat H, Tournier-Lasserve E, Vahedi K, et al: Autosomal dominant migraine with MRI white matter abnormalities mapping to the CADASIL locus. *Neurology* 45:1086–1091, 1995.
30. Welch KMA, Levine SK, D'Andrea G, Helpern JA: Brain pH in migraine: An in vivo phosphorus-31 magnetic resonance spectroscopy study. *Cephalalgia* 8:273–277, 1988.
31. Welch KMA, Levine SR, D'Andrea G, et al: Preliminary observations on brain energy metabolism in migraine studied by in vivo phosphorus 31 NMR spectroscopy. *Neurology* 39:538–541, 1989.
32. Ramadan NM, Halvorson H, Vande-Linde AMQ, et al: Low brain magnesium in migraine. *Headache* 29:590–593, 1989.
33. Mauskop A, Altura BT, Ciullo RQ, Altura BM: Intravenous magnesium sulfate relieves migraine attacks in patients with low serum ionized magnesium levels: A pilot study. *Clin Sci* 89:633–636, 1995.
34. Mauskop A, Altura BT, Cracco RQ, Altura BM: Intravenous magnesium sulfate relieves cluster headaches in patients with low serum ionized magnesium levels. *Headache* 35:597–600, 1995.
35. Montagna P, Cortelli P, Monari L, et al: 31P-Magnetic resonance spectroscopy in migraine without aura. *Neurology* 44:666–669, 1994.
36. Schoenen J, Lenaerts M, Bastings E: High-dose riboflavin as a prophylactic treatment of migraine: Results of an open pilot study. *Cephalalgia* 14:328–329, 1994.
37. Sorensen GA, Tievsky AL, Ostergaard L, et al: Contrast agents in functional MR imaging. *JNRI* 7:47–55, 1997.
38. Cutrer FM, Sorensen AG, Weisskoff RM, et al: Brain perfusion defects during spontaneous migrainous aura identified by echo-planar magnetic resonance imaging. *Cephalalgia* 17:254, 1997.
39. Cao Y, Welch KMA, Aurora SK, Vikingstad E: Functional MRI (BOLD) of visually-triggered headache in migraine patients. *Cephalalgia* 17:254, 1997.
40. Cherry SR, Phelps ME: Positron emission tomography: Methods and instrumentation, in Sandler MP, Patton JA, Coleman RE, et al (eds): *Diagnostic Nuclear Medicine,* vol 1. Baltimore, Wilkins & Wilkins, 1996, pp 139–143.
41. Garnic JD, Schellinger D: Arterial spasm as a finding intimately associated with the onset of vascular headache. *Neuroradiology* 24:273–276, 1983.
42. Schulman EA, Hershey B: An unusual angiographic picture in status migrainous. *Headache* 31:396–398, 1991.
43. Shuaib A, Hachinski VC: Migraine and the risks from angiography. *Arch Neurol* 45:911–912, 1988.
44. Kudrow L: Cluster headache, in Goadsby PJ, Silberstein SD (eds): *Headache.* Boston, Butterworth-Heinemann, 1977, p 227.
45. Moskowitz MA: Cluster headache: Evidence for a pathophysiologic focus in the superior pericarotid cavernous sinus plexus. *Headache* 28:584–586, 1988.
46. Russell D, Nakstad P, Sjaastad O: Cluster headache—pneumoencephalographic and cerebral computerized axial tomography findings. *Headache* 18:272–273, 1978.
47. Sjaastad O, Rinck P: Cluster headache: MRI studies of the cavernous sinus and base of the brain. *Headache* 30:350–351, 1990.
48. Ekbom K, Greitz T: Carotid angiography in cluster headache. *Acta Radiol Diagn* 10:177–186, 1970.
49. Waldenlind E, Ekbom K, Torhall J: MR-angiography during spontaneous attacks of cluster headache: A case report. *Headache* 33:291–295, 1993.
50. Gawel MJ, Krajewski A, Luo YM, Ichise M: The cluster diathesis. *Headache* 30:652–655, 1990.
51. Sianard-Gainko J, Milet J, Ghuysen V, Schoenen J: Increased parasellar activity on Gallium SPECT is not specific for active cluster headache. *Cephalalgia* 14:132–133, 1994.
52. Montagna P, Lodi R, Cortelli P, et al: Phosphorus magnetic resonance spectroscopy in cluster headache. *Neurology* 48:113–118, 1997.
53. Kudrow L: Plasma testosterone levels in cluster headache: Preliminary results. *Headache* 16:28–31, 1976.
54. Tajti J, Sas K, Szok D, et al: Clusterlike headache as a first sign of brain metastases of lung cancer. *Headache* 36:259–260, 1996.
55. Gridley T: Notch, stroke and dementia. *Nature* 383:673, 1996.
56. Chabriat H, Vahedi K, Iba-Zizen MT, et al: Clinical spectrum of CADASIL: A study of 7 families. *Lancet* 346:934–938, 1995.
57. Hirano M, Pavlakis SG: Mitochondrial myopathy, encephalopathy, lactic acidosis, and stroke-like episodes (MELAS): Current concepts. *J Child Neurol* 9:4–13, 1994.
58. Clark JM, Marks MP, Adalsteinsson E, et al: MELAS: Clinical and pathologic correlations with MRI, Xenon/CT, and MR spectroscopy. *Neurology* 46:223–227, 1996.
59. Matthews P, Tampieri D, Berkovic S, et al: Magnetic resonance imaging shows specific abnormalities in the MELAS syndrome. *Neurology* 41:1043–1046, 1991.
60. Morita K, Ono S, Fukunaga M, et al: Increased accumulation of N-isopropyl-p-(^{123}I)-iodoamphetamine in two cases with mitochondrial encephalomyopathy with lactic acidosis and stroke-like episodes (MELAS). *Neuroradiology* 31:358–361, 1989.
61. Seyama K, Suzuki K, Mizuno Y, et al.: Mitochondrial encephalomyopathy with lactic acidosis and stroke-like episodes with special reference to the mechanism of cerebral manifestations. *Acta Neurol Scand* 80:561–568, 1989.
62. Martinuzzi A, Bartolomei L, Carrozzo R, et al: Correlation between clinical and molecular features in two MELAS families. *J Nucl Med* 31:1740–1742, 1990.
63. Grunwald F, Zierz S, Broich K, et al: HMPAO-SPECT imaging resembling Alzheimer-type dementia in mitochondrial encephalomyopathy with lactic acidosis and stroke-like episodes (MELAS). *J Nucl Med* 31:1740–1742, 1990.
64. Suzuki T, Koizumi J, Shiraishi H, et al: Mitochondrial encephalomyopathy (MELAS) with mental disorder CT, MRI and SPECT findings. *Neuroradiology* 32:74–76, 1990.

65. Satoh M, Ishikawa N, Yoshizawa T, et al: N-isopropyl-p-(^{123}I)iodoamphetamine SPECT in MELAS syndrome: Comparison with CT and MRI imaging. *J Comput Assist Tomogr* 15:77–82, 1992.
66. Matthews P, Andermann F, Silver K et al: Photon MR spectroscopic characterization of differences in regional brain metabolic abnormalities in mitochondrial encephalomyopathies. *Neurology* 43:2484–2490, 1993.
67. Barkovich A, Good W, Koch J, Berg B: Mitochondrial disorders: Analysis of their clinical and imaging characteristics. *AJNR* 14:1119–1137, 1993.
68. Pavlakis SG, Phillips PC, DiMauro S, et al: Mitochondrial myopathy, encephalopathy, lactic acidosis, and stroke-like episodes: A distinctive clinical syndrome. *Ann Neurol* 16:481–488, 1984.
69. Kotagal S, Peterson PL, Marten ME, et al: Impaired NADH-COQ reductase activity in a child with moyamoya syndrome. *Pediatr Neurol* 4:241–244, 1988.
70. Rassmussen BK: Epidemiology, in Olesen J, Tfelt-Hansen P, Welch KMA (eds): *The Headaches.* New York, Raven Press, 1993, pp 15–20.
71. Rooke Ed: Benign exertional headache. *Med Clin North Am* 52:801–808, 1968.
72. Symonds C: Cough headache. *Brain* 79:557–568, 1956.
73. Williams B: Cough headache due to craniospinal pressure dissociation. *Arch Neurol* 37:226–230, 1980.
74. Rushton JG, Rooke ED: Brain tumor headache. *Headache* 2:147–152, 1962.
75. Raskin N: Headaches associated with organic diseases of the nervous system. *Med Clin North Am* 62:459–466, 1978.
76. Saper JR, Silberstein SD, Gordon CD, Hamel RL: *Handbook of Headache Management.* Baltimore, Williams & Wilkins, 1993, p 31.
77. Forsyth PA, Posner JB: Headache in patients with brain tumors: A study of 111 patients. *Neurology* 43:1678–1683, 1993.
78. Lipton RB, Ferara ER, Weiss G, et al: Headache and HIV-1-related disorders. *Headache* 31:518–522, 1991.
79. Ramadan NM: Unusual causes of headache. *Neurology* 48:1494–1499, 1997.
80. Arboix A, Massons J, Oliveres M, et al: Headache in acute cerebrovascular disease: A prospective clinical study in 240 patients. *Cephalalgia* 14:37–40, 1994.
81. Edmeads JG: Headache as a symptom of organic diseases. *Curr Opin Neurol* 8:223–236, 1995.
82. Melo TP, Pinto AN, Ferro JM: Headache in intracerebral hematomas. *Neurology* 47:494–500, 1996.
83. Caplan LR, Stern BJ, Diringer M, et al: *Continuum: Vascular Diseases.* Cleveland, Advanstar Communications, 1996, p 73.
84. Weir B: Headache from aneurysms. *Cephalalgia* 14:79–87, 1994.
85. Leblanc R: The minor leak preceding subarachnoid hemorrhage. *J Neurosurg* 66:35–39, 1987.
86. Jakobsson KE, Saveland H, Hillman J, et al: Warning leak and management outcome in aneurysmal subarachnoid hemorrhage. *J Neurosurg* 85:995–999, 1996.
87. Day JW, Raskin NH: Thunderclap headache: Symptoms of unruptured cerebral aneurysm. *Lancet* 2:1247–1248, 1986.
88. Walton JN: *Subarachnoid Hemorrhage.* Edinburgh, E & S Livingstone, 1956.
89. van Gijn J, van Dongen KJ: The time course of aneurysmal hemorrhage on computed tomograms. *Neuroradiology* 23:153–156, 1982.
90. Wijdicks EFM, Kerkhoff H, vanGijn J: Long-term followup of 71 patients with thunderclap headache mimicking subarachnoid hemorrhage. *Lancet* 2:68–70, 1988.
91. Raps EC, Rogers JD, Galetta SL, et al: The clinical spectrum of unruptured intracranial aneurysms. *Arch Neurol* 50:265–268, 1993.
92. deBruijn SF, Stam J, Kapelle LJ: Thunderclap headache as the first symptom of cerebral venous sinus thrombosis. *Lancet* 348:1623–1625, 1997.
93. Dodick DW, Wijdicks EFM, Pituitary apoplexy presenting as thunderclap headache. *Neurology* 50:1510–1511, 1998.
94. Monteiro JMP, Rosas MJ, Correia AP, Vaz AR: Migraine and intracranial vascular malformations. *Headache* 33:563–565, 1993.
95. Morales F, Mostacero E, Marta J, Sanchez S: Vascular malformation of the cerebellopontine angle associated with SUNCT syndrome. *Cephalalgia* 14:301–302, 1994.
96. Ott D, Bien S, Kraszai L: Embolization of a tentorial dural arteriovenous fistula presenting as atypical trigeminal neuralgia. *Headache* 33:503–508, 1993.
97. Chiba S, Nishioka H, Saitoh M, et al: Cervical dural arteriovenous malformation presenting with right-sided occipitalgia: Before and after successful treatment by embolization. *Headache* 34:234–236, 1994.
98. Rozen TD, Swanson JW: Post gamma knife headache: A new headache syndrome? *Headache* 37:180–183, 1997.
99. Mokri B: Headache in spontaneous carotid and vertebral artery dissections, in Goadsby PJ, Silberstein SD (eds): *Headache.* Boston, Butterworth-Heinemann, 1992, pp 327–354.
100. Schievink WI, Mokri B, Whisnant JP: Internal carotid artery dissection in a community: Rochester, Minnesota 1987–1992. *Stroke* 24:1678–1680, 1993.
101. D'Anglejan-Chatillon J, Ribeiro V, Mas JL, et al: Migraine: A risk factor for dissection of cervical arteries. *Headache* 29:560–561, 1989.
102. Mokri B, Sundt TM, Houser W, Piepgras DG: Spontaneous dissection of the cervical internal carotid artery. *Ann Neurol* 19:126–30, 1986.
103. Mokri B: Traumatic and spontaneous extracranial internal carotid artery dissections. *J Neurol* 237:356–361, 1990.
104. Silbert PL, Mokri B, Schievink WI: Headache and neck pain in spontaneous internal carotid and vertebral artery dissections. *Neurology* 45:1517–1522, 1995.
105. Mokri B, Houser W, Sandok BA, Piepgras DG: Spontaneous dissection of the vertebral arteries. *Neurology* 38:880–885, 1988.
106. Russell DS, Rubinstein W: *Pathology of Tumors of the Nervous System,* 4th ed. Baltimore, Williams & Wilkins, 1977.
107. Young WB, Silberstein SD: Paroxysmal headache caused by colloid cyst of the third ventricle: Case report and review of the literature. *Headache* 37:15–20, 1997.
108. Kelly R: Colloid cysts of the third ventricle: Analysis of 29 cases. *Brain* 74:23–65, 1951.
109. Young WB, Packard RC: Posttraumatic headache and posttraumatic syndrome, in Goadsby PJ, Silberstein SD (eds): *Headache.* Boston, Butterworth-Heinemann, 1997, p 277.

110. Pfeller JD, Chibralt JT, Duckro PN: Postconcussion symptoms and cognitive functioning in posttraumatic headache patients. *Headache* 34:503–507, 1994.
111. Rimel RW, Giordani B, Barth JT, et al: Disability caused by minor head injury. *Neurosurgery* 9:221–228, 1981.
112. Weiss HD, Stern BJ, Goldbert J: Posttraumatic migraine: Chronic migraine precipitated by minor head or neck trauma. *Headache* 21:451–456, 1986.
113. Evans RW: The postconcussion syndrome and the sequelae of mild head injury. *Neurol Clin* 10:815–847, 1992.
114. Silberstein S, Marcelis J: Pseudotumor cerebri without papilledema. *Headache* 30:304, 1990.
115. Jensen OK, Nielsen FF: The influence of sex and pretraumatic headache on the incidence and severity of headache after head injury. *Cephalalgia* 10:285–293, 1990.
116. Yamaguchi M: Incidence of headache and severity of head injury. *Headache* 32:427–431, 1992.
117. Rutherford WH: Postconcussion symptoms, in Levin HS, Eisenberg HM, Berton AZ (eds): *Mild Head Injury.* New York, Oxford University Press, 1989, p 217.
118. Kelly AB, Snow RB, Zimmerman RD, et al: Comparison of magnetic resonance imaging and computed tomography in the evaluation of head injury. *Neurosurgery* 18:45–52, 1986.
119. Levin HS, Amparo E, Eisenberg HM, et al: Magnetic resonance imaging and computerized tomography in relation to the neurobehavioral sequelae of mild and moderate head injuries. *J Neurosurg* 66:706–713, 1987.
120. Masdeu JC, Abdel-Dayhem H, Van Heertum RL: Head trauma: Use of SPECT. *J Neuroimaging* 5:S53–7, 1995.
121. Report of the Therapeutics and Technology Assessment Subcommittee of the American Academy of Neurology: Assessment of brain SPECT. *Neurology* 46:278–285, 1996.
122. Rao N, Turski PA, Polcyn RE, et al: 18F Positron emission computed tomography in closed head injury. *Arch Phys Med Rehabil* 65:780–785, 1984.
123. Lay CL, Campbell JK, Mokri B: Low cerebrospinal fluid pressure headache, in Goadsby PJ, Silberstein SD (eds): *Headache.* Boston, Butterworth-Heinemann, 1997, pp 355–367.
124. Schaltenbrand G: Normal and pathological physiology of the cerebrospinal fluid circulation. *Lancet* 1:805, 1953.
125. Murros K, Fogelholm R: Spontaneous intracranial hypotension with slit ventricles. *J Neurol Neurosurg Psychiatry* 46:1149–1151, 1983.
126. Mokri B, Krueger BR, Miller GM, Piepgras DG: Meningeal gadolinium enhancement in low-pressure headache. *J Neuroimaging* 3:11, 1993.
127. Hochman MS, Naidich TP, Kobetz SA, Fernandez-Maitin A: Spontaneous intracranial hypotension with pachymeningeal enhancement on MRI. *Neurology* 42:1628–1630, 1992.
128. Fishman RA, Dillon WP: Dural enhancement and cerebral displacement secondary to intracranial hypotension. *Neurology* 43:609–611, 1993.
129. Maytal J, Bienkowski RS, Patel M, Eviatar L: The value of brain imaging in children with headaches. *Pediatrics* 96:413–416, 1995.
130. Wober-Bingol C, Wober C, Prayer D, et al: Magnetic resonance imaging for recurrent headache in childhood and adolescence. *Headache* 36:83–90, 1996.
131. Diamond S, Dalessio DJ: Additional studies are sometimes necessary in investigating headache, in *The Practicing Physician's Approach to Headache,* 2nd ed. Baltimore, Williams & Wilkins, 1978, pp 39–50.
132. Sargent JD, Solbach P: Medical evaluation of migraineurs: Review of the value of laboratory and radiologic tests. *Headache* 23:62–65, 1983.
133. NIH Consensus Development Panel: Computed tomographic scanning of the brain, in *Proceedings from the National Institutes of Health Consensus Development Conference Summary,* vol 4 (2). Bethesda, MD: National Institutes of Health, U.S. Government Printing Office, 1982.
134. Akpek S, Arac M, Atilla S, et al: Cost-effectiveness of computed tomography in the evaluation of patients with headache. *Headache* 35:228–230, 1995.
135. Demaerel P, Boelaert I, Wilms G, Baert AL: The role of cranial computed tomography in the diagnostic workup of headache. *Headache* 36:347–348, 1996.
136. Kuhn MJ, Shekar PC: A comparative study of MRI and CT in evaluation of migraine. *Comput Med Imaging Graphics* 14:149–152, 1990.
137. Practice parameter: The utility of neuroimaging in the evaluation of headache in patients with normal neurologic examinations (summary statement): Report of the Quality Standards Subcommittee of the American Academy of Neurology. *Neurology* 44:1353–1354, 1994.
138. Frishberg BM: The utility of neuroimaging in the evaluation of headache in patients with normal neurologic examinations. *Neurology* 44:1191–1197, 1994.
139. Fitzpatrick R, Hopkins A: Referrals to neurologists for headaches not due to structural disease. *J Neurol Neurosurg Psychiatry* 44:1061–1067, 1981.

SECTION THREE

DISORDERS OF THE SPECIAL SENSES

CHAPTER 5

DISTURBANCES OF VISION, OCULAR MOVEMENT, AND PUPILLARY FUNCTION

Carl Ellenberger, Jr.

INTRODUCTION

Neuro-ophthalmology had its beginnings when the brain was almost a "black box" to diagnostic neuroimaging. The available noninvasive studies—skull films, electroencephalography (EEG), and nucleotide brain scans—rarely revealed a diagnosis. That was done through a careful analysis of symptoms, precise measurement of vision, and reasoning. Then, 25 years ago, computed tomography (CT) and magnetic resonance imaging (MRI) eliminated many of these diagnostic problems.

At one level of practice all patients with uncorrectable blurred vision or diplopia can be referred for neuroimaging, but that is a costly strategy. If the clinical problem is not understood, the results of a scan can be difficult to interpret. The topic addressed in this chapter is the rational selection and application of imaging techniques on the basis of the provisional clinical diagnosis to obtain the best diagnostic information. The best results are obtained when both the physician who examines the patient and the physician who interprets the images are familiar with the clinical problem, in particular the differential diagnosis, and know the diagnostic capabilities and limitations of each neuroimaging modality.

SYMPTOM-BASED APPROACH TO NEUROIMAGING DIAGNOSIS

Skillful clinical history-taking from patients with visual symptoms has not been outmoded by new technology; that is still the most important and revealing part of the diagnostic evaluation in the quest for clinical localization and differential diagnosis. Because of its complexity, the visual system (for the purposes of this chapter, including the ocular motor system) responds to dysfunction in a wide variety of ways, ranging from a solitary flash caused by a retinal tear to a complex visual hallucination, but its precise topographic organization allows symptoms to be assigned to a specific level (retina, chiasm, optic radiations, etc.). Because a myriad of transient disturbances occur, localization of lesions through an analysis of symptoms may provide the only clue to their origin.

Transient Visual Symptoms

In general, the diagnosis of the cause of transient visual symptoms relies on a thorough description from the patient of the onset, character, duration, and time pattern of recurrence. Transient symptoms express transient disturbance of function, and if vision is normal between episodes, the results of neuroimaging also may be normal. However, to the extent that an episode is atypical, the chance of discovering an unusual cause increases: For example, an hourlong or repetitive fortification pattern resembling migrainous visual loss may actually result from a brain infarction, such as a "strokelike" episode in a patient with mitochondrial encephalopathy.[1] Similarly, a 2-h episode of transient monocular blindness, which typically is a 5-min symptom, suggests an unusual cause (see below) or the possibility of an accompanying brain infarction in the carotid vascular territory.

Monocular Transient Visual Symptoms

Flashes and floaters are the designations given to momentary bright (flashes) or small dark and floating images that originate from vitreoretinal pathology, such as vitreous separation or opacities, and retinal tears, holes, and detachment. They are usually brief, like fireworks, and do not gradually expand or travel over minutes, as do migrainous visual symptoms. Most important, their cause can best be seen by a skilled fundoscopist using an indirect instrument or slit lamp biomicroscopy. Office ultrasound enables the examiner to view these lesions in depth, but only on the rare occasions when papilledema is the cause[2] is CT or MRI valuable in investigating them.

"Amaurosis Fugax" (Transient Monocular Blindness) Like other transient ischemic attacks, amaurosis fugax (AF) indicates an increased risk of stroke. However, in general, the risk is smaller than it is after most other types of transient ischemia (even among patients with significant carotid stenosis[3]) only partly because most series of patients with AF include younger patients who have a variety of nonatherosclerotic causes for this symptom,[4–8] including those with antiphospholipid antibodies.[9] Only about two-thirds of patients with AF have stenotic carotid disease, reflecting the diversity of mechanisms and circumstances of causation: (1) embolic,[10] (2) vasospastic,[11,12] and (3) hemodynamic. Ulceration of stenotic carotid plaques may be a particularly important risk factor,[13] whereas cardiogenic embolism may not.[14] Clinical distinction may be difficult in any individual case.[15]

Ultrasound examination of the carotid arterial bifurcations has proved to be a useful and increasingly accurate noninvasive screening test for carotid stenosis that should be applied to patients with AF that is suspected of having an atherosclerotic cause.[16–19] Numerous studies have validated the sensitivity and accuracy of Doppler testing of carotid flow, but reliability still varies among individual laboratories. Percutaneous angiography remains the most sensitive and accurate means of evaluating the lumen of the carotid artery, but improved MR angiography shows promise of eventually replacing it (Fig. 5-1).[18,20–23] New techniques such as magnetization transfer contrast (MTC), multiple overlapping thin slab acquisitions (MOTSA), and gadolinium enhancement improve image quality, demonstrate the relationship of vessels and adjacent tissues, and provide three-dimensional images that can be viewed from any angle.[23,24] A combination of Doppler ultrasound followed by MR angiography holds promise of providing a balance between the risk of percutaneous angiography and the accuracy needed to make informed therapeutic decisions.[25,26] Spiral CT angiography also holds promise in evaluating carotid stenosis.[27]

Atypical, especially prolonged, AF suggests that a cerebral infarct may have occurred "silently"[28] or gives a clue to one of the rare mechanisms, including some that might visualize by neuroimaging techniques: dural arteriovenous malformation,[29,30] ethmoid artery arteriovenous malformation,[31] orbital lesions (causing gaze-evoked monocular blackouts),[32,33] and pituitary tumors.[34]

Another rare variation of AF is "unilateral visual loss in bright light," a prolonged cloudiness of vision that occurs when an individual enters a bright environment from relative darkness. In these patients, ischemia from reduced ipsilateral carotid perfusion may prolong retinal light adaptation.[35,36] When it is bilateral, this syndrome may be confused with occipital ischemia.[37] The "ocular ischemic syndrome" (monocular visual loss, often with a "red eye," related to reduced perfusion of the globe) provides a warning of serious cardiovascular or cerebrovascular complications.[38]

Monocular or Binocular Transient Visual Symptoms

Transient visual obscurations (TVOs) are momentary binocular or monocular "grayouts" or "blackouts" of vision that last only seconds, often in response to assuming an upright position.[39] Optic nerve axons, usually swollen by papilledema, are confined by the rigid walls of the scleral canal in the globe, creating increased cross-sectional pressure that reduces arterial circulation. When systemic arterial pressure falls, usually as a result of orthostasis, the optic nerve head becomes momentarily ischemic. Not all patients with papilledema have TVOs; those who do not probably have congenitally larger scleral canals, as evidenced by a generous-size physiologic optic cup when the disc is not swollen. Occasionally drusen, the debris in the optic disc of axons destroyed by chronic papilledema or by a congenitally small scleral canal, may be visible on CT or MRI,[40] but the view through the ophthalmoscope is better and more diagnostic.

MRI has aided the delineation of the syndrome of "orthostatic headaches and diffuse pachymeningeal

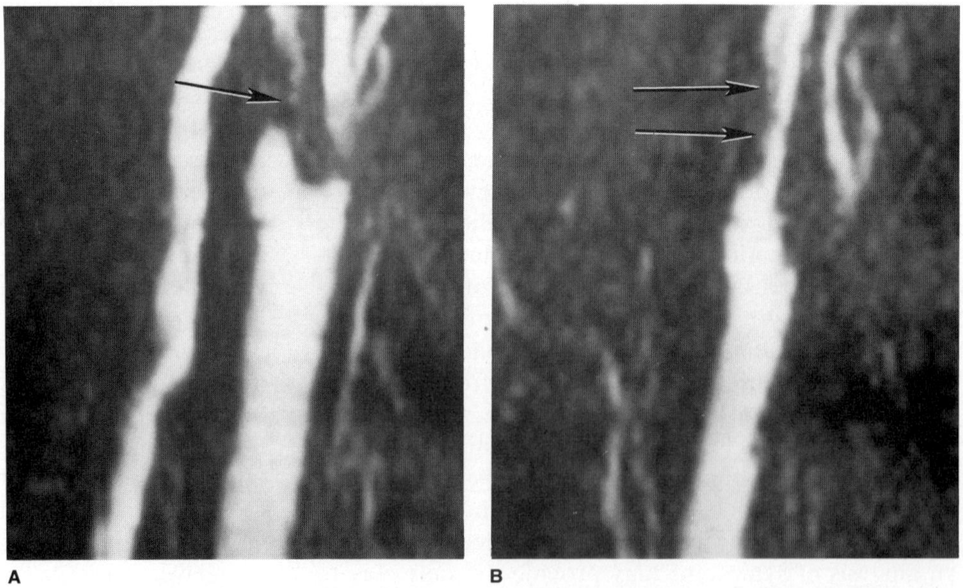

A B

Figure 5-1
MR angiography of internal carotid artery stenosis: **(A)** *>95 percent stenosis of the origin of the right internal carotid artery (arrow) and a dominant right vertebral artery (to the left);* **(B)** *80 to 90 percent stenosis of the long segment of the left internal carotid artery (arrows). Both external carotid arteries (to the right) are severely stenotic.*

server can distinguish with high accuracy the white matter lesions of MS from those caused by other conditions.[95] This degree of accuracy is not always achieved in community practice. Variability exists among observers even in the estimation of the number of white matter lesions.[96] It is unfortunate when a patient with visual or neurologic symptoms is discovered to have white matter lesions on MRI and is labeled erroneously with the diagnosis of MS.

Another problem is that limited follow-up studies so far have not totally clarified the meaning of MRI white matter lesions. Clearly, the incidence and number of focal cerebral white matter lesions among patients with initial monosymptomatic optic neuritis exceed those in the general population. Prospectively, Frederiksen and colleagues[97] found focal white matter lesions on MRI in 63 percent of patients with an initial episode of optic neuritis. Seven (14 percent) of the patients with an abnormal MRI developed clinical MS by 20 months; none with normal MRI did. Jacobs and colleagues[98] found 42 of 74 patients (57 percent) with isolated monosymptomatic optic neuritis to have 1 to 20 brain lesions by MRI. All the brain lesions were clinically silent and had characteristics consistent with MS. None of these patients had ever experienced neurologic symptoms before the episode of optic neuritis. During 5.6 years of follow-up, 21 patients (28 percent) developed definite MS on clinical grounds. These authors concluded that finding an abnormal MRI at the time of optic neuritis was significantly related to the subsequent development of MS on clinical grounds, but abnormal IgG levels in the CSF correlated even more strongly than did abnormal MRIs with the subsequent development of clinically definite MS. Similarly, long-term follow-up of 388 patients who entered the optic neuritis treatment trial showed a cumulative 5-year probability of developing MS of 30 percent (irrespective of treatment group),[99] with that probability ranging from 16 percent in patients with no MRI brain lesions at the onset of optic neuritis to 51 percent in patients with more than three. Lack of pain, the presence of optic disc swelling, and mild loss of visual acuity were features associated with the lowest risk of MS among patients with no MRI lesions.

Uhthoff's symptom (worsening of vision with a rise in body temperature) in patients with an abnormal MRI seems to indicate a greater risk of recurrent optic neuritis and other symptoms of MS.[100]

Ischemic optic neuropathy (ION) is signaled by sudden monocular visual loss (usually segmental) accompanied by pale swelling of the optic disc; therefore, it is sometimes called "anterior" ION. The more common nonarteritic form probably results from the compounding of age-related circulatory changes in the anterior part of the optic nerve and anatomic constriction of the nerve and its circulation as they pass through a congenitally "tight" scleral canal in the ocular globe.[101–103] Transient systemic arterial hypotension—after blood loss, aggressive treatment of malignant hypertension, or even a dip in pessure during sleep—may be a pathogenetic factor that occasionally can be reversed to restore vision.[104] Neuroimaging is not necessary to establish this clinical diagnosis.

However, it is interesting to speculate that the lesion of ION, a small ischemic one, shares some characteristics with the common focal white matter lesions that are almost ubiquitous on MRI examinations of the brains of older individuals. Both share the same risk factors of diabetes and hypertension and have a similar histopathologic appearance.[105,106] One small study investigating the prevalence of focal white matter MRI lesions[107] among 11 patients with ION did not find an increased prevalence. A later study using more rigorous statistics did among 13 patients who presented with nonarteritic ION.[108] Optic neuropathy is a surprisingly rare (0.5 percent) accompaniment of stroke caused by carotid occlusion,[109] and in these cases the pale disc swelling of ION has not been observed, probably because the lesion occurs posteriorly.

Less commonly, "arteritic" anterior ION complicates giant-cell (temporal) arteritis because the extradural arteries that supply the optic nerve contain an elastic layer that is vulnerable in that condition. The diagnosis should be suspected in patients over age 50 years who have associated symptoms, including muscle aches (polymyalgia rheumatica) and new-onset temporal headache. If the optic disc is not tight (i.e., it has a generous optic cup), the diagnosis of the arteritic form of ION is more likely. An elevated sedimentation rate is further suggestive, and the diagnosis has been confirmed by biopsy of a temporal artery. Because of a small chance of false-negative biopsies resulting from "skip areas" of noninvolvement, the tradition of bilateral biopsy has prevailed. However, there are drawbacks to biopsy (stroke, skin necrosis, facial paralysis), as noted by Schmidt and colleagues, who achieved an accurate diagnosis with color duplex ultrasonography of the temporal arteries.[110] Confirmation of this new application of ultrasonography will be necessary.

Retinal stroke [central retinal artery occlusion (CRAO)] causes symptoms indistinguishable from those of ischemic optic neuropathy: sudden, usually painless, monocular visual loss. Examination discloses an afferent pupillary defect; sectoral, arcuate, or complete visual field loss; and retinal infarction. The same risk factors apply that are found with amaurosis fugax,[111] and an embolic pathogenesis is likely, usually emboli from a stenotic carotid bifurcation.[112]

Ultrasound examination of the carotid bifurcations is an easily available, noninvasive initial study in patients who have experienced retinal strokes, and its accuracy is increasing.[17] The sensitivity and specificity of MR angiography for carotid stenosis are also increasing (see above and Fig. 5-1).

Another form of retinal stroke, central or branch retinal venous occlusion, may cause a sudden monocular visual deficit. The diagnosis is based on its appearance. Retinal venous occlusion shares risk factors with retinal arterial occlusion: systemic arterial hypertension and diabetes.[113,114] Apart from its rare association with dural arteriovenous fistula,[115,116] no neuroimaging correlates have been discovered.

Other Causes of Acute Optic Neuropathy A wide variety of far less common causes of sudden optic neuropathy have been described, many of them presenting in a manner similar to that of the more common optic neuritis but all distinguished from it only by serendipitous discovery by neuroimaging. These cause include mucocele of the sphenoid sinus.[117–119] Delayed radionecrosis of the optic nerves may cause abrupt monocular visual loss and is demonstrable with gadolinium-enhanced MRI (Fig. 5-9).[120] Optic neuropathy with drusen may progress with sudden, stepwise visual loss,[121] and sudden visual loss may follow surgical relief of increased intracranial pressure in patients with papilledema.[122] Although intracranial mass lesions, including aneurysms, usually cause progressive visual loss, the rare examples of sudden loss, such as those which occur when a supraclinoid carotid aneurysm[123–125] or craniopharyngioma[126] suddenly expands to compress only one optic nerve, should not be mistaken for optic neuritis. Similarly, pituitary apoplexy in a patient with a postfixed optic chiasm may cause a monocular visual syndrome that is clinically indistinguishable from optic neuritis.[127,128] Other causes of acute optic neuropathy (a parasellar cavernous angioma, for example[129]) or lymphoma,[130] are too rare to list, but their combined total is significant enough to warrant consideration of MRI in most patients who experience sudden monocular visual loss at the time of its onset or after an interval of weeks if vision does not improve, with the timing based on the individual clinical presentation.

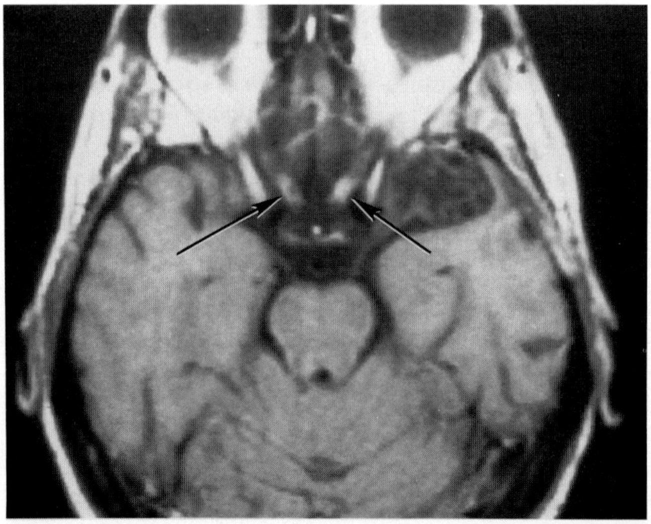

Figure 5-9
Axial spin echo T1 image after the administration of Gd-DTPA of a patient with binocular visual deficit after receiving more than 6000 Gy of radiation to treat a glioma in the temporal lobe. The prechiasmal segments of both optic nerves enhance after contrast administration (arrows). (Reprinted by permission of Little, Brown and Company, Publishers.)

The rare Leber optic neuropathy, which is recognized by its male sex-linked inheritance, characteristic parapapillary microangiopathy, and close sequential involvement of both eyes, may be difficult to distinguish from the more common demyelinative optic neuritis, especially when multifocal white matter lesions appear on MRI of the brain, as they do more often than can be accounted for by chance.[131] This association suggests to some researchers a mitochondrial genetic component in the etiology of MS.[132–134] An enlarged optic nerve sheath may suggest Leber optic neuropathy,[135,136] and point mutations in mitochondrial DNA may establish the diagnosis.[131,137]

Binocular Acute Visual Loss

Bitemporal Hemianopia Bitemporal hemianopia reliably indicates a chiasmal lesion if the field defect is truly hemianopic, that is, has a sharp border anywhere on the vertical meridian of the visual field. Because most chiasmal lesions are suprasellar tumors that grow slowly, the more common diagnostic challenge is to detect their insidious impairment of the visual fields, which sometimes is not noticed by patients and doctors alike. However, chiasmal field defects occasionally occur or advance suddenly, and then the differential diagnosis includes (1) pituitary apoplexy, (2) intrachiasmal angioma, (3) lymphocytic adenohypophysitis, and (4) demyelinating disease, in rough order of incidence. Other causes are rare enough to warrant a case report, such as a thrombosed aneurysm of the anterior communicating artery[138] and mucocele of the sphenoid sinus.[139] The capability of sagittal and coronal imaging, in addition to variability of signal characteristics and enhancement properties, makes MRI the clear diagnostic modality of choice.

Pituitary apoplexy, a life-threatening event, typically presents with sudden headache, visual loss (including diplopia and blindness), meningismus, and sometimes prostration.[140–142] Hemorrhage into an adenoma of any size can cause sudden expansion of the tumor, chiasmal compression, ocular motor dysfunction,[143] endocrine insufficiency, and circulatory collapse. The stress of surgery or general anesthesia,[144] the diagnostic use of gonadotrophin-releasing hormone,[145] the delivery of a baby (Sheehan syndrome),[146] and even certain medications, such as isosorbide,[147] sometimes seem to be the reason for hemorrhage into a previously silent macroadenoma. MRI is particularly helpful in demonstrating and dating hemorrhage within the tumor and defining

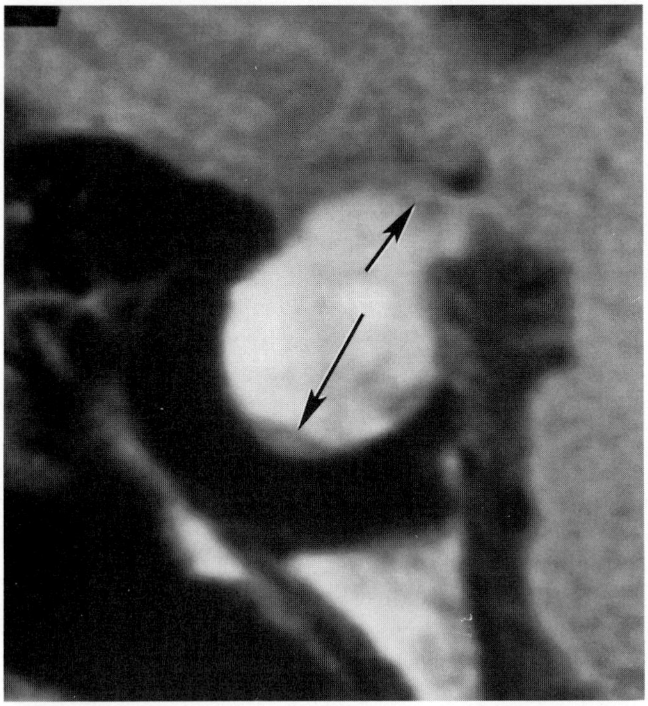

Figure 5-10
Sagittal T1 image without contrast of a 32-year-old man with sudden headache and bitemporal hemianopia showing a large hemorrhagic pituitary adenoma that depresses the sellar floor and elevates the optic chiasm (short arrow). A fluid-fluid level (arrow) indicates the cystic nature of the lesion. Anteriorly, the proteinaceous supernatant fluid shows marked T1 shortening. The dependent portion where cellular blood products accumulate also has high signal as a result of T1 shortening of methemoglobin.

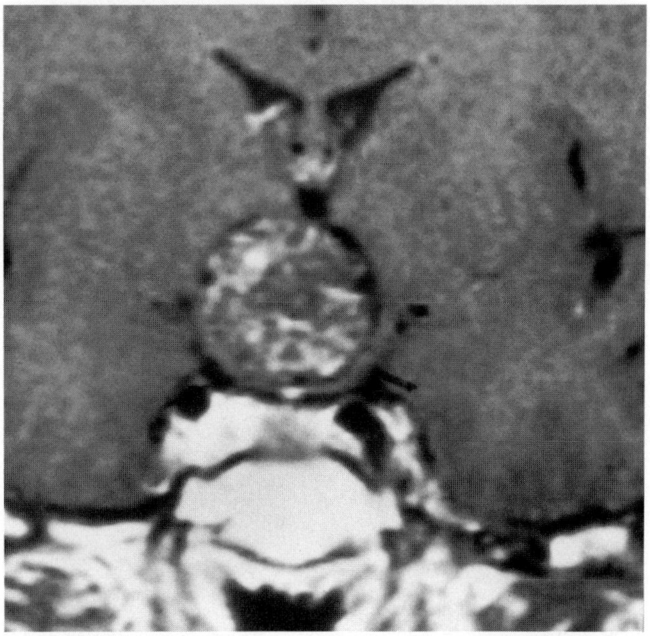

Figure 5-11
Coronal T1 postgadolinium image of a 22-year-old woman with bitemporal hemianopia showing a large suprasellar lesion. Enhancement of blood pool spaces confirms the diagnosis of a cavernous angioma.

the extent of its superior and lateral expansion, particularly its effect on the optic chiasm, and is useful for closely monitoring patients for whom nonoperative management has been selected (Fig. 5-10).[148] Hemorrhage and necrosis can occur in as many as 10 percent of pituitary adenomas without causing symptoms.[149–151] MRI reliably detects the rare intrasellar aneurysm masquerading as an apoplectic expansion of a solid tumor.[138]

Cavernous angioma or another type of vascular malformation may reside within the optic chiasm and cause sudden bitemporal hemianopia if it hemorrhages.[152–154] On CT the hemorrhagic lesion is a hyperdensity within the enlarged chiasm (Fig. 5-11). Each sudden worsening of the visual deficit, caused by recurrent hemorrhage, may be followed by substantial spontaneous improvement. Surgical intervention may subvert this natural healing process but also may decompress the chiasm by removing hemorrhagic necrosis.

Before MRI, cavernous angiomas ("cryptic" vascular anomalies that often are invisible on an angiogram) created diagnostic dilemmas and occasional biopsy attempts met with disaster. However, their appearance on MRI is usually diagnostic (Fig. 5-12).[155] They occur

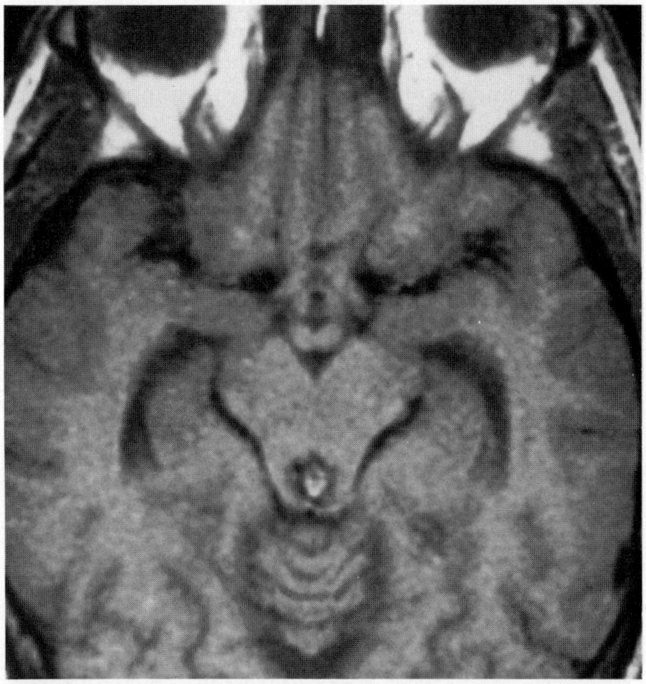

Figure 5-12
Axial spin echo T1 image of an 18-year-old man with biliateral fourth cranial neuropathy showing a typical cavernous angioma dorsal to the aqueduct at the level of the trochlear nuclei. The hypointensity represents hemosiderin.

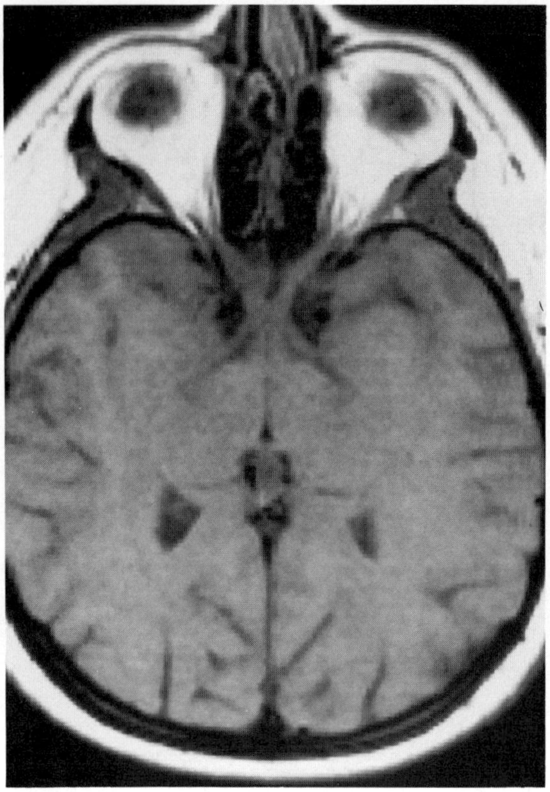

Figure 5-13
Axial T1 spin echo view showing the optic chiasm, optic nerves, and optic tracts. Large lesions lateral to the chiasm can compress all three structures.

anywhere in the brain and, when multiple, may be familial, especially in Hispanic individuals.[156]

Lymphocytic adenohypophysitis may be the cause of a relatively rapid onset of monocular or bitemporal visual impairment in a pregnant woman.[157–159] Perhaps through an autoimmune mechanism, chronic inflammation of the anterior pituitary gland may present as an intrasellar mass that compresses the anterior visual pathways, in some cases causing hypopituitarism and, if untreated, posing a genuine threat of permanent visual impairment. In most but not all[160] cases, corticosteroids reduce the size of the mass and restore vision. The sella turcica usually is not enlarged, helping to distinguish this entity from a pituitary adenoma.

Demyelinative chiasmal lesions are most notable for their rarity.[161–163] MRI is the ideal way to exclude more common causes of the chiasmal syndrome and confirm a diagnosis of demyelinating disease by detecting multiple other white matter lesions in the cerebrum.

Homonymous Hemianopia The hallmark of the optic tract syndrome is "grossly incongruous" homonymous hemianopia[164] (see also Ellenberger[165]). The main reason for the incongruity is involvement of the ipsilateral optic nerve, as well as the optic tract (Fig. 5-13), by a lesion lateral to the chiasm, and so the defect in the ipsilateral visual field is actually a combined hemianopic and monocular defect (and an ipsilateral afferent pupillary defect[166]) that localizes the lesion lateral to the optic chiasm. These extra-axial lesions include giant aneurysms, craniopharyngiomas, and AVMs in the ambient cistern.[162,164,167] Infarctions and demyelinating lesions are the common intra-axial causes of a sudden optic tract syndrome.

Lesions that cause sudden disturbance of conduction in the lateral geniculate nucleus and optic radiation are mostly vascular. Lesions in one hemisphere cause hemianopia; isolated hemianopia usually indicates an occipital lesion in the territory of a posterior cerebral artery (Fig. 5-14). Bilateral lesions cause bilateral hemianopia

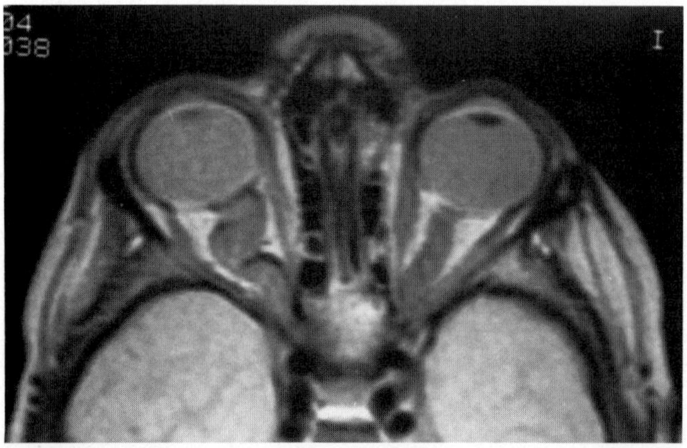

A

Figure 5-14
Axial proton-density image of an 8-year-old boy with type 1 neurofibromatosis showing **(A)** *bilateral diffuse enlargement of both optic nerves by an optic glioma.* **(B)** *coronal T2 image of the same patient showing enlargement of the optic chiasm (arrow).*

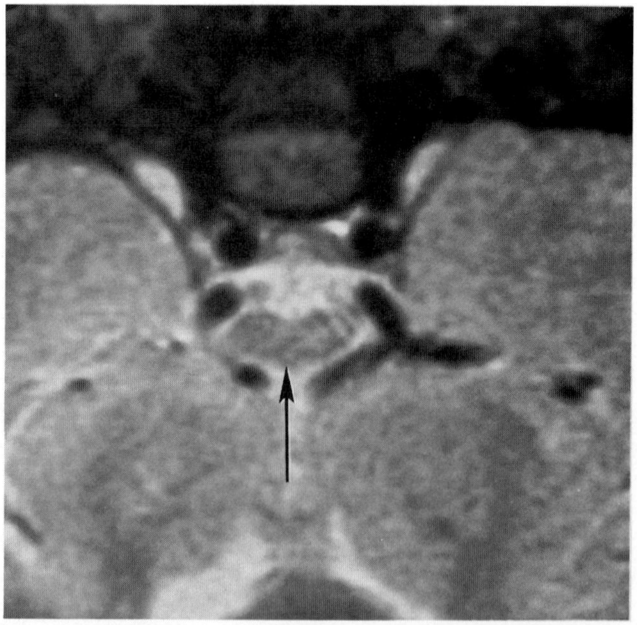

B

or "cortical," "cerebral," or "geniculocalcarine" blindness and result from the common origin of the blood supply to both occipital lobes, the basilar artery.

Neuroimaging has improved the definition of several vascular syndromes that include hemianopia:

Middle Cerebral Artery and Branches

1. *Anterior choroidal branch.* Infarction in this territory may cause hemianopia, hemiplegia, and hemianesthesia by infarction in the optic tract or the lateral geniculate nucleus.[168,169] CT shows an area of reduced density in the posterior limb of the internal capsule, sparing the thalamus medially and encroaching on the tip of the globus pallidus laterally, corresponding to the distribution of the anterior choroidal artery.[170,171] Analysis of risk factors suggests that the mechanism in most cases is small vessel disease. Rarely, the hemianopia may be isolated, erroneously suggesting posterior cerebral arterial (PCA) infarction.[172]
2. *Inferior division of the right middle cerebral artery.* Infarction in this territory may cause left homonymous hemianopia, left visual neglect, constructional apraxia, and an agitated confusional state characterized by hyperactivity, restlessness, and easy distractibility. Motor and sensory abnormalities are not severe or persistent. The most common mechanism is cardiogenic embolism.[173]
3. *Entire middle cerebral artery.* Infarction causes a typical contralateral hemiparetic syndrome, including hemianopia, in 30 percent of patients with long tapering occlusions of the middle cerebral artery (MCA) or its major divisions.[174] Hemianopia is just as likely to result from carotid occlusion as it is from middle cerebral artery occlusion.

Posterior Cerebral Artery

1. *Perimesencephalic portion or cortical branches.* Sudden isolated homonymous hemianopia most commonly indicates occipital infarction caused by embolic occlusion (Fig. 5-14).[175] Pessin and coworkers[176] studied 35 patients with CT-documented occipital infarction; most also had arteriography. Although embolism was the most common stroke mechanism, the list of causes was heterogeneous: cardiac source embolism (10 patients), vertebrobasilar atheroma with local embolism (6), migraine (5), systemic illness with presumed coagulopathy (3), and "unknown source embolism" after negative cardiac investigation (11 patients). A rare fetal PCA branching from the carotid artery may cause an exception.[176] When the patient is confused[177] or amnesic[178] as well, the infarction is likely to be on the left.
2. *Proximal branch.* Less commonly, hemianopia results from occlusion of the posterior choroidal artery that supplies part of the lateral geniculate nucleus. Bogousslavsky and associates[179] considered these cases and others that defined four ischemic thalamic syndromes to be caused by lacunar and embolic infarcts.
3. *Both posterior cerebral arteries.* Bilateral homonymous hemianopia (cortical, cerebral, or geniculocalcarine blindness) usually begins suddenly because it almost always results from the fact that both occipital lobes receive a common blood supply through the basilar artery. Thus, ischemia is a common mechanism by which a wide variety of etiologies cause cortical blindness, including vasospasm,[180] angiographic contrast material,[68] hemodialysis,[79] hypoglycemia,[77] hepatic encephalopathy,[78] seizures,[70] cyclosporine toxicity,[67] ornithine transcarbamoylase deficiency,[181] and hydrocephalus,[74] among countless others.[76] MRI almost always shows an occiptal abnormality.

   CT and MRI have confirmed the traditional clinical observations that (a) "macular sparing" (preservation of 5 to 10° of vision around the fixation point in a hemianopic field) results from collateral flow to the occipital poles via MCA branches, remaining patent after occlusion of the PCA, (b) sparing of a "temporal crescent" of the visual field indicates sparing of an anterior portion of the calcarine cortex,[182] and (c) the geniculocalcarine pathways are topographically organized with precision.[183] However, MRI studies of two patients suggest that the area of calcarine cortex that subserves central vision is larger than the traditional map drawn by Gordon Holmes.[184]
4. *"Top of the basilar" syndrome* is most often due to an embolus. Infarction of rostral brainstem and cerebral hemispheral regions fed by the distal basilar artery causes visual, ocular motor, and behavioral abnormalities and sometimes somnolence, vivid hallucinations, and dreamlike behavior, often without significant motor dysfunction. Temporal and occipital infarctions may cause hemianopia with fragments of Balint syndrome, amnestic dysfunction, and agitated behavior.[185]
5. *Thalamic hemorrhage* causes hemianopia in 40 percent of cases.[186] Weisberg studied 50 patients with thalamic hemorrhage by CT; 84 percent were hypertensive. Five patients had hematomas less than 8 mm and signs that resolved within 4 days; they could have been miscontrued to have had transient ischemic attacks (TIAs). Nineteen had a larger hemorrhage and intraventricular hemorrhage, impaired consciousness, hemiparesis, and pupillary abnormalities; 12 had vertical gaze impairment, and all 19 of these patients died.

Progressive Visual Loss

Monocular Progressive Visual Loss

In general, progressive, uncorrectable monocular visual loss (in the absence of ocular causes such as glaucoma, retinal diseases, and opacities in the ocular media) is caused by progressively expanding lesions, mainly tumors, intrinsic to, surrounding, or compressing the optic nerve. Central vision is impaired early, and tests of visual function reveal central defects in the visual fields, impaired color vision, and an afferent pupillary defect.

Optic and Chiasmatic-Hypothalamic Glioma Since the observations of Verhoeff in 1922 and then those of Hoyt and Baghdassarian,[187] it has been apparent that some of these tumors may not inexorably progress (even though they are probably not hamartomas, as Verhoeff suggested[188]). That observation or, more accurately, the variable aggressivity of these tumors, which is partly related to age at onset and location, created controversy regarding their management. The controversy has been mitigated by modern neuroimaging techniques that permit close observation of the progress of the tumors, allowing intervention by surgery, radiotherapy, and chemotherapy when progression is detected, especially when the tumor threatens to extend beyond the orbit (Fig. 5-15). MRI, utilizing fat-supression techniques and contrast enhancement, is the current method of choice. A substantial proportion of patients with optic or chiasmal gliomas have neurofibromatosis, a possibly favorable prognostic factor.[189,190] However, in these patients optic glioma should raise the suspicion of other central nervous system (CNS) neoplasms.[191] In adults, gliomas of the anterior visual pathways are inevitably aggressive and fatal.[192]

Meningioma Very slowly progressive monocular visual loss (over years) is the hallmark of a meningioma compressing the optic nerve from the sphenoid wing, tuberculum sellae, planum sphenoidale, or elsewhere in the neighborhood of the anterior visual pathways. A pale congested optic disc and optociliary veins indicate that the tumor has invaded the perioptic meninges and is strangling the optic nerve.[193,194] Total excision of a meningioma within the meninges is next to impossible. Gadolinium-enhanced MRI is the most sensitive method of detecting almost inevitable postoperative residual bone and intracranial dural involvement as well as frequent tumor recurrence, and radiation therapy may halt progression[195] or delay recurrence.[196,197]

MRI is becoming the neuroimaging method of first choice, again with fat-suppression techniques, because most of the optic nerve is surrounded by orbital fat. Enhanced images are proving to be the best way to detect intracranial extension of orbital tumors and orbital extension of intracranial tumors.[198] CT is still an alternative (Fig. 5-16) and has the advantage of demonstrating calcium in a substantial number of cases.[199] Sarcoidosis involving the optic nerve,[200] Tolosa-Hunt syndrome,[201] and lymphoma of the optic nerve (Fig. 5-17)[202,203] may be difficult to distinguish from meningioma in the orbit or orbital apex.

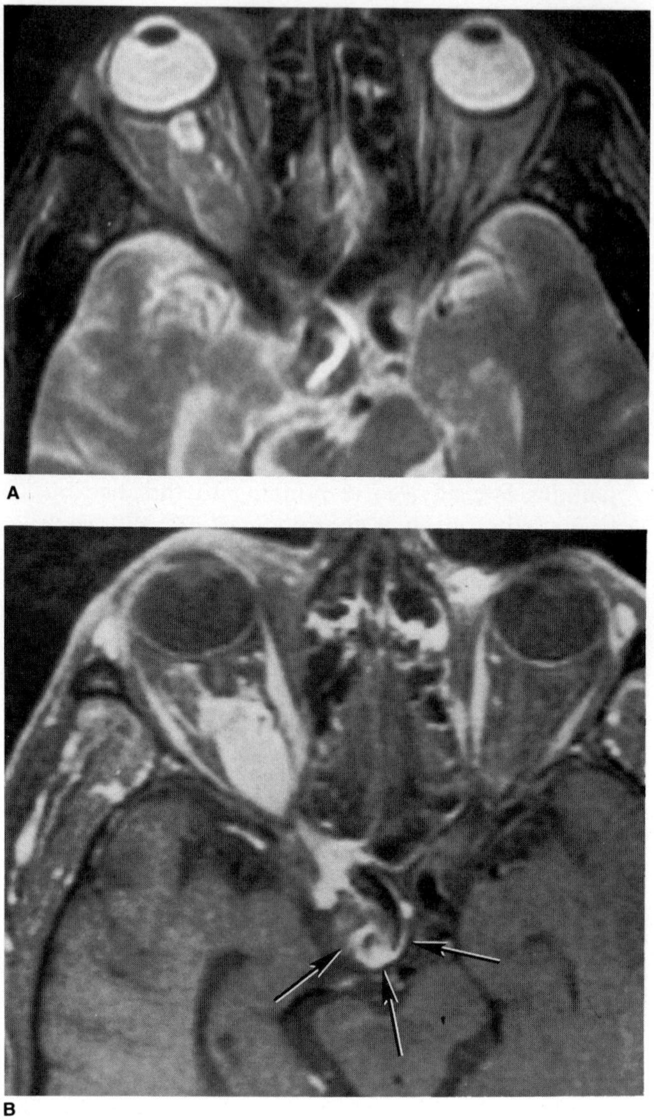

Figure 5-15
MRIs of a 58-year-old man with progressive loss of vision of the right eye. **(A)** *Axial T2 image shows fusiform low-intensity soft tissue (meningioma) along the axis of the right optic nerve.* **(B)** *Postgadolinium axial T1 image demonstrates diffuse enhancement of the meningioma extending proximally into the optic chiasm. Note the presence of a curvilinear signal void of a giant aneurysm of the supraclinoid carotid artery (arrows), also seen in* **A.**

Binocular Progressive Visual Loss

Bitemporal Hemianopia

"Empty Sella"

No particular set of symptoms suggests the "empty sella syndrome," and so the term *syndrome* may not be ap-

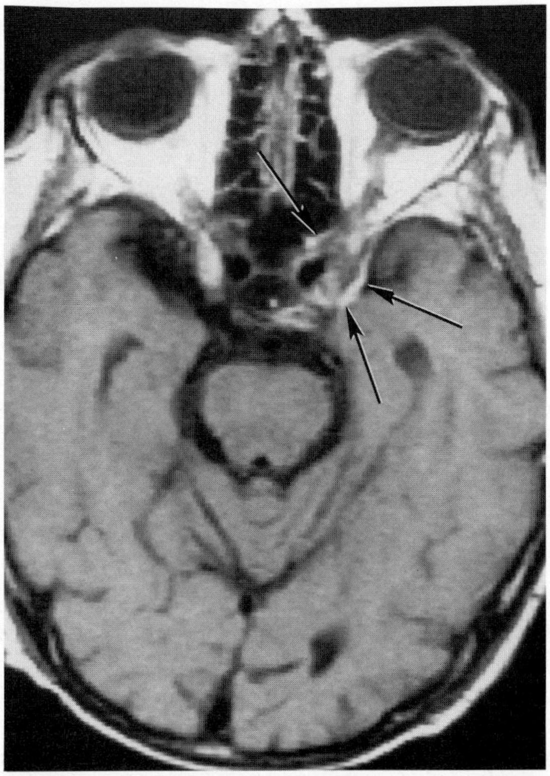

Figure 5-16
Axial T1 spin echo MRI after the administration of Gd-DTPA showing an ill-defined, partially enhancing lesion involving the prechiasmal and intracanalicular portions of the optic nerve and the orbital apex (arrows). The lesion, in a patient with lymphoma, responded to corticosteroids.

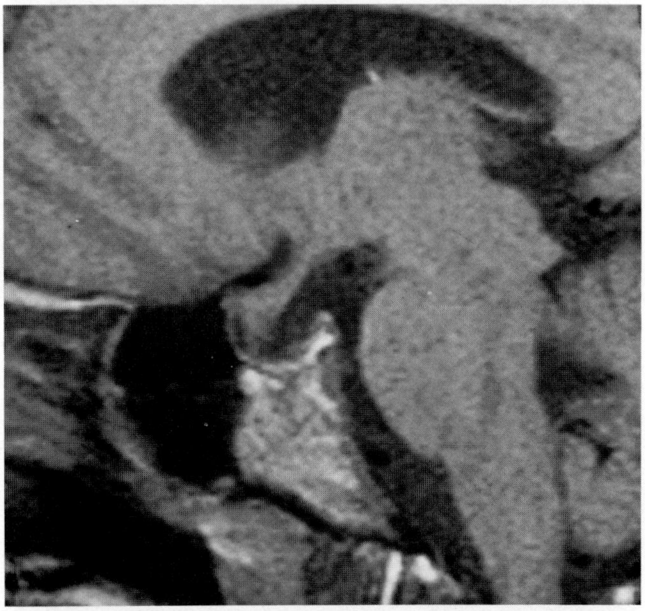

A

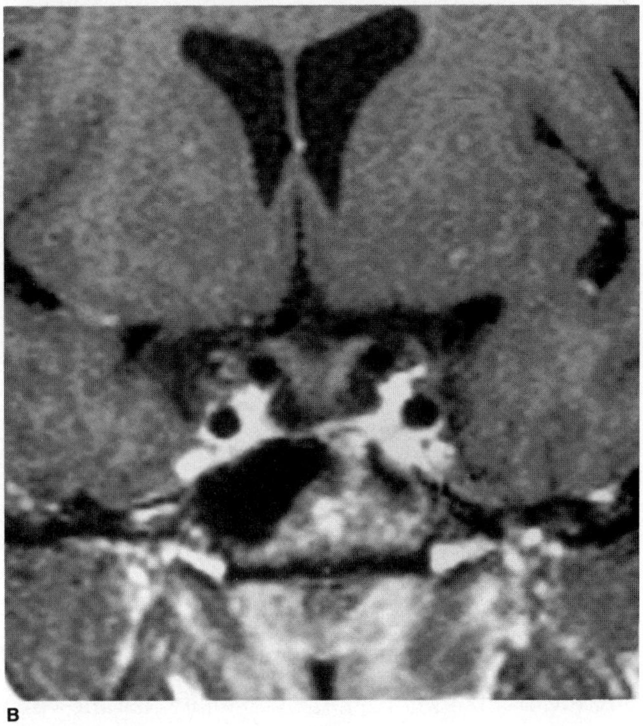

B

Figure 5-17
Sagittal **(A)** *and coronal* **(B)** *T1 MRIs of a 34-year-old woman with an empty sella turcica resulting from ischemic necrosis of the pituitary gland causing prolapse of the optic chiasm almost to the sellar floor.*

propriate for that reason and because an empty sella can be a part of several other syndromes. An empty sella is most often an incidental finding on neuroimaging studies. Confusion is introduced into reports of patients with an empty sella because of the mixing of patients with enlarged and empty sellas and patients with normal-sized, partially empty sella turcicas; the latter usually are benign variants of the norm.

The fact that an enlarged and empty sella can result from long-standing increased intracranial pressure has been established, explaining its frequent discovery among overweight young women with pseudotumor cerebri.[204–206] Also established is the fact that spontaneous involution, mainly resulting from infarction and necrosis of pituitary adenomas, can leave a large empty sella that often is associated with endocrine defects.[207–209] The remaining patients have empty sellas from a variety of causes, including congenital factors such as an incompetent diaphragma sellae.[208]

Visual symptoms associated with an empty sella are rare.[210] One suspects that they more often relate to residual effects of chiasmal compression by an involuted pituitary adenoma than to later "herniation" of the anterior visual pathways into the sella,[211,212] although such herniation may result from pituitary apoplexy. Additional symptoms, such as headache, probably do not relate to the empty sella per se but instead to the cause of it, including chronic increased intracranial pressure. Occasionally, an empty sella can be associated with CSF rhinorrhea.[213] When a patient has had symptoms suggesting subarachnoid hemorrhage or meningitis and

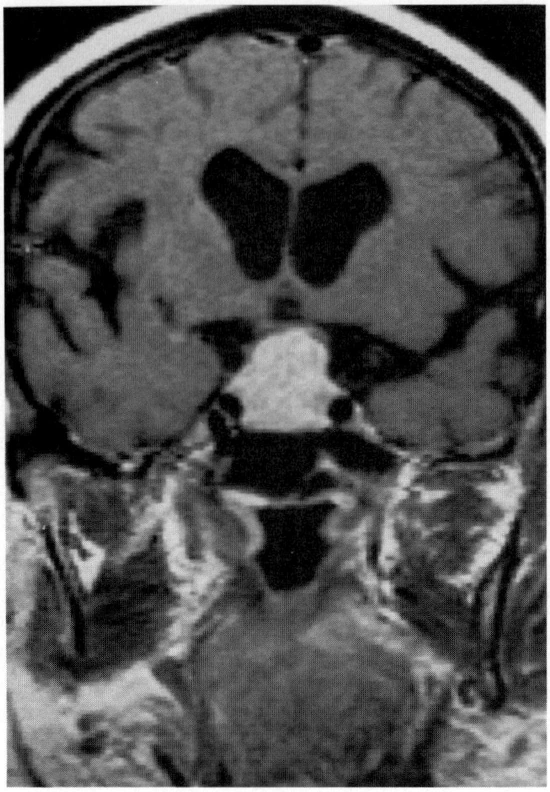

Figure 5-18
Coronal T1 spin echo MRI after administration of Gd-DTPA showing a medium-size uniformly enhancing macroadenoma of the pituitary gland just beginning to elevate the optic chiasm. The tumor widens the sella turcica but does not extend into the cavernous sinuses.

neuroimaging studies disclose an empty sella, pituitary apoplexy may have occured.[214]

When an empty sella is discovered by neuroimaging (Fig. 5-18), the patient should be studied, if that is clinically indicated, for increased intracranial pressure and its various causes and for endocrinologic defects that might have resulted from pituitary apoplexy or hypothalamic dysfunction. Children with an empty sella may have a deficiency in growth hormone.[215,216] The presence of an empty sella, a relatively common finding, should not divert attention from the possibility that the visual loss may related to other common causes, such as glaucoma.[217] Occasionally, successful treatment of intracranial hypertension will allow the pituitary gland to reexpand and fill an empty sella.[218]

Pituitary adenoma is a common resident of the sella turcica that most often declares itself by its endocrinologic misbehavior. Less often, especially when the tumor does not secrete prolactin or another hormone, suprasellar expansion of a pituitary adenoma may be revealed as the cause of slowly progressive uncorrectable visual loss, which often is not recognized because of its slow progression. In general, the bitemporal hemianopia caused by suprasellar extension of pituitary adenomas is binocularly symmetrical; variations from this common pattern result from the variable position of the optic chiasm in relation to the sella and from the occasional asymmetrical tumor. Bitemporal hemianopia indicates that the tumor has reached a substantial size and has elevated and stretched the chiasm.

MRI has several advantages in detecting and demonstrating the full extent of these intrasellar tumors: Sagittal views show sellar enlargement and contents, and coronal views display the relationship of the tumor to the visual pathways and the cavernous sinuses.[219] Most "macroadenomas" (larger than 1 cm) enhance after the administration of paramagnetic agents (Fig. 5-19), but "microadenomas" are distinguishable from surrounding normal pituitary tissue because they do not immediately enhance after a small dose of contrast agent (Fig. 5-20).[220,221] New dynamic techniques of rapid acquisition MRI during bolus contrast infusion have improved the sensitivity for the diagnosis of a small microadenoma.[222] The development of three-dimensional volume imaging has led to a further improvement in sensitivity for small lesions of the sella, and inferior petrosal sinus sampling increases specificity and sensitivity in the diagnosis of secreting tumors.[222]

Craniopharyngioma causes a greater variety of bitemporal hemianopic visual field defects that are less likely to be bilaterally symmetrical and occasionally monocular or homonymous defects. The tumor should be suspected in the presence of a cystic sellar or suprasellar lesion, especially when the sella turcica is not enlarged. MRI is the method of choice for the reasons listed above, although CT may better demonstrate calcium within the tumor. The signals emitted by cysts are variable on T1-weighted sequences and relate to concentrations of protein, lipid, and iron (Fig. 5-21). Paramagnetic contrast agents improve the detection of fleshy parts and "active" cysts. Sometimes helpful to the diagnosis—but not specific—is the "moustache" on axial CT or MRI views caused by perifocal edema in the hypothalamus adjacent to the intraventricular tumor, the optic tracts, and the posterior limbs of the internal capsules.[223] Rarely, a craniopharyngioma may appear to be within the optic chiasm itself.[224,225]

Meningioma can produce a chiasmal syndrome, expanding from a base on the tuberculum sellae or the neighboring meninges (Fig. 5-22).

Rathke's cleft cysts are a less common cause of visual loss than are either pituitary adenomas or craniopharyngiomas, probably because they occur less frequently and remain small. Found in the anterior sella or suprasellar region, they contain fluid with CSF signal characteristics (Fig. 5-23).[226–228]

Aneurysms of the supraclinoid portion of the carotid artery or the anterior communicating artery may cause slowly progressive bitemporal hemianopia (Fig. 5-24).[125,229,230] MRI provides a single method of distinguishing these aneurysms from the more common offenders, particularly pituitary adenoma.

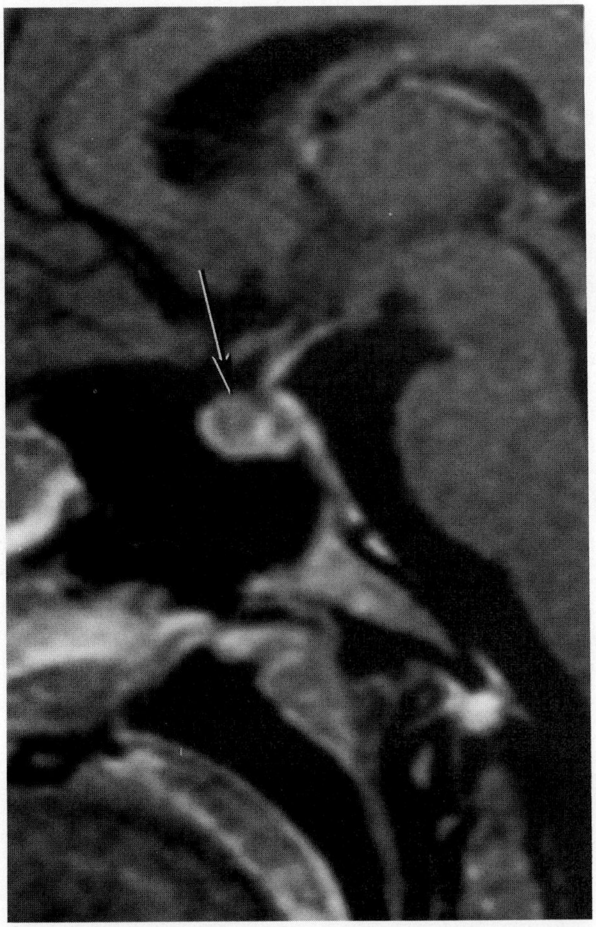

A

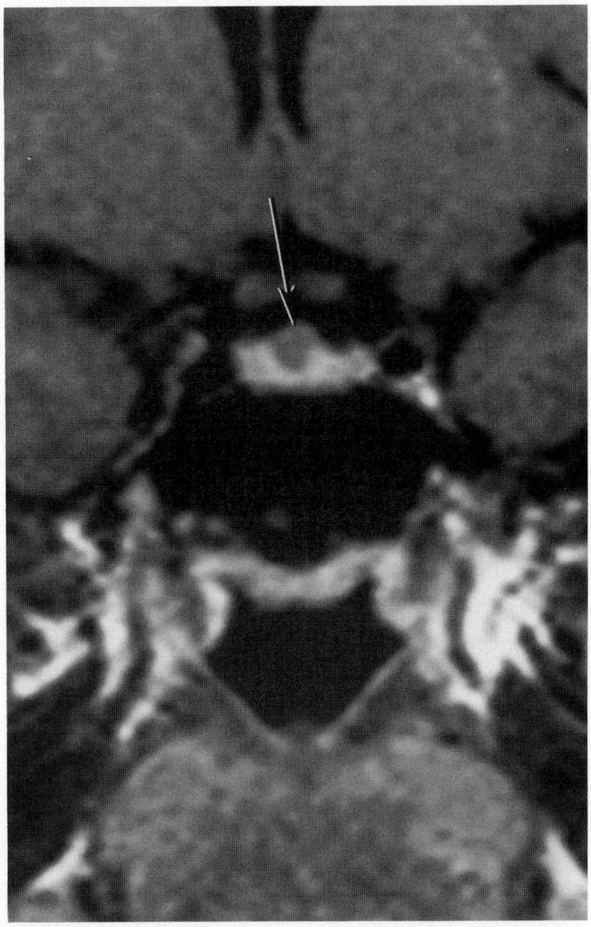

B

Figure 5-19

Sagittal **(A)** *and coronal* **(B)** *spin echo MRIs after the administration of Gd-DTPA showing an 8-mm spherical microadenoma in the superior aspect of the pituitary gland (arrow). Immediately after contrast administration, the normal gland enhances; the tumor does not.*

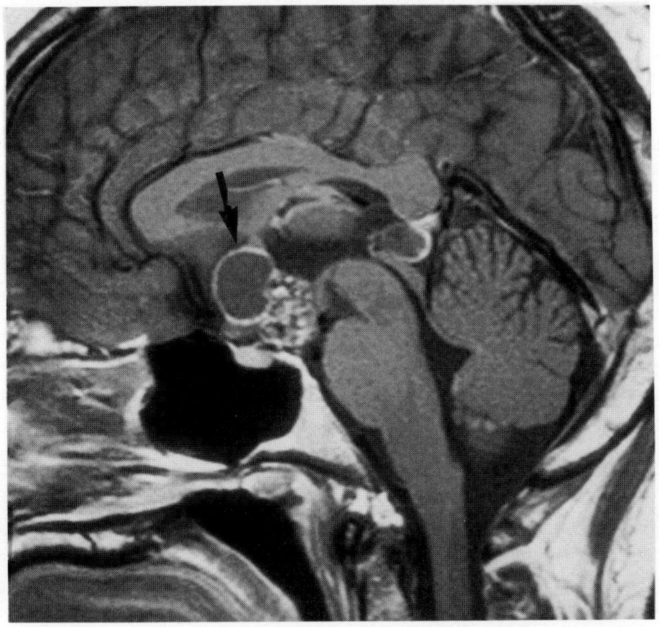

Figure 5-20

Sagittal T1 MRI after gadolinium administration of a 35-year-old man with inferior bitemporal quadrantanopia showing a suprasellar mass with both cystic and solid components, a craniopharyngioma. The cystic component lies superior to the optic chiasm (arrow). Small punctate signal voids within the solid component are foci of calcium. Note the incidental pineal cyst.

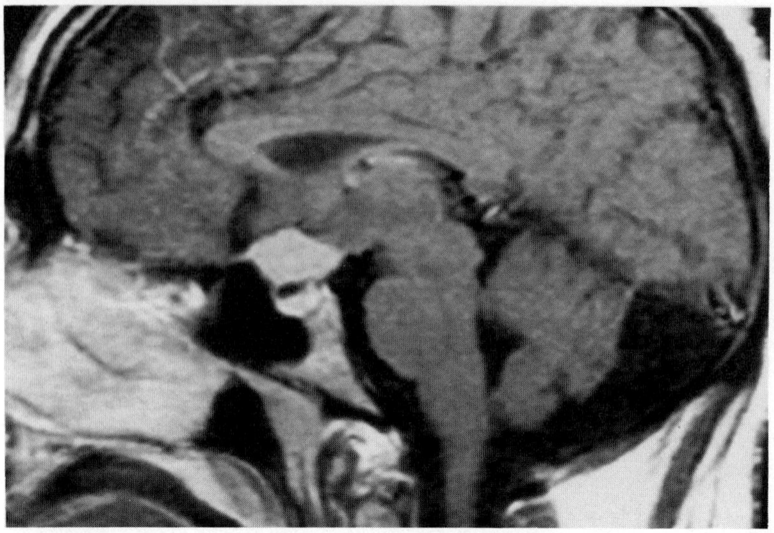

A

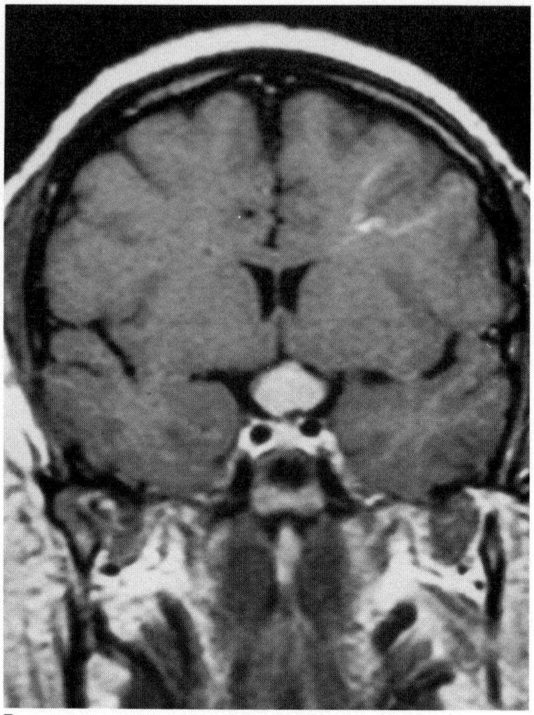

B

Figure 5-21
Sagittal **(A)** *and coronal* **(B)** *T1 spin echo MRIs after the administration of Gd-DTPA showing an enhancing lesion expanding into the suprasellar region from the tuberculum sellae, elevating the optic chiasm. Excisional biopsy diagnosed a meningioma.*

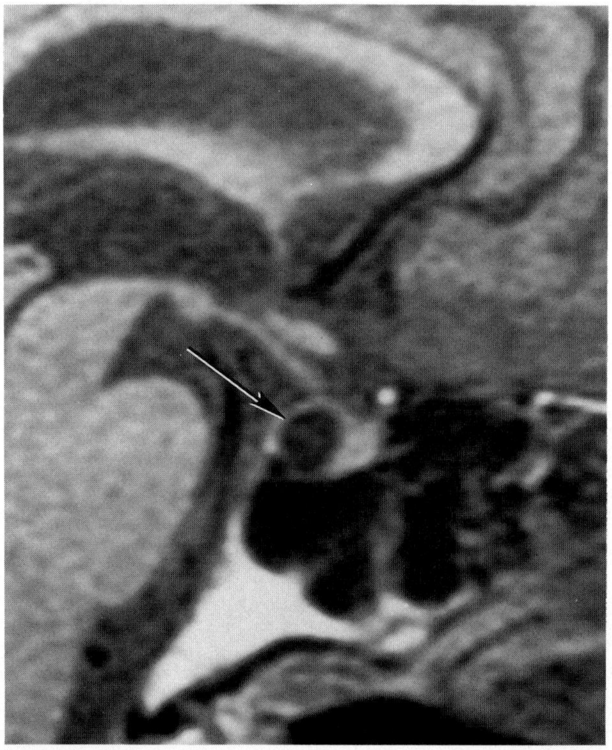

Figure 5-22
Sagittal T1 postgadolinium MRI of a 33-year-old woman with galactorrhea and amenorrhea showing a cystic lesion, isointense with CSF, posterior to the normally enhancing anterior pituitary gland (arrow). The anteriorly displaced infundibulum places this lesion in the pars intermedia, the characteristic site for a Rathke's cleft cyst.

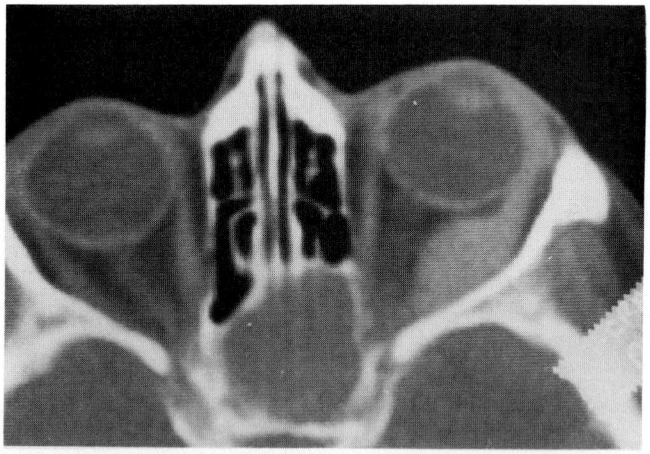

Figure 5-23
Axial Ct view of an enlarged sphenoid sinus filled with inflammatory material (mucocele). Lateral expansion may cause compressive optic neuropathy; superior expansion may cause a chiasmal syndrome. Note that the associated myositis expanding the left lateral rectus muscle extends into its insertion on the ocular globe.

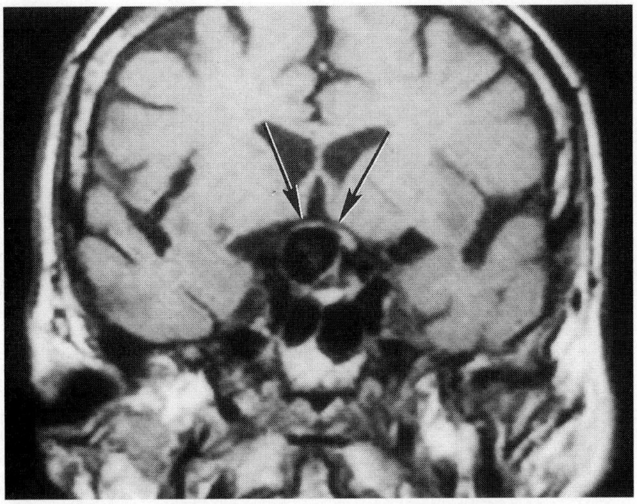

Figure 5-24
A giant aneurysm, probably originating from the supraclinoid portion of the internal carotid artery, elevating the optic chiasm (arrows). Only the uncrossed fibers of the left optic nerve are still capable of conduction.

Mucocele of the sphenoid sinus may cause a chiasmal syndrome that now is easily distinguished from the more common causes of this syndrome by neuroimaging (Fig. 5-25).[139,231]

Other chiasmal lesions are too numerous and various to discuss but much less common than the entities discussed above. A suprasellar dermoid tumor is just one example (Fig. 5-26).

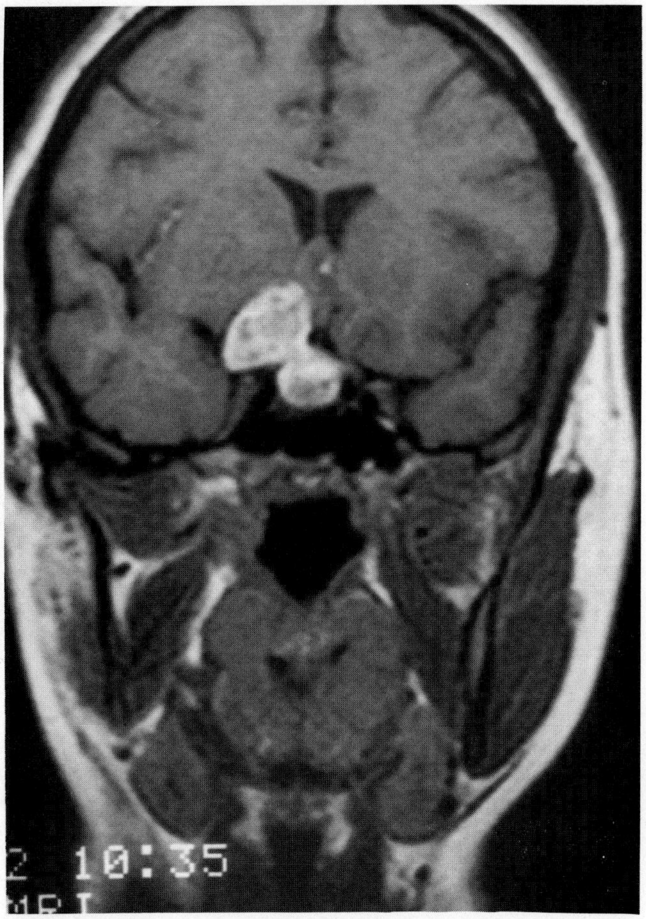

Figure 5-25
Coronal T1 spin echo noncontrast MRI showing a hyperintense intrasellar lesion expanding into the suprasellar space and right inferior frontal lobe. The hyperintensity suggests that the lesion contains fat. Excisional biopsy disclosed a dermoid tumor.

Homonymous Hemianopia Progressive homonymous hemianopia reliably indicates expanding retrochiasmal lesions that span the entire gamut from enlarging aneurysms to benign and malignant tumors of all kinds. Pregeniculate lesions are more likely to cause "incongruous" visual field defects (different pattern in each eye) and postgeniculate lesions are more likely to cause "congruous" defects, but the degree of congruity in each case is not by itself a reliable indicator of the location or type of the lesion.

Because of their location, the optic tract and lateral geniculate nuclei are more vulnerable to extra-axial lesions such as aneurysms, meningiomas, craniopharyngiomas, asymmetric adenomas, and a host of less common tumors, such as a medially expanding temporal lobe astrocytoma or an enlarging pineal region tumor.

Progressive lesions affecting the optic radiations are more likely to be intra-axial, such as glioma and metastatic tumors, and if the hemianopia is not complete, these lesions cause "sloping borders" on the advancing edge of the defect.[165] Binocular altitudinal field defects ("quadrantanopia") may indicate a lesion confined to the upper or lower bank of the calcarine fissure, a characteristic that most often is attributable to infarction, especially if the horizontal borders are sharply delineated, but occasionally an expanding lesion in the extrastriate visual areas of the occipital cortex (areas V2 and V3) causes this defect.[232] MRI with contrast enhancement is the neuroimaging procedure of first choice.

Functional neuroimaging in patients with hemianopia is still in its infancy. The most promising work has been done by Raichle and his group, who found that local increases in functional activity (as occur when one views an image) are best reflected in parallel increases in *blood flow,* not in glucose or oxygen consumption. With this method, Raichle confirmed by functional imaging—with an accuracy of 3 mm—that the retinotopic organization of the living human visual cortex is very similar to that already mapped in animals.[233] Raichle also found by positron emission tomography (PET) that certain areas in the left medial extrastriate visual cortex can be activated by visually presented pseudowords that obey English spelling rules, as well as by actual words, but not by nonsense strings of letters or letter-like forms.[234] Thus, visual word-form computations are based on learned distinctions between words and nonwords.

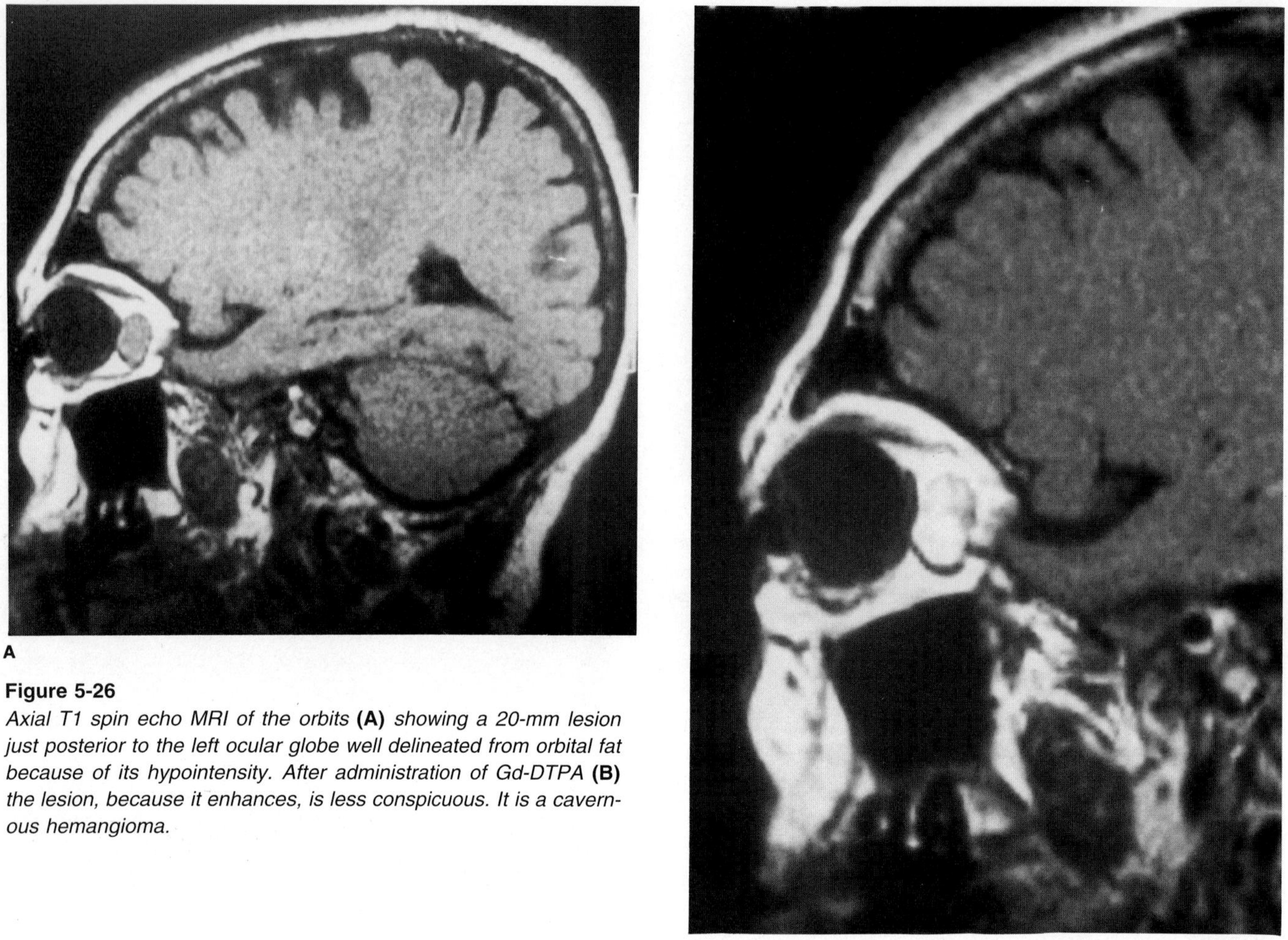

A

B

Figure 5-26
Axial T1 spin echo MRI of the orbits **(A)** *showing a 20-mm lesion just posterior to the left ocular globe well delineated from orbital fat because of its hypointensity. After administration of Gd-DTPA* **(B)** *the lesion, because it enhances, is less conspicuous. It is a cavernous hemangioma.*

Diplopia

Diplopia is the cardinal symptom of disturbances in the infranuclear portion of the ocular motor system, including the ocular muscles. It is a very sensitive and early indicator of ocular motor disturbance because it disrupts the precise ocular alignment necessary for normal binocular vision. In one sense, diplopia must always begin suddenly, because the eyes either are aligned or are not. However, progressive lesions may first cause intermittent diplopia that gradually becomes persistent. Acute lesions, such as microinfarcts in one of the ocular motor nerves, usually cause immediate wide separation of images; progressive lesions may initially cause a small separation the gradually widens.

The "diplopia history" often yields information that permits localization of the impaired ocular muscle or nerve and the formulation of a differential diagnosis. For guidance in the initial evaluation of patients with diplopia and other disorders of ocular movement, the reader is referred to the latest edition of *The Neurology of Eye Movements.*[235] Neuroimaging is valuable for detecting, characterizing, or excluding structural lesions in the orbits and along the course of the ocular motor pathways. For neuroimaging of orbital lesions by CT, MRI, and ultrasound, the reader is referred to *Radiology of the Eye and Orbit.*[236]

On initial examination in the office or at the bedside, common causes of diplopia should be investigated, including ocular myasthenia, thyroid-related eye disease, decompensation of congenital strabismus, orbital retraction syndromes, and tendon sheath syndrome, among others.[235] Transient lesions can be investigated by taking a careful history, and myasthenia can be diagnosed by testing with edrophonium chloride. Orbital lesions and thyroid ophthalmopathy usually can be recognized by the associated orbital signs (see below). If the diplopia can be attributed to dysfunction in the field of action of a single ocular motor nerve, the differential diagnosis can be narrowed to those lesions with a predilection for each nerve.[235] When the possibility of a structural lesion remains after the initial office or bedside diagnostic evaluation, a "neuroimaging" differential diagnosis of diplopia includes lesions in the following areas:

Orbit, inside or outside of the muscle cone, usually localized by unilateral orbital signs such as proptosis, displacement of the globe, and ocular congestion

Orbital apex–superior orbital fissure, suggested by a combination of ocular motor and optic nerve dysfunction and sometimes signs of orbital congestion

Cavernous sinus–parasellar, suggested by a combination of dysfunction of one or more ocular motor nerves, the fifth cranial nerve, oculosympathetic paralysis, pain, and venous congestion of the glove and periocular tissues

Clivus–petrous bone, impairing conduction in the sixth cranial nerve as it courses along the clivus and through Dorello's canal, usually by a malignant or infectious process that has invaded the clivus or petrous apex

Subarachnoid space, impairing conduction in the ocular motor nerves, usually a single nerve, by extrinsic compression, such as by an aneurysm at the junction of the posterior communicating and internal carotid arteries

Ocular motor nerves intra-axially, most often microinfarcts in the intracavernous or subarachnoid segments that cause isolated mononeuropathy

Brainstem, often affecting ascending or descending pathways and other functions in the same segmental level

Orbit

MRI is ideal for displaying masses of all types (Fig. 5-27) and the enlarged ocular muscles of thyroid-related ophthalmopathy (Fig. 5-28) and orbital pseudotumor.[236]

Orbital Apex

Meningiomas, Tolosa Hunt syndrome, sarcoidosis, lymphoma (Fig. 5-17), and metastatic tumors can occupy this region. All are discussed above.

The Tolosa Hunt syndrome (THS) is painful ophthalmoplegia caused by steroid-responsive inflammation in the cavernous sinus.[201] High-resolution CT or MRI with contrast, which is necessary to exclude tumors, may show a characteristic enhancing abnormality in the cavernous sinus, often extending into the orbital apex,[237] but it may not be diagnostic enough to exclude other, more specific causes of this syndrome, including sarcoidosis and lymphoma. Steroid responsiveness (clinical and imaging improvement after treatment) suggests THS, but lymphoma and sarcoidosis also may respond. Some evidence suggests that even the THS itself is heterogeneous.[238] Imaging is useful for long-term follow-up in order to detect alternatives to THS that may have reponded to steroids only temporarily.

Cavernous Sinus

Meningioma within the cavernous sinus, in addition to its typical clinical and imaging hallmarks, is suggested

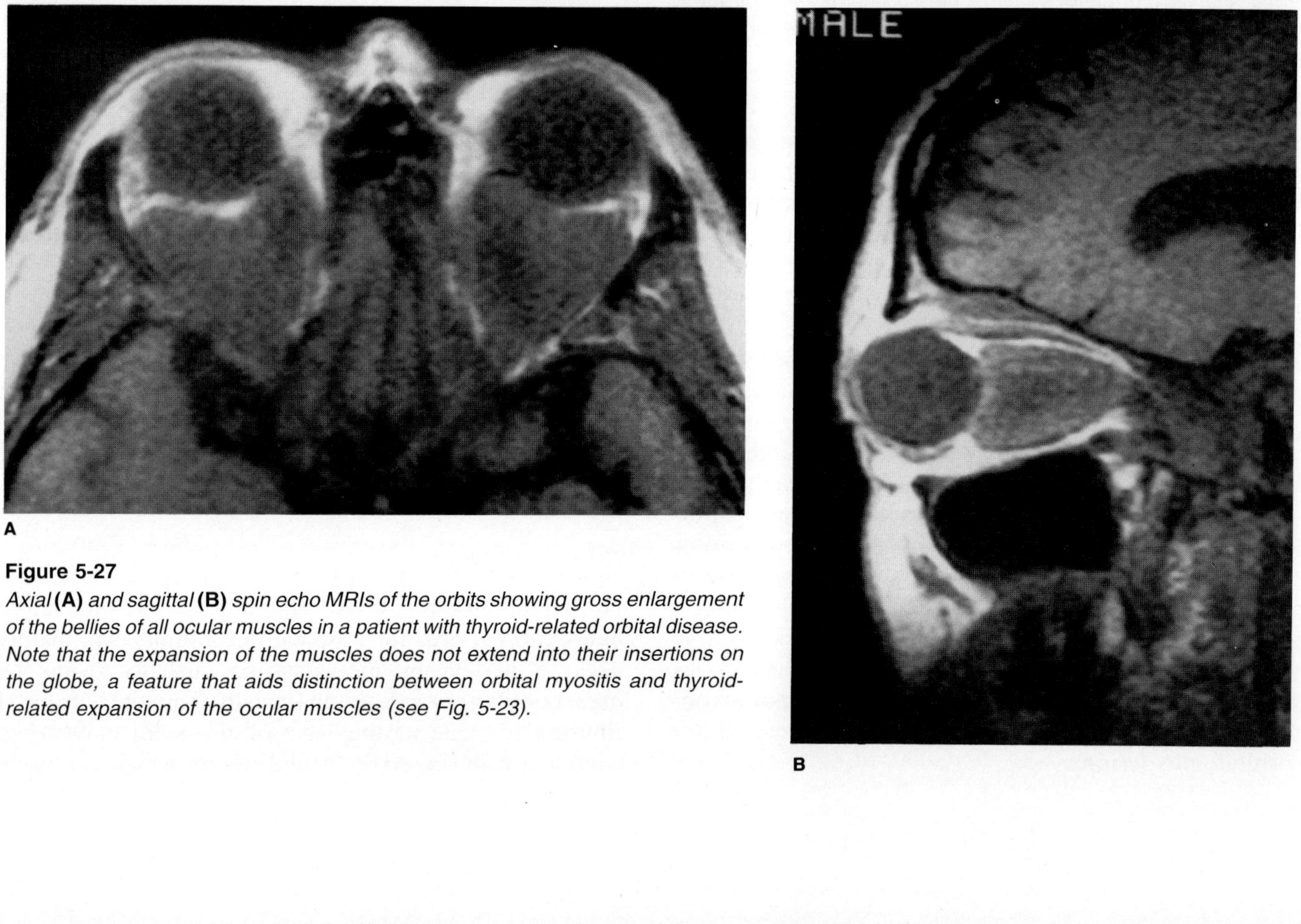

A

B

Figure 5-27
Axial **(A)** *and sagittal* **(B)** *spin echo MRIs of the orbits showing gross enlargement of the bellies of all ocular muscles in a patient with thyroid-related orbital disease. Note that the expansion of the muscles does not extend into their insertions on the globe, a feature that aids distinction between orbital myositis and thyroid-related expansion of the ocular muscles (see Fig. 5-23).*

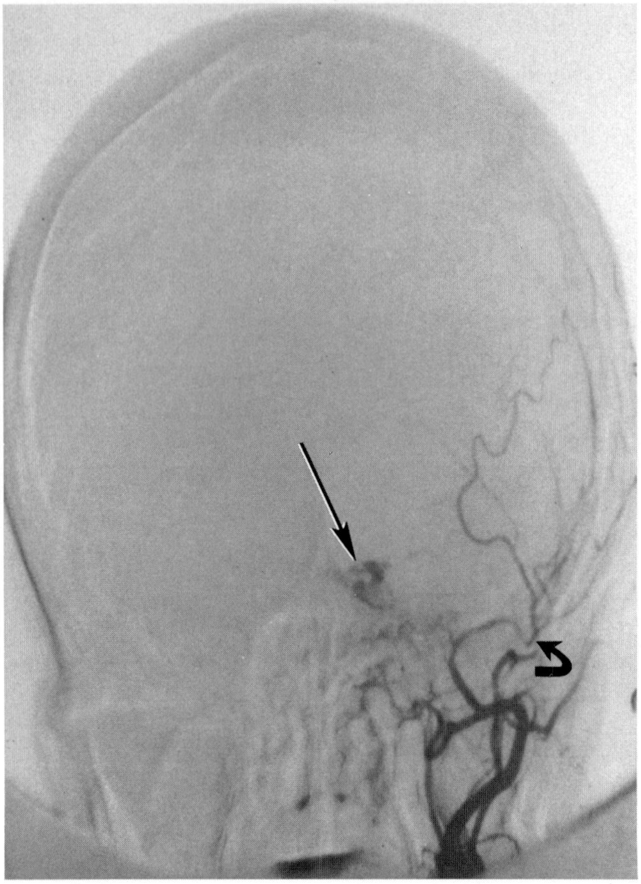

Figure 5-28
Selective external carotid conventional angiogram showing early appearance of contrast material in the cavernous sinus (straight arrow), simultaneous with opacification of the superficial temporal artery (curved arrow). The 56-year-old woman had a spontaneous external carotid-cavernous sinus dural fistula.

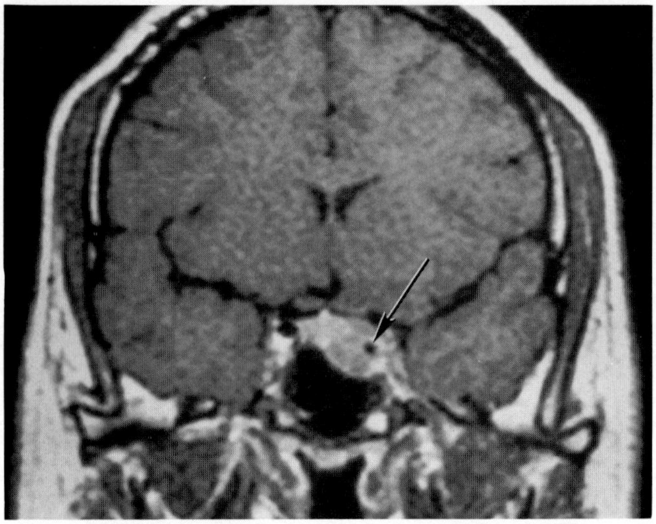

Figure 5-29
Coronal T1 spin echo MRI after administration of Gd-DTPA showing a pituitary macroadenoma centered in the left side of the sella turcica expanding into the left cavernous sinus and surrounding the carotid artery (arrow).

by signs related to primary aberrant regeneration of the third cranial nerve.[239,240] Its very slow progression results in simultaneous destruction and misdirection of regenerated nerve fibers to the wrong ocular muscle. Inexplicably, the ocular motor weakness caused by intracavernous meningiomas and aneurysms may seem to respond to anticholinesterase inhibitors.[241]

Spontaneous extradural carotid-cavernous sinus fistula may present with sudden or subacute painful diplopia and a variety of other signs implicating the cavernous sinus.[242] Because these are low-flow shunts, the full-blown picture of carotid-cavernous fistula usually is not present, that is, ocular congestion and pulsating proptosis. Linear hyperintensity in the intercavernous sinuses on MRI, suggesting abnormal flow, provides a clue to the presence of a fistula, but selective catheterization of the external carotid system is necessary for definitive diagnosis (Fig. 5-29). On MRI, enlarged ocular muscles resulting from the increased venous pressure may erroneously suggest thyroid-related ophthalmopathy or other orbital apex lesions.

Pituitary tumors (see also the discussion above) may expand laterally into the cavernous sinus and cause ocular motor dysfunction and other signs, usually signaling that pituitary apoplexy has occurred, but the orbital signs are not always present.[243] Coronal MRI is ideally suited to demonstrate the extent of this lateral expansion (Fig. 5-30).

Aneurysms along the course of the ocular motor nerves are perhaps the most threatening diagnostic possibilities among patients with sudden painful ophthalmoplegia. In many instances MRI, combined with careful clinical evaluation, can relieve this concern and forestall invasive diagnostic studies.

Intracavernous aneurysms may cause ocular motor dysfunction along with other signs implicating the cavernous sinus[244,245] but rarely rupture.[246] MRI is clearly superior to CT for the initial detection and diagnosis, as it is with all lesions that enlarge the cavernous sinus (Fig. 5-31).[247,248] Thin-section T1 views are the most sensitive and informative. A midposition, poorly reactive pupil is suggestive of cavernous sinus lesions but is not reliably diagnostic by itself.[249] A variety of interventional techniques have been described for cases that require treatment.[250]

Clivus–Skull base

Horizontal diplopia, when related to sixth cranial nerve neuropathy, raises the suspicion of a neoplasm, mainly because neoplasms metastasizing (usually from the breast or lung) or extending (usually from the paranasal sinuses) to bone at the base of the skull may affect conduction in the sixth cranial nerve, which is closely

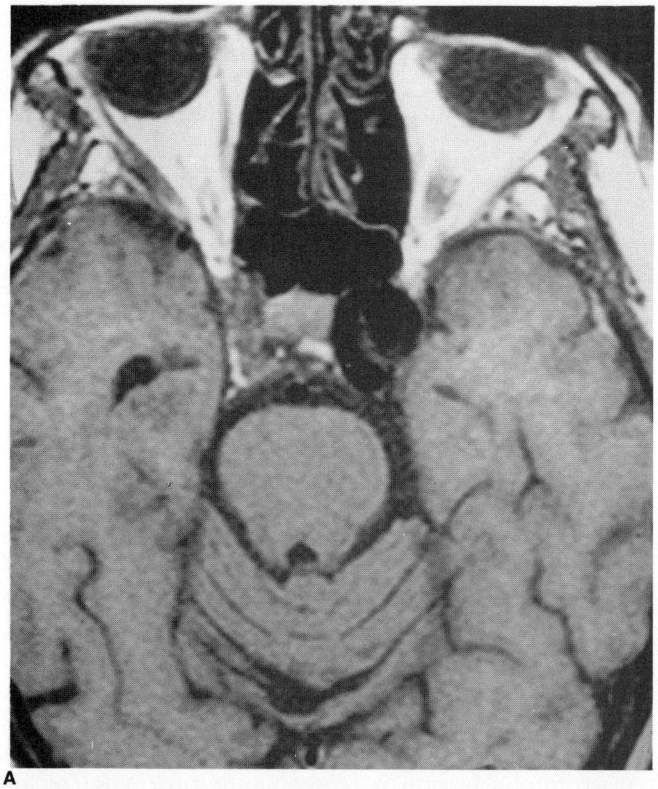

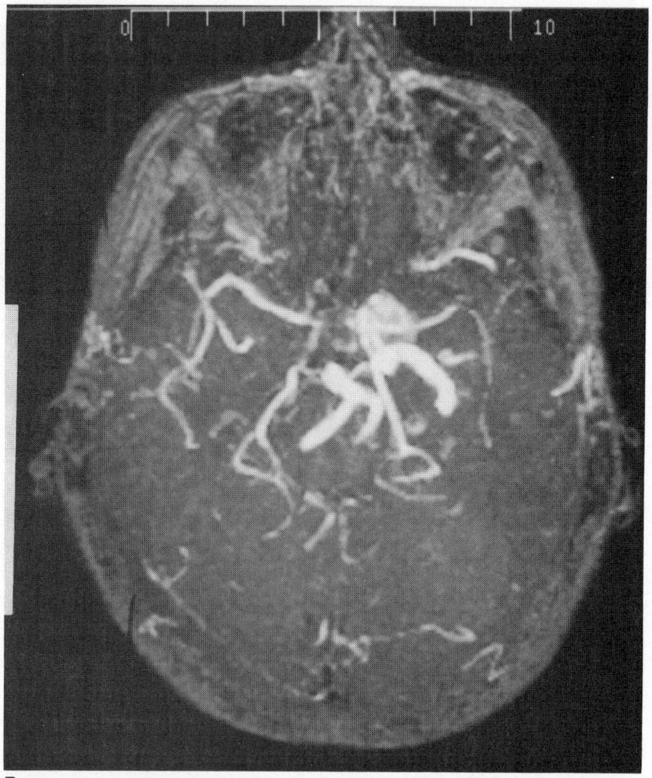

Figure 5-30

MRIs of a 78-year-old woman with transient right hemispheric ischemia. **(A)** *Axial T1 image showing an oval signal void in the region of the cavernous portion of the left carotid artery. Isointensity of the lumen of the right internal carotid artery indicates occlusion by fibrin and platelets and few red blood cells.* **(B)** *MRA (three-dimensional time-of-flight) also shows the aneurysm; intensity is reduced because its large size causes prolonged transit time and slow flow within the lumen, resulting in saturated arterial spins (arrow).*

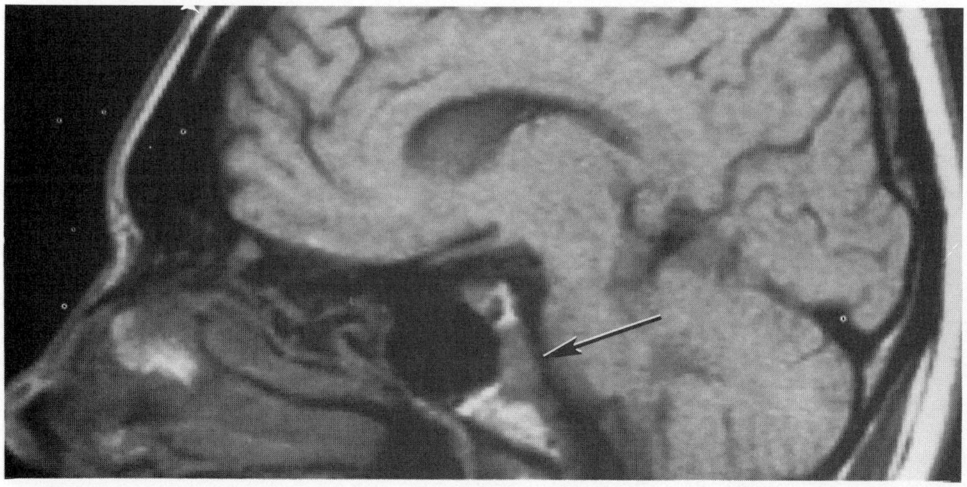

Figure 5-31

Sagittal T1 spin echo MRI of a 42-year-old man with breast cancer and recent sixth cranial nerve neuropathy showing replacement of marrow in the clivus by a metastatic lesion (arrow) that enhanced after contrast administration.

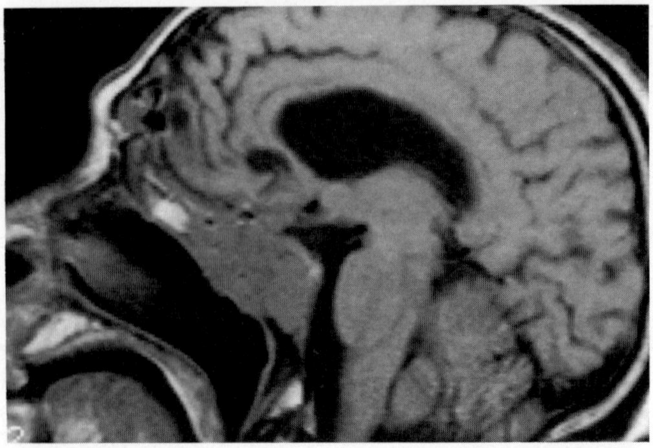

Figure 5-32
Sagittal T1 spin echo MRI showing a nasopharyngeal carcinoma centered in the sphenoid sinus and invading the cortical bone of the clivus in the region of the sixth cranial nerve.

related to the clivus along much of its course (Figs. 5-32 and 5-33).

Mucocele of the sphenoid sinus may present as sudden painful ophthalmoplegia (Fig. 5-25).[139,251]

Subarachnoid Space

Aneurysms at the junction of the internal carotid–posterior communicating arterial junction may compress the third cranial nerve. Before the increased sensitivity of high-resolution noninvasive techniques, the involvement of the pupil was a critical, if not totally reliable,[252] sign that distinguished a microinfarct in the third nerve ("medical" third nerve paresis with pupillary "sparing") from compression by the aneurysm ("surgical" paresis with a larger pupil). Kissel and associates[253] observed that the pupil may be spared initially by a compressing aneurysm, and so equal pupils on the first observation should not give one total confidence in the absence of an aneurysm. Despite some clinical rules developed in an exchange of letters to the editors of the same journal in response to the Kissel article (December 1983),[254–256] most observers agree today that the clinical sign of "pupillary sparing" is too unreliable to obviate neuroimaging (MRI) in almost all patients with paresis of the third cranial nerve.[257] High-resolution MRI, particularly thin-section T1 sequences, is usually adequate to detect or exclude an aneurysm (Fig. 5-34), but conventional arteriography is required preoperatively and also when the suspicion of an aneurysm is high.

Basilar meningitis is another process that can affect the subarachnoid portion of the ocular motor nerves. Usually that diagnosis is made on clinical grounds and confirmed by examination of CSF, but occasionally enhancement of one or more of the cranial nerves will lead to its serendipitous discovery.[258]

Nerve sheath tumors enhance brightly and may be located on any cranial nerve (Fig. 5-35).[259] Hence, contrast administration is recommended for MRI of any patient with chronic or unexplained cranial neuropathy.

Other neoplasms may affect the subarachnoid course of the ocular motor nerves (Fig. 5-36), including meningioma and chordoma.

Brainstem

Intra-axial lesions of the brainstem, including infarcts, demyelinating plaques, and neoplasms, are best evalu-

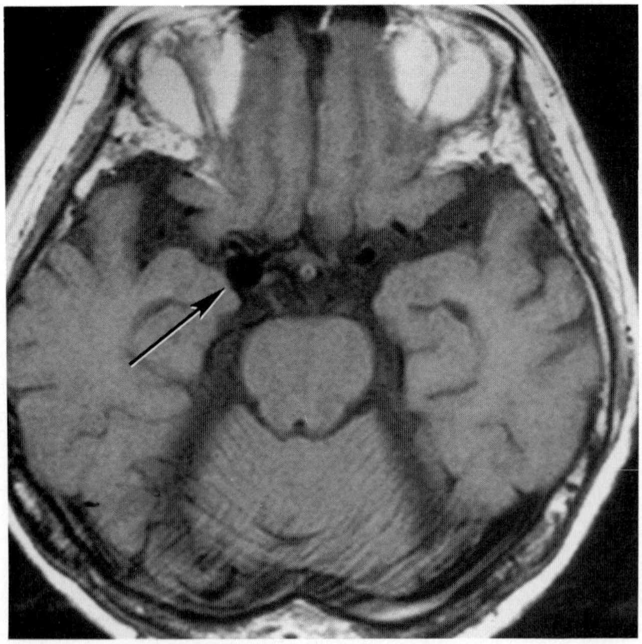

A

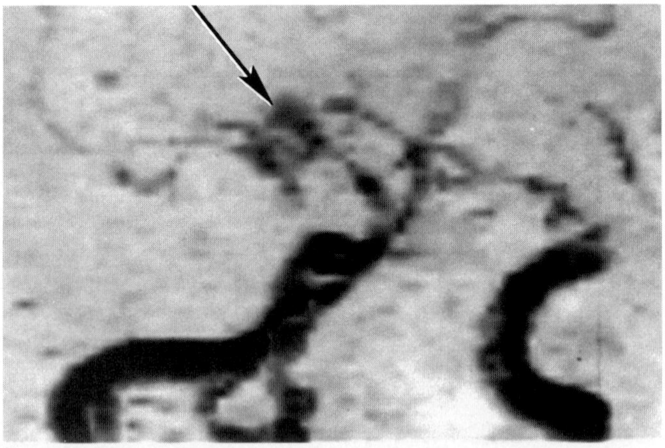

B

Figure 5-33
MR images of a 79-year-old woman with right third cranial neuropathy. **(A)** *Axial T1 image showing an aneurysm arising from the right posterior communicating artery compressing the subarachnoidal segment of the third nerve (arrow).* **(B)** *MRA (three-dimensional, time-of-flight) shows the aneurysm (arrow).*

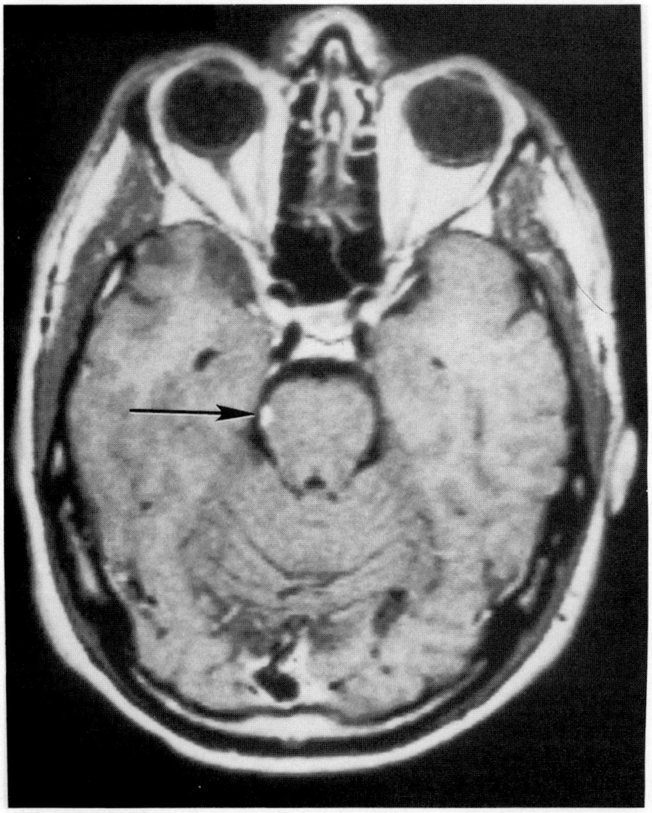

Figure 5-34
Axial T1 spin echo MRI of a 42-year-old man who had weakness of the left superior oblique muscle for 6 months. A small lesion appeared along the perimesencephalic course of the right trochlear nerve after contrast administration (arrow), probably a small nerve sheath tumor. (Reprinted with permission of Little, Brown and Company, Publishers).

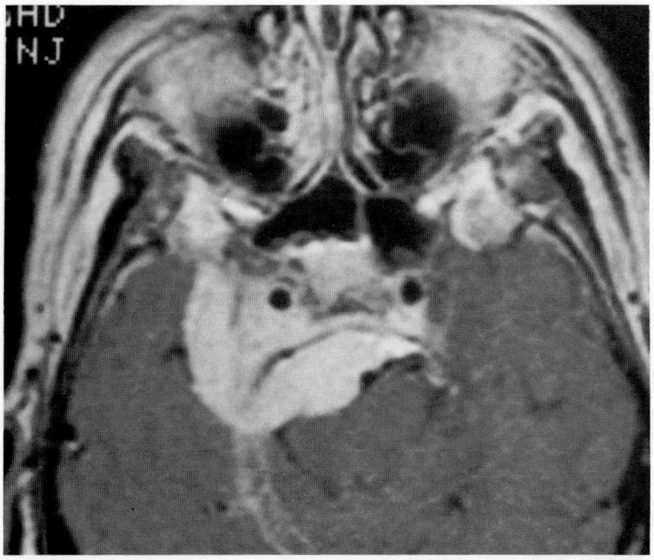

Figure 5-35
Axial T2 spin echo MRI of a 72-year-old woman with paresis of the right third cranial nerve. The extraaxial mass between the brainstem and clivus and surrounding the basilar artery is suspected to be a meningioma.

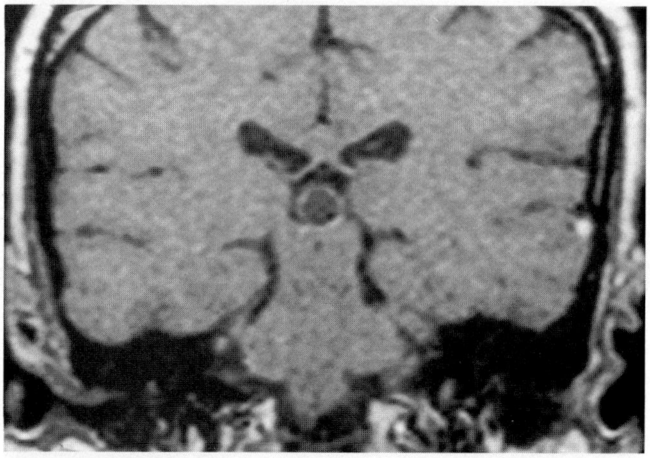

Figure 5-36
Axial T1 spin echo MRI after the administration of Gd-DTPA showing a 2-cm cyst superior to the quadrigeminal plate, a relatively common incidental and usually asymptomatic finding.[263]

ated by MRI because of its multiplanar capability, absence of artifact caused by bone, and variable signal characteristics.

Pineal region tumors, by compressing the midbrain tectum through the quadrigeminal plate, may cause the classic "Parinaud" or "sylvian aqueduct" syndrome of convergence-retraction nystagmus, midposition poorly reactive pupils, and upgaze paralysis, but often diplopia is the symptom that is most troublesome to the patient. These tumors are best detected by the multiplanar capability of MRI, which defines their size, location, and relation to normal structures, such as the third ventricle. Imaging characteristics of these tumors—germinomas, pineocytomas, pineoblastomas, astrocytomas, teratomas, choriocarcinomas, mixed germ cell tumors, ependymoma, meningioma, and metastases—are heterogeneous (by MRI and histopathologic examination) and nonspecific,[260–262] and so the differential diagnosis must be further narrowed by considering the age and sex of the patient and tumor markers, particularly α-fetoprotein and human chorionic gonadotropin–β subunit. Gadolinium-DTPA may[260] or may not[261] increase the specificity of the diagnosis, but contrast definitely better delineates the tumor margins, demonstrates cystic components of the neoplasm, and demonstrates tumor seeding along the neuraxis. Stereotactic biopsy may be necessary for a definitive diagnosis. The more common benign pineal region cysts, which are more common in young women, must be differentiated from tumors because most are asymptomatic and nonprogressive (Fig. 5-37).[263–265]

Oscillopsia

Oscillopsia, the false sense of motion, signals disturbance in the vestibular system. Usually combined with

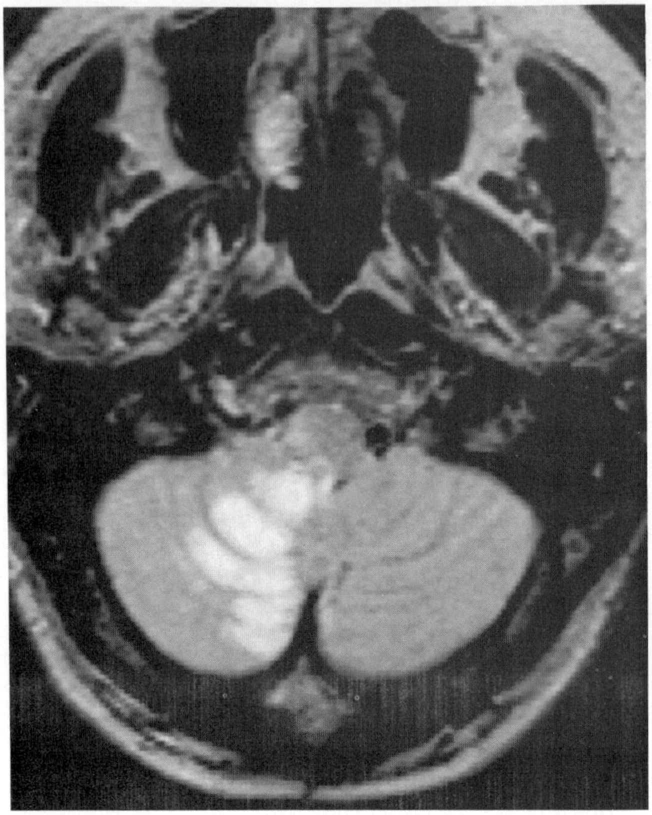

Figure 5-37
Axial T2 spin echo MRI showing an infarction in the territory of the right posterior inferior cerebellar artery.

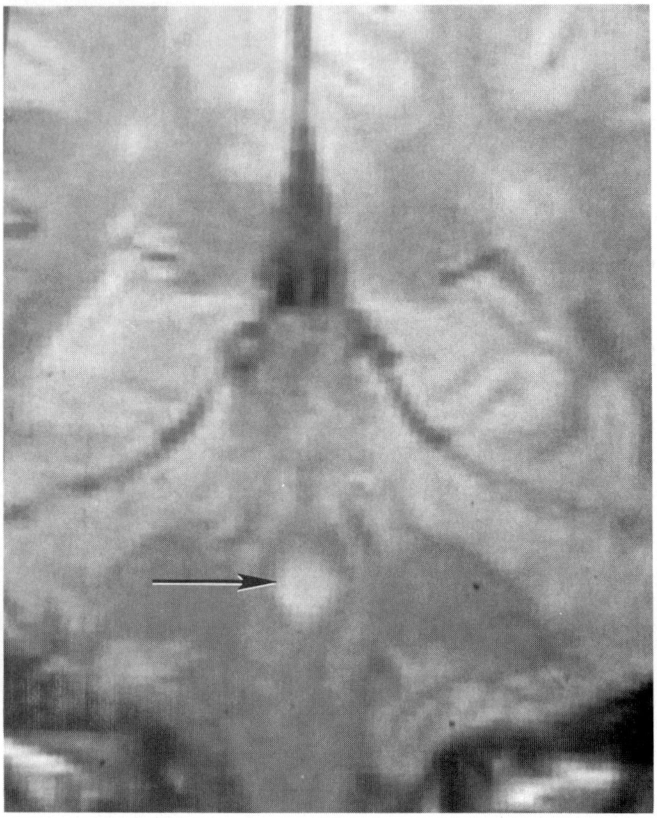

Figure 5-38
Coronal proton density spin echo MRI of a young woman with internuclear ophthalmoplegia showing a diamond-shaped hyperintense demyelinating lesion in the pontine tegmentum affecting conduction in both medial longitudinal fasciculi.

dysequilibrium, oscillopsia indicates loss of the normal bilateral balance of vestibular sensory input as a result of unilateral dysfunction of the end organs in the inner ear, eighth cranial nerve, or vestibulocerebellar pathways in the brainstem or cerebellum.[235] Among its common causes are the following.

Ischemia is caused by infarction in the vertebrobasilar territory. These lesions, which often are too small for visualization and are obscured by bone artifact on CT, are best demonstrated by MRI (Fig. 5-38).

Demyelinating disease is a common cause of oscillopsia, vertigo, and diplopia in younger individuals when it attacks the brainstem or cerebellum (Fig. 5-39).

Acoustic neuroma, which also causes sensorineural hearing loss, is no longer a challenge to demonstrate by neuroimaging, because even small and entirely intracanalicular tumors enhance brilliantly after the administration of Gd-DTPA (Fig. 5-40).

Other posterior fossa tumors of any kind, including ependymoma of the fourth ventricle (Fig. 5-41) and cerebellar hemangioblastoma (Fig. 5-42), can present with oscillopsia and vertigo.

Chiari malformation, a congenital malformation that may present at birth, may also cause symptoms in

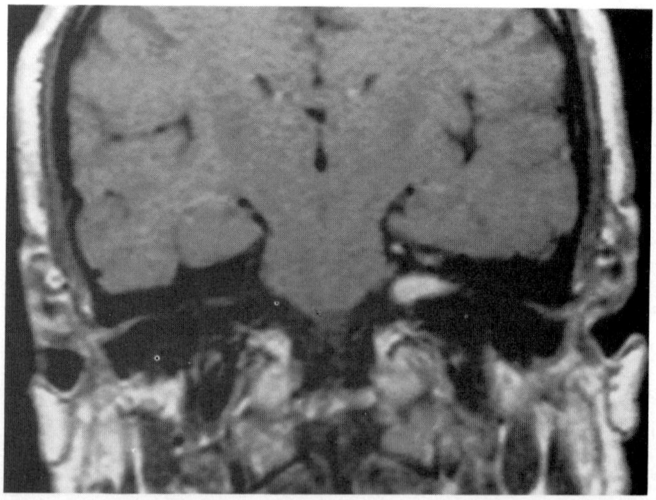

Figure 5-39
Coronal T1 spin echo MRI after the administration of Gd-DTPA showing a small enhancing lesion along the course of the left eighth cranial nerve extending through the internal auditory meatus, an acoustic neuroma.

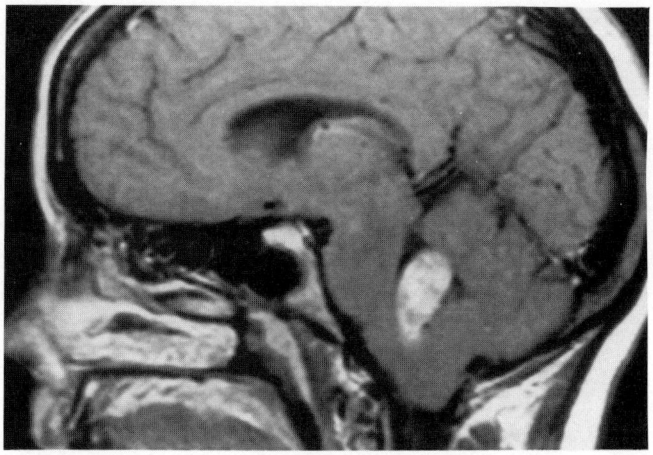

Figure 5-40
Sagittal T1 spin echo MRI after the administration of Gd-DTPA of a 36-year-old woman who presented with vertigo and dysequilibrium showing an enhancing lesion in the fourth ventricle that proved to be an ependymoma when excised.

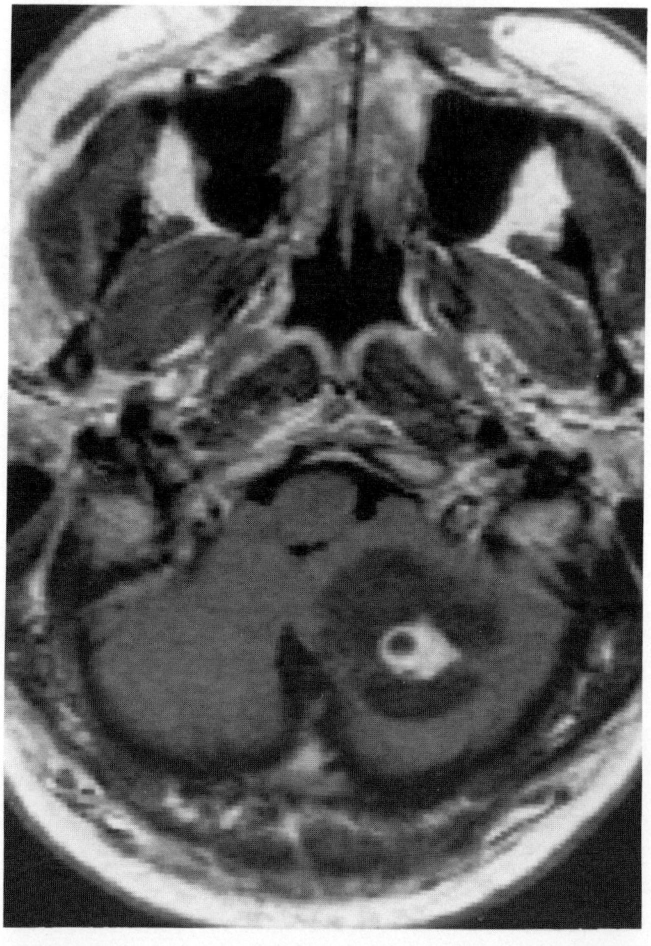

Figure 5-41
Axial T1 spin echo MRI after the administration of Gd-DTPA showing a large cystic lesion in the left cerebellar hemisphere with an enhancing nodule on a pedicle at its center. Typically, this hemangioblastoma does not extend to the cerebellar cortical surface.

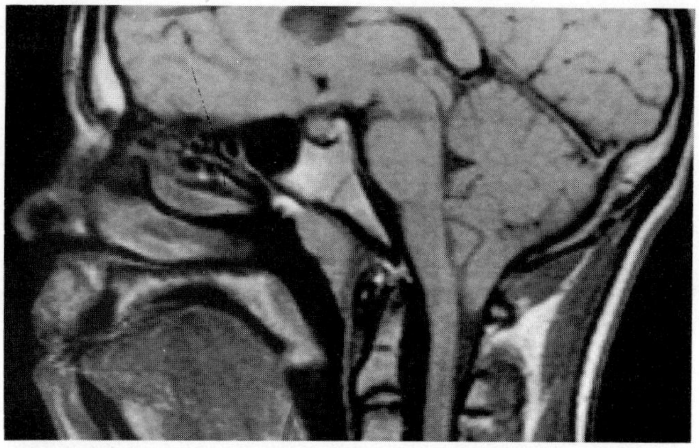

Figure 5-42
Sagittal T1 spin echo MRI showing herniation of the cerebellar tonsils into the upper cervical spinal canal, a Chiari I malformation. The patient presented with symptoms referable to a thoracic syrinx.

adults, particularly vertigo, dysequilibrium, occasionally "cough headache," and diplopia caused by internuclear ophthalmoplegia, along with symptoms referable to the involvement of other cranial nerves. On examination, downbeating nystagmus may be the clue to its presence.[266] Because other conditions, including ischemia, demyelinating disease, and spinocerebellar degeneration, may cause a similar syndrome, neuroimaging is necessary to establish the diagnosis. A Chiari anomaly is not an uncommon incidental finding, and clinical examination is necessary to determine whether it is symptomatic. Formerly difficult to demonstrate, the herniated cerebellar tonsils are exquisitely shown by sagittal MRI views (Fig. 5-42),[267,268] which also detect syringomyelia in 40 percent of patients with a Chiari malformation, a predictor of a less favorable surgical outcome.[268] The greater the extent of the tonsilar herniation, the more likely it is that the patient will experience symptoms.

CONCLUSION

The increasing variety of pulse sequences and scan planes available for MRI make it important to tailor each examination to the differential diagnosis or suspected site of the lesion in each patient. Investigation of a third nerve palsy requires high-resolution thin section images that include the midbrain, interpeduncular cistern, and cavernous sinuses; hemianopia or cortical blindness should be evaluated by a different technique directed to the occipital cortex, posterior arterial circulation, and dural sinuses. Close collaboration between the examining clinician and the neuroimager (if they are not the same individual) will result in an optimal diagnostic yield.

REFERENCES

1. Montagna P, Gallassi R, Medori R, et al: MELAS syndrome: Characteristic migrainous and epileptic features and maternal transmission. *Neurology* 38:751–754, 1988.
2. Orcutt JC, Page NGR, Sanders MG: Factors affecting visual loss in benign intracranial hypertension. *Ophthalmology* 91:1303–1312, 1984.
3. Streifler JY, Eliasziw M, Benavente OR, et al: The risk of stroke in patients with first-ever retinal vs hemispheric transient ischemic attacks and high-grade carotid stenosis: North American Symptomatic Carotid Endarterectomy Trial. *Arch Neurol* 52:246–249, 1995.
4. Appleton R, Farrell K, Buncic JR, et al: Amaurosis fugax in teenagers: A migraine variant. *Am J Dis Child* 142:331–333, 1988.
5. O'Sullivan F, Rossor M, Elston JS: Amaurosis fugax in young people *Br J Ophthalmol* 76:660–662, 1992.
6. Poole CJ, Ross RR, Harrison P, et al: Amaurosis fugax under the age of 40 years. *J Neurol Neurosurg Psychiatry* 50:81–84, 1987.
7. Tippin J, Corbett JJ, Kerber RE, et al: Amaurosis fugax and ocular infarction in adolescents and young adults. *Ann Neurol* 26:69–77, 1989.
8. Adams HJ, Putman SF, Corbett JJ, et al: Amaurosis fugax: The results of arteriography in 59 patients. *Stroke* 14:742–744, 1983.
9. Digre KB, Durcan FJ, Branch DW, et al: Amaurosis fugax associated with antiphospholipid antibodies. *Ann Neurol* 25:228–232, 1989.
10. Fisher CM: Observations of the fundus oculi in transient monocular blindness. *Neurology (Minneap)* 9:333–347, 1959.
11. Burger SK, Saul RF, Selhorst JB, et al: Transient monocular blindness caused by vasospasm. *N Engl J Med* 325:870–873, 1991.
12. Ploner CJ, Valdueza JM, Villringer A: Vasospastic amaurosis fugax in a patient with overlap collagenosis treated with nimodipine. *Neurol Res* 17:66–69, 1995.
13. Perez-Burkhardt JL, Gonzalez-Fajardo JA, Rodriguez E, et al: Amaurosis fugax as a symptom of carotid artery stenosis: Its relationship with ulcerated plaque. *J Cardiovasc Surg (Torino)* 35:15–18, 1994.
14. Smit RL, Baarsma GS, Koudstaal PJ: The source of embolism in amaurosis fugax and retinal artery occlusion. *Int Ophthalmol* 18:83–86, 1994.
15. Goodwin JA, Gorelick PB, Helgason CM: Symptoms of amaurosis fugax in atherosclerotic carotid artery disease. *Neurology* 37:829–832, 1987.
16. Sergott RC, Flaharty PM, Lieb WJ, et al: Color Doppler imaging identifies four syndromes of the retrobulbar circulation in patients with amaurosis fugax and central retinal artery occlusions. *Trans Am Ophthalmol Soc* 90:383–398, 1992.
17. Bluth El, Merritt CR: Doppler color imaging: Carotid and vertebral arteries. *Clin Diagn Ultrasound* 27:61–96, 1992.
18. Polak JF, Bajakian RL, O'Leary DH, et al: Detection of internal carotid artery stenosis: Comparison of MR angiography, color Doppler sonography, and arteriography. *Radiology* 182:35–40, 1992.
19. Hill SL, Donato AT: Ability of the carotid duplex scan to predict stenosis, symptoms, and plaque structure. *Surgery* 116:914–920, 1994.
20. Wilkerson DK, Keller I, Mezrich R, et al: The comparative evaluation of three-dimensional magnetic resonance for carotid artery disease. *J Vasc Surg* 14:803–809, 1991.
21. Anderson CM, Saloner D, Lee RE, et al: Assessment of carotid artery stenosis by MR angiography: Comparison with x-ray angiography and color-coded Doppler ultrasound. *AJNR* 13:989–1003, 1992.
22. Anderson CM, Haacke EM: Approaches to diagnostic magnetic resonance carotid angiography. *Semin Ultrasound CT MR* 13:246–255, 1992.
23. Levy RA, Prince MR: Arterial-phase three-dimensional contrast-enhanced MR angiography of the carotid arteries. *AJR* 167:211–215, 1996.
24. Heiserman JE, Drayer BP, Fram EK, et al: Carotid artery stenosis: Clinical efficacy of two-dimensional time-of-flight MR angiography. *Radiology* 182:761–768, 1992.
25. Vanninen R, Manninen H, Soimakallio S: Imaging of carotid artery stenosis: Clinical efficacy and cost-effectiveness. *AJNR* 16:1875–1883, 1995.
26. Obuchowski NA, Modic MT, Magdinec M, et al: Assessment of the efficacy of noninvasive screening for patients with asymptomatic neck bruits. *Stroke* 28:1330–1339, 1997.
27. Simeone A, Carriero A, Armillotta M, et al: Spiral CT angiography in the study of the carotid stenoses. *J Neuroradiol* 24:18–22, 1997.
28. Bogousslavsky J, Regli F: Cerebral infarct in apparent transient ischemic attack. *Neurology* 35:1501–1503, 1985.
29. Bogousslavsky J, Vinuela F, Barnett HJ, et al: Amaurosis fugax as the presenting manifestation of dural arteriovenous malformation. *Stroke* 16:891–893, 1985.
30. Xiong L, Li J, Jinkins JR: Amaurosis fugax caused by a dural arteriovenous fistula from the ophthalmic artery. *AJNR* 14:191–192, 1993.
31. Fritz W, Klein HJ, Schmidt K: Arteriovenous malformation of the posterior ethmoidal artery as an unusual cause of amaurosis fugax: The ophthalmic steal syndrome. *J Clin Neuro Ophthalmol* 9:165–168, 1989.
32. Brown GC, Shields JA: Amaurosis fugax secondary to presumed cavernous hemangioma of the orbit. *Ann Ophthalmol* 13:1205–1209, 1981.
33. Manor RS, Ben SI, Odel JG, et al: Amaurosis fugax at downward gaze [clinical conference]. *Surv Ophthalmol* 31:411–416, 1987.
34. Dirr LY, Troost BT, Elster AD, et al: Amaurosis fugax due to pituitary tumor. *J Clin Neuro Ophthalmol* 11:254–258, 1991.
35. Furlan AJ, Whisnant JP, Kearns TP: Unilateral visual loss in bright light: An unusual symptom of carotid artery occlusive disease. *Arch Neurol* 36:375–376, 1979.
36. Brigham RA, Youkey JR, Clagett GP, et al: Bright-light amaurosis fugax: An unusual symptom of retinal hypoperfusion corrected by external carotid revascularization. *Surgery* 97:363–368, 1985.
37. Wiebers DO, Swanson JW, Cascino TL, et al: Bilateral loss of vision in bright light. *Stroke* 20:554–558, 1989.
38. Mizener JB, Podhajsky P, Hayreh SS: Ocular ischemic syndrome. *Ophthalmology* 104:859–864, 1997.

39. Lepore FE: Visual obscurations: Evanescent and elementary. *Semin Neurol* 6:167–175, 1986.
40. Turner RM, Gutman I, Hilal SK, et al: CT of drusen bodies and other calcific lesions of the optic nerve: Case report and differential diagnosis. *AJNR* 4:175–178, 1983.
41. Mokri B, Piepgras DG, Miller GM: Syndrome of orthostatic headaches and diffuse pachymeningeal gadolinium enhancement. *Mayo Clin Proc* 72:400–413, 1997.
42. Schievink WI, Meyer FB, Atkinson JL, et al: Spontaneous spinal cerebrospinal fluid leaks and intracranial hypotension. *J Neurosurg* 84:598–605, 1996.
43. Gass A, Barker GJ, Riordan-Eva P, et al: MRI of the optic nerve in benign intracranial hypertension. *Neuroradiology* 38:769–773, 1996.
44. Brodsky MC, Glasier CM: Magnetic resonance visualization of the swollen optic disc in papilledema. *J Neuro Ophthalmol* 15:122–124, 1995.
45. Manfre L, Lagalla R, Mangiameli A, et al: Idiopathic intracranial hypertension: Orbital MRI. *Neuroradiology* 37:459–461, 1995.
46. Jinkins JR, Athale S, Xiong L, et al: MR of optic papilla protrusion in patients with high intracranial pressure. *AJNR* 17:665–668, 1996.
47. Pasquale LR, Moster ML, Schmaier A: Dural sinus thrombosis with abnormalities of protein S and fibrinogen. *Arch Ophthalmol* 108:644, 1990.
48. Horton JC, Seiff SR, Pitts LH, et al: Decompression of the optic nerve sheath for vision-threatening papilledema caused by dural sinus occlusion. *Neurosurgery* 31:203–211, 1992.
49. Karahalios DG, Rekate HL, Khayata MH, et al: Elevated intracranial venous pressure as a universal mechanism in pseudotumor cerebri of varying etiologies. *Neurology* 46:198–202, 1996.
50. Sugerman HJ, DeMaria EJ, Felton WL 3rd, et al: Increased intra-abdominal pressure and cardiac filling pressures in obesity-associated pseudotumor cerebri. *Neurology* 49:507–511, 1997.
51. Sacks O: *Migraine.* Berkeley, University of California Press, 1992.
52. Hupp SL, Kline LB, Corbett JJ: Visual disturbances of migraine. *Surv Ophthalmol* 33:221–236, 1989.
53. Weinstein JM, Appen RE, Houston L, et al: Recurrent scintillating scotoma and homonymous hemianopia due to metastic melanoma. *J Cin Neuro Ophthalmol* 7:155–160, 1987.
54. Troost BT, Newton TH: Occipital lobe arteriovenous malformations: Clinical and radiologic features in 26 cases with comments on differentiation from migraine. *Arch Ophthalmol* 93:250–256, 1975.
55. Caplan LR: Migraine and vertebrobasilar ischemia. *Neurology* 41:55–61, 1991.
56. Bogousslavsky J, Regli F, Van Melle G: Migraine stroke. *Neurology* 38:223–227, 1988.
57. Rothrock JF, Walicke P, Swenson MR: Migrainous stroke. *Arch Neurol* 45:63–67, 1988.
58. Lewis RA, Vijayan N, Watson C, et al: Visual field loss in migraine. *Ophthalmology* 96:321–326, 1989.
59. Ferbert A, Busse D, Thron A: Microinfarction in classic migraine? A study with magnetic resonance imaging findings. *Stroke* 22:1010–1014, 1991.
60. Igarashi H, Sakai F, Kan S, et al: Magnetic resonance imaging of the brain in patients with migraine. *Cephalalgia* 11:69–74, 1991.
61. De Benedittis G, Lorenzetti A, Sina C, et al: Magnetic resonance imaging in migraine and tension-type headache. *Headache* 35:264–268, 1995.
62. Osborn RE, Alder DC, Mitchell CS: MR imaging of the brain in patients with migraine headaches. *AJNR* 12:521–524, 1991.
63. Ziegler DK, Batnitzky S, Barter R, et al: Magnetic resonance image abnormality in migraine with aura. *Cephalalgia* 11:147–150, 1991.
64. Hauser RA, Lacey DM, Knight MR: Hypertensive encephalopathy: Magnetic resonance imaging demonstration of reversible cortical white matter lesions. *Arch Neurol* 45:1078–1083, 1988.
65. Maleki M, Kirkham TH: Arteriovenous malformations of the posterior cerebral hemispheres. *Can J Ophthalmol* 18:22, 1983.
66. Newman DS, Levine SR, Curtis VL, et al: Migraine-like visual phenomena associated with cerebral venous thrombosis. *Headache* 29:82–85, 1989.
67. Rubin AM: Transient cortical blindness and occipital seizures with cyclosporine toxicity. *Transplantation* 47: 572–573, 1989.
68. Lantos G: Cortical blindness due to osmotic disruption of the blood-brain barrier by angiographic contrast material: CT and MRI studies. *Neurology* 39:567–571, 1989.
69. Duncan R, Hadley D, Bone I, et al: Blindness in eclampsia: CT and MR imaging. *J Neurol Neurosurg Psychiatry* 52:899–902, 1989.
70. Ramani V: Cortical blindness following ictal nystagmus. *Arch Neurol* 42:191–192, 1985.
71. Sadeh M: Postictal blindness in adults. *Bull Clin Neurosc* 48:173, 1983.
72. Sethi PK, Kumar BR, Madan VS, et al: Appearing and disappearing CT scan abnormalities and seizures. *J Neurol Neurosurg Psychiatry* 48:866, 1985.
73. Klopstock T, May A, Seibel P, et al: Mitochondrial DNA in migraine with aura. *Neurology* 46:1735–1738, 1996.
74. Tychsen L: Hydrocephalus and transient cortical blindness. *Am J Ophthalmol* 98:819–820, 1984.
75. Pantin CFA, Young RAL: Postprandial blindness. *Br Med J* 281:1686, 1980.
76. Beck L, Stiller RJ, Leone-Tomaschoff S: Postpartum pulmonary embolism as an unusual cause of cortical blindness. *Am J Obstet Gynecol* 162:696–697, 1990.
77. Mukamel M, Weitz R, Nissenkorn H, et al: Acute cortical blindness associated with hypoglycemia. *Brief Clin Lab Observ* 98:583–584, 1981.
78. Naparstek Y, Shouval D, Auerbach E, et al: Transient cortical blindness in hepatic encephalopathy. *Isr J Med Sci* 15:854–856, 1979.
79. Moel DI, Kwun YA: Cortical blindness as a complication of hemodialysis. *J Pediatr* 93:890–891, 1978.
80. Siegel RK: Hallucinations. *Sci Am* 237:132–141, 1977.
81. Lepore FE: Spontaneous visual phenomena with visual loss: 104 patients with lesions of retinal and neural and afferent pathways. *Neurology* 40:444–447, 1990.
82. Shedlack KJ, McDonald WM, Laskowitz DT, et al: Geniculocalcarine hyperintensities on brain magnetic

resonance imaging associated with visual hallucinations in the elderly. *Psychiatry Res* 54:283–293, 1994.
83. Lessell S, Lessell IM, Glaser JS: Topical diagnosis: Retrochiasmal visual pathways and higher cortical function, in: Duane TD, Jaeger EA (eds): *Clinical Ophthalmology,* vol 2. Philadelphia, Lippincott, 1988, pp: 1–24.
84. Kelliher TR, Sabin T: Senile visual hallucination: A case report and review of the literature. *Neurol Chronicle* 213–15, 1993.
85. Crystal HA, Wolfson LI, Ewing S: Visual hallucinations as the first symptoms of Alzheimer's disease. *Am J Psychiatry* 145:1318, 1988.
86. Pfeiffer RF, Kang J, Graber B, et al: Clozapine for psychosis in Parkinson's disease. *Mov Disord* 5:239–242, 1990.
87. Lance JW, Smee RI: Partial seizures with visual hallucinations treated by radiotherapy of cavernous hemangioma. *Ann Neurol* 26:782–785, 1989.
88. Penfield W, Perot P: The brain's record of auditory and visual experience. *Brain* 86:595–596, 1963.
89. Benson MT, Rennie IG: Formed hallucination in the hemianopic field. *Postgrad Med J* 65:756–757, 1989.
90. Kölmel HW: Complex visual hallucinations in the hemianopic field. *J Neurol Neurosurg Psychiatry* 48:29–38, 1985.
91. Fleishman JA, Beck RW, Linares OA, et al: Deficits in visual function after resolution of optic neuritis. *Ophthalmology* 94:1029–1035, 1987.
92. Guy J, Mancuso A, Quisling RG, et al: Gadolinium-DTPA-enhanced magnetic resonance imaging in optic neuropathies. *Ophthalmology* 97:592–599, 1990.
93. Guy J, Mao J, Bidgood W Jr, et al: Enhancement and demyelination of the intraorbital optic nerve: Fat suppression magnetic resonance imaging. *Ophthalmology* 99:713–719, 1992.
94. Tourbah A, Deschamps R, Stievenart JL, et al: Magnetic resonance imaging using FLAIR pulse sequence in white matter diseases. *J Neuroradiol* 23:217–222, 1996.
95. Yetkin FZ, Haughton VM, Papke RA, et al: Multiple sclerosis: Specificity of MR for diagnosis. *Radiology* 178:447–451, 1991.
96. Yetkin FZ, Haughton VM, Fischer ME, et al: High-signal foci on MR images of the brain: Observer variability in their quantification. *AJR* 159:185–188, 1992.
97. Frederiksen JL, Larsson HB, Olesen J, et al: MRI, VEP, SEP and biothesiometry suggest monosymptomatic acute optic neuritis to be a first manifestation of multiple sclerosis. *Acta Neurol Scand* 83:343–350, 1991.
98. Jacobs LD, Kaba SE, Miller CM, et al: Correlation of clinical, magnetic resonance imaging, and cerebrospinal fluid findings in optic neuritis. *Ann Neurol* 41:392–398, 1997.
99. Optic Neuritis Study Group: The 5-year risk of MS after optic neuritis. *Neurology* 49:1404–1413, 1997.
100. Scholl GB, Song HS, Wray SH: Uhthoff's symptom in optic neuritis: Relationship to magnetic resonance imaging and development of multiple sclerosis. *Ann Neurol* 30:180–184, 1991.
101. Ellenberger CJ, Keltner JL, Burde RM: Acute optic neuropathy in older patients. *Arch Neurol* 28:182–185, 1973.
102. Beck RW, Savino PJ, Repka MX, et al: Optic disc structure in anterior ischemic optic neuropathy. *Ophthalmology* 91:1334–1337, 1984.
103. Feit RH, Tomsak RL, Ellenberger CJ: Structural factors in the pathogenesis of ischemic optic neuropathy. *Am J Ophthalmol* 98:105–108, 1984.
104. Horton JC, Fishman RA: Neurovisual findings in the syndrome of spontaneous intracranial hypotension from dural cerebrospinal fluid leak. *Ophthalmology* 101:244–251, 1994.
105. Kawamoto A, Shimada K, Matsubayashi K, et al: Factors associated with silent multiple lacunar lesions on magnetic resonance imaging in asymptomatic elderly hypertensive patients. *Clin Exp Pharmacol Physiol* 18:605–610, 1991.
106. Chimowitz MI, Estes ML, Furlan AJ, et al: Further observations on the pathology of subcortical lesions identified on magnetic resonance imaging. *Arch Neurol* 49:747–752, 1992.
107. Jay WM, Williamson MR: Incidence of subcortical lesions not increased in nonarteritic ischemic optic neuropathy on magnetic resonance imaging. *Am J Ophthalmol* 104:398–400, 1987.
108. Arnold AC, Hepler RS, Hamilton DR, et al: Magnetic resonance imaging of the brain in nonarteritic ischemic optic neuropathy. *J Neuro Ophthalmol* 15:158–160, 1995.
109. Bogousslavsky J, Regli F, Zografos L, et al: Optico-cerebral syndrome: Simultaneous hemodynamic infarction of optic nerve and brain. *Neurology* 37:263–268, 1987.
110. Schmidt WA, Kraft HE, Vorpaul K, et al: Color duplex ultrasonography in the diagnosis of temporal arteritis. *N Engl J Med* 337:1336–1342, 1997.
111. Knabben H, Wolf S, Solbach U, et al: Risk factors in patients with amaurosis fugax. *Klin Monatsbl Augenheilkd* 208:142–144, 1996.
112. Ellenberger C, Epstein AD: Ocular complications of atherosclerosis: What do they mean? *Semin Neurol* 6:185–193, 1986.
113. Rath EZ, Frank RN, Shin DH, et al: Risk factors for retinal vein occlusions: A case-control study. *Ophthalmology* 99:509–514, 1992.
114. Elman MJ, Bhatt AK, Quinlan PM, et al: The risk for systemic vascular diseases and mortality in patients with central retinal vein occlusion. *Ophthalmology* 97:1543–1548, 1990.
115. Barke RM, Yoshizumi MO, Hepler RS, et al: Spontaneous dural carotid-cavernous fistula with central retinal vein occlusion and iris neovascularization. *Ann Ophthalmol* 23:11–17, 1991.
116. Komiyama M, Yamanaka K, Nagata Y, et al: Dural carotid-cavernous sinus fistula and central retinal vein occlusion: A case report and a review of the literature. *Surg Neurol* 34:255–259, 1990.
117. Yasuda Y, Morita T, Akiguchi I, et al: Sphenoid sinus mucocele with recurrent visual disturbance. *Eur Neurol* 32:225–227, 1992.
118. Casteels I, De Loof E, Brock P, et al: Sudden blindness in a child: Presenting symptom of a sphenoid sinus mucocele. *Br J Ophthalmol* 76:502–504, 1992.
119. Weisman JS, Hepler RS, Vinters HV: Reversible visual loss caused by fibrous dysplasia. *Am J Ophthalmol* 110: 244–249, 1990.

CHAPTER 6

DEAFNESS, DIZZINESS, AND DISORDERS OF EQUILIBRIUM

Alfred L. Weber
Laura Vitale Romo

INTRODUCTION[1]

Deafness, dizziness, and disorders of equilibrium are common manifestations of disease entities that require investigation with various imaging modalities, such as computed tomography (CT) and magnetic resonance imaging (MRI).

Hearing loss comprises three types: (1) conductive, (2) sensorineural, and (3) central. *Conductive hearing loss* is most commonly secondary to inflammatory disease and/or cholesteatoma of the middle ear cavity and less frequently secondary to trauma, otosclerosis, and congenital anomalies of the tympanic bone, including the ossicular structures. High-resolution CT is the modality utilized for evaluation of conductive hearing loss. *Sensorineural hearing loss* is caused by abnormalities of the cochlea or the cochlear division of the eighth nerve complex. *Central hearing loss* is less often encountered and is secondary to lesions in the cochlear nuclei and their connections with the primary area for hearing in the anterior transverse temporal gyrus of Heschl. Magnetic resonance imaging with gadolinium is the method utilized for assessment of central and retrolabyrinthine sensorineural hearing loss.

Dizziness is a general term that covers various complaints. In the context of this chapter, dizziness implies vertigo, which refers to subjective and objective perception of motion or position and may be caused by diseases in the labyrinth and vestibular nerve, and the brainstem. The radiologic modality for evaluation of vertigo is MRI with or without the introduction of gadolinium.

Tinnitus, or ringing in the ears, is often associated with hearing loss and vertigo. It is defined as any sensation of sound for which there is no external source. It is encountered in diseases of the inner ear, tumors of the temporal bone, including the jugular fossa, and vascular lesions, such as carotid artery stenosis, basivertebral artery tortuosity and stenosis, and dural venous malformations.

Equilibrium disorders may arise within the vestibule, brainstem, and cerebellum. As in vertigo, MRI with gadolinium is the preferred method of examination.

IMAGING METHODS

The primary imaging methods for patients with disorders of hearing and equilibrium are high-resolution CT and MRI. Both of these methods have advantages and disadvantages, and their selection is based on the underlying clinical problem and the type of lesion that is suspected.

Computed tomography is indicated when the primary abnormality involves the bony structures and air spaces of the temporal bone.[2] Such abnormalities include conductive hearing loss secondary to middle ear and mastoid infections, trauma, tumors, and congenital malformations. Also, CT is indicated in the presurgical evaluation of patients for cochlear implantation.[3] The temporal bone is examined in the axial and coronal planes with thin slices 1 to 2 mm in thickness. With these slices, detailed images of the ossicular chain and the inner ear structures can be obtained. Such information is valuable in patients with infection and/or cholesteatoma with erosion of the scutum or ossicular chain.

Recently, the introduction of *spiral CT*[4] has allowed the rapid acquisition of three-dimensional-volume images in seconds. This is accomplished with continuous movement of the CT table along with simultaneous, circular (slip-ring) movement of the x-ray beam. The acquired volumetric data can be used to construct thin, single slices or three-dimensional reconstructions in any plane.

This faster technique has particular application in temporal bone imaging,[5] especially in patients who are too ill to tolerate conventional, longer scan times. Spiral CT is also useful in the pediatric age group, since such patients must often be sedated to obtain a high-resolution CT study. With the short spiral scan times, little or no sedation may be required.

Spiral CT has recently been combined with maximum intensity projection (MIP) algorithms. The use of this technique, followed by the injection of intravenous contrast medium, can produce high-quality angiographic images in various parts of the body, including the neck and posterior fossa.[6] This method has certain advantages over both conventional and magnetic resonance angiography (MRA). The acquisition time is much shorter than with MRA, and, compared to conventional angiography, it is relatively noninvasive.

Just as CT scanning represented a major advance in imaging of the bony anatomy of the temporal bone, MRI has revolutionized the diagnosis of tumors of the vestibulocochlear system. The most important advantage of MRI is the superior soft tissue and contrast resolution. While CT scanning relies on only one tissue parameter (x-ray attenuation) for image formation, MRI has several tissue parameters that affect image contrast and resolution. These MRI parameters include spin density and T1, and T2 relaxation times. The relaxation times are intrinsic to the tissues, and each may be emphasized by using the appropriate pulse sequence. This is important because a lesion may be apparent on one pulse sequence (e.g., a T2-weighted sequence) but may be difficult or impossible to visualize on alternative pulse sequences.

In some cases, tumors are isointense with the surrounding tissues on all pulse sequences and are nearly impossible to detect unless they distort the surrounding anatomy. In such cases, it is useful to introduce a gadolinium-based contrast agent intravenously. Gadolinium is a paramagnetic agent that causes marked T1 shortening, reflected by increased signal intensity in tissues with contrast material accumulation.

The imaging protocol for evaluation of sensorineural hearing loss, especially when an acoustic neurinoma is suspected, includes sagittal T1- and axial T2-weighted images of the entire brain. These studies are followed by 3-mm coronal T1-weighted sections through the temporal bone before the introduction of contrast medium and cerebellopontine (CP) angle and 3-mm axial and coronal T1-weighted sections after the introduction of gadolinium. If an intracranial lesion is suspected, the entire brain is examined with MRI, and a study is also performed after the introduction of contrast medium. If the patient has had surgery for a previous acoustic neuroma, it may be difficult to distinguish between postoperative fat packing of the porous acousticus and recurrent or residual disease. In these cases, fat suppression techniques[7] allow differentiation of the darkened fat from any residual enhancing tumor.

Magnetic resonance imaging is also the optimal imaging modality for demonstration of pathologic conditions of the CP angle. Lesions of this area include meningioma, epidermoid and cholesterol cysts, lipoma, and metastasis.[8] They may affect hearing by involving the eighth nerve complex in the CP angle. Such lesions are best identified by MRI because of the ability to provide contrast between the tumor, bone, and cerebrospinal fluid (CSF). Furthermore, MRI can demonstrate the central auditory pathway in the medulla, midbrain, and temporal lobes and exclude intra-axial pathologic processes.

The recent development of *"fast-spin echo" sequences* has significantly shortened imaging times while increasing image quality.[9,10] In addition, the availability of *high-resolution, three-dimensional data acquisition* has expanded the uses of MRI in the temporal bone and brain.[11,12] These techniques are, for the most part, variations of gradient echo sequences. Very thin slice thickness can be obtained with these techniques, which may allow detailed study of small structures, such as the cochlea or ossicular chain.[9,13,14] Malformations of the inner ear can be assessed with this technique.

In conjunction with the development of gradient echo and three-dimensional imaging techniques, MRA has been developed. This technique provides an image of flowing blood and has been shown to be an excellent noninvasive screening tool in the detection of carotid artery stenosis, intracranial aneurysms of the circle of Willis, large arteriovenous malformations, and certain vascular anomalies.[15]

The major disadvantage of MRI in the temporal bone is that many of the landmarks are small bony structures, which appear as areas of signal void due to the lack of moving water protons.

Unfortunately, because of the strong magnetic field used in imaging systems (1- to 1.5-tesla field strengths), patients with pacemaker devices, aneurysmal clips, and intraocular metallic foreign bodies should not be imaged, since the metal may move in the magnetic field, causing complications for the patient.[16]

PATHOLOGIC ENTITIES

Temporal Bone

Labyrinthine Lesions

Heretofore, the labyrinth was evaluated with high-resolution CT, which is still the modality of choice to detect bony abnormalities of the labyrinth, such as otospongiosis. However, some lesions of the labyrinth can be visualized with MRI, including hemorrhage, congenital malformations of the inner ear, and neurinomas in the cochlea and vestibule, detected with contrast MRI.[17]

Labyrinthine hemorrhage occurs in patients with coagulopathies, leukemia, and invasion by lesions such as hemangioma, cholesterol granuloma, or malignant tumor. In subacute hemorrhage, MRI demonstrates high signal intensity on the T1- and T2-weighted images.[18]

Labyrinthitis may be caused by a number of viruses, including rubella, mumps, herpes, or measles. It may also be secondary to bacterial infections or syphilis, or may follow meningitis, in which case the disease is bilateral. These agents cause an inflammatory process of the membranous labyrinth, which leads to enhancement of the cochlea or vestibule on contrast MRI[19] (Fig. 6-1). The evolution of enhancement may coincide with the patient's symptoms, and enhancement may recede with resolution of the inflammatory process. In some pa-

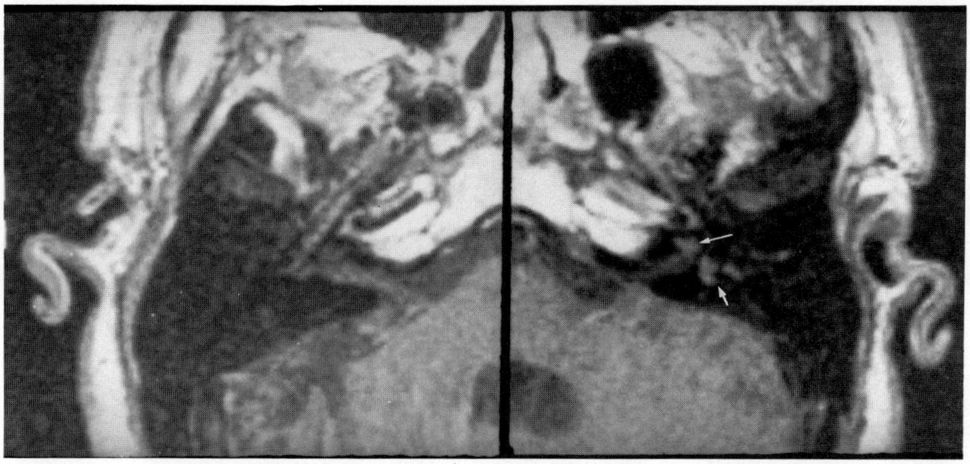

Figure 6-1
Labyrinthitis. Axial T1-weighted image (after gadolinium introduction) reveals diffuse enhancement of the cochlea and vestibule (arrows). (Case from Dr. Alexander S. Mark, Department of Radiology, Washington Hospital Center, Washington, D.C.)

tients, the location of enhancement correlates with the frequency level of the hearing loss, for example, enhancement of the basal turn of the cochlea with high-frequency hearing loss and enhancement of the apical turn in patients with low-frequency hearing loss.[17]

Labyrinthine schwannomas[20,21] are the most common benign neoplasms of the labyrinth. They are more commonly found in the vestibule and less frequently in the cochlea. These schwannomas are histologically identical to their counterparts in the internal auditory canal and CP angle, and present with sensorineural hearing loss and/or vertigo. On contrast MRI, a markedly enhancing mass is demonstrated in the cochlea or vestibule.[22] These lesions may expand the bone within the vestibule and cochlea.

Otosclerosis (Otospongiosis)

Otosclerosis is characterized by the replacement of normal, ivory-like endochondral bone with foci of spongy, vascular, irregular, new bone on the CT study. This spongy bone is indicated by ill-defined, low-attenuation areas within the dense labyrinthine bone.[23]

Otosclerosis is divided into two major forms: (1) fenestral otosclerosis and (2) retrofenestral, or cochlear, otosclerosis. In the *fenestral type*, the lateral wall of the labyrinth, including the promontory, and both the oval and round window niches are involved. Involvement of the oval window leads to fixation of the stapes, with subsequent conductive hearing loss (Fig. 6-2A). The *cochlear type* of otosclerosis may occur as a primary isolated focus but most often is an extension of fenestral otosclerosis. On CT, variably sized, low-attenuation areas are encountered around the cochlea[24](Fig. 6-2B). Cochlear otosclerosis is associated with sensorineural hearing loss.

Middle Ear Diseases

Various middle ear diseases cause conductive hearing loss. In these conditions, the ossicular chain is interrupted, and, depending on the degree of fixation or destruction, significant conductive hearing loss approaching 30 dB and more may ensue. The most common conditions leading to interruption of the conduction mechanism are inflammatory processes associated

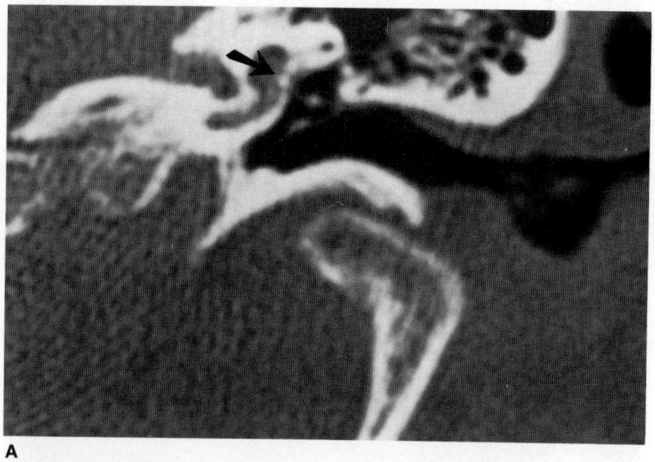

A

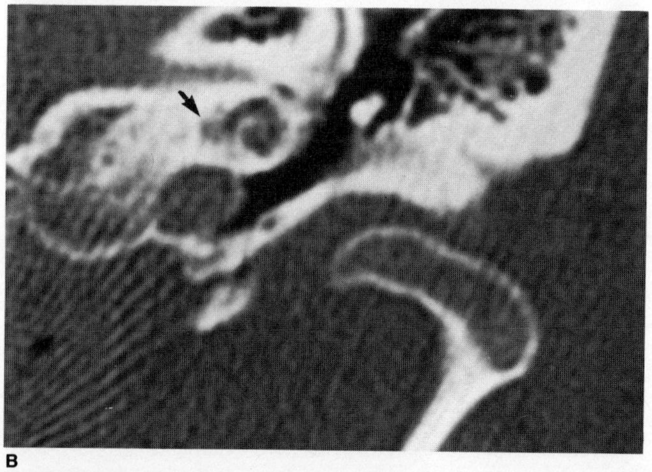

B

Figure 6-2
Otospongiosis. **(A)** *Coronal CT section demonstrates occlusion of the oval window by oteospongeotic bone (arrow).* **(B)** *Coronal CT section illustrates oteospongeotic bone around the cochlea, reflected by lucent areas (arrow).*

with fluid, edema, fibrosis, and cholesteatomas[25] (Fig. 6-3A and B). Inflammatory disease and/or secondary cholesteatoma cause erosion of the ossicular chain, especially the long process of the incus, with consequent interruption of the conduction mechanism (Fig. 6-4A,B,C, and D). Primary cholesteatoma arises from entrapped epidermoid cells within the temporal bone. Primary middle ear cholesteatoma manifests as a whitish mass behind an intact tympanic membrane. A well-

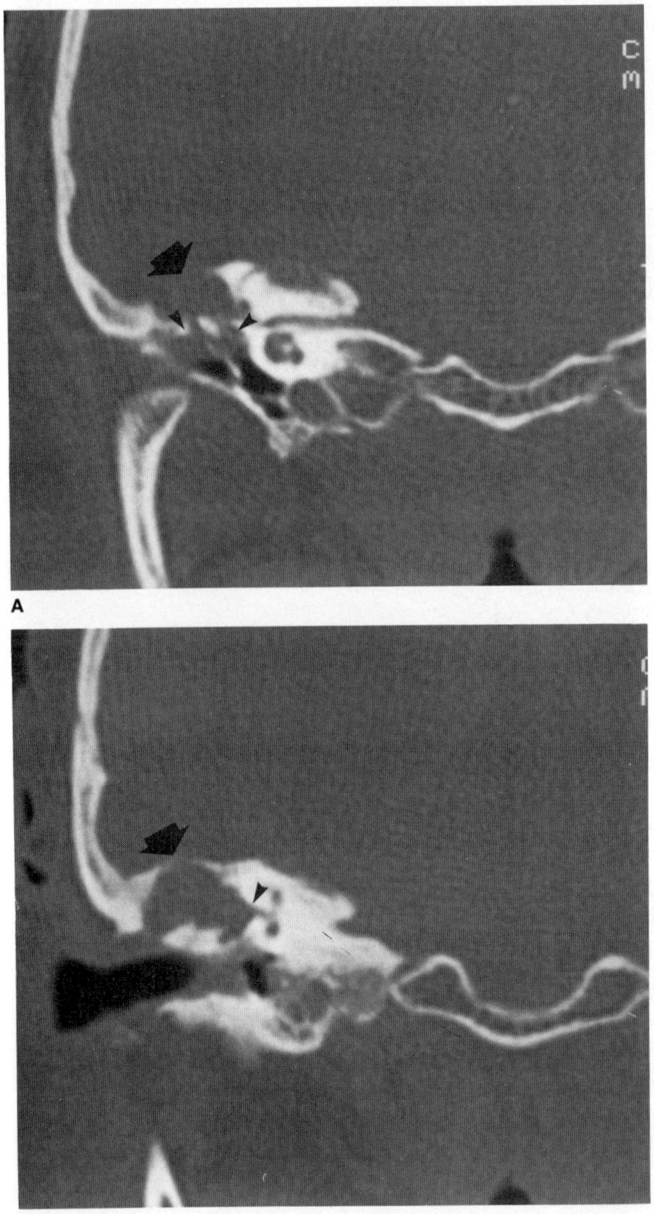

Figure 6-3
Right cholesteatoma. **(A)** *Coronal CT section demonstrates a right-sided cholesteatomatous mass in the bony external canal and middle ear cavity (arrowheads). Also, note the defect in the tegmen and involvement of the mastoid air cells (arrow).* **(B)** *Second coronal section demonstrates expansion of the right mastoid antrum by cholesteatoma (arrow) and fistula of the horizontal semicircular canal (arrowhead).*

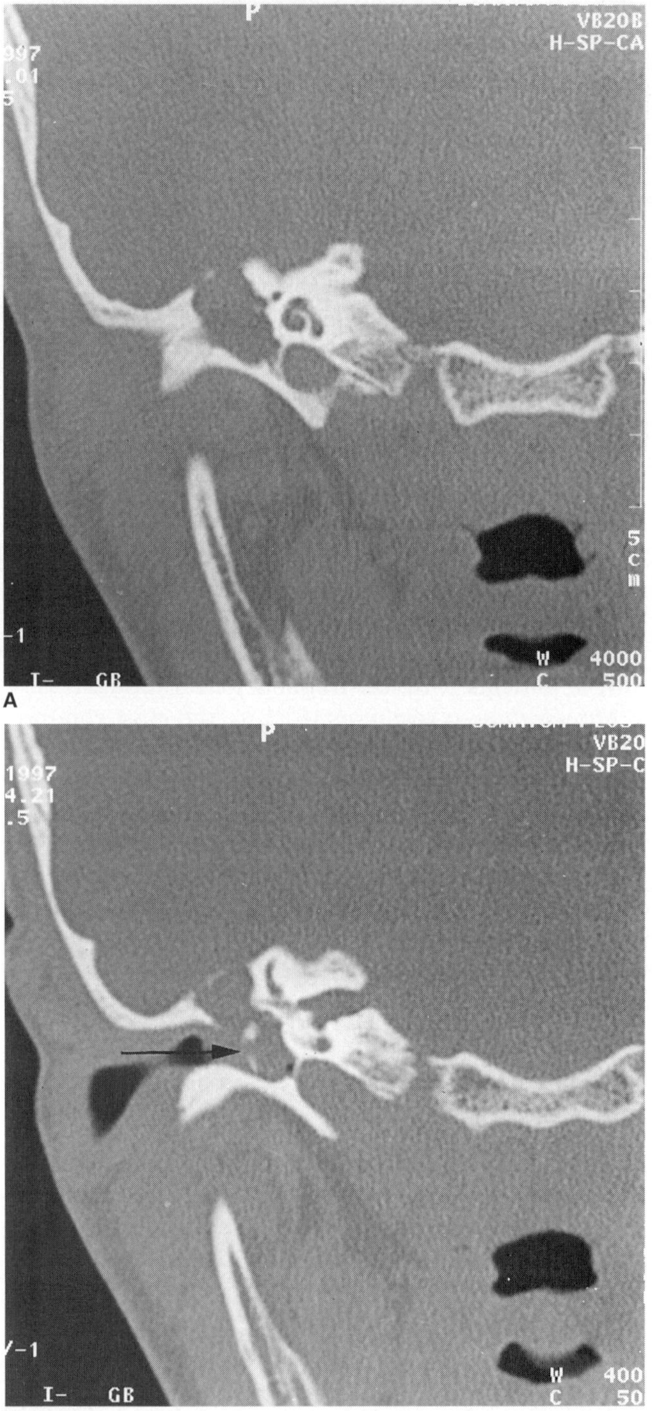

Figure 6-4
Cholesteatoma of the right temporal bone. **(A)** *Coronal CT section through the right middle ear cavity at the level of the cochlea reveals an expansile mass with sharply defined bony margins in the middle ear cavity, epitympanic recess, and adjacent mastoid.* **(B)** *Coronal CT section at the level between the cochlea and vestibule demonstrates the cholesteatoma with erosion of the spur and ossicles. Remnants of ossicles are noted within the cholesteatomatous mass (arrow).*

defined or ill-defined mass is recognized on the CT scan (Fig. 6-5).

Various types of benign and malignant tumors are associated with hearing loss by virtue of mechanical interference. A large variety of these lesions may arise within the middle ear cavity or extend secondarily into the middle ear cavity from the bony external canal or jugular fossa (glomus jugulare tumor)[26] (Fig. 6-6).

Congenital abnormalities may involve the ossicular

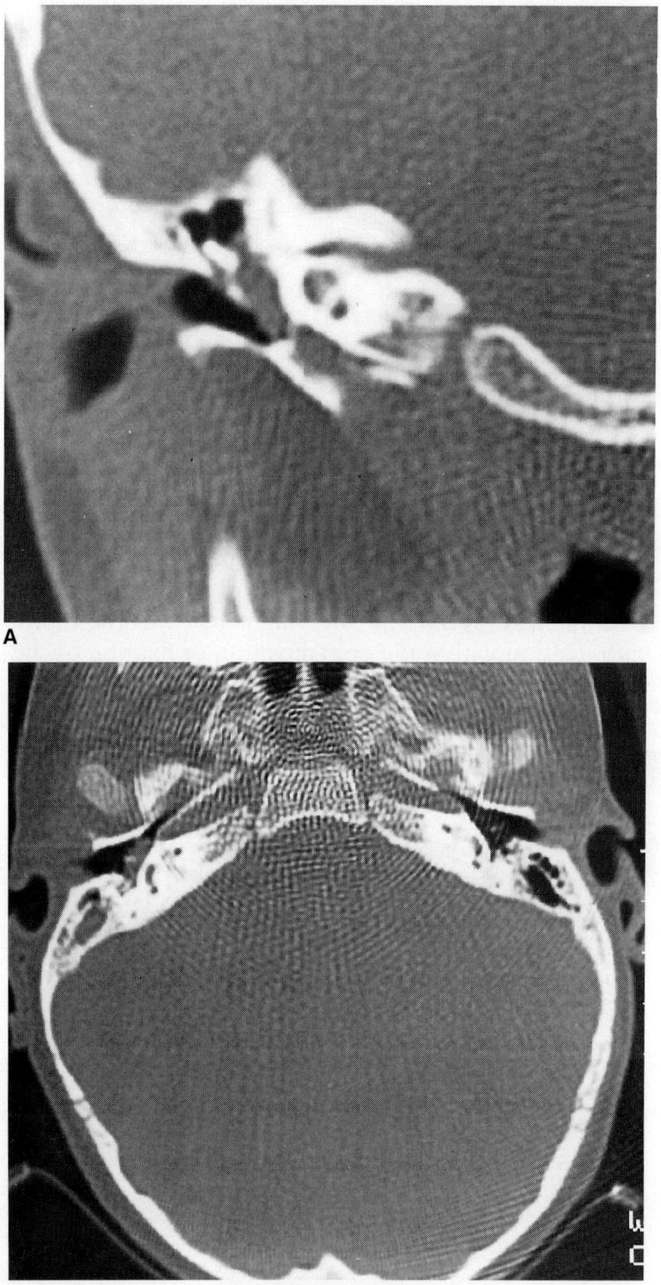

A

B

Figure 6-5

Primary cholesteatoma of the right middle ear cavity. **(A)** *Coronal CT section at the cochlear level demonstrates a well-defined, homogeneous mass in the right middle ear cavity and epitympanic recess medial to the slightly displaced lateral malleus.* **(B)** *Axial CT section through the middle ear cavity demonstrates the oval-shaped mass in the middle ear cavity medial to the malleus. Note slight sclerosis of the right mastoid and nonspecific soft tissue densities in the remaining air space.*

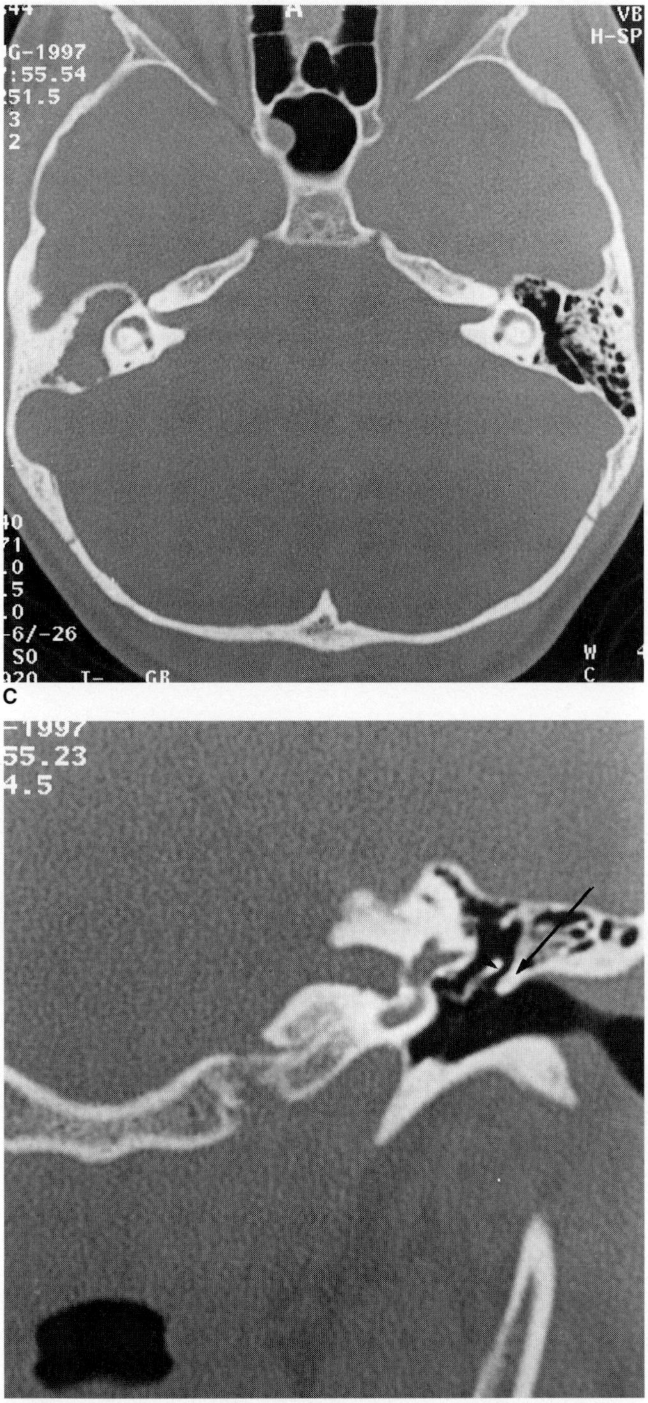

C

D

(C) *Axial CT section through the right temporal bone reveals the expansile cholesteatoma in the middle ear cavity, epitympanic recess, and mastoid. The visualized remaining mastoid is sclerotic.* **(D)** *Normal left ear for comparison, demonstrating the bony external canal, spur (arrow), incus (arrowhead), middle ear cavity, epitympanic recess, and inner ear structures.*

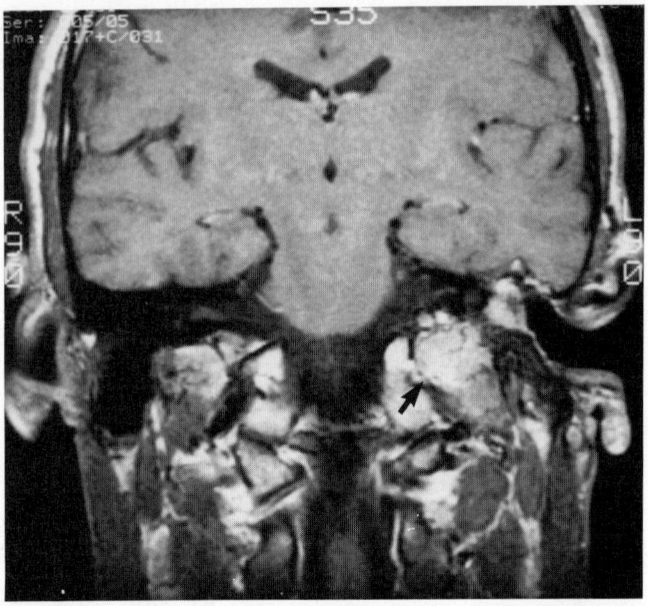

Figure 6-6
Glomus jugulare tumor. Coronal T1-weighted image (after gadolinium introduction) reveals an enhancing tumor mass in the jugular fossa and upper neck (arrow) with extension into left middle ear cavity.

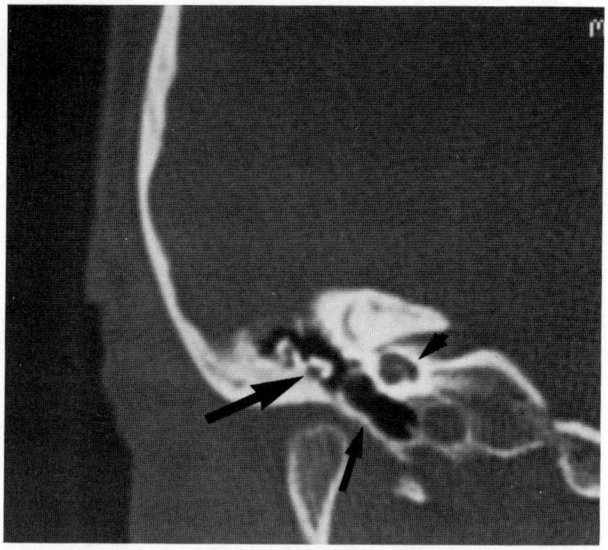

Figure 6-7
Right middle ear malformation. Coronal CT section through the right temporal bone reveals an atresia plate (small arrow) with a malformed malleus (large arrow). Note the normal cochlea (arrowhead).

structures and are characterized by malformation in development, especially of the long process of the incus, with fixation within the epitympanum or fixation of the stapes within the oval window. Ossicular deformities are also encountered in association with maldevelopment of the tympanic bone[27] (Fig. 6-7). In these ear malformations, the tympanic bone is underdeveloped, with hypoplasia or absence of the external auditory canal and formation of an atresia plate of variable thickness, underdevelopment of the middle ear cavity and epitympanic recess, and associated underdevelopment of the mastoid (Fig. 6-8A,B, and C). In most of these cases, the inner ear structures are normal, and no sensorineural

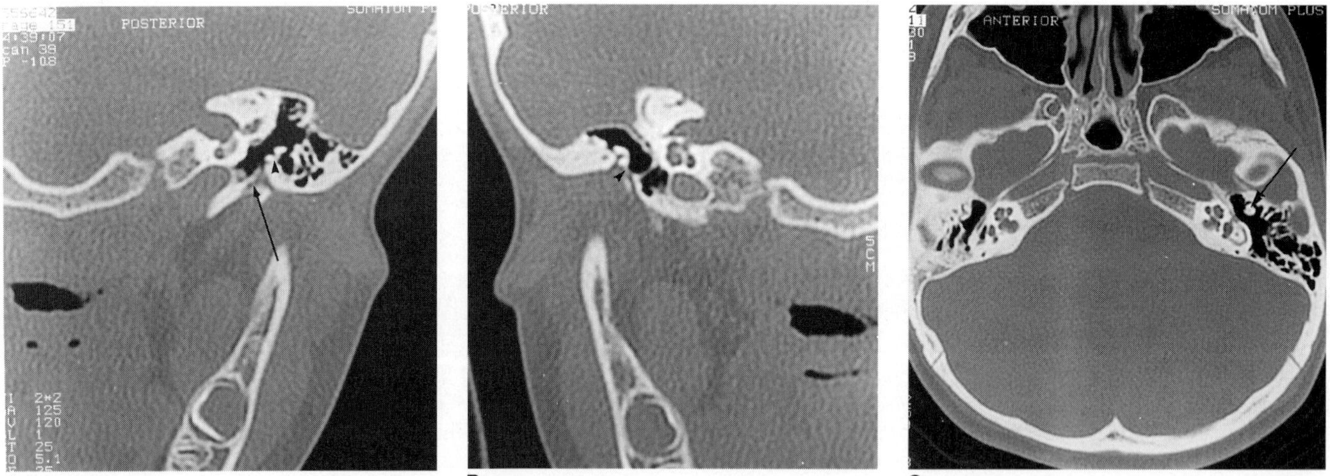

A B C

Figure 6-8
Bilateral aural atresia. **(A)** *Coronal CT section through the left ear at the level of the internal auditory canal demonstrates absence of the external auditory canal, irregularly shaped atresia plate (arrow), and deformed ossicles (arrowhead) fused to the upper margin of the atresia plate.* **(B)** *CT section at the level of the right cochlea demonstrates a thin atresia plate with deformed ossicles fused to the atresia plate (arrowhead). The external auditory canal is absent.* **(C)** *Axial CT section through the temporal bones demonstrates a normally pneumatized left mastoid but an underpneumatized, sclerotic right mastoid. There is slight to moderate diminution in the size of the right middle ear cavity and epitympanic recess and a normal-sized left middle ear cavity and epitympanic recess. Note the fused, deformed malleus and incus in the left epitympanic recess (arrow).*

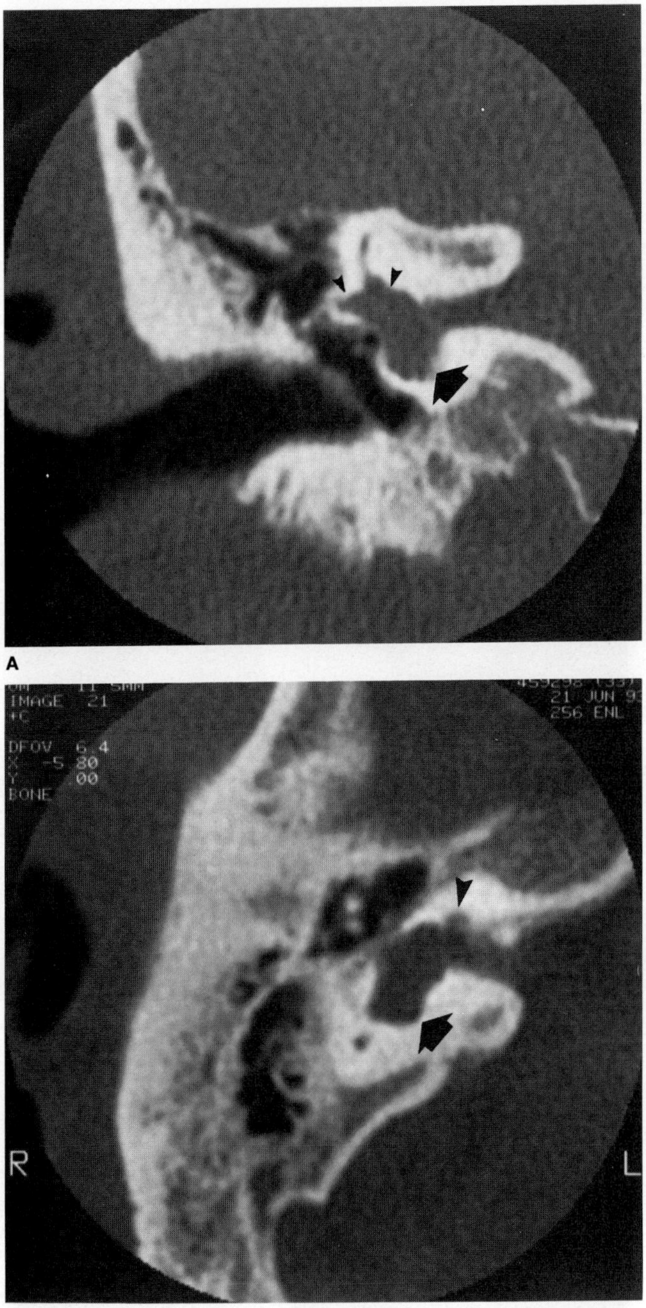

Figure 6-9

Mondini malformation. **(A)** *Coronal CT section through the temporal bones reveals a saccular cochlea (arrow) with loss of turns along with dilatation of the vestibule (arrowheads) and lateral semicircular canal.* **(B)** *Axial CT section through the right temporal bone reveals saccular deformation of the cochlea (arrowhead) with dilatation of the vestibule (arrow).*

hearing loss is present. Sensorineural hearing loss may be caused by malformation of the inner ear, which includes complete aplasia of the inner ear (Michele deformity), deficiency or absence of the turns of the cochlea (Mondini malformation) (Fig. 6-9A and B), or severe underdevelopment of the bony internal auditory canal.

Inflammatory diseases, tumors within the temporal bone, and congenital malformations are optimally evaluated with high-resolution CT in the axial and coronal planes. Extraosseous extensions of tumors or inflammatory proccesses are optimally evaluated with contrast MRI.

Vascular Lesions[28]

Vascular lesions are less common and consist of a variety of abnormalities, such as ectopic carotid artery, high jugular bulb, and aberrant and tortuous arteries. The *ectopic carotid artery* is situated more laterally and posteriorly than the normal artery and presents as a pinkish, middle ear mass (Fig. 6-10A and B). A *high jugular bulb* may protrude into the middle ear cavity via a dehiscence in the floor of the hypotympanum and manifest as a bluish mass in the tympanic cavity (Fig. 6-11A and B). Both entities may cause conductive hearing loss. These aberrant vascular structures are optimally evaluated by CT in conjunction with MRA (Figs. 6-10 and 6-11).

Other vascular abnormalities include *elongation, tortuosity*, and *dilatation of the vertebral basilar artery complex*. Elongation of the basilar artery may be considered to be present if any portion of the vessel extends lateral to the margin of the clivus or the dorsum sellae or if the artery bifurcates above the plane of the suprasellar cistern. The vertebral basilar arterial system is optimally demonstrated on T2-weighted imaging utilizing constructive interference in the steady state (CISS) or complemented by three-dimansional time-of-flight MRA

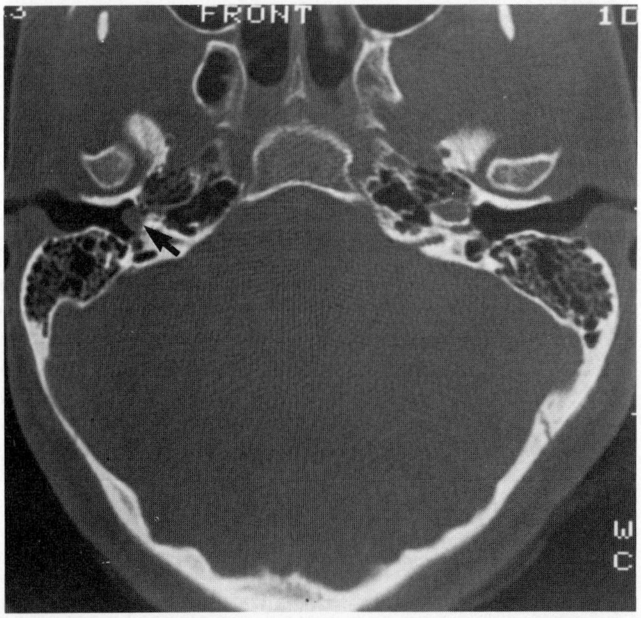

Figure 6-10

Right ectopic carotid artery. Axial high-resolution CT section (bone window setting) demonstrates ectopic right carotid artery in right hypotympanum (arrow).

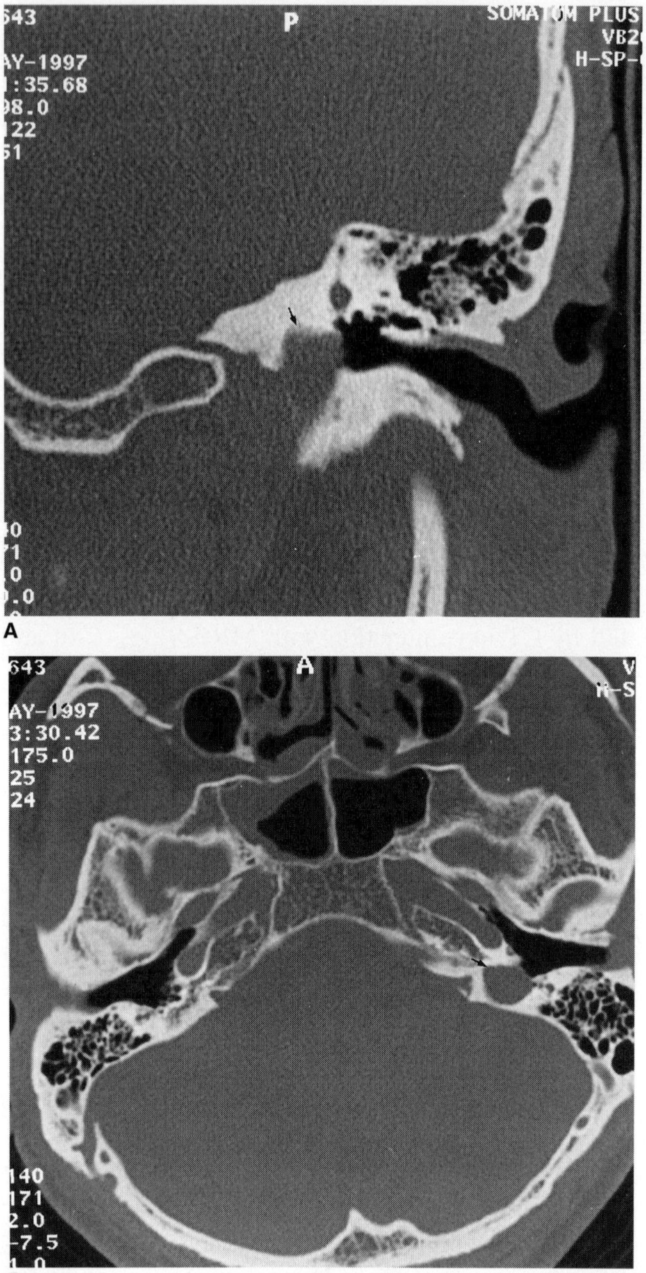

A

B

Figure 6-11
Dehiscent right jugular bulb. **(A)** *Coronal CT section through the left temporal bone at the level of the vestibule demonstrates a high jugular bulb (arrow) bulging into the epi- and mesotympanum. Note the absence of the bony wall at the margin of the protruding bulb.* **(B)** *Axial CT section through the temporal bones at the level of the mesotympanum demonstrates a high jugular bulb (arrow) and absence of the bony wall medially at the level of the mesotympanum.*

(Fig. 6-12A and B). The most common symptoms reported are hemifacial spasm, and/or facial paresis and trigeminal neuralgia. Hearing loss, tinnitus, and vertigo, however, may occur occasionally.

Vascular loops and *aneurysms* are other types of vascular anomalies. A relatively common type is a tortuous anterior inferior cerebellar artery, which is located in the CP angle cistern and may extend into the medial internal auditory canal. Hearing loss and vertigo may ensue.

Rarely, *aneurysms* of the anterior inferior cerebellar artery have been reported.[29] Other aneurysms may originate from the vertebral and basilar arteries (Fig. 6-13), including their branches, and extend into the CP angle cistern, mimicking a mass lesion. Aneurysms may be partially or completely thrombosed. On CT, they demonstrate an enhancing rim or an isodense, nonenhancing

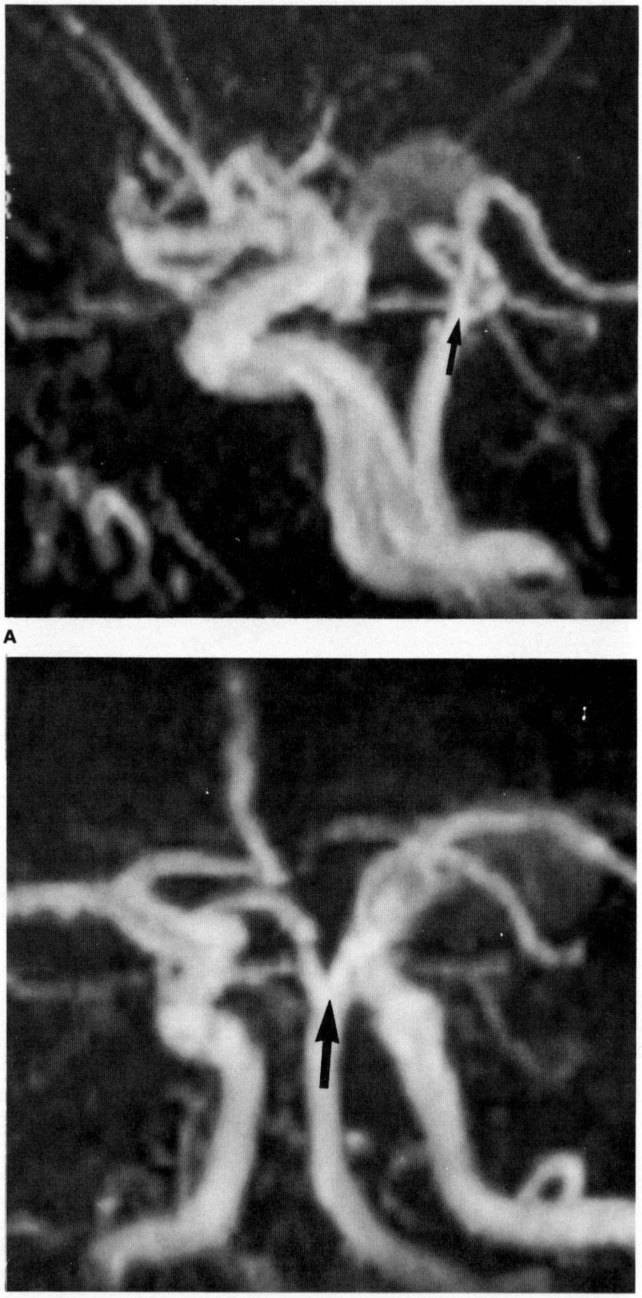

A

B

Figure 6-12
Normal carotid arteries and basilar artery. Three-dimensional MRA displays the normal carotid arteries and basilar artery and bifurcation into posterior cerebral arteries in **(A)** *the lateral view (arrow) and* **(B)** *the anteroposterior view.*

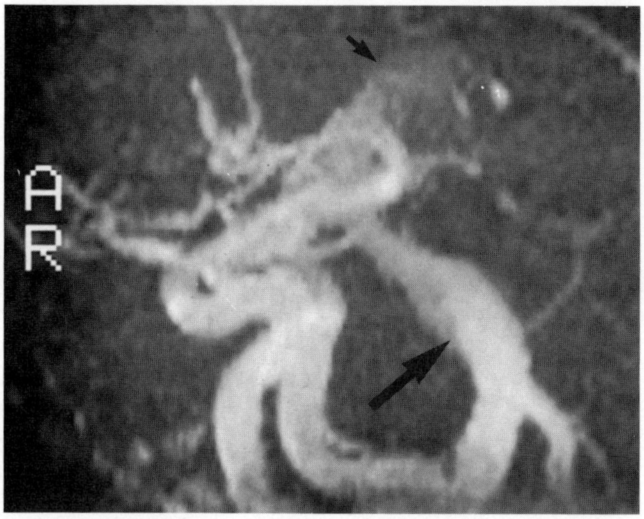

Figure 6-13
Tip basilar artery aneurysm. Three-dimensional time-of-flight MRI angiogram demonstrates a tortuous dilated basilar artery (large arrow) with a partially thrombosed aneurysm at the tip of the basilar artery (small arrow).

mural thrombus of varible size. Following the introduction of contrast material, the nonthrombosed portion of the aneurysm reveals enhancement of the lumen. A calcific rim may be present in the wall of the aneurysm. In some cases, the neck of the aneurysm of the respective vessel can be demonstrated. On MRI, T1- and dual echo T2-weighted sequences demonstrate the various blood degradation products within the thrombus and in the wall and adjacent area of the aneurysm. Flowing blood is characterized by flow voids, or enhancement on contrast MRI. Aneurysms are optimally evaluated with three-dimensional or two-dimensional time-of-flight MRA.

Temporal Bone Trauma[30]

Temporal bone fractures have been classified into fractures along the long axis of the petrous bone (longitudinal) or across the longitudinal axis of the petrous bone (transverse) (Fig. 6-14). Some fractures have components of both the transverse and the longitudinal type, particularly in severe trauma. The symptoms caused by temporal bone fractures include vertigo, dizziness, sensorineural hearing loss, conductive hearing loss, and facial palsy.

Longitudinal fractures represent 70 to 90 percent of temporal bone fractures. These fractures parallel the long axis of the temporal bone and extend from the occipital region and mastoid through the external canal and then continue to the middle ear cavity, petrous apex, foramen lacerum, and carotid canal. Frequently, there is dislocation and/or interruption of the ossicular structures, with variable degrees of conductive hearing loss. Complete incus dislocation from the malleoincudal and incudostapedial articulation is the most common type of ossicular derangement. In about 20 percent of cases, facial paresis is present. These dislocations are best illustrated on 1- to 2-mm axial and coronal high-resolution CT sections. Fractures of the stapes arch are also common, while fractures of the malleus neck are less common.

Transverse fractures are less common and occur in 10 to 30 percent of trauma cases. The fracture lines traverse the petrous bone perpendicular to the long axis, most commonly at the level of the labyrinth. There is a high percentage of facial paralysis (40 to 50 percent). This type of fracture usually spares the ossicular structures. The fracture line may pass through the bony labyrinth and damage the cochlea and vestibular apparatus, with consequent complete hearing loss. Such fractures may also transect the internal auditory canal and eighth nerve complex. Temporal bone fractures may be followed by severe vertigo with spontaneous nystagmus. The sensorineural hearing loss may result from damage to the cochlear end organ or transection of the cochlear nerve within the internal auditory canal. Vertigo is usually the result of injury to the vestibule, vestibular nerve, or vestibular aqueduct. A perilymph fistula may complicate these fractures. Hearing loss and vertiginous symptoms may also be caused by a concussion of the inner ear structures with no demonstrable fracture. The preferred modality for demonstration of these transverse fractures is high-resolution CT in the axial and coronal planes. Magnetic resonance imaging may be of value in the diagnosis of labyrinthine hemorrhage. The signal intensities depend on the blood degradation products and their respective paramagnetic affects.

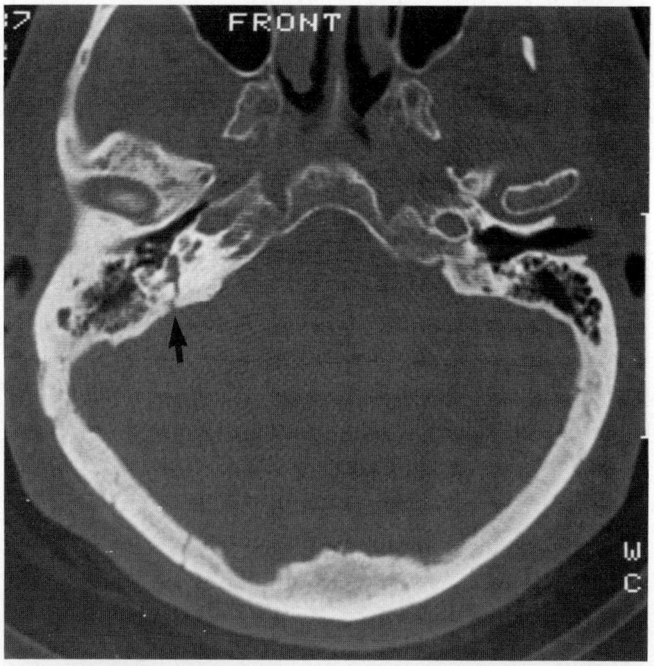

Figure 6-14
Right transverse fracture. Axial CT section through both temporal bones reveals a linear transverse fracture extending into the right vestibule (arrow).

Cerebellopontine Angle Cistern Lesions

The most common CP angle lesions, in order of frequency, are (1) *acoustic neurinoma* (70 to 80 percent), (2) *meningioma* (6 to 10 percent), (3) *epidermoid* and *cholesterol cyst* (6 to 7 percent), (4) *nonacoustic neurinoma* (4 to 5 percent), and (5) other miscellaneous lesions, including *arachnoid cyst, leptomeningeal carcinomatosis, metastases, extensions of glomus jugulare tumors,* and *lateral extension of brainstem lesions.*[31]

Acoustic Neurinoma (Schwannoma)

Magnetic resonance imaging of the temporal bone is employed for the clinical evaluation of a vestibular schwannoma (acoustic neuroma).[32,33] The examination typically consists of whole brain sagittal T1-weighted images, as well as axial proton-weighted and T2-weighted images. T1-weighted axial images using 3-mm thick slices through the internal auditory canals are obtained before contrast adminstration, followed by 3-mm thick T1-weighted axial and coronal images after gadolinium administration.[34–37] Recently, high-resolution T2-weighted imaging or three-dimensional Fourier transform constructive interferance in steady state (CISS) imaging has been studied as an alternative to contrast-enhanced T1-weighted imaging.[38,39] Both of these sequences show focal eighth nerve lesions as dark signals in contrast to the surrounding T2-hyperintensity of cerebrospinal fluid (CSF)[33,38–41] (Fig. 6-15A,B, and C). In general, both of these sequences are felt to be effective, but indeterminate scans should be followed by the more conventional T1-weighted contrast-enhanced images.

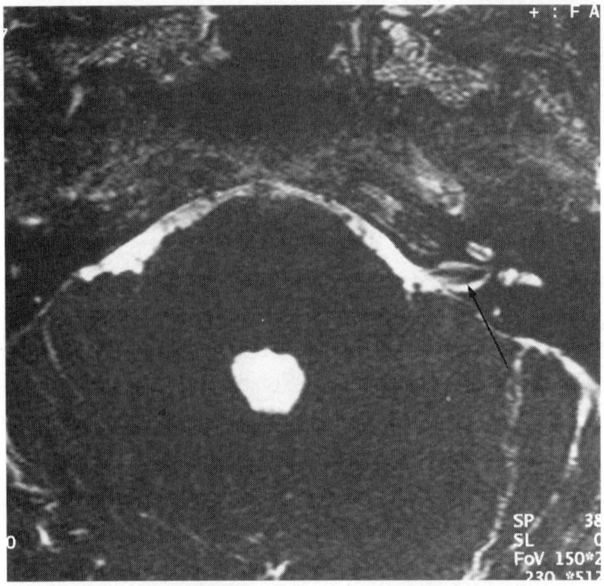

A

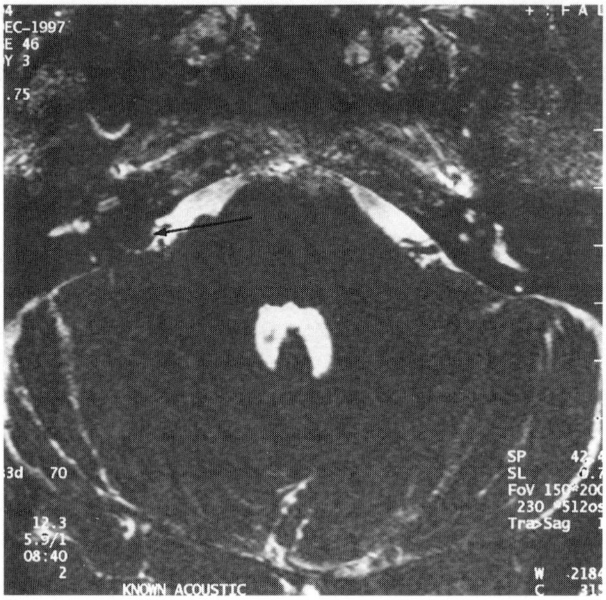

B

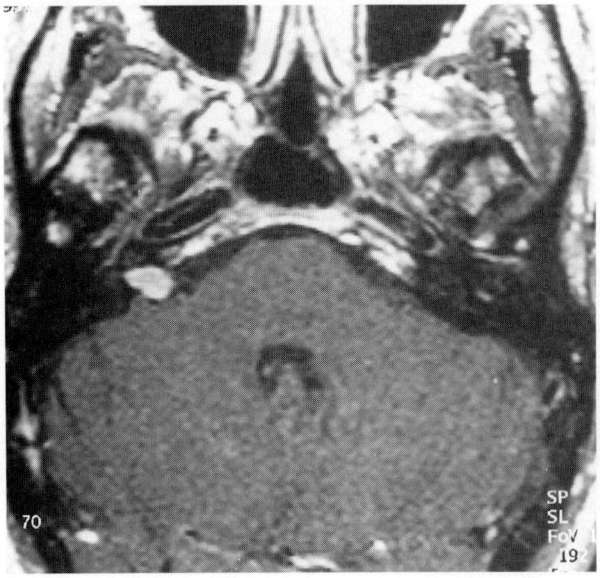

C

Figure 6-15

Normal left internal auditory canal (CISS technique). **(A)** *Axial T2-weighted image (CISS) through the left internal auditory canal demonstrates the vestibular nerve (posteriorly) and the cochlear nerve (anteriorly) surrounded by CSF (arrow).* **(B)** *Axial T2-weighted image (CISS) through the right internal auditory canal reveals a low-intensity mass obliterating the CSF space within the canal and the adjacent CP angle cistern. The medial contour of this tumor is sharply delimited (arrow).* **(C)** *Axial contrast MRI image through the right internal auditory canal reveals a homogeneously enhancing, sharply defined acoustic neuroma within the canal and the adjacent cistern corresponding to the mass demonstrated in B.*

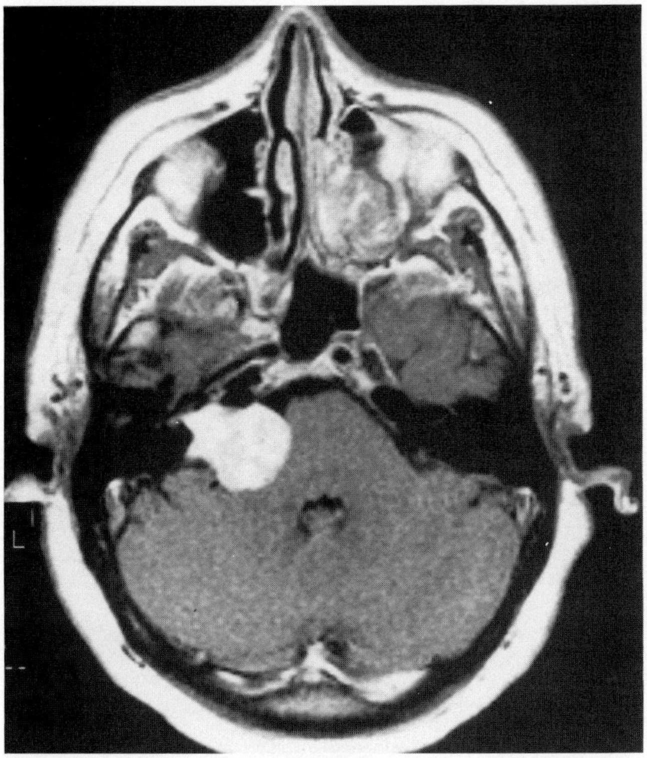

Figure 6-16

Right acoustic neuroma. Axial T1-weighted image (after gadolinium introduction) through the temporal bones reveals an acoustic neuroma that involves the internal auditory canal, CP angle cistern, and vestibule on the right.

In patients with known vestibular schwannomas who have been imaged previously with MRI, an abbreviated study may be performed. The precontrast thin section T1-weighted images may be eliminated and postcontrast thin-section T1-weighted axial and coronal images obtained directly. In patients with a history of surgical resection of a vestibular schwannoma, precontrast thin-section T1-weighted images should be obtained through the internal auditory canals. The post-gadolinium thin-section T1-weighted axial and coronal images through the internal auditory canals should be obtained with fat saturation in order to avoid confusion between fat packing, commonly used in the resection of vestibular scwhannomas, and contrast enhancement.

In those patients for whom MRI is contraindicated, contrast-enhanced CT scanning of the temporal bone is recommended. One- to 2-mm axial and coronal images using bone algorithm and soft tissue review in both planes are obtained.

On the T1-weighted images, schwannomas are usually isointense or mildly hypointense relative to the pons and hyperintense to CSF. On T2-weighted images, they are mildly hyperintense relative to the pons and nearly isointense or hypointense to CSF. On these T2-weighted images, smaller lesions may be completely obscured by the isointense CSF. Likewise, intracanalicular lesions, especially in the fundus portion of the canal, may be difficult to detect with either T1- or T2-weighted images.

Acoustic neurinomas enhance intensely after the intravenous administration of gadolinium-DTPA on T1-weighted spin echo images[42,43](Fig. 6-16). Intracanalicular tumors as small as 1 mm may be detected with gadolinium enhancement (Fig. 6-17). Acoustic neuromas are benign, slow-growing, encapsulated tumors. They constitute about 70 to 80 percent of CP angle lesions. The intracanalicular lesions are a few millimeters in size, while the extracanalicular tumors can grow to 5 to 6 cm in diameter.[44]

Acoustic neuromas are cylindrical in shape and have a convex medial border. The CP angle component is often lobulated and forms an acute angle at the interface between the tumor and the medial aspect of the petrous bone (Fig. 6-18). This is in contrast to meningiomas, which usually are broad based, along the medial aspect of the petrous bone. If there are cystic areas within the tumor, heterogeneous enhancement occurs. The fourth ventricle may be compressed, deformed, and displaced away from the tumor site. These lesions rarely herniate into the middle cranial fossa via the incisura. Large acoustic neurinomas may be associated with edema of the brain, and, rarely, are large enough to cause hydrocephalus. Occasionally, intratumoral hemorrhage is detected by signal characteristics specific for various blood degradation products.

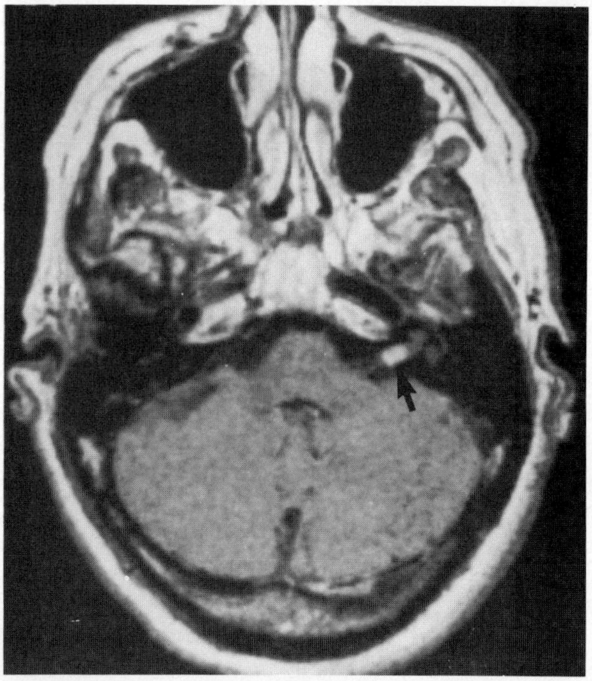

Figure 6-17

Left intracanalicular schwannoma. Axial T1-weighted image (after gadolinium introduction) reveals an intracanalicular enhancing schwannoma (arrow).

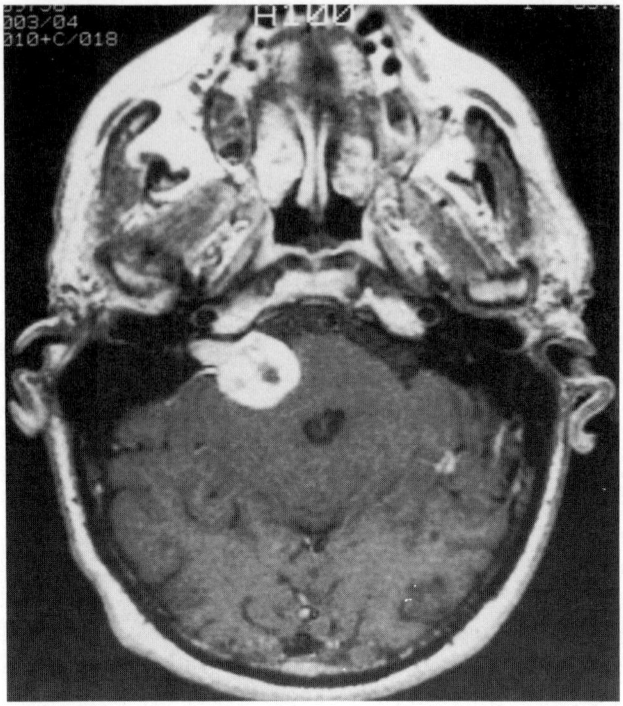

Figure 6-18
Acoustic neuroma. Axial T1-weighted image (after gadolinium introduction) reveals an intracanalicular schwannoma with extension into the right CP angle and indentation of the adjacent pons.

Nonacoustic Neuroma

Nonacoustic neuromas comprise cranial nerve schwannomas, which arise from the third to the twelfth cranial nerves. The most common nonacoustic schwannomas represent the facial nerve and fifth nerve schwannomas.[45,46,47] Facial neuromas may arise within the internal auditory canal, geniculate ganglion area (Fig. 6-19A and B), tympanic cavity, and mastoid.[47] Large tumors may extend into the middle or posterior cranial cavity, depending on their location. The first clinical symptom of a facial nerve neuroma within the internal auditory canal may be hearing loss secondary to compression of the cochlear nerve.[48]

Progressive gradual facial nerve paresis is the predominant clinical finding. Computed tomography is indicated for assessment of bony remodeling, together with enlargement of the facial nerve canal, geniculate fossa, and internal auditory canal (Fig. 19A and B). Contrast MRI delineates the enhancing tumor within the temporal bone and brain in cases with extraosseous extension.

The trigeminal nerve schwannoma originates in the region of Meckel's cave (Fig. 20A and B). Large tumors straddle the cerebellar incisura, with components of tumor in the middle and posterior fossa. The most common clinical finding is hypesthesia and paresthesia in the distribution of the branches of the trigeminal nerve.

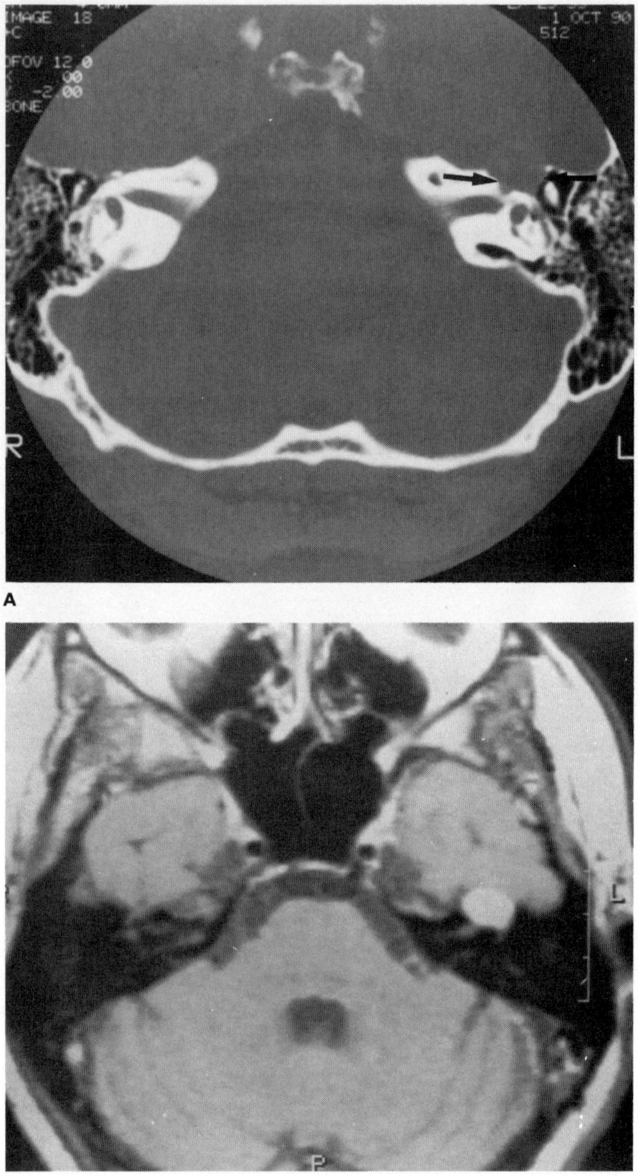

Figure 6-19
Schwannoma of left geniculate ganglion. **(A)** *Axial CT study with bone window setting reveals a bony defect in the region of the right geniculate ganglion secondary to a schwannoma (arrows).* **(B)** *Axial T1-weighted image (after gadolinium) reveals marked enhancement of the geniculate ganglion schwannoma.*

Meningioma

Meningiomas arise from meningothelial arachnoid cells and are usually eccentric to the internal auditory meatus. They are broad based against the dural surface of the posterior medial petrous bone. Most meningiomas are hemispherical in shape and reveal an obtuse angle at the interface of the tumor and the posterior surface of the petrous bone. A few meningiomas have a plaque-like configuration, and occasionally they are round, mimicking an acoustic neurinoma.

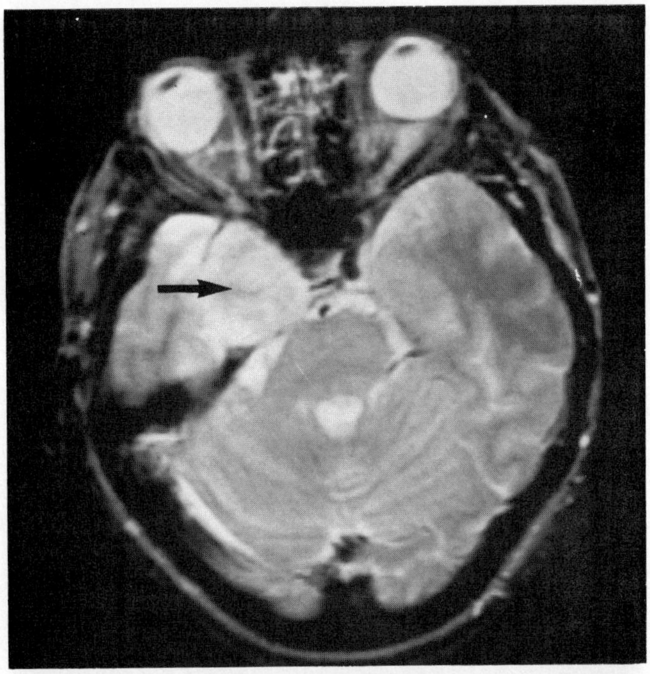

A

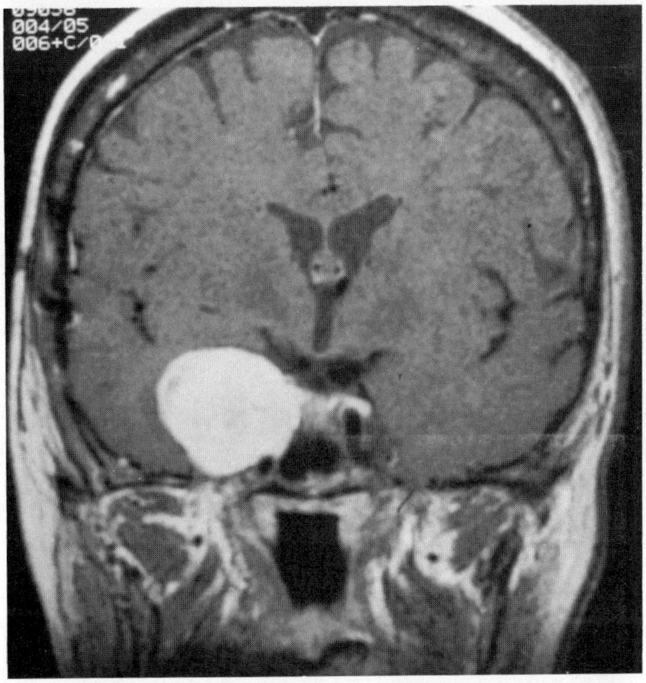

B

Figure 6-20
Trigeminal schwannoma. **(A)** *Axial T2-weighted image reveals a high-signal-intensity, well-demarcated tumor in the right parasellar area bulging into the preopontine and adjacent CP angle cistern via the incisura (arrow).* **(B)** *Coronal T1-weighted image (after gadolinium introduction) reveals marked enhancement of the tumor.*

Less commonly, meningiomas may cause hyperostosis or lytic bone destruction of the adjacent temporal bone. A rare location of meningioma is within the temporal bone, frequently within the middle ear cavity. These tumors probably arise from ectopic meningothelial cells. On CT and MRI, these tumors are often manifested as a nonspecific soft tissue density. Cystification of meningiomas is occasionally encountered, along with perifocal edema of variable degree.

On CT, meningiomas are isodense or hyperdense relative to brain tissue and may calcify in up to 25 percent of cases. These calicifications may be coarse and speckled or may be manifested as psammomatous calcifications, which are reflected by diffuse, homogeneous high density on the CT image.

On MR, meningiomas are hypointense to isointense to gray matter on the T1-weighted images and are low to high in signal intensity on the T2-weighted images. The wide spectrum of T2-weighted signal intensities is due to the diversity of the histopathologic tumor composition. At the tumor margin, blood vessels manifested as surface flow voids may be seen. Meningiomas demonstrate homogeneous intense enhancement following the infusion of gadolinium[49] (Fig. 6-21A and B).

Epidermoid Cyst

Epidermoid cysts are usually congenital and arise from ectodermal cell rests. The cyst wall is lined by stratified squamous epithelium with desquamated keratin on the surface and within the lumen. These cysts may reach considerable size within the CP angle, but they usually cause few symptoms. They insinuate into crevices of the brain and may extend to the contralateral CP angle cistern via the prepontine cistern. Their shape and contour are quite variable, and their surface tends to be lobulated.[50]

On CT, they approach CSF density and show no enhancement following introduction of contrast material (Fig. 6-22A and B). Rarely, they may be hyperdense relative to CSF and reveal rim calcification. These cysts may be confined to the intracranial cavity, but some epidermoids arise within the base of skull, especially in the region of the petrous apex and adjacent clivus, causing a sharply defined bony defect. Such epidermoid cysts project from the base of skull over a variable distance into the adjacent posterior or middle cranial fossa.[51]

On MRI,[52] epidermoids are slightly nonhomogeneous, isointense or slightly hyperintense to CSF on the T1-weighted images, and hyperintense to CSF on T2-weighted images (Fig. 6-23A and B). There is no enhancement following the introduction of gadolinium, although slight enhancement of the rim may occur, probably due to compressed reactive tissue.

Cholesterol Cyst

The cholesterol cyst,[53] occasionally referred to as a cholesterol granuloma, possesses a fibrous lining that contains multinucleated giant cells, along with cholesterol crystals, blood vessels, hemosiderin, and chronic inflammatory cells. The content of these cysts is a yellow-

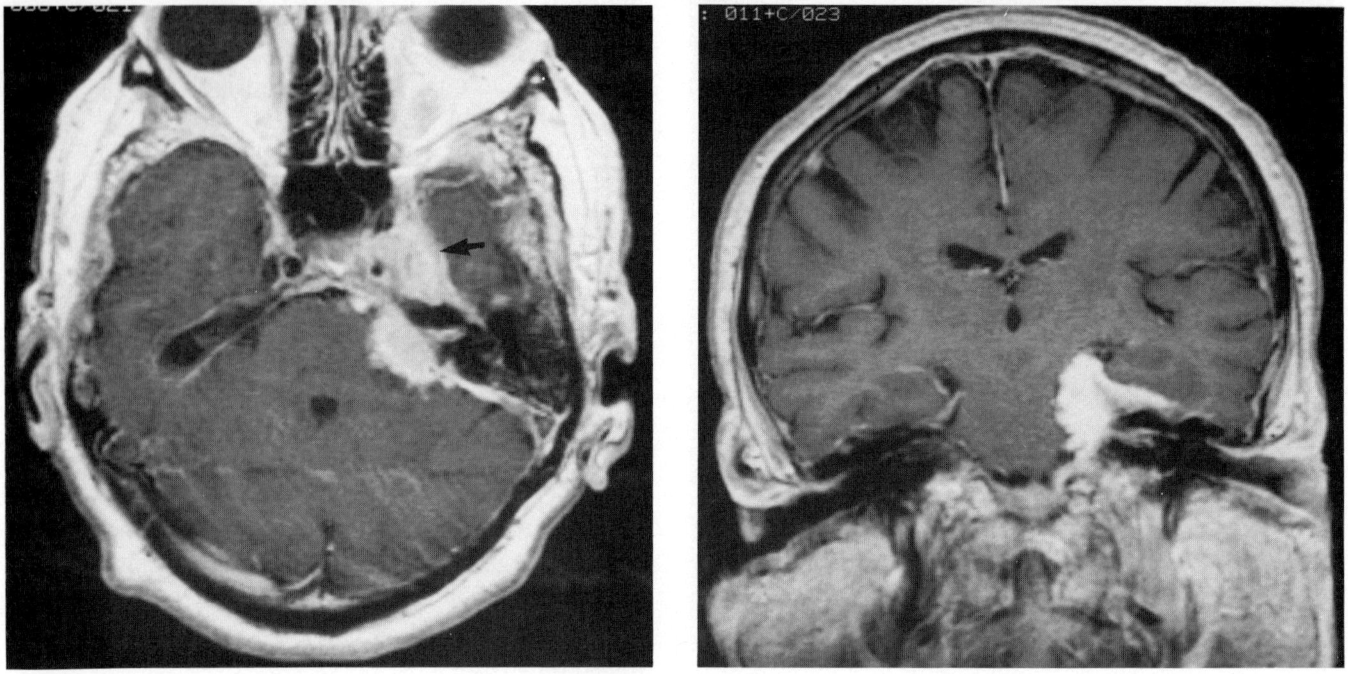

A B

Figure 6-21

Left CP angle meningioma. **(A)** *Axial T1-weighted image (after gadolinium introduction) shows an enhancing broad-based lesion adjacent to the medial aspect of the petrous bone with no extension into the internal auditory canal, which is normal in size and configuration. The meningioma extends into the left cavernous sinus and medial aspect of the left middle cranial fossa (arrow).* **(B)** *Coronal T1-weighted image (after gadolinium introduction) reveals an enhancing lesion around the petrous apex and within the left CP angle cistern, causing indentation of the adjacent pons. The left internal auditory canal is normal.*

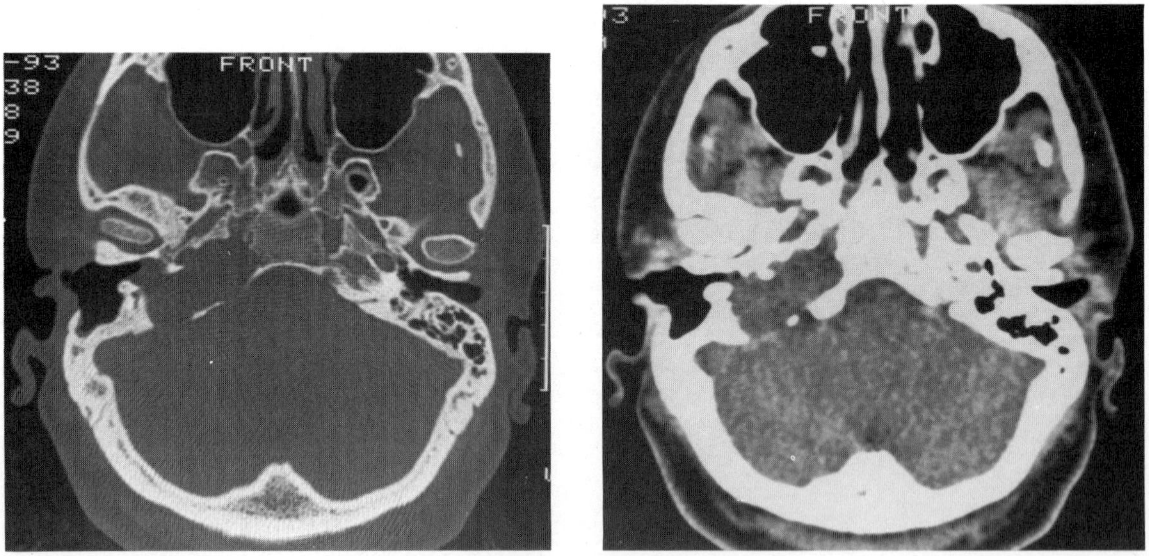

A B

Figure 6-22

Right epidermoid cyst. **(A)** *Axial CT section of the base of the skull demonstrates a sharply defined, lytic lesion in the right petrous apex and adjacent base of the skull.* **(B)** *Axial CT section (after introduction of contrast) demonstates a lesion in the right petrous apex, which is isointense with brain tissue and reveals no enhancement (epidermoid).*

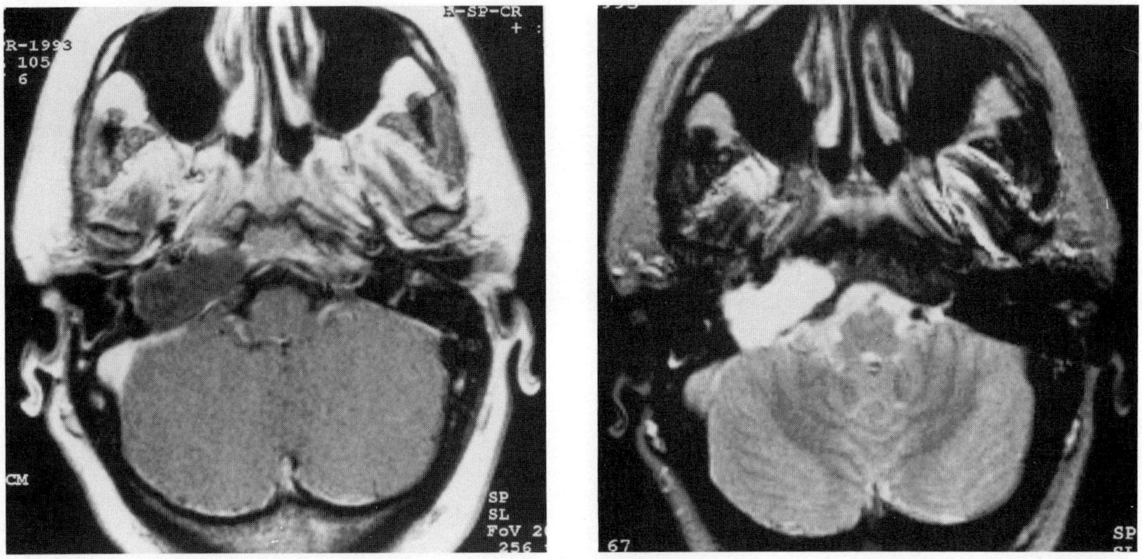

A B

Figure 6-23
Right epidermoid cyst. **(A)** *Axial T1-weighted image demonstrates a well-defined low-intensity epidermoid cyst within the right petrous apex, which is slightly hyperintense relative to the CSF in the prepontine cistern. There was no enhancement with gadolinium.* **(B)** *Axial T2-weighted image displays hyperintensity of the cyst, which is slightly greater than that of the CSF.*

ish-brown liquid. They occur in young and middle-aged adults of both sexes and are of variable size.

On CT, cholesterol cysts are sharply marginated and frequently have an ovoid configuration. They are usually localized in the base of skull, causing a sharply defined bony defect. This defect involves the petrous apex, with resultant erosion. Cholesterol cysts may extend to the adjacent middle cranial fossa and clivus. On CT, they are isodense with the adjacent brain tissue.

On MR, the majority of these lesions are strongly hyperintense on both T1- and T2-weighted images and may contain nonhomogeneous substances within the liquid, causing a mixed hyperintensity pattern (Fig. 6-24A and B). Some of these cysts reveal a hypointense

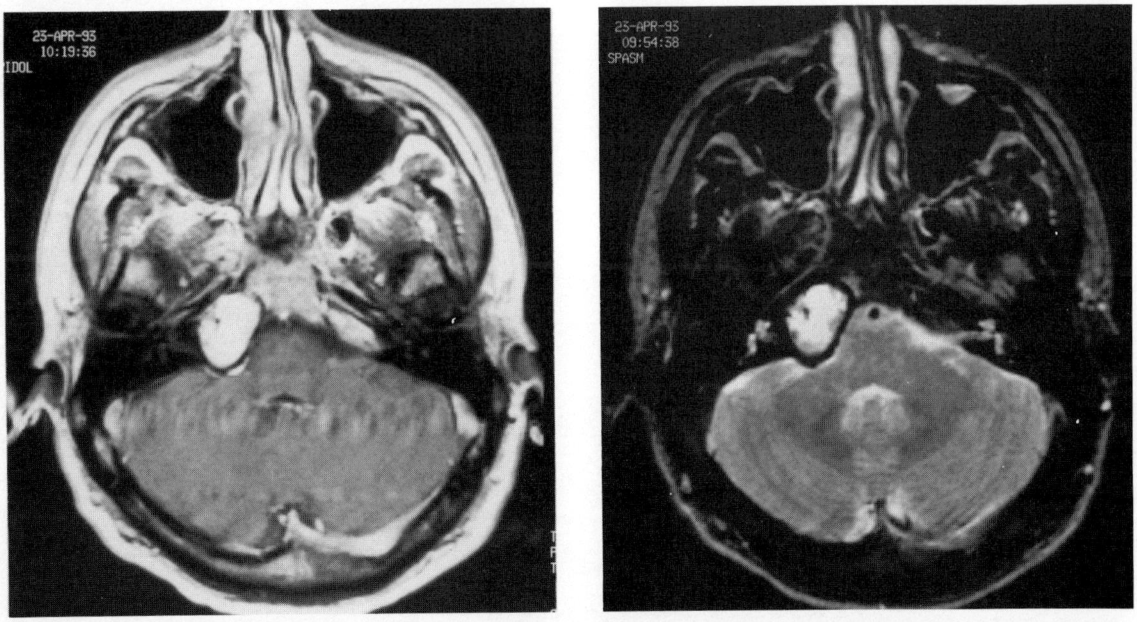

A B

Figure 6-24
Right cholesterol cyst. **(A)** *Axial T1-weighted image (after gadolinium introduction) reveals a high-intensity sharply defined cystic lesion in the right petrous apex containing some low-signal-intensity areas. There is no enhancement with gadolinium.* **(B)** *Axial T2-weighted image demonstrates the same lesion, revealing hyperintensity interspersed with some low-signal-intensity areas.*

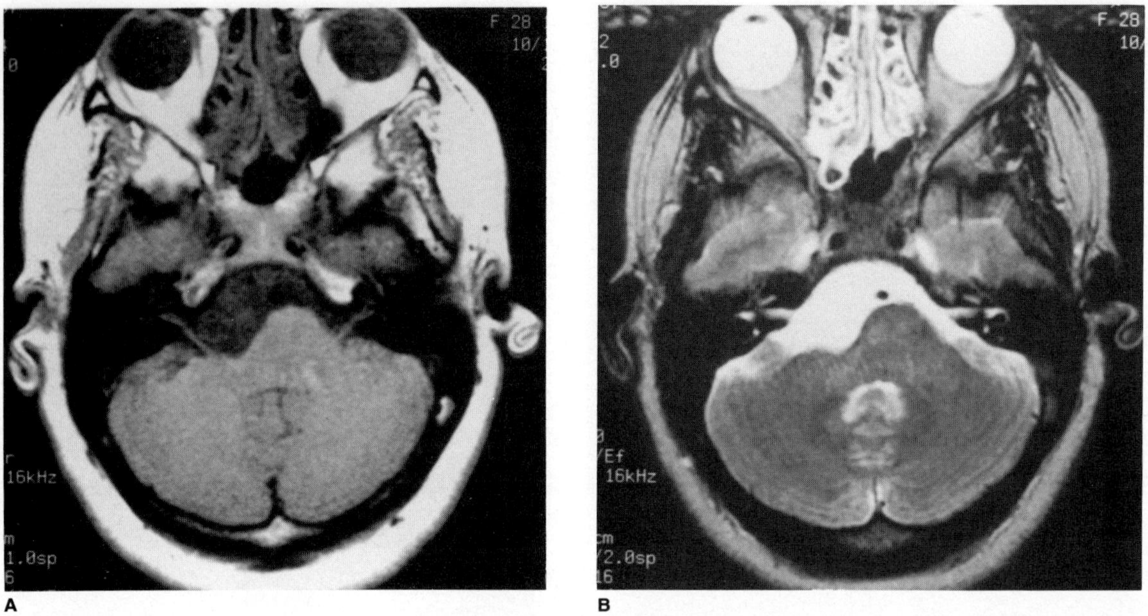

Figure 6-25
Arachnoid cyst. **(A)** *Axial T1-weighted image outlines a slightly expansile arachnoid cyst in the right CP angle cistern and adjacent prepontine angle cistern that is isointense with CSF. The cyst causes indentation of the adjacent pons and encroaches upon the right eighth nerve complex.* **(B)** *Axial T2-weighted image reveals the high signal intensity of the cyst, which is isointense with CSF.*

rim on both T1- and T2-weighted images, probably due to hemosiderin deposits (Fig. 6-24B). After the introduction of gadolinium, there is no enhancement of the cyst content, but there may be slight enhancement of the cyst rim.

Miscellaneous Lesions

Arachnoid cysts are congenital CSF-filled collections. They are similar in intensity to CSF and are situated within the cisterns.[54] The CP angle cistern is a relatively common location, in addition to cisterns in the middle cranial fossa and in the suprasellar and quadrigeminal areas. The arachnoid cyst tends to be a single, expansile lesion that is molded by the surrounding structures. These cysts are differentiated from normal cisterns by their ability to expand with indentation of the brain (Fig. 6-25A andB).

Glomus jugulare tumors are the most frequent tumors arising within the jugular fossa. They cause irregular, lytic bone destruction and may grow into the middle ear cavity and posterior fossa, causing conductive hearing loss. Characteristically, they reveal undulating channel-like flow voids, especially on T2-weighted images (Fig. 6-26). Following gadolinium introduction, there is moderate to marked enhancement.

Other, rarer lesions that may involve the CP angle include *lipoma,*[55] *melanoma,*[56] *metastases*, *leptomeningeal carcinomatosis,*[57] *brainstem glioma*, and *ganglioneuroblastoma,*[58] especially *ependymoma,*[59,60] and *astrocytoma* that extends laterally into the CP angle cistern. Magnetic resonance imaging with gadolinium defines and characterizes these lesions.

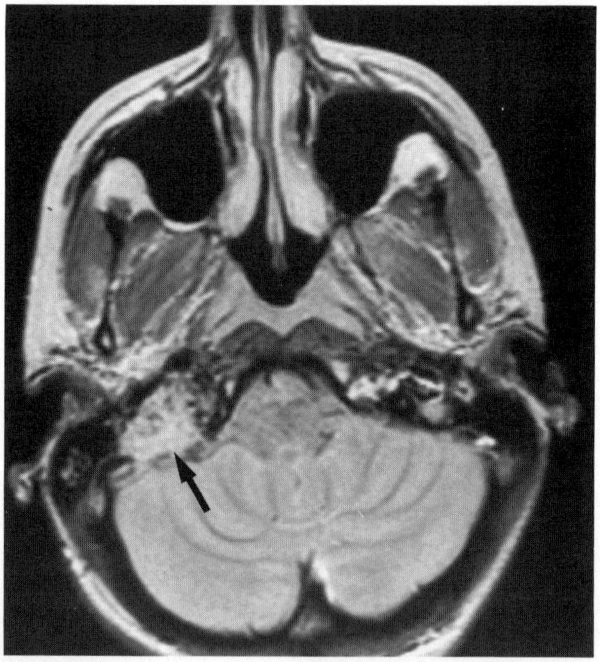

Figure 6-26
Glomus jugulare tumor. Axial T2-weighted image reveals a high-intensity mass in the right jugular fossa, with dark channels representing increased vascularity (arrow).

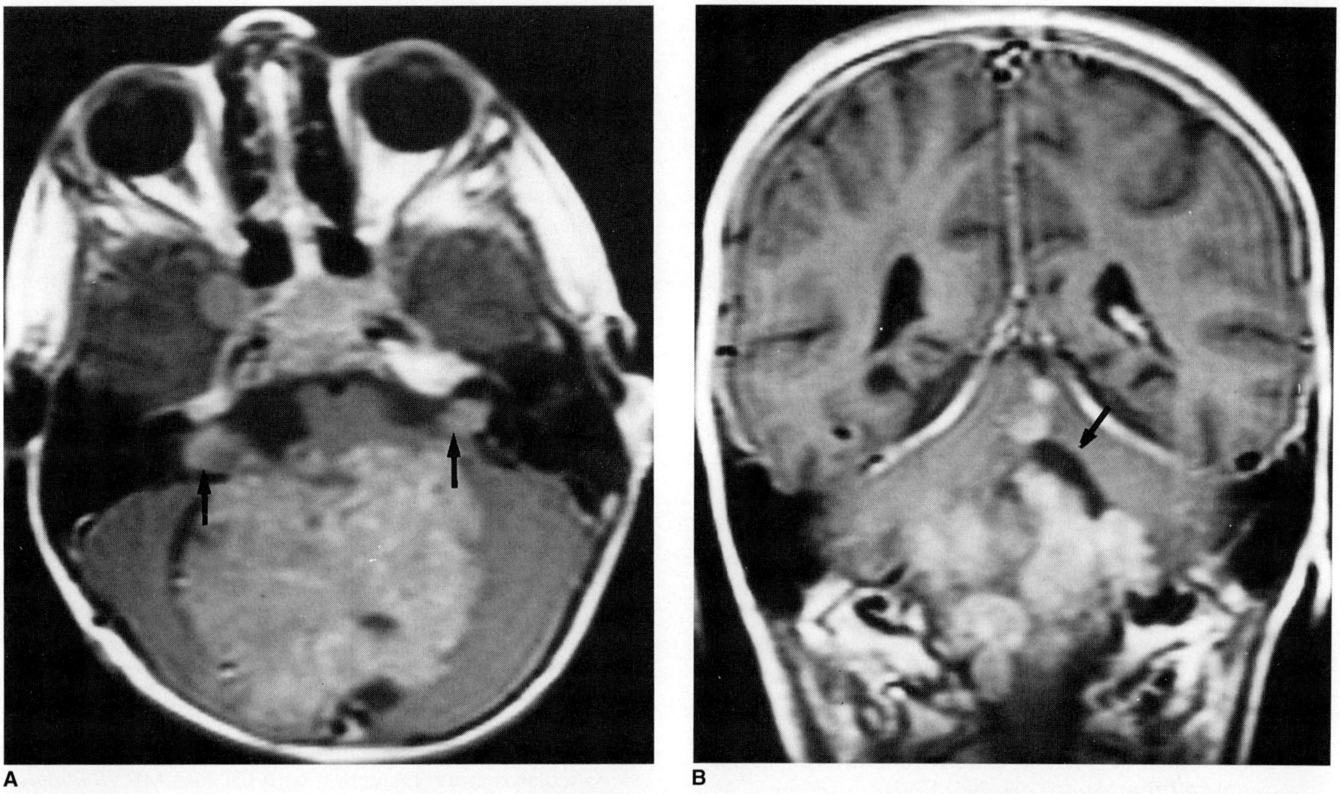

Figure 6-27
Medulloblastoma. **(A)** *Axial T1-weighted image, after gadolinium introduction, through the posterior fossa reveals a large tumor mass in the brainstem with extension into the left and right cerebellar hemispheres. There is tumor extension bilaterally into the CP angle cisterns at the level of the internal auditory canals (arrows). The tumor reveals slight to moderate, heterogeneous enhancement. There is nodular density, presumably metastatic disease, in the anterior lateral portion of the right cavernous sinus.* **(B)** *Coronal postcontrast T1-weighted image through the brainstem demonstrates heterogeneous enhancement of the tumor within the brainstem with extension into the CP angle and perimedullary cisterns. Deformity and some dilatation of the fourth ventricle (arrow) can be seen.*

Brainstem and Cerebellum

Lesions in the brainstem and cerebellum may cause equilibrium disturbances in addition to cranial nerve abnormalities, including sensory and motor disturbances. However, dizziness, deafness, and equilibrium disturbances are usually not the principal findings.

Various types of tumors occur in the brainstem and cerebellum. They include benign and malignant lesions, such as hemangioblastoma, medulloblastoma (Fig. 6-27), ependymoma, brainstem glioma, astrocytoma, and metastastic lesions. Some of these tumors may extend laterally into the CP angle cisterns, notably the ependymoma.

Multiple Sclerosis

Multiple sclerosis (MS) is a chronic inflammatory disease of myelin with a relapsing and remitting course. It commonly causes dizziness and disorders of equilibrium. Magnetic resonance imaging is the principal modality in the diagnostic evaluation and follow-up of the disease.

Other lesions that cause dizziness, disorders of equilibrium, and, rarely, central sensorineural hearing loss include such lesions of the brainstem and cerebellum as vascular malformations, tumors, and infarcts.

Arteriovenous (AV) malformations are encountered in the brainstem. They present as a tangle of abnormal vessels with a central nidus. If these lesions are very small, they are referred to as cryptic malformations. These malformations often bleed and reveal signal characteristics of blood degradation products. On MRI, heterogeneous signal intensities are a reflection of the mixture of various tissue components, such as glial tissue, hemosiderin, and vascular structures.

The cavernous hemangioma presents as a mass with a heterogeneous signal intensity and enhancement with the introduction of contrast material.

Infarcts occur frequently in the brainstem. They are optimally visualized with MRI.[61] Their signal intensities and enhancement pattern depend on the stage of evolution.

REFERENCES

1. Adams RD, Victor M: *Principles of Neurology,* 4th ed. New York, McGraw-Hill, 1989.
2. Swartz JD, Swartz NG, Korsvik H, et al: Computerized tomographic evaluation of the middle ear and mastoid for posttraumatic hearing loss. *Ann Otol Rhinol Laryngol* 94:263–266, 1985.
3. Klein H-M, Bohndorf K, Hermes H, et al: Computed tomography and magnetic resonance imaging in the preoperative work-up for cochlear implantation. Eur J Radiol 15:89–92, 1992.
4. Kalender WA, Seissler W, Klotz E, Volk P: Spiral volumetric CT with single breath hold technique, continous transport, and continous scanner rotation. *Radiology* 176:181–183, 1990.
5. Suojanen JN, Mulkerji SK, Dupuy DE, et al: Spiral CT in the evaluation of head and neck lesions: Work in progress. *Radiology* 183:281–283, 1992.
6. Napel S, Marks MP, Rubin GD, et al: CT scintrigraphy with spiral CT and maximum intensity projection. *Radiology* 185:607–610, 1992.
7. Tien RD: Fat suppression MR imaging in neuroradiology: Technique and clinical applications. *AJR* 158:369–379, 1992.
8. Schuhmann MU, Ludemann WO, Schreiber H, Samii M: Cerebellopontine angle lipoma: A rare differential diagnosis. *Skull Base Surg*7:199–205, 1997.
9. Tien RD, Felsberg GJ, Macfall J: Fast spin echo high resolution MR imaging of the inner ear. *AJR* 159:395–398, 1992.
10. Jones KM, Malkern RV, Schwartz RR, et al: Fast spin echo imaging of the brain and spine: Current concepts. *AJR* 158:1313–1320, 1992.
11. Brogan M, Chakeres DW, Schmalbrock P: High resolution 3 DFT imaging of the endolymphatic duct and soft tissues of the otic capsule. *AJNR* 12:1–11, 1991.
12. Tanioka H, Shirakawa T, Machida T, Sasaki Y: Three-dimensional reconstructed MR imaging of the inner ear. *Radiology* 178:141–144, 1991.
13. Lee JN, King BD, Parker DL,et al: High resolution 3D imaging of the inner ear with a modified fast spin-echo pulse sequence. *J Magn Reson Imaging* 6:223–225, 1996.
14. Phelps P: Fast spin echo MRI in otology. *J Laryngol Otol* 108:383–394, 1994.
15. Edelman RR: MR angiography: Present and future. *AJR* 161:1–11, 1993.
16. Shellock FG: Bioeffects and safety considerations, in Atlas SW (ed): *Magnetic Resonance Imaging of the Brain and Spine.* New York, Raven Press, 1991, chap 6, pp 87–107.
17. Mark AS, Seltzer S, Nelson-Drake J, et al: Labyrinthine enhancement on gadolinium-enhanced magnetic resonance imaging in sudden deafness and vertigo: Correlation with audiologic and electronystagmographic studies. *Ann Otol Rhinol Laryngol* 1001:459–464, 1992.
18. Sando I, Egami T: Inner ear hemorrhage and endolymphatic hydrops in a leukemic patient with sudden hearing loss. *Ann Otol Rhinol Laryngol* 86:518–524, 1977.
19. Mark AS, Fitzgerald D: Segmental enhancement of the cochlea on contrast-enhanced MR: Correlation with the frequency of hearing loss and possible sign of perilymphatic fistula and autoimmune labyrinthinitis. *AJNR* 14:991–996, 1993.
20. Babin RW, Harker LA: Intralabyrinthine acoustic neuromas. *Otolaryngol Head Neck Surg* 88:455–461, 1980.
21. DeLozier HL, Gacek RR, Dana ST: Intralabyrinthine schwannoma. *Ann Otol Rhinol Laryngol* 88:187–191, 1979.
22. Mafee MF, Lachenauer CS, Kumar A, et al: CT and MR imaging of intralabyrinthine schwannoma: Report of two cases and review of the literature. *Radiology* 174:395–400, 1990.
23. Wiet RJ, Raslan W, Shambaugh GE Jr: Otosclerosis 1981 to 1985: Our four year review and current perspective. *Am J Otol* 7:221–228, 1986.
24. Blakely BW, Hilger PA, Taylor S, Hilger J: Computed tomography in the diagnosis of cochlear otosclerosis. *Otolaryngol Head Neck Surg* 94:434–438, 1986.
25. Martin N, Sterkers O, Nahum H: Chronic inflammatory disease of the middle ear cavities: Gd-DTPA enhanced MR imaging. *Radiology* 76:399–405, 1990.
26. Phelps PD: Glomus tumors of the ear: An imaging regime. *Clin Radiol* 41:301–305, 1990.
27. Swartz JD, Harnsberger HR: Temporal bone vascular anatomy, anomalies, and diseases emphasizing the clinical-radiological problems of pulsatile tinnitus, in: *Imaging of the Temporal Bone.* 2d ed. New York, Thieme Medical Publishers, 1992, pp 154–191.[17]
28. Lo WWM, Shelton C, Waluch V, et al. Intratemporal vascular tumors: Detection with CT and MR. *Radiology* 171:445–449, 1989.
29. Dalley RD, Robertson WD, Nugent RA, et al: Computed tomography of anterior-inferior cerebral artery aneurysm mimicking an acoustic neuroma. *JCAT* 10:881–884, 1986.
30. Swartz JD, Harnsberger HR: Trauma, in: *Imaging of the Temporal Bone,* 2d ed. New York, Thieme Medical Publishers, 1992, pp 247–262.
31. Valvassori GE: Cerebellopontine angle tumors. *Otolaryngol Clin North Am* 21:337–348, 1988.
32. Curtin HD: Rule out eighth nerve tumor: Contrast-enhanced T1-weighted or high resolution T2-weighted MR? *AJNR* 18:1834–1838, 1997.
33. Shelton C, Harnsberger HR, Allen R, King B: Fast spin echo magnetic resonance imaging: Clinical application in screening for acoustic neuroma. *Otolaryngol Head Neck Surg* 144:71–76, 1996.
34. Clifton AG, Phelps PD, Lloyd GAS: The investigation of acoustic neuroma. *Clin Radiol* 44:232–235, 1991.
35. Curati W, Graif M, Kingsley D, et al: Acoustic neuromas: Gd-DTPA enhancement in MR imaging. *Radiology* 158:447–451, 1986.
36. Daniels D, Millen S, Meyer G, et al: MR detection of tumor in the internal auditory canal. *AJNR* 8:249–252, 1987.
37. Press G, Hesselink J: MR imaging of cerebellopontine angle and internal auditory canal lesions at 1.5T. *AJNR* 9:241–251, 1988.
38. Casselman JW, Khuweide R, Deimling M, et al: Constructive interference in steady state-3DFT MR imaging of the inner ear and cerebellopontine angle. *AJNR* 14:47–57, 1993.
39. Fukui MB, Weissman JL, Curtin HD, Kanal E: T2-weighted MR characteristics of internal auditory canal masses. *AJNR* 17:1211–1218, 1996.
40. Pfeiderer AG, Evans KL, Grace ARH, Lloyd GAS: A

screening protocol used for the detection of acoustic neuromas: A clinical evaluation. *Clin Otolaryngol* 13:145–151, 1988.

41. Allen RW, Harnsberger R, Shelton C, et al: Low-cost high-resolution fast spin-echo MR of acoustic schwannoma: An alternative to ehanced spin-echo MR. *AJNR* 17:1205–1210, 1996.
42. Stuckey SL, Harris AH, Mannolini SM: Detection of acoustic schwannoma: Use of constructive interference in the steady state three-dimensional MR. *AJNR* 17:1219–1225, 1996.
43. Bassi P, Piazza P, Cusmano F, et al: MR cisternography of the cerebellopontine angle and internal auditory canal in diagnosis of intracanalicular acoustic neuroma. *Neuroradiology* 31:486–491, 1990.
44. Lhuillier FM, Doyon DL, Halimi PM, et al: Magnetic resonance imaging of acoustic neuromas: Pitfalls and differential diagnosis. *Neuroradiology* 34:144–149, 1992.
45. O'Donoghue GM: Tumors of the facial nerve, in Brackmann DE, Jackler RK (eds): *Neurotology.* St. Louis, Mosby, 1994, pp 1321–1332.
46. Weber PC, Osguthorpe JD: Facial nerve neuroma management. *Skull Base Surg* 8:51–55, 1998.
47. Weber AL, McKenna M: Radiological evalulation of the facial nerve. *Isr J Med Sci*28:186–192, 1992.
48. McMenomey SO, Glasscock ME, Minor LB, et al: Facial nerve neuromas presenting as acoustic tumors. *Am J Otol* 15:307–312, 1994.
49. Zimmerman RD, Fleming CA, Saint-Louis LA, et al: Magnetic resonance imaging of meningiomas. *AJNR* 1985; 6:149–157.
50. Gao P-Y, Osborn AG, Smirniotopoulos JG, et al: Radiologic-pathologic correlation: Epidermoid tumor of the cerebellopontine angle. *AJNR* 13:863–872, 1992.
51. Samii M, Tatagiba M, Piquer J, Carvalho GA: Surgical treatment of epidermoid cysts of the cerebellopontine angle. *J Neurosurg* 84:14–19, 1996.
52. Steffey DJ, DeFilipp GJ, Spera T, Gabrielson TO: MR imaging of primary epidermoid tumors. *JCAT* 12:438–440, 1988.
53. Clifton AG, Phelps PD, Brookes GB: Cholesterol granuloma of the petrous apex. *Br J Radiol* 63:724–726, 1990.
54. Wiener SN, Pearlstein AE, Eiber A: MR imaging of intracranial arachnoid cysts. *JCAT* 11:236–241, 1987.
55. Cohen TI, Powers SK, Williams DWI: MR appearance of intracanalicular eighth nerve lipoma. *AJNR* 13:1188–1190, 1992.
56. Vasdev A, David P, Villemot D, et al: Apparently primary malignant melanoma of the cerebellpontine angle: One case. *J Neuroradiol* 17:152–156, 1990.
57. Sceats D, Quisling R, Rhoton A, et al: Primary leptomeningeal glioma mimicking an acoustic neuroma: Case report with review of the literature. *Neurosurgery* 19:649–654, 1986.
58. Sohma T, Tuchita H, Kitami K, et al: Cerebellopontine angle ganglioneuroblastoma. *Neuroradiology* 34:334–336, 1992.
59. Fukui MB, Hogg JP, Martinez AJ: Extraaxial ependymoma of the posterior fossa. *AJNR* 18:1179–1181, 1997.
60. Wagle W, Jaufman B, Mincy J: Intradural extramedullary ependymoma: MR-pathologic correlation. *JCAT* 12:705–707, 1988.
61. Fox AJ, Bogousslavsky J, Carey LS, et al: Magnetic resonance imaging of small medullary infarctions. *AJNR* 7:229–233, 1986.

SECTION FOUR

EPILEPSY AND DISORDERS OF CONSCIOUSNESS

CHAPTER 7

NEUROIMAGING AND EPILEPSY

Michael R. Sperling
Maromi Nei

INTRODUCTION

Technological advances in brain imaging have revolutionized neurological practice. Diagnoses are made with ease and rapidity, interventions are safer and more accurate, and the effectiveness of therapy is better judged. Imaging techniques have also expanded beyond the traditional realm of brain anatomy. Cerebral blood flow and metabolism are measured readily in surface and deep gray matter. This chapter will focuses on magnetic resonance imaging (MRI), functional MRI (fMRI), magnetic resonance spectroscopy (MRS), positron emission tomography (PET), and single photon emission computed tomography (SPECT) and their use in diagnosing and treating people with epilepsy. Magnetic resonance imaging reveals brain structure with detail greatly surpassing that of computed tomography (CT)[1–4] and so has largely supplanted the latter technique. In addition, PET, fMRI, MRS, and SPECT noninvasively evaluate the physiology from of deep and superficial brain structures. These methods are important, since physiologic derangements are the sine qua non of epilepsy.

The epilepsy syndromes can be broadly divided into two groups: the idiopathic, or inherited, epilepsies, and symptomatic, or cryptogenic, epilepsies. By definition, people with idiopathic partial and generalized epilepsies (e.g., childhood absence epilepsy, juvenile myoclonic epilepsy, and benign childhood epilepsy with centrotemporal spikes) have normal structural imaging studies. Imaging is rarely indicated in those conditions, except for research purposes. A structural anomaly in someone with idiopathic epilepsy is either incidental and unrelated, or, if deemed related to the epilepsy, suggests that the diagnosis should be altered to that of a symptomatic syndrome. Functional imaging of cerebral blood flow, metabolism, and receptor binding are still of academic interest in idiopathic epilepsy and have no known clinical application. In contrast, people with symptomatic (or cryptogenic) epilepsy might have structural abnormalities, and do merit investigation with neuroimaging techniques. Unfortunately, the symptomatic epilepsy syndromes are more likely to resist treatment. Since academic centers usually gather patients with refractory seizures, patients with more troublesome symptomatic or cryptogenic epilepsy predominate in literature studies. Indeed, most articles have a decided emphasis on the application of imaging methods to the surgical treatment of epilepsy.

STRUCTURAL (ANATOMIC) IMAGING

The invention of safe, noninvasive anatomic brain imaging was perhaps the most important advance in neurological diagnosis in the latter part of this century. Since most epilepsies are acquired or symptomatic, anatomic imaging has an important role in diagnosing patients with epilepsy. Most of the images in this chapter are made with MRI, given its superior resolution. Other chapters in this text illustrate CT examples of structural lesions, and, with rare exception, little is to be gained by recapitulating those pictures here. A few CT illustrations are shown where advantage is to be gained from them.

Magnetic resonance imaging provides remarkably detailed images of brain anatomy.[3,5–7] Images are easily reconstructed in any plane desired, and coronal images, which cannot be obtained with CT, are especially helpful in evaluating some forms of epilepsy. The integrity of the blood-brain barrier is easily assessed with paramagnetic contrast agents. Magnetic resonance imaging uses no ionizing radiation, and poses no demonstrable health risk.[8]

Studies of Patients

Magnetic resonance imaging is now the preferred test when anatomic brain imaging is required in patients with epilepsy.[2,4,9–23] Tumors, vascular malformations, and cortical dysplasias are clearly displayed, and atrophic lesions are clearly seen.

Abnormalities Seen in Epilepsy

Neoplasms Seizures are sometimes the only symptom of a brain tumor. In epilepsy, tumors are usually indolent and the findings of the neurologic examination are often normal. Magnetic resonance imaging can detect neoplastic lesions in patients whose CT scans appear normal[2,4,5,17,22,24–27] and has a particular advantage for middle fossa lesions, where CT is usually obscured by bone artifact (Figs. 7-1 and 7-2).[5] Surgical epilepsy series report tumors in 10 to 25 percent of patients with intractable epilepsy,[4,16,26] but these percentages must overestimate the incidence of tumors in the general population of people with epilepsy. There are two reports[13,28] of CT-detected lesions missed by older MRI devices, but this phenomenon probably does not occur with modern equipment.

The most common tumors are gangliogliomas, low-grade astrocytomas, oligodendrogliomas, arteriovenous

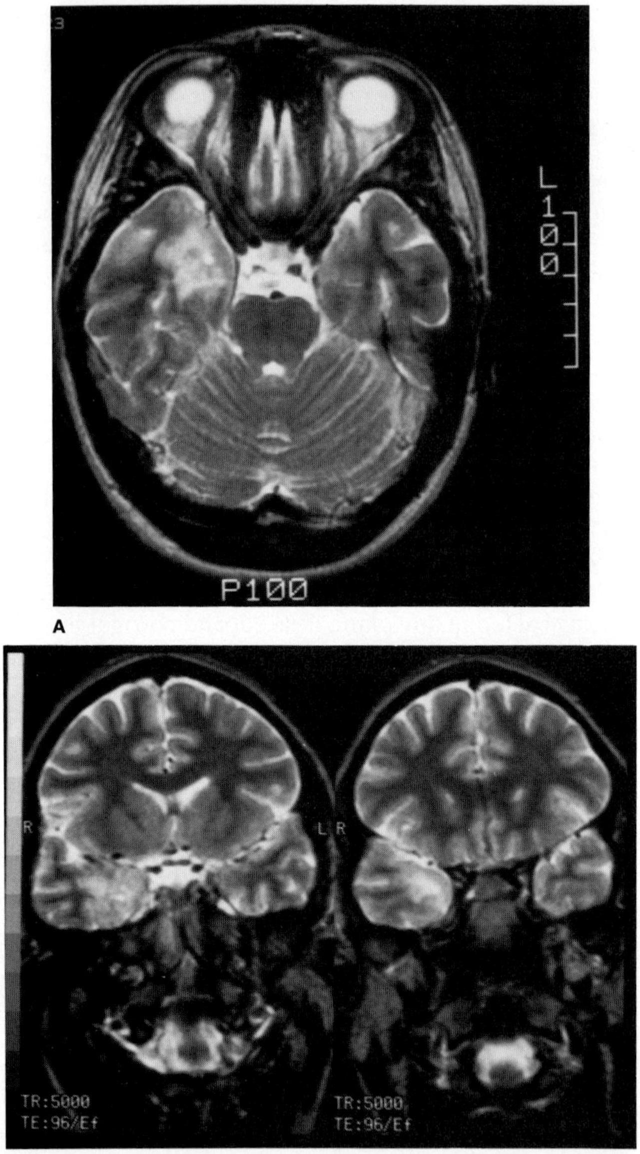

A

B

Figure 7-1
(A) *Axial MRI (TR 4283, TE 108) showing a fibrillary astrocytoma in the right mesial temporal lobe. Note the irregular increased signal intensity and disruption of normal cortical architecture. This patient had a 3-year history of simple partial and complex partial seizures.* **(B)** *Coronal MRI (TR 5000, TE 96) in the same patient, demonstrating the same lesion.*

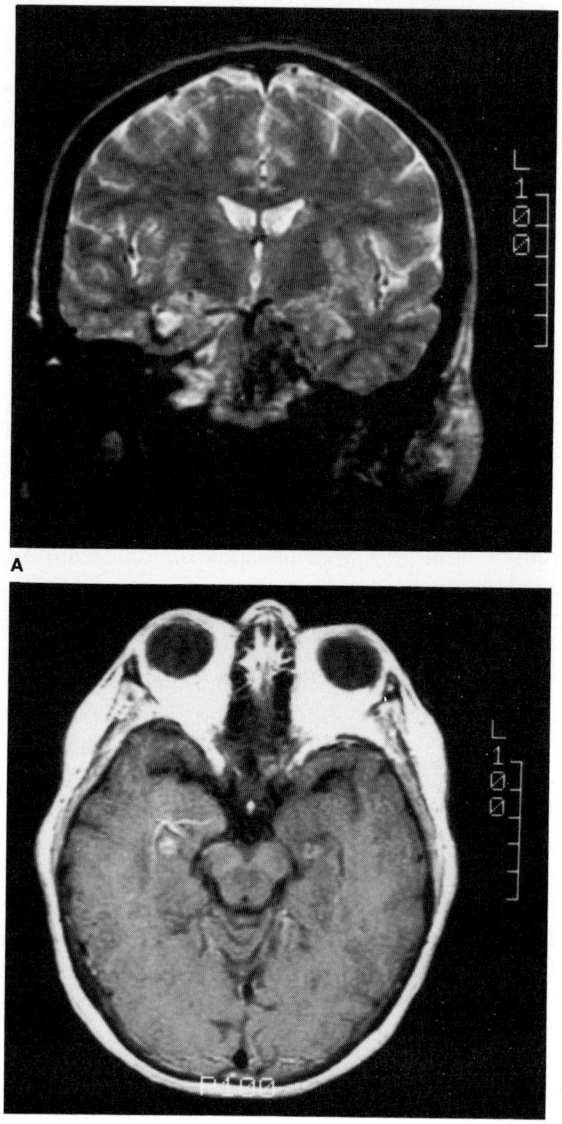

A

B

Figure 7-2
(A) *Coronal MRI (TR 4000, TE 17) of a cavernous hemangioma in the right mesial temporal lobe in a woman with chronic refractory complex partial seizures. Note the hypointense rim surrounding the lesion. This scan is somewhat rotated so the right temporal lobe appears artifactually small.* **(B)** *Axial MRI image (TR 500, TE 15) after contrast injection showing enhancement of the hemangioma and draining veins. The slight enhancement in the contralateral temporal lobe is choroid plexus in the temporal horn of the lateral ventricle.*

malformations, and hamartomas. Tumors are characterized by abnormal signal intensity, particularly in T2-weighted images, and disruption of normal brain architecture. The tumors typically have no associated edema or midline shift. Paramagnetic contrast agents do not improve tumor detection in epilepsy.[29] Meningiomas are not uncommon in the elderly, and may present with seizures (Fig. 7-3). They are typically well demonstrated with CT. Vascular malformations may also present with epileptic seizures, and many have MRI evidence of prior unsuspected hemorrhage (Figs. 7-2 and 7-4).

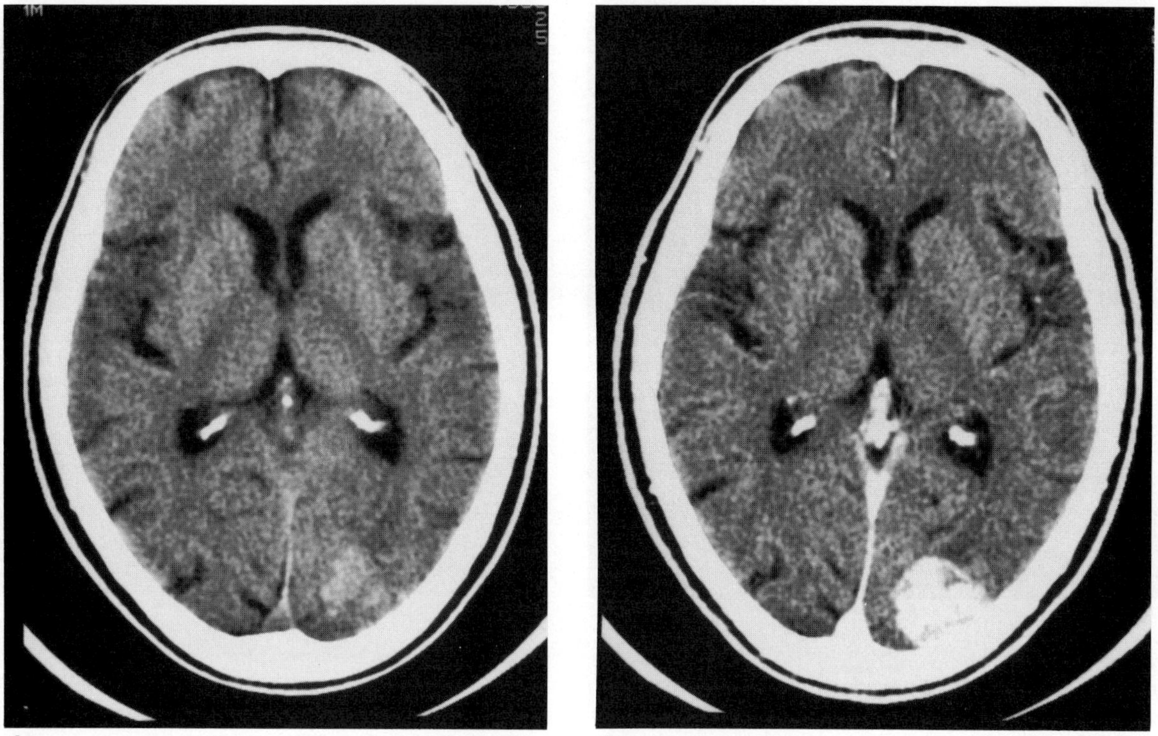

A B

Figure 7-3

(A) *CT scan without contrast injection demonstrating an irregular area of increased signal intensity (caused by calcification) in the left occipital lobe.* **(B)** *CT scan with contrast showing marked homogeneous enhancement of this dural-based meningioma. Such tumors are not uncommon in the elderly and often present with seizures. (Courtesy of Dr. Michael Brooks.)*

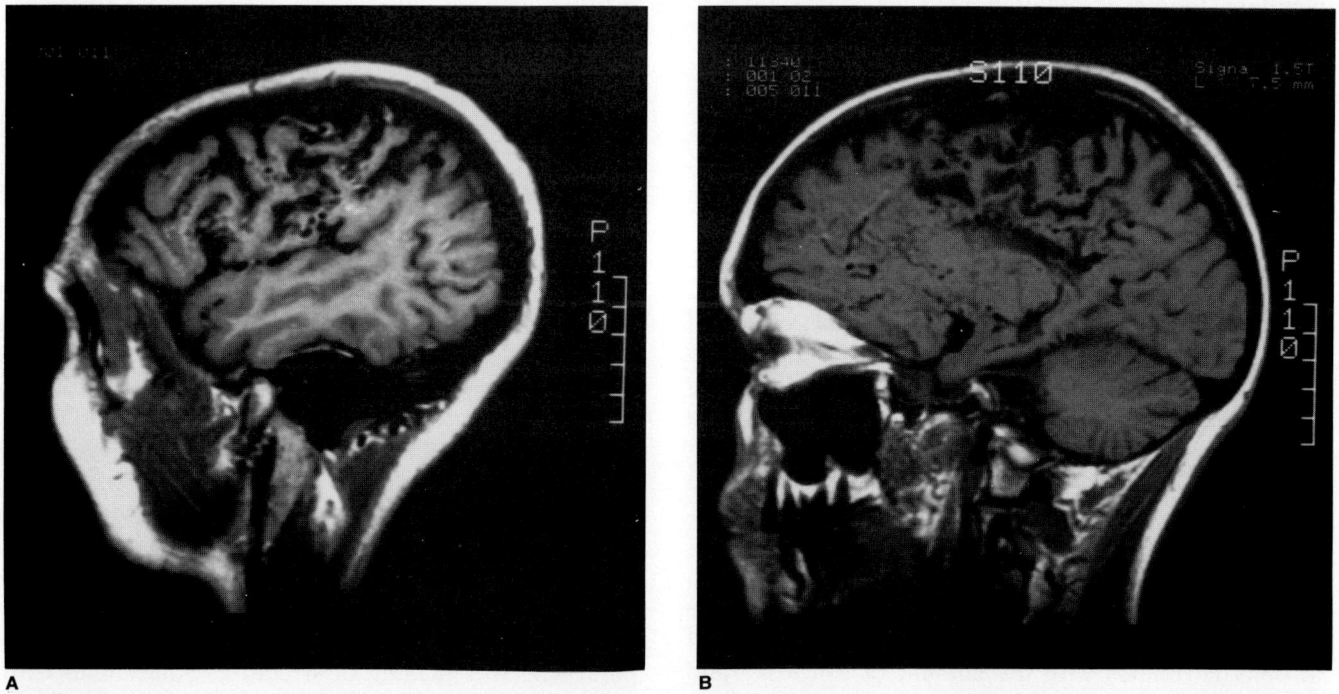

A B

Figure 7-4

(A and B) *Sagittal MRI (TR 550, TE 15) before contrast injection (T1- weighted image) showing the malformation with enlarged veins. The punctate spots are draining veins seen in cross-section. Note the atrophy of surrounding gyri and sparing of the temporal and occipital lobes. Note the multiple draining veins in cortex and deep white matter.* *(continued)*

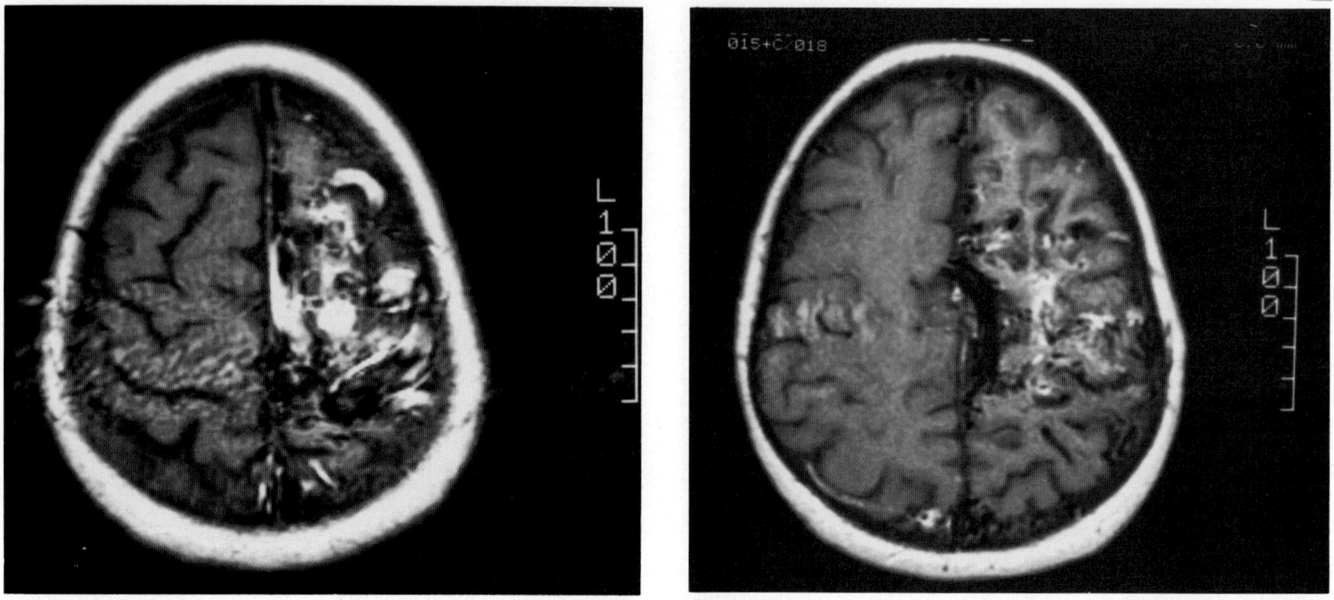

C D

Figure 7-4 *(continued)*
(C and D) *Axial MRI (TR 500, TE 19) after contrast injection showing widespread left frontal and parietal enhancement in a pattern characteristic of a vascular malformation. Note the enlarged veins with increased venous drainage in the left hemisphere. Angiography demonstrates an angiomatous arteriovenous malformation. This patient has a slowly progressive right hemiparesis and aphasia, with recurrent complex partial seizures.*

Dysplasia Although CT shows large heterotopias and dysplasias, more subtle developmental disorders are seen with MRI.[10,11,19,20,30,31] Small regions of dysplastic gray matter are found in the cortex, white matter, or in subependymal regions.[32–38] Migrational anomalies, gyral malformations, and abnormal clefts may be associated with epilepsy (Figs. 7-5, 7-6, and 7-7). Some dysplasias are successfully treated with surgery,[20,39] and MRI delineation of the structural abnormality is perhaps more important than the electroencephalogram (EEG) when planning a resection.

Changes in Tissue Volume and Gliosis Qualitative and quantitative MRI studies show focal atrophy in the hippocampus (Figs. 7-8 and 7-9) in 70 to 90 percent of patients with temporal lobe epilepsy.[12,15,40–48] The atrophy is almost always found in the temporal lobe responsible for the seizures, rare cases of contralateral hippocampal atrophy have been noted. In patients with complex partial seizures, the atrophy is more often restricted to the anterior hippocampus, whereas more diffuse hippocampal volume loss occurs in patients with frequent secondarily generalized seizures.[43] Atrophy is best seen when the coronal slice acquisition angle is orthogonal to the plane of the hippocampus. The degree of hippocampal atrophy correlates with the amount of cell loss[41] and may predict a more favorable outcome after epilepsy surgery.[44] Generalized cortical atrophy (Fig. 7-10) and cerebellar atrophy (Fig. 7-11) also commonly occur in epilepsy.

Trauma (Fig. 7-12) and infarction (Fig. 7-13) may produce focal gliosis and encephalomalacia, which may lead to seizures. Compensatory enlargement of the lateral ventricles sometimes accompanies a focal cortical scar.

In addition to atrophy, enlargement of structures has been noted in epilepsy. Conlon and Trimble found that the corpus callosum was thicker in patients with generalized seizures than in control subjects.[49]

Nonneoplastic Alteration in Signal Intensity A high T2- weighted signal is found on visual inspection of the MRI in 20 to 40 percent of cases of mesial temporal sclerosis.[9,16,18,24,25,50–52] However, abnormal brightness in a T2- weighted image is meaningful only in the presence of hippocampal atrophy or other structural changes. In isolation, it correlates poorly with EEG localization[18] and the precise location of pathologic changes.[16] Quantitative mapping (relaxometry) of T2 relaxation times may also be used to detect sclerotic hippocampi. Relaxation times of sclerotic hippocampi are increased (range 118 to 154 ms) compared with those of controls (range 99 to 106 ms).[45] Fluid attenuated inversion recovery (FLAIR) pulse sequence imaging is a technique that nulls the signal of CSF, thus improving the imaging of structures adjacent to CSF. Thus, FLAIR imaging can be especially useful in evaluation of the temporal lobes, particularly when epilepsy surgery is being considered (Fig. 7-14).[53,54]

Focal frontoparietal white matter hyperintensities

have also been noted in patients with partial epilepsy.[55] These are of usually uncertain significance.

Infections Although uncommon in the United States, parasitic infections are an important cause of epilepsy in underdeveloped countries. A particularly common parasite causing epilepsy is *Taenia solium,* or pork tapeworm. Larval stages of this organism may spread throughout the body, including the brain, causing a condition known as cysticercosis. The dead larvae provoke an inflammatory response, with subsequent tissue calcification. The lesions are most common at the gray-white junction (Fig. 7-15).

Miscellaneous Uses of Neuroimaging Techniques in Epilepsy

Both CT and MRI are used in the stereotactic placement of intracranial electrodes.[56] The location of implanted depth electrodes and subdural electrodes can be verified by use of CT or MRI (Fig. 7-16). Similarly, x-rays are used for assessing intracranial placement of subdural electrodes (Fig. 7-17). Stereotaxis with MRI may be used to guide mesial temporal excision (amygdalohippocampectomy) and in stereotactic lesionectomies.[57]

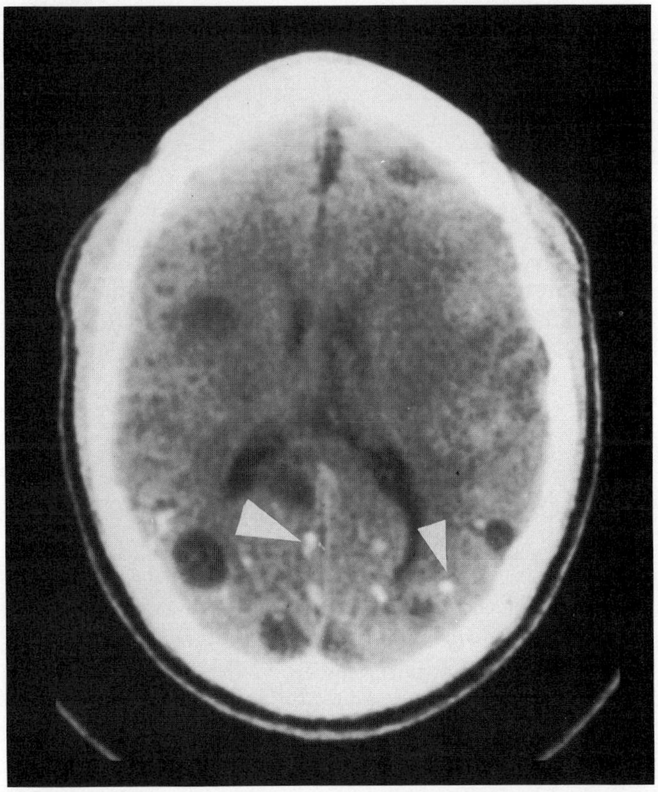

Figure 7-15
Axial CT scan showing multiple calcifications (arrows), mainly in the occipital lobes, typical of cysticercosis. The large lucent lesions were not biopsied but were believed to be echinococcal cysts in this patient, who had multiple parasitic infections. (Courtesy of Dr. Michael Brooks.)

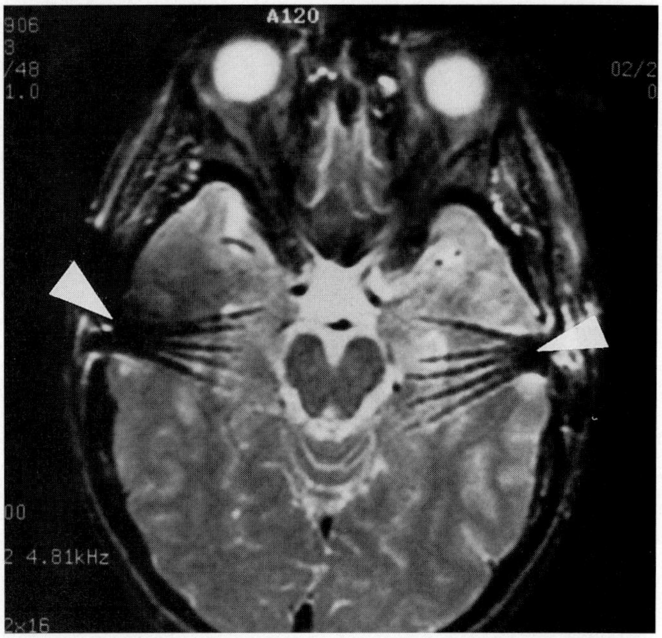

Figure 7-16
Axial MRI (TR3000, TE90) demonstrating depth electrodes (arrows) in the bilateral temporal lobes of a 32-year-old man with epilepsy.

In addition, MRI can accurately assess the completeness of surgery after resective surgery (Fig. 7-18) and corpus callosotomy.[58–60]

Clinical Management

Both CT and MRI are essential tools for diagnosing and treating people with epilepsy. Magnetic resonance imaging is the test of first choice, and CT should be reserved for circumstances in which MRI is unavailable or unsafe. When should imaging be performed? (See the algorithm for neuroimaging in epilepsy, Fig. 7-19.) All patients who have symptomatic partial or generalized epilepsy should have an MRI ordered at the time of initial evaluation. Patients whose seizures prove refractory to antiepileptic medications or whose seizure type, seizure frequency, or neurologic examination findings change should also have an MRI, even if a prior CT or MRI was normal. Unless there is an incomplete response to medication or an atypical feature in the history, patients with well-defined benign genetic epilepsy syndromes do not require MRI scans. In selected cases, PET and SPECT scans may help, particularly when epilepsy surgery is being considered or to aid in classification.

If a neoplasm is detected, its clinical relevance must be determined. Tumors such as astrocytomas and hamartomas often cause seizures, whereas arachnoid cysts and venous angiomas may be incidental. Only when epileptiform EEG abnormalities correspond to the MRI lesion can one presume, without certainty, that the lesion is related to the epilepsy. Therapy can then be

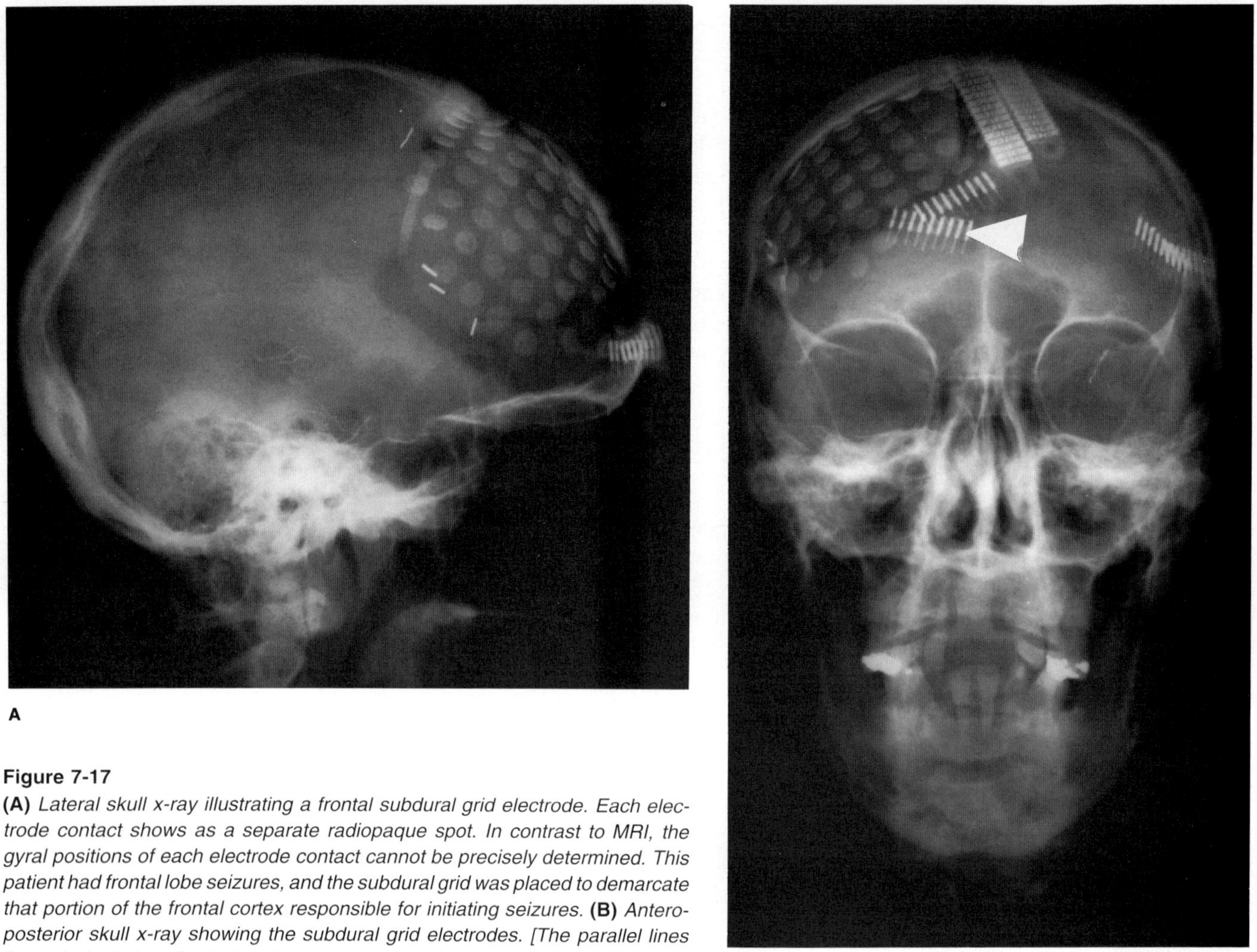

Figure 7-17
(A) *Lateral skull x-ray illustrating a frontal subdural grid electrode. Each electrode contact shows as a separate radiopaque spot. In contrast to MRI, the gyral positions of each electrode contact cannot be precisely determined. This patient had frontal lobe seizures, and the subdural grid was placed to demarcate that portion of the frontal cortex responsible for initiating seizures.* **(B)** *Anteroposterior skull x-ray showing the subdural grid electrodes. [The parallel lines (arrow) clustering about the grid are connector plugs over the scalp.]*

planned based upon the nature of the lesion, the history, and the neurologic examination. Some patients with well-controlled epilepsy and a benign lesion may be followed conservatively with yearly MRI scans and office examinations. Should seizures persist or change in character, an MRI should be repeated, and surgery should be considered.

Focal atrophy usually has little relevance to patients' management outside of the surgical realm. However, the presence of atrophy may help confirm a diagnosis of symptomatic epilepsy.

Future Directions

The range of possible MRI applications is enormous, and one can foresee advances in both structural and physiologic imaging. Current methods are being upgraded for improved structural imaging. For example, gradient echo techniques now being explored allow contiguous thin-section T1-weighted images with 1-mm resolution.[61] These techniques should lead to better understanding of neuronal migration abnormalities. In addition, there have been great advances in functional MRI as well as MRS; these are discussed in the next section.

PHYSIOLOGIC IMAGING

Positron Emission Tomography

Positron emission tomography can be used to examine a variety of physiologic processes in vivo, including glucose consumption, cerebral blood flow, blood volume, oxygen extraction, oxygen metabolism, pH, protein synthesis, and receptor binding.[62–66] Most studies of epilepsy have focused on cerebral glucose metabolic rates, although blood flow, oxygen metabolism, and receptor binding also have been measured. Since PET is expensive and has limited clinical applications at present, its use is restricted to a relative handful of academic centers.

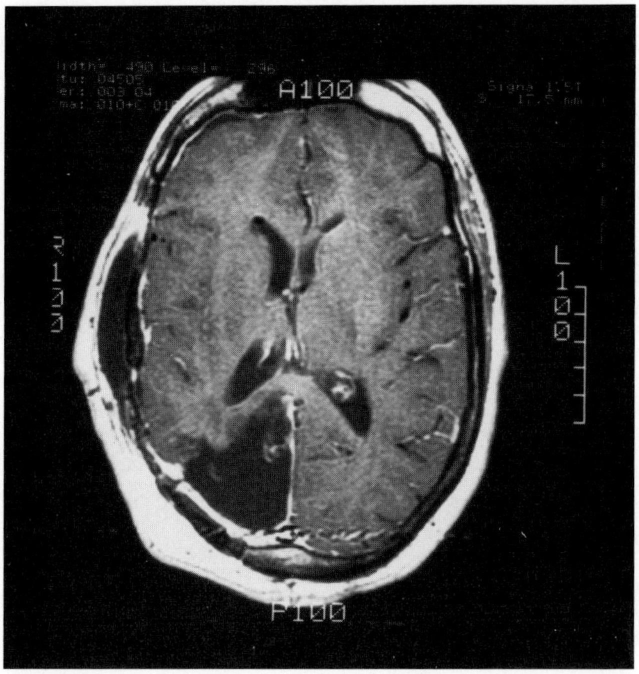

Figure 7-18
Axial MRI (TR 500, TE 15 plus gadolinium) after resection of gliotic tissue from the right occipital lobe. This scan documents the extent of the resection, and the residual space now contains CSF. This 35-year-old man had intractable complex partial and secondarily generalized seizures. Pre-operative visual field testing showed a dense left homonymous hemianopsia; thus, surgery could be performed without risking further visual deficit.

Studies of Patients

Metabolic Studies Interictal PET studies with 18-F-fluorodeoxyglucose (FDG) show focal reduced glucose uptake, also known as hypometabolism, in patients with partial epilepsy.[4,22,27,67–74] This is often accompanied by diminished blood flow.[75–77] Fifty-five to eighty percent of patients with temporal lobe epilepsy have unilateral temporal lobe hypometabolism (Fig. 7-20). Although the pathologic abnormality, mesial temporal sclerosis, is confined to the limbic cortex, the area of hypometabolism usually involves the entire temporal lobe.[4,74,78] However, some patients have restricted mesial temporal hypometabolism (Figs. 7-21, and 7-22), and others may have multilobar hypometabolism (Fig. 7-23). Patients with extratemporal epilepsy often have extensive hypometabolic regions as well.[27,79]

Interictal PET-FDG studies are helpful in choosing patients for epilepsy surgery.[80] The presence of interictal unilateral temporal lobe hypometabolism may predict a good result after epilepsy surgery.[81]

Reduced glucose uptake is present elsewhere in the brain in temporal lobe epilepsy, including subcortical nuclei.[60,82–84] Distant hypometabolism may be caused by either diminished afferent activity or greater inhibition of cortical activity.

In addition, PET-FDG has been used in frontal lobe epilepsy. Focal decreased FDG uptake is reported, but the yield of PET is probably lower in frontal lobe epilepsy.[85]

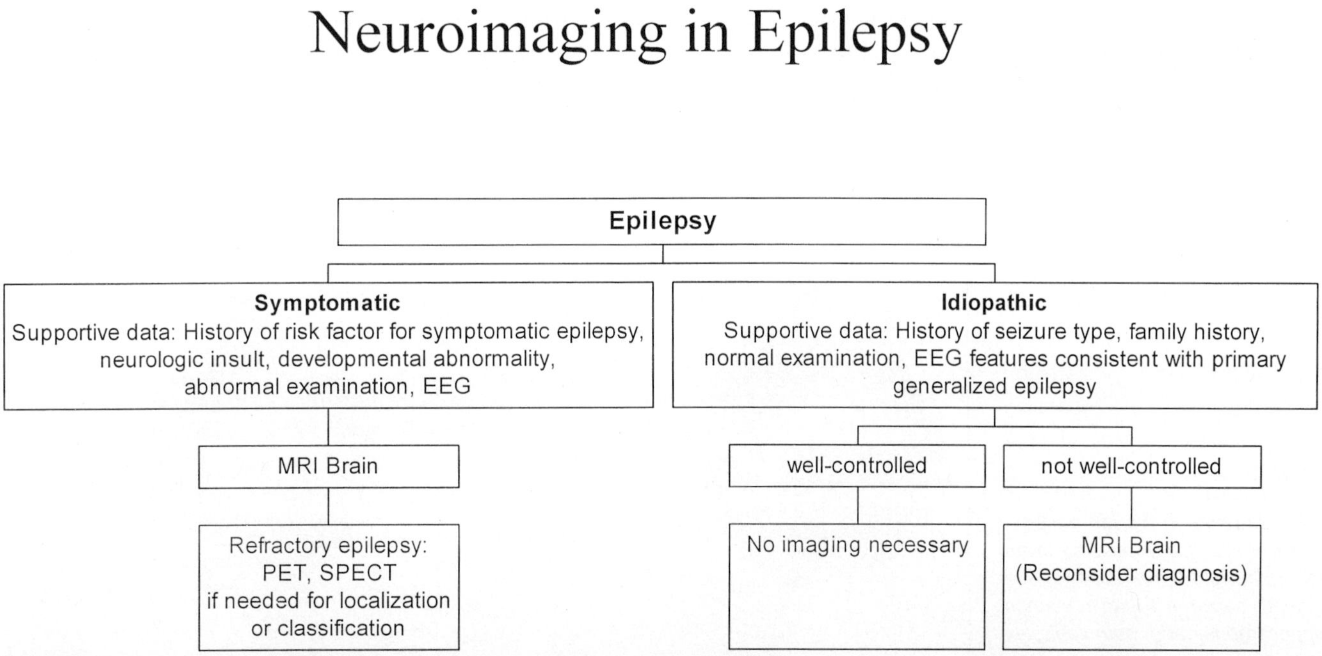

Figure 7-19
Algorithm for neuroimaging in epilepsy.

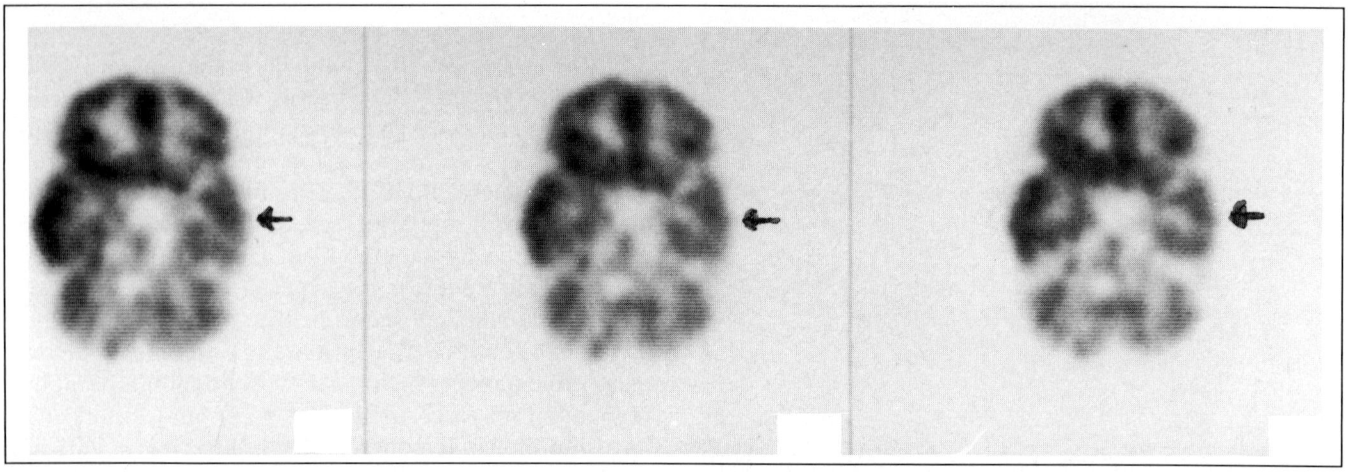

Figure 7-20
PET-FDG scan showing interictal hypometabolism of the entire left temporal lobe (arrows) in three sequential axial scans. This man had complex partial seizures originating in the left temporal lobe. His MRI scan showed no hippocampal atrophy with volumetric measurements.

During partial seizures, energy requirements are increased; thus, increased FDG uptake is seen (Fig. 7-24).[86] The hypermetabolic zones may be highly restricted or multifocal, involving distant regions where seizures spread. Ictal PET studies are not useful because of the complex metabolic patterns and logistical difficulties of obtaining an ictal scan.

Also, PET-FDG has been used in patients with generalized epilepsy. In the Lennox-Gastaut syndrome, a variety of interictal hypometabolic patterns have been described, including multilobar and bihemispheric hypometabolism.[87–89] These hypometabolic areas at times indicate areas of underlying cortical dysplasia and heterotopias. In addition, PET has been used to help select infants with intractable epilepsy for surgery.[90] Patients with idiopathic generalized epilepsy have also been evaluated.[91–94] Interictal metabolism appears normal, and the spike wave discharge has been noted to have variable effects on metabolic rates.

Antiepileptic medications depress cerebral metabolism.[95] Phenobarbital lowers metabolism more than do phenytoin, carbamazepine, and valproic acid, and some authors speculate that this may correlate with cognitive impairment.

Receptor Studies Neuroreceptor binding can also be explored in epilepsy. The mesial temporal lobe shows diminished benzodiazepine receptor binding in patients with partial epilepsy.[96–99] This decrease most likely indicates neuronal loss in that area. Opiate receptors are increased in temporal lobe neocortex but appear normal in mesial structures.[100,101]

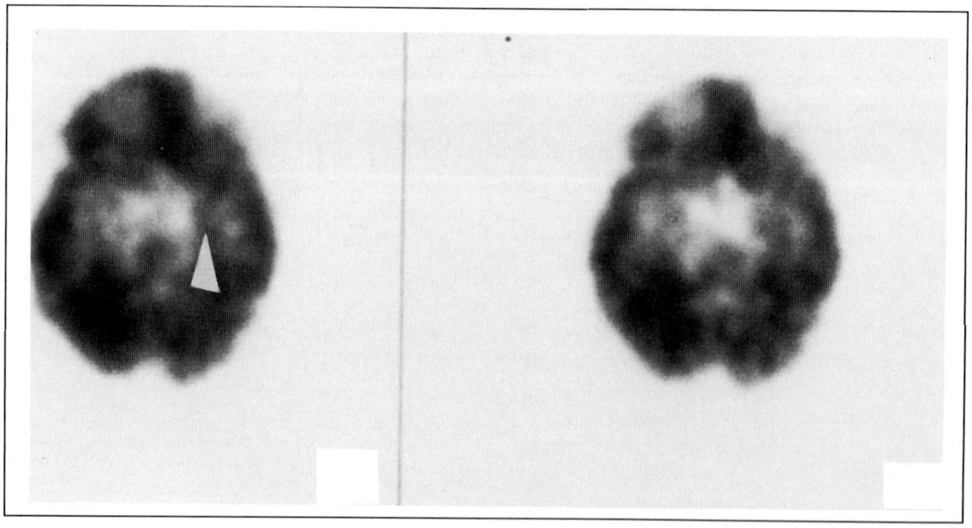

Figure 7-21
Interictal PET-FDG scan showing restricted right mesial temporal hypometabolism. Note the medial rim of FDG uptake in the left temporal lobe (arrow); this is missing in the abnormal right temporal lobe. This patient's seizures began in the right hippocampus, and pathologic examination of his resected temporal lobe showed hippocampal sclerosis.

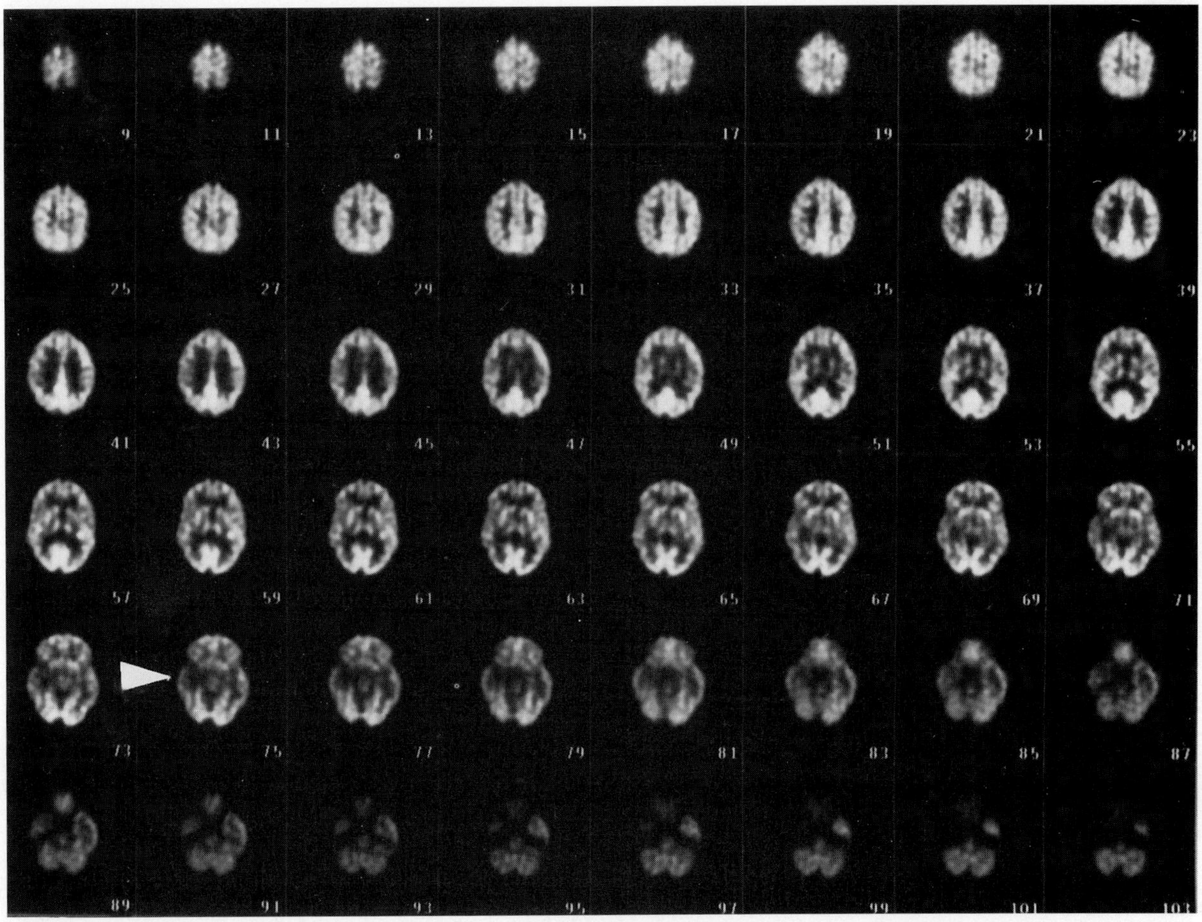

Figure 7-22
Interictal FDG-PET scan showing right temporal lobe hypometabolism (arrow) in a 41-year-old woman with intractable temporal lobe epilepsy. This patient subsequently underwent a right anterior temporal lobectomy and has been seizure-free since surgery.

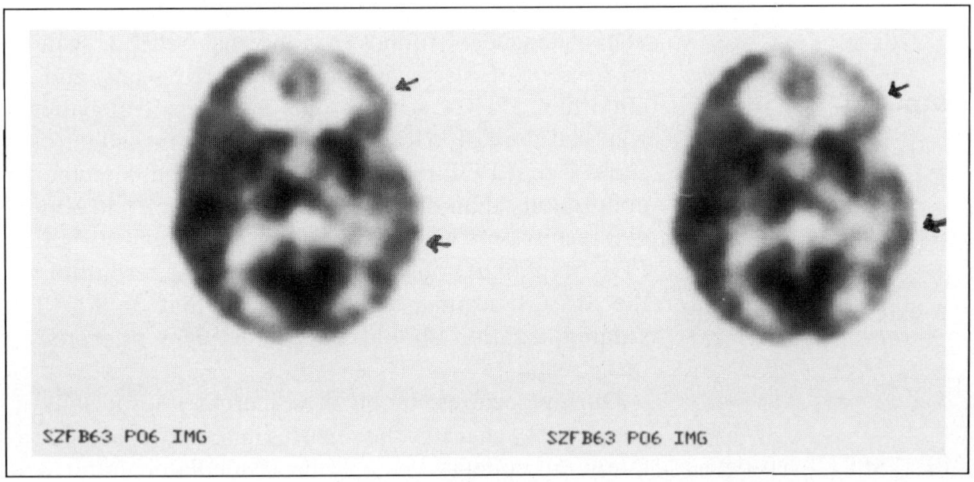

Figure 7-23
Interictal PET-FDG scan showing left frontal and temporal hypometabolism in a patient with temporal lobe epilepsy. Multilobar hypometabolism may also occur in patients with multifocal conditions such as Lennox-Gastaut syndrome, and this scan resembles PET scans seen in that illness.

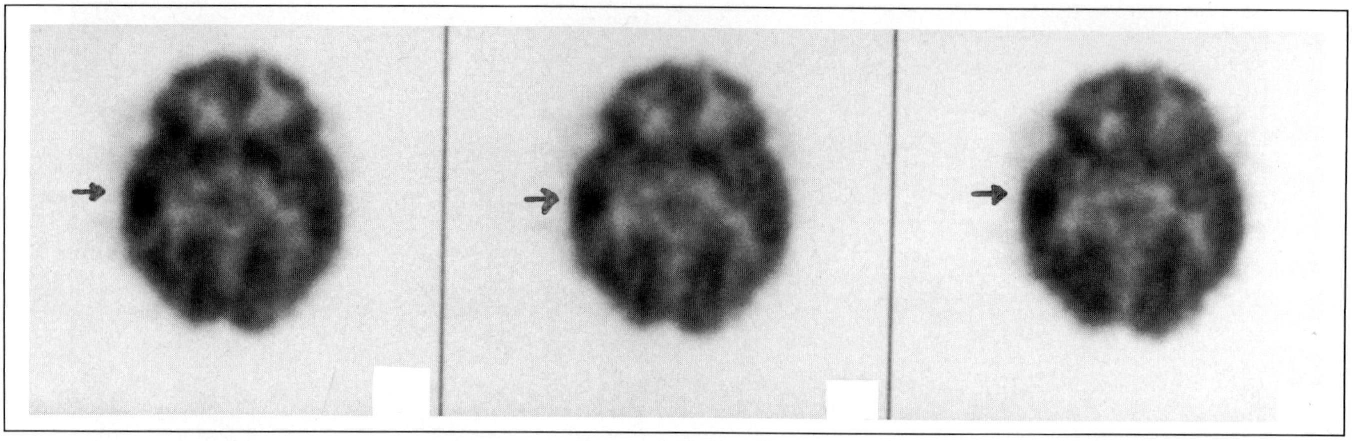

Figure 7-24
PET-FDG study taken during a right temporal lobe seizure. Note the area of increased FDG uptake (arrows) in lateral temporal lobe cortex. Ictal hypermetabolism is transient but may last for several minutes after a seizure has ended.

Clinical Management

To date, PET is worthwhile only for planning epilepsy surgery. Studies utilizing PET-FDG help delineate tissue to be excised. They are used most often in temporal lobe epilepsy and Lennox-Gastaut syndrome. Although premature conclusions should not be drawn, benzodiazepine receptor studies have great potential. They, too, may prove useful in patients considered for surgery.

Future Directions

Much of the early promise of PET in epilepsy remains unfulfilled. Newer studies are using PET to study cerebral blood flow during a variety of behavioral tasks. However, advances in MRI may limit the use of PET as a research and clinical technique. Magnetic resonance imaging offers the prospect of superior imaging of cerebral blood flow. Studies must compare PET-FDG and MRI to learn how these techniques complement each other. Receptor studies may prove to be the chief application of PET, pending the development of MRI ligands.

Single Photon Emission Computed Tomography

Single photon emission computed tomography is a physiologic imaging technique that is far less expensive and complicated than PET. Because of that, SPECT is widely employed. It was originally developed to study cerebral blood flow and has been extensively applied in epilepsy.

Studies of Patients

Cerebral Perfusion Studies Like PET, SPECT has been used mostly with patients being evaluated for epilepsy surgery. A variety of radioisotopes can be used, including ^{123}I-*N*-isopropyl-iodoamphetamine (IMP), ^{123}I-hydroxyiodopropyldianine (HIPDM), ^{133}Xe,[102–107] ^{99m}Tc-label hexamethyl propyleneamine oxime (HMPAO), and Tc ethyl cysteinate dimer (ECD). While SPECT-HMPAO has gained broadest acceptance, ^{99m}Tc ECD SPECT has the practical advantage of having increased radiochemical stability and prolonged intracerebral retention,[108,109] thus extending the time period during which an image can be obtained. Interictal studies show varying patterns of hypoperfusion in 40 to 70 percent of patients with focal epilepsy and West syndrome.[110–127]

In temporal lobe epilepsy, interictal studies do not have a satisfactory yield. While focal temporal lobe hypoperfusion is sometimes seen, many scans are normal, and multilobar reductions in flow are common. Quantitative analysis does not improve interictal SPECT localization.[123] When a hypoperfused region is present, it usually contains the epileptic area. Hypoperfusion is shown in SPECT-HMPAO studies more often when the MRI result is abnormal than when it is normal. Ryvlin and colleagues[128] found an abnormal SPECT scan in 86 percent of cases with abnormal MRI scans, and an abnormal SPECT scan in only 18 percent of patients who had normal MRI results. The same investigators[129] showed that PET-FDG studies more often detected an abnormality than did SPECT studies, which had abnormal results only with patients with "pronounced" PET-FDG hypometabolism. Since the spatial resolution of the SPECT scanner was inferior to that of the PET scanner, caution should be exercised in interpreting these results.

During seizures, blood flow increases, especially in cortex that generates the seizures in temporal and extratemporal epilepsy.[121,122,124,130–132] Immediately after seizures, epileptogenic cortex remains hyperperfused, and surrounding cortex is markedly hypoperfused.[122,133,134] Difference images obtained from subtraction of interictal from ictal or postictal scans may reveal areas of relatively increased cerebral perfusion even more clearly (Fig. 7-25).[143] Ictal and immediate postictal SPECT scanning with HMPAO may have a localization accuracy as high as 80 percent in temporal lobe epilepsy.[121,124,131,133]

In addition, SPECT-HMPAO scans have been used in partial status epilepticus and epilepsia partialis continua.[135,136] Discrete areas of hyperperfusion appear, localizing the area responsible for seizures and helping to confirm the diagnosis (Fig. 7-26).

Intra-arterial HMPAO injections show the distribution of amobarbital during the Wada test.[137] This lipophilic compound binds to tissue directly supplied by the internal carotid artery. Intravenous HMPAO injection during the Wada test shows the area of brain that is functionally inactivated by the amobarbital.[138]

Receptor Studies I-iomazenil, or RO 16–0154, binds to central benzodiazepine receptors. Small numbers of patients with temporal lobe epilepsy have been studied with this ligand.[112,139–142] As with flumazenil, iomazenil binding is diminished in the mesial temporal lobe in temporal lobe epilepsy.

Clinical Management

Clinically, SPECT perfusion scans are useful in the medical and surgical diagnosis of epilepsy. Interictal studies may help clarify the diagnosis, and ictal studies may help confirm whether a behavior is epileptic when the EEG is equivocal. The mediocre sensitivity and specificity of interictal SPECT perfusion scanning limits its utility as a surgical diagnostic tool. Interictal iomazenil scanning has potential, however. Ictal and postictal SPECT-HMPAO studies are helpful in localizing an epileptic focus in people with intractable temporal lobe

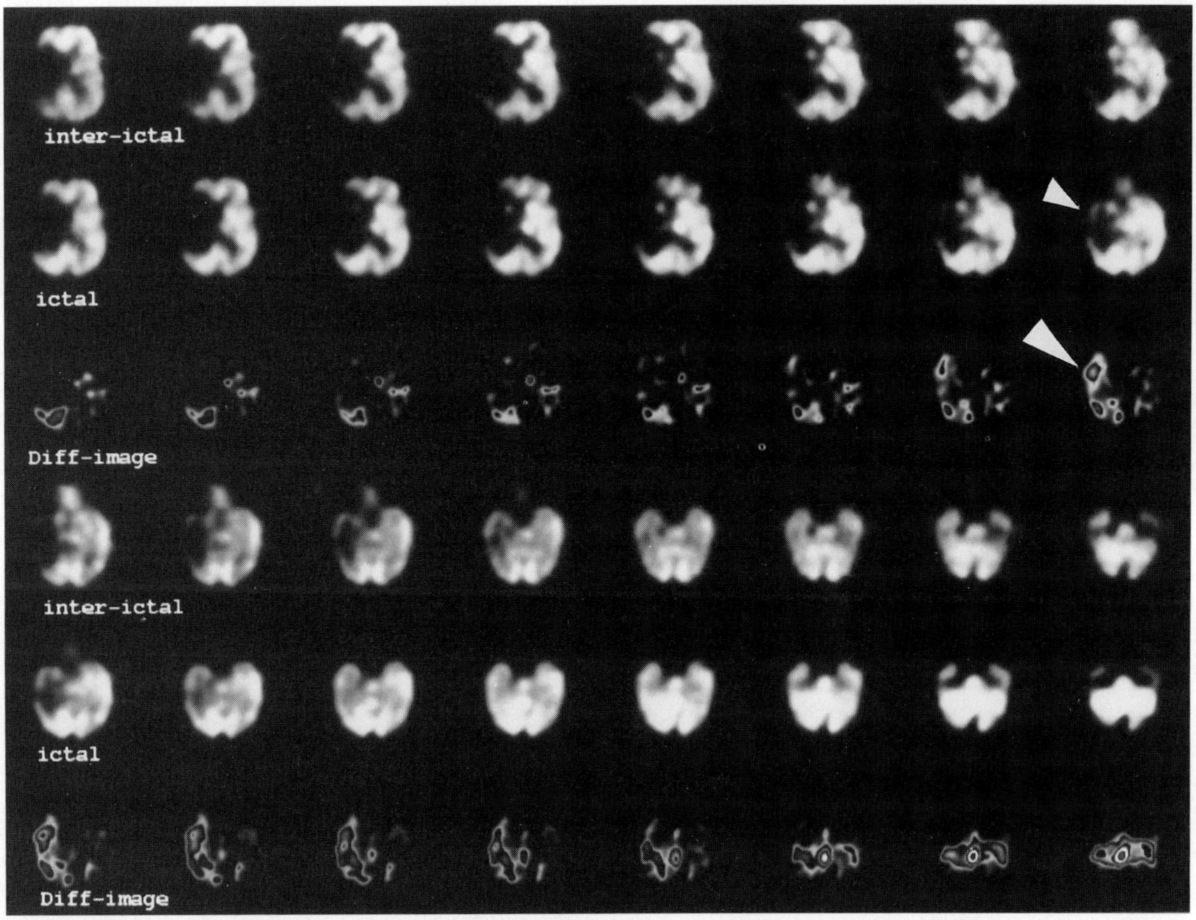

Figure 7-25

Axial ^{99m}Tc ECD SPECT scans obtained in a 45-year-old woman with a right middle cerebral artery distribution infarction and epilepsy. Interictal images (first and fourth lines) reveal hypoperfusion in the area of infarction. Ictal images (second and fifth lines) continue to reveal an area of hypoperfusion in the area of infarction but also shows an area of relative hyperperfusion in the right temporal lobe (small arrow). This area (large arrow) is more clearly seen in the difference images (third and sixth lines), which are obtained by subtracting interictal images from ictal images.

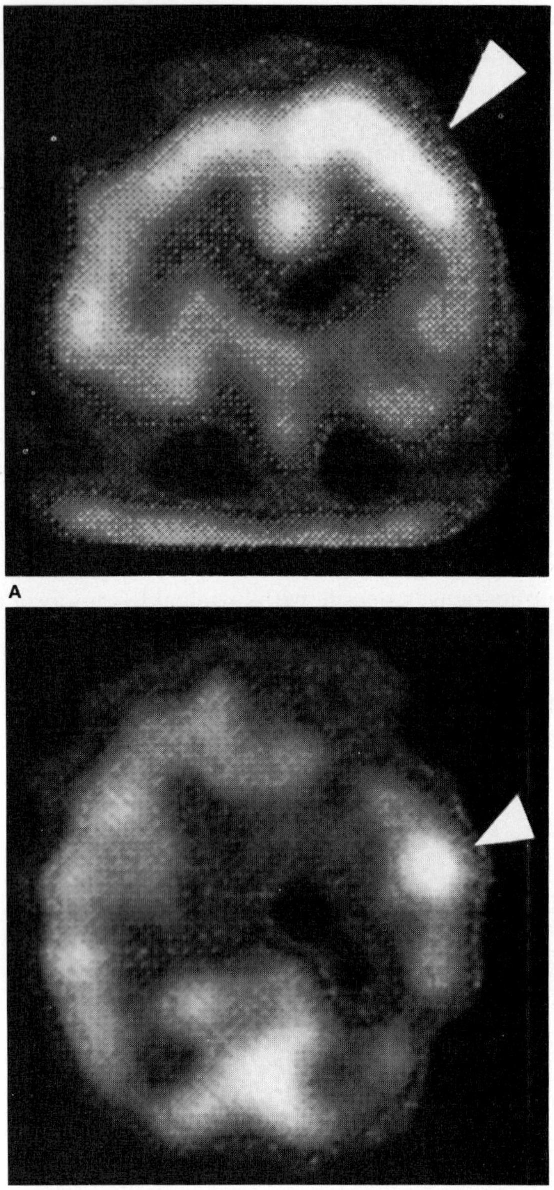

Figure 7-26
(A) *Coronal SPECT-HMPAO scan showing increased perfusion in the left frontal lobe (arrow) in a patient with epilepsia partialis continua from Rasmussen's encephalitis.* **(B)** *Axial SPECT-HMPAO scan showing the same area of hyperperfusion.*

epilepsy. However, seizures must be relatively frequent to obtain these studies, and a trained team capable of immediate response must be ready.

Future Directions

Ictal and postictal SPECT must be compared with modern MRI techniques. One hopes that detailed anatomic imaging and functional imaging will be proven nonredundant. Should cerebral perfusion be easily measured with MRI, interictal SPECT perfusion studies may become completely irrelevant.

Some very preliminary evidence suggests that SPECT scanning with iomazenil may help localize an epileptic focus in partial epilepsy. However, more patients must be evaluated to ascertain the sensitivity and specificity of this ligand.

Functional MRI

Functional MRI (fMRI) is sensitive to changes in cerebral blood flow and volume that occur during seizures. Focal increases in cortical ictal blood flow have been demonstrated during seizures by this technique with patients with frequent seizures and focal status epilepticus. [144,157,158] Studies using fMRI can identify both cortical and subcortical regions of activation and may aid in the understanding of subcortical connections involved in seizure activation and propagation (Fig. 7-27).[145] The identification of areas of focal brain activation during seizures may aid in the planning of epilepsy surgery. However, the usefulness of this application is limited by the need for frequent seizures in order to obtain images and by the difficulty in acquiring data during seizures if they produce movement.

In the future, EEG-triggered echoplanar fMRI may help to resolve some of these issues by enabling acquisition of data during brief or subclinical seizures[146] and possibly may aid in identifying areas of brain activation during interictal spikes. However, fMRI is more likely to be useful when planning epilepsy surgery. It may aid in language localization.[147–149] Moreover, functional mapping of movement, sensation, and memory may improve the safety of neurosurgical procedures.

Magnetic Resonance Spectroscopy

Magnetic resonance spectroscopy (MRS) is emerging as a potentially useful imaging technique in epilepsy. Proton (^{1}H) MRS is more easily performed and has greater signal-to-noise ratio and better spatial resolution than does ^{31}P MRS. It is currently the primary technique used in epilepsy studies.

Proton MRS has been mostly used to study temporal lobe epilepsy. Reductions of *N*-acetylaspartate (NAA) and NAA/[(choline ([Cho]) + creatine ([Cr)]]) ratios in the epileptogenic temporal lobes suggest that there is neuronal dysfunction or loss (decreased NAA) and possibly increased gliosis (increased [Cho + Cr] and thus decreased NAA/[Cho + Cr]ratio) in these regions.[150] These abnormalities may help to lateralize the epileptogenic zone in patients who are being considered for epilepsy surgery,[151] particularly in the absence of evidence of hippocampal atrophy on MRI.[152] Correct lateralization has been reported between 55 to nearly 100 percent with current techniques.[151,153–155] In addition, MRS is useful in identifying bilateral abnormalities,[151,154] reflecting bilateral neuronal dysfunction, which is commonly found in patients with temporal lobe epilepsy. Recent studies reveal that reductions in NAA/[Cho +

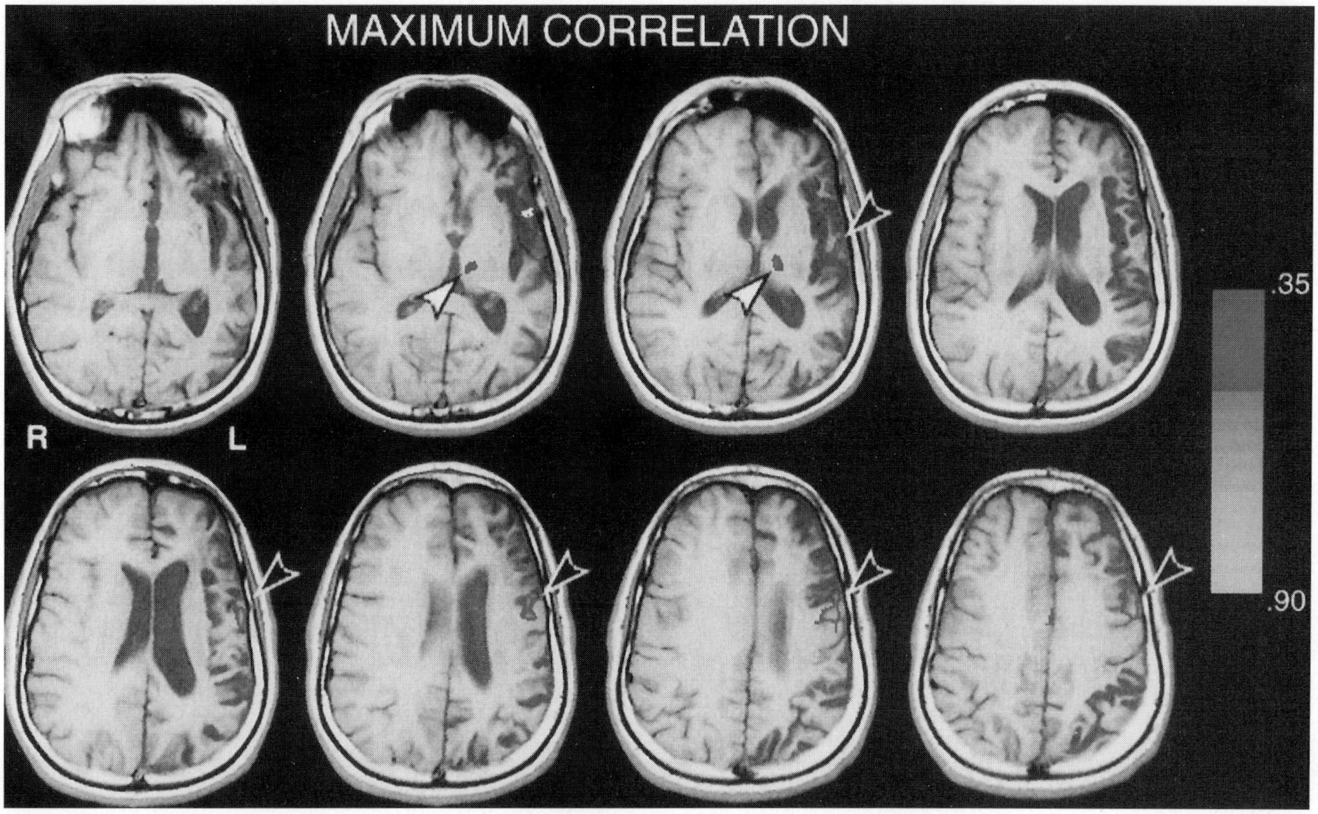

Figure 7-27 (Plate 16)
Axial fMRI depicting functional activation images of eight contiguous slices showing the maximum cross-correlation value versus cortical seizure-signal profile taken from the region of earliest onset of the cortical event. Color scale r values range from 0.35 to 0.9. The left frontal seizure focus is clearly evident (black arrows). The apparent absence of the cortical activity in the fourth slice is an artifact of the thresholding and filtering parameters chosen. Highly correlated activity is seen in the ipsilateral thalamus (white arrows). No other signal changes are correlated with the cortical event. (Reprinted with permission from Detre JA, Alsop DE, Aguirre GK, Sperling MR.)

Cr] ratios in remaining tissue may be reversible after temporal lobectomy for epilepsy, suggesting that neuronal function may improve after surgery.[153]

Also, MRS may become a useful technique for localization of epileptogenic foci in extratemporal epilepsy, but this application requires further investigation. Studies of seizures, status epilepticus, and an early postictal state have revealed changes in NAA and lactate that may correspond with the epileptogenic focus.[156] At this time, MRS appears to hold promise mainly in improving our understanding of the pathophysiology of epilepsy.

CONCLUSION

While MRI and CT show structural lesions and their extent, PET and SPECT reveal the extent of functional disruption. In fact, anatomic and physiologic data may not be as disparate as would appear at first glance. Anatomic lesions usually cause physiologic derangements, and physiologic derangements, although more extensive, often reflect an underlying microscopic structural abnormality. Studies utilizing MRS reveal chemical changes in the brain that may further aid in identification of abnormal brain tissue. Functional MRI techniques will be further developed to aid in localization of function and assessing cognitive organization. They may ultimately aid in targeting surgical therapy more effectively and with decreased risk.

For routine clinical purposes, MRI and EEG are the primary tools that supplement the history and physical examination when diagnosing patients with epilepsy. However, physiologic imaging should prove ultimately useful for reasons other than surgical localization. In the future, SPECT, PET, and fMRI may be used in concert with EEG and MRI to characterize and classify epileptic cognitive and behavioral alterations.

REFERENCES

1. Becker H, Vogelsang H, and Schwarzrock R: Comparative MR and CT research in selected neuroradiological problems. *ROFO* 142:23–30, 1985.
2. Bergen D, Bleck T, Ramsey R, et al: Magnetic resonance imaging as a sensitive and specific predictor of neoplasms

removed for intractable epilepsy. *Epilepsia* 30:318–321, 1989.

3. Bydder GM, Steiner RE, Young IR, et al: Clinical NMR imaging of the brain: 140 cases. *Am J Roentgenol* 139: 215–236, 1982.
4. Sperling MR, Wilson G, Engel J Jr, et al: Magnetic resonance imaging in intractable partial epilepsy: Correlative studies. *Ann Neurol* 20:57–62, 1986.
5. Aaron J, New PF, Strand R, et al: NMR imaging in temporal lobe epilepsy due to gliomas. *J Comput Assist Tomogr* 8:608–613, 1984.
6. Pykett IL, Newhouse JH, Buonanno FS, et al: Principles of NMR imaging. *Radiology* 143:157–168, 1982.
7. Young IR, Burl M, Clarke GJ, et al: Magnetic resonance properties of hydrogen: Imaging the posterior fossa. *Am J Roentgenol* 2:487–493, 1981.
8. Budinger TF: Nuclear magnetic resonance (NMR) in vivo studies: Known thresholds for health effects. *J Comput Assist Tomogr* 5:800–811, 1981.
9. Avrahami E, Cohn DF, Neufeld M, et al: Magnetic resonance imaging (MRI) in patients with complex partial seizures and normal computerized tomography (CT) scan. *Clin Neurol Neurosurg* 89:231–235, 1987.
10. Barkovich AJ, Kjos BO: Gray matter heterotopias: MR characteristics and correlation with developmental and neurological manifestations. *Radiology* 182:493–499, 1992.
11. Barkovich AJ, Kjos BO: Non-lissencephalic cortical dysplasia: Correlation of imaging findings with clinical deficits. *Am J Neuroradiol* 13:85–94, 1992.
12. Berkovic SF, Andermann F, Olivier A, et al: Hippocampal sclerosis in temporal lobe epilepsy demonstrated by magnetic resonance imaging. *Ann Neurol* 29:175–182, 1991.
13. Gerard G, Shabas D, Rossi D: MRI in epilepsy. *Comput Radiol* 11:223–227, 1987.
14. Imakita S, Nishimura T, Yamada N, et al: Cerebral vascular malformations: Applications of magnetic resonance imaging to differential diagnosis. *Neuroradiology.* 31: 320–325, 1989.
15. Jackson GD, Berkovic SF, Tress BM, et al: Hippocampal sclerosis can be reliably detected by magnetic resonance imaging. *Neurology* 40:1869–1875, 1990.
16. Kuzniecky R, de la Sayette V, Ethier R, et al: Magnetic resonance imaging in temporal lobe epilepsy: Pathological correlations. *Ann Neurol* 22:341–347, 1987.
17. Latack JT, Abou-Kahlil BW, Seigel GJ, et al: Patients with partial seizures: Evaluation by MR, CT, and PET imaging. *Radiology* 159:159–163, 1986.
18. McLachlan RS, Nicholson RL, Black S, et al: Nuclear magnetic resonance imaging: A new approach to the investigation of refractory temporal lobe epilepsy. *Epilepsia* 26:555–562, 1985.
19. Palmini A, Andermann F, Olivier A, et al: Focal neuronal migration disorders and intractable partial epilepsy: A study of 30 patients. *Ann Neurol* 30:741–749, 1991.
20. Palmini A, Andermann F, Olivier A, et al: Focal neuronal migration disorders and intractable partial epilepsy: Results of surgical treatment. *Ann Neurol* 30: 750–757, 1991.
21. Stefan H, Pawlik G, Bocher-Schwarz HG, et al: Functional and morphological abnormalities in temporal lobe epilepsy: A comparison of interictal and ictal EEG, CT, MRI, SPECT and PET. *J Neurol* 234:377–384, 1987.
22. Theodore WH, Dorwart R, Holmes M, et al: Neuroimaging in refractory partial seizures: Comparison of PET, CT, and MRI. *Neurology* 36:750–759, 1986.
23. Theodore WH, Holmes MD, Dorwart RH, et al: Complex partial seizures: Cerebral structure and cerebral function. *Epilepsia* 27:576–82, 1986.
24. Franceschi M, Triulzi F, Ferini-Strambi L, et al: Focal cerebral lesions found by magnetic resonance imaging in cryptogenic nonrefractory temporal lobe epilepsy patients. *Epilepsia* 30:540–546, 1989.
25. Jabbari B, Gunderson CH, Wippold F, et al: Magnetic resonance imaging in partial complex epilepsy. *Arch Neurol* 43:869–872, 1986.
26. Laster DW, Penry JK, Moody DM, et al: Chronic seizure disorders: Contribution of MR imaging when CT is normal. *Am J Neuroradiol* 6:177–180, 1985.
27. Swartz BE, Halgren E, Delgado-Escueta AV, et al: Neuroimaging in patients with seizures of probable frontal lobe origin. *Epilepsia* 30: 547–558, 1989.
28. Ormson MJ, Kispert DB, Sharbrough FW, et al: Cryptic structural lesions in refractory partial epilepsy: MR imaging and CT studies. *Radiology* 160:215–219, 1986.
29. Cascino GD, Hirschorn KA, Jack CR, et al: Gadolinium-DPTA-enhanced magnetic resonance imaging in intractable partial epilepsy. *Neurology* 39:1115–1118, 1989.
30. Kuzniecky R, Andermann F, et al: Bilateral central macrogyria: Epilepsy, pseudobulbar palsy, and mental retardation: A recognizable neuronal migration disorder. *Ann Neurol* 25: 547–554, 1989.
31. Ricci S, Cusmai R, Fariello G, et al: Double cortex: A neuronal migration anomaly as a possible cause of Lennox-Gastaut syndrome. *Arch Neurol* 49: 61–64, 1992.
32. Barkovich AJ, Guerrini R, Battaglia G, et al: Band heterotopia: Correlation of outcome with magnetic resonance imaging parameters. *Ann Neurol* 36:609–617, 1994.
33. Huttenlocher PR, Taravath S, Mojtahedi S: Periventricular heterotopia and epilepsy. *Neurology* 44:51–55, 1994.
34. Palmini A, Andermann F, Olivier A, et al: Focal neuronal migration disorders and intractable partial epilepsy. *Ann Neurol* 30:750–751, 1991.
35. Raymond AA, Halpin SF, Alsanjari N, et al: Dysembryoplastic neuroepithelial tumor: Features in 16 patients. *Brain* 117:461–475, 1994.
36. Kuzniecky R, Andermann F, Guerrini R: The epileptic spectrum in the congenital bilateral perisylvian syndrome: CBPS Multicenter Collaborative Study. *Neurology* 44:379–385, 1994.
37. Koeller KK, Dillon WP: Dysembryoplastic neuroepithelial tumors: MR appearance. *Am J Neuroradiol* 13:1319–1325, 1992.
38. Lehericy S, Dormont D, Semah F, et al: Developmental abnormalities of the medial temporal lobe in patients with temporal lobe epilepsy. *Am J Neuroradiol.* 16:617–626, 1995.
39. Palmini A, Gambardella A, Andermann F, et al: Operative strategies for patients with cortical dysplastic lesions and intractable epilepsy. *Epilepsia* 35(suppl 6):S57–S71, 1994.
40. Ashtari M, Barr WB, Schaul N, and Bogerts B: Three-dimensional fast low-angle shot imaging and computerized volume measurement of the hippocampus in patients with chronic epilepsy of the temporal lobe. *Am J Neuroradiol* 12:941–947, 1991.

41. Cascino GD, Jack CR, Parisi JE, et al: Magnetic resonance imaging-based studies in temporal lobe epilepsy: Pathological correlations. *Ann Neurol* 30: 31–36, 1991.
42. Cendes F, Andermann F, Gloor P, et al: MRI volumetric measurement of amygdala and hippocampus in temporal lobe epilepsy. *Neurology* 43:719–725, 1993.
43. Cook MJ, Fish DR, Shorvon SD, et al: Hippocampal volumetric and morphometric studies in temporal and frontal lobe epilepsy. *Brain* 115:1001–1015, 1992.
44. Jack CR Jr, Sharbrough FW, Cascino GD, et al: Magnetic resonance image-based hippocampal volumetry: Correlation with outcome after temporal lobectomy. *Ann Neurol* 31:138–146, 1992.
45. Jackson GD, Berkovic SF, Duncan JS, Connelly A: Optimizing the diagnosis of hippocampal sclerosis using MRI. *Am J Neuroradiol* 14:753–762, 1993.
46. Arruda F, Cendes F, Andermann F, et al: Mesial atrophy and outcome after amygdalohippocampectomy or temporal lobe removal. *Ann Neurol* 40:446–450, 1996.
47. Van Paesschen W, Connelly A, Johnson C, Duncan JS: The amygdala and intractable temporal lobe epilepsy: A quantitative magnetic resonance imaging study. *Neurology* 47:1021–1031, 1996.
48. Spencer SS, McCarthy G, Spencer DD: Diagnosis of medial temporal lobe seizure onset: Relative specificity and sensitivity of quantitative MRI. *Neurology* 43:2117–2124, 1993.
49. Conlon P, Trimble MR: A study of the corpus callosum in epilepsy using magnetic resonance imaging. *Epilepsy Res* 2:122–126, 1988.
50. Grant R, Hadley DM, Condon B, et al: Magnetic resonance imaging in the management of resistant focal epilepsy: Pathological case report and experience of 12 cases. *J Neurol Neurosurg Psychiatry* 50:1529–1532, 1987.
51. Lesser RP, Modic MT, Weinstein MA, et al: Magnetic resonance imaging (1.5 tesla) in patients with intractable focal seizures. *Arch Neurol* 43:367–371, 1986.
52. Sostman HD, Spencer DD, Gore JC, et al: Preliminary observations on magnetic resonance imaging in refractory epilepsy. *Magn Reson Imaging* 2:301–306, 1984.
53. Bergin PS, Fish DR, Oatridge A, et al: Magnetic resonance imaging in partial epilepsy: Additional abnormalities shown with the fluid attenuated inversion recover (FLAIR) pulse sequence. *J Neurol Neurosurg Psychiatry* 58:439–443, 1995.
54. Jack C, Rydberg C, Krecke K, et al: Mesial temporal sclerosis: Diagnosis with FLAIR versus spin-echo MR imaging. *Radiology* 199:367–373, 1996.
55. Awad IA, Johnson PC, Spetzler RF, Hodak JA: Incidental subcortical lesions identified on magnetic resonance in the elderly: II. Postmortem pathologic correlations. *Stroke* 17:1090–1097, 1986.
56. Olivier A, de Lotbiniere A, Peters T, et al: Combined use of digital subtraction angiography and MRI for radiosurgery and stereoencephalography. *Appl Neurophysiol* 50:92–99, 1987.
57. Kelly PJ, Sharbrough FW, Kall BA, Goerss SJ: Magnetic resonance imaging-based computer-assisted stereotactic resection of the hippocampus and amygdala in patients with temporal lobe epilepsy. Mayo Clin Proc 62:103–108, 1987.
58. Jack CR Jr, Sharbrough FW, Marsh WR: Use of MR imaging for quantitative evaluation of resection for temporal lobe epilepsy. Radiology 169:463–468, 1988.
59. Gazzaniga MS, Holtzman JD, Deck MD, et al: MRI assessment of human callosal surgery with neuropsychological correlates. *Neurology* 35:1763–1766, 1985.
60. Sussman NM, Scanlon M, Garfinkle W, et al: Magnetic resonance imaging after corpus callosotomy. *Neurology* 37:350–354, 1987.
61. Brant-Zawadzki M, Gillan G, Nitz WR: MP RAGE: A three-dimensional, T1 weighted, gradient-echo sequence-initial experience in the brain. *Radiology* 182: 769–775, 1992.
62. Phelps ME, Barrio JR, Huang SC, et al: The measurement of amino acid incorporation into protein with PET. *Ann Neurol* 15:S5192–S5202, 1984.
63. Phelps ME, Huang SC, Hoffman EJ, et al: Tomographic measurements of local cerebral metabolic rate in humans with (^{18}F)-fluorodeoxyglucose: Validation of method. *Ann Neurol* 6:371–388, 1979.
64. Phelps ME: Positron computed tomography studies of cerebral glucose metabolism in man: Theory and application in nuclear medicine. *Semin Nucl Med* 11:32–49, 1981.
65. Rottenberg DA, Ginos JZ, Kearfott KJ, et al.: In vivo measurement of regional brain tissue pH using positron emission tomography. *Ann Neurol* 15(suppl):S98–S102, 1984.
66. Sokoloff L, Reivich M, Kennedy C, et al: The (^{14}C) deoxyglucose method for the measurement of local cerebral glucose utilization: Theory, procedure and normal values in conscious and anesthetized albino rat. *J Neurochem* 28:897–916, 1977.
67. Abou-Khalil BW, Siegel GJ, Sackellares JC et al: Positron emission tomography studies of cerebral glucose metabolism in chronic partial epilepsy. *Ann Neurol* 22: 480–486, 1987.
68. Engel J Jr., Kuhl DE, Phelps ME, et al: Interictal cerebral glucose metabolism in partial epilepsy and its relation to EEG changes. *Ann Neurol* 12:510–517, 1982.
69. Engel J Jr., Kuhl DE, Phelps ME, et al: Comparative localization of epileptic foci in partial epilepsy by PCT and EEG. *Ann Neurol* 12:529–537, 1982.
70. Henry TR, Mazziotta, Engel J Jr, et al: Quantifying interictal metabolic activity in human temporal lobe epilepsy. *J Cereb Blood Flow Metab* 10: 748–757, 1990.
71. Holmes MD, Kelly K, Theodore WH: Complex partial seizures: Correlation of clinical and metabolic features. *Arch Neurol* 45:1191–1193, 1988.
72. Sackellares JC, Siegal GJ, Abou-khalil BW, et al: Differences between lateral and mesial temporal metabolism interictally in epilepsy of temporal lobe origin. *Neurology* 40:1420–1426, 1990.
73. Theodore WH, Newmark ME, Sato S, et al: (^{18}F) Fluorodeoxyglucose positron emission computed tomography in refractory complex partial seizures. *Ann Neurol* 14:429–437, 1983.
74. Theodore WH, Katz D, Kufta C, et al: Pathology of temporal lobe foci: Correlation with CT, MRI, and PET. *Neurology* 40:797–803, 1990.
75. Bernardi S, Trimble MR, Frackowiak RS, et al: An interictal study of partial epilepsy using positron emission tomography and the oxygen-15 inhalation technique. *J Neurol Neurosurg Psychiatry* 46:473–477, 1983.

76. Gallhofer B, Trimble MR, Frackowiak R, et al: A study of cerebral blood flow and metabolism in epileptic psychosis using positron emission tomography and oxygen. *J Neurol Neurosurg Psychiatr* 48:201–206, 1985.
77. Kuhl DE, Engel J Jr., Phelps ME, et al: Epileptic patterns of local cerebral metabolism and perfusion in humans determined by emission computed tomography of ^{18}FDG and $^{13}NH_3$. *Ann Neurol* 8:348–360, 1980.
78. Engel J Jr., Brown WJ, Kuhl DE, et al: Pathological findings underlying focal temporal lobe hypometabolism in partial epilepsy. *Ann Neurol* 12:518–528, 1982.
79. Henry TR, Sutherling WW, Engel J Jr, et al: Interictal cerebral metabolism in partial epilepsies of neocortical origin. *Epilepsy Res* 10:174–182, 1991.
80. Engel J Jr, Henry TR, Risinger MW, et al: Presurgical evaluation for partial epilepsy: Relative contributions of chronic depth-electrode recordings versus FDG-PET and scalp-sphenoidal ictal EEG. *Neurology* 40:1670–1677, 1990.
81. Theodore WH, Sato S, Kufta C, et al: Temporal lobectomy for uncontrolled seizures: The role of positron emission tomography. *Ann Neurol* 32:789–794, 1992.
82. Henry TR, Mazziotta JC, Engel J Jr: Interictal metabolic anatomy of mesial temporal lobe epilepsy. *Arch Neurol* 50:582–589, 1993.
83. Sperling MR, Gur RC, Alavi A, et al: Subcortical metabolic alterations in partial epilepsy. *Epilepsia* 31:145–155, 1990.
84. Theodore WH, Fishbein D, Deitz M, Baldwin P: Complex partial seizures: Cerebellar metabolism. *Epilepsia* 28:319–323, 1987.
85. Savic I, Thorell JO, Roland P: [^{11}C]flumazenil positron emission tomography visualizes frontal epileptogenic regions. *Epilepsia* 36:1225–1232, 1995.
86. Engel J Jr, Kuhl DE, Phelps ME, et al: Local cerebral metabolism during partial seizures. *Neurology* 33:400–413, 1983.
87. Chugani HT, Mazziotta JC, Engel J Jr, Phelps ME: The Lennox-Gastaut syndrome: Metabolic subtypes determined by 2-deoxy-2[^{18}F]fluoro-Dd-glucose positron emission tomography. *Ann Neurol* 21:4–13, 1987.
88. Miyauchi T, Nomura Y, Ohno S, et al: Positron emission tomography in three cases of Lennox-Gastaut syndrome. *Jpn J Psychiatry Neurol* 42:795–804, 1988.
89. Theodore WH, Brooks RD, Patronas N, et al: Positron emission tomography in the Lennox-Gastaut syndrome. *Neurology* 34(Suppl 1):106–107, 1984.
90. Chugani HT, Shewmon DA, Peacock WJ, et al: Surgical treatment of intractable neonatal-onset seizures: The role of positron emission tomography. *Neurology* 38:1178–1188, 1988.
91. Engel J Jr, Lubens P, Kuhl DE, Phelps ME: Local cerebral metabolic rate for glucose during petit mal absences. *Ann Neurol* 17:121–128, 1985.
92. Ochs RF, Gloor P, Tyler JL, et al: Effect of generalized spike-and-wave discharge on glucose metabolism measured by positron emission tomography. *Ann Neurol* 21:458–464, 1987.
93. Theodore WH, Brooks R, Margolin R, et al: Positron emission in generalized seizures. *Neurology* 35:684–690, 1985
94. Savic I, Pauli S, Thorell JO, Blomqvist G: In vivo demonstration of altered benzodiazepine receptor density in patients with generalised epilepsy. *J Neurol Neurosurg Psychiatry* 57:797–804, 1994.
95. Theodore WH: Antiepileptic drugs and cerebral glucose metabolism. *Epilepsia* 29(suppl 2):S48–S55, 1988.
96. Savic I, Persson A, Roland P, et al: In-vivo demonstration of reduced benzodiazepine receptor binding in human epileptic foci. *Lancet* 2:863–866, 1988.
97. Debets RM Chr, Sadzot B, van Isselt JW, et al; Is ^{11}C-flumazenil PET superior to ^{18}FDG PET and ^{123}I-iomazenil SPECT in presurgical evaluation of temporal lobe epilepsy? *J Neurol Neurosurg Psychiatry* 62:141–150,1997.
98. Koepp MJ, Richardson MP, Labbe C, Brooks DJ, et al: ^{11}C-flumazenil PET, volumetric MRI, and quantitative pathology in mesial temporal lobe epilepsy. *Neurology* 49:764–773, 1997.
99. Savic I, Svanborg E, Thorell JO: Cortical benzodiazepine receptor changes are related to frequency of partial seizures: A positron emission tomography sutdy. *Epilepsia* 37:236–244, 1996.
100. Frost JJ, Mayberg HS, Fisher RS, et al: Mu-opiate receptors measured by positron emission tomography are increased in temporal lobe epilepsy. *Ann Neurol* 23:231–237, 1988.
101. Mayberg HS, Sadzot B, Meltzer CC, et al: Quantification of mu and non-mu opiate receptors in temporal lobe epilepsy using positron emission tomography. *Ann Neurol* 30:3–11, 1991.
102. Biersak HJ, Penin H, Hartmann A, et al: Cerebral emission computed tomography (SPECT) with ^{123}-I-labelled amphetamines. *Dtsch Med Wochenschr* 109:1155–1159, 1984.
103. Bonte FJ, Stokely EM, Devous MD, et al: Single photon tomographic determination of regional cerebral blood flow. *Am J Neuroradiol* 4:544–546, 1983.
104. Fazio F, Lenzi GL, Gerundini P, et al.: Regional cerebral perfusion with SPECT and I-123-trimethylpropanediamine (HIPDM). *J Cereb Blood Flow Metab* 3(suppl): S158–S159, 1983.
105. Kuhl DE, Barrio JR, Huang SC, et al: Quantifying local cerebral blood flow with *N*-isopropyl-*p*-^{123}I-amphetamine tomography. *J Nucl Med* 23:196–203, 1982.
106. Magistretti R, Uren RF, Parker JA, et al: Monitoring of regional cerebral blood flow by single photon emission tomography of ^{123}I-*N*-isopropyl-iodoamphetamine in epileptics. *Ann Radiol* 26:68–71, 1983.
107. Sanabria E, Chauvel P, Askienazy S, et al: Single photon emission computed tomography (SPECT) using I-123-isopropyl-iodo-amphetamine (IAMP) in partial epilepsy, in Baldy-Moulinier M, Ingvar DH, Meldrum BS (eds). *Current Problems in Epilepsy: Cerebral Blood Flow, Metabolism, and Epilepsy*. London, John Libbey, 1983, pp 82–87.
108. Lancman ME, Morris HH, Raja S, et al: Usefulness of ictal and interictal ^{99m}Tc ethyl cysteinate dimer single photon emission computed tomography in patients with refractory partial epilepsy. *Epilepsia* 38:466–471, 1997.
109. Oku M, Matsumoto M, Hashikawa K, et al: Intra-individual differences between technetium-99m-HMPAO and technetium-99m-ECD in the normal medial temporal lobe. *J Nucl Med* 38:1109–1111, 1997.
110. Adams C, Hwang P, Gilday DL et al: Comparison of SPECT, EEG, CT, MRI, and pathology in partial epilepsy. *Pediatr Neurol* 8:97–103, 1992.

111. Chiron C, Raynaud C, Jambaque I et al: Xe brain SPECT imaging in cryptogenic West syndrome: Correlations between regional CBF defects and neuropsychological disorder. *J Nucl Med* 28:592, 1987.
112. Cordes M, Henkes H, Ferstl F, et al: Evaluation of focal epilepsy: a SPECT scanning comparison of 123-I iomazenil versus HM-PAO. AJNR 13:249–253, 1992.
113. Denays R, Rubinstein M, Ham H, et al: Single photon emission computed tomography in seizure disorders. *Arch Dis Child* 63:1184–1188, 1988.
114. English R, Soper N, Shepstone BJ, et al: Five patients with Rasmussen's syndrome investigated by single-photon-emission computed tomography. *Nucl Med Commun* 10:5–14, 1989.
115. Grunwald F, Durwen HF, Bockisch A, et al: Technetium-99m-HMPAO SPECT in medically intractable temporal lobe epilepsy: A post-operative evaluation. *J Nucl Med* 32:388–394, 1991.
116. Homan RW, Paulman RG, Devous MD, et al: Cognitive function and regional cerebral blood flow in partial seizures. *Arch Neurol* 46:964–970, 1989.
117. Jibiki I, Kubota T, Fujimoto K, et al: Regional relationships between focal hypofixation images in ^{123}I-IMP single photon emission computed tomography and epileptic EEG foci in interictal periods in patients with partial epilepsy. *Eur Neurol* 31:360–365, 1991.
118. LaManna MN, Sussman NM, Harner RN, et al: Initial experience with SPECT imaging of the brain using I-123 *p*-iodoamphetamine in focal epilepsy. *Clin Nucl Med* 14:428–430, 1989.
119. Lee BI, Markand ON, Siddiqui AR, et al.: Single photon emission computed tomography (SPECT) brain imaging using *N,N,N'*-trimethyl-*N'-(2-hydroxy-3-methyl-5-*^{123}I-isobenzyl)-1,3-propanediamine 2 HCl (HIPDM): Intractable complex partial seizures. Neurology 36:1471–1477, 1986.
120. Lee BI, Markand ON, Wellman HN, et al: HIPDM single photon emission computed tomography brain imaging in partial onset secondarily generalized tonic-clonic seizures. *Epilepsia* 28:305–311, 1987.
121. Markand ON, Shen W, Park HM, et al: Single photon imaging computed tomography (SPECT) for localization of epilepgenic focus in patients with intractable complex partial seizures. *Epilepsy Res* (suppl) 5: 121–126, 1992.
122. Rowe CC, Berkovic SF, Austin MC, et al: Patterns of postictal cerebral blood flow in temporal lobe epilepsy: Qualitative and quantitative analysis. *Neurology* 41:1096–1103, 1991.
123. Rowe CC, Berkovic SF, Austin MC, et al: Visual and quantitative analysis of interictal SPECT with technetium-99m-HMPAO in temporal lobe epilepsy. *J Nucl Med* 32:1688–1694, 1991.
124. Rowe CC, Berkovic SF, Sia STB, et al: Localization of epileptic foci with postictal single photon emission computed tomography. *Ann Neurol* 26:660–668, 1989.
125. Ryding E, Rosen I, Elmqvist D, et al: SPECT measurements with ^{99m}Tc-HM-PAO in focal epilepsy. *J Cereb Blood Flow Metab* 8:S95–S100, 1988.
126. Shen W, Lee BI, Park HM, et al: HIPDM-SPECT brain imaging in the presurgical evaluation of patients with intractable seizures. *J Nucl Med* 31:1280–1284, 1990.
127. Stefan H, Kuhnen C, Biersack HJ, et al: Initial experience with ^{99m}Tc-hexamethyl-propylene amine oxime (HM-PAO) single photon emission computed tomography (SPECT) in patients with focal epilepsy. *Epilepsy Res* 1:134–138, 1987.
128. Ryvlin P, Garcia-Larrea L, Philippon B, et al: High signal intensity on T2-weighted MRI correlates with hypoperfusion in temporal lobe epilepsy. *Epilepsia* 33:28–35, 1992.
129. Ryvlin P, Philippon B, Cinotti L, et al: Functional neuroimaging strategy in temporal lobe epilepsy: A comparative study of 18FDG-PET with ^{99m}Tc-HMPAO-SPECT. *Ann Neurol* 31:250–255, 1992.
130. Marks DA, Katz A, Hoffer P, et al: Localization of extemporal epileptic foci during ictal single photon emission computed tomography. *Ann Neurol* 31:250–255, 1992.
131. Newton MR, Berkovic SF, Austin MC, et al: Postictal switch in blood flow distribution and temporal lobe seizures. *J Neurol Neurosurg Psychiatry* 55:891–894, 1992.
132. Ramsay SC, McLaughlin AF, Greenough R, et al: Comparison of independent aura, ictal and interictal cerebral perfusion. *J Nucl Med* 33:438–440, 1992.
133. Lee BI, Markand ON, Wellman HN, et al: HIPDM-SPECT in patients with medically intractable complex partial seizures: Ictal study. *Arch Neurol* 45:397–402, 1988.
134. Hogan RE, Cook MJ, Binns DW, et al: Perfusion pattern in postictal ^{99m}Tc-HMPAO SPECT after coregistration with MRI in patients with mesial temporal lobe epilepsy. *J Neurol Neurosurgery Psychiatry* 63:235–236, 1997.
135. Katz A, Bose A, Lind SJ, et al: SPECT in patients with epilepsia partialis continua. *Neurology* 40:1848–1850, 1990.
136. Tatum WO, Sperling MR, Jacobstein JG: Epileptic palatal myoclonus. *Neurology* 41: 1305–1306, 1991.
137. Jeffery PJ, Monsein LH, Szabo Z, et al: Mapping the distribution of amobarbital sodium in the intracarotid Wada text by use of Tc-99m HMPAO with SPECT. *Radiology* 178:847–850, 1991.
138. Biersak HJ, Linke D, Brassel LF, et al: Technetium-99m HM-PAO brain SPECT in epileptic patients before and during unilateral hemispheric anesthesia (Wada test): Report of three cases. *J Nucl Med* 28:1763–1767, 1987.
139. Beer HF, Blauenstein PA, Hasler PH, et al: In vitro and in vivo evaluation of iodine-123-Ro 16–0154: A new imaging agent for SPECT investigations of benzodiazepine receptors. *J Nucl Med* 31:1007–1014, 1990.
140. Haldemann RC, Bicik I, Pfeiffer A, et al: ^{123}I-iomazenil: A quantitative study of the central benzodiazepine receptor distribution. *Nucl Med* 31:91–97, 1992.
141. Johnson EW, de Lanerolle NC, Kim JH, et al: "Central" and "peripheral" benzodiazepine receptors: Opposite changes in human epileptogenic tissue. *Neurology* 42:811–815, 1992.
142. Schubiger PA, Hasler PH, Beer-Wohlfahrt H, Bekier A, et al: Evaluation of a multicentre study with Iomazenil: A benzodiazepine receptor ligand. *Nucl Med Commun* 12: 569–582, 1991.
143. Zubal IG, Spencer SS, Imam K, et al: Difference images calculated from ictal and interictal technetium-99m-HMPAO SPECT scans of epilepsy. *Nucl Med* 36:684–689,1995.
144. Warach S, Levin JM, Schomer DL, et al: Hyperperfusion of ictal seizure focus demonstrated by MR perfusion imaging. *Am J Neuroradiol* 15:965–968, 1994.

145. Detre J, Alsop DC, Aguirre GK, Sperling MR: Coupling of cortical and thalamic ictal activity in human partial epilepsy: Demonstration by funtional magnetic resonance imaging. *Epilepsia* 37:657–661, 1996.
146. Warach S, Ives JR, Schlaug G, et al: EEG-triggered echoplanar functional MRI in epilepsy. *Neurology* 47: 89–93, 1996.
147. Binder JR, Swanson SJ, Hammeke TA, et al: Determination of language dominance using functional MRI: aA comparison with the Wada test. *Neurology* 46: 978–984, 1996.
148. Desmond JE, Sum JM, Wagner AD, et al: Functional MRI measurement of language lateralization in Wada-tested patients. *Brain* 118:1411–1419, 1995.
149. Hertz-Pannier L, Gaillard WD, Mott SH, et al: Noninvasive assessment of language dominance in children and adolescents with functional MRI: A preliminary study. *Neurology* 48:1003–1012, 1997.
150. Connelly A: Proton MRS in epilepsy. *Epilepsia* 38(suppl 10): 33–38, 1997.
151. Connelly A, Jackson GD, Duncan JS, et al: Magnetic resonance spectroscopy in temporal lobe epilepsy. *Neurology* 44:1411–1417, 1994.
152. Hetherington H, Kuzniecky R, Pan J et al: Proton MRS in human temporal lobe epilepsy at 4.1 T. *Ann Neurol* 38:396–404,1995.
153. Cendes F, Andermann F, et al: Normalization of neuronal metabolic dysfunction after surgery for temporal lobe epilepsy. *Neurology* 49:1525–1533, 1997.
154. Cross JH, Gordon I, Connelly A, et al: Interictal $^{99}Tc^{m}$ HMPAO SPECT and ^{1}H MRS in children with temporal lobe epilepsy. *Epilepsia* 38:338–345, 1997.
155. Hugg JW, Laxer KD, Matson GB, et al: Neuron loss localizes human temporal lobe epilepsy by in vivo proton magnetic resonance spectroscopic imaging. *Ann Neurol* 34:788–794, 1993.
156. Najm IM, Wang Y, Hong SC, et al: Temporal changes in proton MRS metabolites after kainic acid-induced seizures in rat brain. *Epilepsia* 38:87–94, 1997.
157. Detre J, Sirven J, O'Connor MJ, French JA: Localization of subclinical ictal activity by functional magnetic resonance imaging: Correlation with invasive monitoring. *Ann Neurol.* 38:618–624,1995.
158. Jackson GD, Connelly A, Cross JH, et al: Functional MRI of focal seizures. *Neurology* 44:850–856, 1994.

SECTION FIVE

DERANGEMENTS OF INTELLECT, BEHAVIOR, AND LANGUAGE DUE TO DIFFUSE AND FOCAL CEREBRAL DISEASE

CHAPTER 8

NEUROIMAGING AND BEHAVIORAL NEUROLOGY

Michael K. Matthews, Jr.
Julie Pickholtz
Holly Shue

INTRODUCTION

This chapter focuses on normal and abnormal neurobehavioral phenomena as revealed by neuroimaging. The material is organized under two main headings. The section on "Neuropsychological Function and Disturbance" treats normal and disordered language, memory, perception, and executive function. Because sufficiently little neuroimaging information concerning apraxia exists, this topic has been omitted, and disorders of emotion are dealt with in other chapters in this book. The section on "Neurobehavioral Syndromes" treats dementia, and head trauma and recovery of function. Discussions of critical issues in behavioral neurology are embedded within topic discussions. These issues include lateralization, the "binding problem" and disconnection, parallel processing in distributed networks, modularity of neuropsychological functions, and the imaging of mental processing.

Behavioral Neurology

The Scope of Behavioral Neurology

Behavioral neurology is the study and treatment of mental and behavioral abnormality caused by neurologic disease. The essential clinical phenomena of behavioral neurology include amnesia (disturbance of memory), aphasia (disturbance of language), apraxia (disturbance of motor skill), agnosia (disturbance of perception), executive dyscontrol (disturbance of frontal lobe functions), and inattention and neglect (disturbances of attentional processes). From another perspective, behavioral neurology focuses upon conditions in which mental abnormality is a major symptom, such as degenerative dementia, intoxication, HIV encephalopathy, and head trauma. Several sources provide a fuller review of the issues and breadth of this field.[1–5]

Clinicoanatomic Correlation in Behavioral Neurology

The rapid advance of behavioral neurology over the last several decades owes a great deal to the increasing sophistication of neuroimaging.[6,7] Before the advent of neuroimaging, understanding of clinicoanatomic-functional relationships required correlating autopsy and intraoperative data with prior clinical observations. The disadvantage of the autopsy approach lies in its post hoc nature: one cannot readily test hypotheses about clinicoanatomic correlations in a deceased patient, even with extensive premortem clinical records. This is especially true for cognitive dysfunction because of the complexity of cognitive phenomena.

The ability to image brain lesions and metabolic function in vivo has allowed clinicians and investigators to ask new questions about brain function, brain damage, and neurobehavioral deficits, and to obtain answers readily. Anatomic imaging, mainly computed tomography (CT) and magnetic resonance imaging (MRI), continues to improve our understanding of the relationships among brain structures and neurobehavioral syndromes such as dementia and aphasia. Specialized template, planimetric, volumetric, and three-dimensional techniques have added extra power to these basic technologies.[8–11]

Functional Brain Analysis

Information about the functioning of the brain at rest and during mental or physical activity can be obtained from three sources: (1) the patient's performance (e.g., on neuropsychological testing),[12] (2) magnetoencephalography and electrophysiology, and (3) functional neuroimaging. Functional neuroimaging, including single photon emission computed tomography (SPECT), positron emission tomography (PET), and functional MRI (fMRI), has become an important tool for studying the functional basis of cognition and cognitive impairment.[13–20] These modalities rely on the correlation between local changes in neuronal activity during mental activities and local changes in metabolism and blood flow in order to generate functional maps of areas of the brain.

Single photon emission computed tomography measures blood flow and brain metabolism by monitoring photons emitted by iodine-labeled monoamine and diamine tracers carried in the blood to the brain. Typical tracers include *N*-isopropyl-*p*-iodoamphetamine labeled with ^{123}I ([^{123}I]IMP), hexamethyl-propyleneamine oxime labeled with technetium 99m (^{99m}Tc-HMPAO), and technetium 99m–ethyl cysteinate dimer (^{99m}Tc-ECD). With the inert gas clearance technique, SPECT can be used to calculate regional cerebral blood flow by measuring the clearance of ^{133}Xe from the blood.[21,22]

In PET, radiopharmaceutical compounds labeled with a positron-emitting radionuclide, usually ^{11}C, ^{13}N, or ^{15}O, are injected systemically. When positrons interact with matter in the body, the positron and the particle it encounters are annihilated, releasing radiation. By reconstructing measurements of the distribution of radioactivity that are taken from multiple angles, the distribution of the compound in organs can be depicted in an image. This method has been adapted to assess brain function in several ways.[23] The regional cerebral metabolic utilization rate of glucose can be measured using [^{18}F]-fluoro-2-deoxy-D-glucose, labeled with $^{15}O_2$ and H_2O_{15}. Presynaptic dopamine terminals can be evaluated using ^{18}F-L-dopa, and postsynaptic dopamine receptors can be studied using ^{18}F-labeled analogues of spiperone and raclopride. Regional cerebral blood flow and oxygen metabolism can be measured by labeling H_2O with ^{15}O. Receptor distribution and binding can be studied with radiolabeled neurotransmitter agonists and antagonists.[21] Finally, more traditional methods of measuring blood flow, such as transcranial doppler,[24] can be used in neurobehavioral clinicoanatomic correlation.

Functional MRI uses rapid scanning speeds and paramagnetism to produce regional cerebral blood flow maps during resting and activated states. The images obtained can be superimposed on high-resolution T1-weighted anatomic MRIs.[25] For all functional imaging modalities, activated states can be produced by sensory stimulation, movement of limbs, or cognitive activities, procedures similar to activating procedures used in neurophysiology.

Electroencephalographic (EEG) brain mapping is performed by a group of quantitative EEG techniques, including EEG frequency analysis, topographic display, and statistical comparisons to a normative database.[26] It can be adapted to generate images that reflect the relative distribution of EEG frequencies in various parts of the brain. These images may be able to distinguish normal brains from those afflicted with a variety of neurobehavioral syndromes, such as dementia, schizophrenia, and bipolar depression.[27,28]

Biomagnetometry or magnetoencephalography, based on the superconducting quantum interference device (SQUID), detects the very small magnetic fields associated with neuronal activity. The data from such recordings can be superimposed upon MRIs to provide localizing information at rest and during activating procedures. This method has been applied to neurobehavioral functions, such as audition[29] and tactile perception.[30]

NEUROPSYCHOLOGICAL FUNCTION AND DISTURBANCE

Language and Aphasia

Normal Language

In Benson's view,[31] language, speech, and thought are the three major components of human communication. He defined *language* as the "encoding and decoding of semantic and syntactic elements used in some aspects of the production and comprehension of a thought or idea." He defined *speech* as the "output of meaningful communication produced by motor effectors," a broad definition that includes oral speech, writing, and gestures. *Thought* can be viewed as "ideas," the content of communication. While communication can be approached from different disciplinary standpoints, Benson's view is one that makes "medical sense." It facilitates the understanding of the clinical phenomenology of aphasia and can help to guide the investigation of the neurophysiological substrate of language. Table 8.1 provides a list of component language functions.

Current understanding of the neurophysiological substrate of language comes from three main sources: (1) the study of aphasia and its associated brain lesions, (2) the investigation of cortical language organization during neurosurgical brain mapping procedures,[32] and (3) the investigation of communication ability in non-brain-damaged individuals using functional neuroimaging. This section focuses on the contribution of neuroimaging to the understanding of basic language function. Several important questions guide work in this area. For example, what brain areas participate in the various components of speech comprehension, such as pitch discrimination, phonetic discrimination, and judgment of meaning? What are the neurologic substrates and neurophysiological mechanisms of word comprehension, word retrieval from memory (the lexicon), and auditory processing?

Brain Structures and Laterality in the Language System A number of brain structures are known to compose the substrate of language functions, damage to which produces aphasia in several forms (see sections on aphasia below). These structures include the supplementary motor cortex, the third frontal convolution and surrounding gray and white matter, components of the thalamus and caudate, face and mouth representations in primary motor and somesthetic cortex, perisylvian gyri (Wernicke's area), the angular and supramarginal gyri in the parietal and temporoparietal area, primary auditory and visual cortices, and white matter interconnections among these areas.[33,34]

For the majority of right-handed individuals, left-sided structures are most important in language, although melodic aspects of language rely on some of the

Table 8-1
Language functions and dysfunctions

Function	*Definition*	*Examples of dysfunction*
Comprehension	Understanding what is said or read	Inability to follow commands or to answer yes-no questions
Fluency	Unimpeded word flow	Short utterances
Grammar	Accurate expression of the relationships among words	Agrammatic speech: loss of connecting words, e.g., *the* and *on*
Prosody	Variability in tone of speech, melodic line	Monotony
Syntax	Correct choice and order of words	Incorrect use of words, paraphasia
Repetition	Reproducing speech just heard	Impaired repetition
Writing		Agraphia
Reading		Alexia
Naming and word retrieval	Recalling words	Anomia
Seriatim speech	Recitation of practiced phrases	Inability to count

Source: Goodglass and Kaplan.[54]

homologues of these structures in the right hemisphere. Emphasizing their role in the language system, several asymmetries between left side language structures and their right side homologues have been identified. For example, the planum temporale contains structures, such as Heschl's gyrus, that are critical in auditory information processing. In right-handed people, the planum temporale is longer on the left than on the right, occupying a greater anteroposterior extent of the left hemisphere than of the right hemisphere, hence, a normal asymmetry.[35,36] Another asymmetry is seen in the pars triangularis in Broca's area. Using volumetric MRI, Foundas et al[37] found leftward asymmetry of this structure in patients known to be left-hemispheric-dominant for language on the basis of intracarotid amobarbital testing (Wada testing). They found rightward asymmetry in one patient with right-sided language dominance.

More recently, functional imaging research in normal subjects has corroborated classical views of language lateralization. Binder et al[38] used fMRI to investigate the regions involved in language processing in right-handed subjects. By comparing a language task requiring phonetic and semantic analysis of speech sounds with a nonlanguage control task involving perceptual analysis of nonlinguistic sounds, they found that activation associated with language processing lateralized to the left hemisphere.

Language and Auditory Information Processing Zatorre et al[39] measured cerebral blood flow changes with PET in their study of auditory language processing. They arranged five auditory stimulus conditions in a hierarchy of increasing complexity. Normal volunteers listened to silence (baseline state) or pressed a key when they heard every other burst of noise (noise condition), every other pair of speech syllables (passive speech condition), pairs of syllables if they shared consonants (phonetic condition), or pairs of syllables if the second of the pair had a higher pitch than the first of the pair (pitch condition). Some of their results are shown in Fig. 8-1 (see figure legend for details) and Table 8-2. Most important, each experimental condition was associated with activation of a different pattern of brain sites. This suggests that the auditory system is composed of separate subsystems that process information relevant to various aspects of language.[39] These results also dovetail with classical lesion work. For example, when subjects made phonetic judgments, Broca's area and surrounding tissue were activated. This is the "mirror image" of the observations that Broca's area lesions cause impaired phonetic judgment as well as impaired fluency,[40,41]

Table 8-2
Main brain areas activated under various experimental conditions

Condition	*Important brain areas activated*
Baseline	
Noise	Primary auditory cortex
Passive speech	Secondary auditory cortex bilaterally
Phonetic	Part of Broca's area on the left
Pitch	Prefrontal cortex on the right

Source: Adapted from Zatorre et al.[39]

Note: Data were obtained by subtracting PET patterns for the condition of interest from the pattern seen in conditions appearing above it in the table. See Fig. 8-8.

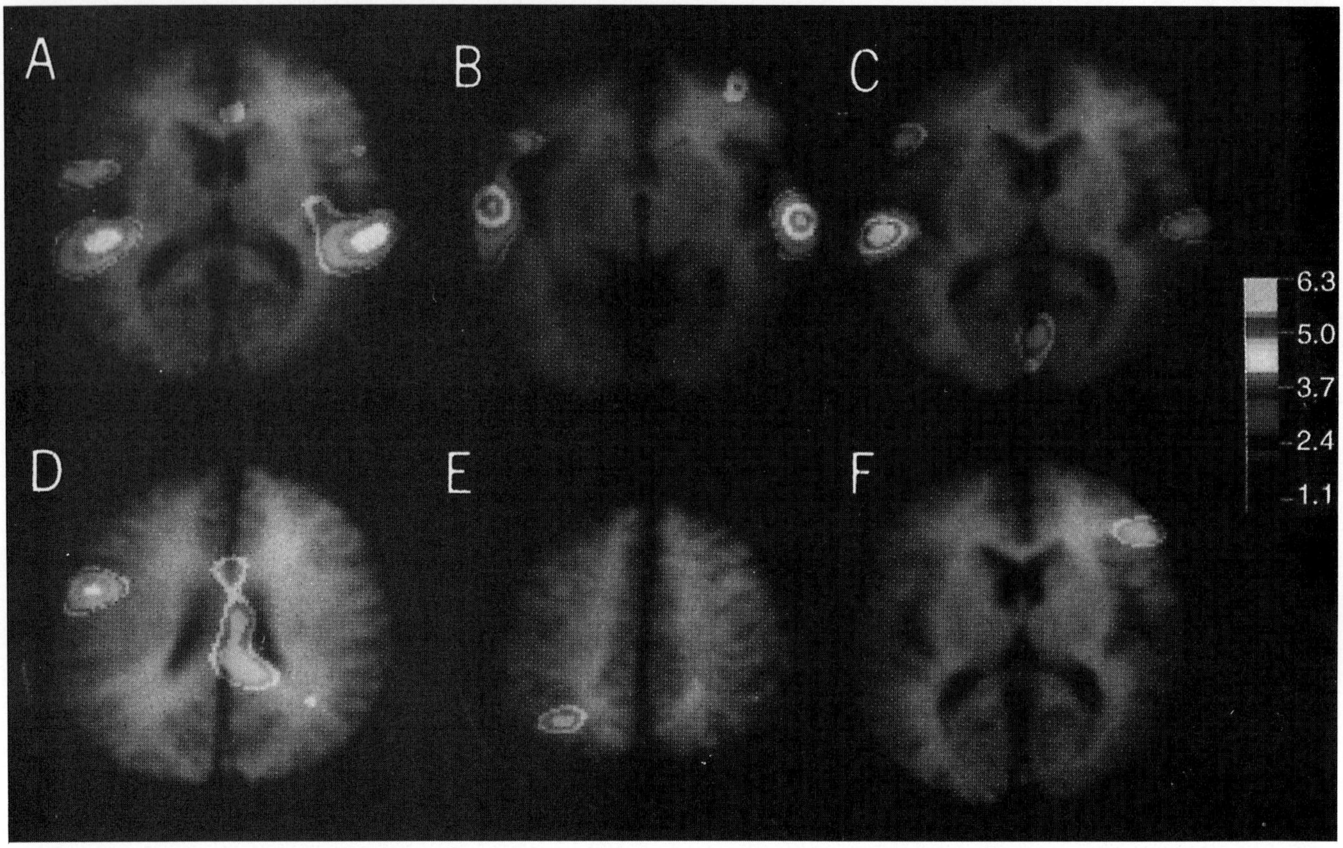

Figure 8-1 (Plate 17)
Averaged PET images (colored areas) superimposed upon MRI transaxial slices, showing significant focal cerebral blood flow increases in each experimental condition of an auditory stimulation experiment (see Table 8-2 and the text for an explanation of experimental conditions). **(A)** *Noise minus baseline condition: flow increase in Heschl's gyrus bilaterally.* **(B and C)** *Passive speech minus noise condition: flow increase in the superior temporal gyrus anterior to Heschl's gyri bilaterally (B), left inferior frontal cortex (B and C), and left posterior temporal area (C; the posterior midline focus on C was not significant).* **(D and E)** *Phonetic minus passive speech condition: flow increase in the superior part of Broca's area (D), left superior parietal lobe (E), and cingulate gyrus (D).* **(F)** *Pitch minus passive speech: flow increase in the right prefrontal cortex. PET scans were acquired with the Scanditronix PC-2048 system using bolus $H_2^{15}O$ methodology to measure the relative distribution of cerebral blood flow in the baseline and activated conditions. (Figure and modified legend from Zatorre et al,[39] copyright 1992 by AAAS. Used by permission.)*

partly because left-side metabolic disturbance may occur in Broca aphasia.[42]

In a similar paradigm, Sergent et al[43] used SPECT to assess focal cerebral activation during music sight-reading, listening, and performance. Their results (Fig. 8-2) show that specific auditory processing tasks are associated with activation of specific areas of the brain. At least one of these areas, the anterior frontal zone, was activated in the language task in the work of Zatorre et al[39] (compare Figs. 8-1 and 8-2). In a task tapping both musical and linguistic functions, Benson et al[44] used fMRI to study auditory cortical activation in normal subjects exposed to pure tones, instrumental music, single words, or discourse. Subtracting baseline data from stimulation data, they recorded signal increases in the supratemporal plane for all stimulus types. These three studies and others like them suggest that cognitive capacities are supported by separate yet partially overlapping neurologic networks that share individual components.[45]

Magnetoencephalographic recordings superimposed upon MRIs have also been used to study localization of auditory information processing. For example, Papanicolaou et al[29] found that magnetic fields evoked by auditory stimulation could be localized to the vicinity of the auditory cortex when projected onto MRIs.

Word Comprehension and Retrieval Wise et al[46] used PET to study the brain substrate of word comprehension and retrieval. They found that thinking of words (the retrieval task) and understanding words (the single-word comprehension task) both activated Wernicke's area in the left perisylvian cortex. In addition, each task activated other, different areas of cortex. Silent word retrieval activated the left dorsolateral prefrontal cortex and supplementary motor area, suggesting that word retrieval requires communication between anterior and posterior language regions. Single-word comprehension tasks activated regions in both temporal lobes plus tissue in the deep left posterior superior temporal gyrus. This

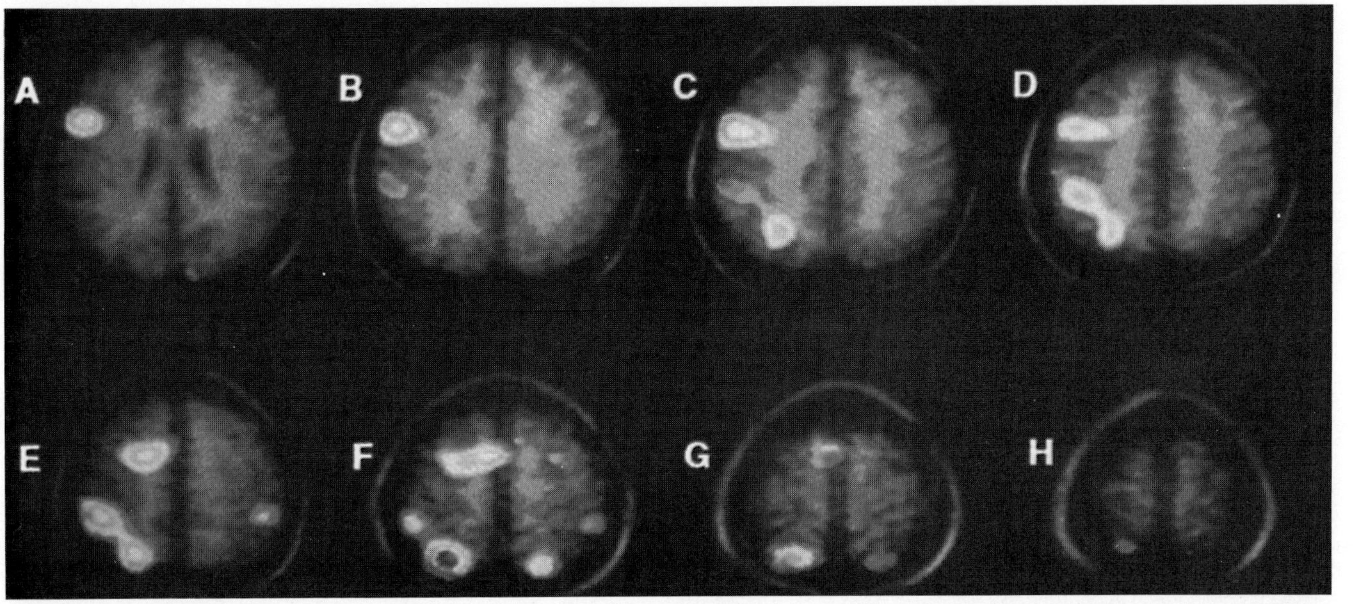

Figure 8-2 (Plate 18)
Averaged PET images (colored areas) depicting cortical activation during musical sight-reading, listening to music, and piano performance. PET data are superimposed on transaxial MRI sections from most inferior to most superior **(A–H)** *(interslice distance 6 mm). PET data were obtained while subjects performed several tasks and were averaged from 10 subjects using subtractive methodology. The left sides of the images correspond to the left side of the brain. Activation in the left anterior hemisphere (area 44, seen in* **A and B,** *and area 6, seen in* **C, D, E, and F***) occurred with right-hand piano performance. Activation of more posterior areas (area 40, supramarginal gyrus, left greater than right) occurred with simultaneous sight-reading and listening to performance of a musical composition. Activation of the most posterior areas (occipitoparietal, seen in* **C** *and* **D,** *and superior parietal lobes, or area 7, seen in* **E, F, and G***) occurred with simultaneous playing, reading, and listening to music, along with activation of the other areas activated in each task individually. This suggests a role for this area of cortex in sensorimotor integration. (Figure and modified legend from Sergent et al,[43] copyright 1992 by AAAS. Used by permission.)*

work complements CT and MRI lesion size and location analysis by showing the importance of posterior temporal areas in language comprehension, and of anterior cortical and subcortical areas in fluency.[8,47]

In a third result, Wise et al[46] found that both word comprehension and nonword sound perception tasks activated nearly identical areas of the posterior temporal lobes. These tasks are sufficiently different from one another that one would expect each to have a different neurophysiologic substrate. Thus, while the PET data showed that these substrates must overlap neuroantomically, it was unable to separate them.

Multiple Routes to Comprehension in the Language System Notions that the comprehension system is strictly localized to discrete zones such as Wernicke's and Broca's areas have been replaced by the concept of overlapping, parallel language comprehension subsystems distributed widely in the brain. An example of the kind of work that supports this view is the analysis of the network substrates of language comprehension in signed versus spoken language. Signed and spoken language comprehension activate overlapping areas of the brain,[48] such as the frontal operculum. This makes neurophysiologic sense because, despite their evident differences, these behaviors are both linguistic.

However, this overlap is not complete. These language tasks also activate different areas in the broadly defined language substrate. It is the *difference* in the brain activation in these two circumstances that reveals the existence of multiple language comprehension pathways. In work done by Soderfeldt et al,[49] people with both intact hearing and sign language skill were presented a narrative in signed as well as spoken language during PET scanning. The information content of the narrative was the same whether it was signed or spoken to them. Results were displayed using a subtraction PET method in which only the differences in brain activation between two language comprehension paradigms are seen. Figure 8-3 shows some of these results. Area A of Fig. 3-8 shows that the comprehension of sign language, in contrast to the comprehension of a visible audible speaker, activated mainly Brodmann's areas 19 and 37. Area B of Fig. 8-3 shows that comprehension of a visible audible speaker, in contrast to comprehension of sign language, activated mainly Brodmann's areas 22 and 43. As in previous work,[48] both conditions activated certain common language areas, especially the left frontal operculum, which is seen indirectly in the lack of differential activation in the zone between the areas representing these two sets of conditions.

The authors interpreted their work as showing that "separate routes exist for visual and auditory input of

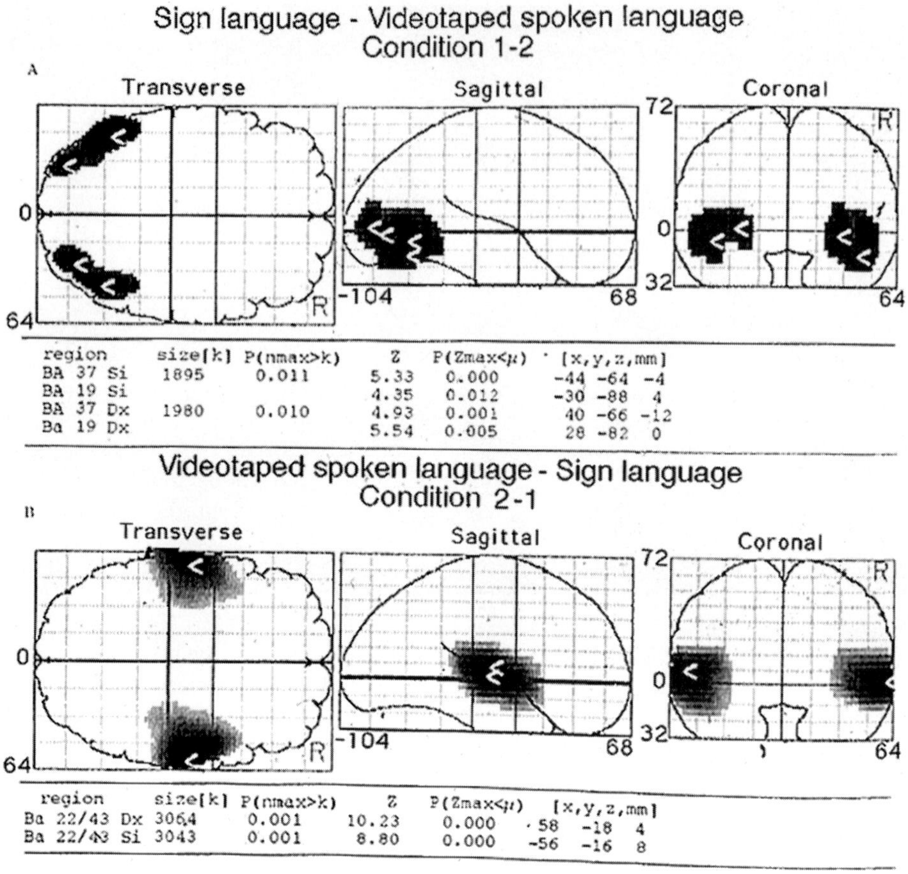

Figure 8-3
Subtraction PET method in which differences in brain activation between two language comprehension paradigms are seen. The top part (labeled A) shows activation in visual system areas 19 and 37 in the sign language comprehension condition. The bottom part (labeled B) obtained during comprehension of spoken visible speech in contrast to comprehension of sign language, activated mainly Brodmann's area 22 and 43. As in previous work,[48] both conditions activated certain common language areas, especially the left frontal operculum, which is seen indirectly in the lack of differential activation in that zone between these two conditions.

language information into higher-order language regions."[49] It shows that the language system is complex in ways that are hard or impossible to discern using lesion methods. This complexity may help to explain some of the individual differences in the quality of the aphasia that occurs with seemingly identical lesions. Some people may rely more heavily than do others on auditory, in contrast to visual, input for language comprehension. For such people, a lesion that affects auditory language subsystems more than visual language subsystems may cause greater overall language impairment than it does for a person with the opposite style of language processing.

Aphasia: Definition and Basic Syndromes

Aphasia is language disorder caused by neurologic disease. Excellent reviews of the topic are available, and Goodglass[34] is especially recommended. Aphasia can be manifested in many ways, depending upon the nature of the neuropathologic process involved (e.g., strokes and degenerative diseases), the location of the lesion (nonfluent aphasia in anterior and fluent aphasia in posterior left hemisphere lesions), and time since brain insult.[50–53] Aphasia can be assessed by neuropsychologic tests such as the Boston Diagnostic Aphasia Battery[50,54] and the Western Aphasia Battery,[55] which determine the degree to which the individual component functions of language are disrupted in individual patients (see Table 8-1). These tests can provide profiles of overall language strengths and weaknesses.

Most aspects of aphasia usually result from left-side disturbances in these structures, although right-side damage can produce aphasia in some left-handed persons and melodic aspects of language can be disrupted by damage in the right temporal area in most right-handed persons.[40] Some patterns of language loss are common and are recognized as specific syndromes of aphasia.[51–53] Typical imaging characteristics of these major types of aphasia are shown in this section; many other examples are available.[56]

Nonfluent Aphasia The dominant feature of nonfluent aphasia, also called expressive or anterior aphasia, is effortful, sparse verbal production with varying degrees of deficits in other language functions.[57] One example is Broca aphasia, characterized by articulatory struggle, speech hesitancy, and telegraphic speech and writing. Another example is transcortical motor aphasia, which is similar to Broca aphasia but with repetition relatively preserved. In these syndromes, lesions tend to occur in the anteriorly located parts of the language structures, hence, the term *anterior aphasia*. The MRI appearance of the posterior frontal and anterior temporoparietal

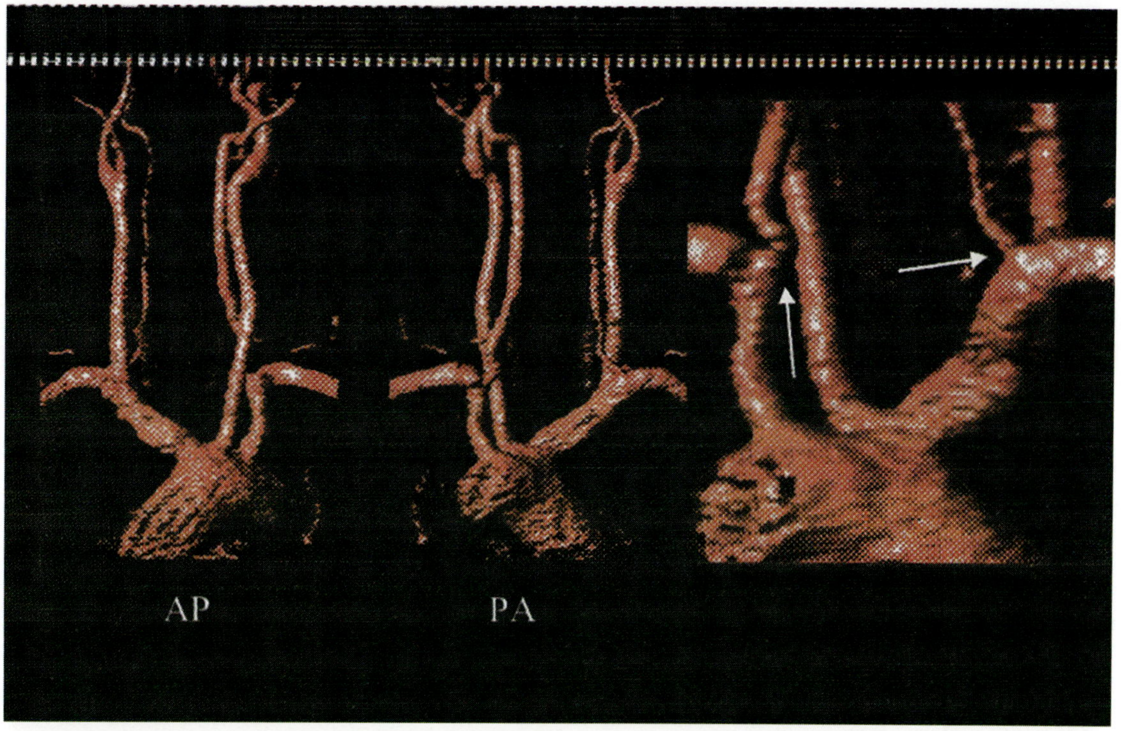

Plate 49 *(Figure 23-45) Volume-rendered display of normal first-pass gadolinium-enhanced 3D TOF MRA of the aortic arch in the same case as depicted in Fig. 23-44. Note the clear depiction of the vertebral artery origins (arrows).*

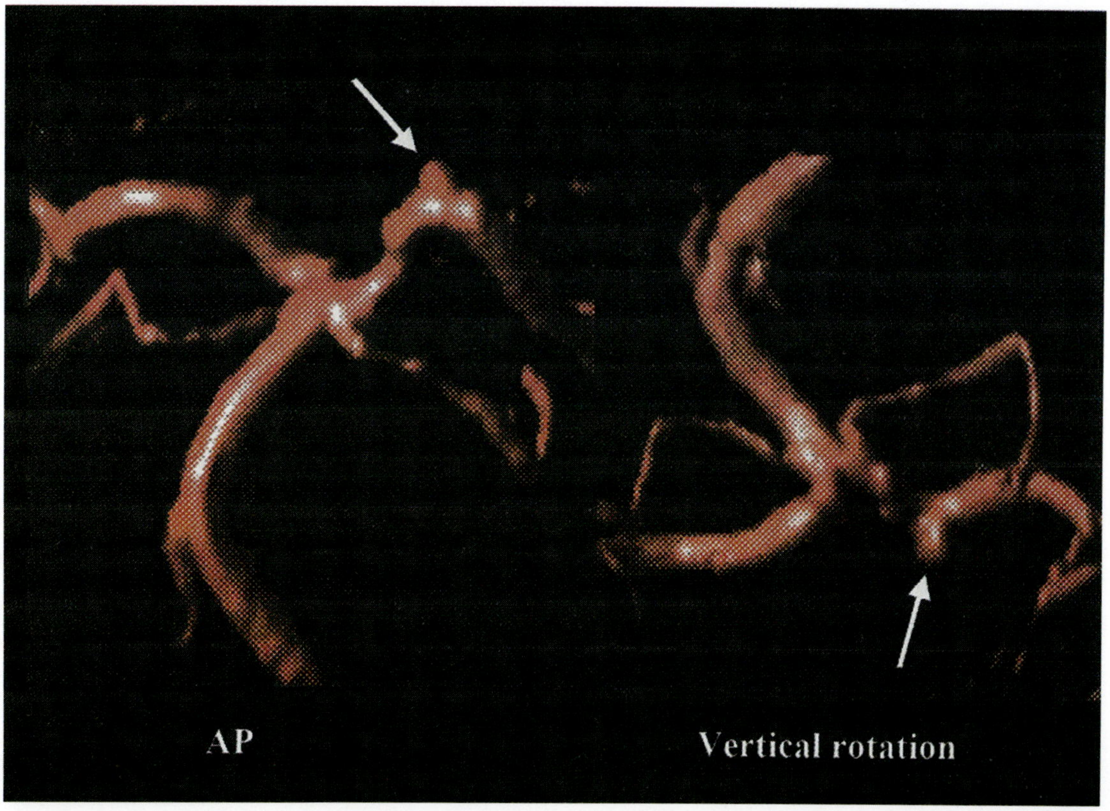

Plate 50 *(Figure 23-60) The volume-rendered reconstruction from 3D TOF MRA, AP view, shows an aneurysm (arrow) in the P2 segment of the left posterior cerebral artery in the same patient as depicted in Fig. 23-59. The vessel has been flipped in the vertical plane, and it continues to show aneurysmal dilatation at the P2 segment on the left (arrow). This aneurysm was confirmed at the time of surgery.*

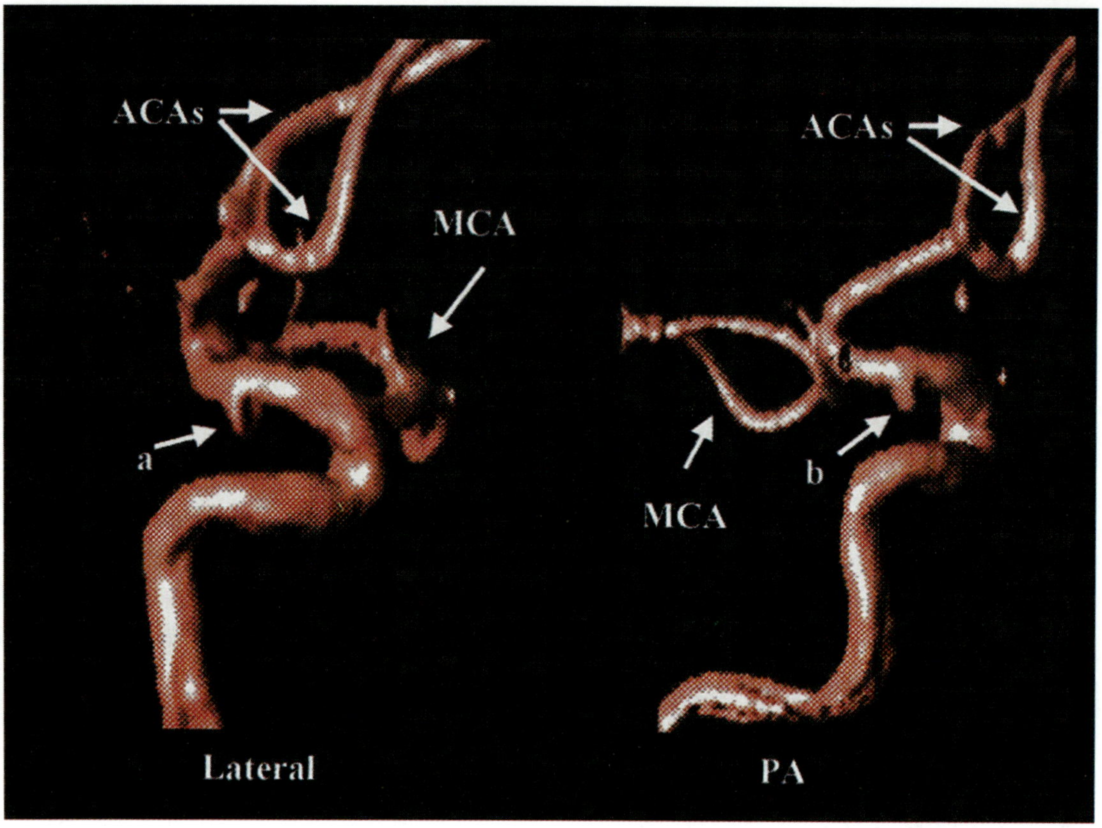

Plate 51 *(Figure 23-62) Vessel loop mimicking an aneurysm in the same patient as depicted in Figs. 23-59 through 23-61. In this volume-rendered reconstruction from 3D TOF MRA of the left carotid and intracranial branches, arrow a in the left view and arrow b in the PA view continue to show a possible aneurysm in the region of the posterior communicating take-off. This was proven to be a tightly wound posterior communicating artery at time of surgery.*

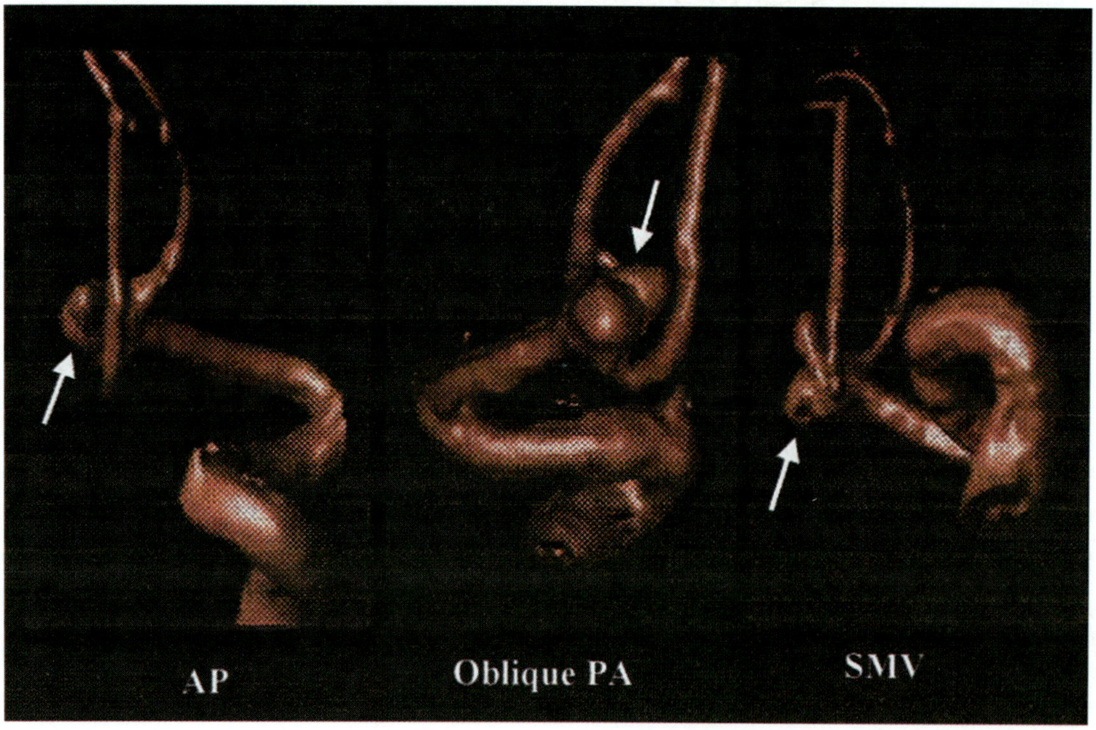

Plate 52 *(Figure 23-65) ACA aneurysm. 3D volume-rendered reconstruction from the targeted MIP of Fig. 23-64 in AP, oblique PA, and SMV views. Note that the aneurysm is clearly defined as bilobed, and its precise relationship to both A2 segments of the anterior cerebral arteries is well defined in this reconstruction.*

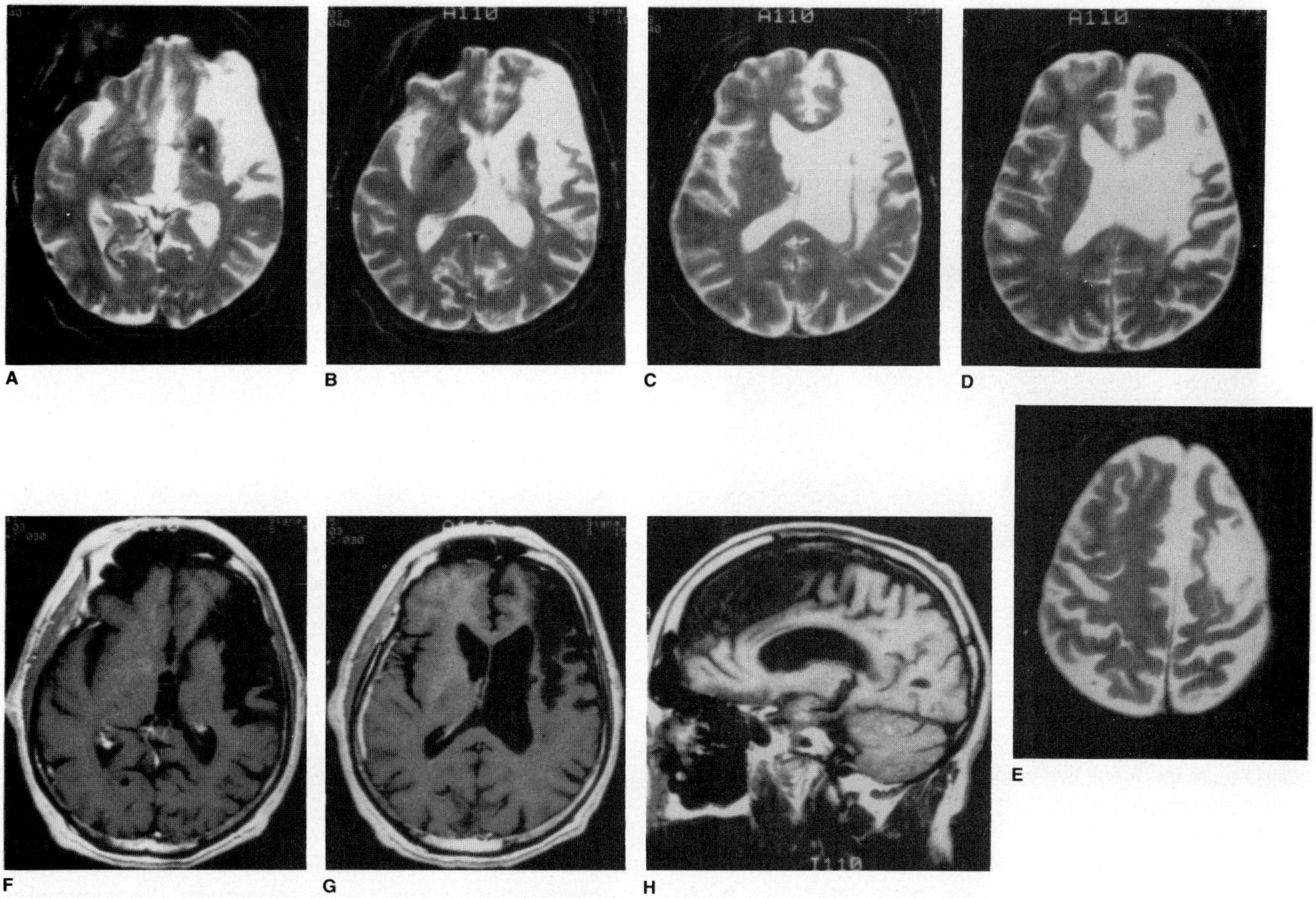

Figure 8-4
MRI of a 61-year-old right-handed man with long-standing nonfluent aphasia. **(A–D)** *Transaxial slices (TR 2700 ms, TE 90 ms, 5-mm slice thickness) showing most of the inferior-superior extent of the lesion.* **(F and G)** *Transaxial slices (TR 650 ms, TE 11 ms 1/1) corresponding to images B and C, respectively.* **(H)** *Sagittal slice (TR 600 ms, TE 17 ms) from several centimeters to the left of midline, giving an improved view of the superior-inferior extent of the lesion. Signal abnormality encompasses much of the dorsolateral frontal lobe on the left, including Broca's area, all of the periventricular white matter adjacent to the superior part of the left lateral ventricle, and white matter that probably includes the medial subcallosal fasciculus on the left. Tissue supplied by the anterior cerebral artery and the posterior language areas are spared. (Courtesy of Dr. Atif Husain).*

lesion that is characteristic of Broca aphasia is shown in Fig. 8-4. As is usual for Broca aphasia, this lesion encompasses more than Brodmann's area 44, the third frontal convolution.

Fluent Aphasia In fluent aphasia, also termed receptive and posterior aphasia, the dominant features are impaired comprehension, relatively preserved fluency, and contamination of speech by paraphasic errors. Paraphasias are incorrect sounds and can be literal (phoneme substitutions) or semantic (morpheme, or whole-word, substitutions or neologisms).[34] Examples of fluid aphasia include Wernicke aphasia and transcortical sensory aphasia, which is similar to Wernicke aphasia except that repetition is relatively preserved. In these syndromes, lesions tend to occur in the posteriorly located parts of the language structures, hence, the term *posterior aphasia*. The CT appearance of the left temporal-parietal lesion usually seen in Wernicke aphasia is shown in Fig. 8-5.

Global Aphasia In global aphasia, all of the components of language (Table 8-1) are significantly disturbed, resulting in loss of the ability to understand most spoken and written speech and failure to initiate speech. Prosodic aspects of language may be relatively preserved. Global aphasia often follows infarction in the distribution of the left middle cerebral artery, a lesion affecting all of the major left-side structures important in language either directly or by depriving them of afferent or efferent connections. These patients usually show a right hemiparesis and right homonomous hemianopsia in addition (but not always; see below) because of the simultaneous involvement of the motor system and visual radiations in the stroke. Figures 8-6 and 8-7 show the CT images of two patients with global aphasia. Large

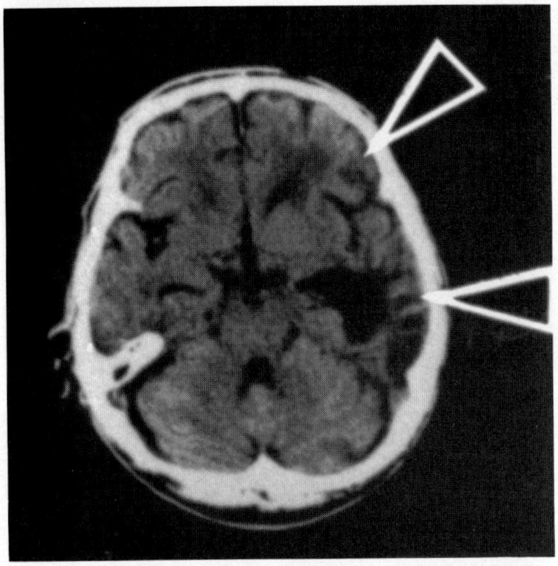

Figure 8-5
Complete transaxial CT study of the brain from a right-handed male patient with two strokes. The earlier stroke (lower arrow) occurred 2 years before the CT was done and appears as a well-organized area of hypodensity with retraction of surrounding tissue in the posterior temporal lobe on the left. It was associated with Wernicke's aphasia. The later stroke (upper arrow) occurred several days before the image was taken. It is much smaller than the first stroke and is located in the left frontal lobe approximately in Broca's area. The two lesions together produced global aphasia without hemiparesis.

amounts of tissue are involved in the frontal, temporal, and parietal cortex as well as in subcortical white matter and nuclei. Figures 8-6 and 8-7 together show some of the variability that can be seen in the extent of lesions in different patients with global aphasia and hemiparesis due to stroke.

The variability in brain lesions that can be seen in global aphasia is emphasized further by the phenomenon of global aphasia without hemiparesis. This occurs most often when multiple lesions occur simultaneously or sequentially in different parts of the brain,[58–64] especially when elements of both posterior and anterior language substrates are involved. Perhaps because less brain tissue is involved in the stroke to begin with, recovery is usually better in global aphasia without hemiparesis. Both of these features of global aphasia without hemiparesis are illustrated by a case studied by Matthews et al,[65] involving a 57-year-old man who had mild residual fluent aphasia from a left temporal infarction 2 years earlier before presenting with acute global aphasia without hemiparesis. Several days after symptom onset, a CT scan of the brain (Fig. 8-5) showed a well-organized area of encephalomalacia in the left temporal lobe consistent with an old stroke, and a smaller area of medium hypodensity in the left lateral frontal lobe near the third frontal convolution (Broca's area), consistent with a new infarction.

Despite the initially global quality of the aphasia, he improved rapidly and by 2 weeks after the stroke a Boston Diagnostic Aphasia Examination showed well-articulated, prosodic, fluent, grammatical speech with paraphasic errors, impaired comprehension, reading, and writing, and preserved repetition, singing, and seriatim speech. This pattern suggested transcortical sensory aphasia (impairment in most aspects of language with relative preservation of ability to repeat).[51,52] At this time a SPECT scan (Fig. 8-8) showed reduced tracer uptake in both the left temporal and left frontal lobes consistent with decreased activity in those areas.

In this case, the addition of a small lesion in the frontal lobe, part of the anterior speech area, to an extant lesion in the posterior speech area produced a syndrome that is characteristic of damage due to a large lesion in the left hemisphere. Rapid improvement to a transcortical sensory aphasia was consistent with the small size of the second lesion.

Conduction Aphasia Some aphasic patients have disproportionate difficulty repeating what they have heard. This has been interpreted as an instance of a "disconnection" syndrome: the isolation of the anterior language area from the posterior language area, preventing what is heard (posterior area) from linking with what one wishes to say (anterior area). The location of the lesion that often accompanies repetition problems, the supramarginal gyrus, seems to support this viewpoint, since the supramarginal gyrus overlies the arcuate fasciculus, a tract connecting the anterior and posterior language areas.[66] There is reason to dispute the disconnection account of this disorder, since other disturbances of language tend to accompany impaired repetition, such as phonemic paraphasias and anomia. Furthermore, lesions outside the arcuate fasciculus can cause the same syndrome.[33,34]

An alternative account of conduction aphasia emphasizes the role of the supramarginal gyrus in perceiving, storing, and reassembling speech sounds so that they can be spoken. In this view, failures of repetition are due not to disconnection of anterior from posterior language areas, but to disruption of these functions of the supramarginal gyrus.[34,67]

Atypical Lesions in Aphasia Aphasic patients may have lesions that are not typically associated with their particular aphasia syndrome.[68,69] An example of this is global aphasia without hemiparesis, discussed above. Similarly, lesions that lie outside of Broca's and surrounding areas can be associated with Broca aphasia. Daffner et al[69] described a patient with Broca aphasia with mainly Wernicke's area lesions seen on CT scan. Subsequent MRI scanning revealed subtle signal abnormalities in the left supplementary motor area, cingulate gyrus, and frontal white matter. While the lesions seen on MRI explained the nonfluent

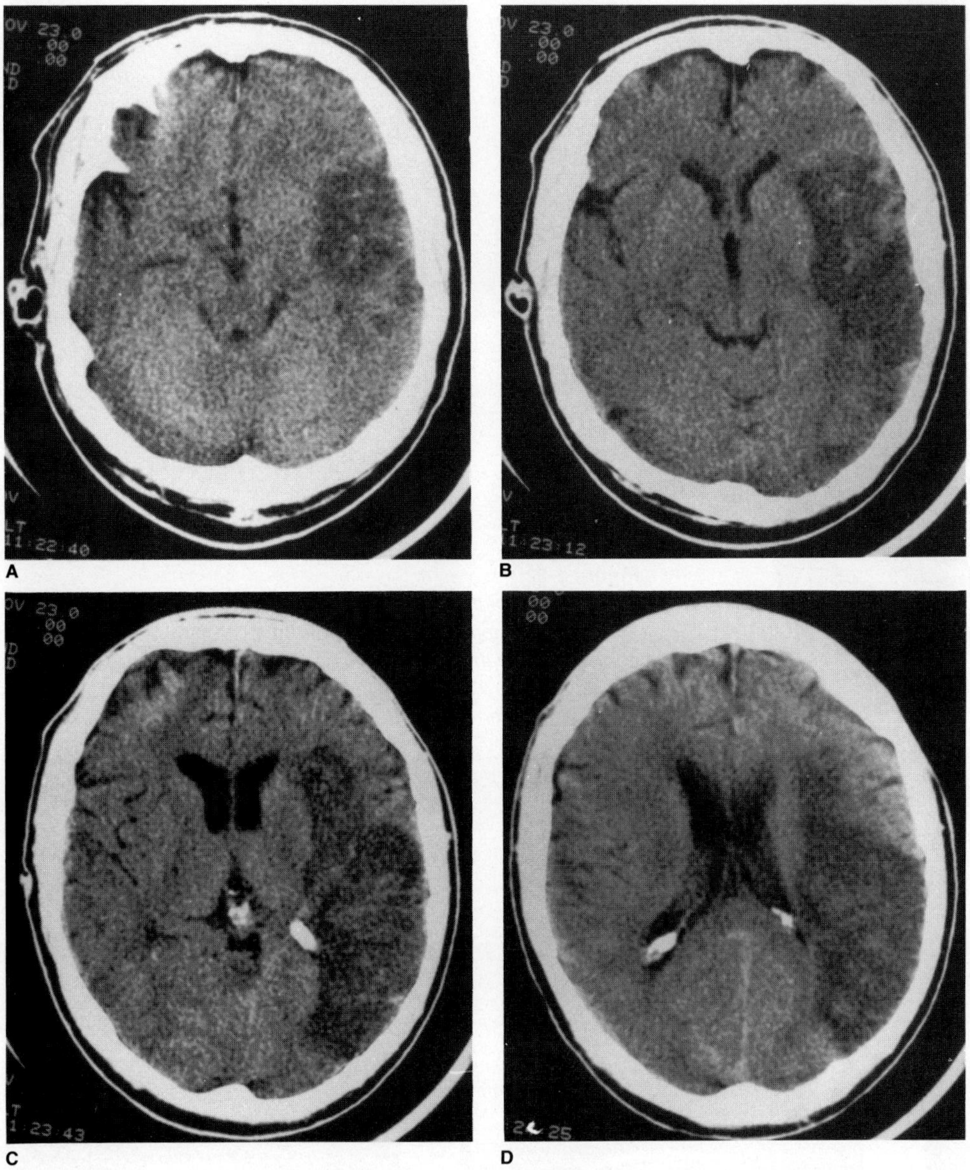

Figure 8-6
Transaxial CT scan of the brain from a 60-year-old right-handed man with long-standing right hemiparesis and global aphasia. A large area of hypodensity includes portions of the frontal, temporal, and parietal lobes, a smaller portion of the occipital lobe, and the insula on the left. Subcortical nuclear structures are mostly spared. Images **A through D** *represent alternate 1-cm slices, providing an approximately 7-cm vertical view.*

aspects of the aphasia, what remained unexplained was why the posterior lesion was not associated with a posterior aphasia. Subsequently, WADA testing suggested that language comprehension was mediated by the right side of the brain, rather than the more usual left-side Wernicke's area.

Another example of a posterior lesion associated with anterior aphasia is seen in Fig. 8-9. This figure is the MRI of a patient with speech hesitancy, articulatory struggle, agrammatism, and relatively preserved comprehension typical of Broca aphasia due to stroke. Most of the signal abnormality is seen in the anterior and posterior temporal lobes, a lesion that might be expected to produce Wernicke aphasia instead. A close look shows subtle signal abnormality in the white matter inferior to the posterior frontal lobe that might have been responsible for much of the nonfluency, explaining this apparently atypical clinicoanatomic correlation.

Functional imaging is especially useful in understanding atypical lesions in aphasia. Metter et al[42] used PET to study cerebral glucose metabolism in patients with Wernicke, Broca, and conduction aphasia. All three of these conditions were associated with left-side hypometabolism. They differed from one another in the location and degree of the left-side disturbance and in the degree of left-right asymmetry. The greatest degree of left-right asymmetry occurred in patients with Broca aphasia, some of whom showed global left hemispheric hypometabolism, even those having relatively posterior lesions on CT images. From the standpoint of CT findings, the latter patients had atypical lesions for mainly nonfluent aphasia. The PET findings showed that, even in these patients, anterior language areas were functionally impaired despite the fact that they appeared anatomically intact on CT images.

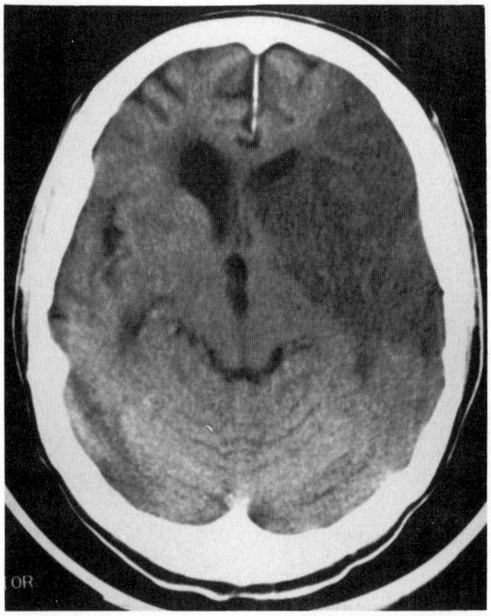

Figure 8-7
One horizontal section from a transaxial CT scan of the brain of a 61-year-old right-handed man with the recent onset of left hemiparesis and global aphasia. A large area of hypodensity includes the frontal, temporal, and parietal lobes, insula, and subjacent nuclear structures on the left. Mild edema, with shift of the medial lateral ventricular wall, is present, consistent with the short period of time elapsed between the stroke and the scan. The level of this image corresponds most closely to the levels represented by slices B and C in Fig. 8-6.

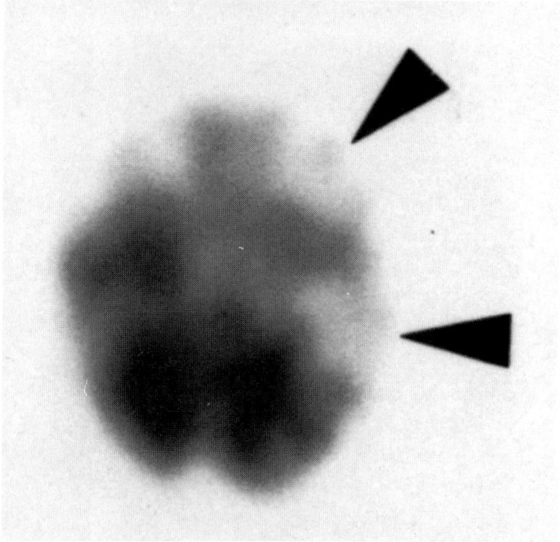

Figure 8-8
SPECT scan of the brain of the patient whose CT scan is shown in Fig. 8-5. The upper arrow points to an area of hyperperfusion that corresponds to the developing area of encephalomalacia marked by the upper arrow in Fig. 8-5. The lower arrow points to the area of hypoperfusion that corresponds to the well-established area of encephalomalacia marked by the lower arrow in Fig. 8-5.

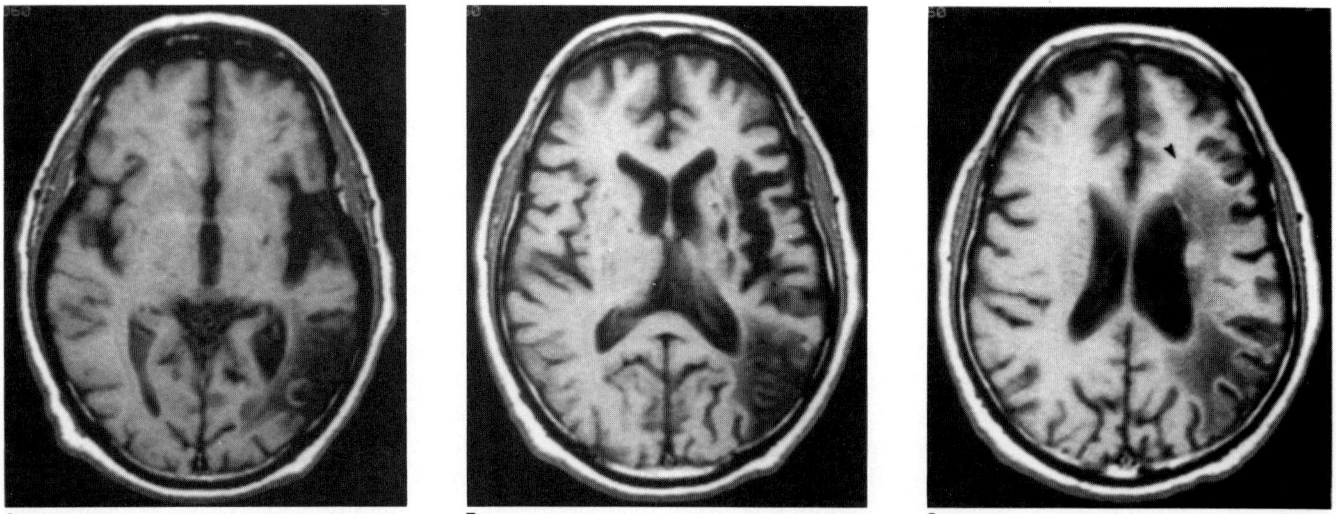

A B C

Figure 8-9
Transaxial MRI (TR 650 ms, TE 11 ms, 5-mm slice thickness) of the brain in a 63-year-old man with nonfluent aphasia that developed after a stroke. Signal abnormality appears mainly in the posterior portions of the language zone. His aphasia was somewhat atypical for the main location of the lesion. The fainter signal abnormality in the frontal white matter (small arrowhead) may explain his nonfluency. (Courtesy of Dr. Atif Husain.)

Several conclusions may be drawn from these observations:

1. There are individual differences in language localization in the brain. Some people have bilateral representation of language capacities that in most people are mediated on the left side only.
2. Lesions that one might expect to see because a patient has a particular kind of aphasia may not appear in one imaging modality but may appear in another. This shows the value of multimodal neuroimaging studies combined with language analysis for understanding aphasic patients.
3. Metabolic abnormalities remote from a zone of infarction (diaschisis) may underlie some atypical findings in aphasia.[42]

In many cases of aphasia, patients show mixtures of deficits that do not conform well to the basic aphasia syndromes summarized above, even when anatomic imaging shows lesions that might be expected to produce "classical" patterns of aphasia. In these cases the aphasia is better understood by specifying the profile of language deficits that the patient shows than by trying to fit the pattern into a discrete category according to existing aphasia terminology. A graphic means of illustrating profiles of linguistic strengths and weaknesses was developed by Goodglass and Kaplan.[50,54]

Recovery from Aphasia

Lesion extent is an important determinant of both the initial severity of aphasia and language recovery in aphasia.[8,47,70] Several quantitative and qualitative techniques of anatomic imaging have been used for measuring the location and extent of brain lesions in aphasia and for predicting functional recovery of language. Damasio and Damasio[56] developed a template method of determining the extent of lesions in aphasia and other neurobehavioral syndromes. A similar method of determining lesion extent in aphasia is described in the next section.

Anatomic Imaging Methods Severe, persistent nonfluent aphasia, in which little productive speech ever recovers, is highly disabling. Naeser and colleagues[8,47,70–72] have developed a CT-based method of lesion size and location analysis for studying the neuroanatomic factors that predict the occurrence of this condition. They acquire CT images 15 to 20° to the canthomeatal line with 10-mm slices separated by 7-mm intervals. Important structures in the language system are numbered according to Brodmann's system, and CT slices are labeled with respect to cortical language areas present on that slice. In slice B, Broca's area is especially well seen, in slice W Wernicke's area is seen, and in slices SM the supramarginal gyrus is represented (Fig. 8-10).[71] On these CT slices, each outlined and labeled

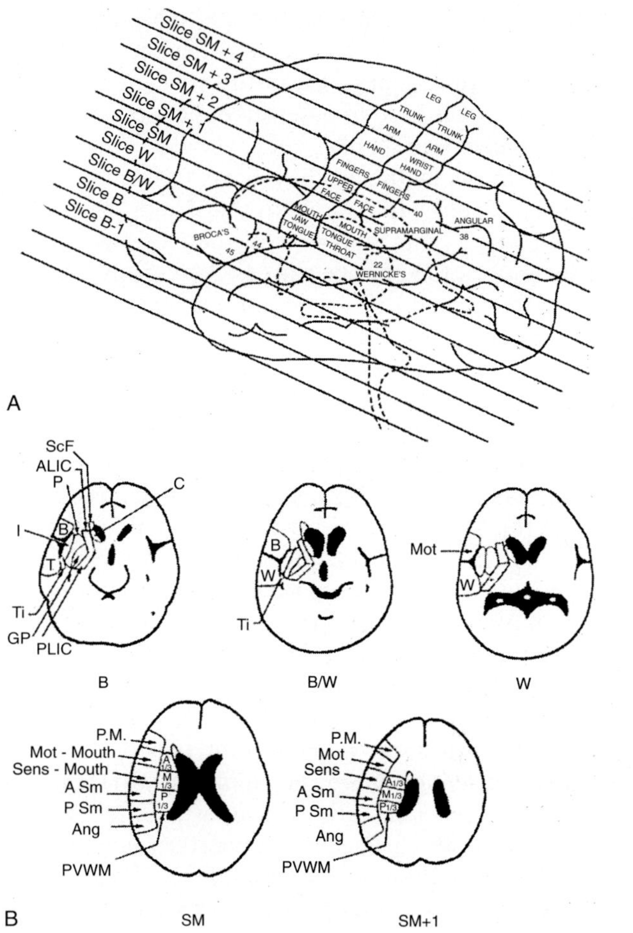

Figure 8-10
CT-based method of lesion size and location analysis for studying the neuroanatomic factors that predict the occurrence of severe persistent nonfluent aphasia. The top part (labeled A) is a lateral diagram of the location of cortical language areas in relationship to the ventricular system (dotted lines). The CT scan slices are marked at 20° to the canthomeatal lines, similar to the angle at which they are acquired. Numbers refer to Brodmann's areas as follows: 44 and 45, Broca's area; 22, Wernicke's area; 40, supramarginal gyrus area; and 39, angular gyrus area. The various parts of the motor and sensory homunculi are labeled for each CT scan slice. The motor-sensory cortex areas for the mouth are located on CT scan slice SM.

The bottom part (labeled B) shows the location of specific neuroanatomic areas that are visually assessed for extent-of-lesion ratings on CT scans (see original article[71] for details). Each neuroanatomic area is examined using a 0- to 5-point scale (0, no lesion; 3, half of area has lesion; 5, entire area has solid lesion; see text). B, Broca's area (45 on slice B; 44 on slice B/W); T, temporal lobe anterior-inferior to Wernicke's area on slice B; Ti, temporal isthmus; I, insular structures, including insula, extreme capsule, claustrum, and external capsule; P, putamen; GP, globus pallidus; ALIC, anterior-limb internal capsule; PLIC, posterior-limb internal capsule; ScF, medial subcallosal fasciculus; C, caudate; W, Wernicke's area (22); Mot, motor cortex; P-M, premotor cortex; Sens, sensory cortex; A Sm, anterior supramarginal gyrus; P Sm, posterior supramarginal gyrus; Ang, angular gyrus, PVWM, periventricular white matter area ($A^{1/3}$, anterior one-third of PVWM; $M^{1/3}$, middle one-third of PVWM; $P^{1/3}$, posterior one-third of PVWM. (Figure and modified caption from Naeser and Palumbo,[71] copyright 1994 by Raven Press. Used by permission. Courtesy of Dr. Margaret A. Naeser.)

anatomic area is measured using a 0- to 5-point involvement scale in which 0 represents no lesion and 5 represents the involvement of the entire structure. An automated method is used to determine the total percentage of left-hemisphere damage.

Using these methods, they have found that global aphasia patients with poor recovery of auditory comprehension 1 to 2 years after a stroke had lesions involving half or more of Wernicke's area. Conversely, recovery was better when only subcortical temporal lobe lesions were present. In patients with persistent nonfluency, the nonfluency was worse and recovery was least when two main structures were damaged: the medial subcallosal fasciculus and the medial third of the periventricular white matter. The medial subcallosal fasciculus connects the cingulate gyrus with the caudate nucleus, and the middle third of the periventricular white matter carries motor cortical fibers that subserve mouth and tongue movements. Both of these structures are important in the initiation of speech, and both can be affected by lesions that include or exclude cortical involvement. From the neurobehavioral standpoint, this emphasizes that subcortical lesions can be even more incapacitating than cortical lesions. Images from two patients with persistent nonfluency are shown in Figs. 8-11 and 8-12. One patient has a mainly cortical lesion, and the other patient has both cortical and subcortical involvement.

Using the method of Naeser et al[8,47,70–72] to study nonfluency in patients with left opercular area stroke, Alexander et al[57] identified three profiles of nonfluency that fall within the general category of Broca's area aphasia. The first profile is impaired articulation and prosody (see Table 8-1 for terms), correlated with damage in the lower motor cortex or the subcortical white matter. The second profile is delayed initiation of speech, sparse utterances, anomia, semantic paraphasias, and preserved repetition and grammatic structure, correlated with lesions of the frontal operculum, sparing the regions affected in patients with the first profile. The third profile is impaired articulation and prosody, and phonemic errors, correlated with lesions in the lower motor cortex, subcortical white matter, and periventricular white matter of the deep to lower motor cortex. These separate features of nonfluency are usually seen together in typical Broca aphasia, but the observations of Alexander et al[57] showed that they can be dissociated and that lesions in various areas are correlated with these dissociations.

Naeser et al[72] have extended this work to an analysis of the imaging features in stroke patients that predict response to the Computer-Assisted Visual Communication program (C-ViC), a method of language remediation. The C-ViC language consists of three icons for verb action (*lift*, *turn*, and *give*) and pictures of objects and people. Patients try to learn this language by using a computer mouse in order to carry out commands, and then they try to communicate with the system. How well they succeed in using C-ViC for communication can be measured using the Visual Index of Communicative Ability. Severely nonfluent stroke patients with bilateral brain lesions were unable to learn the C-ViC language. Of those patients who could learn and use the system, lesions in several areas led to special difficulty initiating language, with better capacity to answer questions using C-ViC. These areas included Wernicke's area, the subcortical temporal isthmus, the supplementary motor area, the cingulate gyrus, and the medial subcallosal fasciculus. This suggests that failure to initiate language

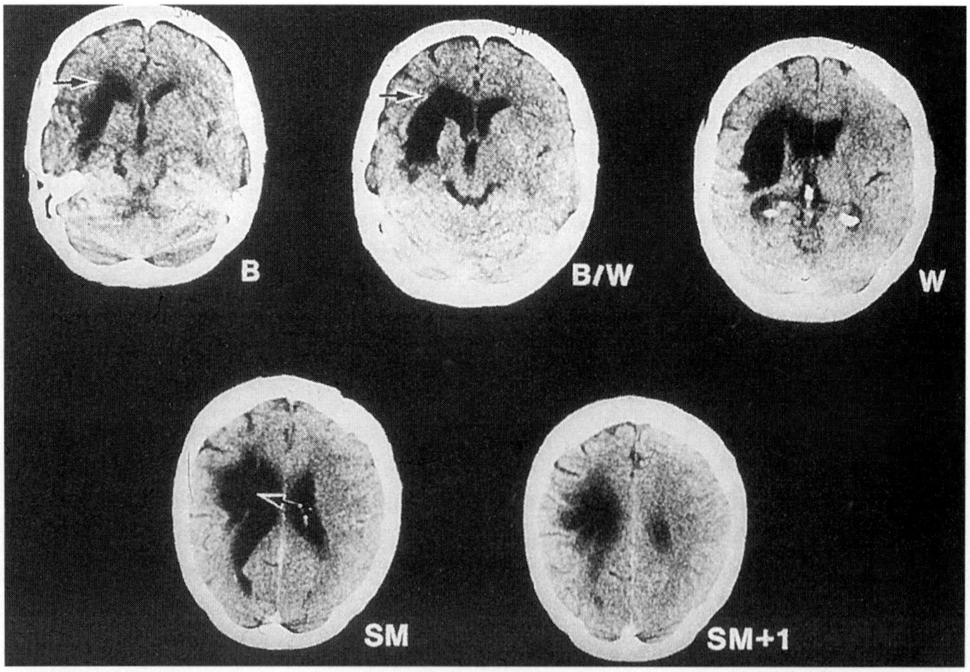

Figure 8-11
CT scan a 35-year-old man who had no speech 2 years after onset. A dense right hemiplegia was present. The left-hemisphere lesion is on the left side of the CT scan. The extent-of-lesion rating for the medial ScF area at slice B was 5; at slice B/W, it was also 5 (arrows); the mean was 5. The extent-of-lesion rating in the $M^{1/3}$ PVWM area at slice SM was 4.95 (arrow); the total extent-of-lesion rating was 9.95. The lesion is primarily subcortical. See also Fig. 8–10. (Figure and modified legend from Naeser and Palumbo,[71] copyright 1994 by Raven Press. Used by permission. Courtesy of Dr. Margaret A. Naeser.)

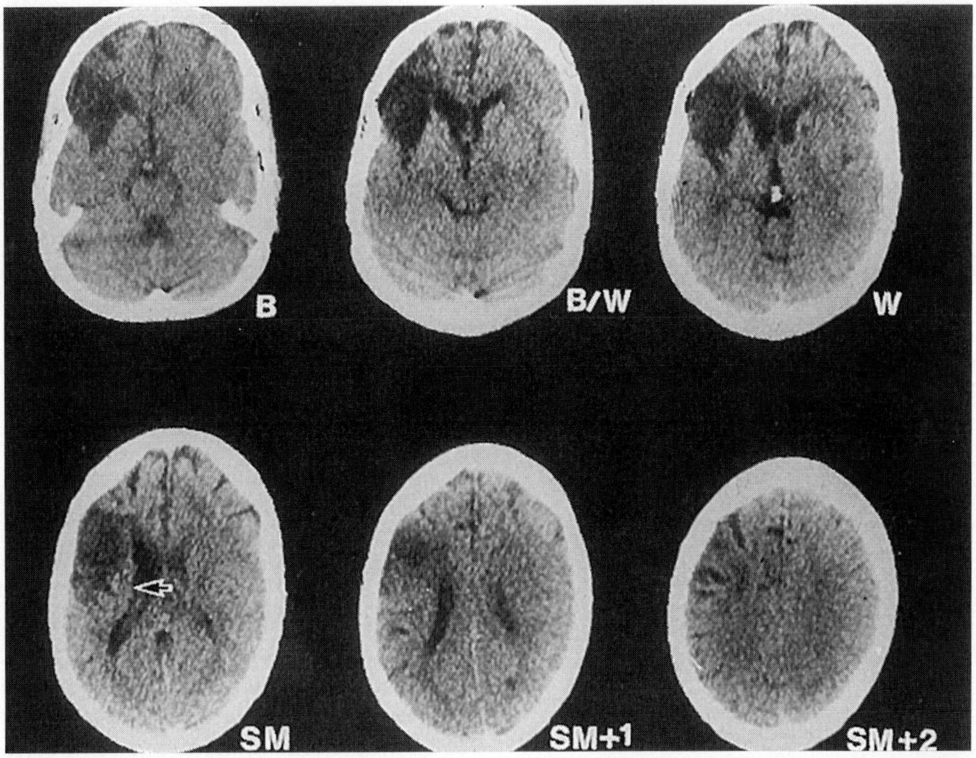

Figure 8-12
CT scan 44 months after onset of lesion, from a 54-year-old man with nonfluent agrammatic speech and Broca aphasia 7 months after onset. A mild hemiparesis was present, and there was good recovery. The extent-of-lesion rating in the medial ScF area at slice B was 4; at slice B/W it was 3.75; the mean was 3.88. The extent-of-lesion rating in the $M^{1/3}$ PVWM area at slice SM was only 2; the total extent-of-lesion rating was 5.88. The arrow at slice SM shows minimal lesion in the $M^{1/3}$ PVWM area that greatly reduced the combined extent-of-lesion ratings to less than 6, a value compatible with the patient's mild limitations in speech. The mild hemiparesis with good recovery was compatible with sparing of the deepest PVWM area immediately adjacent to the body of the lateral ventricle at slices SM and SM + 1, which contains, in part, the descending pyramidal tract pathways. See with Figs. 8-10 and 8-11. (Figure and modified legend from Naeser and Palumbo,[71] copyright 1994 by Raven Press. Used by permission. Courtesy of Dr. Margaret A. Naeser.)

may not be just a matter of impaired oral production but may also include a failure to initiate language function in either the visual or auditory modality.

Functional Imaging Methods Functional imaging and transcranial doppler have been applied in the prognostication of aphasia. Silvestrini et al[24] used transcranial doppler to study language recovery in patients rendered aphasic by a left middle cerebral artery (MCA) stroke. All patients initially had similar degrees of nonfluent aphasia, as measured by the Western Aphasia Battery, and all were enrolled in a program of aphasia rehabilitation (described as a "standard regimen of aphasia rehabilitation"), but they varied in how much fluency they eventually recovered. Both before and after a 2-month period of rehabilitation, mean flow velocities in the left MCA were measured at rest and during a word fluency task. The patients who performed better on this task, and hence the ones who had shown better recovery, showed greater increases in left MCA flow during the task both before and after the course of remediation and an increase in flow in the right MCA after remediation. In addition to the potential usefulness of this method in predicting aphasia recovery, Silvestrini et al[24] interpreted their data as suggesting that the degree of potential residual activation in the language substrate is one mechanism by which language recovery can occur after stroke.

This potential activation can be more directly measured by functional imaging methods. Using SPECT, Bushnell et al[73] found that smaller blood flow deficits in the zone of infarctions were associated with better general neurologic and language recovery in aphasia than were larger flow deficits. Nagata et al[74] analyzed PET images in patients with aphasia after left-hemispheric stroke and suggested that this methodology may help to clarify the role of the undamaged right hemisphere in recovery from aphasia. Subsequently, Ohyama et al[75] studied aphasic patients engaged in a repetition task designed to activate residual language areas. They observed activation in right-sided homologues to left-sided language areas during the task. Heiss et al[76] acquired PET measurements of the cerebral metabolic rate of glucose utilization in left-hemisphere stroke patients with aphasia. They found that two PET measurements of metabolism were correlated positively with recovery from aphasia: (1) resting metabolism of the left hemisphere outside the zone of the infarct and (2) the increase in metabolism due to spontaneous speech in residual language-related areas. Using PET, Karbe et al[77] measured cerebral metabolic rates of glucose utilization in language-relevant areas soon after stroke. They found that subnormal metabolism, even in areas of the brain remote from left MCA lesions as seen on CT scans, predicted poor eventual recovery of language function.

Several conclusions about recovery of function in aphasia are suggested by these studies. First, dysfunction in language substrate remote from areas of tissue death (diaschisis) can contribute to aphasia. This is likely to be the case when relatively small, subcortical lesions exert marked effects on language (see the discussion of critical infarct dementia below). Second, both lesion location and lesion volume can play a role in determining the severity of aphasia and the degree of recovery possible. Third, functional imaging methods can help to gauge success in aphasia intervention programs.

Dyslexia

Dyslexia is a developmental disorder of language ability that manifests in impaired reading, spelling, and writing. The precise deficit responsible for dyslexia is not yet clear. Traditionally it has been viewed as a relatively isolated language problem, with other elements of basic intelligence being preserved.[78] Evidence now suggests that this view may be too narrow. Dyslexia may be a disorder of visual information processing, a disorder of language and/or sound processing, or a more general disorder of information processing.[79–82] Dyslexia may represent a family of separate but related information processing disorders rather than a unitary disorder.

Dyslexia may be caused by abnormal organization of the visual system, a prominent manifestation of which, in a reading society, is difficulty reading (the condition might not be recognized otherwise). For example, dyslexics report "visual confusions" in which small letters blur and seem to move.[83] These confusions may be due, not to a specific reading deficit, but, rather, to impairments in the processing of rapidly presented or moving visual targets. This function appears to rely especially heavily upon a component of the visual system called the magnocellular, or M, pathway that originates in the magnocellular region of the lateral geniculate nucleus and ends in the posterior parietal cortex.[82,84] This visual subsystem may be specialized for processing motion, while other visual subsystems are involved in processing of color and form[82] (see "Visual Perception" and "Visual Agnosia," below).

Functional Imaging and Dyslexia The neurophysiologic basis of dyslexia has been studied using PET, functional MRI, and magnetoencephalography.[82,84–89] Some of these studies point to dysfunction in auditory information processing, and some point to dysfunction in visual information processing as the basis of dyslexia. Hagmann et al[88] compared PET profiles of cortical activation in dyslexic adults with those of control subjects during auditory processing tasks. Dyslexic subjects showed higher absolute and relative rates of brain metabolism along an anterior-posterior gradient in the medial temporal lobe than did controls. This observation supports the hypothesis that dyslexia is related to abnormal cerebral processing of auditory data.[88] Rumsey et al[87] made similar observations, finding that dyslexic men showed language-specific abnormalities in left temporal activation on PET scans.

Paulesu et al[90] used PET to study dyslexic adults who were required to use visually presented letters in order to perform a rhyming and short-term memory task. They found abnormal activation of brain regions known to be involved in the performance of these tasks by nondyslexics. In particular, the insula was not activated in these tasks in dyslexics. The authors speculated that developmental dyslexia could be a disconnection syndrome due to an inadequate anatomic bridge between anterior and posterior components of the language system. In similar work using magnetoencephalography, Salmelin et al[89] found that dyslexics showed delayed word-specific responses in the inferior temporooccipital region during passive viewing of single words. These studies suggest that dyslexia is mainly a visual information processing disorder.

Support for the view that dyslexia represents defective functioning in the M stream of visual information processing was provided by Demb et al.[84] They used functional MRI to show that dyslexics had reduced activity in visual areas that are believed to receive a strong M input. Furthermore, activation of this network was correlated with reading ability. Eden et al[82] used functional MRI to show that, when presented with moving stimuli, dyslexics did not show normal activation in the magnocellular visual system. In contrast, when presented with stationary patterns, they did show normal cerebral activation patterns. The study by Eden et al[82] suggests that dyslexia may reflect a general disturbance in visual functioning.

Anatomic Imaging and Dyslexia Abnormal function does not necessarily imply abnormal gross morphologic structure, but such abnormality has been documented in dyslexia. Increased symmetry and even reversal of normal asymmetry of the planum temporale (see the section above on the anatomy of the language system) has been seen in dyslexics.[91–93] In addition, using high-resolution MRI, Leonard et al[80] found three main types of cortical abnormalities in dyslexics: an abnormally large proportion of tissue in the planum temporale shifted to the parietal lobe (parietal shift), unusual terminations of sylvian fissures on the left, and duplicated Heschl's gyri on both right and left. Figure 8-13 shows high-resolution MRIs of normal subjects and dyslexics illustrating some of these features.[80] The work of Leonard et al[80] suggests that standard MRI plane angle and slice thickness may be insensitive to subtle anomalies that may underlie dyslexia.

It has been speculated that dyslexia is linked to abnormal cerebral lateralization, to left-handedness, and to immune disorders by a common factor such as elevated prenatal testosterone.[94,95] In view of the functional imaging work discussed above, it is tempting to speculate that an early disorder of insular development could cause abnormal lateralization. Dyslexia may be due to abnormal cell migration in the insula or other structures during development. This might produce abnormal gyri and a microstructure that is incapable of supporting fully the computational activity of normal linguistic and/or visual-spatial functioning.[81]

The notion that dyslexia is at least partly a disorder of lateralization is reinforced by findings of abnormal corpus callosum morphology in dyslexics. Rumsey et al[96] made quantitative MRI measurements of the corpus callosum in dyslexic men. They found that the area of the splenium and isthmus was larger in dyslexic than in nondyslexic men. The two groups did not differ in anterior callosal morphology. The investigators suggested that this abnormality reflected abnormal lateralization of function in posterior regions of the brain bilaterally.

In summary, recent advances in the conceptualization of dyslexia have been driven to a large degree by advances and application of quantitative anatomic and functional imaging methodologies. These research tools may be ultimately adaptable to the clinical diagnosis of dyslexia.

Memory and Amnesia

The Nature of Memory

The term *memory* is used to refer to many phenomena at various levels of analysis. It is intimately related to terms that label other modules of cognitive functioning such as *attention, language, executive function,* and *perception.* For the purposes of this discussion, *memory* is defined as the way in which an organism notices, initially engages and judges, acquires, stores, modifies, interlinks, and retrieves information or knowledge. *Information or knowledge* can be defined as symbols or representations of reality. Since memory is essential for thought and adaptive behavior, it is an essential part of any unified theory of cognition.[97] Conceptions of memory are fluid, and what we present here is a distillation of several current views, which experience shows are likely to evolve.

Benson[31] has framed the aspects of memory that hold particular interest for neurologists in three axioms, or postulates:

1. Memory is an essential element for thinking and consists of several functional processes.
2. Specific memory processes rely on separate neuroanatomic bases. While some anatomic sites are shared among various functions, these sites are organized into a discrete network for each discrete memory function.
3. Each memory function participates in thought, but one or more memory functions may be fully or partially inoperable without impairing other aspects of memory.

The Multiple Components of Memory A complete account of memory must go beyond older accounts of memory as being composed of short, intermediate, and long-term aspects. Memory now is viewed from several perspectives, and evidence shows that these several perspectives are all correct in some respect, touching as they do upon various aspects of memory. What binds these views together is the same overriding concept taking shape in cognitive neuroscience in general: that of serial and parallel information processing. This issue with respect to memory is reviewed frequently, and there are several recent treatments of the topic.[98–101] Particularly useful is the excellent brief review by Duffy.[98]

Serial processing in memory refers to the sequence of events that begins in the memory substrate when new data are received. Most treatments of serial processing in memory view memory as a three-component process: iconic memory (short-lived sensory "echos" of data), working memory, and long-term memory. From the standpoint of *parallel processing*, memory can be viewed from two additional perspectives: that of the modality in which information is represented and that of the nature of the knowledge one has. This implies the existence of at least two sets of parallel memory systems. The first set (modality set) includes parallel systems for verbal information and for visual-spatial information, with the substrates for each located mainly in the left and right hemispheres, respectively. The second set (nature of knowledge set) includes parallel systems for conscious knowledge (knowing that something is the case, or declarative or explicit memory) and for unconscious knowledge (knowing how to do something, or procedural or implicit memory).

These sets of parallel systems are linked in several ways. First, serial processing occurs in each of these parallel processes. Second, these parallel processing functions can work upon the same information, each managing different aspects of the information. A central challenge is to identify the distributed neural networks

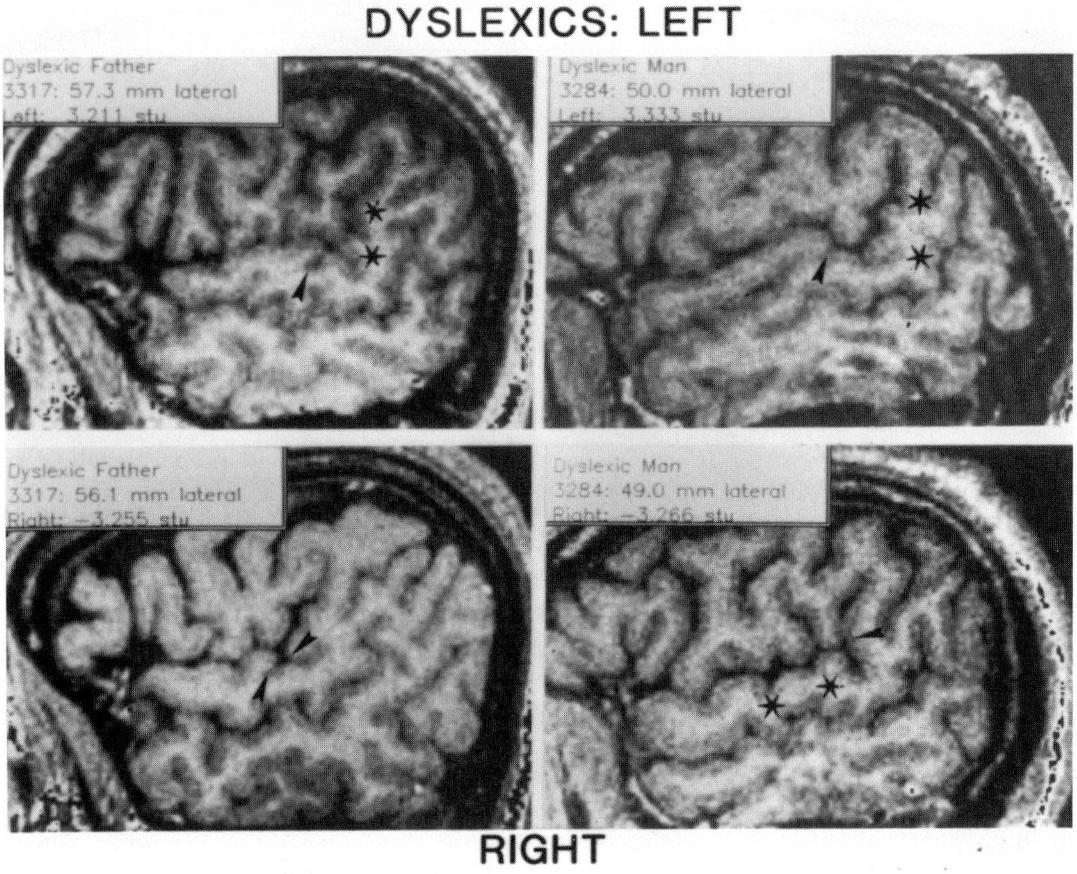
DYSLEXICS: LEFT
Dyslexic Father
3317: 57.3 mm lateral
Left: 3.211 stu
Dyslexic Man
3284: 50.0 mm lateral
Left: 3.333 stu
Dyslexic Father
3317: 56.1 mm lateral
Right: −3.255 stu
Dyslexic Man
3284: 49.0 mm lateral
Right: −3.266 stu
RIGHT

A

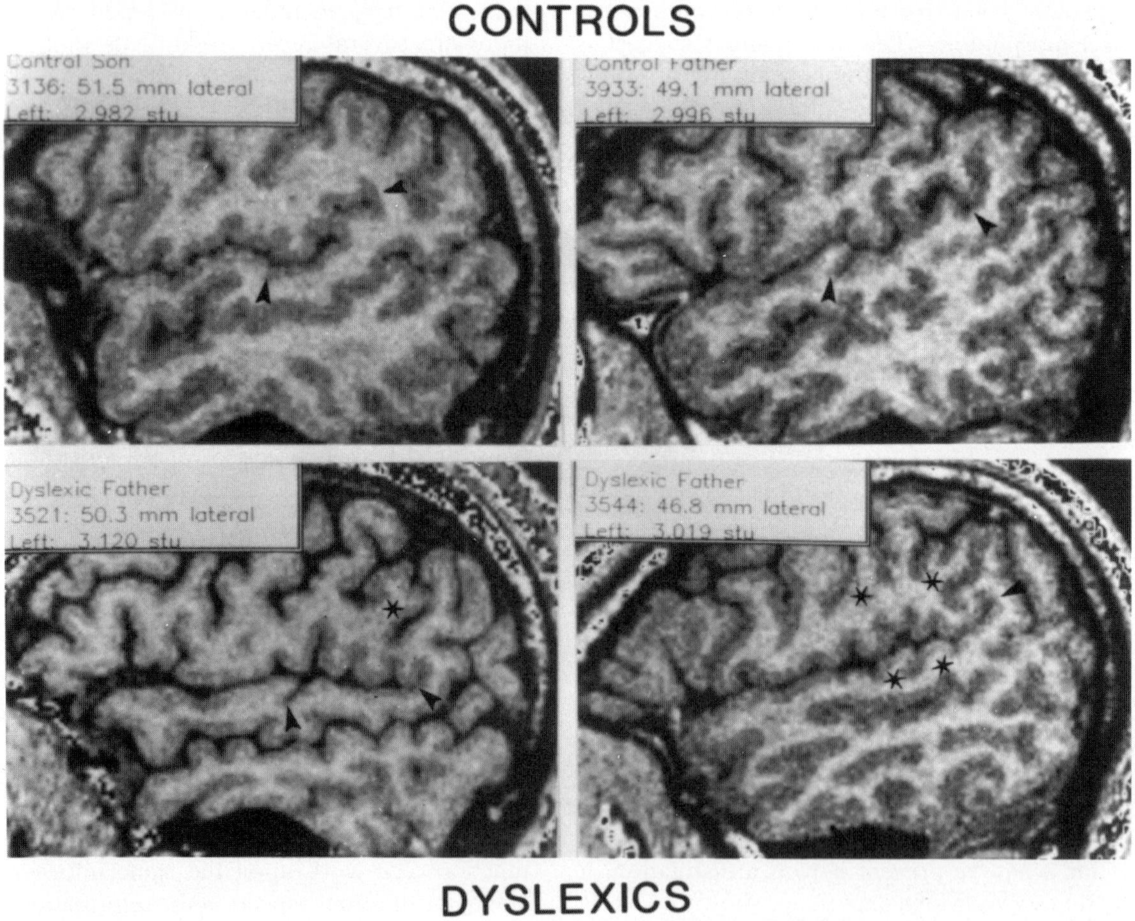
CONTROLS
Control Son
3136: 51.5 mm lateral
Left: 2.982 stu
Control Father
3933: 49.1 mm lateral
Left: 2.996 stu
Dyslexic Father
3521: 50.3 mm lateral
Left: 3.120 stu
Dyslexic Father
3544: 46.8 mm lateral
Left: 3.019 stu
DYSLEXICS

B

that underlie these serial, parallel, and interrelated functions. Each of these aspects of memory is discussed below, with an emphasis on the contributions of neuroimaging to the understanding of these network substrates.

Serial Processing: Working Memory and Long-Term Memory A real-time process of active attention to information that has been labeled *working memory* can be distinguished from a related but separate function termed *long-term memory*.[98,100,102] In many respects the notion of working memory has supplanted the older, although still used term *short-term memory*. Working memory is a "system that temporarily stores information as part of the performance of complex tasks."[102] It is admixed with perceptual and with executive information processing. It may involve the simultaneous storage and processing of information and has both visual-spatial and phonological (i.e., linguistic) components. This system is limited in carrying capacity, and information carried there must be attended to continuously, as when one rehearses a new telephone number, or else it rapidly decays and is lost. This topic is discussed further in the treatment of the executive functions; the bulk of this section is devoted to the second aspect of memory: long-term memory.

Long-term memory refers to the acquisition and storage of information for a variable period of time (minutes to years) that exceeds the limited span of short-term memory. Material from working memory must be processed correctly in order for it to enter long-term memory. Long-term memory can exist in two forms, represented by two parallel systems and processes: explicit memory and implicit memory.[98,99,103] Greiner et al[104] have published a short but clear explanation of these functions.

Figure 8-13
Sagittal MRIs in dyslexia (1.0- to 1.25-mm slice thicknesses, either TR 22 ms and TE 6 ms, or TR 10 ms and TE 4 ms; see original source for detailed imaging parameters).[80] **(A)** *Two subjects with dyslexia, subject 1 left top and bottom, subject 2 right top and bottom. Arrowheads mark Heschl's sulcus. Top images are from the left hemisphere and show extra gyri in the parietal bank of the planum temporale for both subjects (asterisks). Bottom images are from the right hemisphere, where subject 1 has an extra gyrus in the parietal bank and a short temporal bank (arrowheads), and subject 2 has a large Heschl's gyrus (asterisk) in the region normally occupied by the temporal bank of the planum.* **(B)** *Single images from each of two control (top) and two dyslexic (bottom) subjects. The top images depict normal anatomy: on the left, the normal sylvian fissure ends in a typical bifurcation; on the right, the sylvian fissure ends in an ascending parietal bank that enters a clearly demarcated supramarginal gyrus. The bottom images depict abnormal anatomy, mainly abnormal sylvian fissures with multiple primary sulci and extra gyri in the parietal operculum (asterisks), and/or multiple Heschl's gyri (asterisk in lower right). On all images, arrowheads mark the borders of the temporal bank of the planum temporale. (Figure and modified legend from Leonard et al,*[80] *copyright 1993 by the American Medical Association. Used by permission. Courtesy of Dr. Christiana Leonard, University of Florida.)*

Parallel Processing: Explicit and Implicit Memory Explicit, or declarative, memory involves intentional or conscious recollection of previous experiences;[105,106] it is memory for facts and is of two kinds. *Semantic explicit memory* is memory for general knowledge of the world, such as people, objects, and events. *Episodic explicit memory* is autobiographical memory, or memory for things that happen (episodes), such as the fact that the Pittsburgh Pirates won the world series in 1960.[107]

Implicit memory refers to unconscious learning and memory;[103,105,108] it is "knowledge without awareness."[98] There are three forms of implicit memory: skill learning, classical conditioning, and priming. *Priming* refers to the increased ease of learning after prior exposure to information without obvious evidence that learning had taken place.[109] In other words, priming is improvement in memory for detecting or identifying recently presented stimuli.[110] *Classical conditioning* occurs after repeated pairings of a signal, such as a bell (the conditional stimulus), with a stimulus that causes a physiological response, such as a puff of air blown onto the eye (unconditional stimulus), which causes an eye blink (unconditional response). Conditional learning occurs when the sound of the bell gains the capacity to elicit the eye blink (which now becomes the conditional response) without the occurrence of the puff of air. *Skill learning* is motor learning, such as gaining skills in gymnastics.

Parallel Processing: Verbal and Visual Knowledge Studies of patients with isolated left or right hemispheric damage have supported the existence of separate memory systems for verbal and visual information. Left-sided lesions predominantly affect verbal learning and recall. Right-sided lesions are more likely to affect visual-spatial learning and recall, and possibly aspects of musical learning and recall as well.[111–114] Studies of patients undergoing WADA testing have partially agreed with these observations, although the applicability of WADA test information from epileptic patients to nonepileptic people is unclear.[115] Functional imaging studies have begun to isolate the components of these two systems. In a series of studies using PET, Gur et al[116,117] found greater left than right midtemporal regional cerebral blood flow (rCBF) increases during a word recognition task and the opposite during a face recognition task. Predominantly unilateral activation has been found also in the parahippocampal gyrus, hippocampus, and amygdala as well, depending on the memory task.[117] What has emerged is a view of left- or right-sided predominance in verbal and spatial learning and memory rather than strict localization of these types of learning either to right- or to left-sided structures (see below).

Brain Structures in Memory There is neuropsychologic and neuroimaging evidence for the existence of all of the abovementioned memory functions. In addition, there is evidence that the neural substrates of these separate functions consist of a neural network of multiple interconnected cortical and subcortical structures arranged in separate but overlapping systems[31] (see above). Considerable information exists about the consequences for memory function of damage in each of these systems[118–120] (see below).

The hippocampus, the cortex adjacent to the hippocampus in the medial temporal lobe, the perirhinal, entorhinal, and parahippocampal cortical areas, the mammillary bodies, the medial thalamus, and connecting structures, such as the fornix, constitute a vital core of the memory system. This limbic-diencephalic memory system, in concert with neocortical systems, may be viewed as most important for explicit (declarative) memory. There appear to be other, parallel memory systems as well in the brain, relying upon some of these but also upon other structures. These systems may include, for example, a neostriatal-neocortical system subserving habit learning and other systems subserving implicit learning, including an amygdala-neocortical system subserving emotional learning, the cerebellum as a participant in classical conditioning, and the posterior neocortex as a participant in perceptual priming.[108,120] Some of the evidence of these multiple systems and substrates of memory is discussed below.

Neuroimaging and Explicit Memory

Working Memory and Long-Term Memory In an effort to separate neural networks subserving long-term versus short-term memory, Grasby et al[121] used PET to compare rCFB in research subjects performing a short-term word list memory task and subjects performing long-term memory tasks. Increased rCBF during the long-term compared with the short-term memory task was observed in the left and right prefrontal cortex, precuneus, and posterior cingulate cortex. An additional rCBF comparison, this time between a group performing a long-term memory task and a group at rest, showed activation of the left anterior cingulate gyrus, thalamus, and cerebellum in the long-term memory task group. The two conditions together showed an extensive network subserving the acquisition of explicit memories.

Expanding on this work, Grasby et al[122] found that the more memory was taxed during an auditory-verbal word list memorization task (memory load measured by word list length), the greater the increase in rCBF in the cerebellum, thalamus, superior and middle frontal gyri, anterior insular regions, anterior cingulate, precuneus, and left and right lateral premotor areas. Some of these results can be seen in Fig. 8-14.

These and similar studies indicate that the circuitry involved in explicit memory has a much larger cortical, subcortical, and cerebellar substrate than had been apparent from earlier lesion studies in animals and studies of brain damage in humans. Within a distributed neural systems framework, auditory-verbal memory function appears to involve the simultaneous operation of over-

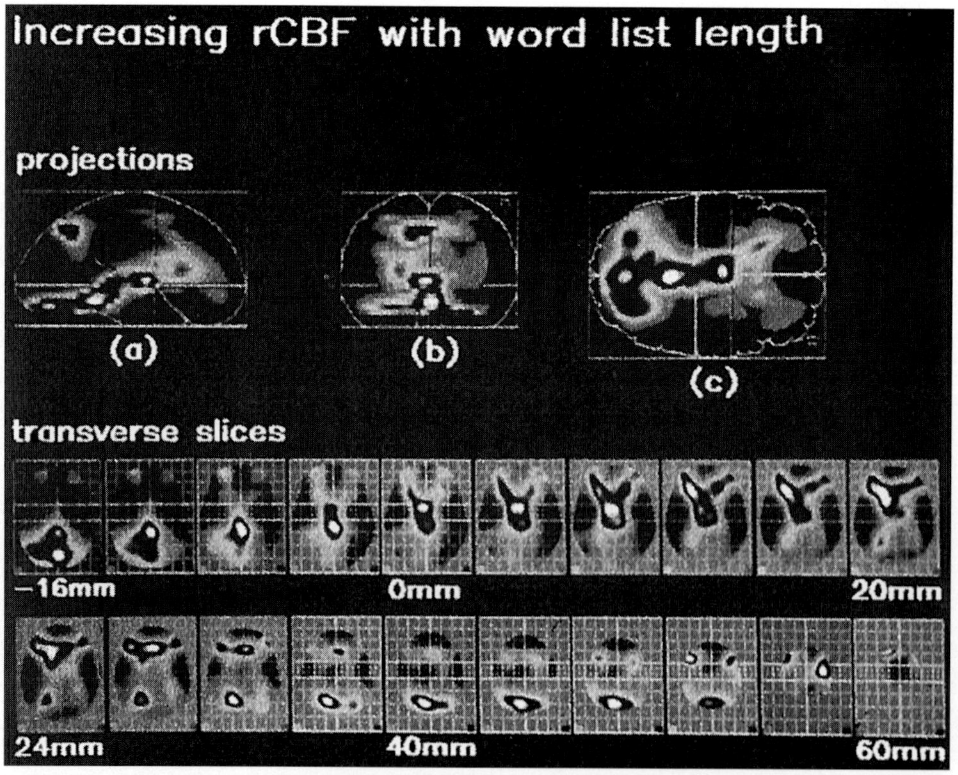

Figure 8-14
Correlations between cerebral perfusion and ability to memorize (memory load). The figure shows the locations of positive correlations of rCBF with word list length. The upper images show the spatial distribution of significant flow increases, shown as integrated projections along sagittal **(A)**, *coronal* **(B)**, *and* **(C)** *transverse views of a brain atlas (see the original article for details).*[122] *The lower images reflect relative blood flow with respect to the anterior cerebral–posterior cerebral (AC-PC) line. Anterior is at the top of each slice. The subject's right is on the right. The superimposed grid provides brain atlas stereotactic coordinates. (Figure and modified legend from Grasby et al,*[122] *copyright 1994 by Oxford University Press. Used by permission.)*

lapping networks that include those for attention and linguistic processing.

Episodic and Semantic Memory Functional neuroimaging work supports the view that these memory processes are both lateralized and subserved by different brain networks. Tasks in which subjects must retrieve information from semantic memory have been associated with left frontal activation, as measured by PET.[123,124] Conversely, tasks in which subjects must retrieve episodic information are associated with right frontal activation.[125–127]

Encoding and Retrieval Normal explicit memory function requires that information first be encoded and then be retrieved when needed. These two processes appear to rely on different but overlapping cortical, subcortical, and paralimbic structures, with these different substrate components having different lateralizing aspects.

Among the neocortical structures, episodic memory encoding has been associated with increased left prefrontal cortical activity regardless of the type of material memorized (e.g., words, objects, odors, or faces).[128] Measurements of rCBF obtained with PET have shown increased activity in the left prefrontal cortex as well as the retrosplenial area of the cingulate cortex during memorization of words (encoding of auditory verbal information).[125,126] Haxby et al[129] found that memorization of faces also produced activation of left prefrontal cortex. To an extent, therefore, the general rule that visual-spatial information is dealt with by right hemispheric structures and auditory-linguistic information is dealt with by left hemispheric structures, may not apply to all aspects of memory: evidence suggests that, during encoding of information in either modality, left frontal cortical activation occurs (see the discussion of laterality in memory below).

In contrast, episodic memory retrieval appears to recruit elements of the right prefrontal cortex.[109,128,130] Retrieval of verbal information has been associated with increased rCBF in the precuneus and the right prefrontal cortex,[125,126] as well as from the left ventrolateral frontal cortex.[127] In the study by Haxby et al,[129] while encoding of faces activated the left prefrontal cortex, recognition of faces (a form of retrieval) activated the right prefrontal cortex. Hence, regardless of the modality in which information is stored, right prefrontal cortical structures are critical components of the network that subserves memory retrieval.

Among the paralimbic structures, the hippocampus probably plays a role in both encoding and storage of information in long-term memory and probably in recognition or retrieval of information as well. Hippocampal memory function may be partially lateralized, with the left hippocampus more active for verbal material and the right hippocampus more active for visual-spatial material. The existence of material-specific amnesias in epileptic patients with hippocampal sclerosis supports this view of hippocampal functional asymmetry (see the discussion of the hippocampus in the amnesia section of this chapter).

Functional imaging in normal subjects also implies hippocampal lateralization. Using PET, Grady et al[131] found evidence of increased rCBF in the right hippocampus and left prefrontal and temporal cortices during both encoding and face recognition tasks, and in the right prefrontal and parietal areas during recognition tasks. Squire et al[110] and Buckner et al[109] found increased rCBF in the right hippocampus and parahippocampal gyrus, in addition to the right prefrontal cortex, during the retrieval stage of a visually presented word recall task. Maguire et al[132] provided PET evidence that the right hippocampus is part of a network of brain regions activated during recall of complex geographic routes but not during recall of nonspatial information. While other work has shown that left-sided structures play some role in spatial memory,[133] it is nonetheless consistent with the view of right hemispheric relative specialization for spatial memory and left hemispheric relative specialization for verbal information.

Despite these findings, uncertainty remains about hippocampal function in encoding and retrieval. In a fMRI study, Stern et al[134] found that, during encoding of novel pictures, fMRI signal increases occurred bilaterally in the posterior hippocampus and other areas. To some extent, this bilaterality may have reflected the use of novel stimuli in the encoding task; exposure to novel stimuli has been found to produce hippocampal activation in an intracranial event-related potential study.[135] Nonetheless, this fMRI result points out uncertainties about the concept of hippocampal lateralization.

Second, while many studies of amnesic patients implicate the hippocampus in explicit memory, hippocampal activation has not been consistently found in functional imaging studies of encoding and retrieval processes. To some degree, this may reflect inherent limitations in the imaging techniques. Both PET and SPECT may be too insensitive to demonstrate consistently task-associated activation of the hippocampus, which may involve only very sparse neuronal activation.[126] As well, cognitive subtraction techniques may fail to demonstrate hippocampal activation if the hippocampus is continually active during experimental and control tasks.[125] In order to compensate for this limitation, graded, rather than subtraction, methods have been used to study hippocampal activation during retrieval, sometimes with better results.[122,136]

Summary: Laterality in Explicit Memory A brief summary of laterality in memory, highly simplified, is as follows. There appears to be relative lateralization of the encoding (left) and the retrieval (right) processes regardless of the modality of the information being learned (i.e., whether verbal or visual-spatial). Orthogonal to this lateralized dichotomy is a tendency toward lateralization of verbal and spatial memory tasks to the left and right hemisphere, respectively.

Neuroimaging and Implicit Memory

Priming While the hippocampal formation has been implicated in explicit memory in studies of brain-damaged amnesic patients, it is thought to be uninvolved in priming. For example, in a PET study Squire et al[110] found increased right hippocampal activity during recall tasks but not during priming conditions. Other brain areas have been implicated in priming in a three-step research paradigm called a stem-completion priming task. In step one (the baseline task), subjects read a list of words, which might include, for example, woman. For purposes of illustration, the list would not include *carpet.* In step two, they are shown three-letter stems, such as *wom* and *car,* which either were (priming condition: *wom*) or were not (baseline condition: *car*) the beginnings of the study word. In step three, during a word association task, they are asked to reveal the first word that comes to mind in response to the stem. During the word association task, only the subjects in the priming condition showed blood flow changes (reductions in this case) in occipitotemporal regions compared to the baseline task.[109,110,137]

Similar decreases in blood flow in the temporal auditory areas have been found in response to priming with auditory material.[128] Similar findings have been obtained with neurophysiologic probes of implicit face memory. During a visual explicit learning task given to partial epilepsy patients, Seeck et al[138] recorded visual evoked potentials from mid- and inferotemporal leads more often than from limbic site leads.

These and other priming studies suggest the following:

1. Prior exposure to a stimulus makes subsequent perceptual processing more efficient.
2. Increased efficiency produces quicker response times and requires less neural activity for word generation. This is reflected in lessened activation in the memory substrate during the association component of priming tasks.[109]
3. Implicit encoding is one function of neocortical association areas.

Classical Conditioning Using PET to compare rCBF before and after conditioning in which a tone (conditional stimulus) was paired with an electrical shock (unconditional stimulus), Hugdahl et al[139] found activation in the *right* dorsolateral, orbitofrontal, and inferior and superior frontal cortices; in the *right* temporal cortex; and in the *left* superior frontal cortex. This finding supports the notion that there is a right hemispheric bias for classical conditioning but stands in uncertain relationship to results from animal studies of fear conditioning, in which the amygdala, thalamus, and hypothalamus have been implicated in classical conditioning.

In another PET study using a classical conditioning paradigm, Blaxton et al[140] paired a tone (conditional stimulus) with an air puff (unconditional stimulus) so that the tone alone could elicit an eye blink. Trained subjects showed increased activity in the cerebellum and amygdala, the *right* frontal and temporoparietal cortex and cingulate gyrus, and the *left* occipital cortex and cingulate gyrus.[140,141] These studies together suggest that the network components of the memory system that are activated during classical conditioning may vary with the experimental paradigm and with the emotional significance of the unconditional stimulus.

Skill Learning Learning of a new motor skill has been found to be associated with increased activity in parietal regions, a possible reflection of a role of spatial attention in motor learning.[142] In contrast, performance of well-learned tasks is associated with increased activity in the primary motor cortex and supplementary motor area.[143] Using fMRI to study subjects training in a motor task, Karni et al[144] found initially decreased activity in the primary motor cortex over the first few weeks of training. Subsequently, increased activity was seen in the same area, and it persisted for several months, suggesting that acquisition of motor skills is associated with a slowly evolving reorganization of the motor cortex that is reflected in increased activity in the area. This notion is supported by the finding of Shadmehr and Holcomb.[145] They used PET to show that, in the early stages of skill learning, prefrontal areas of the brain were preferentially activated. Within 6 h of completion of training, increased activity had shifted to premotor, posterior parietal, and cerebellar cortical strucures. Based on these findings, the investigators suggested that task learning entails the construction of an internal model of the task. The brain can use this internal model to "predict and compensate for mechanical behavior." According to this notion, as time passes after practice, even though practice has ended, the neural representation of the internal model undergoes solidification and ramification. This is the concept of dynamic memory based upon malleable brain substrates of memory.

The Amnestic Syndrome

The amnestic syndrome is characterized by impaired ability to learn new information (anterograde amnesia) and impaired recall of old memories (retrograde amnesia). There also may be positive phenomena, such as confabulation in amnesia.[146] Amnestic patients may have relative preservation of other intellectual capacities and of implicit memory processes.[101,108,147,148] There are many causes of amnesia, including stroke, anoxia, trauma, dementing illnesses, infections, epilepsy, electroconvulsive therapy, medications and recreational substances, metabolic encephalopathy, neoplasm, and demyelination. The differential distribution, extent, and nature of brain structures involved in these conditions explains the different patterns of amnesia seen, such as the dominantly anterograde amnesia of alcoholic Korsakoff's syndrome (mammillary body disease) and the more generalized amnesia of Alzhheimer disease (hippocampal and neocortical disease).[149,150] In general, the most severe amnestic syndromes follow bilateral cerebral, especially limbic, damage.[151]

Brain Structures in Amnestic Syndromes A large number of brain structures have been implicated in amnestic syndromes.[101] Amnesia often follows medial temporal cortex damage that occurs with herpes simplex encephalitis, epilepsy surgery,[152,153] trauma, and stroke. When it is unilateral, temporal damage can produce material-specific amnesias: amnesia for verbal materials with left temporal damage, and amnesia for visual-spatial information with right temporal damage.[101] Diencephalic damage appears to underlie Korsakoff's amnesia, with involvement of the mammillary nuclei of the hypothalamus and nuclei of the thalamus.[154] Focal mammillary body damage may be associated with amnesia; Tanaka et al[155] reported deficits in delayed recall after surgical removal of a craniopharyngioma that left mostly local mammillary atrophy. Damage to orbitofrontal cortex after rupture of anterior communicating artery aneurysms has been associated with an amnestic syndrome. Damage to the fornix, hippocampus, and thalamus is associated with amnesia as well, and these structures are discussed below.

Fornix The fornix projects from the hippocampus to the mammillary body, connecting two important structures in memory. Because the fornix is long and narrow and lesions that damage it selectively are uncommon, whether fornix damage alone could cause amnesia has been difficult to determine.[156] Furthermore, studies of fornicotomy patients have not always supported an important role for the fornix in memory.[157]

Better imaging has made it clearer that fornix damage can cause amnesia. This has been seen in patients who have had surgical removal of third ventricular cysts. The fornix abuts the third ventricle where these cysts are found and can be damaged during cyst removal while other brain structures in the memory system remain relatively intact. Gaffan et al[158] studied two patients who developed amnesia after transcallosal removal of a colloid cyst via the left lateral ventricle. When compared to another group of patients with stroke-related amnesia, the post-operative group showed similar patterns of anterograde memory loss in standard memory tests such as scene recognition. The patient bearing bilateral fornix lesions was more severely affected than the patient with a unilateral right-side fornix lesion. In the postoperative group, MRIs verified that the fornix was damaged, while the thalamus, mammillothalamic tract, hippocampus, amygdala, and parahippocampal areas were intact. Figure 8-15 shows a third ventricular colloid cyst and its proximity to the fornix.

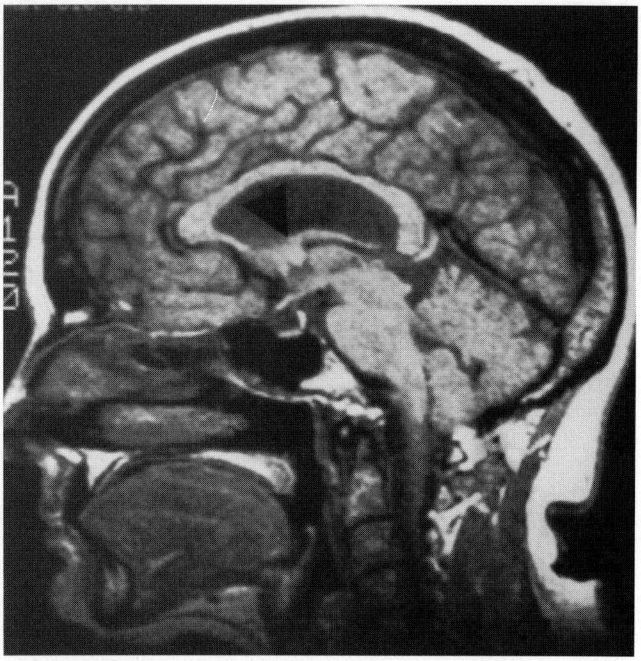

Figure 8-15
Sagittal MRI (TR 800 ms, TE 15 ms, 8-mm slice thickness) at the level of the midline, showing an abnormal high-signal mass (colloid cyst) abutting the fornix; the fornix is marked by the lower tip of the black triangle, with the high-signal colloid cyst immediately below. (Courtesy of Dr. Jack Greenberg, Philadelphia.)

Several other case reports reinforce the observation that fornix lesions produce anterograde amnesias. D'Esposito et al[159] reported a patient with traumatic brain injury (TBI) who had persistent anterograde amnesia. His CT scan showed a lesion only in the proximal posterior portions of both fornices. Calabrese et al[157] studied a patient who had sustained relatively focal fornix damage during a retrochiasmal astrocytoma removal. Subsequently, the patient exhibited an anterograde verbal and nonverbal amnesia, with relative preservation of implicit memory processes and other intellectual functions.

Thalamus Lesions restricted to the thalamus can cause severe amnesia; different forms of amnesia can result from discrete lesions in different parts of the thalamus. As in the case of the fornix, identifying the role of each thalamic structure in human memory has been difficult because, until recently, lesions affecting specific thalamic nuclei have been difficult to document. Mennemeier et al[160] studied a patient with a thalamic lesion who showed difficulty incorporating new items into long-term memory and impaired ability to process multiple bits of information simultaneously. Working from

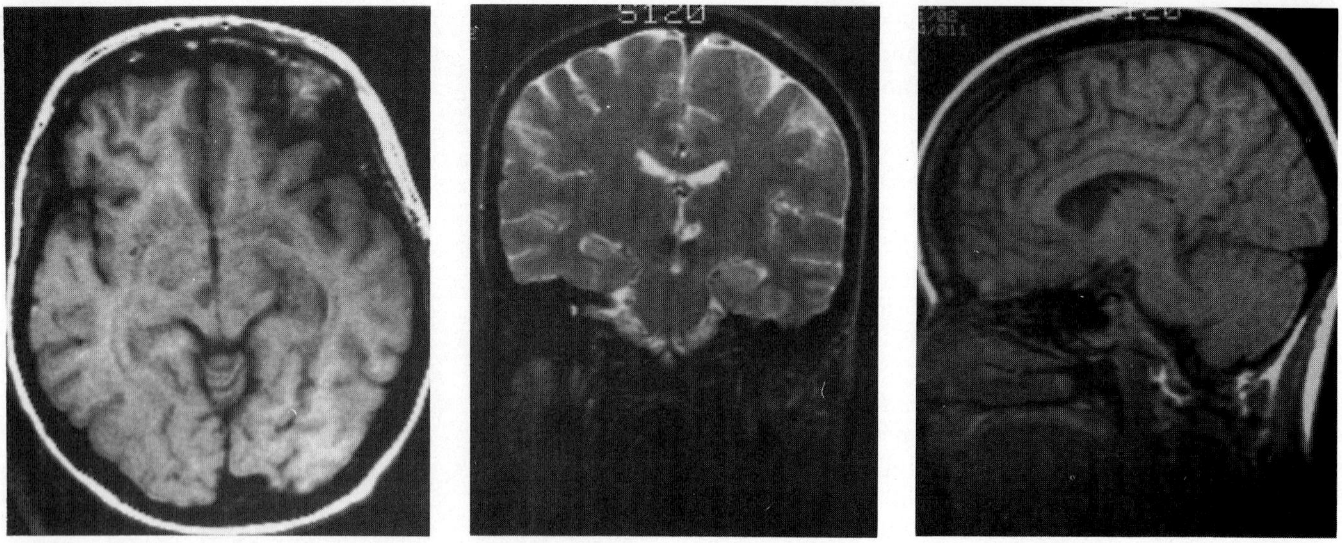

Figure 8-16
MRI of the head showing a thalamic infarction. (Left) Transaxial slice (TR 2000 ms, TE 80 ms, 2/2). (Middle) Coronal slice (TR 2400 ms; TE 80 ms, 2/2. (Right) Sagittal slice (TR 600 ms; TE 20, 1/1). See also Fig. 8-17. (Figure and modified legend from Mennemeier et al,[160] copyright 1992 by the American Medical Association. Used by permission.)

coronal, sagittal, and horizontal MRI images, they mapped the lesion onto a stereotactic atlas, finding that the lesion affected the caudal intralaminar and medial nuclei of the left thalamus and the mesencephalic gray matter. Nuclei that are generally viewed as especially important in memory, including the mammillary bodies, mammillothalamic tract, anterior thalamic nuclei, and most mediodorsal thalamic nuclei, were undamaged. This is depicted in Figs. 8-16 and 8-17.

Consistent with the imaging data, their patient's amnesia was not characterized by the severe encoding deficits that may be seen with lesions in the latter areas. Rather, they concluded that the patient's memory problem was due to distractibility. Based on these findings, they suggested that there are at least two types of memory disturbance associated with diencephalic lesions. One is characterized by an encoding deficit, seen in patients with lesions of structures such as the mammillary bodies. For example, this type of deficit is seen in Korsakoff's syndrome and the amnesia of fornix lesions. The other type of diencephalic amnesia is characterized by the inability to withstand distractions, which inhibits the operation of otherwise intact encoding functions. This is seen in patients with intralaminar and medial thalamic nuclear lesions.

Malamut et al[161] studied a 28-year-old man who sustained acute thalamic lesions (probably infarctions related to a lupus anticoagulant). Several years after recovery from the acute illness, he continued to show severe anterograde amnesia on neuropsychological testing while he remained intact in other areas of cognition. Reconstructing the MRI image of the thalamic lesion on a brain atlas, the investigators found that the lesion involved the inferior thalamic peduncle and mammillothalamic tracts. These two structures connect the hippocampus to the diencephalon. This case suggests that these connections are vital for the explicit recall of new facts and events, and that their patient's amnesia was due to a disconnection between the diencephalon and hippocampus. Their patient's lesion did not affect most of the structures affected in the case of Mennemeier et al.[160] Therefore, the amnestic syndrome in these two cases differed.

Hippocampus Hippocampal degeneration is characteristic of Alzheimer disease and probably explains the prominence of amnesia in this disease. Temporary hippocampal dysfunction may underlie transient global amnesia[151] (see below). Epilepsy has been associated with memory impairments attributed to hippocampal sclerosis. In epileptic patients who undergo temporal lobectomy for intractable seizures, left hippocampal dysfunction is associated with verbal memory impairments (verbal material-specific amnesia), while right hippocampal dysfunction is associated with visual-spatial memory impairments.[162] Volumetric measurements obtained with MRI have shown a positive correlation between verbal memory impairment and left hippocampal volume loss in epileptic patients.[163] This work dovetails with histologic work showing that hippocampal pyramidal cell density in patients with medically refractory epilepsy is related to preoperative performance on verbal memory tests.[164]

Transient Global Amnesia Transient global amnesia (TGA) is the sudden onset, usually in people older than 50 years of age, of a temporary global anterograde amnesia.[165] Affected patients are unable to learn new infor-

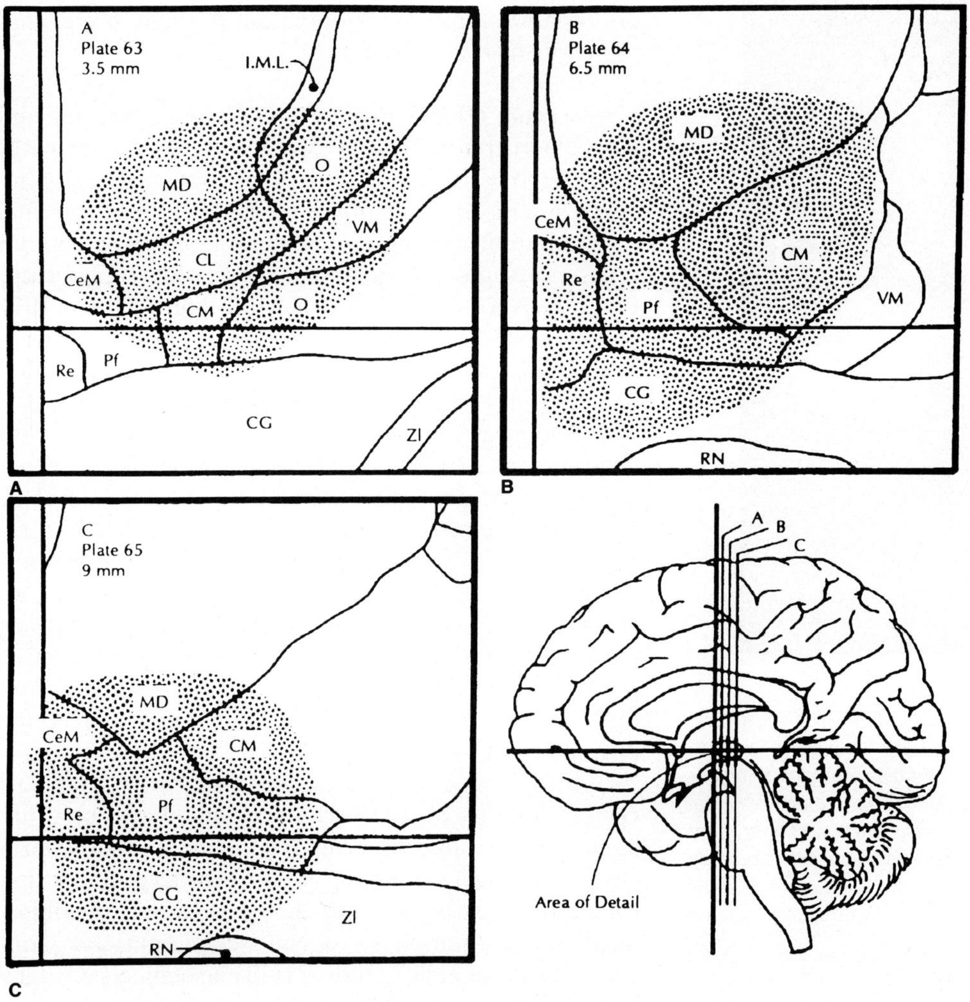

Figure 8-17

Line drawing showing the thalamic lesion seen on MRI in Fig. 8-16, plotted on sections from a stereotactic atlas that correspond to the three orientations of view of Fig. 8-16. Dark lines in **A, B, and C** *correspond to Y (horizontal grid) and Z (vertical grid) axes. Dark lines in the brain drawing represent X (horizontal) and Z (vertical) axes. Speckled area on* **A, B, and C** *represents the lesion. CG, central gray; CL, central lateral nucleus; CM, central median nucleus; CeM, central medial nucleus; MD, mediodorsal nucleus; O, oralis (principal ventral medial nucleus); Pf, parafascicular nucleus; Re, reuniens (medioventral nucleus); RN, red nucleus; VM, ventral medial; ZI, zona incerta. Measurements in millimeters under plate numbers indicate the distance of the plane of the section posterior to the point midway between the anterior and posterior commissures (Figure and legend modified from Mennemeier et al,[160] copyright 1992 by the American Medical Association. Used by permission.)*

mation or to recall recent events and are often anxious and confused. When the condition resolves several hours later, they are left with a retrograde amnesia for the event. Several causes of TGA have been suggested, including seizures, stress, migraine, and ischemia in the distribution of the posterior cerebral arteries. Neuroimaging evidence exists for several different localizations for TGA, including the hippocampus and anterior temporal structures,[166,167] thalamus,[168] temporal or temporoparietal lobes,[169,170,171] and left prefrontotemporal cortex/lentiform nucleus.[172] Some functional imaging studies have shown a variety of structures involved in TGA, differing from patient to patient.[173] The multiplicity of structures found to be involved in cases of TGA raises the issue of multiple routes to TGA or even multiple forms of TGA.[172]

Perhaps because of the transience of the acute amnestic syndrome in TGA, anatomic imaging rarely can be done during an episode. When performed afterward, imaging usually shows no lesion. When MRI or functional imaging can be brought to bear in a timely manner in these patients, reversible abnormalities sometimes can be seen. Figure 8-18 shows an MRI done during an episode of TGA in a 68-year-old woman. Compared to the rest of the brain, an increased signal is seen in the hippocampus, most prominently on the right. A follow-up MRI (not available) done 2 weeks later, after recovery, no longer showed signal asymmetry in the hippocampus. This reversible change may have been caused by hippocampal vascular or migrainous phenomena.

Perception, Agnosia, and Neglect

Normal perception requires the assembly of sensory data into meaningful wholes so that visual, auditory, and somesthetic phenomena can be recognized. Recognition exists when a person can identify a stimulus array, feel a subjective familiarity with the array, and behave in an adaptive way toward the array.[174] Much of what is known about the brain substrate of recognition comes from the study of patients with failures of recognition, or agnosia, due to brain damage (see "Visual Agnosia," below). Because the bulk of neuroimaging work on agnosia concerns visual agnosia, the discussion in this chapter concentrates on normal and abnormal visual perception.

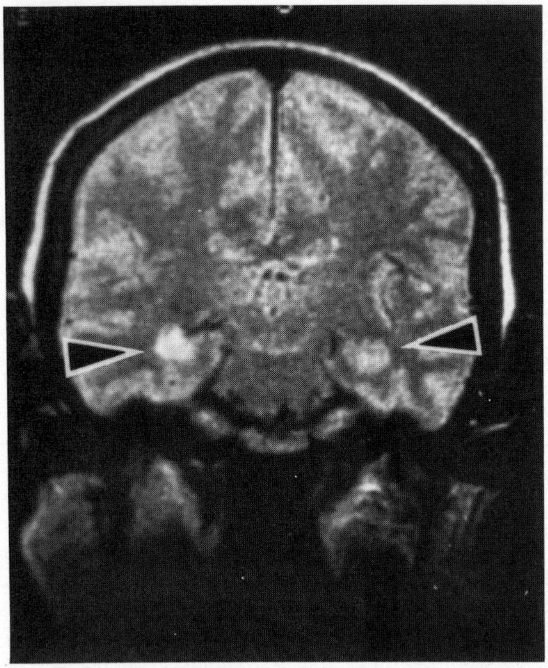

Figure 8-18
Transaxial MRI (TR 1500 ms, TE 80 ms, 5-mm slice thickness) obtained during an episode of transient global amnesia in a 68-year-old woman. The signal intensity in the right hippocampus is higher compared to the left. Arrows mark the relative hyperintensity of signal in the right compared to the left hippocampus. Two weeks later, after resolution of the attack, the signal asymmetry has resolved. (Courtesy of Dr. Jack Greenberg, Philadelphia.)

Visual Perception

Visual perception requires the normal functioning of a large array of brain structures, including the retina; lateral geniculate thalamic nucleus; visual radiations; striate cortex, or area 17; and visual association cortex, or areas 18 and 19. Additional temporal, parietal, and frontal areas participate in visual perception as well as in other types of neuropsychological information processing. A new understanding of how these structures interact in supporting normal visual perception has followed the development of functional imaging.

Visual perception is not a homogeneous neuropsychological function. Rather, it seems to consist of several interrelated visual functions distinguished by the nature of the visual information being processed. First, processing of information about the identity of an object (what it is) is somewhat separate from the processing of information about its spatial location (where it is). Second, information about the color of an object seems to be processed differently from information about its form. Third, while faces are objects, processing of faces differs from that of other objects, possibly because the critical social importance of faces was an evolutionary selection pressure for according face analysis special consideration in the visual system. The brain structures that form the substrates of these perceptual functions are organized into overlapping but partially segregated networks of brain structures.[175]

Face versus Object Perception Face perception and object perception both involve ventral-temporal pathways. Studies of disordered perception in brain-damaged patients and functional imaging studies in normal research subjects suggest that general object perception relies more upon left-sided structures, while face perception relies more upon right-sided structures. Using PET Haxby et al[176,177] found that face perception tasks were associated with increased activity in the right frontal and temporal lobes and bilaterally in the occipital areas. This finding is consistent with studies of patients with prosopagnosia (deficits in face perception and/or recognition), in whom lesions tend to involve bilateral or right-sided temporooccipital structures.[178,179] When research subjects are challenged with tests of object perception, subtraction studies using PET have shown increased rCBF in left occipital, left temporal, and left parietal areas when compared with face perceptual tasks.[180,181] In addition, bilateral activation in the occipital,[182] parietal,[180] and frontal areas[181,183] has been found during object perception tasks.

Object Identity and Object Location Functional imaging studies support a distinction between the processing of object identity information by a ventral occipitotemporal pathway and the processing of object location information by dorsal occipitoparietal pathways.[175] Kohler et al[182] studied rCBF in subjects engaged in tasks that required them to focus either on the location of an object or on what the object was. They found that, when the rCBF signature of an "object–spatial location" condition was subtracted from an that of an "object-identity" condition (a data manipulation designed to show brain activation that is unique to the process of identifying objects), increased temporal activity was found. This finding is consistent with the reduction of rCBF in ventral temporooccipital cortex that has been seen in patients with visual agnosia.[184] In contrast, when an object-identity condition was subtracted from an object-spatial location condition (a data manipulation designed to show brain activation that is unique to the process of determining where objects are in the visual space), increased activity was detected in parietal regions. This supports the notion of two separate streams of information analysis in the visual system.

The concept of dual perceptual streams is still being modified as some challenges are posed to the dual-stream hypothesis. Kraut et al[175] presented subjects with objects, some that were recognizable and real and some that were composites of real objects that formed a nonobject, such as a jet aircraft with the outline of a wrench where one wing should be (Fig. 8-19A). Distinguishing objects from nonobjects seemingly poses no challenge to the part of the visual system that determines spatial

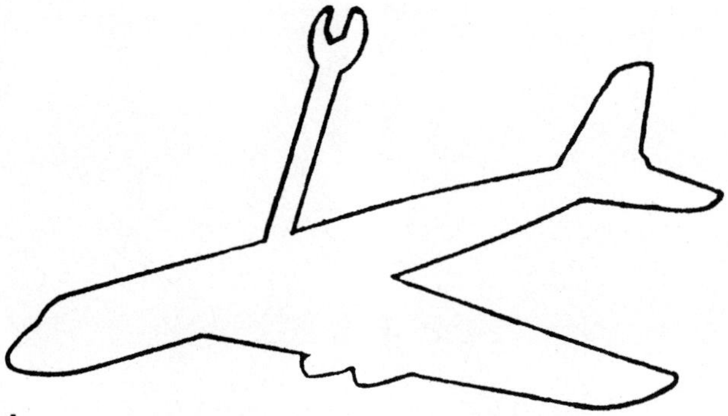

A

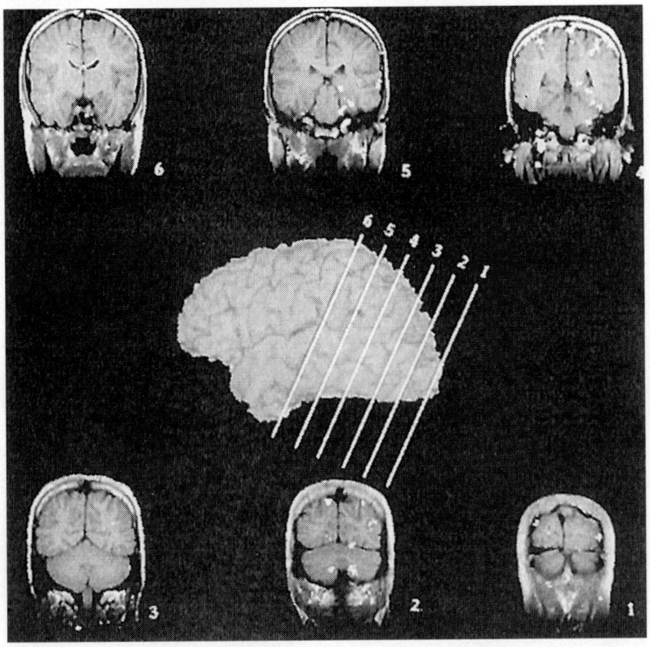

B

Figure 8-19
(A) *Drawing used in object shape processing experiment. This is a nonobject, a jet aircraft with the outline of a wrench in the location where one would expect to see the right wing.* **(B)** *Functional MRI data from one of the subjects in the experiment. In the center of the figure is a surface rendering of the brain. The lines superimposed on the surface rendering indicate the locations and angles of the sections from which fMRI data were gathered. The sections are angled perpendicular to the intercommissural line. The images arrayed around the periphery show the loci of fMRI signal changes superimposed on the T1-weighted anatomic template images gathered at the same locations. Subjects' left is to the right side of the figure. There are signal changes in regions corresponding to both the dorsal and the ventral pathways. Scattered regions of signal change outside the cerebral parenchyma are of unknown origin (perhaps reflecting vascular pulsation artifact) and were not consistently seen either within or across subjects. (Figure and modified legend from Kraut et al,[175] copyright 1997 by Lippincott-Raven. Used by permission.)*

location. Based on the dual-stream concept of visual processing, the expected result would be activation in the ventral object recognition ("what") pathway but not in the dorsal spatial location ("where") pathway. In actuality, investigators found that elements of both pathways were activated (Fig. 19B). The authors suggested that some ostensibly object-identification tasks can recruit the dorsal spatial-location visual processing stream when the object to be identified requires spatial analysis in itself. That is, odd and unexpected objects must be analyzed using a spatial-search strategy, which is done using the spatial-search substrate. This finding may require expansion of the notion of what spatial search means in the visual system and has implications for the nature of forms of agnosia. For example, simultanagnosia may sometimes represent loss of the ability to apply spatial-search strategies to a whole object in order to determine what it is.

Color versus Form Perception The processing of luminance, or brightness, of a percept seems to involve structures different from those involved in the processing of color. Processing of both of these aspects of visual experience seems separable from processing of form. In a PET study, Lueck et al[185] found increased activity in the lingual and fusiform gyri in the visual cortex when subjects were stimulated with a multicolored abstract display, compared to a condition where subjects viewed equiluminous shades of gray. This activity was greater in the left than in the right hemisphere. Other studies have identified predominantly left-sided rCBF increases in normal subjects during the performance of color compared to form discrimination tasks.[186] Functional imaging studies performed in patients with deficits in color processing (achromatopsia), however, have revealed nonlateralizing deficits in the visual cortex.[187] Thus, the picture of lateralization of color, brightness, and form perception remains unclear.

Summary Enough consistent data exist to support the view that visual perception recruits partially separable neural networks in which processing of different stimulus dimensions occurs simultaneously and in parallel. There may be a further synthetic function that assembles all of this processing in order to generate the perception of a whole object. Alternatively, the perception of the whole may be an emergent property of the simultaneous activity of parallel visual analytic circuits.

Visual Agnosia

Agnosia and the "Binding Function" To a degree, failures of a synthetic function that serves to bind the separate threads of perceptual function into a meaningful percept may underlie the phenomenon of agnosia.[188] Agnosia is said to exist when a patient fails to recognize a stimulus array despite having intact basic sensory systems and a normal level of arousal.[101] Agnosia usually is modality specific; visual, auditory, and somesthetic agnosia can occur independently of one another. Sudden and dramatic agnosia usually is caused by stroke and trauma. A more insidious onset of agnosia suggests a degenerative process, and a wide range of pathologic processes can produce agnosia.[174]

Phenomenology of Visual Agnosia Several phenomena are subsumed under the general category of visual agnosia. *Alexia* is the failure to recognize written words. When uncomplicated by other higher cognitive abnormalities, alexia implies a lesion in the distribution of the left posterior cerebral artery interrupting posterior callosal fibers.[189] Although often accompanied by a left homonymous visual field defect, alexia is not due to visual loss. It is an agnosia because affected patients can see and describe letters but cannot recognize them. *Prosopagnosia* is the inability to recognize familiar faces and often is accompanied by bilateral cerebral lesions, especially affecting anterior inferior occipital regions, the visual association cortex.[190,191] The bilaterality of the lesions in prosopagnosia is somewhat at variance with functional imaging work suggesting a right-hemispheric preponderance in the processing of face information. Some work does show bilateral cerebral activation when experimental subjects are engaged in face analysis tasks (see above).[178,179]

In *visual object agnosia* patients fail to recognize a wide range of objects, not just faces. It implies bilateral temporooccipital junction lesions.[192] This is illustrated in a case of a 66-year-old right-handed man who presented with stroke manifested by the sudden onset of aphasia and visual agnosia. Two years beforehand he had sustained a right occipital infarct that produced an isolated left homonymous hemianopsia. The aphasia caused by his second stroke was marked by impaired repetition, variable fluency, moderately impaired comprehension, and difficulty naming objects by vision alone. Naming was improved by touching the object, suggesting visual anomia or optic aphasia. Agnosia was marked by alexia, impaired ability to demonstrate use of objects, and loss of subjective familiarity with many simple objects. At times visual recognition suddenly occurred, a phenomenon called unblocking or static visual agnosia.[190,193] His MRI scan (Fig. 8-20) shows bilateral lesions in the inferior temporo-occipital areas.

The effect on perception of damage in the superior visual association cortex is generally different from that which occurs with more inferiorly placed lesions. Inferiorly placed lesions may produce disorders of object spatial analysis, such as simultanagnosia (piecemeal visual recognition or inability to perceive the whole of a visual array),[194] impaired depth discrimination, and Balint's syndrome (simultanagnosia; optic ataxia, or deficit of visual reaching; and ocular apraxia, or deficit of visual scanning).[190]

The variability of outcomes of damage to the superior and inferior visual association cortices supports several key points about the anatomic basis of visual perception and agnosia that are implied by functional imaging studies in normal perception (see above). First, the visual analytic system appears to be bipartite, with a dorsal, or superior, part responsible for spatial aspects of vision and a ventral, or inferior, part responsible for object

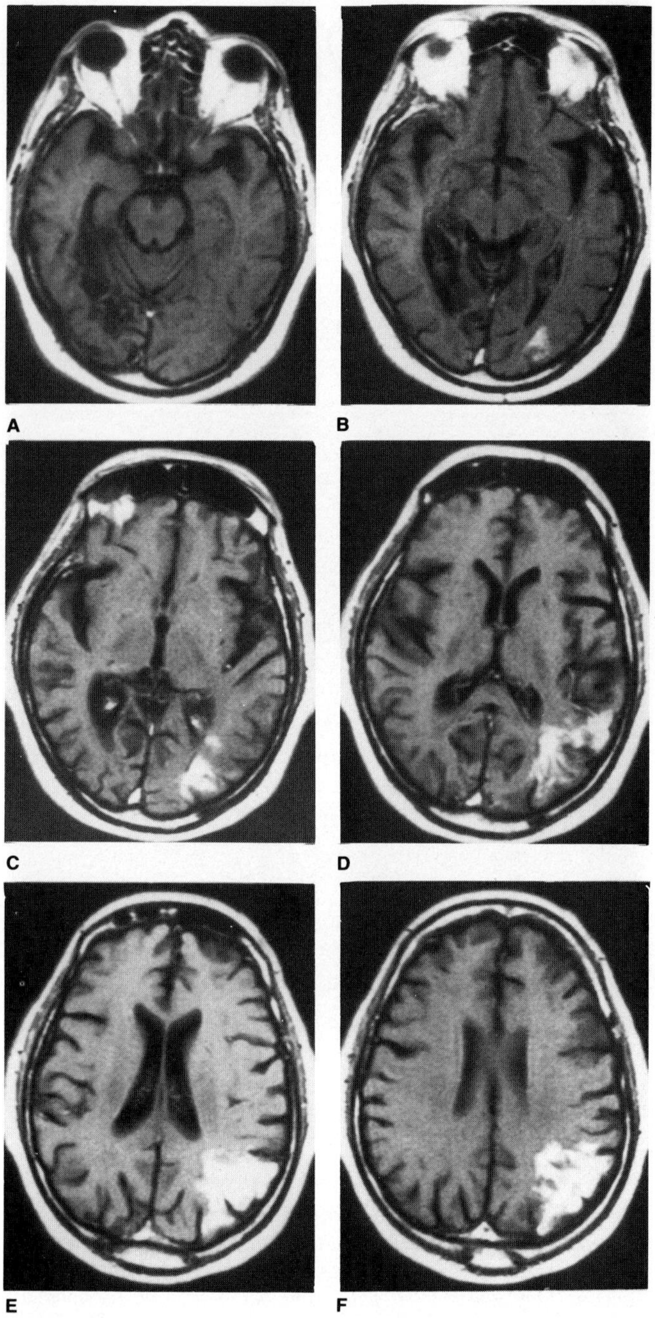

Figure 8-20
MRI in visual agnosia. Transaxial slices (TR 750 ms, TE 20 ms, 13 mL gadolinium). More superior slices **(D–F)** *show an area of enhancement in the left parieto-occipital area highlighting a recent infarction. More inferior slices* **(A–C)** *show a low-signal nonenhancing area in the right frontotemporoparietal area produced severe visual agnosia. The right-side lesion alone was associated with left homonymous hemianopsia. The left-side lesion combined with the right-side lesion was associated with conduction aphasia, visual anomia, and visual agnosia.*

identification.[195] Second, the visual work of spatial analysis and object recognition may occur simultaneously, that is, by parallel processes.[194]

In some patients with agnosia, PET or SPECT has demonstrated neurophysiologic abnormalities that were not suspected based upon the anatomic images. Milner et al[196] studied a patient with visual form agnosia, characterized by impaired visual recognition and discrimination of shape, reflectance, and orientation. An MRI showed signal abnormality in the bilateral lower occipital regions and in the globus pallidus. A SPECT study showed reduced cortical blood flow in the left posterior parietal, temporooccipital, and frontal regions, showing the presence of metabolic abnormalities distant from the zone of damage as seen on the MRI. Milner et al[196] suggested that their patient's deficits stemmed from disconnection of visual information from a central processor and from damage to the magnocellular visual pathway (M pathway; see above).

Neglect

Some patients with unilateral brain damage behave as if objects are not present in the contralesional space despite the lack of a primary sensory deficit.[197,198] This behavior is called hemineglect. The most striking hemineglect is of the left side after damage to the right parietal lobe, mainly the inferior parietal lobule. Striatal and thalamic lesions can also produce contralesional neglect,[199,200] and left frontal lesions can produce a milder right hemineglect.[201] Several bedside tests have been developed in order to assess severity of neglect for clinical and research purposes. This includes, for example, line and letter cancellation tasks (patients must cross out, or cancel, lines or letters arrayed across a sheet; ignored targets are typically in the negelected part of space)[190] and line bisection tests (bisecting a line to left of center implies right hemineglect).[202]

Several major issues guide the study of neglect:[203]

1. Is neglect caused by disruption of sensory-attentional, internal representational, or motor-intentional processes?[198,204–206]
2. To what degree is neglect due to loss of functions subserved by a particular brain area, hypofunction of distal intact structures that have lost critical input from damaged areas (diaschisis), or disconnection of important components of perceptual systems from one another?
3. Are there different syndromes of hemineglect depending upon which part of the brain is damaged?

Addressing the latter question, Binder et al[208] used the template system of Damasio and Damasio[56] to study CT scans of patients with right-hemispheric stroke. They divided their patients into three main groups based on clinical findings: a neglect group showing mainly line bisection errors and sometimes cancellation errors (neglect-bisection group), a neglect group showing cancellation errors only (neglect-cancellation group), and a group showing no evidence of neglect. The CT templates of patients within each group separately were superimposed on one another to produce composites of lesions associated with each clinical pattern. They found that the neglect-cancellation group had mainly frontal or deep subcortical lesions. The neglect-bisection group had mainly posterior parietal lesions, while in patients without neglect these areas were spared.

Based upon these and prior findings, Binder et al[208] interpreted their results as supporting a multicomponent model of attention. In their model, both frontal and parietal structures mediate various component functions in the service of overall attentional functions. Whether these component functions are perceptual, executive, motor exploratory, or of some other nature remains unclear.

The latter question was addressed by Kim et al[206] in the context of a study of motor neglect (poverty of action within the neglected field). Their patient had right frontotemporoparietal infarction (see Fig. 8-21) and left hemineglect manifested by left-side extinction during double simultaneous tactile stimulation and by neglect of left-sided targets during a line cancellation test. They compared eye movements during a line bisection test in the patient to those shown by normal subjects. Control subjects initially directed their gaze to the left end of the line to be bisected, then scanned to the right, and then looked back toward the center when finished. In contrast, the patient initially directed his attention to the right end of the line to be bisected without looking toward the left initially and without a final look to the center of the line when finished. They concluded that their patient had a directional ocular motor intention deficit, a form of motor neglect. They pointed out, however, that his abnormal ocular scanning may not be seen in all patients with neglect, especially in those with sensory-attentional or representational forms of neglect.

In work relevant to the issue of diaschisis in neglect, Vallar et al[209] used SPECT to study patients who developed neglect after subcortical stroke. In the early stages of recovery after stroke, their patients with neglect showed cortical hypoperfusion. As neglect waned over time, perfusion patterns returned toward normal. This suggests that one mechanism of subcortical neglect may be cortical diaschisis,[207] producing a disconnection syndrome.[36] The results of Bogousslavski et al[210] also support disconnection as one mechanism of neglect. Their patients had infarction restricted to the internal capsule and had contralesional hemineglect. A SPECT study showed hypoperfusion in the parietal cortex superior to the internal capsule, suggesting that functional, rather than anatomic, disturbance of the parietal lobe caused the neglect.

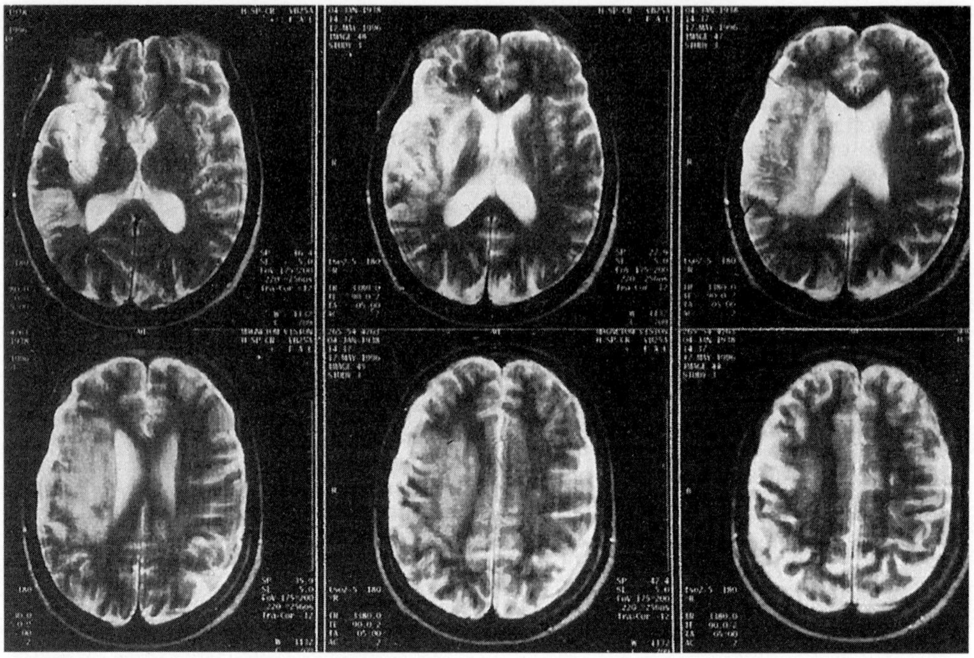

Figure 8-21
MRI of the experimental subject in Kim et al[206] showing diffuse middle cerebral arterial territory infarction involving the frontotemporoparietal area. (Figure and modified legend from Kim et al,[206] copyright 1997 by Lippincott-Raven. Used by permission.)

The Executive Functions

The Nature of Executive Functioning

Neurobehavioral operations, such as language, memory, perception, and skilled movements (praxis), must be organized and directed in order for a person to engage in adaptive behavior. The capacities that perform this function have come to be called the executive functions because of the supervisory role they appear to have.[211–213] An excellent summary of the nature of executive cognition was provided by Duffy and Campbell:[214] "Executive cognition refers to the organizing principles necessary to navigate the fluctuating and ambiguous challenges confronted in autonomous social behavior. These "metacognitive" functions are necessary to produce context-appropriate, goal-oriented behavior, including motivation, planning, self-regulation, and self-monitoring. A deficit in any of these supervisory mental processes will result in a breakdown in autonomous behavior and render the individual incapable of generating self-determined rather than environmentally determined (stimulus-bound) behavior."

The prefrontal cortex forms much of the neuroanatomic substrate for these functions, and thus the terms *frontal lobe functions* and *executive functions* are sometimes used interchangeably. While playing a central role in executive functioning, the frontal lobes are not the sole substrate of executive functioning. This chapter distinguishes between executive functioning as a neuropsychological process and the distributed network consisting of the frontal lobes and other brain structures that forms the substrate for executive functioning. The term *frontal lobe syndrome* is reserved for the syndromes of executive dysfunction that occur with frontal lobe disease. This chapter emphasizes, as other authors have done, that signs of executive dysfunction occur across a wide landscape of brain disease.[214]

The Core of Executive Functioning Most theorists would probably agree that executive functioning is evident when someone shows planning, initiation, and sustained execution of behavior or thought. During such behavior, executive functioning manifests in monitoring of the internal and external environment both locally and globally, taking into account the broad picture. Behavior guided in this manner is then steered around obstacles and toward advantageous paths. Executive control results in termination of the behavior when a goal is met and in assessment of the outcome of the behavior.

A large list of executive neuropsychological abilities and events, including the ones just listed, can be assembled. Which of these capacities is believed to lie at the center of executive activity and how these capacities are defined varies among various conceptions of executive function.

Conceptions of Executive Functioning According to Luria, executive functioning is represented by the programming, regulation, and verification of behavior. Impaired executive functioning causes poor performance on complex, conflicting, and unusual tasks.[215] Goldman-Rakic and Friedman[216] suggest that executive functioning is the guidance of behavior through representations of the outside world. These representations are the product of working memory. To Hecaen and Albert,[217] executive functioning is the regulation of intentions, programming of complex activity, and monitoring of activity. Goldberg and colleagues[218,219] suggest that the executive functions help to promote a balance between set maintenance (ability to be guided by internal representations) and set shifting (ability to respond to environmental changes). Shallice and Burgess[213] suggest that the executive functions act as a supervisory system responsible for error monitoring and correction and for adapting to novelty. They act mainly in situations in which no routine solutions exist to problems and thus creative solutions are demanded. Based on the observation that frontal-lobe–damaged patients are impaired in novel decision making, Godefroy and Rousseaux[220] suggest that novel decision making requires the creation of internal referents. These internal references associate a desired event with the information processing that must be done in order to obtain it. Baddeley[102] (see the discussion of working memory above) suggested that working memory plays a role not only in immediate information storage but also in the coordination of all mental resources via a central executive.[214] Fuster[221] saw the essence of executive functioning as motor-sensory integration producing purposeful behavior. It is especially needed when novel and complex behavior is needed. Mesulam[222] focused on the activation, inhibition, and integration of the outputs of ideomotor and sensorimotor distributed neural networks as the essence of executive functioning.

Writing from a cognitive rehabilitation perspective, Levin[223] suggested that problems in behavioral self-regulation are the essence of executive dysfunction. Impaired self-regulation leads to loss of autonomy after head injury. He lists the key features of behavioral self-regulation as "problem identification; generation of alternative solutions; selection, initiation, evaluation, and revision of solutions according to environmental consequences." In this view, key to the operation of these executive functions is "zoom navigation," the "process by which individuals observe their impact upon the environment and its effect upon their own behavior and subjective world." Zoom navigation is shifting of attention among perspectives ranging from most broad to most narrow. Hence, in Levin's view, distribution of attention is a vital aspect of executive functioning.

A central role for attention is provided in Barkley's view[224] of executive functioning as well. Writing about attention deficit disorder, he also suggests that the essence of executive functioning is behavioral self-regulation. There are four executive functions: (1) behavioral inhibition that prevents interference with adaptive behavior; (2) working memory that shifts behavior away from environmental control and toward internal control; (3) the appraisal of past events held in working memory; and (4) the manipulation of the information held in working memory so that it can be reconstituted in the service of behavioral diversity, flexibility, and creativity.

While they differ in terminology and emphasis, these views have in common the notion of *guidance* of behavior. Good behavioral guidance depends on a wide array of brain structures.

Brain Substrates of Executive Functioning It has already been stated that the frontal lobes are central components in a distributed network forming the executive substrate. It has been suggested that three parallel frontal-subcortical circuits form this substrate.[225] These circuits may share structures but encompass different parts of those structures. Two circuits link frontal lobes, caudate, globus pallidus, substantia nigra, and thalamus. The dorsolateral prefrontal circuit mediates the solution of complex problems, activation of remote memories, self-direction, shifting and maintenance of "sets," and verbal guidance of behavior. The orbitofrontal circuit mediates social behavior. The third circuit, the anterior cingulate circuit, links Brodmann area 24, striatum, olfactory tubercle, thalamus, and cingulate cortex, and mediates motivated behavior.

Considerable evidence from stroke and trauma patients supports the existence of these networks. More recently, functional imaging work has begun to illuminate the distributed network of executive functioning as well. In particular, several studies have found activation of networks of structures, including the frontal cortex, during working memory tasks. D'Esposito et al,[159] studying working memory, required subjects to perform non-working-memory tasks and working memory tasks. The non-working-memory tasks involved semantic judgment and mental rotation. The working memory task required the subjects to perform the two non-working-memory tasks simultaneously. This is a working memory task because of the need to hold information from one modality in active consideration while performing the task based on the other modality. This latter task would be expected to demand considerable deployment of mental resources, a key aspect of executive function. They found that only during dual task performance was there activation of the prefrontal cortex. This is illustrated in Fig. 8-22.

Jonides et al[226] used PET to identify substrates of working memory using a common research paradigm, the "*n*-back" task. Here, subjects are presented with a series of letters. For each letter presented, they must decide whether it matches the one presented *n* items earlier in the series. The higher the value of *n*, the greater the load placed on working memory. They found that, as *n* increased, activation increased in the dorsolateral prefrontal and posterior parietal cortex, as well as the thalamus and cerebellum. There was no increase in activation in areas mediating perception and verbal

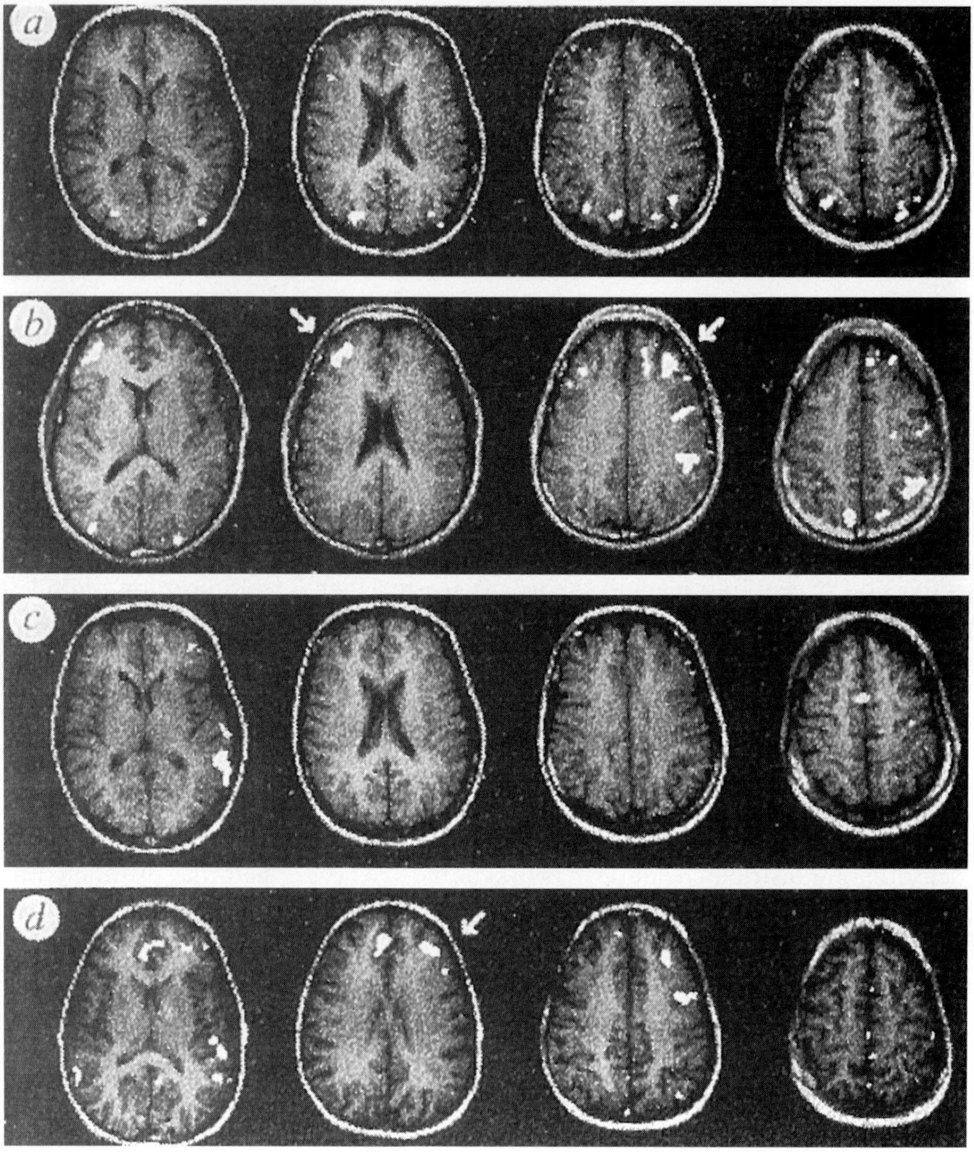

Figure 8-22 (Plate 19)
Functional MRI from the experiment of D'Esposito et al.[159] The figure depicts regions significantly activated under single- and dual-task conditions in individual subjects. Single-task activations are from the same subject; dual-task activations are from two different subjects. Comparison of the single-task and baseline conditions shows activation in the bilateral parieto-occipital regions for the spatial judgment task **(A)** *and the left temporal region for the semantic judgment task* **(C)**. *Regions significantly activated during the dual-task versus single-task conditions are shown in* **B** *and* **D**. *In the first comparison (dual-task minus semantic-task), activation is seen in prefrontal cortex anterior cingulate and premotor cortex* **(B)**. *In addition, activation is seen in bilateral parieto-occipital regions, which represents activation during the spatial judgment. In the second comparison (dual task minus spatial task), activation again is seen in prefrontal cortex and anterior cingulate* **(D)**. *In addition, activation is seen in bilateral superior temporal gyri, which represents activation during the semantic judgment task. See the original article for technical details of the fMRI procedure. (Figure and modified legend from D'Esposito et al,[159] copyright 1995 by Nature. Used by permission.)*

response. These studies emphasize the intimate link between working memory and executive functioning, a link that includes a common neurologic substrate.

Executive Dysfunction

Depending on the circumstances, executive dysfunction can be manifested by a wide range of maladaptive behavior, such as perseveration, impersistence, impaired planning, failure to be guided by feedback, "environmental dependency" (slavish response to the environment rather than being guided by internal plans), poor performance on tasks of novel decision making,[220] and poor self-control. Many general treatments of executive dysfunction are available, some containing extensive lists of the types of behavioral disturbances seen in executive dysfunction.[211–213, 215–219, 227–234] These deficits often occur in patients with frontal lobe damage and form some of the signs of the frontal lobe syndrome. These deficits also can occur with damage to frontosubcortical circuits of the executive system and to many other parts of the brain as well.

Frontal Lobes and Executive Dysfunction

The location of a lesion within the frontal lobes is an important determinant of the characteristics of the resulting executive dysfunction. For example, Truelle et al[235] classified movement errors made by patients with frontal lobe lesions into three main types: (1) simplification, in which only part of a required activity was performed (a planning deficit); (2) deautomatization, in which component movements of a whole behavior were not linked correctly (a sequencing deficit); and (3) disin-

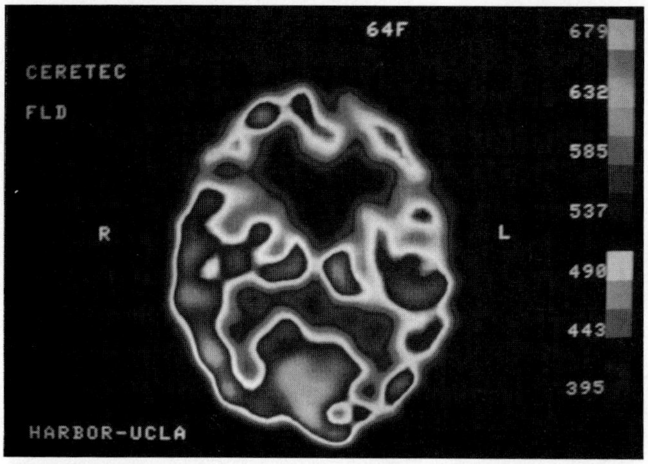

Figure 8-27 (Plate 21)
^{99m}Tc HMPAO transaxial SPECT image at the level of the basal ganglia from an AD patient. Minimal blood flow is depicted by colors at the bottom of the scale, with flow increasing progressively with colors toward the top of the scale. There is temporoparietal hypoperfusion, with relative preservation of frontal perfusion. Compare to Fig. 8-28. (Courtesy of Dr. Bruce L. Miller, University of California at Los Angeles.)

A fuller discussion of frontal dementia and AD is presented below.

Multiple Sclerosis Multiple sclerosis (MS) can produce a wide range of motor and cognitive abnormalities, both transient and fixed.[254] When accompanied by impaired performance on tests of executive function, these patients may show PET-demonstrated hypometabolism in frontal and other brain areas.[255,256]

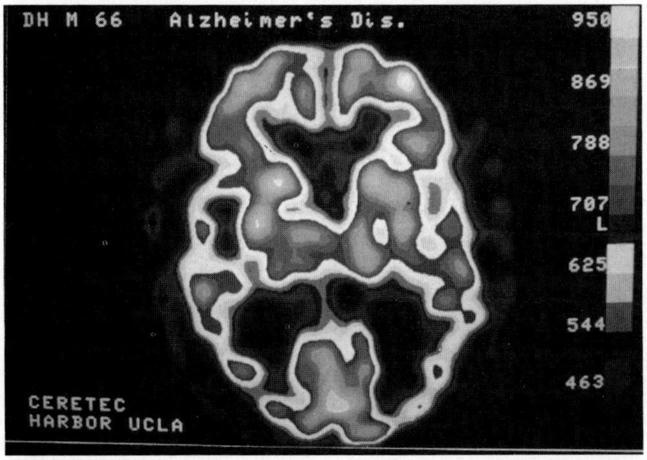

Figure 8-28 (Plate 22)
^{99m}Tc HMPAO transaxial SPECT image at the level of the basal ganglia from a patient with frontal lobe dementia. The hues on the color scale differ from those seen in the SPECT image in Fig. 8-27. As in Fig. 8-27, minimal blood flow is depicted by colors at the bottom of the scale, with flow increasing progressively with colors toward the top of the scale. There is frontal hypoperfusion with relative preservation of temporoparietal perfusion, the reverse of what is seen in Fig. 8-27. (Courtesy of Dr. Bruce L. Miller, University of California at Los Angeles.)

Closed Head Injury When the frontal lobes are damaged in head trauma, executive dysfunction frequently results.[257,258] Writing from a cognitive rehabilitation perspective, Levin[223] suggested that problems in behavioral self-regulation, that is, executive dysfunction, lie at the core of the loss of autonomy that occurs after head injury; this notion was discussed above in the treatment of concept of executive function. Since head trauma often causes damage in other areas of the brain as well, determining the relative contribution of frontal damage to executive dysfunction requires controlling for the effects of lesions in nonfrontal areas. Levin et al[257] described a subtractive MRI method designed for this purpose. In that study, MRI images from various patients with head trauma were overlapped in order to produce composites of lesions from different patients. They found that the most severe manifestations of executive dysfunction occurred with frontal lesions. Trauma is discussed further in the section on recovery of function, below.

Psychosurgery The ability to induce the behavioral changes of a frontal lobe syndrome, especially the calming aspects of the abulic state, was applied to agitated psychiatric patients using frontal leukotomies.[259] This operation interrupts the efferent and afferent supply of the frontal lobes, disconnecting the frontal lobes from other brain structures. Figure 8-31 shows the location of white matter damage in a patient many years after this procedure. Benson et al[260] discussed the long-term effects of these operations.

A contemporary psychosurgical procedure, stereotactic subcaudate tractotomy, is done in order to relieve severe symptoms of affective disorders, including unipolar depression, bipolar disorder, and obsessive-compulsive disorder (OCD). The volume of tissue destroyed is relatively small and aims to avoid the severe executive impairment that occurs in the frontal leukotomy. In their study of this procedure, Kartsounis et al[261] showed that postoperative impairment in tests of frontal lobe function (e.g., as the Modified Card Sorting Test) were correlated with widespread frontal edema visualized by MRI. When the MRI evidence of edema resolved, performance on these tests returned to preoperative levels. The MRI images supported their contention that the short-lived frontal dysfunction was due to edema rather than to substantial permanent damage to or disconnection of the frontal lobes from other parts of the brain.

Obsessive-Compulsive Disorder Obsessive-compulsive disorder is often characterized by intense intrusive thoughts and/or repetition of rituals such as checking or hand washing that accomplish little of practical value.[262] Several observations suggest that these behaviors repre-

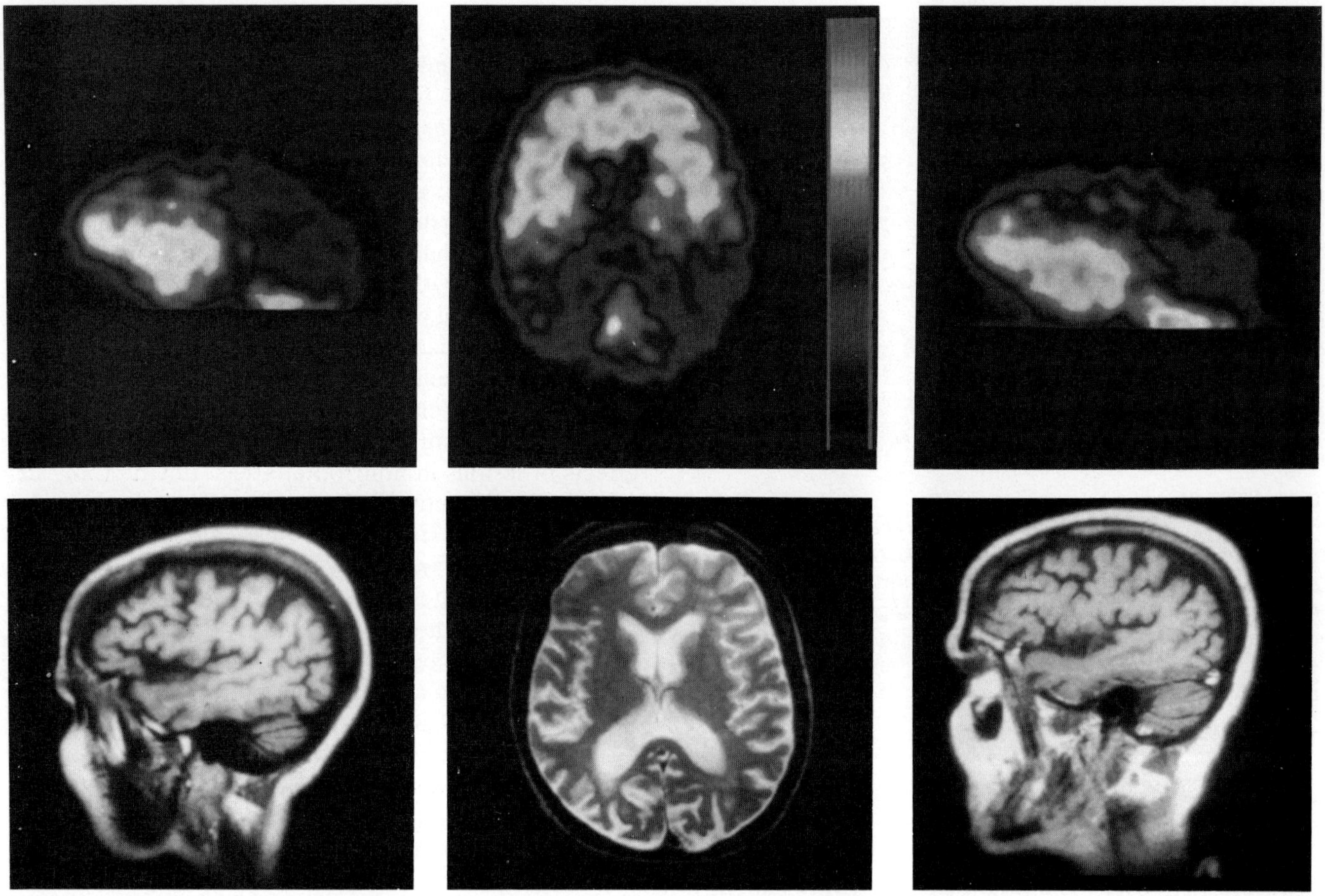

Figure 8-29 (Plate 23)

PET and MRI study of a 59-year-old woman with probable AD who presented with mild difficulties in memory, visual processing, and word finding that progressed to include profound comprehension deficits. Sagittal views of the left hemisphere (leftmost image) and the right hemisphere (rightmost image) on her MRI scan suggest the possibility of parietal atrophy. The sagittal PET images of the left hemisphere (leftmost image) and the right hemisphere (rightmost image) demonstrate reduced cortical functioning in parietal and posterior temporal cortices. The transaxial PET image (middle scan, oriented so that the left hemisphere is on the right of the image) emphasizes relative cortical dysfunction in left and right parietal and posterior temporal regions with relatively preserved functioning in primary visual cortex. High perfusion is represented by colors at the top of the scale. (Courtesy of Dr. Murray Grossman, University of Pennsylvania.)

sent a form of executive dysfunction. First, the repetitiveness of these behaviors is reminiscent of the perseveration that may occur in syndromes of executive dysfunction. Hollander and Wong[263] hypothesized that OCD involves aberrant assessment of harm in some patients. This may be due to accentuation of activity in frontal subcortical systems that makes it difficult for OCD patients to relinquish preferential sets (a way of viewing perseveration).

Second, subsets of OCD patients, such as patients with obsessional slowness,[264] may be impaired on tests of executive function, such as set shifting.

Third, evidence suggests that OCD may stem from abnormal serotonergic and dopaminergic activity in frontal cortical-basal ganglionic systems.[263,265] This idea is consistent with functional imaging data showing abnormal metabolic activity in the frontal lobes and subjacent basal ganglia in patients with OCD. It is consistent also with the ability of serotonin reuptake blockers to normalize neuropsychological function and frontosubcortical flow abnormalities seen in OCD patients.[263,266,267]

Both increased and decreased flow in frontosubcortical systems have been reported in OCD. Using PET, Baxter et al[268,269] found evidence of increased glucose metabolism in the orbital gyrus and possibly in the caudate nuclei in acute OCD patients. Using PET, Sawle et al[270] (see also for review) studied patients with obsessional slowness. They measured regional cerebral oxygen metabolism with ^{15}O and assessed the presynaptic nigrostriatal system with [^{18}F]-6-fluorodopa (^{18}F-dopa). They found hypermetabolism in the orbital frontal cortex and in the premotor and midfrontal cortices. These studies support the view that OCD may stem from overactivity in a frontosubcortical circuit.[218] In this respect,

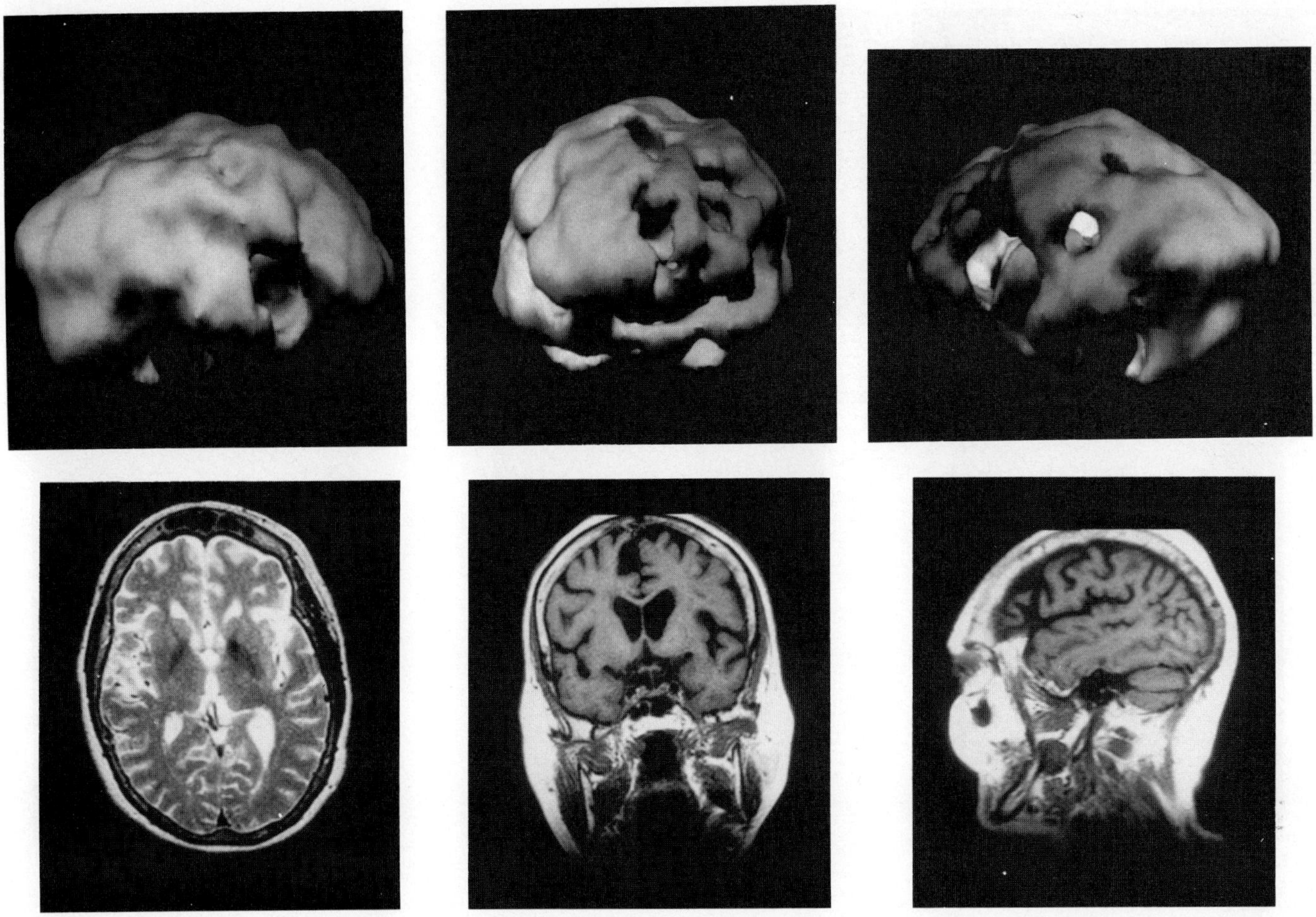

Figure 8-30 (Plate 24)
SPECT and MRI studies of a 63-year-old woman with probable Pick disease. She demonstrated progressive difficulty initiating speech as well as other activities over the past 6 years that more recently included episodic memory difficulty and bizarre behaviors. A sagittal view of her left hemisphere on MRI (leftmost image) demonstrates relative atrophy in frontal and anterior temporal structures. Coronal and transaxial views (oriented so that the left hemisphere is on the right of the image) also indicate relative frontotemporal atrophy that is most prominent in the left hemisphere. A three-dimensional reconstruction of her SPECT scan revealed prominent hypoperfusion throughout the left frontal lobe and anterior portions of the left temporal lobe on the left sagittal view (leftmost image). An anterior view of her SPECT scan (middle image, oriented so that the left hemisphere is on the right of the image) emphasizes the relative hypoperfusion in the left frontal lobe compared to the right frontal lobe. A sagittal view of the right hemisphere on the SPECT scan (rightmost image) reveals right anterior temporal hypoperfusion as well. (Courtesy of Dr. Murray Grossman, University of Pennsylvania.)

OCD may represent the opposite of the impulsivity seen in orbitofrontal stroke patients.

Some OCD patients show frontal hypometabolism[270] rather than hypermetabolism. The precise conditions under which frontal hypermetabolism and frontal hypometabolism occur in OCD remain to be defined.

Some forms of OCD may be caused by primary disease of the basal ganglia. Weilberg et al[271] described a man with OCD and impaired performance on tests of executive function (Stroop test and go/no-go tests).[252] He had a striatal lesion seen on MRI and CT scans. They noted the similarities between their patient's behavior and that of patients with Huntington disease and Tourette's syndrome. All three conditions are marked by varying degrees of executive dysfunction, obsessions and compulsions, and a movement disorder.

Attention Deficit Hyperactivity Disorder Attention deficit hyperactivity disorder (ADHD) in children is characterized by easy distractibility, impulsivity, failure to complete tasks, and restlessness. Perhaps its most bothersome manifestation in inability to maintain focus, especially in school.[272] Attention deficit hyperactivity disorder may persist into adulthood (residual adult attention deficit disorder, or ADD) and then can be manifested by poor job ratings because of task incompletion, inefficiency, and nonproductivity despite the expending of great energy at work.[273]

While inattention has been viewed as the essential difficulty in ADHD, increasingly it is being viewed more broadly as an inefficiency of executive functioning. It may represent a family of disorders with varying degrees of impaired vigilance, systematic search, and ability to

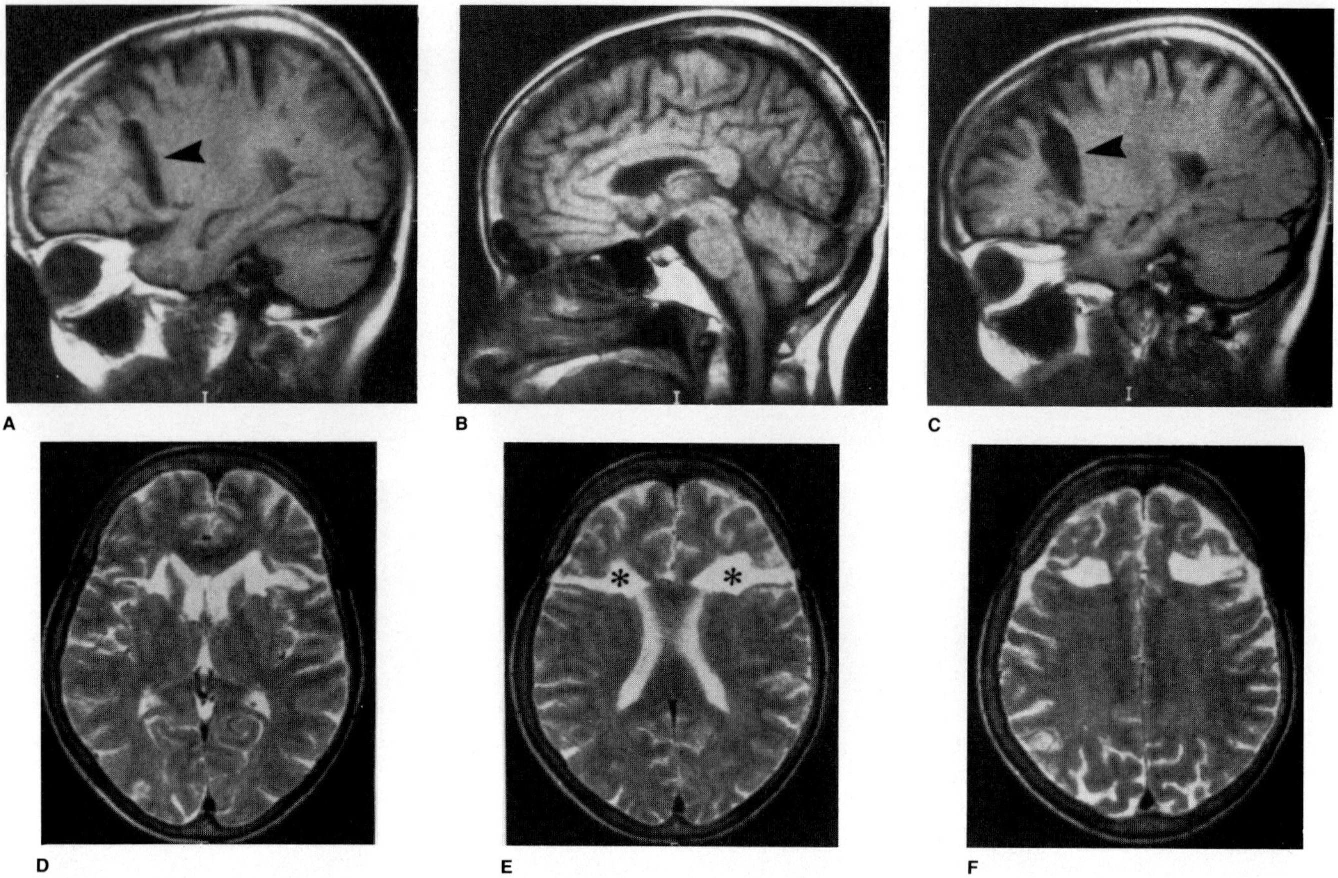

Figure 8-31

MRI of a patient with frontal leukotomy many years previously. **(A–C)** *Sagittal slices (TR 500 ms, TE 30 ms, 5.1-mm slice thickness). Arrowheads indicate low-signal areas reflecting white matter tissue loss.* **(D–F)** *transaxial sections (TR 3000 ms, TE 80 ms, 5.1-mm slice thickness). Areas of white matter tissue loss are seen as high-signal areas (indicated by asterisks in* **E***). (Courtesy of Dr. Jack Greenberg, Philadelphia.)*

inhibit inappropriate responses and perceptions.[224,272,273] There is some neuroimaging support for this idea. Several studies have found resting hypofunctioning of frontal structures in ADHD that normalized with methylphenidate (see Pennington for a review of these studies).[272]

These observations imply that ADHD may be a "mirror-image" disorder compared to OCD. Excess activity in frontosubcortical systems might produce perseverationlike behavior in OCD (stability bias).[236] This would contrast with deficient activity in frontosubcortical systems producing environmental dependency in ADHD (plasticity bias).[236] In view of the hypothesis of lateralized frontosubcortical functions, it is further possible that OCD represents either overactivity of left-side or underactivity of right-side frontosubcortical circuitry. The converse could be true with ADHD.

Not all functional imaging data clearly implicate frontosubcortical system dysfunction in ADHD. In a fMRI study, Sunshine et al[274] challenged subjects on a visual vigilance test, an executive-attentional test. They found activation in regions that are usually activated in non-ADDH people during such tasks, including bilateral middle frontal gryi, superior parietal lobules, and inferior parietal lobules. In the ADHD subjects, there may have been slight excess activation in the right inferior and left superior parietal lobules.

NEUROIMAGING AND NEUROBEHAVIORAL SYNDROMES

Dementia

Definition

Dementia is the global deterioration of mental and behavioral capabilities that occurs in the absence of focal deficits such as aphasia, developmental mental abnormalities such as dyslexia, and acute impairments in level of consciousness such as obtundation and delirium.[275] There are several standardized definitions of dementia. For example, according to the fourth edition of the *Diagnostic and Statistical Manual of Mental Disorders*,[276] dementia is manifested by impairment in social and occupational functioning and in memory and other cognitive capacities, in the absence of a delirium or axis I psychiatric disorder. Clinical criteria for the dementia resulting from specific diseases, such as AD[277] and vascular disease,[278,279] have been formulated also.

Patients with dementia can have a wide range of deficits in language, memory, visual-spatial skills, calculation, executive functioning, speed of cognitive processing, personality, mood, speech, and motor abilities.[275,280,281] The profile of mental and behavioral abnormalities seen in dementia varies with the main location of brain disturbance. Three dementia profiles are especially common and have received the most attention in clinical research: the temporoparietal pattern exemplified by AD, the frontotemporal pattern typified by Pick disease, and the subcortical pattern typified by multi-infarct dementia. Each of these patterns is discussed below. For more detail, the reader may consult many reviews of dementia written from behavioral neurologic and neuropsychological viewpoints.[2,5]

Imaging and Dementia

Anatomic Imaging Computed tomography and MRI can help to distinguish Pick disease from AD by the different distribution of gyral narrowing that tends to occur in each condition: frontotemporal in Pick disease[282] and temporoparietal in AD[283,284] (see Figs. 8-27 through 8-30). Anatomic imaging can identify infarctions and diffuse white matter disease (multi-infarct dementia) associated with cognitive decline.[285] The diffuse cerebral cortical and basal ganglia variant of Creutzfeldt-Jakob disease may be suggested by the combination of rapidly progressive dementia and high signal in the basal ganglia on long relaxation time (TR) MRI images. Figure 8-32 presents an MRI of a patient with Creutzfeldt-Jakob disease.

Functional and Planimetric Anatomic Imaging Usually neither the specificity nor the sensitivity of conventional anatomic imaging is sufficiently high to permit a definitive diagnosis in dementia solely on the basis of neuroimaging. In AD, MRI or CT scans can be normal, can show abnormalities common to aging regardless of mental state, or can show white matter abnormalities similar to those seen in multi-infarct dementia.[287–289] Functional imaging and high-resolution volumetric and planimetric CT and MRI are better able to distinguish between the brains of patients with some of these dementing illnesses and the brains of normal people of the same age.[290,291] These techniques eventually may be relied upon for definitive diagnosis in dementia. Functional imaging studies in dementia have encountered problems because of signal averaging across the cerebrospinal fluid (CSF)–parenchymal border zone in

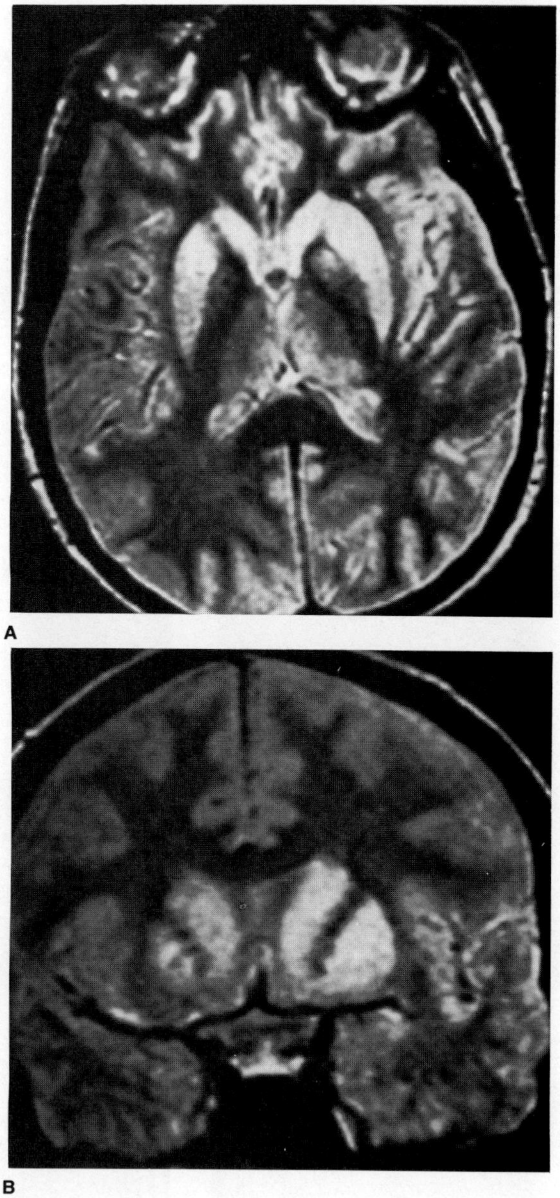

Figure 8-32
MRI of a patient with Cretuzfeldt-Jakob disease. **(A)** *Transaxial slices (TR 3000 ms, TE 30 ms).* **(B)** *Coronal slices (TR 3000 ms, TE 30 ms) at the level of the basal ganglia, showing an abnormally high signal in the basal ganglia, including the capsular gray matter bridges. No contrast agent was administered. This suggests gray matter disease. (Figure and modified legend from Milton et al,[286] copyright 1991 by Little, Brown. Used by permission.)*

atrophic cortex; attempts have been made to correct functional imaging data for atrophy.[292]

Spectroscopic Imaging Some forms of dementia, such as AD, are associated with neuronal loss. Anatomic and functional imaging provide little information about this variable other than the indirect evidence of neuronal loss seen in atrophy. Using atrophy as the sole measure of in vivo neuronal loss invites error, since glial replace-

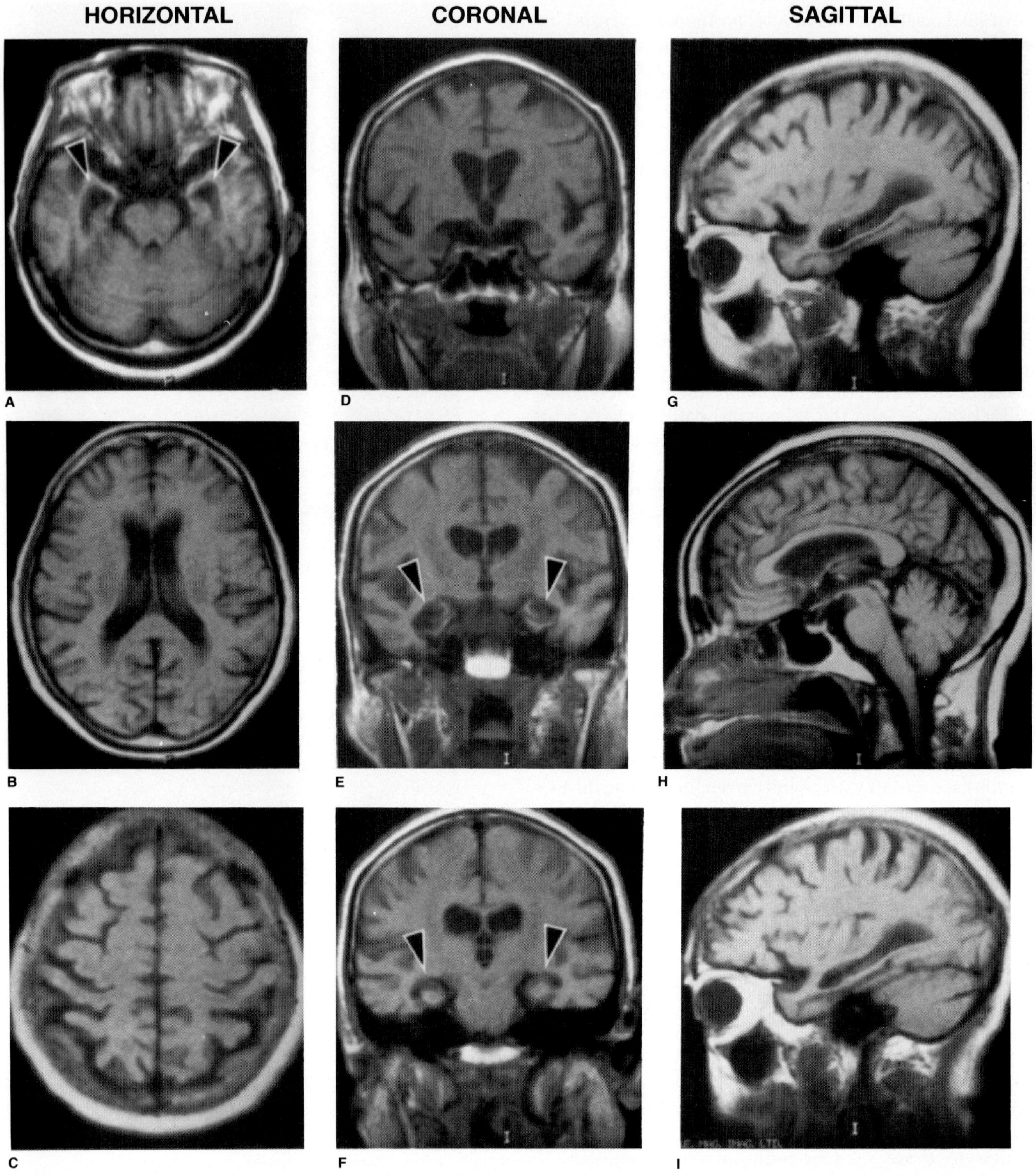

Figure 8-33

MRI in clinically diagnosed AD. **(A–C)** *Transaxial sections showing moderate sulcal and ventricular enlargement with disproportionate enlargement of the temporal horns of the lateral ventricles (arrows).* **(D–F)** *Coronal sections at the level of the hippocampus, demonstrating hippocampal atrophy (arrows).* **(G–I)** *Sagittal sections at the level of the temporal horns on the left* **(G)** *and right* **(I)**, *and midline* **(H)**. *The diagonally oriented areas of low signal in* **G** *and* **I** *represent the enlarged temporal horns. (All sections TR 600 ms, TE 30 ms, 10-mm slice thickness.) (Courtesy of Dr. Jack Greenberg, Philadelphia.)*

ment of vanished neurons can minimize macroscopically evident atrophy. Proton magnetic resonance spectroscopy (^{1}H MRS) and ^{1}H MRS imaging (^{1}H MRSI) can provide a measure of neuronal preservation that helps to circumvent this problem. It can detect cerebral constituents, including *N*-acetyl aspartate (NAA), an amino acid found in neurons but not in glia.[293] An example of this is provided below in the sections on AD and HIV dementia.

Alzheimer Disease

Alzheimer disease is a degenerative condition characterized by the accumulation in the brain of abnormal structures, mainly senile plaques and neurofibrillary tangles. Errant processing of the amyloid precursor protein and the TAU protein are major contributors to this accumulation.[281,294] Other neuropathologic features of AD include congophilic angiopathy, Hirano bodies, granulovacuolar degeneration, and neuronal loss. The main site of neuropathology in AD is in the temporal lobes, especially in the hippocampus. Patients with AD can display a wide array of mental and behavioral symptoms and signs, such as amnesia, apraxia, agnosia, aphasia, delusions, and abnormal behaviors, suggesting predominantly temporal and parietal dysfunction.[281]

Several attempts have been made to identify a neuroimaging signature of AD. Magnetic resonance imaging and CT planimetric and volumetric measurements of structures, such as the hippocampus, that are affected in AD; measurements of CSF space and gray matter volume; and functional imaging of cerebral metabolism and blood flow have been studied for this purpose.[10,292,295–299]

Hippocampus The hippocampus tends to be atrophied out of proportion to other brain structures in AD. This condition is associated with the impairment of episodic memory that is typical of AD.[300] Figure 8-33 shows the MRI of a woman with the clinical diagnosis of AD. When the coronal view of Fig. 8-33 is compared to a similar view in Fig. 8-45 (MRI of a patient with HIV dementia), the hippocampus is atrophied out of proportion to atrophy elsewhere in the patient with AD. The hippocampus is not atrophied in the patient with HIV-related dementia.

High-resolution quantitative MRI techniques have been developed for measuring hippocampal atrophy and ventricular enlargement in patients with AD. Kesslak et al[298] measured hippocampal atrophy in AD with MRI, acquiring 5-mm coronal slice thicknesses with 2.5-mm intervening gaps. Pixels within regions of interest (ROI) were counted, providing a quantitative estimate of hippocampal, parahippocampal gyral, and striatal volumes. They found volume loss in the hippocampus and entorhinal cortex when compared to the striatum in patients with a clinical diagnosis of AD. These volume losses correlated well with scores on the mini-mental state examination. This suggests that this technique may prove to be clinically useful for diagnosing early AD when mental abnormalities first appear but before gross changes in the brain become evident with conventional anatomic brain imaging.

Jack et al[299] developed an MRI-based technique for measuring volumes in the anterior temporal lobe and hippocampus. They acquired images with 4-mm slice thicknesses without intervening gaps. The ROI were identified with borders defined by CSF-brain interface. Pixels within the ROI were counted, and normalized volume measures in the ROI were derived using measurements of total intracranial volume. They found that (1) the normalized volumes of anterior temporal lobe and hippocampus decreased with age in AD patients and age-matched control subjects, (2) 85 percent of AD patients had smaller normalized volumes for these structures than did normal age-matched control subjects, and (3) measures of hippocampal volume were superior to measures of anterior temporal volume in distinguishing AD patients from normal control subjects.

Refining this methodology, Jack and colleagues[291] derived volume measurements of the hippocampus, parahippocampal gyrus, and amygdala from 1.6-mm thick contiguous slices in early AD patients and elderly control subjects. They found that the volume of each of these medial temporal lobe structures was smaller in AD patients than in control subjects. Total hippocampal volume was superior to the other measurements for distinguishing normal elderly individuals from early AD patients. One of their comparisons between a normal elderly subject and an early AD patient is seen in Fig. 8-34.

The epsilon 4 allele at APOE, the polymorphic locus for apolipoprotein E, is a risk factor for AD. Hippocampal volume, as measured by volumetric MRI, has been found to be smaller in patients with the epsilon 4 allele, even before cognitive impairment has developed.[301] This suggests that the combination of APOE genotyping and volumetric MRI (and perhaps functional imaging as well) may provide combined diagnostic power in AD. Combining quantitative MRI and MRS may also provide extra predictive power in AD (see below).[293]

There are several limitations to the use of these techniques for the clinical diagnosis of AD. First, as Jack et al[299] note, there is overlap in ROI measurements between AD patients and normal subjects (although technical refinements may lessen the impact of this overlap).[291] Second, visual inspection of ROI, one way in which these techniques might be used routinely in a clinical setting, may not generate the same results as do quantitative methods, since the latter use mathematical adjustments. Third, neuronal loss, a key feature of AD,

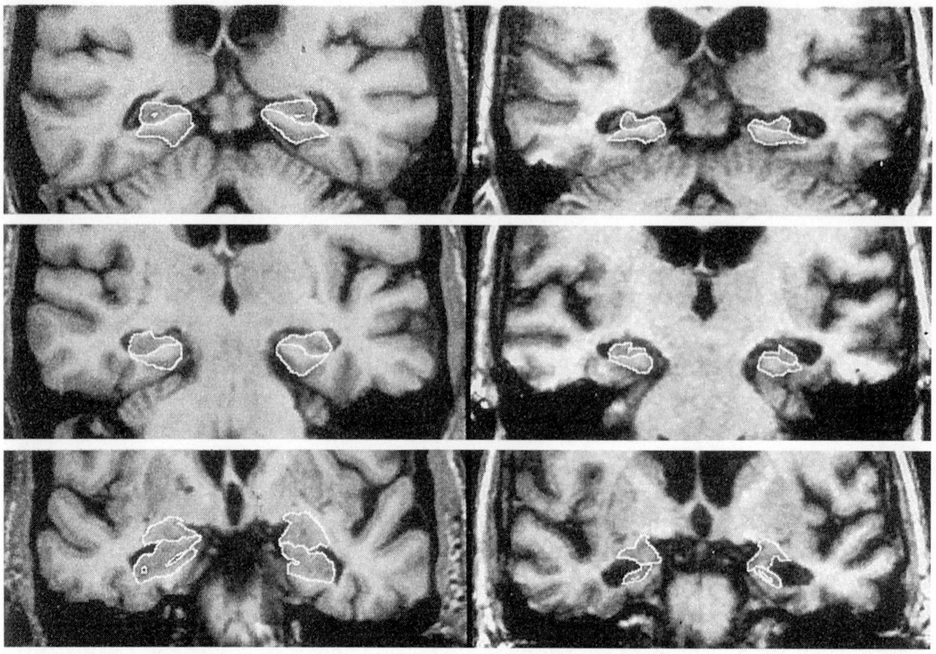

Figure 8-34

Method of defining neuroanatomic boundaries for obtaining volumetric measures. Two columns of images are presented: cropped oblique coronal MRIs through the temporal lobes of a 75-year-old female control subject (left) and images from a 73-year-old female AD patient (right). Each column contains three images. From top to bottom, they represent sections at the level of the hippocampal tail, hippocampal body, and hippocampal head. The anatomic outlines of the hippocampus and parahippocampal gyrus are indicated on images of the hippocampal head and hippocampal body. The outlines of the amygdala and hippocampus are indicated in the bottom image of the hippocampal head. See the original article for neuroanatomic criteria employed when tracing the boundaries of these.[291] (Figure and modified legend from Jack et al,[291] copyright 1997 by Lippincott-Raven. Used by permission.)

may be underestimated in cases in which lost neurons are replaced by glial cells.

The latter problem can be addressed by the use of MRS. Schuff et al[293] studied the hippocampus in AD patients and normal control subjects using both volumetric MRI and MRS. In AD patients, NAA (see "Spectroscopic Imaging," above) concentrations were lower in the hippocampus, hippocampal volume was less, and the two measurements used together discriminated AD patients from normal control subjects better than did either measurement alone. Some of this work is shown in Fig. 8-35.

Ventricular Volume Some investigators have found that absolute measures of ventricular volume are subnormal in AD and can distinguish AD patients from nondemented subjects.[297] Others have found that ventricular volumes can overlap considerably between normal aged people and patients with AD.[295] The rate at which ventricular enlargement occurs in aging may be a more suitable marker for AD than measurements of absolute volume. Using volumetric CT, DeCarli et al[302] measured ventricular volume in patients with AD and in age-matched control subjects. Images were oriented parallel to the orbitomeatal line, with a slice thickness of 1 cm and an interslice distance of 7 mm. Images were analyzed by altering window settings to establish the ventricular ROI; the investigator traced the outline of the depicted ventricle and then calculated the ventricular volume. Repeating these measurements over time for patients with AD and for nondemented control subjects, the investigators found an accelerated rate of lateral ventricular enlargement in the AD patients. Absolute measurements of ventricular volume did not distinguish well between AD and non-AD patients.

Gray and White Matter Since AD is mainly a disease of gray matter, knowing whether the appearance of atrophy on anatomic imaging represents mainly gray matter or mainly white matter loss might help in the differential diagnosis of dementia. Rusinek et al[297] developed a volumetric MRI method to compensate for the volume averaging that causes signal mixing between gray and white matter in conventional MRI. They found that the percentage of total brain substance represented by gray matter in AD patients was lower than that in control subjects (44.9 versus 50.2 percent). Unlike the findings of DeCarli et al,[302] ventricular volume also was greater in AD patients than in control subjects, while white matter volume was the same in both groups. This suggests that the ventricular enlargement seen in AD patients may be due to neuronal loss. Discrepancies between the results of Decarli et al[302] and Rusinek et al[297] may be due to methodologic differences.

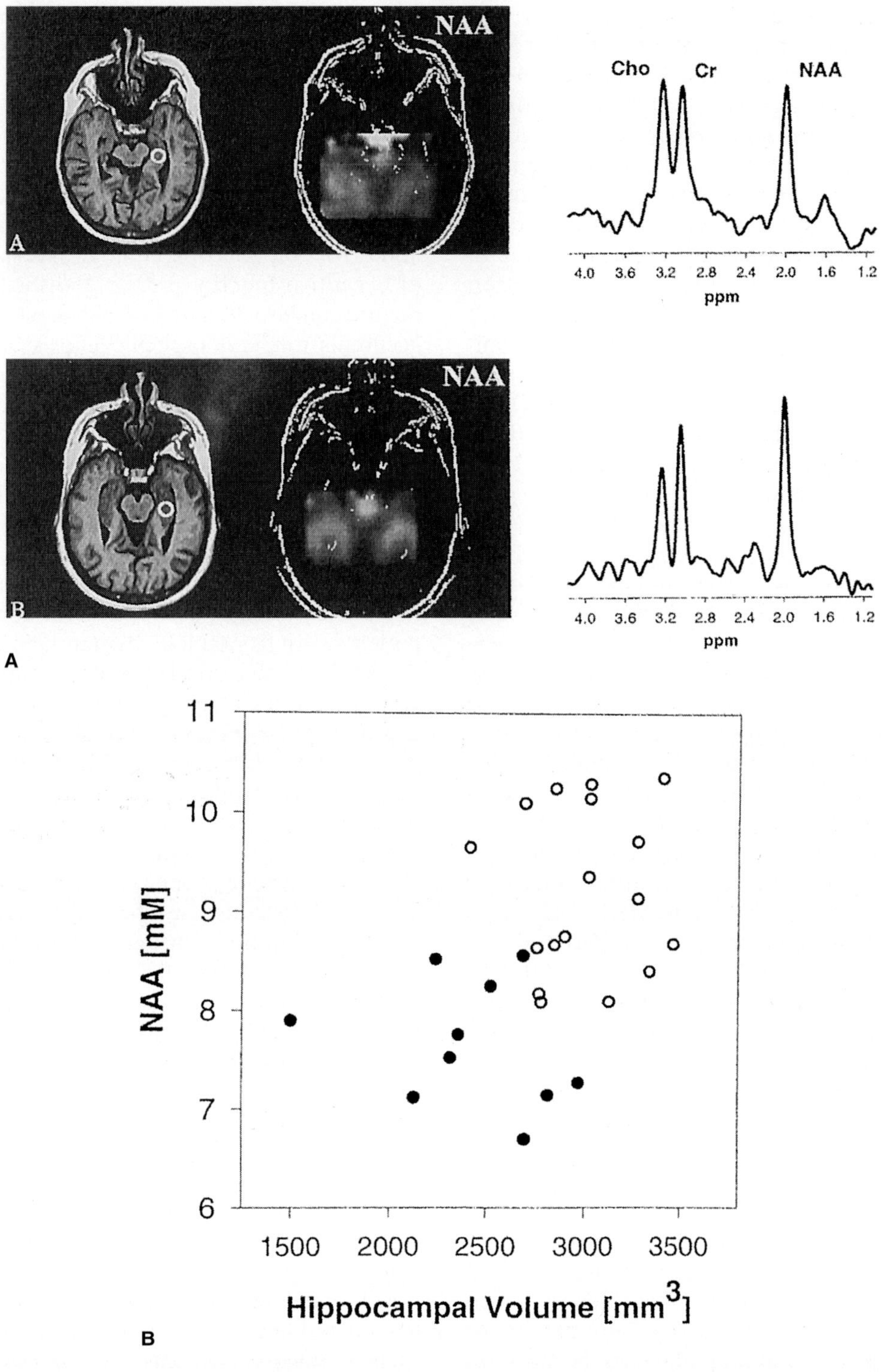

Figure 8-35

(A) *On the left side of the figure, axial MRI from an 80-year-old AD patient (A) and a 74-year-old control subject (B) at the position of the hippocampus. To the immediate right of the MRIs are placed the corresponding* N*-acetyl aspartate (NAA) images from this region, restricted to the sensitive area of the preselected ROI. MRI contours are superimposed on the NAA image for better anatomic reference. Note that MRI and NAA images have different fields of view. On the far right are shown representative proton MRI spectra selected from the hippocampal body (location indicated by a circle in the MRI). Reduction of NAA in the AD patient with respect to the control subject becomes apparent when the NAA peak intensity in each spectrum is compared with creatine (CR). Cho, choline.*

(B) *Summary data for patients as depicted in* **A:** *atrophy-corrected hippocampal NAA as a function of normalized hippocampal volume from each of the 10 AD patients (black dots) and 16 control subjects (white dots) with complete MRI and MRS imaging examination in the series of Schuff et al.*[293] *NAA and volume are mean values of the right and left hippocampus. (Figure and modified legend from Schuff et al,*[293] *copyright Lippincott-Raven. Used by permission.)*

Although AD is mainly a disease of gray matter, AD patients often show white matter abnormalities on MRI that can add to the symptoms of AD.[303] Harrell et al[287] studied MRI findings in depressed AD patients, nondepressed AD patients, and nondepressed older people. All groups showed areas of high signal in the periventricular white matter on proton-density-weighted images. Neuropsychological test performance tended to be worse for AD patients who had the greatest degree of signal abnormality in the periventricular white matter. The investigators concluded that these white matter changes were not specific enough to be used for definitive diagnosis but that they may predict poorer performance in AD patients who have them than in AD patients who do not have them. The meaning of these white matter signal abnormalities on MRI in AD has received considerable attention.[287,289,304]

Cerebral Metabolism Images obtained with PET, SPECT, and fMRI have been used to characterize patients with dementia as well as to identify the areas of the brain that are affected in dementia.[15,18,305,306] Generally, what is seen is a tendency for temporoparietal hypoperfusion and/or hypometabolism to occur in AD patients, and for frontal hypoperfusion and/or hypometabolism to occur in frontal dementias such as Pick disease.[251,303,306,307] Figure 8-29 shows PET and MRI studies of a woman with probable AD. There is mild parietal atrophy on MRI and reduced functioning in the parietal and posterior temporal cortex. In contrast, Fig. 8-30 shows three-dimensional SPECT and MRI studies of a patient with probable Pick disease. The MRI shows frontotemporal atrophy, which is more prominent than the temporoparietal atrophy seen in the patient with AD (Fig. 8-29). The SPECT study shows corresponding hypoperfusion in the frontal and temporal lobes, most prominent in the left hemisphere.

Focal neuropsychological deficits have been found to correlate with focal hypoperfusion in AD. Using SPECT in AD patients, O'Brien et al[305] found positive correlations between cerebral blood flow (1) in the right parietal area and praxis, perception, object assembly, and block design; (2) in the left posterior temporal area and memory; and (3) in the left hemisphere and language ability. Meguro et al[308] used PET to measure the rate of [^{18}F]6-fluoro-l-dopa (^{18}F-dopa) uptake into the striatum (the K_i value) in AD patients. The K_i value correlated with glucose utilization in the anterior frontal, inferior frontal, and temporal lobes. Both K_i and glucose utilization were lower in patients with more severe dementia, and both were lower in patients with a greater tendency to wander. Based on these findings, the investigators suggested that the striatum is part of a functional neural network involving the frontal and temporal lobes and that dysfunction of this network impaired behavioral regulation, causing wandering behavior. This illustrates that, in some forms of AD or perhaps in later AD, symptoms and signs can overlap with those of frontal dementias.

Frontal Dementia

Degenerative Frontal Dementia Neurobehaviorally, patients with frontal dementia show varying degrees of personality change, apathy, disinhibition, perseveration, and errors on neuropsychological tests of memory and of executive function.[251,309–311] Neuropathologically, this picture can be associated with Pick disease,[310] Lewy body accumulation,[312] nonspecific gliosis and neuronal loss (dementia lacking distinctive histology),[311] and other conditions.[311] Studies utilizing CT and MRI in frontal dementia sometimes show disproportionate frontal and/or temporal sulcal enlargement and gyral narrowing.[282,311,313–317] Studies utilizing PET and SPECT in frontal dementia may show frontal lobe hypoperfusion and hypometabolism[251,316–318] (see Figs. 8-27 and 8-30).

Probably the best characterized of the frontal dementias is Pick disease, accounting for about 20 percent of patients with frontal lobe dementia in one series.[319] Pick disease is characterized by circumscribed, mainly frontal and/or temporal atrophy, absence of neurofibrillary tangles and senile plaques in the atrophic cortex, neuronal inclusions (Pick bodies), and ballooned neurons found mainly in the atrophic areas.[251,311,319,320] Figure 8-30 shows the frontal hypoperfusion that can be seen in Pick disease on SPECT scanning.

Whether frontal dementia with ultrastructural inclusions (e.g., Pick disease), frontal dementia with atrophy and gliosis but no inclusions, or other conditions affecting the frontal lobes disproportionately should be included within the same nosologic classification remains unclear. Kumar and Gottlieb[309] have proposed the term *frontotemporal dementia* as a label for the neurobehavioral syndrome of frontotemporal progressive dysfunction, distinguishing the syndrome from the possible underlying causative disease entities. They suggest diagnostic criteria for frontotemporal dementia that rely mostly on neurobehavioral disturbances but that are supported by functional imaging criteria.[251] These imaging criteria include evidence of decline in either cerebral blood flow or glucose metabolism, mainly in the frontal and anterior temporal lobes, and the absence of such findings in the parietal and posterior regions of the brain.

Acquired Frontal Dementia Predominantly frontal lobe atrophy may occur in pathologic states other than degenerative processes. For example, frontal atrophy is also associated with cocaine use.[11] Using planimetric CT to calculate indices of atrophy, Pascual-Leone et al[11] found a positive relationship between duration of cocaine use and degree of atrophy in the frontal lobes in patients without alcohol abuse, HIV seropositivity, or other neurologic conditions (Figs. 8-36, 8-37, and 8-38).

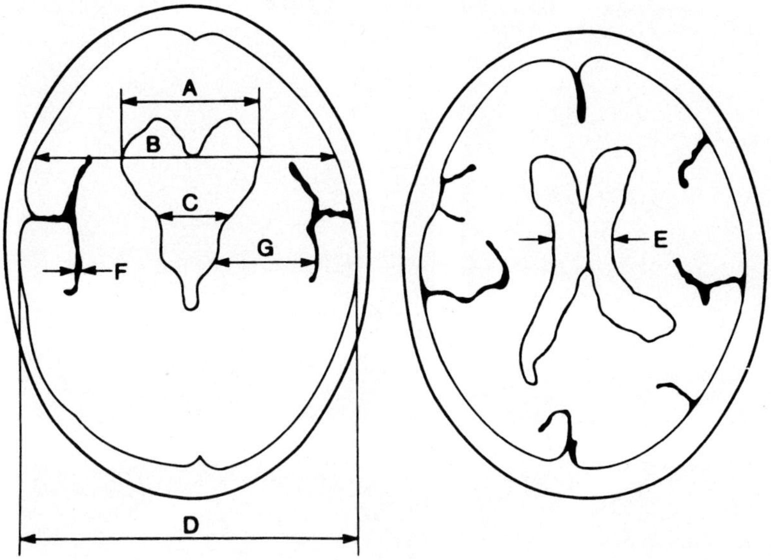

Figure 8-36
Linear measurements taken on axial CT slices in a planimetric CT study of the brain in cocaine abusers. **(A)** *Maximal width of the frontal horns of the lateral ventricles.* **(B)** *Frontal brain width.* **(C)** *Minimal intercaudate distance.* **(D)** *Maximal width of the brain.* **(E)** *Minimal width of the ventricular bodies.* **(F)** *Maximal width of the sylvian fissure.* **(G)** *Mean distance between the third ventricle and the sylvian fissure. See in conjunction with Figs. 8-37 and 8-38. (Figure and modified legend from Pascual-Leone et al.[11] Used by permission.)*

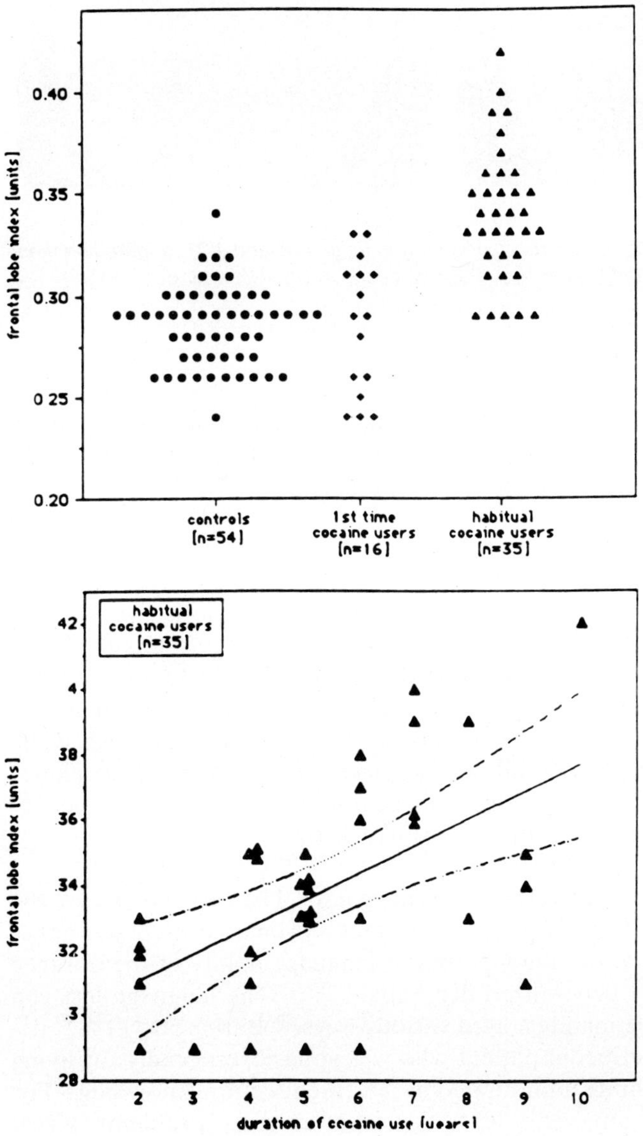

Figure 8-37
Data derived from a planimetric CT study of the brain in cocaine abusers. The "frontal lobe index" was calculated from parameters defined in Fig. 8-36 as A/B. (Top) Distributions of frontal lobe indices for non-cocaine-using control patients with headache, first-time cocaine users, and habitual cocaine users. (Bottom) Regression line and 90-percent confidence bands for the true mean of the frontal lobe index in habitual cocaine abusers. See in conjunction with Figs. 8-36 and 8-38. (Figure and modified legend from Pascual-Leone et al.[11] Used by permission.)

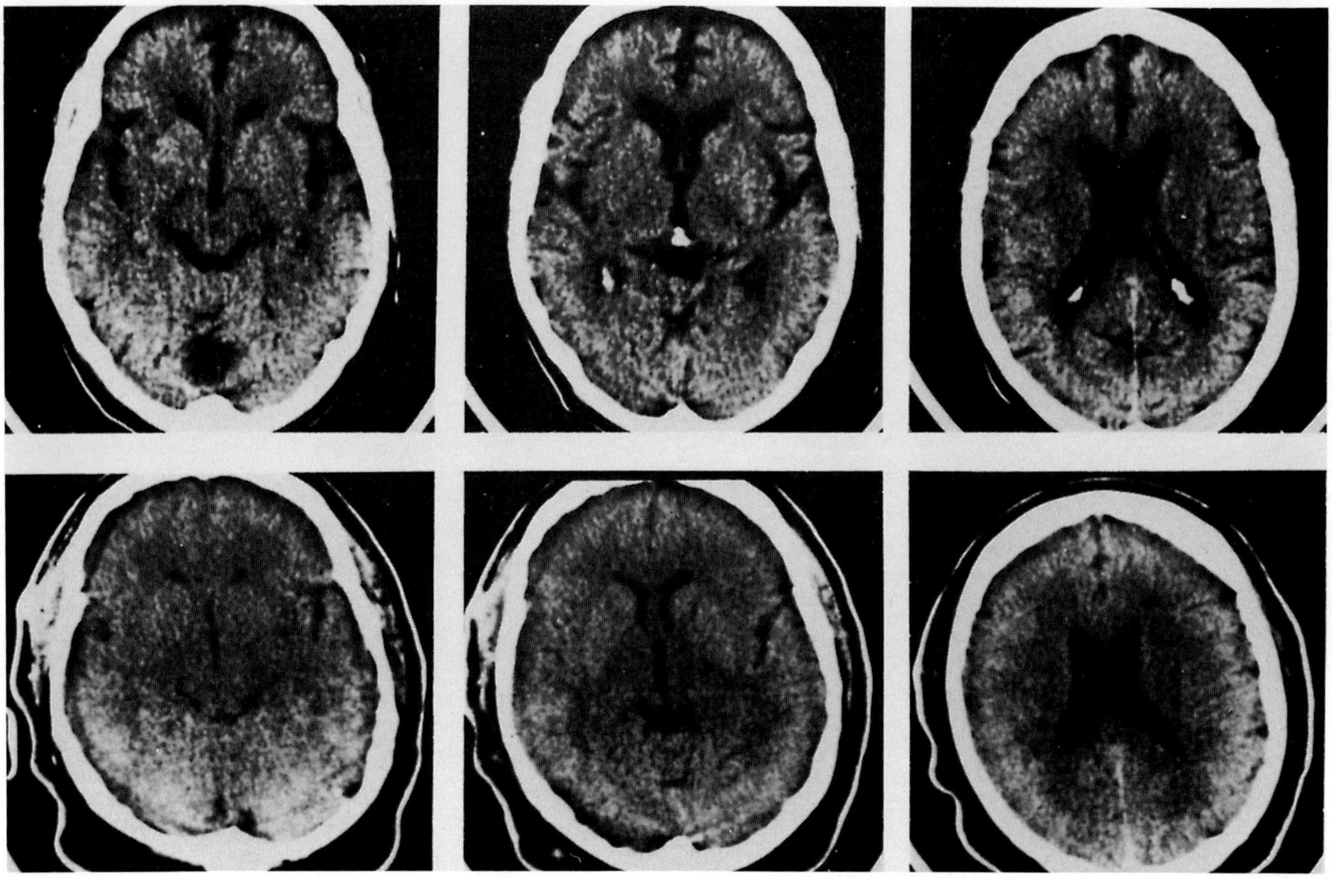

Figure 8-38
CT scans from a planimetric CT study of the brain in cocaine abusers. (Top row) CT scans from a 27-year-old man with 9 years of habitual cocaine use. (Bottom row) CT scans from a 29-year-old control patient. See in conjunction with Figs. 8-36 and 8-37. (Figure and modified legend from Pascual-Leone et al.[11] Used by permission.)

This suggests that chronic cocaine use might be associated with a frontal dementia. Consistent with these results is the demonstration with SPECT of frontotemporal perfusion deficits in cocaine users.[321]

Asymmetric Cortical Degeneration Syndromes

Since Mesulam[322] described the syndrome of primary progressive aphasia, several other syndromes of focal progressive neurobehavioral dysfunction have been described, including progressive amusia and aprosody,[323] Gerstmann syndrome,[324] visual agnosia,[325] right parietal lobe syndrome,[326] and apraxia.[327] While patients with these syndromes may show demonstrable asymmetry in cortical involvement, some have a more diffuse pathologic condition in addition to the more focal areas responsible for the focal neurobehavioral syndrome. Consequently, Caselli and Jack[328] proposed the term *asymmetric cortical degeneration syndrome* for these conditions.

The asymmetric cortical degeneration syndromes are probably pathologically heterogenous. Some appear to reflect the early-stage focal onset of degenerative conditions that later generalize to other parts of the brain. Other cases may represent a truly focal degenerative condition that does not generalize.[328,329] Based on their own series of patients, Caselli and Jack[328] divided these syndromes into three classes, each with two subclasses: (1) aphasia (fluent and nonfluent); (2) perceptuomotor dysfunction (left and right parietal lobe syndromes); and (3) neuropsychiatric disorder manifested by abulia, perseveration, pseudobulbar affect, and dependency (with and without spasticity). Neuroimaging has fostered the understanding of these syndromes, especially because it allows the process of asymmetric degeneration and of neurobehavioral deterioration to be observed simultaneously over time.[329]

Left-Hemisphere Syndromes The best known of the left-hemisphere syndromes is primary progressive aphasia, the gradual loss of language ability in the absence of generalized dementia.[322,328–333] The language loss can be manifested in various ways.[328] Barbarotto et al[334] described a patient who was aphasic, especially for living things, famous people, and architectural knowledge. For many years after the onset of these problems, visual and verbal information about other categories of knowledge, such as knowledge about tools, vehicles, and furniture, was spared. Studies utilizing MRI showed predominantly right-sided temporal lobe atrophy as well as disease in the basal neocortex, hippocampus, and parahippocampal gryi.

While most cases of primary progressive aphasia are characterized by predominantly left-sided dysfunction, aphasic dementias occasionally occur with predominantly right-sided disease, possibly because of atypical cerebral dominance. Progressive aphasia may be pathologically heterogeneous. Cases have been described with nonspecific gliosis and spongiform change,[329,335,336] swollen achromasic neurons,[337] neuronal depletion and gliosis,[336] the pathologic conditions of Creutzfeldt-Jakob disease,[338] Pick disease,[313,339] and AD.[340] Based upon their own patients and the literature, Snowden et al[329] suggested that most cases of progressive aphasia represent clinically heterogeneous presentations of non-Alzheimer lobar atrophy.

Using SPECT, McDaniel et al[330] found unilateral left hypoperfusion in two patients with progressive aphasia, contrasting their findings with the more typically bilateral patterns of hypoperfusion seen in AD.[306] Findings obtained with SPECT of left focal hypoperfusion in primary progressive aphasia should be interpreted with caution, since predominantly left-sided hypoperfusion on SPECT images has also been found in patients clinically diagnosed with AD.[305] Figure 8-39 shows PET and MRI studies of a patient with primary progressive aphasia and relatively intact performance on tests of memory and visual functioning. Hypofunctioning is seen in the left hemisphere and is most prominent in the anterior and inferior portions of the temporal lobe.

Karbe et al[332] compared the language deficits in AD patients and those of patients with primary progressive aphasia. In patients with primary progressive aphasia, the dominant feature of the aphasia in the early stages was impaired fluency and anomia. In contrast, AD patients had more global deterioration of language. Figure 8-40 shows typical MRI findings from patients.

Right-Hemisphere Syndromes Confavreux et al[323] studied a patient with progressive impairment of singing and storytelling caused by loss of ability to convey emotion in her voice (amusia and aprosody). Her deficits

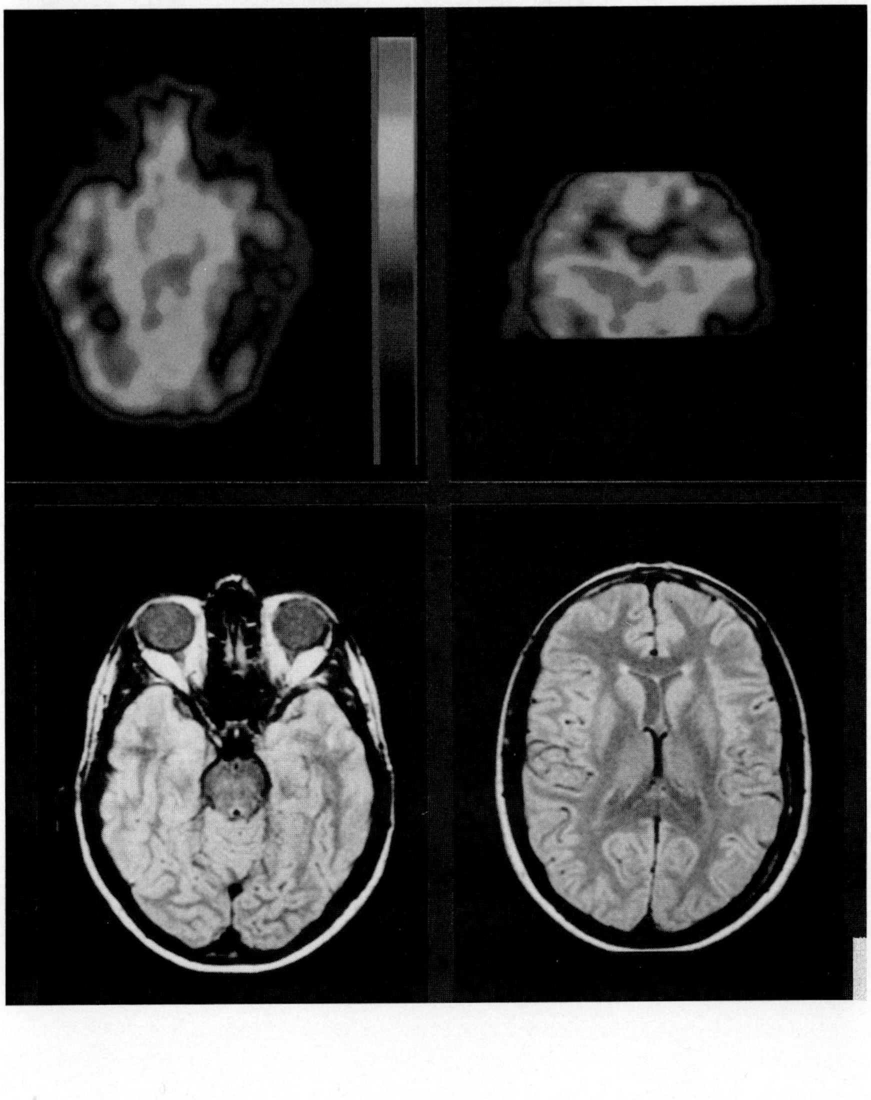

Figure 8-39 (Plate 25)
MRI and PET studies of a 54-year-old patient with primary-progressive aphasia. She showed significant language impairment that progressed over 5 years despite relatively normal episodic memory and visual functioning. Her pattern of language impairment was most notable for agrammatic expression in oral and written spontaneous expression, difficulty understanding grammatically complex sentences, and a repetition deficit. Her MRI scan (oriented so that the left hemisphere is on the right of the image) appears to be normal. Her PET scan (oriented so that the left hemisphere is on the right of the image) reveals reduced cortical functioning throughout the left hemisphere that is most prominent in the anterior and inferior portions of the left temporal lobe. (Courtesy of Dr. Murray Grossman, University of Pennsylvania.)

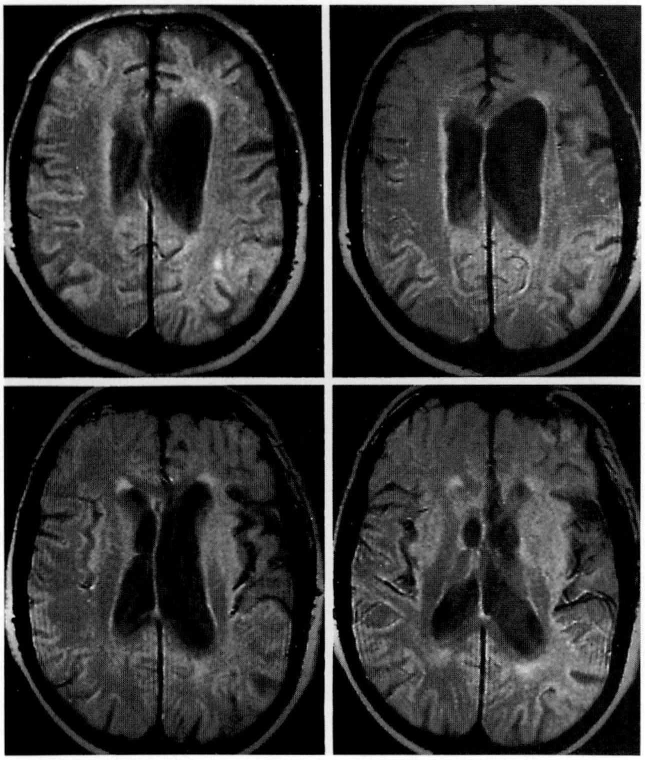

Figure 8-40

Transaxial MRI of the brain in a patient with primary progressive aphasia, showing disproportionate enlargement of the left lateral ventricle and sulcal enlargement mainly in the left frontal and perisylvian cortex. (Figure and modified legend from Karbe et al.[232] Copyright 1993 by the American Medical Association. Used by permission.)

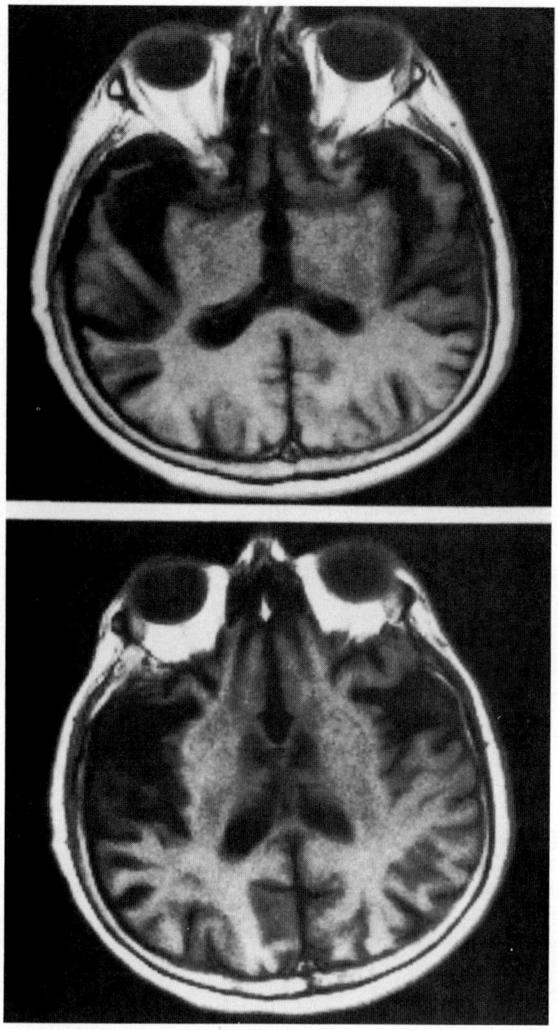

Figure 8-41

Transaxial MRI (TR 500 ms, TE 21 ms) at the level of the insular cortex, showing bilateral sulcal enlargement in the temporoinsular cortex, more pronounced on the right, in a patient with progressive amusia and aprosody. Compare to Fig. 8-40. (Figure and modified legend from Confavreux et al.[323] Copyright 1992 by the American Medical Association. Used by permission.)

remained mostly restricted to amusia and aprosody for several years before she began a more rapid progression to impairments in speech initiation and in activities of daily living. During the period of relatively restricted amusia and aprosody, SPECT and MRI scans demonstrated abnormalities in the right anterotemporal area (Figs. 8-41 and 8-42). The fact that she later developed global dementia suggests that the condition eventually generalized to other areas of the cortex.

Focal Symmetric Syndromes Chapman et al[341] reported a patient with a progressive motor speech loss with preservation of language functions. The posterior frontal lobes were affected symmetrically. There was a family history of similar problems, and analysis suggested that this was an autosomal dominant condition. Chapman et al[341] discussed a number of other cases of speech impairment, noting that few cases of motor-speech decline as the dominant symptom in progressive speech and language loss have been described. They speculated that more careful attention to the distinction between speech and language deficits in patients believed to have primary progressive aphasia may reveal more such cases. Figures 8-43 and 8-44, from Chapman et al,[341] show the MRI and SPECT images for this patient. This case may be viewed as a unique type of frontal lobe syndrome.

Subcortical Dementia

The term *subcortical dementia* has been applied to the neuropsychological profile consisting of slowed cognition, impaired visual-spatial skills, executive dysfunction, apathy, depression, and impaired information retrieval and working memory. Capacities such as language and praxis are preserved.[280,342–344] As with the clinical syndrome of frontotemporal dementia, this neurobehavioral syndrome is neuropathologically heterogeneous, occurring in conditions such as the multi-

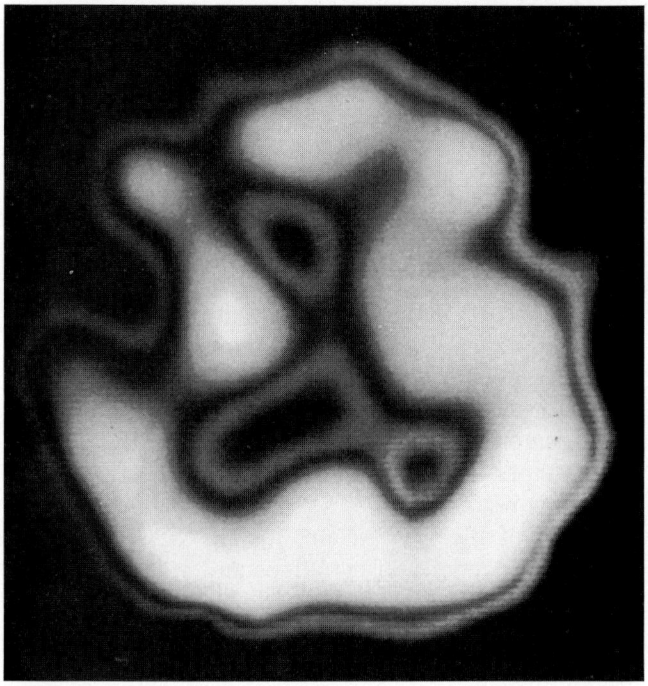

Figure 8-42

SPECT study of progressive amusia and aprosody. Horizontal SPECT image of cerebral uptake of ^{99m}Tc HMPAO, horizontal plane, showing reduced tracer uptake mainly in the right anterior temporal area, consistent with decreased blood flow and metabolism. The zone of abnormal tracer uptake corresponds with the zone of predominantly sulcal enlargement seen on MRI in Fig. 8-41. (Figure and modified legend from Confavreux et al,[323] copyright 1992 by the American Medical Association. Used by permission.)

infarct state (multi-infarct or vascular dementia),[345,346] MS,[254,256] some cases of Parkinson disease (PD),[347,348] HIV infection,[349,350] and progressive supranuclear palsy (PSP).[343,351,352] The probable mechanism by which dementia is produced in these conditions is cortical-subcortical and cortical-cortical disconnection. This may especially lead to varying degrees of isolation of the frontal lobes, explaining why affected patients resemble those with frontal-temporal dementia neurobehaviorally.[280,353,354]

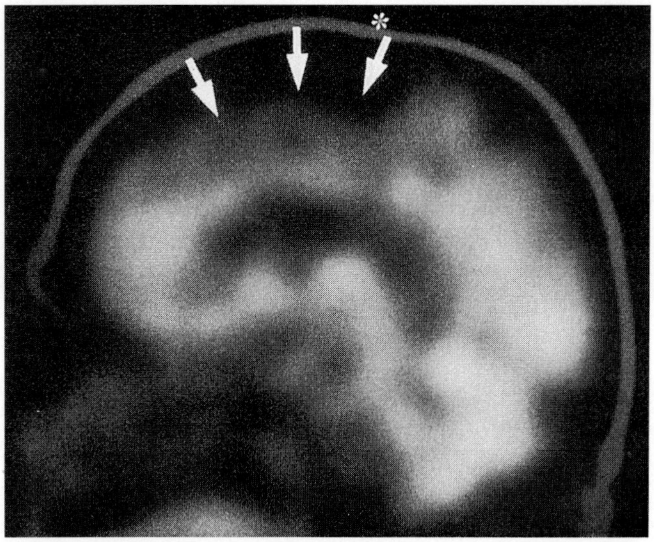

Figure 8-44

SPECT study of the patient whose MRI is shown in Fig. 8-43. SPECT at age 68 indicates areas of hypoperfusin corresponding to the atrophic regions identified on MRI and confirms involvement in the cingulate gyrus. The arrows indicate marked reduction in regional cerebral blood flow in the superior frontal lobes extending to the anterior parietal and superior temporal lobes (shown by an asterisk). (Figure and modified legend from Chapman et al,[341] copyright 1997 by Lippincott-Raven. Used by permission.)

The term *subcortical dementia* is somewhat controversial; there are doubts that it represents a distinct dementia syndrome.[355] One reason for doubt may be that some patients with conditions such as MS can show cognitive deficits typical of subcortical dementia yet may not display the degree of disability needed in order to meet formal definitions of dementia. If the view is adopted that the cognitive deficits seen in patients with these conditions lie along a continuum from normal functioning to severe dementia,[356] the term may lose some of its controversial character. This same issue figures prominently in definitions of vascular dementia (see "Vascular Dementia," below).

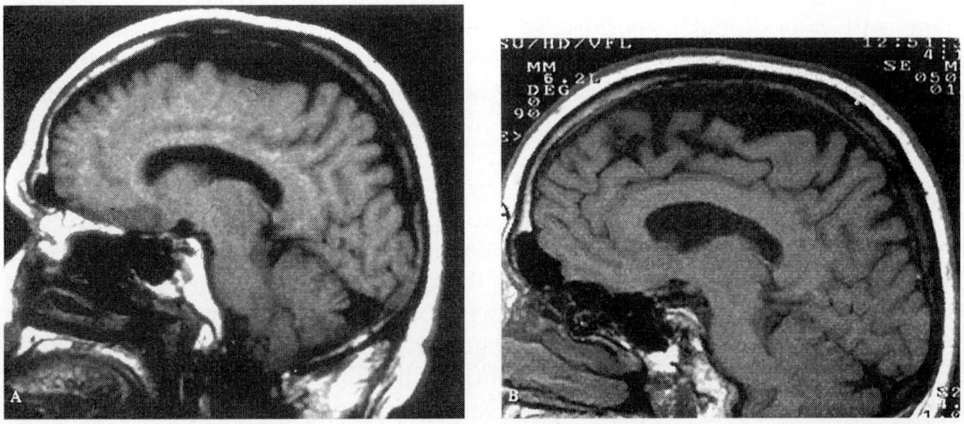

Figure 8-43

MRI of a patient with progressive motor speech loss with preserved language function. **(A)** *Sagittal view of the patient's MRI at age 66 and* **(B)** *at age 68. The images show progression of atrophy in the posterior frontal and anterior parietal lobes extending into the cingulate cortex in the later image. See also Fig. 8-44. (Figure and modified legend from Chapman et al,[341] copyright 1997 by Lippincott-Raven. Used by permission.)*

Difficulties with the term *subcortical dementia* may stem as well from confusion about whether it is being used as a descriptive label or as an anatomic explanation of cognitive deficits. When used as a label, it is a way of summarizing a group of cognitive impairments. When used as an explanatory concept, it implies dementia caused by disease in subcortical structures.[353] Being clear about which is the case may help to eliminate some uncertainty. Nonetheless, the boundaries between cortical and subcortical dementia are not clear-cut. Some patients with conditions associated with subcortical dementia and with the clinical profile of subcortical dementia also have impairments usually thought of as reflecting cortical impairment, such as aphasia, apraxia, and agnosia.[357]

The following sections review several conditions that have been associated with a subcortical pattern of dementia. One such condition is vascular dementia; because of some unique issues with the concept of vascular dementia, we treat it separately from the other conditions.

Parkinson Disease While many patients with PD are relatively cognitively intact, a number have cognitive impairments.[347,348,358] These deficits are not uniform from patient to patient. Some patients bear relatively restricted neurobehavioral deficits, such as cognitive slowing, depression, and impairments on tests of executive function such as set shifting.[348] Others are globally impaired in a fashion resembling AD.[359,360] Functional and anatomic imaging studies suggest that PD patients with dementia have pathologic conditions in multiple extranigral areas, a conclusion supported by neuropathologic studies.[361] These conditions may extend to the frontal lobes, helping to account for some of the frontosubcortical pattern of cognitive deficits seen in many patients with PD.

In SPECT studies, PD patients with neurobehavioral deficits resembling those seen in AD tend to have reduced temporoparietal blood flow and metabolism of the sort seen in AD.[360,362,363] Using SPECT, Jagust et al[360] showed that the severity and type of neurobehavioral problems in PD were related to the severity and location of perfusion deficits: (1) PD patients with poor global functioning had bilateral temporal hypoperfusion similar to that seen in AD; (2) PD patients not meeting criteria for dementia yet showing impairments in construction and executive functions had temporal perfusion measurements that were intermediate between those of the AD patients and the control subjects; and (3) depressed PD patients performed more poorly than did nondepressed PD patients on tests of global cognitive function and on specific tests of frontal function.[360] These patients tend to show decreased perfusion and metabolism in the frontal lobes on functional imaging studies. In addition, PET studies have found evidence of frontal dysfunction in PD, although sometimes not in the same parts of the frontal lobe where SPECT has found dysfunction.[364] Possible reasons for discrepancies between SPECT and PET studies have been discussed by Jagust et al.[360]

HIV Dementia Infection with HIV can be associated with a wide range of neurobehavioral abnormalities.[349,350,365] Both cortical and subcortical patterns of dementia occur, with a subcortical pattern perhaps predominating.[366] The impairments may be caused by a direct effect of the HIV virus upon the brain; by opportunistic infections and neoplasms, such as syphilis, toxoplasmosis, and lymphoma; or by a combination of these factors. The direct effects of HIV infection on the brain may be mediated by several factors, including the virulence of the HIV strain, toxicity of HIV gp 120 antigen, the activity of cytokines and arachidonic acid metabolites, blood-brain barrier changes, and actions of nitric oxide and quinolinic acid.[367]

Neuroimaging plays an important role in the clinical and investigational study of cognitive impairment in this condition.[368] Studies using CT and MRI with routine and double-dose contrast enhancement are especially valuable for finding opportunistic lesions that may be responsible for cognitive impairment. Tuite et al[369] studied an HIV-positive patient with progressive cognitive decline who had abnormal patterns of enhancement on gadolinium-enhanced T1 MRI images (Fig. 8-45). Subsequent investigation led to the diagnosis of neurosyphilis, the probable cause of both the cognitive impairment and the abnormal enhancement on MRI. Treatment of neurosyphilis reversed the cognitive decline.

Cognitive impairment can occur in HIV infection in the absence of demonstrable opportunistic disease. This has been termed *HIV-1–associated dementia complex, HIV encephalopathy*, and *AIDS-related dementia.*[349,350,370] Neurobehaviorally, affected patients tend to have a frontosubcortical pattern of deficits.[349,350,365,371] The neuropathologic basis of HIV-related cognitive impairment and of some aspects of HIV-related dementia may involve both neuronal loss due to direct HIV infection and disconnection of one cortical area from another because of HIV-related white matter disease.

A major challenge in this area is to devise imaging techniques that can detect the neuropathologic signature of HIV infection in the absence of opportunistic infections. In HIV-related dementia, routine CT and MRI study results are often normal or only mildly abnormal in a nonspecific way.[372,373] Figure 8-46 presents typical MRI findings in a patient with HIV dementia. This 36-year-old man had severe dementia manifested by extreme apathy and slowing of responses. The image shows moderate cortical atrophy. Notably, there is relative preservation of the hippocampus, in contrast to the pattern seen in AD (compare to Fig. 8-33).

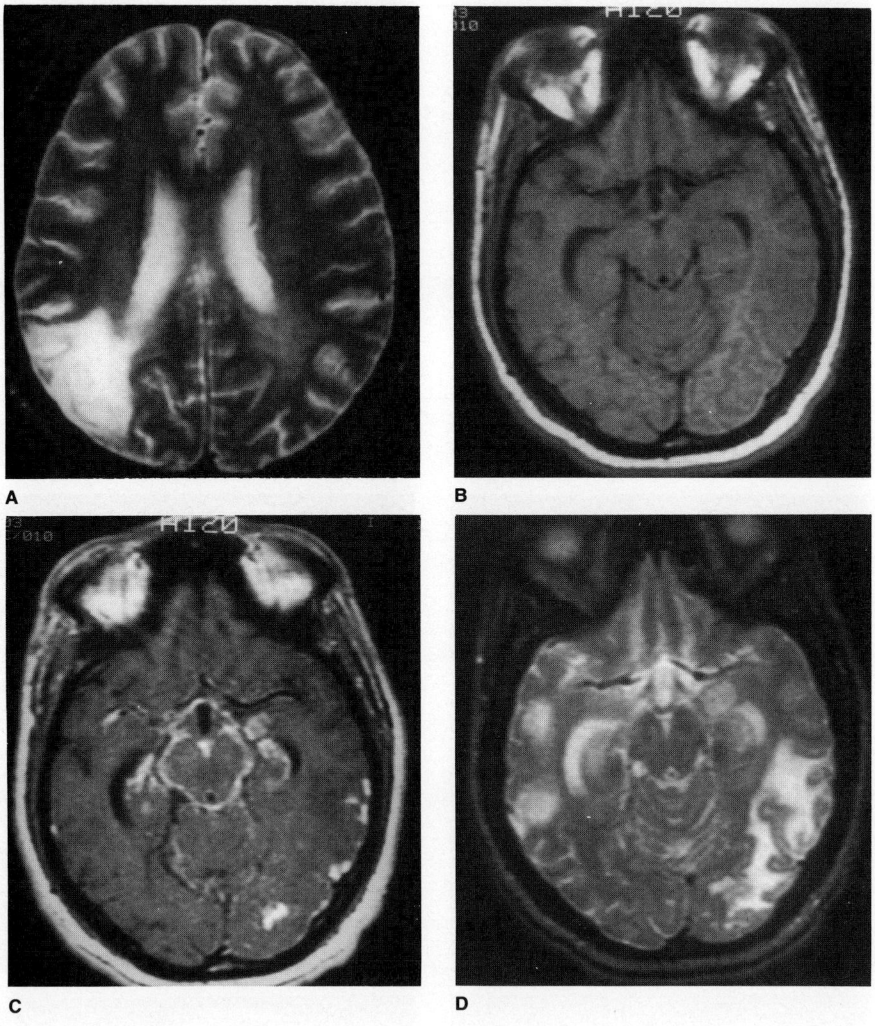

Figure 8-45
Transaxial MRI of HIV-infected patient with progressive cognitive decline, positive serum RPR, and CSF lymphocytosis. **(A)** *Noncontrast image (TR 2000 ms, TE 80 ms) showing high-signal area consistent with infarction (arrow).* **(B and C)** *Pre-* **(B)** *and post-contrast* **(C)** *images (TR 600 ms, TE 20 ms) showing enhancing basilar meninges (arrow in* **C***) and parenchymal areas (arrowhead in* **C***).* **(D)** *Noncontrast image (TR 2000 ms, TE 80 ms) at the level of the midbrain shows high-signal areas consistent with white matter edema (arrows) surrounding parenchymal lesions. These findings were consistent with meningovascular neurosyphilis. (Figure and modified legend from Tuite et al,[369] copyright 1993 by the American Society of Neuroradiology. Courtesy of Dr. Leena Ketonen, University of Rochester Medical Center, Rochester, N.Y.)*

Dooneief et al[373] applied quantitative methods to routine T2-weighted and heavily T2-weighted MRI scans in order to measure brain water content in homosexual men and in intravenous-drug-using men with and without HIV positivity. A surprising number (97 percent) of all subjects showed evidence of mild or moderate cerebral atrophy, a finding also reported in intravenous drug users[11] (see above, including Figs. 8-36, 8-37, and 8-38). Neither measures of atrophy nor measures of water content were related to neuropsychological functioning or global performance ratings. Measures of intracranial water content tended to distinguish HIV-positive from HIV-negative subjects, but the significance of that finding is unclear. Relatively negative results were also obtained by Cohen et al,[372] who found no significant MRI differences between HIV-positive non-AIDS patients and HIV-negative subjects, and no relationship between MRI abnormalities and cognitive performance.

Other MRI techniques are proving to be more successful in revealing brain abnormalities in these patients. Meyerhoff et al[374,375] used MRI and water-suppressed proton MRS to measure brain NAA and choline in cognitively impaired and nonimpaired HIV-infected patients. In the cognitively impaired patients, NAA signal intensity, and NAA/choline and NAA/creatine ratios were reduced. This suggested that neuronal loss could explain at least some of the cognitive deficits in these patients. Neuronal loss in HIV infection may be mediated through macrophage-induced neurotoxicity.[376] Figures 8-47 and 8-48 illustrate some of the spectroscopic findings and methods used by Meyerhoff et al.[375]

Both SPECT and PET can show abnormalities in subcortical gray matter structures and in the cerebral cortex in patients with HIV-related dementia.[368] Using PET, Rottenberg et al[377] demonstrated decreased rates of glucose metabolism in the cortex in HIV patients with impaired performance on tests of verbal fluency and mental tracking. In addition, in patients with HIV infection and cognitive impairment, SPECT studies have shown reduced perfusion in cerebral cortex[378] and in subcortical gray matter.[379,380] The latter is consistent with the occurrence of macrophage and monocyte infiltrates that have been seen in some patients with HIV

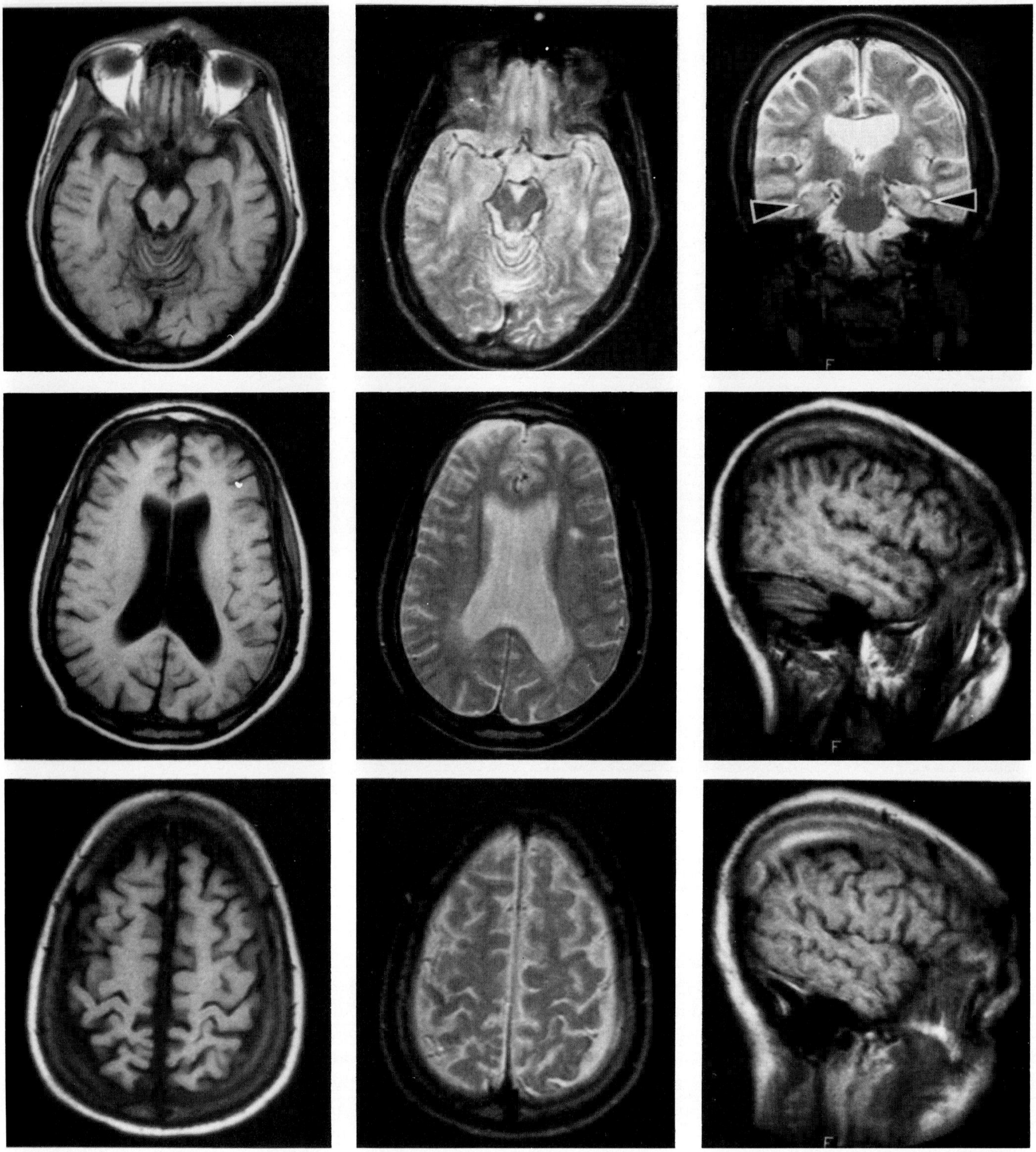

Figure 8-46

MRI of HIV-related dementia. (Left column) Transaxial slices (TR 750 ms, TE 20 ms, 8-mm slice thickness) showing mild ventricular and sulcal enlargement. (Middle column) Transaxial slices (TR 2450 ms, TE 100 ms, 8-mm slice thickness) showing a few areas of signal abnormality in the white matter. (Right column, top image) Coronal slice at the level of the hippocampus, which appears to be normal in size (arrows; TR 2450 ms, TE 100 ms, 10-mm slice thickness). In contrast to AD patients with similar degrees of ventricular and sulcal enlargement (see Figs. 8-29 and 8-33), the hippocampus is not disproportionately affected. (Right column, middle and bottom images) Sagittal slices (TR 750 ms, TE 20 ms, 8-mm slice thickness) showing the left and right sylvian fissures. Disproportionate perisylvian atrophy of the kind seen in asymmetric cortical degeneration is not present (compare to Figs. 8-39, 8-40, and 8-41).

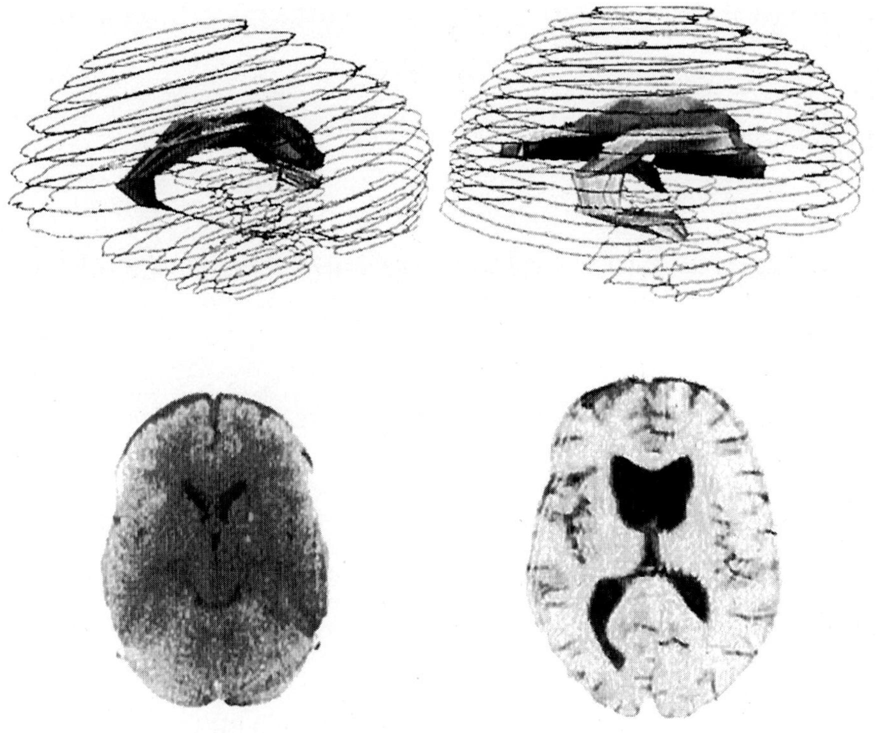

Figure 8-50
Method of depicting ventricular enlargment in chronic TBI. (Top) Three-dimensional lateral view of ventricular dilation on the day-of-injury CT scan (left) compared with the postinjury MRI (right). (Bottom) Axial day-of-injury CT (left) and postinjury MRI (right) at the level of the anterior horns. See the original article for methologic details.[409] (From Anderson and Bigler,[409] copyright 1995 by the American Psychiatric Press. Used by permission.)

cally present surface areas of brain structures and to separate gray matter, CSF, and white matter. Using a three-dimensional image analysis method described by Bigler,[411] a two-dimensional DOI CT and postinjury MRI can be extrapolated onto a three-dimensional image. An example of this is seen in Fig. 8-50. Bigler[406] used this method to depict cortical encephalomalacia after TBI. The figure also illustrates the tendency for trauma to damage the frontal and temporal lobes disproportionately because of their association with bony promontories against which they can be flung during trauma.[382] This helps to explain the frequency with which TBI is associated with executive, attentional, and memory deficits.[412]

Ventricular Volumetry The technique of multispectral segmentation, which yields whole-brain values of gray matter, white matter, and CSF, can be combined with ROI tracing and pixel counting to quantify volumes of brain structures in MRIs.[413] Using this method, Bigler et al[413] showed that atrophy in the hippocampus and the temporal horns manifested between 71 and 210 days post-TBI. Left temporal horn volume predicted verbal IQ, while right temporal horn volume predicted pictorial IQ. Both left and right hippocampus volume correlated with verbal memory function. This is illustrated in Fig. 8-51.

Functional Imaging and TBI

Prognosis after TBI While anatomic MRI scans may reveal small focal abnormalities that are not present on a corresponding SPECT scan, functional imaging tends to be more sensitive than anatomic imaging in depicting brain abnormalities after TBI. For example, Ichise et al[414] studied patients with both minor and major TBI, finding that SPECT scans were more likely to show abnormalities than were MRI scans; both SPECT and MRI were more sensitive than CT. Figure 8-52 shows a SPECT scan done on a 40-year-old woman 2.4 years after major head injury. She showed impairments in memory under interference conditions, in information processing ability, and in attention. The SPECT scan shows a mild to moderate perfusion deficit in the right inferior temporal lobe that was not correlated with findings on the MRI scan.

A normal initial SPECT scan has been shown to predict a favorable outcome after mild to moderate TBI.[415] In contrast, an abnormal SPECT scan after TBI can herald persistent deficits. Quantitative SPECT measurements may be especially useful for prognosis in TBI. One such measurement is the anterior-posterior perfusion ratio (APR).[414] The APR is measured on a midsagittal SPECT image by drawing a radius centered on the thalamus, extending perpendicular to the canthomeatal line. This divides the sagittal section into roughly equal anterior and posterior segments. Four ROIs anterior and four ROIs posterior to the radius are identified. Then, the sum of the SPECT activities in the four anterior ROIs is divided by the sum of the activities in the four posterior ROIs. This generates the APR. This method is illustrated in Fig. 8-53. In their series of 29 TBI patients, Ichise et al found that APR correlated with more neuropsychological measurements of out-

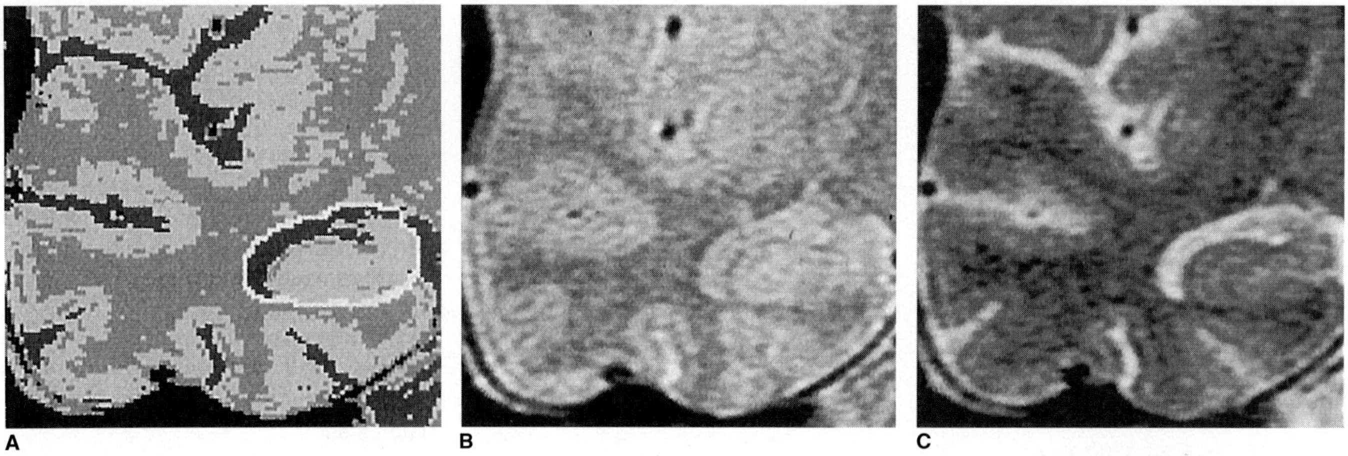

Figure 8-51.
Volumetric method based on multispectral segmention. **(A)** *Close-up of segmented image reduced to three tissue types depicting the loosely traced outline of the hippocampus defining the ROI. Once the ROI is identified, the outer boundary of the hippocampus is traced. A pixel count is then taken based on gray matter pixels. A similar method is used to obtain temporal horn pixels based on their CSF classification within the ROI.* **(B)** *Original intermediate-weighted MRI.* **(C)** *T2-weighted MRI. (From Bigler et al,[413] copyright 1997 by the American Society of Neuroradology. Used by permission.)*

come (in memory, attention, and executive function) than did VBR (see above),[416] although the correlations were somewhat weak.[414]

There are at least two potential contributors to APR reduction in TBI: the disproportionate tendency of frontotemporal areas to be damaged in TBI and deafferentation effects stemming from DAI, causing reduced regional cortical perfusion.[414] Low APR is not specific for TBI, however, since TBI patients can be depressed, and depression has been linked to frontal lobe hypoperfusion.[417] Studies utilizing PET also may provide prognostic information after TBI. For these purposes, timing of the PET scan is important; the results of a study by Worley et al[418] suggest that PET performed within 12

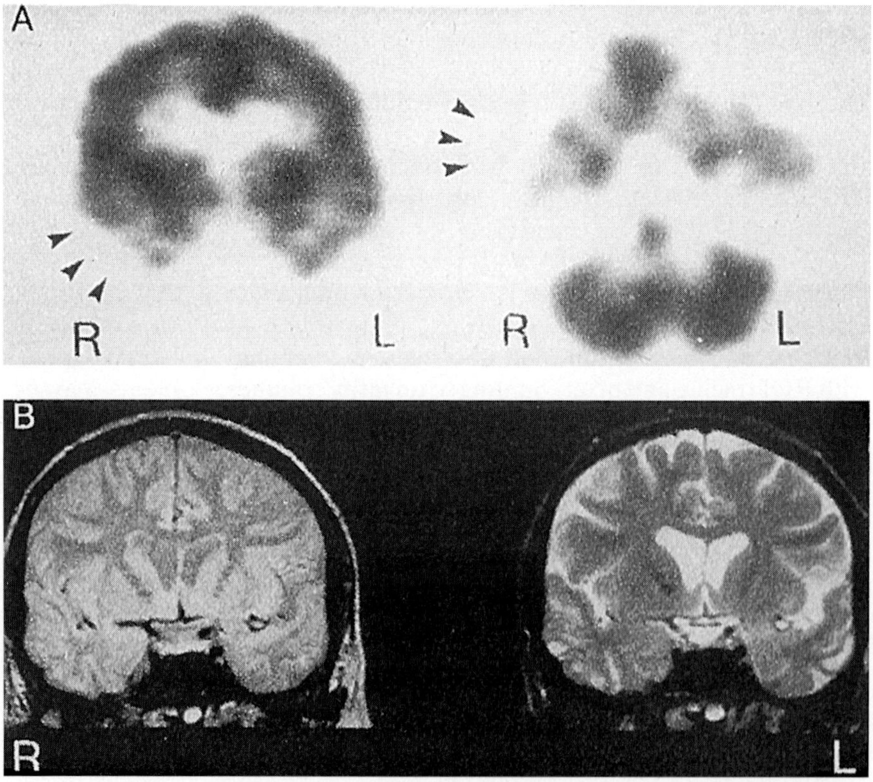

Figure 8-52
MRI and SPECT studies in the evaluation of TBI. (Top) HMPAO SPECT images. (Bottom) MRI. The SPECT study includes a coronal view through the basal ganglia (left) and a transaxial image at the inferior temporal lobe level (right). The perfusion of the right inferior temporal lobe is decreased (arrowheads). The corresponding coronal MRI scans (proton density on the left and T2-weighted on the right) show mild ventricular enlargement but no other abnormalities. See the text for details on the patient. (Figure and modified legend from Ichise et al,[414] copyright 1994 by the Journal of Nuclear Medicine. Used by permission.)

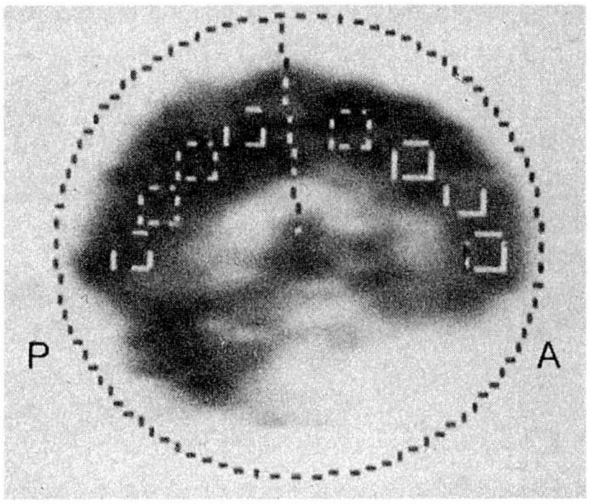

A

Figure 8-53
(A) *Method of determining the anterior-posterior perfusion ratio (APR) in SPECT. A mid-sagittal HMPAO SPECT image shows eight square ROIs. A circular ROI is placed encompassing the midsagittal brain (dotted line border). Its radius is positioned perpendicular to the canthomeatal line, which has been determined from the planar-lateral image obtained prior to the SPECT study. Two sets of four square ROIs are then placed anterior and posterior to this radius, respectively. A, anterior; P, posterior.* **(B)** *Two mid-sagittal HMPAO SPECT images with normal (0.950 left) and decreased (0.886 right) anteroposterior perfusion ratios. A, anterior; P, posterior. (Figure and modified legend from Ichise et al.*[414] *Used by permission.)*

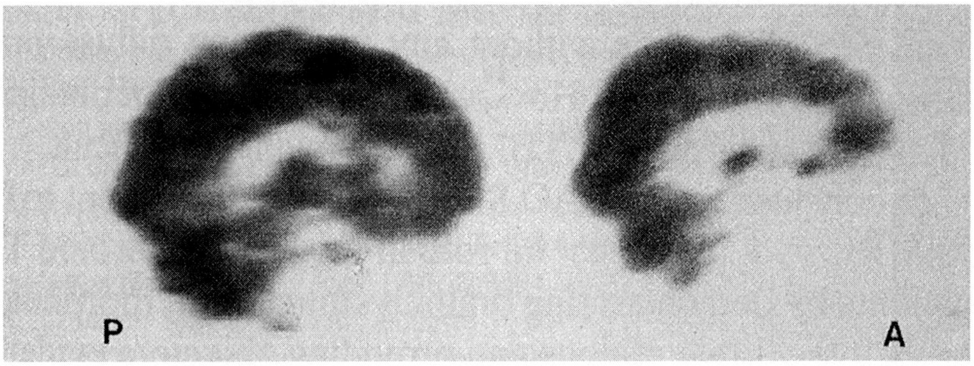

B

weeks postinjury is a more reliable predictor of outcome than is PET performed soon after injury. However, MRI and CT measurements were as predictive as PET measurements in that study.

Neuroimaging and Recovery of Function in TBI Recovery of function after TBI depends on a variety of factors, including severity, location, and cause of injury; immediate postinjury events at the neurophysiologic and neuropsychological level of analysis; and possibly response to programs of pharmacotherapy and cognitive remediation.[419–421] One remaining uncertainty is the mechanism by which brain recovery, and hence cognitive recovery, proceeds after TBI. Functional imaging is playing a role in elucidating these processes. Dobkin[422] treats this issue extensively, listing a number of ways in which functional neuroimaging can illuminate the process of recovery of function after brain injury, including (1) studying its natural history; (2) determining readiness for rehabilitation; (3) predicting recovery; (4) analyzing mechanisms of recovery; (5) understanding remote effects of lesions; (6) comparing brain activity differences between TBI patients and normal subjects; (7) tracking brain response to rehabilitation interventions and medications; and (8) testing interventions for their ability to recruit or to suppress uninjured areas of the brain.

Levin et al[423] studied a 17-year-old male who sustained a traumatic right temporal hemorrhage at age 7 months. Studies with MRI at age 16 years had shown occipital horn dilation and right parietal cortical atrophy.[423] When examined at age 17, he demonstrated mild left hemiparesis and hyperreflexia, dyscalculia, dyslexia, and impaired attention span but otherwise exhibited normal social behavior. Functional MRIs acquired while he performed tests of calculation showed predominantly left-hemisphere frontal and posterior parietal activation with marked reduction in activation in the right hemisphere relative to the left hemisphere. In contrast, performance of the same task by normal control subjects caused bilateral activation of the supramarginal gyrus. Because he showed no evidence of visuospatial impairment and visual neglect, which are characteristic of right parietal injury in adults, Levin et al[423] suggested that these functions had been transferred to the homologous left parietal regions. A crowding effect may have compromised the normal functions subserved by the left parietal region, the consequence of which was dyscalculia and dyslexia.

This illustrates one of the proposed mechanisms by which recovery of function occurs after brain damage: the appropriation of a brain system by a function that formerly was organized elsewhere. While this and other putative mechanisms of brain recovery are debated, functional imaging will probably play a large role in identifying the mechanism of recovery of function after TBI and other brain injury mechanisms.

CONCLUSION

One of the first imaging studies relating brain structure to cognitive function, published by McRae et al,[424,425] was a pneumoencephalogram that showed a correlation between hemispheric asymmetry and hand preference. In the short time that has elapsed since then, the landscape of imaging tools has changed considerably, altering our view of the relationship between brain and cognition. Hazy pneumoencephalographic images have given way to images that rival anatomic specimens in their gross anatomic detail. Neuroimaging now plays a vital role in posing and helping to answer critical questions about brain structure-function relationships.

One such central issue is the "binding problem," the issue of how distant brain areas are linked to produce emergent properties of awareness and cognition. Functional imaging addresses this issue by showing the sequential and simultaneous activation of separate areas of the brain during specific tasks. These areas can be viewed as components of distributed networks that form the substrates of cognitive function and that function in parallel to perform subtasks, which themselves combine to form the whole of a perceptual-motor-cognitive event. The concept of parallel processing in distributed networks may be a solution to the classic problem of localization of function versus equipotentiality in brain-behavior relationships.

Imaging also helps to illuminate what might be thought of as the converse of binding: disconnection. Many of the symptoms and signs of neurobehavioral dysfunction can be viewed as a consequence of disconnection of brain regions from one another.[66,426] Disconnection is a common theme in many neurobehavioral syndromes discussed above, such as nonfluency in aphasia, strategic infarct dementia, subcortical dementia, and amnesia due to focal lesions of the fornix. Disconnection may be responsible for some instances of diaschisis,[207] a concept that helps to explain the phenomenon of disproportionate neurobehavioral effects of relatively small lesions. This phenomenon can sometimes be visualized by functional imaging methods.[42,242]

Imaging illuminates the fundamental problem of modularity in neurology and neuropsychology. Modularity is the reification of cognitive functioning in discrete modules (e.g., language and memory). Modular thinking in neuropsychology seems to be demanded by some clinical observations of behavioral neurology. While clinically useful, as Goldberg[427] suggests, such observations may have held too much sway in the attempt to understand brain-behavior relationships. Both clinical observation and experimental evidence can be interpreted as showing that one cognitive function blends gradually and almost seamlessly into another. Goldberg[427] suggests that this is no accident, but, rather, that the neocortex represents a neurophysiologic shift away from modularity toward integrated emergent cognitive functioning.

For example, while information retrieval can be viewed as an issue of memory, it is clearly one of language as well. The problem of retrieving semantic information is not one of memory or of language alone, but is an adaptive requirement that draws on functioning in distributed networks. Information encoded in these networks is processed simultaneously in parallel and also sequentially, in the formulation of a goal directed behavior.

Functional imaging of neocortical and subcortical areas during cognitive tasks, showing the participation of the same parts of neocortex in widely different tasks, supports this view. Neuroimaging, therefore, serves both as a critical clinical tool in behavioral neurology and as a heuristic device in the study of brain-behavior relationships.*

REFERENCES

1. Mesulam M-M: *Principles of Behavioral Neurology*. Philadelphia, F.A. Davis, 1985.
2. Heilman KM, Valenstein E (eds): *Clinical Neuropsychology,* 3d ed. New York, Oxford Univesity Press, 1993.
3. Pincus JH, Tucker GJ: *Behavioral Neurology*, 3d ed. New York, Oxford University Press, 1985.
4. Brumback RA (ed): *Behavioral Neurology: Neurologic Clinics*, vol 11. Philadelphia, Saunders, 1993.
5. Feinberg TE, Farah MJ (eds): *Behavioral Neurology and Neuropsychology*. New York, McGraw-Hill, 1997.
6. Pritchard JW, Brass LM: New anatomical and functional imaging methods. *Ann Neurol* 32:395–400, 1992.
7. Kertesz A (ed): *Localization and Neuroimaging in Neuropsychology*. San Diego, Academic Press, 1994.
8. Naeser MA, Palumbo CL: How to analyze CT/MRI scan lesion sites to predict potential for long-term recovery in aphasia, in Kirschner H (ed): *Handbook of Neurologic Speech and Language Disorders*. New York, Marcel Dekker, 1994.
9. Damasio AR, Frank R: Three-dimensional in vivo mapping of brain lesions in humans. *Arch Neurol* 49:137–143, 1992.
10. Jagust WJ, Eberling JL: MRI, CT, SPECT, PET: Their use in diagnosing dementia. *Geriatrics* 46:28–35, 1991.
11. Pascual-Leone A, Dhuna A, Anderson DC: Cerebral atrophy in habitual cocaine abusers: A planimetric CT study. *Neurology* 41:34–38, 1991.
12. Jones-Gotman M: Localization of lesions by neuropsychological testing. *Epilepsia* 5:S41-S52, 1991.

*Thanks to Mary Wolfe, Linda Wellner, and Bethany Matthews for valuable contributions to this edition.

13. Boivin MJ, Giordani B, Berent S, et al: Verbal fluency and positron emission tomographic mapping of regional cerebral glucose metabolism. *Cortex* 28:231–239, 1992.
14. Alavi A, Hirsch LJ: Studies of central nervous system disorders with single photon emission computed tomography and positron emission tomography: Evolution over the past 2 decades. *Semin Nucl Med* 21:58–81, 1991.
15. Mazziotta JC, Frackowiak RSJ, Phelps ME: The use of positron emission tomography in the clinical assessment of dementia. *Semin Nucl Med* 22:233–246, 1992.
16. Caplan LR: Question-driven technology assessment: SPECT as an example. *Neurology* 41:187–191, 1991.
17. Tikofsky RS, Hellman RS: Brain single photon emission computed tomography: Newer activation and intervention studies. *Semin Nucl Med* 21:40–57, 1991.
18. Bonte FJ, Hom J, Tintner R, Weiner MF: Single photon tomography in Alzheimer's disease and the dementias. *Semin Nucl Med* 20:342–352, 1990.
19. Van Heertum RL, O'Connell RA: Functional brain imaging in the evaluation of psychiatric illness. *Semin Nucl Med* 21:24–39, 1991.
20. Prichard JW, Cummings JL: The insistent call from functional MRI. *Neurology* 48:797–800, 1997.
21. Kung HF, Ohmomo Y, Kung M-P: Current and future radiopharmaceuticals for brain imaging with single photon emission computed tomography. *Semin Nucl Med* 20:290–302, 1990.
22. Holman BL, Devous MD: Functional brain SPECT: The emergence of a powerful clinical method. *J Nucl Med* 33:1888–1904, 1992.
23. Ter-Pogossian MM: The origins of positron emission tomography. *Semin Nucl Med* 22:140–149, 1992.
24. Silvestrini M, Troisi E, Matteis M, et al: Correlations of flow velocity changes during mental activity and recovery from aphasia in ischemic stroke. *Neurology* 50:191–195, 1998.
25. Belliveau JW, Kennedy DN, McKinstry RC, et al: Functional mapping of the human visual cortex by magnetic resonance imaging. *Science* 254:716–719, 1991.
26. American Academy of Neurology Therapeutics and Technology Assessment Subcommittee: Assessment: EEG brain mapping. *Neurology* 39:1100–1101, 1989.
27. John ER, Prichep LS, Fridman J, Easton P: Neurometrics: Computer-assisted differential diagnosis of brain dysfunctions. *Science* 239:162–169, 1988.
28. Duffy FH: Clinical value of topographic mapping and quantified neurophysiology. *Arch Neurol* 46:1133–1136, 1989.
29. Papanicolaou AC, Baumann S, Rogers RL, et al: Localization of auditory response sources using magnetoencephalography and magnetic resonance imaging. *Arch Neurol* 47:33–37, 1990.
30. Yang TT, Gallen CC, Schwartz B, et al: Detailed somatosensory homunculus mapping using a large array biomagnetometer. *Neurology* 43(suppl):A158, 1993.
31. Benson DF: *The Neurology of Thinking.* New York, Oxford University Press, 1994, p 143.
32. Ojemann GA: Cortical stimulation and recording in language, in Kertesz A (ed): *Localization and Neuroimaging in Neuropsychology.* San Diego, Academic Press, 1994, pp 35–55.
33. Alexander P: Aphasia: Clinical and anatomic aspects, in Feinberg TE, Farah MJ (eds): *Behavioral Neurology and Neuropsychology.* New York, McGraw-Hill, 1997, chap 9, pp 133–150.
34. Goodglass H: *Understanding Aphasia.* San Diego, Academic Press, 1993.
35. Geschwind N: Cerebral dominance and anatomic asymmetry. *N Engl J Med* 287:194–195, 1972.
36. Geschwind N, Levitsky W: Human brain: Left-right asymmetries in temporal speech region. *Science* 161:186–187, 1968.
37. Foundas AL, Leonard CM, Gilmore RL, et al: Pars triangularis asymmetry and language dominance. *Proc Natl Acad Sci U S A* 93:719–722, 1996.
38. Binder JR, Frost JA, Hammeke TA, et al: Human brain language areas identified by functional magnetic resonance imaging. *J Neurosci* 17:353–362, 1997.
39. Zatorre RJ, Evans AC, Meyer E, Gjedde A: Lateralization of phonetic and pitch discrimination in speech processing. *Science* 256:846–849, 1992.
40. Alexander MP: Aphasia: Clinical and anatomic aspects, in Feinberg TE, Farah MK (eds): *Behavioral Neurology and Neuropsychology.* New York: McGraw-Hill, 1994, chap. 9, pp 133–149.
41. Benson DF, Geschwind N: Aphasia and related disorders: A clinical approach, in Mesulam M-M (ed): *Principles of Behavioral Neurology*. Philadelphia, F.A. Davis, 1985, chap 5, pp 193–238.
42. Metter EJ, Kempler D, Jackson C, et al: Cerebral glucose metabolism in Wernicke's, Broca's, and conduction aphasia. *Arch Neurol* 46:27–34, 1989.
43. Sergent J, Zuck E, Terriah S, MacDonald B: Distributed neural network underlying musical sight-reading and keyboard performance. *Science* 257:106–109, 1992.
44. Benson RR, Kwong KK, Belliveau JW, et al: Functional MRI of human auditory cortex. *Neurology* 43(suppl): A159, 1993.
45. Churchland PS, Sejnowski TJ: Neural representation and neural computation, in Nadel L, Cooper LA, Culicover P, Harnish RM (eds): *Neural Connections, Mental Computation.* Cambridge, MIT Press, 1990, chap. 1, pp 15–48.
46. Wise R, Chollet F, Hadar U, et al: Distribution of cortical neural networks involved in word comprehension and word retrieval. *Brain* 114:1803–1817, 1991.
47. Naeser MA, Palumbo CL, Helm-Estabrooks N, et al: Severe nonfluency in aphasia: Role of the medial subcallosal fasciculus and other white matter pathways in recovery of spontaneous speech. *Brain* 112:1–38, 1989.
48. Soderfeldt B, Ronnberg J, Risberg J: Regional cerebral blood flow in sign language users. *Brain Lang* 46:59–68, 1994.
49. Soderfeldt B, Ingvar M, Ronnberg J, et al: Signed and spoken language perception studied by positron emission tomography. *Neurology* 49:82–87, 1997.
50. Goodglass H, Kaplan E: *The Assessment of Aphasia and Related Disorders*, 2d ed. Philadelphia, Lea & Febiger, 1983.
51. Albert ML, Helm-Estabrooks N: Diagnosis and treatment of aphasia: I. *JAMA* 259:1043–1047, 1988.
52. Albert ML, Helm-Estabrooks N: Diagnosis and treatment of aphasia: II. *JAMA* 259:1205–1210, 1988.

53. Damasio AR: Aphasia. *N Engl J Med* 326:531–439, 1992.
54. Goodglass H, Kaplan E: *Boston Diagnostic Aphasia Examination.* Philadelphia, Lea & Febiger, 1972.
55. Kertesz A: *Western Aphasia Battery.* New York, Grune & Stratton, 1982.
56. Damasio H, Damasio AR: *Lesion Analysis in Neuropsychology.* New York, Oxford University Press, 1989.
57. Alexander M, Naeser M, Palumbo C: Broca's area aphasias: Aphasia after lesions including the frontal operculum. *Neurology* 40:353–362, 1990.
58. Deleval J, Leonard A, Mavroudakis N, Rodesch G: Global aphasia without hemiparesis following prerolandic infarction. *Neurology* 39:1532–1535, 1989.
59. Legatt AD, Rubin MJ, Kaplan LR, et al: Global aphasia without hemiparesis: Multiple etiologies. *Neurology* 37: 201–205, 1987.
60. Tranel D, Biller J, Damasio H, et al: Global aphasia without hemiparesis. *Arch Neurol* 44:304–308, 1987.
61. Tranel D, Biller J, Damasio H, Adams H: Global aphasia without hemiparesis. *Neurology* 36(suppl 1):318, 1986.
62. Van Horn G, Hawes A: Global aphasia without hemiparesis: A sign of embolic encephalopathy. *Neurology* 32: 403–406, 1982.
63. Van Horn G: Global aphasia without hemiparesis. *Neurology* 37:1691, 1987.
64. Ferro JM: Global aphasia without hemiparesis. *Neurology* 33:1106, 1983.
65. Matthews MK, Glosser G: Language recovery in global aphasia without hemiparesis. *Neurology* 41(suppl 1): 410, 1991.
66. Geschwind N: Disconnexion syndromes in animals and man: I and II. *Brain* 88:237–294, 585–644, 1965.
67. Damasio H, Damasio AR: *Neuroanatomy and Neuropsychological Disorders: Neuroimaging Procedures and Problems.* New York, Oxford University Press, 1989.
68. Basso A, Lecours AR, Moraschini S, Vanier M: Anatomoclinical correlations of the aphasias defined through computerized tomography: exceptions. *Brain Lang* 26: 201–229, 1985.
69. Daffner KR, Schomer DL, Cosgrove R, et al: Broca's aphasia following damage to Wernike's area: For or against traditional aphasiology? *Arch Neurol* 48:766–768, 1991.
70. Naeser MA: Quantitative approaches to computerized tomography in behavioral neurology, in Mesulam MM (ed): *Principles of Behavioral Neurology.* Philadelphia, F.A. Davis, 1985, chap 11, pp 363–383.
71. Naeser MA, Palumbo CL: Neuroimaging and language recovery in stroke. *J Clin Neurophys* 11:150–174, 1994.
72. Naeser MA, Baker EH, Palumbo CL, et al: Lesion site patterns in severe, nonverbal aphasia to predict outcome with a computer-assisted treatment program. *Arch Neurol* 55:1438–1449, 1998.
73. Bushnell DL, Gupta S, Mlcoch AG, Barnes WE: Prediction of language and neurologic recovery after cerebral infarction with SPECT imaging using *N*-isopropyl-*p*-(I 123) iodoamphetamine. *Arch Neurol* 46:665–669, 1989.
74. Nagata K, Watahiki Y, Satoh Y, et al: Role of right hemisphere function during recovery from aphasia due to cerebral infarction. *Ann Neurol* 30:238, 1990.
75. Ohyama M, Senda M, Kitamura S, et al: Role of the nondominant hemisphere and undamaged area during word repetition in poststroke aphasics: A PET activation study. *Stroke* 27:897–903, 1996.
76. Heiss W-D, Kessler J, Karbe H, Fink G: Recovery of poststroke aphasia is related to glucose metabolism at rest and during activation. *Ann Neurol* 32:237, 1992.
77. Karbe H, Kessler J, Herholz K, et al: Long-term prognosis of poststroke aphasia studied with positron emission tomography. *Arch Neurol* 52:186–190, 1995.
78. Galaburda AM: Neuroanatomic basis of developmental dyslexia. *Neurologic Clin* 11:161–173, 1993.
79. Rosenberger PB: Dyslexia:I Is it a disease? *N Engl J Med* 326:192–193, 1992.
80. Leonard CM, Voeller KKS, Lombardino LJ, et al: Anomalous cerebral structure in dyslexia revealed with magnetic resonance imaging. *Arch Neurol* 50:461–469, 1993.
81. Leonard CM, Williams CA, Nicholls RD, et al: Angelman and Prader-Willi syndrome: A magnetic resonance imaging study of differences in cerebral structure. *Am J Med Genet* 46:26–33, 1993.
82. Eden GF, VanMeter JW, Rumsey JM, et al: Abnormal processing of visual motion in dyslexia revealed by functional brain imaging. *Nature* 382:66–69, 1996.
83. Stein J, Walsh V: To see but not to read: The magnocellular theory of dyslexia. *Trends Neurosci* 20:147–152, 1997.
84. Demb JB, Boynton GM, Heeger DJ: Brain activity in visual cortex predicts individual differences in reading performance. *Proc Natl Acad Sci U S A* 94:13363–13366, 1997.
85. Elliott T, Chugani HT, Messa C, Phelps ME: Developmental dysphasia studied with positron emission tomography. *Ann Neurol* 30:483, 1991.
86. Rumsey JM: The biology of developmental dyslexia. *JAMA* 268:912–915, 1992.
87. Rumsey JM, Andreason P, Zametkin AJ, et al: Failure to activate the left temporoparietal cortex in dyslexia: An oxygen 15 positron emission tomographic study. *Arch Neurol* 49:527–534, 1992.
88. Hagman JO, Wood F, Buchsbaum MS, et al: Cerebral brain metabolism in adult dyslexic subjects assessed with positron emission tomography during performance of an auditory task. *Arch Neurol* 49:734–739, 1992.
89. Salmelin R, Service E, Kiesila P, et al: Impaired visual word processing in dyslexia revealed with magnetoencephalography. *Ann Neurol* 40:157–162, 1996.
90. Paulesu E, Frith U, Snowling M, et al: Is developmental dyslexia a disconnection syndrome? Evidence from PET scanning. *Brain* 119:143–157, 1996.
91. Duara R, Kushch A, Gross-Glenn K, et al: Neuroanatomic differences between dyslexic and normal readers on magnetic resonance imaging scans. *Arch Neurol* 48: 410–416, 1991.
92. Hynd GW, Semrud-Clikeman M, Lorys AR, et al: Brain morphology in developmental dyslexia and attention deficit disorder/hyperactivity. *Arch Neurol* 47:919–926, 1990.
93. Galaburda AM: The planum temporale. *Arch Neurol* 50:457, 1993.
94. Geschwind N, Galaburda AM: *Cerebral Lateralization: Biological Mechanisms, Associations, and Pathology.* Cambridge, MIT Press, 1987.

95. Tonnessen FE, Lokken A, Hoien T, Lundberg I: Dyslexia, left-handedness, and immune disorders. *Arch Neurol* 50:411–416, 1993.
96. Rumsey JM, Casanova M, Mannheim GB, et al: Corpus callosum morphology, as measured with MRI, in dyslexic men. *Biol Psychiatry* 39:769–775, 1996.
97. Newell A: *Unified Theories of Cognition*. Cambridge, Harvard University Press, 1990.
98. Duffy CJ: Implicit memory: Knowledge without awareness. *Neurology* 49:1200–1202, 1997.
99. Gordon B: Neuropsychology and advances in memory function. *Curr Opin Neurol* 10:306–312, 1997.
100. Verfaellie M, Keane MM: The neural basis of aware and unaware forms of memory. *Semin Neurol* 17:153–161, 1997.
101. Bauer RM, Tobias B, Valenstein E: Amnestic disorders, in Heilman KM, Valenstein E (eds): *Clinical Neuropsychology*, 3d ed. New York, Oxford University Press, 1993, chap 15, pp 523–602.
102. Baddeley A: Working memory. *Science* 255:556–559, 1992.
103. Perani D, Bressi S, Cappa SF, et al: Evidence of multiple memory systems in the human brain. *Brain* 116:903–919, 1993.
104. Greiner F, English S, Dean K, et al: Expression of game-related and generic knowledge by dementia patients who retain skill at playing dominoes. *Neurology* 49:518–523, 1997.
105. Shacter DL, Chiu C, Ochsner KN: Implicit memory: A selective review. *Ann Rev Neurosci* 16:159–182, 1993.
106. Roskies AL: Mapping memory with positron emission tomography. *Proc Natl Acad Sci U S A* 91:1989–1991, 1994.
107. Farah MJ, Grossman M: Semantic memory impairments, in Feinberg TE, Farah MK (eds): *Behavioral Neurology and Neuropsychology*. New York, McGraw-Hill, 1997, chap 37, pp 473–477.
108. Tulving E, Schachter DL: Priming and human memory systems. *Science* 247:301–306, 1990.
109. Buckner RL, Peterson SE, et al: Functional anatomical studies of explicit and implicit memory retrieval tasks. *J Neurosci* 15:12–29, 1995.
110. Squire LR, Ojemann JG, Miezin FM, et al: Activation of the hippocampus in normal humans: A funtional anatomical study of memory. *Proc Natl Acad Sci U S A* 89: 1837–1841, 1992.
111. Smith ML, Milner B: The role of the right hippocampus in the recall of spatial location. *Neuropsychologicia* 19: 781–793, 1981.
112. Heil M, Rosler F, Hennighausen E: Topographically distinct cortical activation in episodic long-term memory: The retrieval of spatial versus verbal information. *Mem Cogn* 24:777–795, 1996.
113. Milner B: Amnesia following operation on the temporal lobe, in Whitty CWM, Zangwil OL (eds): *Amnesia*. London, Butterworths, pp 109–133, 1996.
114. Saykin AJ, Gur RC, Sussman NM, Gur RE: Memory deficits before and after temporal lobectomy: Effect of laterality and age of onset. *Brain Cogn* 9:191–200, 1989.
115. Perrine K, Gershengorn J, Brown ER, et al: Material-specific memory in the intracarotid amobarbital procedure. *Neurology* 43:706–711, 1993.
116. Gur RC, Jaggi JL, Ragland JD, et al: Effects of memory processing on regional brain activation: Cerebral blood flow in normal subjects. *Int J Neurosci* 72:31–44, 1993.
117. Gur RC, Ragland D, Mozley LH, et al: Lateralized changes in regional cerebral blood flow during performance of verbal and facial recognition tasks: Correlations with performace and "effort." *Brain Cogn* 33:388–414, 1997.
118. Goldman-Rakic PS, Friedman HR: The circuitry of working memory revealed by anatomy and metabolic imaging, in Levin HS, Eisenberg HM, Benton AL (eds): *Frontal Lobe Function and Dysfunction*. New York, Oxford University Press, 1991, chap 4, pp 72–91.
119. Zola S: Amnesia: Neuroanatomc and clinical aspects, in Feinberg TE, Farah MK (eds): *Behavioral Neurology and Neuropsychology*. New York, McGraw-Hill, 1997, chap 35, pp 447–462.
120. Knowlton BJ, Mangels JA, Squire LR: A neostriatal habit learning system in humans. *Science* 273:1399–1402, 1996.
121. Grasby PM, Frith CD, Friston KJ, et al: Functional mapping of brain areas implicated in auditory-verbal memory function. *Brain* 116:1–20, 1993.
122. Grasby PM, Frith CD, Friston KJ, et al: Activation of the human hippocampal formation during auditory-verbal long-term memory function. *Neurosci Lett* 163:185–188, 1993.
123. Kapur S, Craik FI, Tulving E, et al: Neuroanatomical correlates of encoding in episodic memory: Levels of processing effect. *Proc Natl Acad Sci U S A* 91: 2008–2011, 1994.
124. Kapur S, Rose R, Liddle PF, et al: The role of the left prefrontal cortex in verbal processing: Semantic processing or willed action? *NeuroReport* 5:2193–2196, 1994.
125. Fletcher PC, Frith CD, Grasby PM, et al: Brain systems for encoding and retrieval of auditory-verbal memory: An in vivo study in humans. *Brain* 118:401–416, 1995.
126. Shallice T, Fletcher P, Frith CD, et al: Brain regions associated with acquisition and retrieval of verbal episodic memory. *Nature* 368:633–635, 1994.
127. Petrides M, Alivisatos B, Evans AC: Functional activation of the human ventrolateral frontal cortex during mnemonic retrieval of verbal information. *Proc Natl Acad Sci U S A* 92:5803–5807, 1995.
128. Tulving E, Kapur S, Markowitsch HJ, et al: Neuroanatomical correlates of retrieval in episodic memory: Auditory sentence recognition. *Proc Natl Acad Sci U S A* 91:2012–2015, 1994.
129. Haxby JV, Ungerleider LG, Horwitz B, et al: Face encoding and recognition in the human brain. *Proc Natl Acad Sci U S A* 93:922–927, 1996.
130. Kapur S, Craik FI, Jones C, et al:Functional role of the prefrontal cortex in tretirval of memories: A PET study. *NeuroReport* 6:1880–1884, 1995.
131. Grady CL, McIntosh AR, Horwitz B, et al: Age-related reductions in human recognition memory due to impaired encoding. *Science* 269:218–221, 1995.
132. Maguire EA, Frackowiak RSJ, Frith CD: Recalling routes around London: Activation of the right hippocampus in taxi drivers. *J Neurosci* 17:7103–7110, 1997.
133. Maguire EA, Burke T, Phillips J, Staunton H: Topographical disorientation following unilateral temporal

lobe lesions in humans. *Neuropsychologia* 34:993–1001, 1996.

134. Stern CE, Corkin S, Gonzalez RG, et al: The hippocampal formation participates in novel picture encoding: Evidence from functional magnetic resonance imaging. *Proc Natl Acad Sci U S A* 93:8660–8665, 1996.
135. Knight R. Contribution of human hippocampal region to novelty detection. *Nature* 383:256–259, 1996.
136. Grasby PM, Frith CD, Friston K, et al: Activation of the human hippocampal formation during auditory-verbal long-term memory function. *Neurosci Lett* 163:185–188, 1993.
137. Schacter DL, Alpert MA, Savage CR, et al: Conscious recollection and the human hippocampal formation: Evidence from positron emission tomography. *Proc Natl Acad Sci U S A* 93:321–325, 1996.
138. Seeck M, Mainwaring N, Cosgrove R, et al: Neurophysiologic correlates of immplicit face memory in intracranial visual evoked potentials. *Neurology* 49:1312–1316, 1997.
139. Hugdahl K, Berardi A, Thompson WL, et al: Brain mechanisms in human classical conditioning: A PET blood flow study. *NeuroReport* 6:1723–1728, 1995.
140. Blaxton TA, Zeffiro TA, Gabrieli JD, et al: Functional mapping of human learning: A PET activation study of eyeblink conditioning. *J Neurosci* 16:4032–4040, 1996.
141. Molchan SE, Sutherland T, McIntosh AR, et al: A functional anatomical study of associative learning in humans. *Proc Natl Acad Sci U S A* 91:8122–8126, 1994.
142. Jenkins IH, Brooks DJ, Nixon PD, et al: Motor sequence learning: A study with positron emission tomography. *J Neurosci* 14:3775–3790, 1994.
143. Grafton ST, Mazziotta JC, Presty S, et al: Functional anatomy of human procedural learning determined with regional cerebral blood flow and PET. *J Neurosci* 12:2542–2548, 1992.
144. Karni A, Meyer G, Jezzard P, et al: Functional MRI evidence for adult motor cortex plasticity during motor skill learning. *Nature* 377:155–158, 1995.
145. Shadmehr R, Holcomb HH: Neural correlates of motor memory consolidation. *Science* 277:821–825, 1997.
146. Benson DF, Djenderedjian A, Miller BL, et al: Neural basis of confabulation. *Neurology* 46:1239–1243, 1996.
147. Symonds C: Disorders of memory. *Brain* 89:24–644, 1966.
148. Benson DF: Amnesia. *South Med J* 71:1221–1228, 1978.
149. Moss MB, Albert MS, Butters N, Payne M: Differential patterns of memory loss among patients with Alzheimer's disease, Huntington's disease, and alcoholic Korsakoff's syndrome. *Arch Neurol* 43:239–246, 1988.
150. Squire LR: Comparisons between forms of amnesia: Some deficits are unique to Korsakoff's syndrome. *J Exp Psychol Learn Mem Cogn* 8:560–571, 1982.
151. Signoret JL: Memory and amnesias, in Mesulam M-M (ed): *Principles of Behavioral Neurology*. Philadelphia, FA Davis, 1985, chap 4 pp 169–192.
152. Sagar HJ, Gabrieli JD, Sullivan EV, Corkin S: Recency and frequency discrimination in the amnesic patient H.M. *Brain* 113:581–602, 1990.
153. Scoville WB, Milner B: Loss of recent memory after bilateral hippocampal lesions. *J Neurol Neurosurg Psychiatry* 20:11–21, 1957.
154. Victor M, Adams RD, Collins GH: *The Wernicke-Korsakoff Syndrome and Related Neurologic Disorders Due to Alcoholism and Malnutrition*, 2d ed. Philadelphia, FA Davis, 1989.
155. Tanaka Y, Miyazawa Y, Akaoka F, Yamada T: Amnesia following damage to the mammillary bodies. *Neurology* 48:160–165, 1997.
156. Garcia-Bengochea F, Friedman WA: Persistent memory loss following section of the anterior fornix in humans: A historical review. *Surg Neurol* 27:361–364, 1987.
157. Calabrese P, Markowitsch HJ, Harders AG, et al: Fornix damage and memory: A case report. *Cortex* 31:555–564, 1995.
158. Gaffan EA, Gaffan D, Hodges HR: Amnesia following damage to the left fornix and to other sites: A comparative study. *Brain* 114:1297–1313, 1991.
159. D'Esposito M, Verfaellie M, Alexander MP, Katz DI: Amnesia following traumatic bilateral fornix transection. *Neurology* 45:1546–1550, 1995.
160. Mennemeier M, Fennell E, Valenstein E, Heilman KM: Contributions of the left intralaminar and medial thalamic nuclei to memory: Comparisons and report of a case. *Arch Neurol* 49:1050–1058, 1992.
161. Malamut BL, Graff-Redford N, Chawluk J, et al: Memory in a case of bilateral thalamic infarction. *Neurology* 42:163–169, 1992.
162. Miller LA, Munoz DG, Finmore M: Hippocampal sclerosis and human memory. *Arch Neurol* 50:391–394, 1993.
163. Kalviainen R, Partanen K, Aikia M, et al: MRI-based hippocampal volumetry and T2 relaxometry: Correlation to verbal memory performance in newly diagnosed epilepsy patients with left-sided temporal lobe focus. *Neurology* 48:286–287, 1997.
164. Sass KJ, Spencer DD, Kim JH, et al: Verbal memory impairment correlates with hippocampal pyramidal cell density. *Neurology* 40:1694–1697, 1990.
165. Fisher CM, Adams RD: Transient global amnesia. *Acta Neurol Scand* 40(suppl 9):7–83, 1964.
166. Melo TP, Ferro JM, Ferro H: Transient global amnesia: A case control study. *Brain* 115:261–270, 1992.
167. Woolfenden AR, O'Brien MW, Schwartzberg RE: Diffusion-weighted MRI in transient global amnesia precipitated by cerebral angiography. *Stroke* 28:2311–2314, 1997.
168. Goldenberg G, Podreka I, Pfaffelmeyer N, et al: Thalamic ischemia in transient global amnesia: A SPECT study. *Neurology* 41:1748–1752, 1991.
169. Laloux P, Brichant C, Cauwe F, Decoster P: Technetium-99m HM-PAO single photon emission computed tomography imaging in transient global amnesia. *Arch Neurol* 49:543–546, 1992.
170. Stillhard G, Landis T, Schiess R, et al: Bitemporal hypoperfusion in transient global amnesia: 99m-Tc-HM-PAOSPECT and neuropsychological findings during and after an attack. *J Neurol Neurosurg Psychiatry* 53:339–342, 1990.
171. Volpe BT, Herscovitch P, Raichle ME, et al: Cerebral blood flow and metabolism in human amnesia. *J Cereb Blood Flow Metab* 3(suppl 2):S5-S6, 1983.
172. Eustache F, Desgranges B, Petit-Taboue MC, et al: Transient global amnesia: Implicit/explicit memory dissocia-

329. Snowden JS, Neary D, Mann DMA, et al: Progressive language disorder due to lobar atrophy. *Ann Neurol* 31: 174–183, 1992.
330. McDaniel KD, Wagner MT, Greenspan BS: The role of brain single photon emission computed tomography in the diagnosis of primary progressive aphasia. *Arch Neurol* 48:1257–1260, 1991.
331. Mendez MF, Zander BA: Dementia presenting with aphasia: Clinical characteristics. *J Neurol Neurosurg Psychiatry* 54:542–545, 1991.
332. Karbe H, Kertesz A, Polk M: Profiles of language impairment in primary progressive aphasia. *Arch Neurol* 50: 193–201, 1993.
333. Hodges JR, Patterson K, Oxbury S, Funnell E: Semantic dementia: Progressive fluent aphasia with temporal lobe atrophy. *Brain* 115:1783–1806, 1992.
334. Barbarotto R, Capitani E, Spinnler H, Trivelli C: Slowly progressive semantic impairment with category specificity. *Neurocase* 1:107–119, 1995.
335. Kirshner HS, Tanridag O, Thurman L, Whetsell WO: Progressive aphasia without dementia: Two cases with focal spongiform degeneration. *Ann Neurol* 22:527–532, 1987.
336. Kobayashi K, Kurachi M, Gyoubu T, et al: Progressive dysphasic dementia with localized cerebral atrophy: Report of an autopsy. *Clin Neuropathol* 9:254–261, 1990.
337. Lippa CF, Cohen R, Smith TW, Drachman DA: Primary progressive aphasia with focal neuronal achromasia. *Neurology* 41:882–886, 1991.
338. Mandell AM, Alexander MP, Carpenter S: Creutzfeldt-Jakob disease presenting as isolated aphasia. *Neurology* 39:55–58, 1987.
339. Holland Al, McBurney DH, Moossy J, Reinmuth OM: The dissolution of language in Pick's disease with neurofibrillary tangles: A case study. *Brain Lang* 24:36–58, 1985.
340. Green J, Morris JC, Sandson J, et al: Progressive aphasia: A precursor of global dementia? *Neurology* 40:423–429, 1990.
341. Chapman SB, Rosenberg RN, Weiner MF, Shobe A: Autosomal dominant progressive syndrome of motor-speech loss without dementia. *Neurology* 49:1298–1306, 1997.
342. Albert ML: Subcortical dementia, in Katzman R, Terry RD, Bick KL (eds): *Alzheimer's Disease: Senile Dementia and Related Disorders.* New York, Raven Press, 1978.
343. Albert ML, Feldman RG, Willis AL: The "subcortical dementia" of progressive supranuclear palsy. *J Neurol Neurosurg Psychiatry* 37:121–130, 1974.
344. Perry RJ, Hodges JR: Spectrum of memory dysfunction in degenertive disease. *Curr Opin Neurol* 9:281–285, 1996.
345. Hachinski VC, Lassen NA, Marshall J: Multi-infarct dementia: A cause of mental deterioration in the elderly. *Lancet* 2:207–210, 1974.
346. Stuss DT, Cummings JL: Subcortical vascular dementias, in Cummings JL (ed): *Subcortical Dementia.* New York, Oxford University Press, 1990, chap 11, pp 145–163.
347. Gibb WRG: Dementia and Parkinson's disease. *Br J Psychiatry* 154:596–614, 1989.
348. Tamaru F: Disturbances in higher function in Parkinson's disease. *Eur Neurol* 38(suppl 2):33–36, 1997.
349. Price RW, Brew B, Sidtis J, et al: The brain in AIDS: Central nervous system HIV-I infection and AIDS dementia complex. *Science* 239:586–592, 1988.
350. Pajeau AK, Roman GC: HIV encephalopathy and dementia. *Psychchiatr Clin North Am* 15:455–466, 1992.
351. Lees AJ: Progressive supranuclear palsy (Steele-Richardson-Olszewski syndrome), in Cummings JL (ed): *Subcortical Dementia.* New York, Oxford University Press, 1990, chap 9, pp 123–131.
352. Salmon E, Van der Linden MV, Franck G: Anterior cingulate and motor network metabolic impairment in progressive supranuclear palsy. *Neuroimage* 5:173–178, 1997.
353. Cummings JL, Benson, DF: Subcortical mechanisms and human thought: in Cummings JL (ed): *Subcortical Dementia.* New York, Oxford University Press, 1990, chap 17, pp 251–260.
354. Cummings JL (ed): *Subcortical Dementia.* New York, Oxford University Press, 1990.
355. Kase C: Multi-infarct dementia: A real entity? *J Am Geriatr Soc* 34:482–484, 1986.
356. Wolfe N, Linn R, Babikian VL, et al: Frontal systems impairment following multiple lacunar infarcts. *Arch Neurol* 47:129–132, 1990.
357. Kramer JH, Duffy JM: Aphasia, apraxia, and agnosia in the diagnosis of dementia. *Dementia* 7:23–26, 1996.
358. Marder K, Mayeux R: The epidemiology of dementia in patients with Parkinson's disease. *Adv Exp Med Biol* 295:439–445, 1990.
359. Ebmeier KP, Calder SA, Crawford JR, et al: Dementia in idiopathic Parkinson's disease: Prevalence and relationship with symptoms and signs of parkinsonism. *Psychol Med* 21:69–76, 1991.
360. Jagust WJ, Reed BR, Martin EM, et al: Cognitive function and regional cerebral blood flow in Parkinson's disease. *Brain* 115:521–537, 1992.
361. Zweig RM, Cardillo JE, Cohen M, et al: The locus ceruleus and dementia in Parkinson's disease. *Neurology* 43: 986–991, 1993.
362. Pizzolato G, Dam M, Borsato N: [^{99m}Tc]-HM-PAO SPECT in Parkinson's Disease. *J Cereb Blood Flow Metab* 8:S101–S108, 1988.
363. Kawabata K, Tachibana H, Sugita M: Cerebral blood flow and dementia in Parkinson's disease. *J Geriatr Psychiatry Neurol* 4:194–203, 1991.
364. Mayberg HS, Starkstein SE, Sadzot B, et al: Selective hypometabolism in the inferior frontal lobe in depressed patients with Parkinson's disease. *Ann Neurol* 28:57–64, 1990.
365. Grant I: The neuropsychiatry of human immunodeficiency virus. *Semin Neurol* 10:267–275, 1990.
366. Brouwers P, Nohr E, Hildebrand K, et al: A novel approach to the determination and characterization of HIV dementia. *Can J Neurol Sci* 23:104–109, 1996.
367. Power C, Johnson RT: HIV-1 associated dementia: Clinical features and pathogenesis. *Can J Neurol Sci* 22:92–100, 1995.
368. Kramer EL, Sanger JJ: Brain imaging in acquired immunodeficiency syndrome dementia complex. *Semin Nucl Med* 20:353–363, 1990.
369. Tuite M, Ketonen L, Kieburtz K, Handy B: Efficacy of gadolinium in MR brain imaging of HIV-infected patients. *Am J Neuroradiol* 14:257–263, 1993.

370. American Academy of Neurology AIDS Task Force: Nomenclature and research case definitions for neurologic manifestations of human immunodeficiency virus-type 1 (HIV-1) infection. *Neurology* 41:778–785, 1991.
371. Navia BA: The AIDS dementia complex, in Cummings JL (ed): *Subcortical Dementia*. New York, Oxford University Press, 1990, chap 13, pp 181–198.
372. Cohen WA, Maravilla KR, Gerlach R, et al: Prospective cerebral MR study of HIV seropositive and seronegative men: Correlation of MR findings with neurologic, neuropsychologic, and cerebrospinal fluid analysis. *Am J Neuroradiol* 13:1231–1240, 1992.
373. Dooneief, G, Bello J, Tadak G, et al: A prospective controlled study of magnetic resonanace imaging of the brain in gay men and parenteral drug users with human immunodeficiency virus infection. *Arch Neurol* 49:38–43, 1992.
374. Meyerhoff DJ, MacKay S, Dillon WP, et al: In vivo evidence of neuron loss in HIV-infected brains. *Neurology* 43:A254, 1993.
375. Meyerhoff DJ, MacKay S, Bachman L, et al: Reduced brain *N*-acetyl aspartate suggests neuronal loss in cognitively impaired human immunodeficiency virus-seropositive individuals: In vivo ^1H magnetic resonance spectroscopic imaging. *Neurology* 43:509–515, 1993.
376. Epstein LG, Gendelman HE: Human immunodeficiency virus type I infection of the nervous system: Pathogenetic mechanisms. *Ann Neurol* 33:429–436, 1993.
377. Rottenberg DA, Moeller JR, Strother SC: The metabolic pathology of the AIDS dementia complex. *Ann Neurol* 22:700–706, 1987.
378. Pohl P, Vogl G, Fill H: Single-photon emission computed tomography in AIDS dementia complex. *J Nucl Med* 29: 1382–1386, 1988.
379. LaFrance ND, Pearlson GD, Schaerf FW: I-123 IMP-SPECT in HIV-related dementia. *Adv Funct Neuroimag* 1:9–15, 1988.
380. LaFrance ND, Pearlson GD, Schaerf FW: SPECT imaging with I-123 isopropyl amphetamine in asymptomatic HIV seropositive persons. *J Nucl Med* 29:742, 1988.
381. Vazeux R, Brousse N, Jarry A, et al: AIDS subacute encephalitis: Identification of HIV-infected cells. *Am J Pathol* 126:403–410, 1987.
382. Adams RD, Victor M, Ropper AH: *Principles of Neurology*, 6th ed. New York, McGraw-Hill, 1997.
383. Grafman J, Litvan I, Stark M: Neuropsychological features of progressive supranuclear palsy. *Brain Cogn* 28: 311–320, 1995.
384. Jacobs DM, Stern Y, Mayeux R: Dementia in Parkinson disease, Huntington disease, and other degenerative conditions, in Feinberg TE, Farah MJ (eds): *Behavioral Neurology and Neuropsychology*. New York, McGraw-Hill, 1997, chap 45, pp 579–587.
385. Foster NL, Gilman S, Berent S, et al: Cerebral hypometabolism in progressive supranuclear palsy studied with positron emission tomography. *Ann Neurol* 24:399–406, 1988.
386. Leenders KL, Frackowiak RSJ, Lees AJ: Progressive supranuclear palsy: Brain energy metabolism, blood flow and fluorodopa uptake measured by positron emission tomography. *Brain* 111:615–630, 1988.
387. Pillon B, Blin J, Vidailhet M, et al: The neuropsychological pattern of corticobasal degeneration: Comparison with progressive supranuclear palsy and Alzheimer's disease. *Neurology* 45:1477–1483, 1995.
388. Rao SM: Neuroposychology of multiple sclerosis: A critical review. *J Clin Exp Neuropsychol* 8:502–542, 1986.
389. Mahler ME, Benson DF: Cognitive dysfunction in multiple sclerosis: A subcortical dementia?, in Rao SM (ed): *Neurobehavioral Aspects of Multiple Sclerosis*. New York, Oxford University Press, 1990, chap 5, pp 88–101.
390. Rao SM (ed): *Neurobehavioral Aspects of Multiple Sclerosis*. New York, Oxford University Press, 1990.
391. Blinkenberg M, Rune K, Jonsson A, et al: Cerebral metabolism in a case of multiple sclerosis with acute mental disorder. *Acta Neurol Scand* 94:310–313, 1996.
392. Bowler JV, Hachinski V: Vascular dementia, in Feinberg TE, Farah MJ (eds): *Behavioral Neurology and Neuropsychology*. New York, McGraw-Hill, 1997, chap 46, pp 589–603.
393. McPherson SE, Cummings JL: Neuropsychological aspects of vascular dementia. *Brain Cogn* 31:269–282, 1996.
394. Hachinski VC, Bowler JV: Vascular dementia. *Neurology* 43:2159–2160, 1993.
395. Desmond DW, Tatemichi TK, Figueroa M, et al: Cognitive dysfunction following lacunar infarction. *Ann Neurol* 32:240, 1992.
396. Figueroa M, Tatemichi TK, Desmond DW, Cross DT: CT correlates of dementia in lacunar infarction. *Ann Neurol* 32:266, 1992.
397. Loeb C, Gandolfo C, Croce R, Conti M: Dementia associated with lacunar infarction. *Stroke* 23:1225–1229, 1992.
398. Kinkel WR, Jacobs L, Polachini I, et al: Subcortical arteriosclerotic encephalopathy (Binswanger's disease). *Arch Neurol* 42:951–959, 1985.
399. Gupta SR, Naheedy MH, Young JC, et al: Periventricular white matter changes and dementia. *Arch Neurol* 45:637–641, 1988.
400. Regli L, Regli F, Maeder P, Bogousslavsky J: Magnetic resonance imaging with gadolinium contrast agent in small deep (lacunar) cerebral infarcts. *Arch Neurol* 50: 175–180, 1993.
401. Boone KB, Miller BL, Lesser IM, et al: Neuropsychological correlates of white-matter lesions in healthy elderly subjects: A threshold effect. *Arch Neurol* 49:549–554, 1992.
402. Shyu WC, Lin JC, Shen CC, et al. Vascular dementia of Binswanger's type: Clinical, neuroradiological and 99mTc-HMPAO SPET study. *Eur J Nucl Med* 23:1338–1344, 1996.
403. Brown SJ, Fann JR, Grant I: Postconcussional disorder: Time to acknowledge a common source of neurobehavioral morbibdity. *J Neuropsychiatry* 6:15–22, 1994.
404. Alexander JP: Mild traumatic brain injury: Pathophysiology, natural history, and clinical management. *Neurology* 45:1253–1260, 1995.
405. Marsh NV, Smith MD: Post-concussion syndrome and the coping hypothesis. *Brain Injury* 9:553–562, 1995.
406. Bigler ED: Brain imaging and behavioral outcome in traumatic brain injury. *J Learn Disabil* 29:515–530, 1996.
407. Wilson JTI, Wyper D: Neuroimaging and neuropsychological functioning following closed head injury:

CT, MRI, and SPECT. *J Head Trauma Rehabil* 7:29–39, 1992.
408. Macnamara SE, Bigler ED, Blatter D, et al: Magnetic resonance identified ventricular dilation in traumatic brain injury: Comparison of pre- and postinjury scan and postinjury results. *Arch Clin Neurol* 7:275–284, 1992.
409. Anderson CV, Bigler ED: Ventricular dilation, cortical atrophy, and neuropsychological outcome following traumatic brain injury. *J Neuropsychiatry* 7:42–48, 1995.
410. Bigler ED, Kurth S, Blatter D, Abildskov T: Day-of-injury CT as an index to pre-injury brain morphology: Degree of post-injury degenerative changes identified by CT and MR neuroimaging. *Brain Injury* 7:125–134, 1993.
411. Bigler ED: Three-dimensional image analysis of trauma-induced degenerative changes: An aid to neuropsychological assessment. *Arch Clin Neuropsychol* 7:449–456, 1992.
412. Katz DI: Neuropathology and neurobehavioral recovery from closed head injury. *J Head Trauma Rehabil* 7:1–15, 1992.
413. Bigler ED, Blatter DD, Anderson CV, et al: Hippocampal volume in normal aging and traumatic brain injury. *Am J Neuroradiol* 18:11–23, 1997.
414. Ichise M, Chung DG, Want P, et al: Technetium-99m-HMPAO-SPECT, CT, and MRI in the evaluation of patients with chronic traumatic brain injury: A correlation with neuropsychological performance. *J Nucl Med* 35:217–226, 1994.
415. Jacobs A, Put E, Ingels M, Bossuyt A: Prospective evaluation of technetium-99m-HMPO-SPECT in mild and moderate traumatic brain injury. *J Nucl Med* 35:942–947, 1994.
416. Levin HS, Williams D, Crofford MJ, et al: Relationship of depth of brain lesions to consciousness and outcome after closed head injury. *J Neurosurg* 69:861–866, 1988.
417. Vanheertum RL, O'Connell RA: Functional brain imaging in the evaluation of psychiatric illness. *Semin Nucl Med* 21:24–39, 1991.
418. Worley G, Hoffman JM, Paine SS, et al: 18-Fluorodeoxyglucose positron emission tomography in children and adolescents with traumatic brain injury. *Devel Med Child Neurol* 37:213–220, 1995.
419. Hamm RJ, Temple MD, O'Dell DM, et al: Exposure to environmental complexity promotes recovery of cognitive function after traumatic brain injury. *J Neurotrauma* 13:41–47, 1996.
420. Stein DG, Brailowsky S, Will B: *Brain Repair*. New York, Oxford University Press, 1995.
421. Kreutzer JS, Wehman PH (eds): *Cognitive Rehabilitation for Persons with Traumatic Brain Injury: A Functional Approach*. Baltimore, Brookes, 1991.
422. Dobkin BH: *Neurologic Rehabilitation*. Philadelphia, FA Davis, 1996.
423. Levin HS, Scheller J, Rickard T, et al: Dyscalculia and dyslexia after right hemisphere injury in infancy. *Arch Neurol* 53:88–96, 1996.
424. McRae DL, Branch CL, Milner B: The occipital horns and cerebral dominance. *Neurology* 18:95–98, 1968.
425. Witelson SF: Cognitive neuroanatomy: A new era. *Neurology* 42:709–713, 1992.
426. Absher JR, Benson DF: Disconnection syndromes: An overview of Geschwind's contribution. *Neurology* 43: 862–867, 1993.
427. Goldberg E: Rise and fall of modular orthodoxy. *J Clin Exp Neuropsychol* 17:193–208, 1995.

SECTION SIX

DISORDERS OF MOOD AND EMOTION

CHAPTER 9

IMAGING IN PSYCHIATRIC DISORDERS

K. Ranga Rama Krishnan
Orest B. Boyko
Kelly N. Botteron
Gary S. Figiel

INTRODUCTION

The search for neuroanatomic substrates of various psychiatric disorders has become a quest for a holy grail in psychiatric research. At first, the only way of assessing pathologic conditions of the brain in psychiatric disorders was by postmortem examination. The initial studies were notoriously difficult and were plagued by a number of methodologic problems, including changes in the brain tissue following death, lack of suitable control subjects, poorly representative samples (usually patients who died in institutions or committed suicide), coexistent medical problems, and confounding effects of treatment. These studies formed the basis of the sometimes erroneous assumption that psychiatric disorders, unlike many neurologic disorders, are not due to pathologic conditions of the brain.

With the advent of modern imaging methodologies, it has become possible to gradually dispel this notion and begin to understand the neuroanatomic substrates of many of these disorders. Structural imaging, such as computed tomography (CT) and magnetic resonance imaging (MRI), has demonstrated numerous changes in various structures in the brains of patients with a variety of psychiatric disorders, including schizophrenia, depression, autism, anorexia nervosa, bulimia nervosa, panic disorder, social phobia, and obsessive compulsive disorder. Functional studies using positron emission tomography and single photon emission CT have not only demonstrated metabolic changes in various regions of the brain but also allowed for the testing of hypotheses relating specific neurochemical transmitters to particular psychiatric disorders. For example, dopamine changes have been observed in schizophrenia.

This chapter focuses on structural changes in the brains of patients with psychiatric disorders and provides an introduction to some of the exciting functional changes reported in these patients. This chapter does not address structural and functional changes in the brains of individuals with substance abuse, including alcohol abuse. Substance abuse constitutes an extensive area of research and is beyond the scope of this chapter.

AFFECTIVE DISORDER

Affective disorders are characterized by impairments in mood, cognition, and neurovegetative symptoms. The two major types of affective disorder are unipolar and bipolar. Unipolar disorder, or major depressive disorder, is characterized by the occurrence of just depressive episodes. When there are repeated episodes, the condition is called recurrent unipolar disorder. Increasing evidence supports the existence of diagnostic heterogeneity within major depression, with some subtypes defined by comorbidity and family history. This remains an area of active research. Bipolar disorder is a type of affective disorder characterized by the occurrence, not just of depressive episodes, but also of hypomanic and manic episodes. Over the last 20 years, there have been a number of imaging studies in major depressive disorder and bipolar affective disorder. These studies have utilized various imaging modalities, including CT, MRI, single photon emission (SPECT), and positron emission tomography (PET). Studies of cerebral morphology in affective disorder and functional imaging studies have begun to help define the neuroanatomic and, to a limited extent, biochemical substrates of this disorder. In particular, studies in elderly depressed individuals have proved useful. Studies across the age span, including a number of studies of elderly depressed subjects, have begun to define differences in morphology and function based on age of onset.

DEPRESSION IN THE ELDERLY

Between 1 and 2 percent of elderly persons who live in the community have major depression.[1,2] The causes of depression in the elderly are poorly understood. The concept that psychological factors and social factors are the primary contributors to the occurrence of depression in later life, although intuitively appealing, is not supported by available evidence. In addition, genetic factors appear to be less significant in patients presenting with depression for the first time in later life. A number of studies—family, twin, and molecular genetic studies—have provided strong evidence of a genetic predisposition to develop affective disorder. The few studies that have examined this in the elderly have found minimal evidence of a genetic basis in patients with depression with onset late in life.[3] Hopkinson found the risk for immediate relatives of patients with first onset of depression after the age of 50 to be substantially lower (8.3 percent) than that for relatives of patients whose episodes started before that age.[4]

There has been considerable speculation that structural changes in the brain are of primary importance in the cause of late-life depression.[7,8,9,10] Post[8] reported that 12 percent of elderly depressed patients showed evidence of focal brain damage. He noted that the prevalence of cerebrovascular brain damage was higher in elderly depressed patients than that reported in surveys of the elderly population. This led Post to suggest that the cerebrovascular damage was a causative factor in the affective disorder and probably played a significant role in precipitating the illness. In addition, he speculated that the aging process itself facilitated the emergence of depression in later life. Post[11] cites a number of studies in support of this hypothesis.[12,13] Further analysis of these hypotheses requires a thorough understanding of the normal and pathologic alterations that occur in the aging brain.

IMAGING STUDIES OF THE AGING BRAIN

Computed Tomography Studies of the Normal Aging Brain

A number of studies have utilized CT to examine changes in the brain with aging. The studies have used various methods to assess changes, including global visual ratings by radiologists; linear measurements; a variety of ratio measures, such as the ventricular brain ratio, bifrontal-bicaudate ratio, and so on; and volumetric methods.[14,15,16,17,18,21] Most of the CT studies indicate that progressive cortical atrophy and enlargement of the lateral ventricles of the brain occur with aging.[22–26] In addition to cortical atrophy and enlargement of the lateral ventricles, an increase in the size of the third ventricle, cerebellar vermian atrophy, and leukoaraiosis[27] with aging have been reported. Hachinski[27] used the term *leukoaraiosis* to describe hypodensities in the cerebral white matter seen in CT scans of elderly patients.[28–31] Others have used other terms, such as *leukoencephalopathy,* to describe this entity.

Magnetic Resonance Imaging Studies of Normal Aging

Magnetic resonance imaging has been used to examine not only changes in cerebrospinal fluid (CSF) volumes and leukoencephalopathy but also morphometric changes in subcortical gray matter of the brain with aging. Grant et al[32] studied CSF volumes using MRI and demonstrated that total cranial CSF volume increased significantly with age in both males and females.

Studies utilizing MRI show a much higher prevalence of leukoencephalopathy than do CT studies.[33–39] These changes are seen as areas of signal hyperintensities on T2-weighted images. The changes are primarily found scattered in the periventricular white matter, deep white matter, basal ganglia, and pons.[34,35] These hyperintensities have also been called unidentified bright objects (UBOs) and, when seen in the gray matter, as subcortical hyperintensities. They are distributed along the noncollateralizing perforating vessels, such as medullary and lenticulostriate arteries.[34]

Like the CT studies, the initial MRI studies suggested that leukoencephalopathy increases with aging. These studies were confounded, however, by inclusion of patients with chronic systemic, cardiac, psychiatric, and neurologic diseases. Subsequent studies examined this issue in normal volunteers. Fazekas et al[40] studied nine healthy elderly control subjects free of any neurologic, psychiatric, or major systemic illness. T1- and T2-weighted axial images were utilized. Periventricular hyperintensities (PVH) were graded as follows: 0, absent; 1, "cap," pencil-thin lining; 2, smooth halo; and 3, irregular PVH extending into the deep white matter. Deep white matter hyperintensities (DWMH) were rated as follows: 0, absent; 1, punctate foci; 2, beginning confluence of foci; and 3, large confluent areas. Three subjects had grade 1 PVH; one had grade 3 PVH. Three subjects had grade 2 DWMH, and two had grade 1 DWMH. One subject had a basal ganglia lesion.

Hendrie et al[41] studied 27 healthy control subjects 63 to 86 years old. There was no relationship between white matter lesions and hypertension, diabetes mellitus, smoking, or cardiac factors. George et al[33] studied 47 normal subjects, 12 of whom were above the age of 45. Leukoencephalopathy was graded as none, minimal, mild, moderate, or severe. In six subjects, the change was minimal; in one it was mild, and in one it was moderate in severity.

Hunt et al[42] studied volunteers above the age of 60 using T1- and T2-weighted images. Thirty-four of 46 subjects had leukoencephalopathy; only 4 individuals had severe changes, 29 percent had moderate changes, and 59 percent had mild changes. Lesions were more severe in the parietal and occipital region than in the frontal or temporal region.

Fazekas[43] noted in a subsequent report that, in 87 volunteers between the ages of 31 and 83 years, lesions in the subcortical and deep white matter increased from 11 percent in the fourth decade to 83 percent in subjects over 70 years of age and were detected more often in individuals with cerebrovascular risk factors ($P < 0.01$). Confluent and early confluent white matter lesions were rare. Leukoaraiosis was seen by Inzitari et al[45] in 12 percent of control subjects (neurologic). They demonstrated that leukoaraiosis was associated with hypertension.

Sullivan et al[46] studied 60 patients with T1- and T2-weighted 5-mm thick axial sections. Deep white matter hyperintensities were graded as follows: 0, absent; 1, punctate foci; 2, beginning confluence of foci; and 3, large confluent areas. In this study, hypertension, transient ischemic attacks (TIAs), cardiac disease, and diabetes did not contribute to the severity of the leukoencephalopathy. The grading systems utilized are important to bear in mind because the pathology of the lesions varies according to both size and location.

Imaging and Pathologic Correlative Studies

Tomlinson et al,[47] in a study of 28 elderly patients without neurologic symptoms (although many had "affective psychoses"), found that over half the older subjects had cortical atrophy and a significant number had ventricular enlargement at autopsy. Cortical atrophy was prominent in the frontal and parietal area. Six of the subjects had infarcts of the basal ganglia. The neuropathologic basis underlying leukoaraiosis is more controversial. Awad et al[48] compared MRIs with neuropathologic studies on 8 postmortem brains. They found that the hyperintensities involved the periventricular white matter, optic radiations, basal ganglia, and centrum semiovale. The most common finding was ectasia of the arterioles with enlargement of the perivascular space. The changes resembled état criblé. État criblé is a condition characterized by round holes (resembling a sieve) in cerebral tissue in each of which a small vessel is seen. Additional changes include myelin pallor and lacunar infarcts. Similar findings were noted by Kilpatrick and Hayman,[49] Braffman et al,[51] and Marshall et al.[50] Larger lesions were noted by Marshall et al to be characterized centrally by necrosis, axonal loss, and demyelination and therefore represented true infarcts.

Sze et al[52] reported that the hyperintensities located anterior to the frontal horns of the ventricle seen in most normal volunteers are due to increased interstitial fluid in the region secondary to patchy loss of ependyma with astrocytic gliosis and a loose network of axons in the region.

Thus, in summary, the periventricular white matter changes, especially those anterior to the frontal horns, appear to be secondary to interstitial fluid accumulation and patchy loss of ependyma. The small punctate foci on MRI appear to be primarily enlargement of the perivascular spaces. The larger foci appear to be infarcts, or lacunae. The clinical significance of lacunae has been described in great detail by Fisher.[53] The lacunae in his series were primarily located in the basal ganglia, pons, and deep white matter. He felt that they were usually secondary to infarction. The location of the lesion was secondary to arterial occlusion of perforating vessels. Lability of mood has been noted in 26 percent of patients who have lacunar disease.

The location of the lacunae is primarily in the watershed zone of the distribution of the perforating vessels. The watershed zone consists of the areas of the brain that receive blood supply from perforating vessels with no other collateral blood supply. These vessels are not only susceptible to hypertension but are also sensitive to hypotension. Hypoperfusion secondary to hypotension often results in infarction in these watershed areas.[15] Hypertension in its severe form can lead to infarction[15] and chronic ischemia secondary to narrowing of the arterioles. This can result in loss of vasoregulation and subsequent cerebral edema, perivascular demyelination, myelin pallor, and gliosis. Hypotension and poor brain perfusion may be responsible for white matter changes seen in individuals who do not have hypertension or other cerebrovascular risk factors.

Morphometric Studies of Aging

There are few MRI studies of specific brain structures in normal aging at this time. Krishnan et al have studied the basal ganglia in 39 normal volunteers.[54] The caudate and putamen steadily decline in size with age. The decline in cerebral hemisphere volume is much smaller than the change in the volume of the basal ganglia. A moderate decline in the midsagittal corpus callosum area has been reported.[56] Autopsy studies confirm many of these findings.[57]

In summary, these studies demonstrate the following structural changes in the brain with aging: (1) enlarged lateral ventricles, (2) increased frequency and severity of leukoencephalopathy and cerebrovascular pathologic conditions, (3) decreased volume of the caudate, and (4) decreased volume of the putamen.

IMAGING STUDIES OF ELDERLY DEPRESSED PATIENTS

Computed Tomography Studies of Elderly Depressed Subjects

Jacoby and Levy[58] studied 41 patients (12 males) admitted to a geropsychiatry unit and 50 control subjects. The patients ranged in age from 63 to 86 years. When the patients were divided into two groups—those with onset of affective illness before the age of 60 (16 patients) and those with onset of depression after the age of 60—and CT measures compared, it was found that 8 of the late-onset patients had enlarged ventricles, whereas only one of the early-onset group had an enlarged ventricle. This finding provides support for the notion that the emergence of depression in the elderly is facilitated by organic pathologic conditions in the brain, although the nature of these conditions remains uncertain. In a subsequent report,[59] the investigators noted increased mortality rates in these patients compared to the control subjects. Of the five patients who had enlarged ventricles, two deaths were due to cerebrovascular accidents.

After this initial study, few have reexamined this issue. The same group reported that CT attenuation numbers were decreased in the elderly depressed patients compared to control subjects.[60] Shima et al[61] studied 45 patients ranging in age from 25 to 77 years and control subjects, and reported that the ventricular brain ratio (VBR) was increased in patients whose onset of depression was before the age of 50. Pearlson et al[62] studied patients over age 60 with major depression and compared them to normal control subjects. The VBR was measured blindly. It was increased in depressed patients both with and without cognitive impairment compared to normal control subjects.

Dolan[63] studied depressed patients and normal control subjects. The mean VBRs for the young patients were similar to those of control subjects. For patients between the ages of 60 and 79, the mean VBR was significantly greater than that of age-matched controls.

These studies do not identify the cause or time of onset of these changes. It is possible that the CT brain abnormalities are life-long in the depressed. There is evidence that ventricular enlargement is seen in young depressed patients. (For discussion, see references 70 and 71.)

There is considerable variability in the VBRs reported in control subjects among the various studies. Depue and Iacono[72] noted that studies reporting ventricular enlargement in patients with major affective disorder have control groups whose VBR was smaller than the VBR reported by studies that did not find any difference in ventricular size.[3]

This does not seem to be the case in the studies reported primarily in elderly subjects. Dolan's study also supports the contention that the enlarged ventricles are primarily seen in older depressives compared to younger patients with depression.

If all the studies of VBR are taken in perspective, it appears that the enlarged ventricles are more commonly and prominently seen in the older patients, and, when seen in younger individuals,[73] it is possible that the enlargement of the ventricles may potentially be secondary to hypercortisolemia.[75] Also see discussion below. CT studies[74] have reported other abnormalities, such as sulcal widening and atrophy of cerebellar vermis.[76,78,78,79,80]

The ventricular enlargement may reflect progressive shrinkage of periventricular white matter and gray matter structures, which leads to secondary ex vacuo expansion of the lateral ventricles. The CT studies demonstrated ventriculomegaly, but only one study addressed the issue of cerebrovascular changes in elderly patients with depression. These studies provide additional support for Post's speculation that age-related changes in the central nervous system are factors that facilitate depression in later life.[8]

Magnetic Resonance Imaging Studies of Leukoencephalopathy and Late-Onset Depression

Since leukoencephalopathy might reflect subtle alterations in cerebrovascular systems and is an index of aging, the occurrence of patchy white matter lesions (leukoencephalopathy) was assessed in 35 patients with depression.[81] The major finding of this study was a high prevalence (72 percent) of patchy white matter lesions in patients with late-onset depression. The lack of control subjects limited the conclusions.

Coffey et al[82] reproduced these findings. They studied 67 elderly depressed patients referred for electroconvulsive treatment (ECT). Thirty-one patients were studied with CT and the rest with MRI. Deep white matter hyperintensities were graded as follows: 0, absent; 1, punctate foci; 2, beginning confluence of foci; and 3, large confluent areas (Fazekas rating scale reference 40). Grade 1 DWMH was seen in 11 patients. Grade 2 DWMH was seen in 11 patients and grade 3 in 5 patients. Computed tomography identified leukoencephalopathy in 69 percent of patients, and MRI identified more lesions than did CT. Subcortical gray matter abnormalities were observed in many of the patients with leukoencephalopathy. Twenty-three of the 31 patients had lacunae in either the basal ganglia, the thalamus, or the pons. Pontine lesions were seen in 13 patients.

Many of the patients had a high risk of cerebrovascular disease. The authors suggested that the leukoencephalopathy was secondary to atherosclerotic changes in the deep penetrating arterioles. The leukoencephalopathy was associated with the occurrence of late-onset (after 60 years of age) depression. However, this study also did not include normal volunteers.

In a subsequent study, Coffey et al[83] expanded the sample to 51 subjects examined with MRI, including normal control subjects, and confirmed many of the earlier findings. Grade 2 and 3 DWMHs were more common in depressed patients (55 percent) than control subjects (14 percent). Basal ganglia lesions were present in 51 percent of depressed patients and in 5 percent of control subjects. The occurrence of lesions was associated with risk factors for cerebrovascular disease. Since vascular risk factors were more prevalent in depressed patients than in control subjects, the potential differences could have been related primarily to differences in risk factors. However, lesions of the deep gray nuclei and large PVH or DWMH (grade 3) were not seen in any of the control subjects, including those with similar risk factors. Thus, although vascular factors may play a role in causing these lesions, the site and size of the lesions may play a role in rendering an individual vulnerable to the risk of depression. In addition to vascular

cance of the finding remains to be clarified. Lithium is the primary medication used to treat bipolar disorder, and it can be measured using MRS.[183,184] Studies have examined the relationship between brain and plasma lithium levels. These studies in general suggest that brain lithium concentrations do correlate with plasma concentrations. The concentration of lithium was found to be lower in the brain than in plasma. The effective serum concentration of lithium is about 0.7 mEq/L for treatment of bipolar disorder, and the effective brain concentration is only 0.2 to 0.3 mEq/L.[183,184] The relevance of this finding and its potential clinical application are currently being evaluated.

Functional Imaging in Affective Disorders

Both PET and SPECT have been used to study affective disorders.[185–195] Studies of major depression have focused predominantly on metabolic changes in specific brain regions, such as the frontal cortex, temporal lobes, limbic structures, and basal ganglia. Early PET studies demonstrated decreased metabolism in the frontal cortex and basal ganglia. More recent studies suggest that various prefrontal cortex regions are specifically affected and involved in the pathophysiology of affective disorders, including the dorsolateral and ventral medial prefrontal cortex (Fig. 9-1).[188,195] Other studies have also implicated limbic lobe structures, such as the amygdala. Cohen et al,[189] in a recent study, demonstrated that the mid-prefrontal cortex is dysfunctional in patients with affective disorder during the performance of an auditory discrimination task. Converging evidence implicates two interconnected corticolimbic circuits, one including the amygdala, mediodorsal nucleus of the thalamus, and ventral prefrontal cortex and the other involving a related limbic-pallidal-thalamic circuit.[195]

Serotonin is the primary neurotransmitter implicated in the pathophysiology of affective disorders. Agren et al,[196,197] using 5-hydroxy-tryptophan (a precursor of serotonin), reported significantly lower uptake in patients with major depression, especially in the region of the prefrontal areas and basal ganglia.

Neuroanatomic Substrates of Affective Disorder

Both the structural and the functional studies described above clearly implicate the prefrontal cortex, basal ganglia, and limbic temporal lobe structures.[198,199] Neuroanatomic models have been developed to facilitate understanding of the pathophysiology of affective disorder.[192] The amygdala is believed to be the primary region involved in evaluating and processing emotional significance of stimuli. The expression of emotion probably involves projections of the amygdala to the basal ganglia, hypothalamus, and brainstem. Projections to the basal ganglia mediate motor components of emotional expression, projections to the hypothalamus mediate neuroendocrine components, and projections to the medial prefrontal cortex and brainstem mediate autonomic components. These regions are integral components of limbic-cortical-striatal-pallidal-thalamic circuits that have been hypothesized by several to be important in the pathophysiology of affective disorders.[192,198–200] Fu-

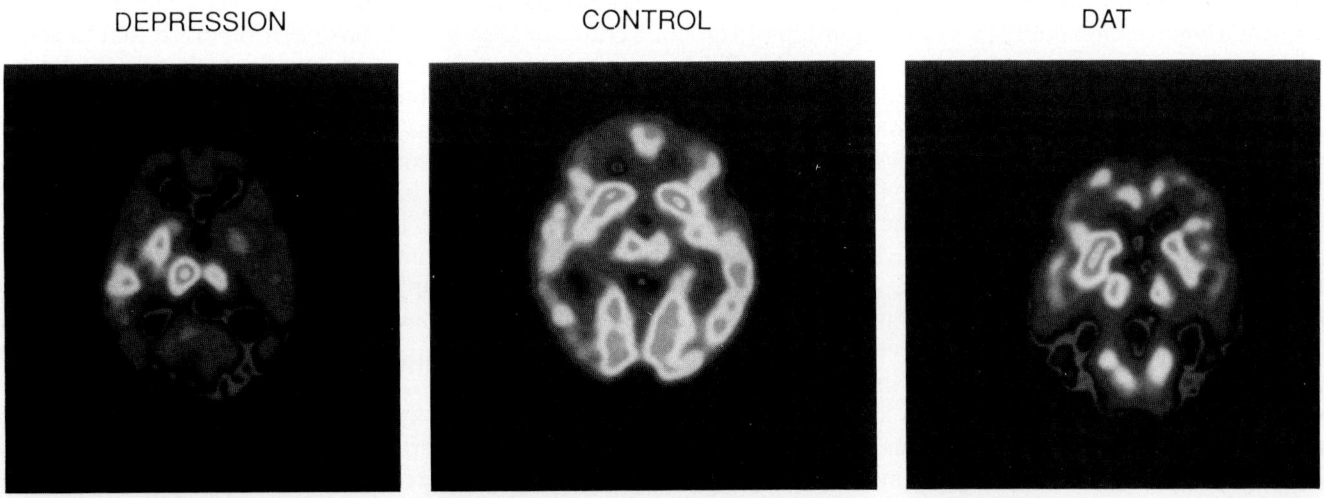

Figure 9-1 (Plate 26)
The figure compares glucose metabolic activity in a subject with late-life depression, a subject with probable Alzheimer disease (DAT), and a healthy age-matched control subject. Note the widespread decline in glucose metabolism in major neocortical and subcortical regions in depression and dementia (DAT) when compared to the healthy control brain. (Courtesy of Dr. Anand Kumar, Dept. of Psychiatry, University of Pennsylvania Medical Center.)

ture studies should clarify both the structural and the biochemical abnormalities in these regions. (For a review, see references 198 and 199.)

SCHIZOPHRENIA

Ventricular Enlargement

Probably the most common abnormality reported in patients with schizophrenia is ventricular enlargement.[201–211] Computed tomography studies using a simple measure of ventricular size, the VBR, first reported that the VBR is increased in patients with schizophrenia. The VBR is defined as the ratio of the ventricular area to intracranial area at the single CT section on which the ventricles are largest. This measure is relatively insensitive and is usually insufficient to detect minor changes in ventricular volume.[212,213]

Although the majority of studies of ventricular volume in patients with schizophrenia have demonstrated ventricular enlargement, there have also been studies with negative results. Over 50 studies have estimated ventricular size in patients with schizophrenia. The results of these studies have been evaluated by a number of investigators.[214–218] Raz and Raz[214] estimated the *effect size* of ventricular enlargement (i.e., the difference in mean ventricular volume between patients and control subjects divided by the pooled standard deviation). The effect size was found to be between 0.5 and 0.7.

Initially, it was thought that ventricular enlargement would be seen primarily in patients with negative (deficit) symptoms, such as flat affect, apathy, and so on; poor premorbid adjustment; and poor response to medication. However, the findings have been extremely variable, and no consistent profile has emerged.[214,218] A particularly intriguing finding is the relationship of ventricular enlargement to a greater extent to males. The enlarged ventricles do not seem to be related to the presence of genetic factors. A bimodal distribution in ventricular enlargement has not been found. In monozygotic twins, ventricles were larger in the affected twin, suggesting a relationship between the disease process and ventricular enlargement. However, in the unaffected twin, the ventricles were also larger than normal.[219] These studies were carried out in a relatively small number of subjects, and more extensive studies need to be carried out to determine the significance of ventricular enlargement in schizophrenia. The ventricular enlargement was seen in patients examined soon after the onset of the illness, suggesting that the change is due to the disease and not to subsequent treatment.

A number of studies have also assessed the possibility that there may be a progression in ventricular enlargement in schizophrenia.[214,220] Follow-up studies for as long as 8 years have not found any evidence of progression of ventricular enlargement.[221] Cross-sectional studies have also not found a relationship between illness duration and ventricular enlargement. The suggested relationship between ventricular enlargement and birth injury is difficult to assess and remains unproven.[218]

Studies of ventricular size in schizophrenia do indeed confirm ventricular enlargement. However, ventricular enlargement is not diagnostic of schizophrenia, since it is observed in a variety of other disorders, including Alzheimer's disease, depression, and others.

Sulcal Enlargement

A number of studies have reported sulcal enlargement.[214,218] These studies have used a variety of assessment techniques. This finding has not been reproduced to the same extent as ventricular enlargement, and the effect size is smaller. A correlation between ventricular enlargement and sulcal enlargement has been observed by some, but not all, studies.

Brain Size

As part of the hypotheses that neuroanatomic changes in schizophrenia are due to prenatal injury, it has been suggested that there is a reduction in brain size in schizophrenia.[222,223] Some investigators have indeed found a reduction not just in brain size but also in head size.[224] However, this has not been replicated in other studies. A recent study using MRI has suggested a global reduction in gray matter volume in patients with schizophrenia.[225]

Septum Pellucidum

The septum pellucidum is a thin sheet, located in the midsagittal line of the brain, that separates the lateral ventricles (Fig. 9-2). It has been reported that in some patients this is malformed. One such abnormality is the cavum septum pellucidum. Cavum septum pellucidum is often regarded as an incidental finding. This abnormality is seen in about 2 percent of the normal population but is present in about 21 percent of patients with schizophrenia.[226-228] This provides further evidence of anomalous development of the limbic system in patients with schizophrenia.

Corpus Callosum

One of the many hypotheses regarding schizophrenia is that there is a disruption in the interhemispheric connections. Thus, there has been much interest in studying the corpus callosum. The corpus callosum is usually studied using the midsagittal image. The area, length, width, and, in many studies, dimensions of segments of the corpus callosum have been examined. Results of these studies have in general been inconsistent.[229–233] Some studies have reported decreased corpus callosal

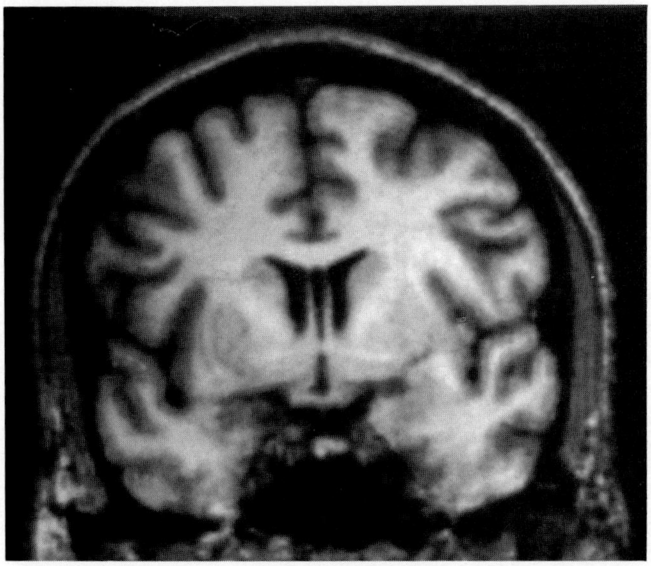
A

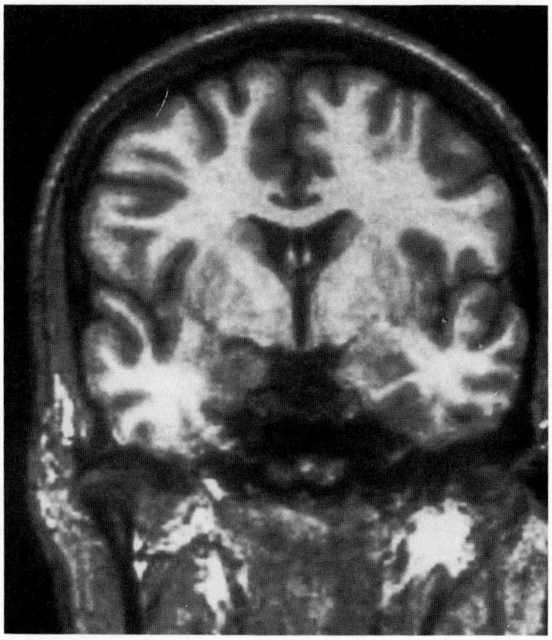
B

Figure 9-2
Cavum septum pellucidum as seen on coronal section in patients with schizophrenia. (Courtesy of Dr. Jeffrey Lieberman, Long Island Jewish Hospital, New York.)

area; others have reported increased area or no difference. A few studies have reported that the corpus callosum area in the middle and anterior segments is increased. One study has reported a reversal in the normal sex difference in schizophrenia. One study has reported that there is a shape distortion of the corpus callosum in patients with schizophrenia.[233]

Cerebellum

The cerebellum has been implicated in cognitive processes in a variety of studies. Early CT studies showed that cerebellar abnormalities are not uncommon in patients with schizophrenia. These changes were primarily indirect assessments, that is, measurements of vermal sulci and fourth ventricle size. With the advent of MRI, it has become possible to easily assess various aspects of the cerebellum. The MRI studies in general have not found any differences in cross-sectional midsagittal cerebellar area, vermal area, or fourth ventricular area.[234–236] Two groups did in fact find a trend for the cerebellar area to be larger in patients with schizophrenia.[235,236]

Basal Ganglia

A number of studies have suggested that the basal ganglia may be involved in the pathophysiology of schizophrenia. Some have suggested that it may be involved in the expression of motivation and is the primary interface of the temporal-limbic structures for the expression of behavior. Thus, it is likely to be related to the occurrence of negative symptoms in schizophrenia. Jernigan et al[237] reported that the lenticular nucleus was larger in patients with schizophrenia, whereas others reported no change. Delisi et al[238] reported that the caudate nucleus was larger in patients with chronic schizophrenia than those evaluated during the first episode. Other investigators have reported negative results. Buchanan et al[239,240] reported that the right caudate nucleus was larger in patients with deficit symptoms and that the caudate may be related to the occurrence of negative symptoms. Swayze et al also reported that the caudate and putamen were larger in male patients with schizophrenia.[241] However, Young et al have reported that patients with marked negative symptoms have smaller caudate nuclei.[208] In addition (as reviewed affective disorder section), there is evidence that typical neuroleptics may be associated with basal ganglia enlargement.[242] Further study of subgroups of patients with schizophrenia is required to delineate the nature of abnormalities in the basal ganglia.

Temporal Lobe and Structures in the Temporal Lobe

Postmortem studies have demonstrated that there are numerous changes in the temporal lobe in patients with schizophrenia. These changes include reduction in the size of the hippocampus, amygdala, superior temporal gyrus, parahippocampus, and entire temporal lobe itself. Magnetic resonance imaging studies have confirmed many of these postmortem findings. Significant asymmetry in many of these findings has been reported.

Temporal Lobe

Suddath et al reported that the temporal lobes, especially the right lobe, are reduced in patients with schizophrenia.[243] The reduction was primarily in temporal lobe gray matter and was associated with enlargement of the lateral ventricles. In a related study of twins discordant for schizophrenia, Suddath noted a similar reduction in temporal lobe volume in the affected twin.[224] Rossi et al[245] also reported that cross-sectional temporal lobe area was reduced more on the left side in patients with schizophrenia. The reduction in temporal lobe size may also be reflected as sylvian fissure enlargement. Dauphinais et al[246] have also reported a reduction in temporal lobe size. However, Shenton et al[247] did not find an overall reduction in temporal lobe size despite reduction in volumes of many temporal lobe structures. The temporal lobe reduction has been related to enlargement of temporal horns.[243]

Hippocampus

Suddath et al[244] showed that the hippocampus was smaller at the level of the pes hippocampi on the left side in 14 of 15 pairs (monozygotic) of twins discordant for schizophrenia and on the right side in 13 of 15 pairs in the twin with schizophrenia compared to the unaffected twin. There were no differences in 7 sets of monozygotic normal twins. Bogerts et al[248,249] also reported that the hippocampal tissue was reduced on the left side in 34 patients with schizophrenia compared to normal control subjects. Barta et al[250] did not find differences in the hippocampus but reported that the amygdala was smaller in patients with schizophrenia. Swayze et al[241] did not demonstrate any changes in the hippocampus, amygdala, or temporal lobe volume in patients with schizophrenia. However, this study used very thick slices, which is likely to have significantly limited the findings. Weinberger et al[251] showed that, in the twin pairs reported by Suddath et al,[244] the hippocampal reduction was related to abnormalities in prefrontal function assessed by regional cerebral blood flow studies. Shenton et al also showed that the left anterior hippocampus and left parahippocampus were reduced in patients with schizophrenia. Brier et al[240] have also reported that both the left and right amygdala/hippocampal complex is reduced in patients with schizophrenia. In this study also, changes were greater in the left hippocampus. Overall, these studies demonstrate more changes in medial temporal gray matter on the left side in patients with schizophrenia than on the right. These changes have been reported to consist of reductions in the hippocampus, parahippocampus, and amygdala. However, these distinctions should be considered preliminary, since discrimination among these structures is still difficult and not completely reliable.

Planum Temporale

Rossi et al[294] reported that, unlike normal subjects, patients with schizophrenia did not have the normal asymmetry in the size of the planum temporale. The authors used a relatively simple index of planum temporale: area. Petty et al[255] also reported reversal of asymmetry of planum temporale in schizophrenia. Other studies have not reported the same finding. The planum temporale is implicated in higher-order cognitive function, and the lack of asymmetry is of great interest and needs to be further pursued.

Superior Temporal Gyrus

In an initial report, Barta et al[250] reported that the volume of the superior temporal gyrus was reduced in patients with schizophrenia. This change was greater on the left side. The reduction in size of the superior left anterior temporal gyrus was correlated with the severity of auditory hallucinations. The superior temporal gyrus is part of the auditory association cortex, and thus this finding is of particular interest. Shenton et al[247] also noted changes in the superior temporal gyrus, although, in their study, the findings were more significant for the posterior segment. These investigators noted that the volume of the left posterior temporal gyrus correlated with thought disorder. Menon et al[256] reproduced the results of Shenton et al.[252] They also found an inverse correlation between thought disorder and gray matter reduction in the left superior temporal gyrus.

Prefrontal Lobe

A number of studies implicate the dorsolateral prefrontal cortex in schizophrenia. Interest in this area is based on functional imaging, primate studies, and neuropsychological impairment in these patients. Andreasen et al[204] reported that the frontal area is reduced in patients with schizophrenia. However, the results of this early study were not reproduced by subsequent studies. These studies were limited in that the dimensions of the prefrontal lobe were not easy to assess by the methods available at that time. When schizophrenics were compared with control subjects, no differences were found in measurements of the frontal lobe, such as bifrontal width, bifrontal ratio, total frontal lobe volume, and prefrontal gray and white matter volume. Similarly, Casanova et al[253] reported no difference in prefrontal lobe shape between schizophrenic patients and control subjects. Zipursky et al,[224] on the other hand, reported that the frontal temporal sulci are widened in these patients, suggesting that there may be some atrophy of the frontal lobes. Postmortem studies have indeed shown changes in the frontal lobes of patients with schizophrenia. Part of the reason that frontal lobe changes were not seen in some early imaging studies may be because they may be related to the occurrence of deficit symptoms. Schlaepfer et al[257] reported a reduction in prefrontal lobe volumes. Buchanan et al[240] have shown that the prefrontal lobes are smaller in patients without deficit symptoms. Further research is needed using methods for assessing individual regions of the prefrontal lobes in these patients to evaluate the nature of the changes in the prefrontal regions in patients with schizophrenia.

Parietal Lobe

The findings with regard to the parietal lobe have not been consistent. Most of the early studies did not report any changes in parietal lobe volumes. Schlaepfer et al,[257] using a relatively rough demarcation, suggested that the inferior parietal lobule (a heteromodal association cortex) was reduced. This result was not reproduced by Shenton et al.[247] This issue needs further evaluation.

Thalamus

A recent study by Andreasen et al[258] has noted a reduction in volume of the thalamus. Buchsbaum et al[259] have confirmed abnormalities in thalamic function. This intriguing finding requires further study.

Qualitative Evaluation of Brain Morphology in Patients with Schizophrenia

The changes described above in patients with schizophrenia have been assessed by quantitative methods. However, these methods are not generally useful for clinical purposes. The radiologist or clinician reading the MRI scan is more interested in changes that can be visually assessed on examining the scan. Thirty percent of patients with acute and 42 percent of patients with chronic schizophrenia are reported to have an abnormal scan. The most common abnormalities are seen in the region of the lateral ventricles and the frontal, parietal, and medial temporal regions.[203] The common changes are usually ventricular enlargement and atrophy of the cortex in these regions. Another change sometimes seen is the enlargement of the cavum septum pellucidum (Fig. 9-2). None of these changes is diagnostic of schizophrenia, and a diagnosis cannot be made solely on the basis of an MRI scan.

Magnetic Resonance Spectroscopy in Schizophrenia

A number of studies have utilized ^{31}P spectroscopy to evaluate phospholipid changes in patients with schizophrenia (Fig. 9-3). The reason for evaluating phospholipid changes in schizophrenia is based on studies that have demonstrated membrane abnormalities in patients with schizophrenia. Since there is evidence implicating the prefrontal lobe in schizophrenia, some studies have examined this region using ^{31}P spectroscopy.[260,261,262] A number of metabolic abnormalities have been observed in these patients, including low concentrations of phosphomonoesters and inorganic phosphate and elevated concentrations of phosphodiesters and adenosine triphosphate (ATP). These findings were noted with neuroleptic-naive first-episode patients with schizophrenia. Similar changes have been observed in more chronic patients by some, but not all, investigators. The phosphomonoester and phosphodiester results suggest that there is a change in phospholipid metabolism, with less synthesis and more breakdown of phospholipids. Calabrese et al[261] evaluated the temporal lobes in patients with schizophrenia. He noted that there was no

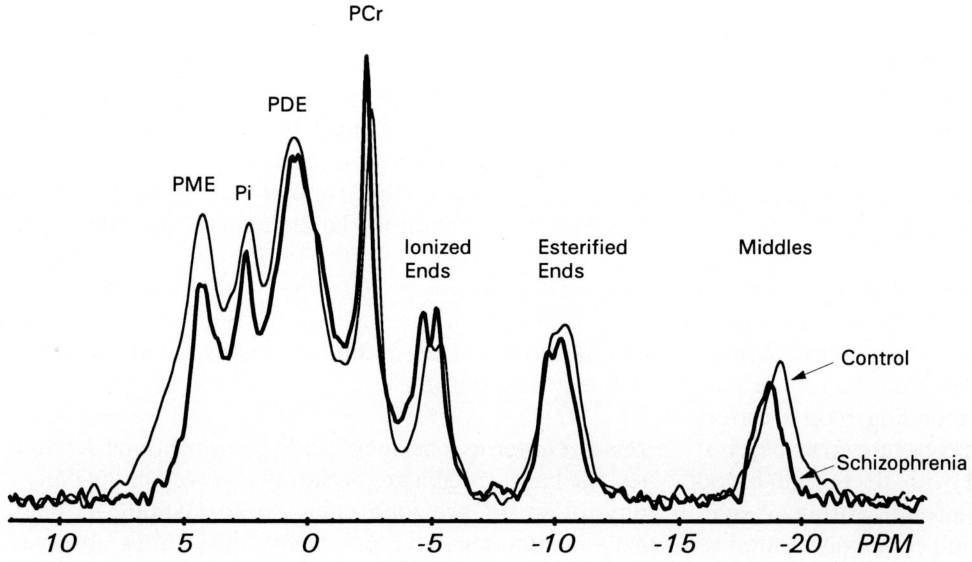

Figure 9-3
^{31}P spectra from a patient with schizophrenia, demonstrating a decrease in phosphomonoesters. (Courtesy of Dr. Matcheri Keshavan, University of Pittsburgh, Pittsburgh, PA.)

asymmetry in phosphorus metabolite ratios. However, phosphocreatinine/β-ATP and phosphocreatinine/inorganic phosphorus ratios appeared to be higher on the right side, whereas the percentage of β-ATP primarily reflected the left side. Proton MRS studies have begun to document reduction in *N*-acetyl aspartate in the temporal lobe and prefrontal cortex. These studies are preliminary and need to be extended. For a detailed discussion, see Keshavan et al.[263]

Positron Emission Tomography Studies in Schizophrenia

A number of PET studies have been conducted in schizophrenia. These studies have used a variety of ligands. Some have examined metabolic function. Others have assessed dopamine function (dopamine is a neurotransmitter in the brain believed to be critically involved in the pathophysiology of schizophrenia).

Metabolic Studies

Metabolic studies using PET have primarily used the tracer 18 fluorodeoxyglucose (FDG). These studies measure the uptake of FDG into the cells. This process is coupled with blood flow and cerebral metabolism. Thus, FDG studies have been used to assess regional metabolism in patients with schizophrenia.

Frontal Lobes Early studies using blood flow measurements suggested that patients with schizophrenia had decreased blood flow in the frontal region of the brain. This was primarily described in patients with chronic schizophrenia who had negative symptoms.[264,265] Initial PET studies using FDG showed that patients with schizophrenia indeed had relative hypofrontality (relative to occipital lobes). Of the studies, some found hypofrontality, a few did not, and one study in neuroleptic-naive patients reported increased blood flow in the frontal lobes.[264-276] There were several reasons for the discrepancy, including (1) neuroleptic effects, which may have been responsible for reducing blood flow in the frontal region; (2) duration of illness (i.e., chronic patients were more likely to exhibit the finding); (3) severity of negative symptoms; and (4) methodological differences (e.g., use of absolute or relative measures or different definitions of resting states).[276]

Recent studies suggest that hypofrontality is primarily related to negative symptoms and that patients with an enduring deficit state have reduced glucose utilization in the frontal region. Liddle et al[277-279] studied 50 chronic patients with schizophrenia. They identified three patterns of blood flow change corresponding to three different syndromes. One syndrome, characterized by psychomotor poverty, was associated with decreased blood flow in the left dorsolateral prefrontal cortex. A syndrome characterized by disorganization was related to the anterior cingulate region. These studies have indicated that the left parahippocampal region is critical for perception of reality but that different syndromes are produced by involvement of other brain systems, such as the dorsolateral prefrontal cortex or anterior cingulate gyrus. All these studies used a resting paradigm. However, because of the variance introduced in these studies, investigators have begun to use perturbation approaches to assess whether patients with schizophrenia show the same pattern of activation as normals.[280] Patients with schizophrenia often have difficulty with tasks that activate frontal lobe function, such as the Wisconsin Card Sort Test.[281,282] Xenon blood flow studies of patients with schizophrenia conducted while they were performing this task showed that the patients failed to activate the frontal lobes. Furthermore, PET studies with the same task have localized the abnormality to the inferior frontal gyrus. A similar abnormality is seen when the study is conducted using a continuous-performance task.[283] Thus, all these studies suggest that there is a frontal lobe dysfunction in patients with schizophrenia.

Parietal Lobes Hypometabolism has been observed in the region of the parietal cortex in several studies.[271,283-285] Hypometabolism in this region has been primarily related to negative symptoms. The finding has been observed both in drug-naive patients and in those on neuroleptics. A reduced activation of the parietal cortex during a continuous-performance task has been observed in patients with schizophrenia.[286] The inferior parietal lobe has been related to cognitive impairment.[287]

Temporal Lobes Many studies have begun to focus on temporal lobe function, based partly on multiple reports of structural changes in the region of the temporal lobes, with more changes on the left side. However, PET studies have not been consistent in demonstrating abnormalities in the temporal lobe in patients with schizophrenia.[286,289,290,291] Some studies have documented hypometabolism in the left temporal lobe, although a few have not reproduced this finding. In addition, PET studies have reported hypometabolism in the region of the posterior superior temporal gyrus region in patients experiencing auditory hallucinations.[292,293] This finding in a region close to that reported by Barta et al[250] as associated with auditory hallucinations provides additional information about the importance of this region in the pathophysiology of auditory hallucination. Liddle related reality distortion to increased left parahippocampal flow.[277] This finding was constant in all of his defined subsyndromes.

Basal Ganglia As suggested by morphometric studies, the basal ganglia are probably involved in the pathophysiology of schizophrenia. Abnormalities in basal ganglia function have not been consistently observed in patients with schizophrenia.[294,295,296] However, many studies have documented an increase in basal ganglia metabolism in patients following the administration of neuroleptics.[291,297,300–305] This change has been related to recovery from psychoses. However, this could be reflective of concomitant change in this region paralleling changes in other regions that may be critical in the pathophysiology of schizophrenia. An abnormality in left globus pallidus function has been reported, but has not been further studied.[299] In addition, Buchsbaum has reported a reduction in thalamic blood flow.[259]

Dopamine Function

The dopamine hypothesis remains the primary biologic hypothesis in schizophrenia. The hypothesis is based on studies demonstrating the efficacy of dopamine antagonists in the treatment of schizophrenia and on postmortem studies. These studies raise the possibility that schizophrenia is characterized by increased D2 receptor function in schizophrenia. Postmortem studies have demonstrated elevations in D2 receptor binding in patients with schizophrenia.

With the advent of PET, it has become possible to examine D2 receptor binding in vivo.[306–316] However, PET studies are limited by a number of considerations. First, binding reflects both B_{MAX} (number of receptor sites) and Kd (affinity), but, to obtain separate estimates of both, multiple studies have to be conducted, which is not feasible because of radiation issues. Second, PET resolution and sensitivity do not permit study of structures such as the prefrontal cortex. Third, multiple factors affect binding of the injected radioligand, including pharmacokinetic factors, blood-brain barrier permeability, and specificity of binding. Since all these factors cannot be easily dealt with, there is considerable controversy on the use of particular ligands, the methods used, and the interpretation of results.

Wong et al,[306] using ^{11}C *N*-methyl spiperone, showed that both B_{MAX} and affinity were increased in the basal ganglia of 10 drug-naive patients with schizophrenia when compared to normal control subjects. Two scans were obtained from each subject, one drug-free and the other on haloperidol. These two scans were then used to calculate B_{MAX}. Binding concentrations, measured as striatal cerebellar ratios, did not show any difference. However, other studies have not reproduced these results. Farde et al,[307] using ^{11}C-raclopride and a two-scan experiment, were unable to confirm Wong's results. Martinot et al[308,309] using bromospiperone, found a trend toward D2 elevation. A number of factors could be responsible for the discrepancy, including (1) different ligands, (2) different population of patients, (3) different duration of illness, and (4) different methodologies and assumptions for calculating B_{MAX}. Future studies will have to resolve these methodologic difficulties to clarify the nature of D2 receptor changes in schizophrenia.

Neuroanatomic Substrates of Schizophrenia

Both functional and structural studies have clearly implicated the temporal lobe structures, such as the hippocampus, parahippocampus, amygdala, thalamus, and, particularly, superior temporal gyrus. The superior temporal gyrus on the left side has been related to the occurrence of auditory hallucinations. Functional studies have also implicated the dorsolateral prefrontal cortex and parietal cortex. Both of these regions are heteromodal association areas and are involved in higher-order sensory and potentially cognitive, processing, functions known to be altered in schizophrenia.

AUTISM

With the advent of MRI, there have been numerous investigations of posterior fossa structures in autism.[317–318] Earlier studies suggested structural changes in the cerebellar vermis; however, there are some inconsistencies in results, and these findings remain controversial. These findings are not diagnostic of autism. Other studies have begun to investigate temporal structures, including the hippocampus, in patients with autism. Gross changes, such as polymicrogyria, macrogyria, and schizencephaly, can be seen. Serotonin synthesis has been shown to be lower in discrete brain regions.

ANOREXIA NERVOSA

Early CT studies demonstrated that many patients with anorexia had cerebral atrophy and ventricular enlargement.[319,320] The cerebral atrophy was shown to be reversible in these patients after recovery from the illness.[321] An MRI study confirmed the presence of cerebral atrophy in these patients.[320] Both ventricular enlargement and sulcal enlargement were observed. Cerebral atrophy in these patients can often be visually observed.[322] However, the finding must still be considered nonspecific and not diagnostic of anorexia.

A study by Husain et al[323] showed that the thalamus is smaller and there are changes in the mesencephalon in these patients. Pituitary volume has also been assessed in these patients. The pituitary gland is smaller in anorectic subjects than in control subjects.[324,325] This reduction in the size of the pituitary gland is related to cessation of menses and probably reflects a reduction in size, and possibly number, of gonadotropin-hormone-secreting cells.

Functional studies using PET have also been conducted in these patients. Relative caudate hypermetabolism has been observed in these patients compared to those with bulimia nervosa.[326,327] (For a review of structural and functional studies, see Black and Botteron.[328])

BULIMIA NERVOSA

As with anorexia nervosa, cerebral atrophy has been demonstrated in patients with bulimia nervosa.[322] An MRI study showed that the sagittal cerebral-to-cranial area was significantly less in the bulimic group than in control subjects.[322] The VBR was unaltered between the two groups.[322] This study suggests that cortical atrophy is more critical in these patients than is ventricular enlargement. The pituitary gland was also noted to be smaller in these patients than in control subjects.[324,325] However, the change was less than that seen in anorexia.

Functional studies have also been conducted in bulimia.[330,331] Positron emission tomography studies using FDG have demonstrated that in bulimia there is a loss of normal right hemisphere activation and that there is temporal lobe hypermatabolism.[330] Unlike anorexia, there is no evidence of increased activation of the caudate nuclei in these patients.[331]

SOCIAL PHOBIA

Social phobia is a disorder characterized by marked social anxiety in all or almost all social situations. Thus, patients with social phobia tend to be socially withdrawn, anxious in parties, anxious about meeting strangers, and fearful of public speaking while being observed. A number of studies have implicated the dopamine system and the basal ganglia in the pathophysiology of social phobia. A recent study of basal ganglia volumes in patients with social phobia showed no evidence of cerebral atrophy.[332] However, the preliminary study suggested that there was a greater rate of atrophy of the putamen with increasing age in patients compared to control subjects. A preliminary study of the basal ganglia using proton MRS found that there was reduced metabolic activity in the region of the basal ganglia.

PANIC DISORDER

Panic disorder is characterized by panic attacks. Panic attacks are acute episodes of anxiety in which the patient experiences a wide variety of symptoms, including palpitations, chest pain, lump in the throat, difficulty breathing, numbness, tingling in the fingers and toes, and a feeling of losing control or dying. Using CT, Uhde et al showed that there was no difference in ventricular size between patients with panic disorder and control subjects.[333] Lepola et al[334] reported that—in general–panic patients had normal CT scans, but about 20 percent had incidental findings, such as cerebral atrophy, enlarged ventricles, or lacunar infarcts. Fontaine et al[336] studied patients with panic disorder using MRI. He found that many of these patients had temporal lobe abnormalities, including abnormal signal intensities and atrophy of the temporal lobe, especially on the right side.

Positron emission tomography studies have produced interesting but controversial findings. Reiman et al[337] demonstrated that patients with panic disorder have a left parahippocampal functional abnormality on PET studies. The brain regions affected during a panic attack have also been studied. These studies suggest activation of a number of regions, including the temporal lobe and the basal ganglia. However, controversy surrounds some of these findings, since there is a question as to whether these changes could be reflective of changes outside the brain, such as clenching of the jaw.[338]

OBSESSIVE COMPULSIVE DISORDER

Obsessive compulsive disorder (OCD) is characterized by obsessions (thoughts that the patient is unable to turn off) and compulsions (repetitive behaviors, e.g., washing, checking, etc., in response to the obsessions). Garber et al[339] reported that the relaxation time was increased in patients with OCD. Harris et al[340] found no structural abnormalities, including no change in the volumes of the basal ganglia. Kellner et al[341] evaluated 12 patients with OCD and control subjects. They examined a number of areas, including the caudate, and did not find any significant differences. However, recently Rosenberg et al reported alteration in the volumes of the basal ganglia.[342]

Functional studies have demonstrated a number of changes in the brain.[343–348] One of the most interesting is the reversible changes in caudate metabolism in OCD patients treated with either medication or behavior therapy.[346] Most, but not all, studies have documented abnormalities in frontal striatal circuits.

ATTENTION DEFICIT HYPERACTIVITY DISORDER

Children with attention deficit hyperactivity disorder (ADHD) are characterized by significant impairment in sustained attention and impulse control and have difficulty with hyperkinesis. They are easily distractible and disorganized and tend to present with significant behavioral problems. Such children are at risk for significant academic, family, and social impairment and have been demonstrated to be at risk for negative outcomes in adolescence and adulthood. A number of imaging studies are now demonstrating alterations in frontal lobe and basal ganglia structures in children and adolescents with ADHD. Early studies using simple measures reported changes in the asymmetry of the frontal lobes in ADHD groups.[349,350] More recent sophis-

151. Hauser PH, Dauphinais D, Berrettini W: Temporal lobe measurement in primary affective disorder by magnetic resonance imaging. *J Neuropsychiatry* 1:128–134, 1989.
152. Johnstone EC, Owens DG, Crow TJ: Temporal lobe structure as determined by nuclear magnetic resonance in schizophrenia and bipolar affective disorder. *J Neurol Neurosurg Psychiatry* 52:736–741, 1989.
153. Altschuler LL, Conrad A, Hauser P: Reduction of temporal lobe volume in bipolar disorder: A preliminary report of magnetic resonance imaging. *Arch Gen Psychiatry* 48:482–483, 1992.
154. Swayze VW, Andreasen NC, Alliger RJ: Subcortical and temporal structures in affective disorder and schizophrenia: A magnetic resonance imaging study. *Biol Psychiatry* 31:221–240, 1992.
155. Coffey CE, Wilkinson WE, Weiner RD, et al: Quantitative cerebral anatomy in depression. *Arch Gen Psychiatry* 50:7–16, 1993.
156. Sapolsky RM, McEwen BS: Why dexamethasone resistance? Two possible neuroendocrine mechanisms, in Schatzbert AF, Nemeroff CB (eds): *The Hypothalamic-Pituitary-Adrenal Axis: Physiology, Pathophysiology and Psychiatric Implications*. New York, Raven Press, New York, 1988.
157. Axelson DA, Doraiswamy PM, McDonald WM, et al: Hypercortisolemia and hippocampal changes in depression. *Psychiatry Res* 47:163–173, 1993.
158. Sheline YI, Want PW, Gado MH, et al: Hippocampal atrophy in recurrent major depression. *Proc Natl Acad Sci U S A* 93:3908–3913, 1996.
159. Pearlson GD, Berta PE, Powers RE, et al: Ziskind-Somerfeld Research Award 1996. Medial and superior temporal gyral volumes and cerebral asymmetry in schizophrenia vs bipolar disorder. *Biol Psychiatry* 41:1–14, 1997.
160. Heath RG, Franklin DE, Walker CF, et al: Cerebellar vermal atrophy in psychiatric patients. *Biol Psychiatry* 17:569–583, 1982.
161. Lippman S, Manshadi M, Baldwin H, et al: Cerebellar vermis dimensions on computerized tomographic scans of schizophrenic and bipolar patients. *Am J Psychiatry* 139:667–668, 1982.
162. Reider RO, Mann LS, Weinberger DR: Computed tomographic scans in patients with schizophrenia, schizoaffective and bipolar affective disorder. *Arch Gen Psychiatry* 40:735–739, 1983.
163. Nasrallah HA, Jacoby CG, McCalley-Whitters M: Cerebellar atrophy in schizophrenia and mania. *Lancet* 1:1102, 1981.
164. Weinberger DR, Delisis LE, Perman GP: Computed tomography in schizophreniform disorder and other acute psychiatric disorders. *Arch Gen Psychiatry* 39:778–783, 1982.
165. Shah SA, Doraiswamy PM, Husain MM, et al: Posterior fossa abnormalities in major depression: A controlled magnetic resonance imaging study. *Acta Psychiatr Scand* 85:474–479, 1992.
166. Escalona PR, MacDonald WM, Doraiswamy PM, et al: Reduction of cerebellar volume in major depression: A controlled MRI study. Manuscript 2000. *Depression* 1:156–158, 1993.
167. Sandyk R, Pardeshi R: The relationship between ECT nonresponsiveness and calcification of the pineal gland in bipolar patients. *Int J Neurosci* 54:301–306, 1990.
168. Hauser PH, Dauphinais D, Berrettini W: Corpus callosum dimensions measured by magnetic resonance imaging in bipolar affective disorder and schizophrenia. *Biol Psychiatry* 26:659–668, 1989.
169. Coffman JA, Nasrallah HA: Brain density patterns in schizophrenia and mania. *J Affect Disord* 6:307–315, 1984.
170. Husain MM, Figiel GS, Lurie SN: MRI of corpus callosum and septum pellucidum in depression. *Biol Psychiatry* 29:300–301, 1991.
171. Dupont RM, Jernigan TL, Butters N, et al: Subcortical abnormalities deteced in bipolar affective disorder using magnetic resonance imaging. *Arch Gen Psychiatry* 47:55–59, 1990.
172. Swayze VW, Andreasen NC, Alliger RJ, et al: Structural brain abnormalities in bipolar affective disorder. *Arch Gen Psychiatry* 47:1057–1059, 1990.
173. Figiel GS, Krishnan KRR, Rao VP, et al: Subcortical hyperintensities on brain magnetic resonance imaging: A comparison of normal and bipolar subjects. *J Neuropsychiatry* 3:18–22, 1991.
174. Strakowski SM, Woods BT, Tohen M, et al: MRI subcortical signal hyperintensities in mania at first hospitalization. *Biol Psychiatry* 33:204–206, 1993.
175. Botteron KN, Vannier MW, Geller B, et al: Magnetic resonance imaging in childhood and adolescent bipolar affective disorder: A pilot investigation. *J Am Acad Child Adoles Psychiatry* 34:742–749, 1995.
176. Dupont RM, Jernigan TL, Heindel W, et al: Magnetic resonance imaging and mood disorders. *Arch Gen Psychiatry* 52:747–755, 1995.
177. Nemeroff CB, Krishnan KRR, Reed D, et al: Adrenal gland enlargement in major depression. *Arch Gen Psychiatry* 49:384–387, 1992.
178. Krishnan KRR, Doraiswamy PM, Lurie SN, et al: Pituitary size in depression. *J Clin Endocrinol Metab* 72:256–259, 1991.
179. Axelson DA, Doraiswamy PM, Boyko OB, et al: In vivo assessment of pituitary volume with magnetic resonance imaging and systematic stereology: Relationship to dexamethasone suppression test results in patients. *Psychiatry Res* 44:63–70, 1992.
180. Kato T, Takahashi S, Shiori T, Inubushi T: Brain phosphorous metabolism in depressive disorders determined by phosphorous 31 magnetic resonance spectroscopy. *J Affect Disord* 26:223–230, 1992.
181. Kato T, Takahashi S, Shion T, Inubushi T: Measurement of brain phosphoinositide metabolism in bipolar patients using in vivo ^{31}P MRS. *J Affect Disord* 22:185–190, 1991.
182. Sharma RP, Subramanian PNV, Barany M, et al: Proton magnetic resonance spectroscopy of the brain, in *New Research Program and Abstracts: 143rd Annual Meeting of the American Psychiatric Association*. Washington, APA, 1990.
183. Kato T, Takahoshi S, Shion T, Inubushi T: Alteration in brain phosphorus metabolism in bipolar disorder detected by in vivo ^{31}P and ^{7}Li magnetic resonance spectroscopy. *J Affect Disord* 27:53–59, 1993.

184. Komoroski RA, Newton JEO, Walker E, et al: In vivo NMR spectroscopy of lithium-7 in humans. *Magn Reson Med* 15:347–356, 1990.
185. Wu JC, Gillin JC, Buchsbaum MS, et al: Effect of sleep deprivation on brain metabolism of depressed patients. *Am J Psychiatry* 149:538–543, 1992.
186. Martinot JL, Hardy P, Feline A, et al: Left prefrontal glucose hypometabolism in the depressed state: A confirmation. *Am J Psychiatry* 147:1313–1317, 1990.
187. Martinot JL, Hardy P, Feline A, et al: Left prefrontal glucose hypometabolism in the depressed state: A confirmation. *Am J Psychiatry* 147:1313–1317, 1990.
188. Baxter LR, Schwartz JM, Phelps ME, et al: Reduction of prefrontal cortex glucose metabolism common to three types of depression. *Arch Gen Psychiatry* 46:243–250, 1989.
189. Cohen RM, Gross M, Nordahl TE, et al: Preliminary data on the metabolic brain pattern of patients with winter seasonal affective disorder. *Arch Gen Psychiatry* 49:545–552, 1992.
190. Hurwitz TA, Clark C, Murphy E: Regional cerebral glucose metabolism in major depressive disorder. *Can J Psychiatry* 35:684–688, 1990.
191. Dolan RJ, Bench CJ, Brown RG: Regional cerebral blood flow abnormalities in depressed patients with cognitive impairment. *J Neurol Neurosurg Psychiatry* 55:768–773, 1992.
192. Drevets WC, Videen TO, Price JL, et al: A functional anatomical study of unipolar depression. *J Neurosci* 12:3628–3641, 1992.
193. Cohen RM, Semple WE, Gross M, et al: Evidence for common alterations in cerebral glucose metabolism in major affective disorders and schizophrenia. *Neuropsychopharmacology* 2:241–254, 1989.
194. Guze BH, Baxter LR Jr, Schwartz JM, et al: Changes in glucose metabolism in dementia of the Alzheimer type compared with depression: A preliminary report. *Psychiatry Res* 40:195–202, 1991.
195. Drevets WC, Price JL, Simpson JR, et al: Subgenual prefrontal cortex abnormalities in mood disorders. *Nature* 386:824–827, 1997.
196. Agren H, Reibring L, Hartvig P, et al: Low brain uptake of L-5-hydroxytryptophan in major depression: A positron emission tomography study on patients and healthy volunteers. *J Acta Psychiatr Scand* 83:449–455, 1991.
197. Hartvig P, Agren H, Reibring L, et al: Positron emission tomography of 5-hydroxytryptophan utilization in the brain of healthy volunteers and a patient with major deprssion. *Acta Radiol Suppl* 376:159–160, 1991.
198. Krishnan KRR: Neuroanatomic substrates of depression in the elderly. *J Geriatr Psychiatry Neurol* 6:39–58, 1993.
199. Botteron KN, Figiel GS: The neuromorphometry of affective disorders, in Krishnan KRR, Doraiswamy PM (eds): *Brain Imaging in Clinical Psychiatry*. New York, Marcel Dekker, 145–184, 1997.
200. Swerdlow NR, Koob GF: Dopamine, schizophrenia, mania and depression: Toward a unified hypothesis of cortico-striato-pallido-thalamic function. *Behav Brain Sci* 10:197–245, 1987.
201. Lewine RR, Risch SC, Risby E, et al: Lateral ventricle-brain ratio and balance between CSF HVA and 5-HIAA in schizophrenia. *Am J Psychiatry* 148:1189–1194, 1991.
202. Flaum M, Arndt S, Andreasen NC: The role of gender in studies of ventricle enlargement in schizophrenia: A predominantly male effect. *Am J Psychiatry* 147:1327–1332, 1990.
203. Lieberman J, Bogerts B, Degreef G, et al: Qualitative assessment of brain morphology in acute and chronic schizophrenia. *Am J Psychiatry* 149:784–794, 1992.
204. Andreasen NC, Ehrhardt JC, Swayze VW 2d, et al: Magnetic resonance imaging of the brain in schizophrenia: The pathophysiologic significance of structural abnormalities. *Arch Gen Psychiatry* 47:35–44, 1990.
205. DeLisi LE, Stritzke P, Riordan H, et al: The timing of brain morphological changes in schizophrenia and their relationship to clinical outcome. *Biol Psychiatry* 31:241–254, 1992.
206. Bachhneff SA: Positron emission tomography and magnetic resonance imaging: A review and a local circuit neurons hypo(dys)function hypothesis of schizophrenia. *Biol Psychiatry* 30:857–886, 1991.
207. Miller R: Computerized tomography in schizophrenia. *Br J Psychiatry* 158:863, 1991.
208. Young AH, Blackwood DH, Roxborough H, et al: A magnetic resonance imaging study of schizophrenia: Brain structure and clinical symptoms. *Br J Psychiatry* 158:158–164, 1991.
209. Blackwood DH, Young AH, Muir WJ, et al: An MRI study in schizophrenia: Relationships with structural imaging, evoked potentials and neurospsychological test results. *Clin Neuropharmacol* 15(suppl 1, part A):114A–115A, 1992.
210. O'Callaghan E, Buckley P, Redmond O, et al: Abnormalities of cerebral structure in schizophrenia on magnetic resonance imaging: Interpretation in relation to the neurodevelopmental hypothesis. *J R Soc Med* 85:227–231, 1992.
211. Risch SC, Lewine RJ, Kalin NH, et al: Limbic-hypothalamic-pituitary-adrenal axis activity and ventricular-to-brain ratio studies in affective illness and schizophrenia. *Neuropsychopharmacology* 6:95–100, 1992.
212. Woods BT, Douglass A, Gescuk B: Is the VBR still a useful measure of changes in the cerebral ventricles? *Psychiatry Res* 40:1–10, 1991.
213. Arndt S, Cohen G, Alliger RJ, et al: Problems with ratio and proportion measures of imaged cerebral structures. *Psychiatry Res* 40:79–89, 1991.
214. Raz S, Raz N: Structural brain abnormalities in the major psychoses: A quantitative review of the evidence from computerized imaging. *Psychol Bull* 108:93–108, 1990.
215. Raz S, Raz N, Bigler ED: Ventriculomegaly in schizophrenia: Is the choice of controls important? *Psychiatry Res* 24:71–77, 1988.
216. Pfefferbaum A, Zipursky RB, Lim KO: Computed tomographic evidence for generalized sulcal and ventricular enlargement in schizophrenia. *Arch Gen Psychiatry* 45:633–640,1988.
217. Pfefferbaum A, Lim KO, Rosenbloom M, et al: Brain magnetic resonance imaging: Approaches for investigating schizophrenia. *Schizophr Bull* 16:453–476, 1990.
218. Lewis SW: Computerized tomography in schizophrenia: 15 years on. *Br J Psychiatry* 157:16–24, 1990.
219. Suddath RL, Casanova MF, Goldberg TE, et al: Temporal lobe pathology in schizophrenia: A quantitative magnetic resonance imaging study. *Am J Psychiatry* 146:464–472, 1989.

220. Nasrallah HA, Olson SC, McCalley-Whitters M, et al: Cerebral ventricular enlargement in schizophrenia: A preliminary follow-up study. *Arch Gen Psychiatry* 43:157–159, 1986.
221. Turner SW, Toone BK, Brett-Jones JR: Computerized tomographic scan changes in early schizophrenia: Preliminary findings. *Psychol Med* 16:219–225, 1986.
222. Pfefferbaum A, Zipursky R: Neuroimaging studies of schizophrenia. *Schizophr Res* 4:193–208, 1991.
223. Pfefferbaum A, Lim KO, Rosenbloom M, et al: Brain magnetic resonance imaging: Approaches for investigating schizophrenia. *Schizophr Bull* 16:453–476, 1990.
224. Zipursky GS, Lim KO, Sullivan EV: Widespread cerebral gray matter volume deficits in schizophrenia. *Arch Gen Psychiatry* 49:195–205, 1992.
225. Gur RE, Mozley PD, Resnick SM, et al: Magnetic resonance imaging in schizophrenia: I. Volumetric analysis of brain and cerebrospinal fluid. *Arch Gen Psychiatry* 48:407–412, 1991.
226. Degreef G, Lantos G, Bogerts B, et al: Abnormalities of the septum pellucidum on MR scans in first-episode schizophrenic patients. *Am J Neuroradiol* 13:835–840, 1992.
227. Degreef G, Lantos G, Bogerts B, et al: Abnormalities of the septum pellucidum on MR scans in first-episode schizophrenic patients. *Arch Gen Psychiatry* 49:531–537, 1992.
228. Mathew RT, Partain CL, Prakash R, et al: A study of the septum pellucidum and corpus callosum in schizophrenia with MR imaging. *Acta Psychiatr Scand* 72:414–421, 1985.
229. Raine A, Harrison GN, Reynolds GP, et al: Structural and functional characterisitcs of the corpus callsoum in schizophrenics, psychiatric controls, and normal controls: A magnetic resonance imaging and neuropsychological evaluation. *Arch Gen Psychiatry* 47:1060–1064, 1990.
230. Lewine RR, Gulley LR, Risch SC, et al: Sexual dimorphism, brain morphology and schizophrenia. *Schizophr Bull* 16:195–203, 1990.
231. Hauser P, Dauphinais ID, Berrettini W, et al: Corpus callosum dimensions measured by magnetic resonance imaging in bipolar affective disorder and schizophrenia. *Biol Psychiatry* 26:659–668, 1989.
232. Gunther W, Petsch R, Steniberg R, et al: Brain dysfunction during motor activation and corpus callosum alterations in schizophrenia measured by cerebral blood flow and magnetic resonance imaging. *Biol Psychiatry* 29:535–555, 1991.
233. Casanova MF, Sanders RD, Goldberg TE, et al: Morphometry of the corpus callosum in monozygotic twins discordant for schizophrenia: A magnetic resonance imaging study. *J Neurol* 53:416–421, 1990.
234. Schwarzkopf SB, Nasrallah HA, Olson SC, et al: Family history and brain morphology in schizophrenia: An MRI study. *Psychiatry Res* 40:49–60, 1991.
235. Vematsu M, Kaiya M: Midsagittal cortical pathology in schizophrenia. *Psychiatry Res* 30:11–20, 1989.
236. Nasrallah HA, Schwarzkopf SB, Olson SC, et al: Perinatal brain injury and cerebellar vermal lobules I-X in schizophrenia. *Biol Psychiatry* 29:567–574, 1991.
237. Jernigan TL, Zisook S, Heaton RK, et al: Magnetic resonance imaging abnormalities in lenticular nuclei and cerebral cortex in schizophrenia. *Arch Gen Psychiatry* 48:881–890, 1991.
238. DeLisi LE, Hoff AL, Schwartz JE, et al: Brain morphology in first-episode schizophrenic-like psychotic patients: A quantitative magnetic resonance imaging study. *Biol Psychiatry* 29:159–175, 1991.
239. Buchanan RW, Breier A, Kirkpatrick B, et al: Structural abnormalities in deficit and nondeficit schizophrenia. *Am J Psychiatry* 150:59–65, 1993.
240. Breier A, Buchanan RW, Elkashef A, et al: Brain morphology and schizophrenia: A magnetic resonance imaging study of limbic, prefrontal cortex and caudate structures. *Arch Gen Psychiatry* 49:921–926, 1992.
241. Swayze VW, Andreasen NC, Alliger RJ: Subcortical and temporal structures in affective disorder and schizophrenia: A magnetic resonance imaging study. *Biol Psychiatry* 31:221–240, 1992.
242. Keshavan MS, Bagwell WW, Haas GL, et al: Changes in caudate volume with neuroleptic treatment. *Lancet* 344:1434, 1994.
243. Suddath RL, Casanova MF, Goldberg TE, et al: Temporal lobe pathology in schizophrenia: A quantitative magnetic resonance imaging study. *Am J Psychiatry* 146:464–472, 1989.
244. Suddath R, Christison G, Torrey E, et al: Anatomical abnormalities in the brains of monozygotic twins discordant for schizophrenia. *N Engl J Med* 322:789–794, 1990.
245. Rossi A, Stratta P, D'Albenzio L, et al: Reduced temporal lobe areas in schizophrenia: Preliminary evidence from a controlled multiplanar magnetic resonance imaging study. *Biol Psychiatry* 27:61–68, 1990.
246. Dauphinais ID, DeLisi LE, Crow TJ, et al: Reduction in temporal lobe size in siblings with schizophrenia: A magnetic resonance imaging study. *Psychiatry Res* 35:137–147, 1990.
247. Shenton ME, Kikinis R, Jolesz FA, et al: Abnormalities of the left temporal lobe and thought disorder in schizophrenia. *N Engl J Med* 327:604–612, 1992.
248. Bogerts B, Ashtari M, Degreef G, et al: Reduced temporal limbic structure volumes on magnetic resonance images in first episode schizophrenia. *Psychiatry Res* 35:1–13, 1990.
249. Bogerts B, Falkai P, Greve B: Evidence of reduced temporolimbic structure volumes in schizophrenia. *Arch Gen Psychiatry* 48:956–958, 1991.
250. Barta P, Pearlson G, Powers R, et al: Auditory hallucinations and smaller superior temporal gyrus volume in schizophrenia. *Am J Psychiatry* 147:1457–1462, 1990.
251. Weinberger DR, Goldberg TE, Torrey EF, Berman KF: Relations between neuropsychological performance and brain morphological and physiological measures in monozygotic twins discordant for schizophrenia. *Psychiatry Res* 55:51–61, 1994.
252. Shenton ME, Kikinis R, Jolesz FA, et al: Abnormalities of the left temporal lobe and thought disorder in schizophrenia: Quantitative magnetic resonance imaging study. *N Engl J Med* 327:604–612, 1992.
253. Casanova MF, Goldberg TE, Suddath RL, et al: Quantitative shape analysis of the temporal and prefrontal lobes of schizophrenic patients: A magnetic resonance image study. *J Neuropsychiatry* 2:363–372, 1990.
254. Rossi A, Stratta P, Mattei P, et al: Planum temporale in schizophrenia: A magnetic resonance study. *Schizophr Res* 7:19–22, 1992.
255. Petty RG, Barta PE, Pearlson GD, et al: Reversal of

asymmetry of the planum temporale in schizophrenia. *Am J Psychiatry* 152:715–721, 1995.

256. Menon RR, Barta PE, Aylward EH, et al: Posterior superior temporal gyrus in schizophrenia: Grey matter changes and clinical correlates. *Schizophr Res* 16:127–135, 1995.
257. Schlaepfer TE, Harris GJ, Tien AY, et al: Decreased regional cortical gray matter volume in schizophrenia. *Am J Psychiatry* 151:842–848, 1994.
258. Andreasen NC, Arndt S, Swayze V 2d, et al: Thalamic abnormalities in schizophrenia visualized through magnetic resonance image averaging. *Science* 266:294–298, 1994.
259. Buchsbaum MS, Someya T, Teng CY, et al: PET an dMRI of the thalamus in never-medicated patients with schizophrenia. *Am J Psychiatry* 153:191–199, 1996.
260. Williamson P, Pelz D, Merskey H, et al: Frontal, temporal and striatal proton relaxation times in schizophrenic patients and normal comparison subjects. *Am J Psychiatry* 149:549–551, 1992.
261. Calabrese G, Deicken RF, Fein G, et al: Phosphorus magnetic resonance spectroscopy of the temporal lobes in schizophrenia. *Biol Psychiatry* 32:26–32, 1992.
262. Waddington JL, O'Callaghan E, Buckley P, et al: MR imaging and spectroscopy in schizophrenia in relation to the neurodevelopmental hypotheses. *Clin Neuropharmacol* 15(suppl 1, part A):118A–119A, 1992.
263. Keshavan MS, Pettegrew JW: Magnetic resonance spectroscopy in schizophrenia and psychotic disorder, in Krishnan KRR, Doraiswamy PM (eds): *Brain Imaging in Clinical Psychiatry,* New York, Marcel Dekker, 1977, pp 318–400.
264. Buchsbaum MS, DeLisi LE, Holcolmb HHY, et al: Anteroposterior gradients in cerebral glucose use in schizophrenia and affective disorders. *Arch Gen Psychiatry* 41:1159–1166, 1984.
265. Farkas T, Wolf AP, Jaeger J: Regional brain glucose metabolism in chronic schizophrenia. *Arch Gen Psychiatry* 41:293–300, 1984.
266. Cohen RM, Semple WE, Gross M, et al: Dysfunction in a prefrontal substrate of sustained attention in schizophrenia. *Life Sci* 40:2031–2039, 1987.
267. Jernigan TL, Sargent T III, Pfefferbaum A, et al: 18-Fluorodeoxyglucose PET in schizophrenia. *Psychiatry Res* 16:317–330, 1985.
268. Kling AS, Metter EJ, Riege WH: Comparison of PET measurement of local brain glucose metabolism and CAT measurement of brain atrophy in chronic schizophrenia and depression. *Am J Psychiatry* 143:175–180.
269. Wolkin A, Jaeger J, Brodie JD, et al: Persistence of cerebral metabolic abnormalities in chronic schizophrenia as determined by positron emission tomography. *Am J Psychiatry* 142:564–571, 1985.
270. Wolkin A, Angrist B, Wolf A, et al: Low frontal glucose utilization in chronic schizophrenia: A replication study. *Am J Psychiatry* 145:251–253, 1988.
271. Cleghorn JM, Garnett ES, Nahmias C, et al: Increased frontal and reduced parietal glucose metabolism in acute untreated schizophrenia. *Psychiatry Res* 28:119–133, 1989.
272. Sheppard G, Gruzelier J, Manchanda R, et al: Positron emission tomographic scanning in predominantly never-treated acute schizophrenic patients. *Lancet* 2:1448–1452, 1983.
273. Buchsbaum MS, Haier RJ, Potkin SG, et al: Frontostriatal disorder of cerebral metabolism in never-medicated schizophrenics. *Arch Gen Psychiatry* 49:935–942, 1992.
274. Cohen RM, Semple WE, Gross M, et al: Evidence for common alterations in cerebral glucose metabolism in major affective disorders and schizophrenia. *Neuropsychopharmacology* 2:241–254, 1989.
275. Gur RE, Resnick SM, Gur RC: Laterality and frontality of cerebral blood flow and metabolism in schizophrenia: Relationship to symptoms specificity. *Psychiatry Res* 27:325–334, 1989.
276. Cleghorn JM, Zipursky RB, List SJ: Structural and functional brain imaging in schizophrenia. *J Psychiatry Neurosci* 16:53–74, 1991.
277. Liddle PF, Friston KJ, Frith CD, et al: Patterns of cerebral blood flow in schizophrenia. *Br J Psychiatry* 160:179–186, 1992.
278. Liddle PF: Regional brain abnormalities associated with specific syndromes of persistent schizophrenic symptoms. *Clin Neuropharmacology* 15(suppl 1, part 1):401A–402A, 1992.
279. Liddle PF, Friston KJ, Frith CD, et al: Cerebral blood flow and mental processes in schizophrenia. *J R Soc Med* 85:224–227, 1992.
280. Frith CD, Friston KJ, Liddle PF, et al: PET imaging and cognition in schizophrenia. *J R Soc Med* 85:222–224, 1992.
281. Weinberger DR, Berman KF, Illowsky BP: Physiological dysfunction of dorsolateral cortex in schizophrenia: III. A new cohort and evidence for a monoaminergic mechanism. *Arch Gen Psychiatry* 45:609–615, 1988.
282. Berman KF, Gold CRJ, Abi-Darghain A: PET studies of frontal lobe function during cognition. *Schizophr Res* 4:399, 1991.
283. Buchsbaum MS, Nuechterlein KH, Haier RJ, et al: Glucose metabolic rate in normals and schizophrenics during the Continuous Performance Test assessed by positron emission tomography. *Br J Psychiatry* 156:216–227, 1990.
284. Buchanan RW, Breier A, Kirkpatrick B, et al: The deficit syndrome: Functional and structural characteristics. *Schizophr Res* 4:400–401, 1991.
285. Cleghorn JM, Szechtman H, Garnett ES, et al: Neuroleptic effects on regional brain metabolism in first episode schizophrenics. *Schizophr Res* 5:208–209, 1991.
286. Buchsbaum MS: The frontal lobes, basal ganglia, and temporal lobes as sites for schizophrenia. *Schizophr Bull* 16:379–389, 1990.
287. Cleghorn JM, Kaplan RD, Nahmias C, et al: Inferior parietal region implicated in neurocognitive impairment in schizophrenia. *Arch Gen Psychiatry* 49:966–974, 1992.
288. DeLisi LE, Buchsbaum MS, Holcomb HH: Increased temporal lobe glucose use in chronic schizophrenic patients. *Biol Psychiatry* 25:835–851, 1989.
289. Gur R, Resnick SM, Gur RC, et al: Regional brain function in schizophrenia: II. Repeated evaluation with positron emission tomography. *Arch Gen Psychiatry* 44:126–129, 1987.
290. Tamminga CA, Thaker GK, Buchanan R, et al: Limbic system abnormalities identified in schizophrenia using positron emission tomography with fluorodeoxyglucose

and neocortical alterations with deficit syndrome. *Arch Gen Psychiatry* 49:522–530, 1992.

291. Friston KJ, Liddle PF, Frith CD, et al: The left medial temporal region and schizophrenia: A PET study. *Brain* 115:367–382, 1992.
292. Cleghorn JM, Garnett ES: Patterns of regional brain metabolism during auditory hallucinations. *Biol Psychiatry* 29:75S, 1991.
293. Cleghorn JM, Franco S, Szechtman B, et al: Toward a brain map of auditory hallucinations. *Am J Psychiatry* 149:1062–1069, 1992.
294. Buchsbaum MS, Wu JC, DeLisi LE et al: Positron emission tomography studies of basal ganglia and somatosensory cortex neuroleptic drug effects: Differences between normal controls and schizophrenic patients. *Biol Psychiatry* 22:479–494, 1987.
295. DeLisi LE, Holcomb HH, Cohen RM: Positron emission tomography in schizophrenic patients with and without neuroleptic medication. *J Cereb Blood Metab* 5:201–206, 1985.
296. Buchsbaum MS, Haier RJ, Potkin SG, et al: Frontostriatal disorder of cerebral metabolism in never-medicated schizophrenics. *Arch Gen Psychiatry* 49:935–942, 1992.
297. Buchsbaum MS, Potkin SG, Siegel BV Jr, et al: Striatal metabolic rate and clinical response to neuroleptics in schizophrenia. *Arch Gen Psychiatry* 49:966–974, 1992.
298. Cleghorn JM, Kaplan RD, Nahmias C, et al: Inferior parietal region implicated in neurocognitive impairment in schizophrenia. *Arch Gen Psychiatry* 49:966–974, 1992.
299. Wolkin A, Sanfilipo M, Wolf AP, et al: Negative symptoms and hypfrontality in chronic schizophrenia. *Arch Gen Psychiatry* 49:959–965, 1992.
300. Buchsbaum MS, Potkin S, Siegel B, et al: PET studies of drug interaction with brain regional glucose metabolism. *Clin Neuropharmacol* 15(suppl 1, part A):472A–473A, 1992.
301. Pickar D, Hsiao JK, Litman RE: Regional brain metabolism as predictors of clozapine response. *Clin Neuropharmacol* 15(suppl 1, part A):399A–400A, 1992.
302. Wood FB, Flowers DL: Hypofrontal vs hypo-sylvian blood flow in schizophrenia. *Schizophr Bull* 16:413–424, 1990.
303. Murphy D, Rapoport LL: PET scanning in schizophrenia, a critical evaluation: Commentary on "The current status of PET scanning with respect to schizophrenia." *Neuropsychopharmacology* 7:59–61, 1992.
304. Bartlett EJ, Wolkin A, Brodie JD, et al: Importance of pharmacologic control in PET studies: Effects of thiothixene and haloperidol on cerebral glucose utilization in chronic schizophrenia. *Psychiatry Res* 40:115–124, 1991.
305. Wik G, Wiese FA, Sjogren I, et al: Effects of sulpiride and chlorpromazine on regional cerebral glucose metabolism in schizophrenic patients as determined by positron emission tomography. *Psychopharmacology* 97:309–318, 1989.
306. Wong DF, Wagner HN Jr, Tune LE, et al: Positron emission tomography reveals elevated D2 dopamine receptors in drug-naive schizophrenics. *Science* 234:1558–1563, 1986.
307. Farde L, Wiesel FA, Stone-Elander S, et al: D2 dopamine receptors in neuroleptic-naive schizophrenic patients: A positron emission tomography study with raclopride. *Arch Gen Psychiatry* 47:213–219, 1990.
308. Martinot JL, Paillere-Martinot ML, Loc'h C, et al: The estimated density of D2 striatal receptors in schizophrenia: A study with positron emission tomography and ^{76}Br bromolisuride. *Br J Psychiatry* 158:346–350, 1991.
309. Martinot JL, Peron-Magnan P, Huret JD, et al: Striatal D2 dopaminergic receptors assessed with positron emission tomography and bromospiperone in untreated schizophrenic patients. *Am J Psychiatry* 147:44–50, 1990.
310. Wong DF: PET studies of neuroreceptors in schizophrenia: Commentary on "The current status of PET scanning with respect to schizophrenia." *Neuropsychopharmacology* 7:69–72, 1992.
311. Sedvall G: The current status of PET scanning with respect to schizophrenia. *Neuropsychopharmacology* 7:41–54, 1992.
312. Martinot JL, Huret JD, Peron-agnan P, et al: Striatal D2 dopaminergic receptor status ascertained in vivo by positron emission tomography and ^{76}Br-bromospiperone in untreated schizophrenics. *Psychiatry Res* 29:357–358, 1989.
313. Lundberg T, Lindstrom LH, Hartvig P, et al: Striatal and frontal cortex binding of ^{11}C-labelled clozapine visualized by positron emission tomography (PET) in drug-free schizophrenics and healthy volunteers. *Psychopharmacology* 99:8–12, 1989.
314. Farde L, Wiesel FA, Nilsson L, et al: The potential of positron-emission tomography for pharmacokinetic and pharmacodynamic studies of neuroleptics. *Psychopharmacology* 7:32–39, 1989.
315. Martinot JL, Dao-Castellana MH: Brain imaging and schizophrenia. *Rev Pract* 41:611–614, 1991.
316. Farde L: Selective D1- and D2-dopamine receptor blockade both induces akathisia in humans—a PET study with SCH 23390 and raclopride. *Psychopharmacology* 107:23–29, 1992.
317. Courchesne E, Yeung-Courchesne R, Press GA, et al: Hypoplasia of cerebellar lobules VI and VII in infantile autism. *N Engl J Med* 318:1349–1354, 1988.
318. Kuperman S, Gaffney GR, Hamdan-Allen G, et al: Neuroimaging in child and adolescent psychiatry. *J Am Acad Child Adoles Psychiatry* 29:159–172, 1990.
319. Krieg JC: Eating disorders as assessed by cranial computerized tomography (CCT, dSPECT, PET). *Fuel Homeostasis Nerv Syst* 223–229, 1991.
320. Kornreich L, Shapira A, Horev G, et al: CT and MR evaluation of the brain in patients with anorexia nervosa. *Am J Neuroradiol* 12:1213–1216, 1991.
321. Hoffman GW, Ellinwood EH, Rockwell WJK, et al: Cerebral atrophy in anorexia nervosa: A pilot study. *Biol Psychiatry* 26:321–324, 1989.
322. Hoffman GW, Ellinwood EH, Rockwell WJK, et al: Cerebral atrophy in bulimia. *Biol Psychiatry* 25:894–902, 1989.
323. Husain MM, Black KJ, Doraswamy PM, et al: Subcortical brain anatomy in anorexia and bulimia. *Biol Psychiatry* 31:735–738, 1992.
324. Doraiswamy PM, Krishnan KRR, Figiel GS, et al: A brain magnetic resonance imaging study of pituitary gland morphology in anorexia nervosa and bulimia. *Biol Psychiatry* 28:110–116, 1990.

325. Doraiswamy PM, Krishnan KR, Boyko OB, et al: Pituitary abnormalities in eating disorders: Further evidence from MRI studies. *Prog Neuropsychopharmacol Biol Psychiatry* 15:351–356, 1991.
326. Krieg J-C, Holthoff V, Schreiber W, et al: Glucose metabolism in the caudate nuclei of patients with eating disorders, measured by PET. *Eur Arch Psychiatry Clin Neurosci* 240:331–333, 1991.
327. Krieg J, Lauer C, Leinsinger G, et al: Brain morphology and regional cerebral blood flow in anorexia nervosa. *Biol Psychiatry* 25:1041–1048, 1989.
328. Black KJ, Botteron KN: Neuroimaging in anorexia nervosa and bulimia nervosa, in Krishnan KRR, Doraiswamy M (eds): *Brain Imaging in Clinical Psychiatry*. New York, Marcel Dekker, 1997, pp 267–295.
329. Hoffman GW, Ellinwood EH, Rockwell WJK, et al: Brain T1 measured by magnetic resonance imaging in bulimia. *Biol Psychiatry* 27:116–119, 1990.
330. Wu JC, Hagman J, Buchsbaum MS, et al: Greater left cerebral hemispheric metabolism in bulimia assessed by positron emission tomography. *Am J Psychiatry* 147:309–312, 1990.
331. Andreason PJ, Altemus M, Zametkin AJ: Regional cerebral glucose metabolismin bulimia nervosa. *Am J Psychiatry* 149:1506–1513, 1992.
332. Potts NLS, Davidson RT, Krishnan KRR, et al: Magnetic resonance imaging in social phobia. *Psychiatry Res* 52:35–42, 1994.
333. Uhde TW, Kellner CH: Cerebral ventricular size in panic disorder. *J Affect Disord* 12:175–178, 1987.
334. Lepola U, Nousiainen U, Puranen M, et al: EEG and CT findings in patients with panic disorder. *Biol Psychiatry* 28:721–727, 1990.
335. Lader MH, Ron M, Petersson F: Computed axial brain tomography in long-term benzodiazepine users. *Psychol Med* 14:203–206, 1984.
336. Fontaine R, Breton G, Dry R, et al: Temporal lobe abnormalities in panic disorder: An MRI study. *Biol Psychiatry* 27:304–310, 1990.
337. Reiman EM, Raichle ME, Robins E, et al: The application of positron emission tomography to the study of panic disorder. *Am J Psychiatry* 143:469–477, 1986.
338. Drevets WC, Videen TO, MacLeod AK, et al: PET images of blood flow changes during anxiety: Correction. *Science* 256:1696, 1992.
339. Garber HJ, Ananth JV, Chiu LC, et al: Nuclear magnetic resonance study of obsessive-compulsive disorder. *Am J Psychiatry* 1461001–1005, 1989.
340. Harris GJ, Rhew EH, Noga T, et al: User-friendly method for rapid brain and CSF volume calculation using transaxial MRI images. *Psychiatry Res* 40:61–68, 1991.
341. Kellner CH, Jolley RR, Holgate RC, et al: Brain MRI in obsessive-compulsive disorder. *Psychiatry Res* 36:45–49, 1991.
342. Rosenberg DR, Keshavan MS, O'Hearn KM, et al: Frontostriatal measurement in treatment-naive children with obsessive-compulsive disorder. *Arch Gen Psychiatry* 54:824–830, 1997.
343. Martinot JL, Allilaire JF, Mazoyer BM, et al: Obsessive-compulsive disorder: A clinical, neuropsychological and positron emission tomography study. *J Acta Psychiatr Scand* 82:233–243, 1990.
344. Swedo SE, Schapiro MB, Grady CL, et al: Cerebral glucose metabolism in childhood-onset obsessive-compulsive disorder. *Arch Gen Psychiatry* 46:518–523, 1989.
345. Rubin RT, Billanueya-Meyer J, Ananth J, et al: Regional xenon 133 cerebral blood flow and cerebral technetium 99m HMPAO uptake in unmedicated patients with obsessive/compulsive disorder and matched normal control subjects: Determination by high resolution single photon emission computed tomography. *Arch Gen Psychiatry* 49:695–702, 1992.
346. Baxter LR Jr, Schwartz JM, Bergman KS, et al: Caudate glucose metabolic rate changes with both drug and behavior therapy for obsessive-compulsive disorder. *Arch Gen Psychiatry* 49:681–689, 1992.
347. Benkelfat C, Nordahl TE, Semple WE, et al: Local cerebral glucose metabolic rates in obsessive-compulsive disorder: Patients treated with clomipramine. *Arch Gen Psychiatry* 47:840–848, 1990.
348. Swedo SE, Pietrini P, Leonard HL, et al: Cerebral glucose metabolism in childhood-onset obsessive-compulsive disorder: Revisualization during pharmacotherapy. *Arch Gen Psychiatry* 49:690–694, 1992.
349. McCarley RW, Shenton ME, O'Donnell BF, et al: Auditory P300 abnormalities and left posterior superior temporal gyrus volume reduction in schizophrenia. *Arch Gen Psychiatry* 50:190–197, 1993.
350. Keshavan MS, Sanders RD, Pettegrew JW, et al: Frontal lobe metabolism and cerebral morphology in schizophrenia: 31P MRS and MRI studies. *Schizophr Res* 10:241–246, 1993.
351. Noga JT, Aylward E, Barta PE, Pearlson GD: Cinculate gyrus in schizophrenic patients and normal volunteers. *Psychiatry Res* 61:201–208, 1995.
352. Hokama H, Shenton ME, Nestor PG, et al: Caudate, putamen and globus pallidus volume in schizophrenia: A quantitative MRI study. *Psychiatry Res* 61:209–229, 1995.
353. Pearlson GD, Barta PE, Powers RE, et al: Medial and superior temporal gyral volumes and cerebral asymmetry in schizophrenia versus bipolar disorder. *Biol Psychiatry* 41:1–14, 1997.
354. Nasrallah HA, Skinner TE, Schmalbrock P, Robitaille PM: Proton magnetic resonance spectroscopy (1H MRS) of the hippocampal formation in schizophrenia: A pilot study. *Br J Psychiatry* 165:481–485, 1994.
355. Buckley PF, Moor C, Long H, et al: ^{1}H-magnetic resonance spectroscopy of the left temporal and frontal lobes in schizophrenia: Clinical and neurodevelopmental, and cognitive correlates. *Biol Psychiatry* 36:792–800, 1994.
356. Baxter LR Jr, Schwartz JM, Bergman KS, et al: Caudate glucose metabolic rate changes with both drug and behavior therapy for obsessive-compulsive disorder. *Arch Gen Psychiatry* 49:681–689, 1992.
357. Swedo SE, Pietrini P, Leonard HL, et al: Cerebral glucose metabolism in childhood-onset obsessive-compulsive disorder: Revisualization druing pharmacotherapy. *Arch Gen Psychiatry* 49:690–694, 1992.
358. Rothfeld JM: Generalized dystonia and obsessive-compulsive disorder associated with bilateral circumscribed magnetic resonance signal changes in the putamen. *J Nerv Ment Dis* 183:113–114, 1995.

PART TWO

THE NEUROLOGY OF AGING

CHAPTER 10

NEUROIMAGING OF NORMAL BRAIN AGING AND DEMENTIA

John B. Chawluk
Abass Alavi

INTRODUCTION

As the twentieth century draws to a close, neuroscientific study and neurologic care are increasingly concerned with issues of brain development, maturation, and senescence. The triumph of medical science over infectious diseases in the first half of this century tremendously reduced childhood mortality and morbidity rates in the industrialized nations of the world. As a result, inherited disorders of brain development have attained a greater prominence in pediatric medicine. Progress in molecular genetics has fueled an attack on these developmental brain diseases, which were heretofore resignedly relegated to descriptive textbook catalogs. Major advances in the treatment and prevention of cancer and atherosclerotic disease have led to a burgeoning population of physically vigorous individuals over age 60. In this setting of excellent health, the ravages of dementia are particularly poignant. Alzheimer disease (AD) now ranks as the fourth leading killer of elderly Americans, after heart disease, cancer, and stroke.

New techniques for imaging the central nervous system have been applied to the investigation of normal brain aging and dementia. X-ray computed tomography (CT), magnetic resonance imaging (MRI), positron emission tomography (PET), and single photon emission computed tomography (SPECT) have greatly advanced the understanding, diagnosis, and treatment of cerebral senescence. These technologies have also substantially enhanced insight into brain development and maturation. Without in-vivo tomographic techniques, knowledge in these two areas could only be inferred from autopsy or animal investigations.

The first part of this chapter reviews the neuroimaging of normal brain development and maturation. Then the imaging of normal brain aging, and finally dementia, are discussed, with emphasis on the diagnostic utility and shortcomings of the various tomographic modalities. Chapter 8 provides a more detailed treatment of behavioral issues in neuroimaging, including behavioral features of dementia.

BRAIN DEVELOPMENT AND MATURATION

A striking figure from Adams and Victor's *Principles of Neurology* (Fig. 7-2, 5th ed., p. 106) illustrates the "evolution of erect stance and gait and of paraplegia in flexion of cerebral origin according to Yakovlev" (Fig. 10-1). The figure legend continues: "The ripening forebrain of the fetus (a) drives the head and body up and moves the individual onward (b through e). When the 'driving brain' (frontal lobe, striatum, and pallidum) degenerates, the individual 'curls up' again (e through h)."[1] Our early studies of cerebral glucose metabolism in normal aging using PET and 18F-fluorodeoxyglucose (FDG)[2] demonstrated a fall-off of frontal metabolism with advancing years and developing dementia, paralleling the degeneration of Yakovlev's "driving brain" (Fig. 10-2). Subsequent FDG PET research by Chugani et al[3] provided metabolic correlates to the first half of Yakovlev's schema, with frontal (and temporoparietal) metabolic activity appearing as a final developmental stage (Fig. 10-3). The heuristic philosophical value of these analogies is undoubtedly greater than their direct scientific clinical utility. Nonetheless, it is intriguing to imagine a genetically programmed sequence of events leading from the embryonic and fetal brain to that of the infant, child, mature adult, normal older individual, and finally the patient afflicted with AD. This progression is especially provocative given some studies suggesting a very high prevalence of AD in the over-80 age group.

Magnetic Resonance Imaging and Normal Brain Development

Before the advent of modern neuroimaging (i.e., the pre-CT era), studies of early human cerebral development were hindered by the lack of appropriate autopsy material as well as the disruptive effects of agonal events upon the postmortem tissue. Serial evaluations of the same individual at different developmental stages were impossible. Even with the CT revolution of the mid-1970s, the harmful effects of ionizing radiation upon

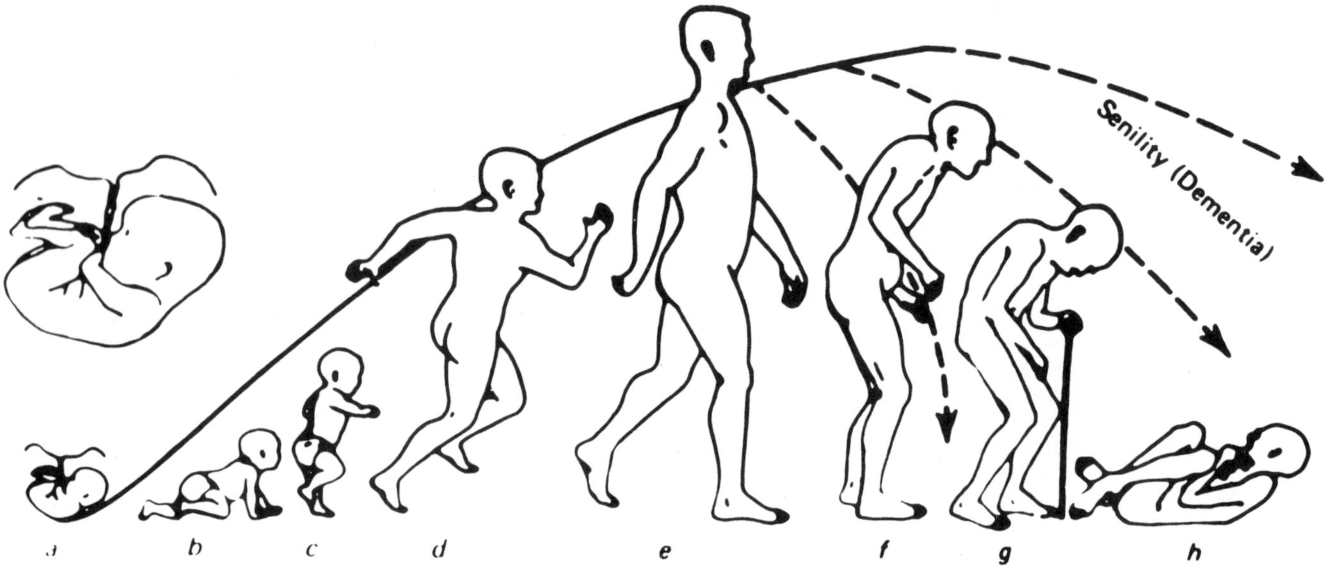

Figure 10-1
Evolution of erect stance and gait according to Yakovlev (see the text). (From Adams and Victor.[1] Used by permission.)

fetuses and infants also limited the use of CT in investigations of normal brain maturation. Moreover, the relatively poor gray matter–white matter discrimination hampered CT evaluation of myelination patterns, while beam-hardening (bone) artifacts[4] obscured subtle but significant ontogenic changes in the cortical ribbon. On the other hand, MRI, with its exquisitely high gray matter–white matter contrast sensitivity, relative absence of cortical artifacts, and low biohazard level, is the ideal tool for examining brain development.

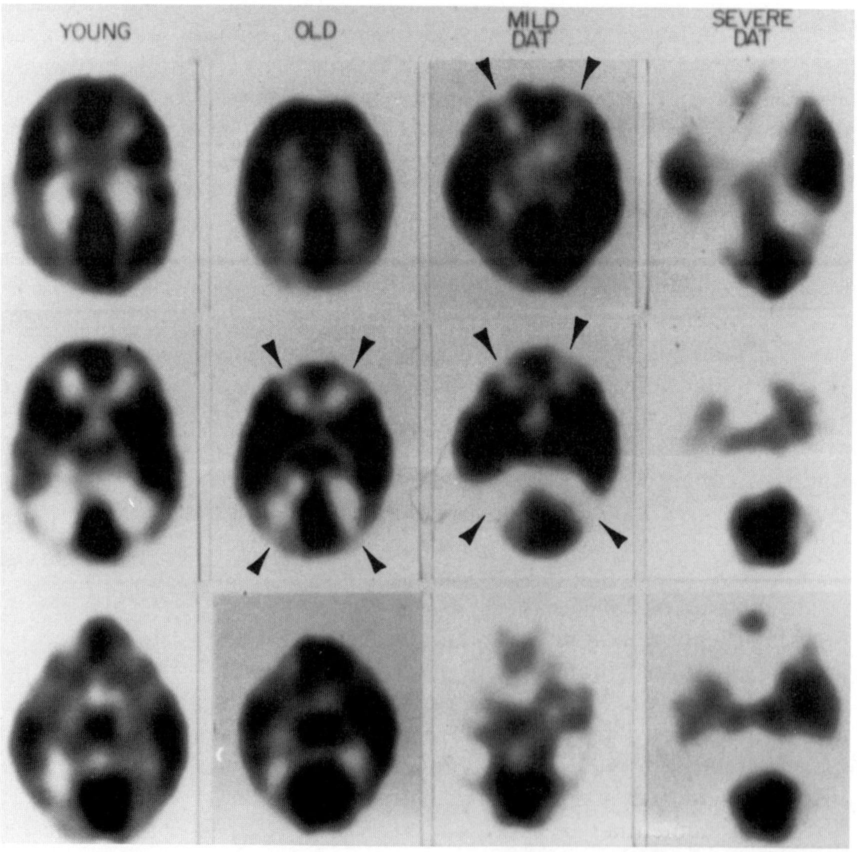

Figure 10-2
Characteristic cerebral glucose metabolic patterns in normal adults of different ages and patients with mild and severe AD. Note declining frontal and temporoparietal metabolism in elderly normals and patients with mild AD (arrowheads). DAT, dementia of the Alzheimer type. (From Chawluk et al.[2] Used by permission.)

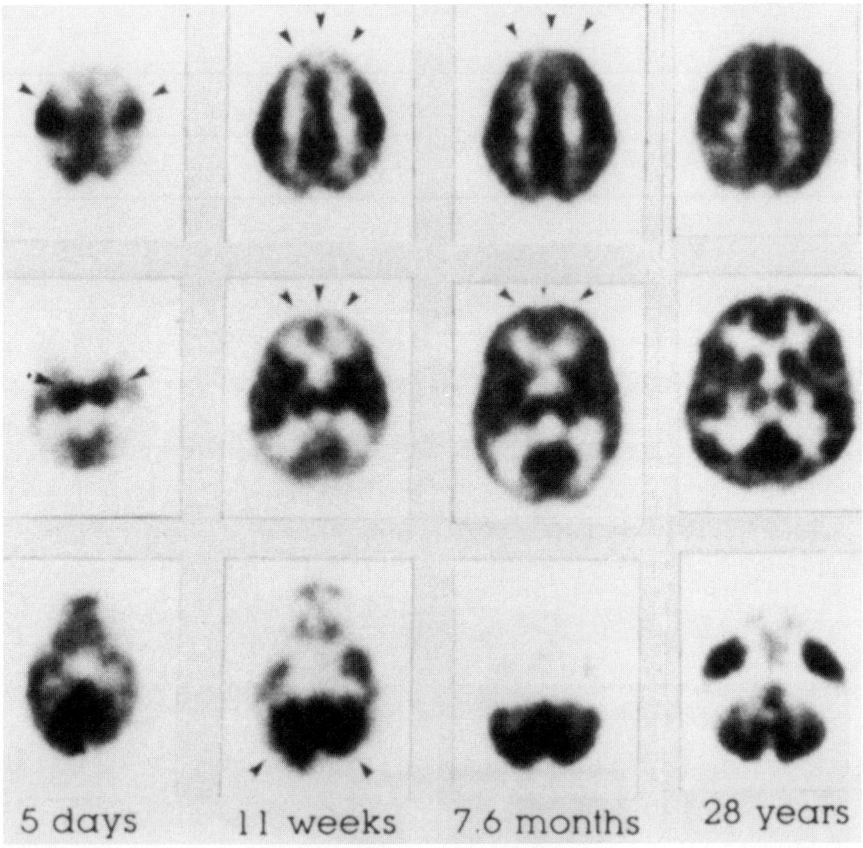

Figure 10-3
Characteristic cerebral glucose metabolic patterns in infants and children of different ages, compared with a 28-year-old adult. In the 5-day-old infant, arrowheads indicate prominent glucose utilization in the sensorimotor cortices (top frame) and thalamus (middle frame). In the 11-week-old and 7.6-month-old infants, arrowheads indicate developing frontal glucose utilization (top and middle frames). In the 11-week-old infant, increasing glucose utilization is also seen in the cerebellar hemispheres (arrowheads, bottom frame). (From Chugani and Phelps.[3] Used by permission.)

The concept that an orderly progression of myelin deposition underlies functional maturation of the developing brain dates back to the work of Flechsig at the turn of the century.[5] It was only with the advent of MRI that this hypothesis could be systematically explored. The developmental stages of brain myelination have been established with reasonable consistency by several authors[6–9] and can be demonstrated with T1- and/or T2-weighted images. Within the brain as a whole, myelination begins in the brainstem and progresses through the cerebellum and the cerebrum. Cerebral myelination commences in occipital regions and proceeds anteriorly, with frontal association white matter the last to myelinate. Myelination in the cerebrum also begins in the deeper, periventricular zones and occurs last in the peripheral cortical gyri.[6]

Although the inversion recovery technique can provide high-contrast-sensitivity T1-weighted images, most protocols scan the infant brain using T1- and T2-weighted spin-echo pulse sequences. The distinctive features of the neonatal brain are, in part, due to much longer T1 and T2 values compared with the adult brain.[7] Since T1 increases with field strength, the staging of myelination patterns using T1-weighted images must take into account the scanner's main magnetic field strength. The lengthening of T1 with higher field strength may also require a longer repetition time (TR) for adequate gray matter–white matter contrast on T2-weighted scans. Changes in brain myelination patterns are seen earlier on T1-weighted images. The increase in white matter signal intensity typically seen on T1-weighted studies of infant brain development may reflect a rise in cholesterol, glycolipid, and/or protein content in the maturing myelin sheaths.[6] A later stage in myelin development is characterized by an increase in phospholipid with a resultant hydrophobic lipid bilayer. There are fewer mobile protons available for excitation in this hydrophobic layer, leading to a decrease in both effective proton density and T2 relaxation. Therefore, the decrease in white matter signal in the developing brain seen with T2-weighted images will occur at a later chronological age than the white matter signal increase noted on T1-weighted scans. The scan weighting (T1: short TR, short TE; T2: long TR, long TE) thus reflects various stages of myelin formation.

Table 10-1 summarizes the normal age ranges for myelin deposition in various parts of the brain as visualized on T1- and T2-weighted images. In the first month of life, myelin is seen in the thalami, cerebellar peduncles, and (nascently) posterior limb of the internal capsule (Fig. 10-4). By 2 to 3 months of age, T1-weighted scans demonstrate high-signal myelin in the anterior limb of the internal capsule, splenium of the corpus callosum, optic radiations, and central semiovale (Fig. 10-5). By 7 months these regions, as well as the genu and rostrum of the corpus callosum, are seen as low-

Table 10-1
Myelination milestones

Gray-white pattern	*Myelination site*	*Age* *T1 images*	*Age* *T2 images*
Infantile	Thalami, cerebellar peduncles	Birth	Birth–2 months
Infantile	Posterior limb internal capsule	Birth	Birth–2 months
Infantile	Anterior limb internal capsule	2–3 months	7–11 months
Infantile	Corpus callosum (splenium before genu and rostrum)	3–6 months	4–8 months
Infantile	Centrum semiovale	2–4 months	7–11 months
Isointense	Parietal and frontal white matter	3–5 months	8–12 months
Early adult	Temporal white matter	4–7 months	10–14 months
Early adult	Branches into peripheral subcortical fibers	10–16 months	18–24 months

Source: Adapted from Barkovich et al[6] *and Dietrich et al.*[7] *Used by permission.*

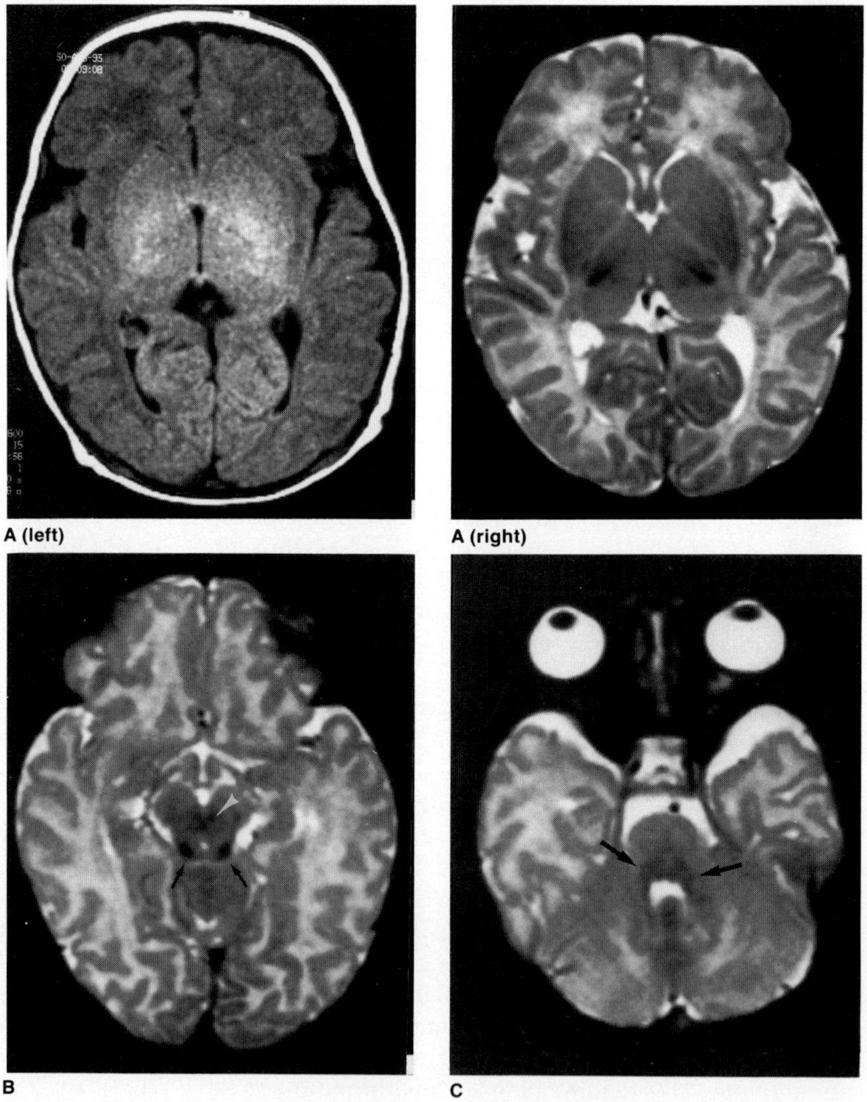

Figure 10-4
MRI scan of a 25-day-old infant. **(A)** *(left) T1-weighted scan with high-signal myelination seen in the thalami and posterior limbs of the internal capsules. (right) Corresponding T2-weighted scan with low-signal thalamic and internal capsular myelin deposition.* **(B)** *T2-weighted scan with dense low-signal myelination in the collicular plate (black arrows) and patchy early myelination of the red nuclei and superior cerebellar penduncle decussation (white arrowhead).* **(C)** *T2-weighted scan with low-signal myelination in the middle cerebellar peduncle (black arrows). (Courtesy of Dr. Robert A. Zimmerman.)*

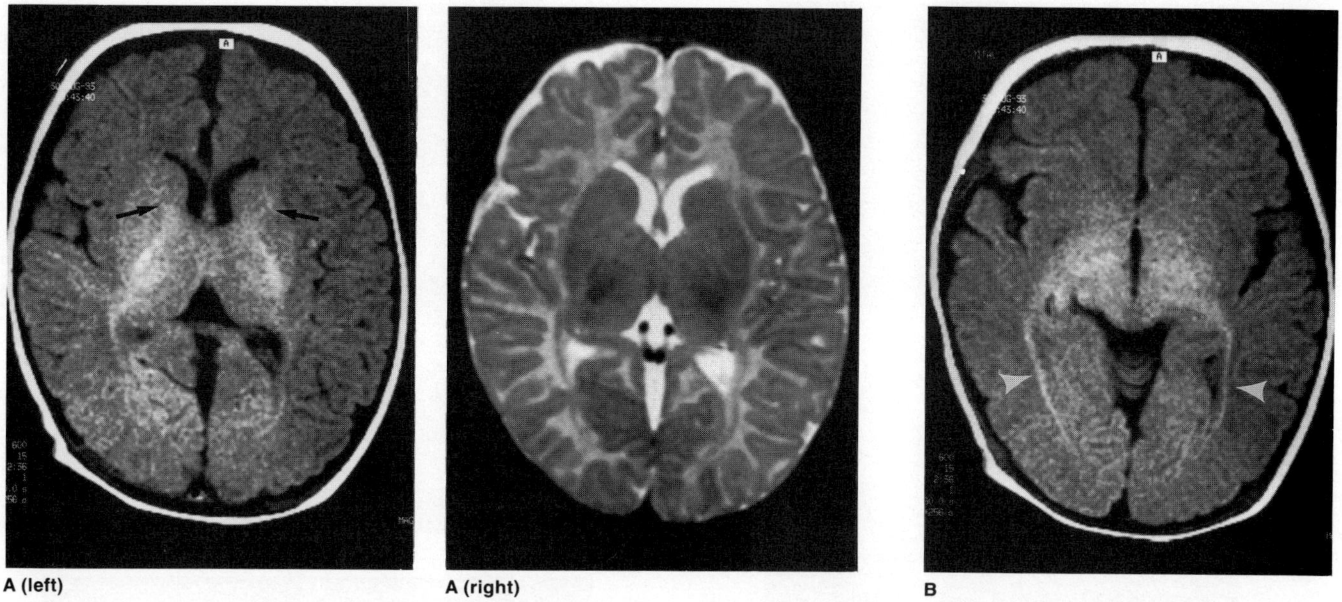

A (left) A (right) B

Figure 10-5

MRI scan of a 2-month-old infant. **(A)** *(left) T1-weighted scan with high-signal myelination beginning in the anterior limbs of the internal capsules (black arrows). The posterior limbs are more densely myelinated. (right) Corresponding T2-weighted scan. Note the absence of low-signal myelination in the anterior limbs of the internal capsules.* **(B)** *T1-weighted image with high-signal myelination in the optic radiations (white arrowheads). (Courtesy of Dr. Robert A. Zimmerman.)*

signal myelinated structures on T2-weighted scans (Fig. 10-6). Up until approximately this age (6 to 8 months), the gray matter–white matter pattern on T2-weighted scans is essentially the reverse of that seen in adults, that is, white matter is relatively *hyperintense* compared with gray matter. This has been termed the "infantile pattern" by Dietrich and Bradley.[7] At 8 to 12 months, T2-weighted scans go through a transitional "isointense phase,"[7] with low gray-white contrast in many regions of the brain (Fig. 10-7). T1-weighted images at this stage, however, demonstrate high gray-white contrast at the corticomedullary interface, and myelinated subcortical U fibers are clearly seen as areas of increased signal intensity (Fig. 10-8). As myelination proceeds peripherally and anteriorly, cerebral white matter becomes hypointense relative to gray matter on T2-weighted scans. The relative gray-white intensities are, therefore, similar to what is seen in the mature brain, hence the appellation "early adult pattern."[7] This pattern is seen in essentially all normal infants older than 12 months.[7]

Cataloging the various stages of myelin development is not a trivial academic exercise. Delayed myelination may result from a number of prenatal and perinatal cerebral insults, including hypoxic-ischemic injury, infection, and inherited disorders of neuronal migration.[7] In infants with developmental delay, the myelination stages (in various brain regions) correspond with developmental age rather than chronological age.[7,8] Serial MRI studies, by demonstrating retarded myelination patterns, may be extremely helpful in documenting and

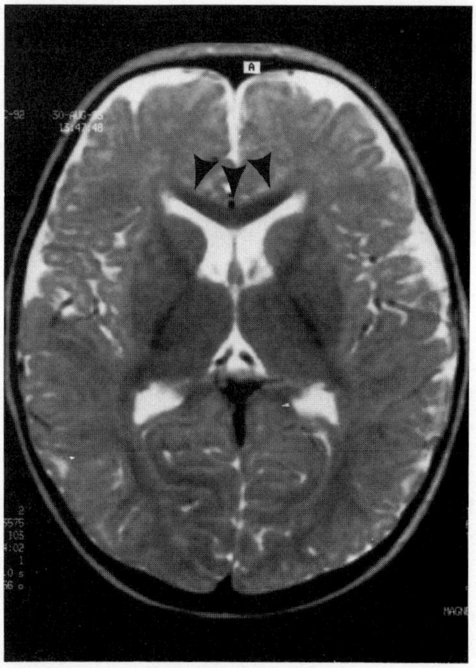

Figure 10-6

MRI scan of a 7-month-old infant. T2-weighted scan reveals low-signal myelination in the anterior and posterior limbs of the internal capsules, as well as the genu of the corpus callosum (arrowheads). (Courtesy of Dr. Robert A. Zimmerman.)

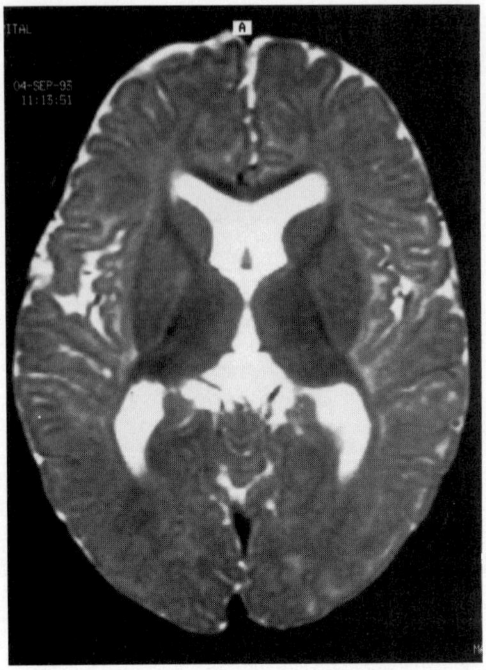

Figure 10-7
T2-weighted MRI scan of a 10-month-old infant. Note loss of gray matter–white matter contrast posteriorly ("isointense phase"). The internal capsules, external capsules, and corpus callosum genu are well myelinated. (Courtesy of Dr. Robert A. Zimmerman.)

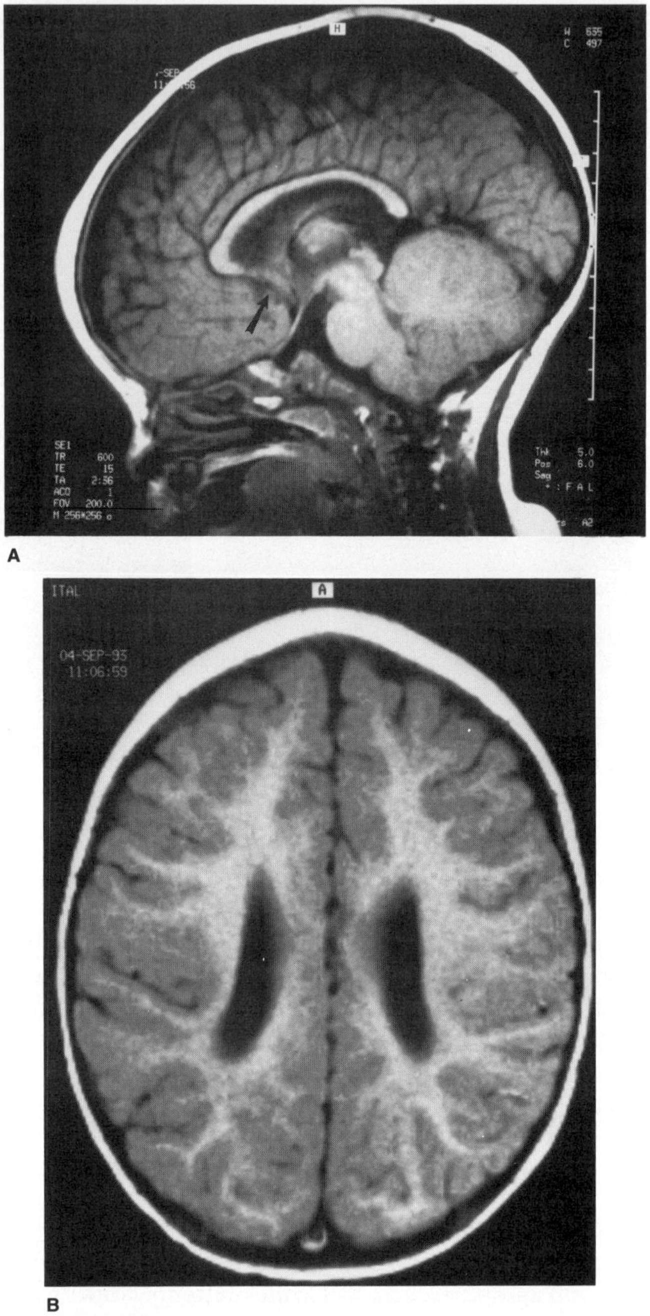

Figure 10-8
T2-weighted MR images of a 10-month-old infant. **(A)** *Midsagittal view demonstrates high-signal myelination of the corpus callosum in its entirety (artifact obscures the signal increase in the rostrum of the callosum; arrow).* **(B)** *Axial scan shows fine high-signal myelin "tentacles" extending into the superficial peripheral subcortical zones. (Courtesy of Dr. Robert A. Zimmerman.)*

monitoring developmental delay. In van der Knaap's study,[8] a strong correlation was found between myelination stage and neurodevelopmental testing (Bayley scales of infant development). About 70 percent of the variance in test performance was related to the degree of myelin maturity.

Before leaving our discussion of MRI and myelin maturation, it is important to point out bilateral triangular areas posterior and superior to the lateral ventricle trigones that myelinate quite slowly. As a result, these areas remain hyperintense on T2-weighted images at a time when the rest of the brain has developed an adult pattern of gray-white contrast (Fig. 10-9). This periventricular hyperintensity should not be mistaken for ischemia, demyelination, or other periventricular pathologic process.[6]

Positron Emission Tomography and Normal Brain Development

Given the pervasive interdependence of anatomy and physiology in biological systems, it is not surprising to see function follow form in human brain development. Moreover, the behavior of an individual organism reflects regional biochemical events that can be tomographically mapped with PET scanning. The relative invasiveness of older techniques of measuring cerebral blood flow and metabolism, as well as the radiation exposure involved, limited their use in studies of infants and children. In contrast, investigators have not hesitated to use these techniques to study brain physiology in normal and demented elderly adults.[10] Pioneering work by the University of California at Los Angeles PET group in the mid-1980s[3,11,12] provided crucial origi-

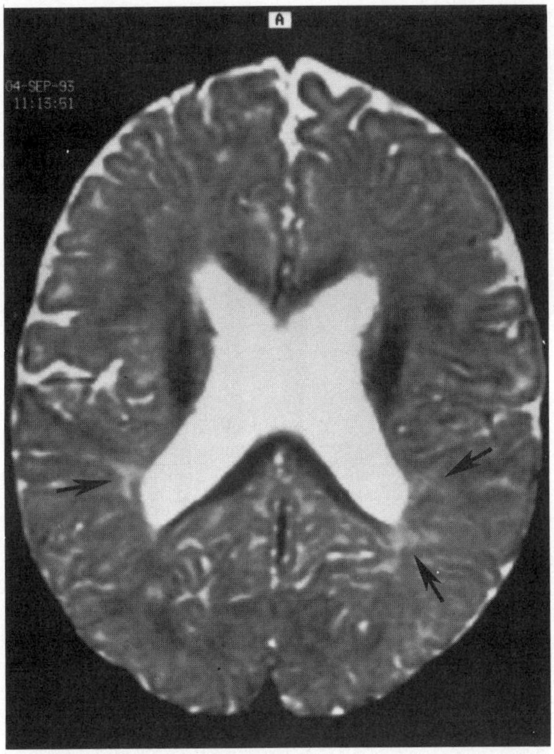

Figure 10-9
T2-weighted MRI scan of a 10-month-old infant. Patchy posterior periventricular zones of relatively increased signal (arrows) represent areas of normally delayed myelination and should not be mistaken for pathologic processes (see the text). (Courtesy of Dr. Robert A. Zimmerman.)

nal information on patterns of regional cerebral metabolism in infants and children at various developmental stages.

Figure 10-3 illustrates these developmental changes in regional cerebral glucose metabolic patterns according to the FDG PET studies of Chugani and Phelps.[3] Normal neonates exhibit a distinctive pattern of regional glucose metabolism. The brainstem, cerebellar vermis, thalami, and sensorimotor cortices (i.e., evolutionarily older areas of the brain) are metabolically active, with other brain regions relatively quiescent. Neonatal behavior is basically limited to reflex responses that can be functionally mapped to these metabolically active structures. The 2- to 3-month-old infant acquires visuospatial and higher-level sensorimotor skills, reflected in increased metabolic activity in the primary visual cortices, cerebellar hemispheres, basal ganglia, and temporoparietal cortical regions. It is not until 7 to 8 months of life that major metabolic activity is seen in the frontal cortex and posterior parietal–anterior occipital cortices. The infant at this age begins to demonstrate more complex behaviors, such as "stranger anxiety," and performs much more effectively on neuropsychologic tests of frontal lobe function.[12] By 1 to 2 years of age, the regional glucose metabolic pattern is similar to that seen in normal adults and remains so during childhood and adolescence. Absolute rates of glucose metabolism in the neocortex rise above adult levels, however, from ages 3 to 9 years and then decline gradually over the next decade.[11] Chugani and coworkers speculate that this elevated glycolytic activity is due to the increased synaptic density (therefore increased surface area of metabolically active neuronal membrane) seen in children in this age range. This synaptic excess may underlie the "plasticity of recovery" demonstrated after brain injury by children under 10 years old. Magnetic resonance imaging studies by Jernigan et al suggest a decrease in gray matter volume in the cerebral cortex generally, most pronounced in frontal and parietal areas, during adolescence.[13] This finding corresponds well with the FDG PET studies of Chugani et al discussed above.

NORMAL BRAIN AGING

Each neuroimaging modality discussed in this chapter—CT, MRI, PET, and SPECT—is plagued by the difficulty of distinguishing between findings not observed on scans of younger adults but seen in older individuals who appear otherwise neurologically normal and changes definitely characteristic of a dementing illness. A tale circulates about an alien from Eternium (a fictitious planet where senescence does not occur) visiting Earth for the first time. The alien sees what we would all consider to be a remarkably healthy octogenarian (sans cosmetic surgery), standing next to his robust 20-year-old grandson. Observing the obvious contrast in physical vigor, the alien concludes that the "healthy octogenarian" must be seriously ill. This vignette illustrates an important generality to keep in mind when imaging the maturing human brain. No matter which neuroimaging technique is being considered, it is often easier to distinguish the scan of a healthy young person from that of a healthy older subject than it is to distinguish a "normal old scan" from a "demented scan." This caveat is especially applicable to everyday clinical scanning. Nevertheless, careful observation and investigation have revealed diagnostic features of the various imaging modalities that permit some discrimination of the major dementing illnesses.

Computed Tomographic Scanning and Normal Brain Aging

Cerebral atrophy has long been recognized by neuropathologists as a prominent feature of the normal aging process as well as dementing illnesses. In a study that opened the modern era of dementia pathology, Tomlinson, Blessed, and Roth observed that severe atrophy occurred only in demented elderly individuals and not in the normal aged.[14] In another autopsy series, however, Miller et al documented a decrease in mean hemispheric volume in normal subjects of 2 percent per decade beginning at age 50.[15] Observations such as these have led to attempts to quantify cerebral atrophy antemortem, enhancing our understanding of the pathophysiology of normal brain aging and dementia while improving diagnostic acumen. In the midportion of this century, senescent cerebral atrophy could be detected invasively via pneumoencephalography. The earliest CT studies proved quite capable of demonstrating brain tissue loss in the elderly.[16] Many investigators were able to document statistically significant correlations between age and both ventricular size[17–20] and extent of cortical atrophy[19,21] even with relatively crude qualitative or semiquantitative estimates of cerebrospinal fluid (CSF) volumes.

As mentioned above, a limitation in CT assessments of generalized cerebral atrophy is the considerable overlap in these estimates between nondemented and demented elderly individuals. Since AD, the single most important dementing illness of the aged, primarily involves degeneration of mesial temporal lobe structures, it makes sense to focus imaging efforts on this anatomic area. Routine CT scans of the brain are performed with slices parallel to the canthomeatal line; such scans therefore image the hippocampus and surrounding structures obliquely (Fig. 10-10). Axial cuts angled at 20° negative to the canthomeatal line will image the choroidal-hippocampal fissure and temporal horns of the lateral ventricles in a single slice (Fig. 10-11). Using such an imaging approach to assess temporal lobe atrophy can identify normal older subjects with a specificity of up to 95 percent; that is, the absence of temporal lobe atrophy strongly suggests the absence of AD.[22] In this study by George and coworkers, hippocampal lucency, presumably due to widening of the choroidal and hippocampal fissures, correctly distinguished 80 percent of AD patients from elderly control subjects (Fig. 10-11).[22] Nevertheless, 55 percent of the normal elderly controls exhibited mild or greater temporal lobe atrophy.

Kido et al examined CT atrophy features in 39 patients with AD and 29 age-matched control subjects.[23] Temporal horn and sylvian fissure size (Fig. 10-10) were assessed by blind subjective ranking and objective measurements. Subjective temporal horn enlargement was noted in 26 of 39 AD patients and only one control subject. A receiver-operator curve analysis detected no significant difference between the subjective and objective appraisals of temporal lobe atrophy. The presence of temporal horn dilatation was clearly a highly specific indicator of AD. Sylvian fissure widening was more sensitive, however, in detecting the presence of primary degenerative dementia. The overall accuracy of these measurements in distinguishing AD from normal brain aging is at least 80 percent.

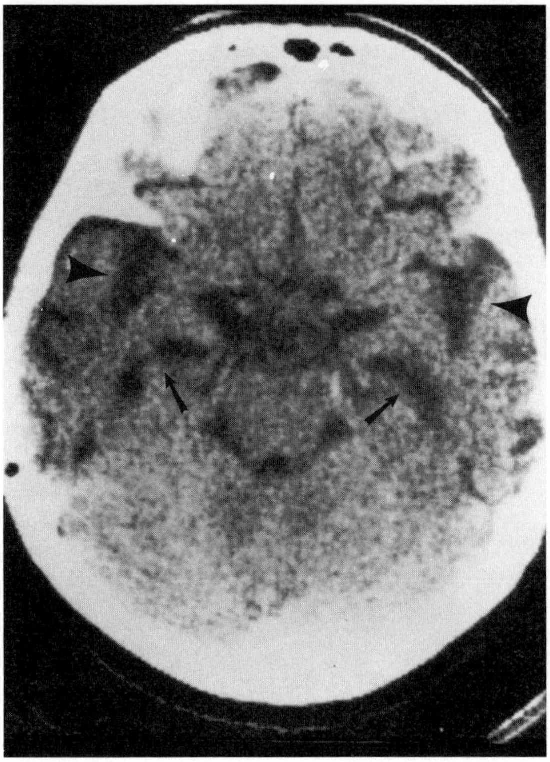

Figure 10-10
A 61-year-old woman with AD. The CT section through the temporal lobes was oriented +15° with respect to the canthomeatal line. There is moderate symmetrical widening of the sylvian fissures (arrowheads) and similar dilatation of the temporal horns (arrows). (From Kido et al.[23] Used by permission.)

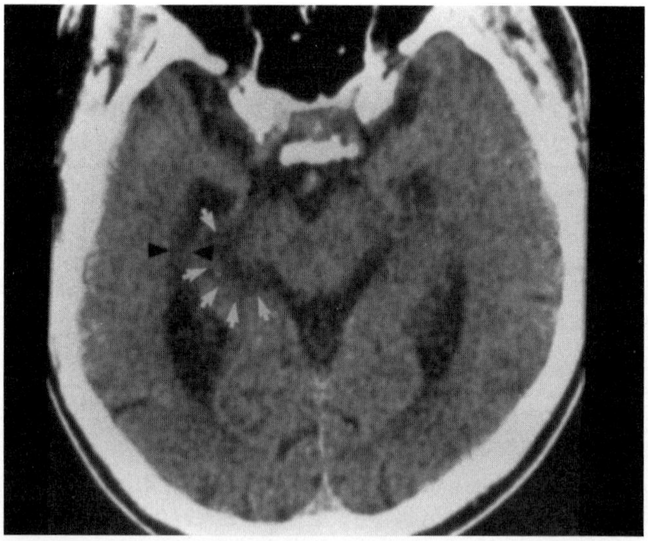

Figure 10-11
A 63-year-old man with presumed mild AD. The CT section through the temporal lobes was oriented −20° to the canthomeatal line. Moderate hippocampal lucency (see the text) is seen on the right (white arrows). Severe temporal horn dilatation is also seen (black arrowheads). (From George et al.[22] Used by permission.)

Jobst and coworkers also used thin-section (2-mm) CT scans oriented transversely through the middle cranial fossa to assess temporal lobe atrophy.[24] Using a selected slice through the midportion of the mesial temporal lobe, simple temporal lobe width measurements were made. The minimum width of the mesial temporal lobe in 44 autopsy-diagnosed AD patients was about one-half of that in 75 nondemented age-matched control subjects. The presence of AD could be detected at a rate of 92 percent, allowing for a 5 percent false-positive rate. This information, combined with age-specific prevalence data, allows the calculation of an odds-likelihood ratio for the diagnosis of AD in an individual based upon the simple temporal lobe width measurement.

Although CT technology has improved dramatically since the first-generation pictures from the mid-1970s, this x-ray technique is still hampered by beam-hardening artifacts[4] in areas encased by cortical bone, such as the middle cranial fossa. However, MRI does not suffer this limitation and is clearly the logical neuroimaging technique for further investigations of temporal lobe atrophy in studies of the aging brain. DeLeon et al used CT and MRI to examine the occurrence of hippocampal atrophy in a research clinic population.[25] Their cohort of 405 individuals included normal elderly subjects, patients with mild memory and cognitive impairments ("benign senescent forgetfulness"), and patients with AD (one mild group and one moderate to severe group). Hippocampal atrophy (HA) was found in 29 percent of normal old people, its frequency increasing with advancing age. In the cognitively impaired individuals, HA prevalence was associated, not with advancing age, but, rather, with degree of cognitive impairment (ranging from 78 percent in the benign senescent forgetfulness group to 96 percent in the moderate to severe AD group). Their data, although somewhat preliminary, did suggest an association between the presence of HA and memory impairment, even in subjects not meeting clinical criteria for the diagnosis of AD. Moreover, HA, when present, may identify individuals at greater risk for the development of clinical and neuropathologic AD.

Magnetic Resonance Imaging and Normal Brain Aging

The ability of MRI to demonstrate cerebral atrophy has been clear from the earliest days of T1-weighted inversion recovery images. Our first atrophy measurements in the early 1980s using T1-weighted MRI scans demonstrated a clear superiority of this technology over CT in assessing cortical tissue loss (increased sulcal volumes).[26] With the rapid realization that T2-weighted spin-echo paradigms were exquisitely sensitive to pathologic insults, attention focused on long TR–long TE pulse sequences in imaging the aging brain. The easily detected presence of multiple hyperintense lesions in the subcortical white matter of the cerebral hemispheres initially appeared to facilitate the diagnosis of multi-infarct dementia (MID). Technology revealed an ephemeral epidemic of MID, however, as it became apparent that these subcortical high-signal changes were also quite common in normal individuals over age 50 (Fig. 10-12). Indeed Yue et al, in their study of 3660 community-living elderly subjects, found greater degrees of sulcal atrophy, ventricular enlargement, and white matter signal changes with increasing age.[27] During a 5-year longitudinal observation of extremely healthy ("successfully aged") older people, Wahlund

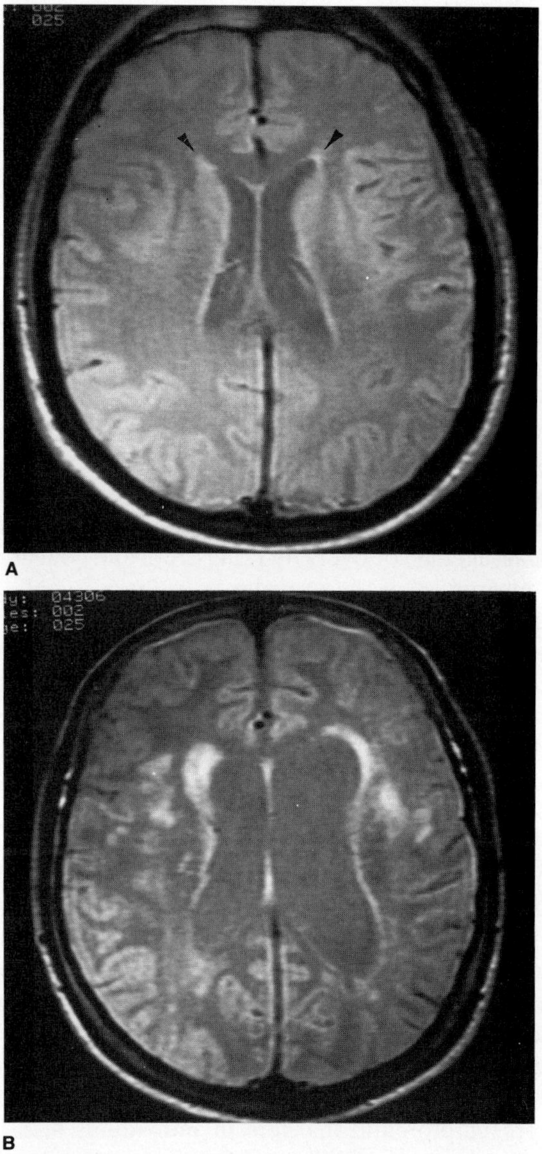

A

B

Figure 10-12
Intermediate-weighted MRI sections (long TR, short TE). **(A)** *Normal 50-year-old man. Faint periventricular "capping" is seen (arrowheads).* **(B)** *Normal 70-year-old man with hypertension. Periventricular "capping" is more prominent. Patchy "early confluent" deep WMHs are seen bifrontally.)*

and coworkers found an increase in frontal and ventricular CSF volumes as well as a mild increase in white matter and basal ganglia high-signal changes.[28]

The proliferation of terms to describe these common, age-related findings on T2-weighted scans confirms the uncertainty over their significance and cause. *Unidentified bright objects, white matter lesions, white matter hyperintensities, periventricular hyperintensities,* and *leukoaraiosis* are but a few of the many appellations for these enigmatic MRI signal changes. Bradley et al were among the first to point out how common these white matter hyperintensities (WMHs) are in the elderly population.[29] Our early investigations into their significance suggested an association with increasing age, vascular risk factors, and presence of dementia, either degenerative or (especially) vascular.[30] A follow-up study with a larger cohort by Fazekas and coinvestigators supported many of these earlier observations.[31] In 101 neurologically intact volunteers ranging in age from 31 to 84 years, WMHs (removed from the ventricular surface) or periventricular hyperintensities (PVHs) were seen in 48 and 45 percent of subjects, respectively. The WMHs were predominantly punctuate, that is, small and discrete, while the PVHs were usually "caps" restricted to the ventricular apices or smooth, relatively thin "lines" surrounding the lateral ventricles. Individuals with more extensive white matter signal abnormalities either had cerebrovascular risk factors (e.g., hypertension, diabetes mellitus, or cardiovascular disease) or were over age 60 (Fig. 10-12B). These findings have been confirmed and extended in a much larger study population (3301 individuals aged 65 or over) by Longstreth and colleagues.[31a] An awareness of the prevalence of these signal abnormalities by decade is useful in clinical scan interpretation. Based on the work of Fazekas et al,[31] a reasonably accurate mnemonic approximation for WMH/PVH prevalence by decade is 20 percent for age 30 to 39, 30 percent for age 40 to 49, 50 percent for age 50 to 59, 60 percent for age 60 to 69, and 70 percent for over age 70.

As important as determining the prevalence of WMHs are the efforts to ascertain their clinical and neuropsychologic significance and pathologic basis. A reasonable consensus is developing that, in normal elderly individuals, cerebral white matter signal changes are indeed associated with advancing age and vascular risk factors.[32–35] Less clear is whether these lesions correlate with cognitive decline or other clinical deficits in the normal aged population and whether they may serve as presymptomatic markers in individuals at risk for the development of degenerative or vascular dementia. From a practical standpoint, it appears that only relatively subtle cognitive impairments are present in subjects with extensive WMH who were otherwise determined to be normal by careful bedside neurologic evaluation.[33,34,36–38] Further studies are needed to prove or discredit the hypothesis that the accumulation of these lesions is a harbinger of clinical dementia. As pharmacotherapeutic means become available to prevent cerebrovascular damage (e.g., antiplatelet drugs and hemorrheologic agents) or brain degeneration (e.g., free radical scavengers and nerve growth factors), the detection of such presymptomatic risk markers becomes increasingly important.

The pathologic basis for these "incidental" white matter lesions has also been controversial and somewhat elusive, although a number of studies have begun providing a limited consensus elucidating the underlying histologic changes. Histopathologic evidence for infarction is an expected finding in patients with vascular dementia. Ischemic damage would not necessarily be expected, however, in individuals suffering from *degenerative* dementia or normal older persons selected for their excellent general health. Kirkpatrick and Hayman examined 15 brains from subjects 52 to 72 years of age with no clinical or autopsy evidence of neurologic disease.[39] Three brains had no lesions at all. Eight of the 12 remaining brains contained zones of atrophic perivascular demyelination (i.e., perivascular fibrosis and gliosis with associated fluid-filled spaces), bilaterally symmetrical in five cases. These abnormalities were found throughout the centrum semiovale. The pathogenesis of atrophic perivascular demyelination is thought to be chronic, low-grade vascular insufficiency. Such changes are more commonly demonstrated in hypertensive subjects with thickened arteriolar walls and resultant impaired nutritive function of these vessels.[40] Braffman et al directly correlated white matter abnormalities seen on MRI with pathologic examination.[41] Magnetic resonance imaging scans, gross pathologic studies, and histopathologic studies were performed on 36 formalin-fixed brains from elderly subjects with and without neurologic symptoms during life. Fourteen lacunar infarctions were seen in seven cases, with five lacunae seen in the supratentorial white matter. Enlargement of the Virchow-Robin perivascular CSF spaces (*état criblé,* Fig. 10-13) in the basal ganglia was seen in four brains. All lesions seen on pathologic examination were identified by MRI, and all patients except one had clinical and/or autopsy evidence of hypertension. *État criblé* had been described earlier by Awad and coworkers as one pathologic basis for subcortical high-signal lesions seen on MRI in the elderly.[42] In a companion study of 23 formalin-fixed brains from patients over age 60 at the time of death, Braffman and colleagues found 15 WMH foci in seven brains.[43] All patients except two had evidence of hypertension. Six lesions were due to completed infarction, two reflected areas of gliosis or noncavitated ("incomplete") infarction, one hyperintense focus represented a small brain cyst, while another was due to a small congenital diverticulum of the lateral ventricle. Three lesions seen on MRI were not found on the corresponding autopsy sections. These authors concluded that most hyperintense white matter changes seen on MRI in the

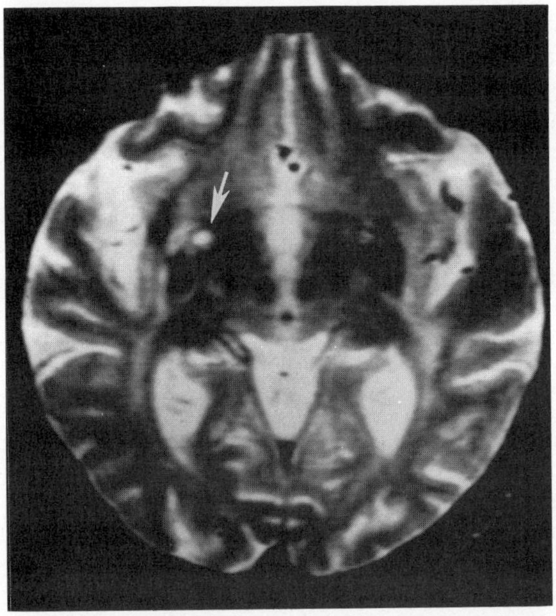

A

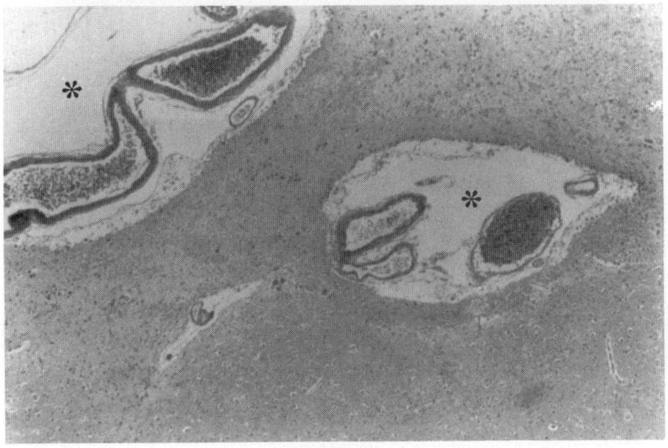

B

Figure 10-13
Dilated perivascular spaces (état criblé). **(A)** *Strongly T2-weighted (long TR, long TE) MRI section demonstrating a large dilated perivascular space in a characteristic location: adjacent to the anterior commissure and globus pallidus (arrow).* **(B)** *Histopathologic section demonstrating état criblé, with separation of the pia-arachnoid from tortuous vessels, resulting in small CSF pockets (asterisks). (From Braffman et al.[41] Used by permission.)*

elderly are the result of chronic vascular insufficiency or frank infarction.

Fazekas et al performed postmortem examinations on the brains of six patients without clinically significant dementia or cerebrovascular disease who had demonstrated incidental white matter hyperintensities on antemortem MRI scans.[44] Magnetic resonance imaging scans were also performed on the formalin-fixed brains before sectioning to assess fixation-induced signal changes, document any agonal alterations, and optimize lesion identification. White matter signal changes were more conspicuous on the premortem scans. Visual inspection of the brain slices revealed an abnormality in only one instance. Histologic examination revealed areas of reduced myelination with thinning of the neuropil around fibrohyalinotic arteries. Perivenous damage was also seen, ranging from spongiform change and scattered demyelinated foci to large perivenous areas with marked rarefaction of myelinated fibers. Fazekas therefore speculated that minor perivascular ischemic damage, but not completed infarction, is the most likely pathologic substrate of WMHs in elderly brains.

Several other autopsy-MRI correlative studies have demonstrated similar findings,[45–47] leading Munoz and colleagues to conclude that the more extensive, confluent (greater than 10 mm) areas of WMH were due to ischemic demyelination and rarefaction of the neuropil, while punctate high-signal lesions were less well defined pathologically, probably representating dilated Virchow-Robin spaces in many instances.[43]

In a study of the CT equivalent of WMH, periventricular white matter lucencies, or leukoaraiosis, (from the Greek, meaning "white matter rarefaction"), Leys et al presented the interesting speculation that these white matter changes may be due to wallerian degeneration.[48] Leukoaraiosis was more prominent in posterior periventricular areas in AD patients and in anterior periventricular zones in patients with Parkinson disease and progressive supranuclear palsy. Two of their AD patients went to autopsy. Areas of white matter lucency demonstrated pallor on myelin stains and mild fibrillary astrocytosis without infarction or hypertensive vascular changes. White matter degeneration was more severe in areas adjacent to cortical regions with the greatest density of neurofibrillary tangles. Leys therefore proposed wallerian degeneration as perhaps another cause of white matter pathology in neurodegenerative disorders associated with brain aging.

Our early investigation of white matter signal abnormalities in normal aging and dementia utilized a ranking scale with 0 for no abnormality, 1 for mild "caps" of high signal at the ventricular apices or punctate hyperintensities in the subcortical white matter, 2 for early confluent high-signal lesions, and 3 for extensive PVHs or deep WMHs.[30] Evidence is now accruing to support the existence of specific underlying pathologic conditions for these changes, although further work still needs to be done. Mild periventricular capping may be explained on the basis of either a mild local myelin rarefaction, ependymal breakdown (ependymitis granularis) with CSF transudation, or centripetal drainage toward the ventricle of increased interstitial fluid (presumably associated with gliosis or other senescent changes in the neuropil). Wong et al have used the technique of magnetization transfer imaging to support the contention that periventricular WMH in the elderly is due to edema and increased intracellular water in reactive astrocytes.[49] In their study of 21 elderly patients with periventricular WMH and 11 control subjects, the periventricular WMH magnetization transfer ratios were much higher than those of demyelinating lesions but similar to those of experimental lesions with only edema. Punctate subcortical hyperintensities may be due to dilated perivascular spaces or small areas of ischemic demyelination and neuropil rarefaction. The more extensive white matter lesions are seen most often at higher ventricular levels that correspond to the distal fields of attenuated medullary arteries. Because of the relative inability of white matter to autoregulate cerebral blood flow (CBF) incomplete infarction with demyelination and gliosis ensues.

Emission Tomography and Normal Brain Aging

Controversy over alterations in CBF and metabolism with normal aging have centered, not on distinguishing normal subjects from demented patients, but on determining whether normal aging is associated with any global or regional physiologic changes. This debate appears to derive from the distinction between usual aging (a neurologically asymptomatic state allowing minor neurologic signs commonly seen in other individuals of the same age) and successful aging (characterized by exceptional physiology differing little from that of younger individuals).[50] Most of the studies contending that brain metabolism in older normal subjects is similar to that seen in younger subjects emanate from the National Institutes of Health or National Institute of Aging. These research institutions have traditionally selected "supernormal" volunteers for their investigations of brain aging. Using the somewhat invasive but pioneering technique of Kety and Schmidt[51] to measure global cerebral blood flow and metabolism, Dastur reported no difference in global CBF or oxygen metabolism ($CMRO_2$) in normal elderly men (mean age 71) compared with young men (mean age 21).[52] A significant 23 percent reduction in glucose metabolism (CMRgl) was noted in the older men, however, suggesting that aging may produce changes in cerebral metabolism, leading to a reduction in CMRgl, with no associated changes in CBF or $CMRO_2$. Approximately 20 years later, using PET technology, Frackowiak et al found a decline in CBF with aging but no such decline in $CMRO_2$.[53] As with early ischemia, the ability of the brain to extract oxygen from the blood (measured as the oxygen extraction fraction) may rise in a compensatory fashion with age so that $CMRO_2$ is maintained at a constant level.

Duara and coinvestigators performed PET scans of regional cerebral glucose metabolism (rCMRgl) in another cohort of NIH supernormal subjects.[54] These scans were performed with the volunteers at rest, eyes covered, and ears plugged (i.e., a relatively sensory-deprived state). Mean hemispheric and regional cerebral metabolic rates for glucose did not decline significantly with advancing age. When these results were analyzed to look at intercorrelations of metabolic rates among brain regions, however, there was a significant loss of integration among parietal and frontal regions.[55]

In an attempt to address the issue of usual versus successful aging, we examined rCMRgl in healthy individuals ranging in age from 18 to 83 measured by FDG PET scans,[56] breaking down the older normal subjects into three groups: those with no medical diseases (successful supernormal subjects), those with minor noncardiovascular diseases (e.g., mild anemia, inactive peptic ulcer disease, or degenerative arthritis), and those with mild cardiovascular disease or risk factors (e.g., controlled hypertension on medications, asymptomatic bundle branch block or other mild electrocardiographic abnormality, or asymptomatic reduction of distal leg pulses). These PET studies were performed with the subjects' eyes open and ears unoccluded in a dimly lit, quiet room. Older volunteers demonstrated a 17 percent reduction in frontal lobe metabolism compared with younger subjects (Fig. 10-14). With rCMRgl values normalized to reduce intersubject variability in absolute metabolic rates, significant relative metabolic decrements were seen in inferior parietal, left superior temporal, and primary sensorimotor areas. No significant differences were seen in rCMRgl values among the three older groups, suggesting that aging is associated with declines in rCMRgl independent of atherosclerotic and other systemic health factors.

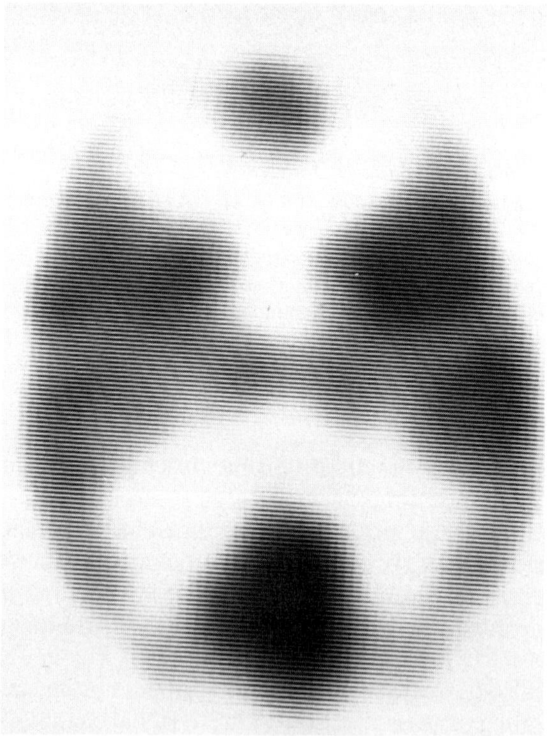

Figure 10-14
FDG PET scan of a neurologically normal 70-year-old man. A pattern of bilateral frontal hypometabolism is occasionally seen in the normal aged population.

In an early FDG PET study of 40 normal volunteers ranging in age from 18 to 78 years, Kuhl et al found a gradual decrease in mean CMRgl with age.[57] Scans were also performed with the subjects' eyes open and ears unoccluded. Superior frontal and posterior inferior frontal regions showed the most rapid decline in CMRgl with age. Yoshii and colleagues also found a decline in rCMRgl with aging, especially in frontal, temporal, and parietal areas.[58] In their cohort of 76 normal subjects, 58 also underwent MRI scanning. It is not surprising that there was a strong relationship between age and brain atrophy. When the effects of brain atrophy were factored out by covariate analysis, age (and gender) no longer had a significant influence upon rCMRgl. We and others have questioned the effects of cerebral atrophy and partial volume averaging on findings in emission tomography studies of brain aging.[59–61] In the only investigation of focal atrophy in PET examinations of older patients and normal volunteers, we found very little frontal lobe atrophy in older normal subjects.[61] If generalized, this suggests that any frontal hypometabolism seen on PET scans of older normal subjects (see Fig. 10-14) is likely to reflect a true decrement in tissue metabolic rate, not a partial volume-averaging artifact of atrophy.

Positron emission tomographic scanning has limitations not shared by CT and MRI, which have impeded its clinical utility. These limitations include equipment and supply expense, relatively high radiation exposure, lower spatial resolution, and complexity of quantitative data analyses. The dynamic, physiologic nature of emission tomography also leads to difficulties with data analysis and comparisons across studies. For example, conflicting results in normal aging investigations (hypofrontality with aging versus no change) could be due to methodologic issues, including the subject's state (sensory deprived or not). The individual's overall health status, "normal" old person or "supernormal," also appears to play a role. Based on PET results to date, it appears safe to conclude that regional metabolic interactions, especially between parietal and frontal association areas, become less tightly linked with normal aging. An actual decline in frontal metabolism is probably a feature of usual aging, corresponding to deterioration of frontal lobe executive functions with age.[62]

ABNORMAL BRAIN AGING: THE NEUROIMAGING OF DEMENTIA

It has become almost a cliché to cite the main value of CT (and now MRI) scanning in the evaluation of patients with dementia: to exclude treatable structural disease. The greater sensitivity of MRI to essentially all disease processes, including infarction, makes it the anatomic imaging procedure of choice in the evaluation of cognitive decline (Figs. 10-15 and 10-16).

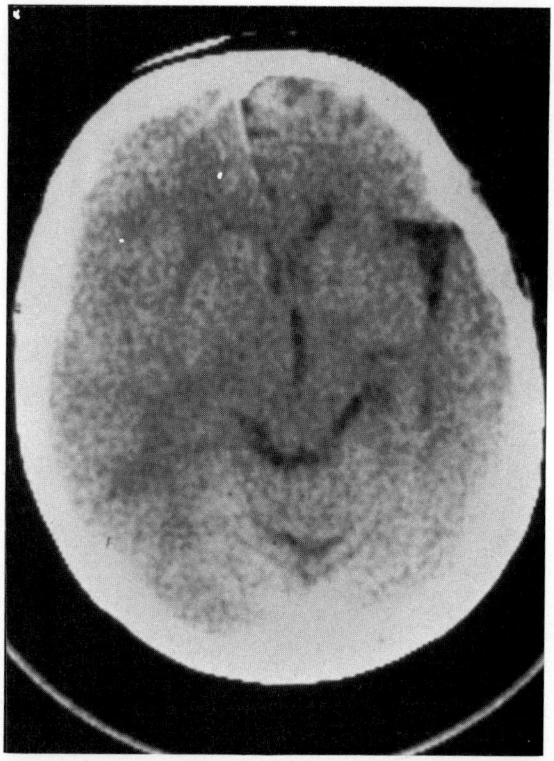

A

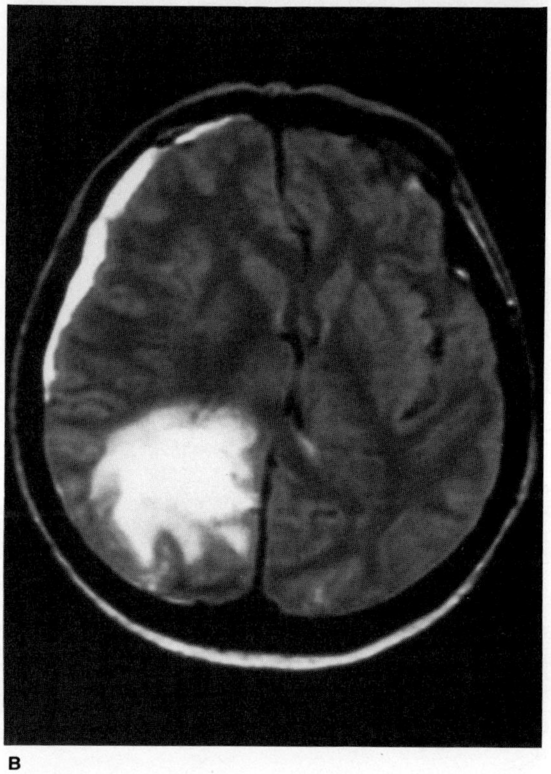

B

Figure 10-15

An 83-year-old patient with mild dementia. **(A)** *CT scan demonstrates right-hemisphere mass effect. The underlying disease process is not evident.* **(B)** *Intermediate-weighted MRI scan shows a subacute posterior parenchymal hemorrhage and associated subdural hematoma, possibly due to amyloid angiopathy (no history of trauma was obtained).*

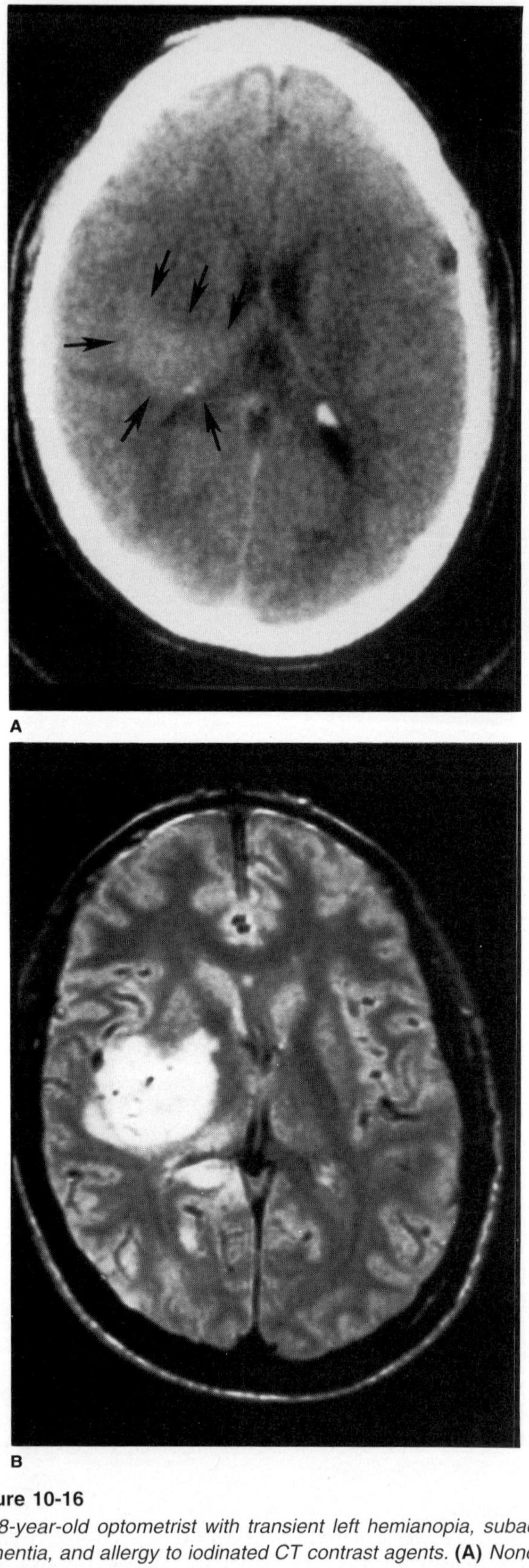

Figure 10-16
A 48-year-old optometrist with transient left hemianopia, subacute dementia, and allergy to iodinated CT contrast agents. **(A)** *Noncontrast CT scan, officially interpreted as normal, demonstrates a subtle, high-density lesion in the deep structures of the right hemisphere (arrows).* **(B)** *The lesion (biopsy-proven glioblastoma multiforme) is flagrantly obvious on the unenhanced intermediate-weighted MRI scan.*

Some might dispute the cost-effectiveness of MRI in dementia workups, given the good ability of CT to demonstrate ischemic stroke, hemorrhage (including subdural hematoma), tumor, hydrocephalus, and other cerebral lesions. These conditions are discussed in detail in their respective chapters (Chaps. 2, 11, 12, and 15). Since reimbursement for MRI continues to decline and regulation of access to medical technology is increasing, the cost issue will become less a factor, and MRI will become the standard imaging technology in routine dementia evaluations. Thus, the discussion of CT scanning in dementing illnesses is brief, and the more current technologies of MRI, PET, and SPECT are emphasized.

Computed Tomographic Scanning and Dementia

The advent of CT scanning in the early 1970s permitted, for the first time, the *noninvasive* visualization of several pathologic processes that could lead to dementia, including subdural hematoma, cerebral infarction, tumors, and hydrocephalus (Figs. 10-15 and 10-16). Erkinjuntti et al combined CT analysis with clinical data in a study of vascular dementia and were able to make this diagnosis with an accuracy of 85 percent.[63] The precise value of CT in the diagnosis of primary degenerative dementia has been less evident, since cerebral atrophy is also part of the normal aging process. The section on "Computed Tomographic Scanning and Normal Brain Aging" discussed several recent studies supporting the value of CT in distinguishing AD from normal aging based on the presence or absence of temporal lobe atrophy.[22–25] As with the imaging of parenchymal disease, MRI is superior to CT in demonstrating loss of temporal lobe brain tissue. Although CT can demonstrate white matter changes with aging (white matter lucencies, or leukoaraiosis), these changes are much more conspicuously and sensitively demonstrated on MRIs (WMHs). At least one study contends that such sensitivity may not always be a clinical advantage. Lopez and colleagues performed a longitudinal evaluation of 27 patients with probable AD for whom both CT and MRI scans had been obtained at baseline.[64] As expected, WMHs were seen more often on MRI (78 percent of patients) than on CT (44 percent of patients). There was no correlation between WMH severity and the presence of abnormal neurologic signs. However, there was a greater frequency of WMH shown on CT scans than on MRI scans at baseline in patients in whom abnormal neurologic signs developed at 12 month follow-up. This finding suggests that CT may be more specific in predicting subsequent symptomatic cerebrovascular disease in AD patients, although MRI appears to be more sensitive in detecting WMHs.

Alzheimer Disease

Magnetic Resonance Imaging and Alzheimer Disease

Routine MRI studies easily demonstrate atrophy of the mesial temporal structures that bear the brunt of Alzheimer-type degenerative changes.[65] Kesslak et al quantified hippocampal and parahippocampal atrophy in 8 patients with probable AD and 7 age-matched controls.[66] AD patients demonstrated an approximately 40 percent volume reduction in the parahippocampal gyrus, and 50 percent reduction in hippocampal volume (Fig. 10-17). There was a high correlation (0.90) between atrophy of these structures and a brief assessment of general cognitive functioning, the Mini-Mental State Examination.[67] Using a relatively simple subjective grading system, Barclay and coworkers found medial temporal atrophy (MTA) to be a specific indicator of Alzheimer dementia.[68] They studied patients with the clinical diagnosis of mixed Alzheimer and multi-infarct dementia (MID) as well. Not unexpectedly, these individuals exhibited *both* MTA *and* ischemic changes on their MRI scans. Scheltens et al, using a similar subjective ranking system for MTA, were also able to distinguish AD patients from age-matched controls.[69] These assessments were more sensitive than specific in their patient cohort, which included older subjects than in Kesslak's or Barclay's series. There was also a significant correlation between objective linear measures of MTA and the visual ranking determinations, validating the subjective appraisals. In patients with AD, the degree of MTA reflected the severity of memory loss as well as overall cognitive deterioration. Scheltens and colleagues appropriately concluded that the presence of MTA, assessed by simple visual inspection of routine MRI scans, strongly supports the clinical diagnosis of AD, especially in individuals under age 75.

Frisoni et al examined the sensitivity of simple linear measurements of frontotemporal atrophy in diagnosing mild AD.[70] Their study population included 31 control subjects, 33 patients with mild AD, and 13 patients with moderately severe AD. Simple linear measurements of hippocampal atrophy alone could discriminate patients with mild AD from control subjects with 83 percent sensitivity and patients with moderate AD from control subjects with 87 percent sensitivity. These findings suggest that linear measurements of hippocampal atrophy can assist in the diagnosis of AD, even in early stages. Jack and coinvestigators arrived at a similar conclusion in a larger study cohort (126 normal control subjects and 94 patients with probable AD), utilizing a volumetric measurement of MTA.[71] At a fixed specificity of 90 percent, the sensitivity of hippocampal volumetric measurements in discriminating control subjects from patients was 72.2 percent for very mild AD and 81.4 percent for mild AD.

An even more intriguing question is whether temporal lobe atrophy revealed by MRI can identify subjects *at risk* for developing AD. In a longitudinal volumetric MRI study of asymptomatic individuals at risk for autosomal dominant familial AD ($n = 7$), Fox and coworkers observed the development of asymmetric hippocampal atrophy *before* the appearance of symptoms in the three at-risk subjects who became symptomatic.[72] Verbal and visual memory measurements declined in parallel with hippocampal loss. A decline of 8 percent per year in hippocampal volume occurred in the 2-year period during which symptoms first appeared. Convit et al, also using temporal lobe volumetric measurements, examined 27 normal elderly individuals, 22 subjects with minimal cognitive impairment (MCI) but not meeting clinical criteria for the diagnosis of AD, and 27 AD patients.[73] Hippocampal volume separated MCI patients

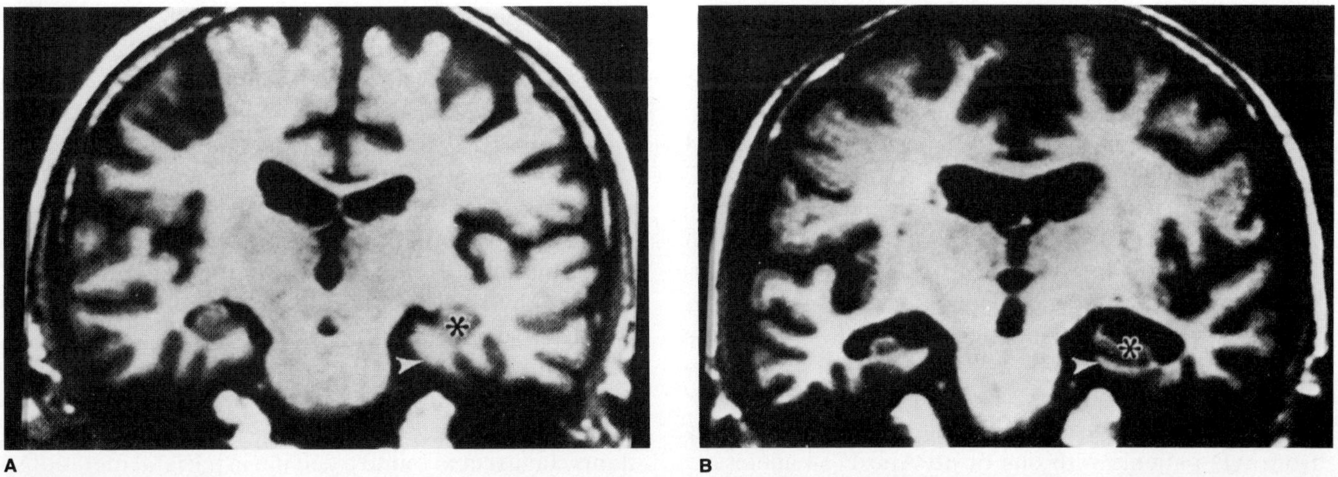

Figure 10-17

Coronal inversion recovery MRIs through the hippocampus (asterisk) and parahippocampal gyrus (arrowhead). **(A)** *Normal elderly control subject.* **(B)** *Marked hippocampal and parahippocampal gyrus atrophy in a patient with moderate severity AD. Note also the diffuse cortical atrophy. (From Kesslak et al.[66] Used by permission.)*

from normal control subjects with a sensitivity of 74 percent. In a combined cohort of normal and MCI subjects, hippocampal volume was the only measurement that correlated with delayed recall memory. Comparing MCI individuals with AD patients, the fusiform gyrus volume (a lateral temporal lobe structure) uniquely improved the ability of the hippocampal volume to distinguish the two groups from 74 to 80 percent. It would therefore appear that, once cognitive function has declined to the point where a clinical diagnosis of AD may be made, not only is the medial temporal lobe atrophic, but lateral temporal structures (specifically the fusiform gyrus) are as well.

Kaye and colleagues similarly concluded that progressive atrophy of temporal association cortex (lateral temporal lobe), superimposed upon a critically atrophic hippocampus, leads to the development of clinical dementia in the "oldest old" (subjects over age 83).[74] Thirty nondemented healthy elderly individuals were compared to 12 initially healthy patients who subsequently exhibited cognitive decline. Both groups suffered progressive hippocampal and parahippocampal atrophy over time, with similar rates of tissue loss. The cognitively impaired patients had significantly smaller hippocampi *when asymptomatic,* however. Significant time-dependent atrophy of the entire temporal lobe was seen only in the cognitively impaired subjects. In this study, time-dependent temporal lobe atrophy was estimated to begin approximately 6 years before the onset of clinically apparent dementia.

A biochemical process essential to the pathophysiology of AD is intracerebral β-amyloid deposition.[75] It might be expected, therefore, that indices of β-amyloid deposition (e.g., reduced CSF βA4 levels) would correlate with measurements of temporal lobe atrophy. In 23 AD patients, Schroder et al found a significant correlation between reduced CSF βA4 levels and temporal lobe volume, but not with any other MRI volumetric measurements.[76] One may therefore hypothesize that cerebral βA4 accumulation contributes to temporal lobe atrophy in AD, supporting the theory that β-amyloid deposition is crucial for the development of AD.

From a molecular genetic perspective, the epsilon 4 allele of apolipoprotein E (Apo E ε4) is a strong risk factor for late-onset AD.[77] In a volumetric MRI study, Lehtovirta and coinvestigators found that patients with AD homozygous for Apo E ε4 had severe MTA compared to heterozygotes or patients without the Apo E ε4 allele.[78] They therefore concluded that AD patients homozygous for the Apo E ε4 allele exhibit severe medial temporal lobe damage early in the disease process and differ pathophysiologically and pathoanatomically from AD patients with one or no Apo E ε4 alleles.

Magnetic resonance imaging studies of AD patients demonstrate not only cerebral atrophy but also the same WMHs seen in the normal aged population. The distinction of AD from normal aging or MID on the basis of white matter signal changes is discussed below (see "Vascular Dementia").

Positron Emission Tomography and Alzheimer Disease

Our earliest investigations of regional cerebral glucose metabolism (rCMRgl) in AD found metabolic rates in dementia patients to be 20 to 30 percent below those of normal elderly control subjects, with the most striking metabolic decrements seen in the frontal lobes.[79] Other PET studies from the early 1980s failed to demonstrate consistent metabolic rate reductions, except in the most severely demented patients.[80–82] A number of factors hindered these first PET assessments of cerebral metabolism in dementia, including low spatial resolution and signal-to-noise capabilities of the scanners at that time, less than stringent subject selection criteria, and data analysis schemes that lacked the sophistication to extract maximal information from this complex technology. For example, the large variance in absolute metabolic rates seen in control subjects as well as demented patients tends to obscure significant regional differences that are evident on visual scan inspection. Using normalization ratios of regional metabolism to the same subject's average whole-brain metabolic rate, or to the metabolic rate of a brain area typically less involved histopathologically (e.g., primary visual or sensorimotor cortex), more reliable metabolic observations can be made with PET. This approach has led to the important and reproducible observation of bilateral temporoparietal regional metabolic deficits in mild to moderate AD[83–88] (Fig. 10-18). Asymmetric reductions of temporoparietal CMRgl are also seen in AD. Some investigators report a preferential susceptibility of left-hemisphere regions when such asymmetries are found,[89,90] while others report no hemispheric preference.[91,92] Hypometabolism in frontal association areas is seen in more severely demented patients.[83,85,87,93–95] In their final stages, AD patients have widespread metabolic defects, with relatively preserved glycolytic activity in the deep nuclei, sensorimotor cortices, and primary visual areas of the brain (Fig. 10-19).

Yamaguchi et al evaluated 13 patients with probable AD using MRI and FDG-PET, to determine the relationship between hippocampal atrophy and rCMRgl.[96] They found a correlation between unilateral hippocampal atrophy and ipsilateral decreased temporoparietal rCMRgl, suggesting a possible functional relationship between the anatomic and physiologic abnormalities.

The PET technique has been used to evaluate the progression of metabolic deficits over time in AD patients. Jagust et al found a decline in parietal metabolism in 5 of 6 AD patients studied over a 1- to 2-year period.[97] The sixth patient, who was more severely demented, developed frontal hypometabolism during that time in-

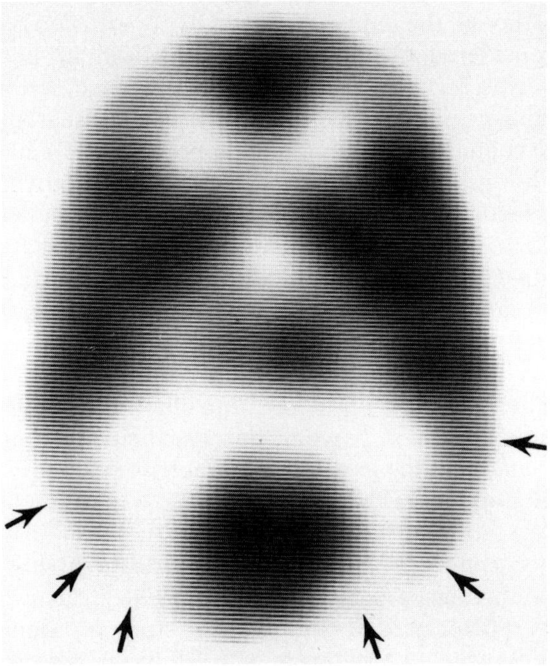

Figure 10-18
FDG PET section demonstrating the typical pattern of bilateral temporoparietal hypometabolism (arrows) seen in mild to moderate AD.

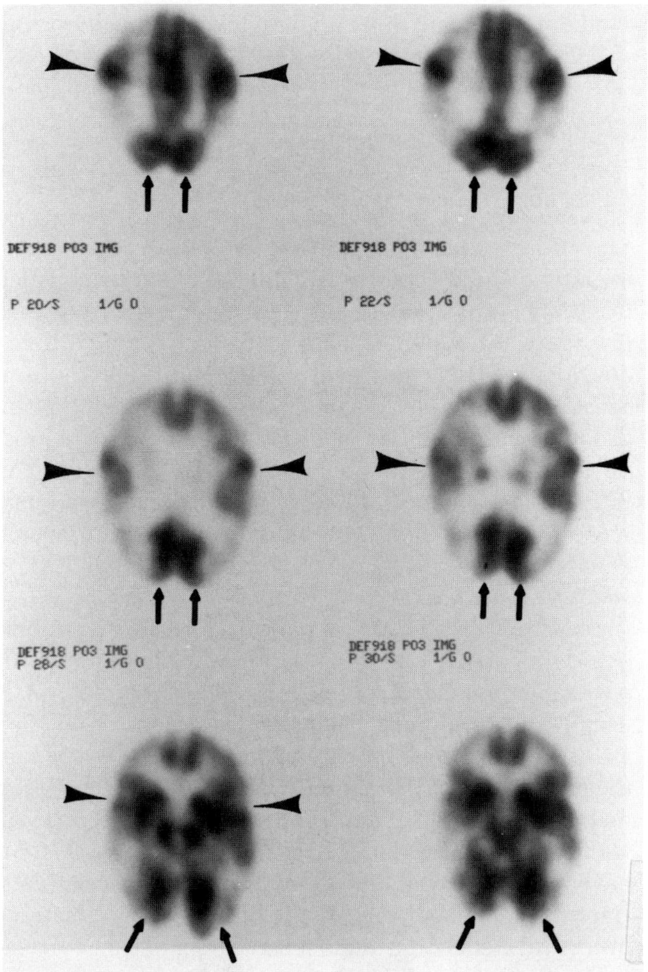

Figure 10-19
FDG PET scan of a patient with severe AD. Note the preserved metabolic activity in the visual cortex (arrows) and primary sensorimotor areas (arrowheads).

terval. A man with familial AD also showed progressive decreases in parietal CMRgl on three PET scans performed at 8-month intervals.[98]

The value of PET imaging in the evaluation of degenerative dementia would lie, it is hoped, in its ability to demonstrate *physiologic* alterations in the brain before *structural* damage is seen on MRI or CT scans. Haxby and associates performed PET scans of rCMRgl in five subjects with mild memory deficits but no apparent difficulties on a battery of language and visuospatial tests.[92] Despite the absence of neocortically mediated cognitive dysfunction, these individuals demonstrated reductions in rCMRgl in parietal association areas and left-right metabolic asymmetries similar to those seen in AD patients with more typical diffuse cognitive impairments. Haxby therefore concluded that physiologic dysfunction may be seen in neocortical association areas before neuropsychologic impairments are evident. Small and colleagues measured rCMRgl in nondemented relatives at risk for familial AD (12 with the Apo E ε4 allele and 19 without the allele).[99] Parietal metabolism was significantly lower and left-right parietal asymmetry significantly higher in at-risk subjects with Apo E ε4 compared to those without the allele. Patients with clinical AD had significantly lower parietal metabolism than did at-risk subjects with Apo E ε4. Polinsky et al similarly found that an asymptomatic individual at risk for familial AD displayed reduced rCMRgl in the left supramarginal gyrus.[100] On the other hand, Cutler and colleagues found memory impairments in a 57-year-old man whose first PET scan of CMRgl was normal but who manifested bilateral parietal lobe hypometabolism on a scan performed about 12 months later.[98] Luxenberg et al evaluated neuropsychologic function and CMRgl in the identical twin of a patient with probable AD.[101] They found abnormalities of visuoperceptual organization and verbal memory in the "unaffected" twin, despite normal global and regional cerebral glucose metabolism. Both PET and careful neuropsychologic assessments have the potential to detect AD at early stages. Discrepancies in the above-mentioned studies are, at least in part, due to the sensitivities of the psychometric batteries and technical characteristics of the PET scanners utilized (spatial resolution, signal-to-noise, data processing, etc.). Tomographic imaging and neuropsychologic testing are complementary in the study of cognitively impaired individuals, as emphasized in Chap. 8. Positron emission tomography does not yet appear to have the power to detect at-risk but definitely asymptomatic AD candidates with anything approaching its sensitivity and specificity in the investigation of Huntington disease (see Chap. 1).

Single Photon Emission Computed Tomography and Alzheimer Disease

The wider availability and relatively low cost of performing SPECT (compared with PET) studies has led to greater utilization of this technology over the past few years. Although SPECT tracers have not yet been developed that can measure cerebral metabolism, SPECT imaging of CBF indirectly reflects metabolism, given the tight coupling of CBF and metabolism in most physiologic and pathologic states. Improvements in SPECT instrumentation now permit routine clinical scans with an in-plane resolution of 6 to 9 mm, which equals that of PET scanners used in the mid- to late 1980s!

As with PET, the typical pattern of regional cerebral blood flow (rCBF) in AD is hypoperfusion of temporoparietal areas. This hypoperfusion may be unilateral, is usually bilateral, and is often asymmetric[102,103] (Fig. 10-20). Frontal hypoperfusion is occasionally seen in the more severely demented AD patients, matching the metabolic pattern seen in PET studies of dementia. As with PET studies of rCMRgl, SPECT scans of rCBF have been correlated with neuropsychologic deficits. Bartenstein and colleagues noted that rCBF reductions in cortical association areas showed a significant correlation with the overall level of cognitive decline.[104] Moreover, region-specific correlations were noted between left temporal hypoperfusion and aphasia, as well as right parietal rCBF decline and constructional apraxia.

Although the temporoparietal hypoperfusion pattern is considered characteristic of AD, similar bilateral posterior cortical defects have also been described in Parkinson disease,[105,106] cerebrovascular disease,[107] hypoglycemia,[108] carbon monoxide poisoning,[108] and rarer conditions (e.g., mitochondrial encephalomyopathy with lactic acidosis and strokelike episodes, also known as MELAS syndrome).[109] The sensitivity, specificity, and positive predictive value of SPECT in AD was examined systematically by Masterman and co-investigators.[110] They found that a pattern of temporoparietal hypoperfusion was seen in most patients with AD but could also be found in other dementing illnesses. The SPECT sensitivity was 75 percent, but specificity was only 52 percent, resulting in a positive predictive value (in their clinic population) of 78 percent.

Two studies have shown that the flow patterns demonstrated by SPECT scan correlate highly with the metabolic patterns revealed by PET.[111,112] Kuwabara et al performed a comparative study in dementia patients with two different SPECT blood flow tracers (^{123}I-IMP and ^{99m}Tc-HMPAO), $H_2{}^{15}O$ PET measurements of CBF, and CMRgl measured by PET and 18F-FDG.[111] The CBF determined by both SPECT blood flow tracers correlated significantly with PET CBF measurements. Both SPECT agents overestimated low-count areas and underestimated high-count areas compared with PET. The SPECT studies also showed diminished parietal lobe–motor cortex and frontal lobe–motor cortex contrast in AD and Pick disease patients compared with PET. Studies with SPECT did not perform as well as did PET studies in detecting mildly affected brain regions. Gemmell and colleagues found a high correlation ($r = 0.81$)

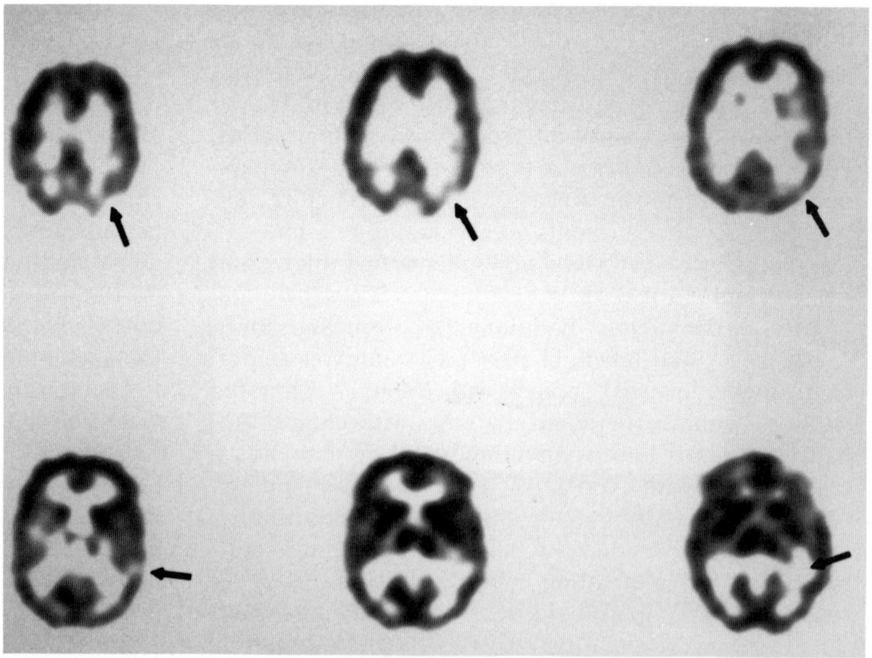

Figure 10-20
HMPAO SPECT scan shows the typical AD pattern of bilateral temporoparietal hypoperfusion, somewhat greater on the left (arrows).

between HMPAO SPECT and ^{15}O PET in normalized quantitative measurements of rCBF.[112]

The ability of SPECT scans to distinguish AD patients from age-matched control subjects has been demonstrated by a number of research groups.[102,113–117] In general, the accuracy of SPECT in making this distinction ranges from 80 to 90 percent. Testa and associates found an 85 percent sensitivity and 85 percent specificity in distinguishing AD patients from patients with "frontal lobe dementia" and progressive supranuclear palsy.[118]

As with PET, a key question is the ability of SPECT to detect pathophysiologic changes in AD before abnormalities are seen clinically or on anatomic scans. Holman et al found that patients with memory loss and a normal SPECT scan had a 19 percent chance of having more widespread cognitive deficits indicating full-blown AD.[119] Patients with memory loss and bilateral temporoparietal perfusion deficits (the "typical" AD pattern), however, had an 82 percent probability of exhibiting full-blown AD. The probability of AD was 57 percent with unilateral temporoparietal defects, 43 percent with frontal defects only, and 18 percent with other large perfusion defects. Patients with memory loss and multiple small cortical defects were never found to have AD.

The relatively low radiation exposure from technetium compounds permits serial studies using SPECT and HMPAO, facilitating the monitoring of drug efficacy in the treatment of AD. Agnoli and colleagues used HMPAO SPECT to assess the response of AD patients to the administration of the selective monoamine oxidase type B inhibitor L-deprenyl.[120] The SPECT measurements of CBF were performed at baseline and after a 60-day trial of L-deprenyl or placebo. Patients who received L-deprenyl and whose cognitive function improved exhibited no changes in rCBF at 60 days compared with baseline. Patients receiving placebo who demonstrated diminished cognitive function also showed a reduction in parietal lobe CBF compared with their baseline cerebral perfusion.

A receptor agent, [^{123}I]3-quinuclidinyl-4-iodobenzilate (IQNB), has been used to study muscarinic receptor activity in aging and AD. Earlier investigations demonstrated a positive correlation between FDG PET and IQNB SPECT in dementia patients, suggesting that IQNB uptake may be strongly related to cerebral blood flow or metabolism, obfuscating the biologic significance of any receptor binding.[121,122] Weinberger and associates recently found only a minimal correlation between rCMRgl and IQNB uptake.[123] In their series, AD patients generally showed larger defects on IQNB SPECT scans than on FDG PET images. A recent study by Kuhl et al used a different SPECT tracer, [^{123}I]iodobenzovesamicol (IBVM), an in vivo marker of the vesicular acetylcholine transporter.[124] FDG-PET was coregistered for metabolic assessment, and MRI was coregistered for atrophy assessment. Cortical IBVM binding correlated inversely with dementia severity in their AD patients. Differences in IBVM binding patterns were seen with early-onset AD patients, late-onset AD patients, and Parkinson disease (PD) patients without dementia. PD patients with dementia had an IBVM binding pattern similar to that of the early-onset AD group. The relative reduction of IBVM binding in affected brain areas was about 30 percent. This indicates that in vivo cholinergic neuronal integrity (assessed by IBVM-SPECT) is not as severely affected as suggested by postmortem measurements of choline acetyltransferase activity (50 to 80 percent).[125,126]

Vascular Dementia

Anatomic Imaging in Vascular Dementia

The autopsy studies of Tomlinson, Blessed, and Roth over a quarter of a century ago suggested that the pathogenesis of multi-infarct dementia (MID) depended largely upon the aggregate volume of infarcted brain tissue.[14] Subsequent reports from the burgeoning CT literature refined our concept of the pathoanatomic correlates of MID diagnosed clinically with the assistance of the Hachinski ischemia scale.[127,128] This scale contains a number of items from a patient's medical history, such as hypertension and history of antecedent stroke, that have been correlated on postmortem examination with the presence of vascular lesions in the brains of demented subjects. Further autopsy studies indicate that patients classified as having AD on the basis of the Hachinski scale are diagnosed correctly 80 to 90 percent of the time.[129,130] The specificity of a clinical diagnosis of MID using the Hachinski scale is considerably lower, however. When the appropriate clinical cutoff is applied, postmortem examination reveals "pure" MID only 25 percent of the time.[130] More commonly, a mixed AD-MID picture is demonstrated.

The CT findings supporting the clinical diagnosis of MID include multiple supratentorial infarctions with a volume of infarcted tissue of at least 50 mL;[14,131] bilateral supratentorial infarctions, especially when involving the thalamus or basal ganglia;[131,132] and diffuse or focal periventricular white matter lucencies with dilatation of the lateral ventricles, suggesting subcortical arteriosclerotic encephalopathy, or Binswanger disease (BD).[133,134] With the realization that MRI demonstrates cerebral ischemic damage much more sensitively than does CT, a new era in the investigation of vascular dementia was born.

Our initial MRI study of white matter abnormalities in AD patients, MID patients, and healthy elderly control subjects found that patients and control subjects could, for the most part, be distinguished on the basis of white matter signal changes.[30] Fifty percent of AD patients had a relatively prominent halo of periventricular hyperintensity (PVH; Fig. 10-21) compared with control subjects, who tended to have either no PVH, very

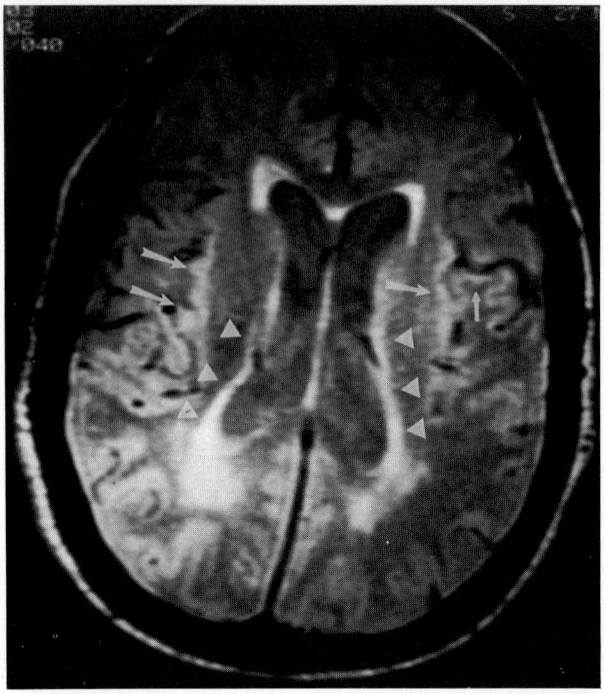

Figure 10-21
A 70-year-old man with mild AD. Note the periventricular "halo" (arrowheads) and bilateral insular cortex hyperintensity (arrows).

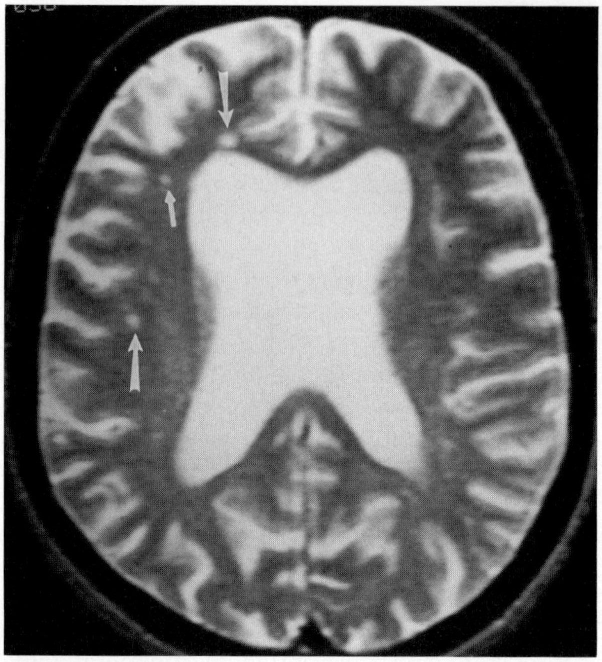

Figure 10-22
Small areas of subcortical hyperintensity (arrows) in a 65-year-old woman with mild AD. Note the ventricular enlargement and mild sulcal prominence. These findings would not be unusual in a normal subject over age 80.

thin rims, or apical "caps" of PVH (see Fig. 10-12). Control subjects and AD patients frequently demonstrated small, or punctate, high-signal changes in the subcortical white matter (Fig. 10-22). In contrast to both control subjects and AD patients, 75 percent of those with clinically diagnosed MID demonstrated more prominent, irregular PVH extending into the deep white matter, or larger confluent subcortical hyperintense lesions (Fig. 10-23). It is not surprising to note that classical infarcts were seen in the MID group but not in the AD cohort. Areas of cortical hyperintensity were seen in both AD and MID patients.

Earlier studies such as ours brought into sharper focus several important questions concerning MRI and CT in the study of normal brain aging and dementia: (1) Does the presence of parenchymal abnormalities (especially in the white matter) on MRI or CT scans distinguish demented patients from control subjects? (2) Can vascular dementia (i.e., MID and BD) be distinguished from degenerative dementia (AD) on the basis of lesions seen on anatomic scans? (3) Does dementia severity correlate with the extent of tissue damage demonstrated by MRI or CT?

Our preliminary observation that PVH on MRI scans distinguishes AD from normal aging has been disputed. Duara, Bowen, and associates reported significant differences in periventricular and subcortical hyperintensity scores when AD patients were compared with age-matched control subjects.[135,136] Other investigators have failed to find a significant difference in the nature or extent of white matter lesions on MRI scans when AD was compared with normal aging.[35,137] Mantyla and coworkers suggest that some of the inconsistencies in MRI studies of WMHs are due to the differences in the visual rating scales.[138] Although there has been some speculation that the studies finding significant white matter lesions in AD have inappropriately included patients with clinically important vascular risk factors, a more reasonable explanation may be pathophysiologic differences between early-onset (presenile) and late-onset (senile) AD.[139,140] Scheltens et al, rating signal hyperintensities in periventricular zones (PVH), subcortical or "lobar" white matter (WMH), basal ganglia (BGH), and infratentorial region (IFTH), found that scores in the first three categories (PVH, WMH, and BGH) were significantly higher in late-onset AD patients than in control subjects.[140] This correlation was not seen in the early-onset AD group. The two AD groups were not distinguishable on the basis of cortical atrophy, leading Scheltens to conclude that early- and late-onset AD differ with respect to white matter pathology but not in the degree of gray matter involvement demonstrable on MRI scans.

The ability to discriminate AD from vascular dementia on the basis of MRI findings has also been questioned. Erkinjuntti and colleagues found both CT and MRI to be effective in making this distinction.[139] White matter abnormalities on MRI scans were seen in all of their patients with vascular dementia (29 patients) but

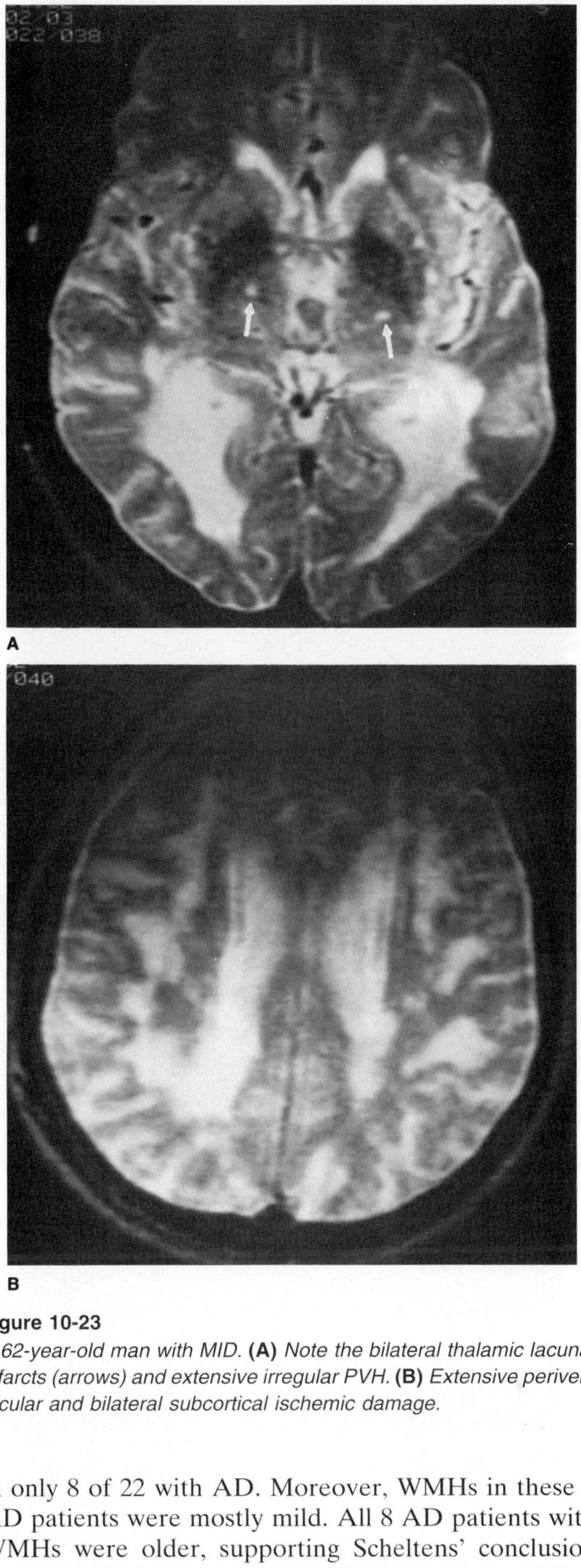

Figure 10-23
A 62-year-old man with MID. **(A)** *Note the bilateral thalamic lacunar infarcts (arrows) and extensive irregular PVH.* **(B)** *Extensive periventricular and bilateral subcortical ischemic damage.*

in only 8 of 22 with AD. Moreover, WMHs in these 8 AD patients were mostly mild. All 8 AD patients with WMHs were older, supporting Scheltens' conclusion that presenile and senile AD exhibit significant differences in white matter involvement.[140] Computed tomography was less sensitive but more specific in establishing a diagnosis of probable vascular dementia, with only 1 of 22 AD patients exhibiting white matter lucencies. Bowen et al considered periventricular, subcortical, and cortical lesions separately in their study of AD and MID.[136] The Hachinski ischemia score correlated significantly with all three categories of signal abnormality, most strongly with the extent of cortical damage, least strongly with the degree of periventricular high-signal change. The prevalence of PVH was similar in the two dementia groups (AD and MID), although PVH was more extensive in the MID patients. Subcortical high-signal lesions were significantly more prevalent and prominent in the vascular dementia patients. A more recent study by Barclay and associates[68] supports the observations of Bowen et al.

Brief clinical scales assessing dementia severity, such as the Mini Mental State Examination,[67] do not seem to correlate with the degree of white matter damage revealed by CT or MRI.[30,35,136,137,139] A number of investigators have correlated WMHs with cognitive dysfunction detected by more sophisticated neuropsychologic batteries, however.[141,142] This issue is discussed in depth in Chap. 8.

At this point we can reasonably attempt to summarize the relevance of the investigations reviewed above to routine scan interpretation in patients over age 50. The clinical neurologist is typically confronted with establishing a specific diagnosis after having determined (usually a straightforward proposition) that a nonmetabolic dementing illness is present. Assuming that treatable structural disease (e.g., subdural hematoma, tumor, or hydrocephalus) has been excluded, the following guidelines may be applied:

1. The presence of mild to moderate PVH on MRI scan may be seen in the normal elderly as well as in patients with AD or vascular dementia, and is therefore not usually a helpful finding.
2. Scattered small subcortical hyperintensities may be seen in normal subjects or dementia patients and are generally not a useful diagnostic observation.
3. In patients 65 years old or less, the presence of medial temporal lobe atrophy (MTA), especially in the absence of prominent parenchymal signal abnormality, strongly supports a diagnosis of AD.
4. Extensive subcortical (white matter or deep gray nuclei, but *not* periventricular) high-signal abnormality, in conjunction with a positive Hachinski ischemia score, suggests a diagnosis of MID.
5. The diagnosis of MID is also more likely if multiple cortical infarcts are seen or if the CT scan demonstrates prominent subcortical lucencies.
6. In patients over age 65, the presence of MTA does not necessarily indicate AD, nor does the presence of moderate WMH establish a diagnosis of vascular dementia.
7. After a diagnosis of vascular dementia is made based on clinical and scan criteria, the possibility of coexistent AD has not been eliminated.

Functional Imaging in Vascular Dementia

Several factors contribute to the limited number of reports describing PET findings in vascular dementia. In comparison with their AD counterparts, a greater proportion of MID patients are severely demented; therefore, relatively fewer MID patients are available who can cooperate during a lengthy and complicated PET scanning session. Until the mid-1980s, many researchers felt that a diagnosis of vascular dementia could be easily and reliably made based on anatomic scan findings and clinical criteria. The preceding section reviews the studies that serve to dispel that notion. Finally, with AD having become the "brain disease of the decade," 1980s investigators channeled their energies into basic AD research, and vascular dementia therefore received less attention.

One of the first reports of PET scanning in dementia examined CBF and oxygen metabolism with ^{15}O.[81] In this study Frackowiak and coworkers found predominantly parietal metabolic and perfusion defects in their MID patients; idiosyncratic patterns of hypometabolism and hypoperfusion reflected individual variation in infarct location. In 1983 (i.e., the pre-MRI era) Benson et al reported three cases of clinical MID with nondiagnostic CT scans but appropriate focal abnormalities on FDG PET images.[93] Kuhl's FDG-PET investigations suggest that MID differs from AD not only on the basis of multifocal metabolic defects (MIDs) versus bilateral temporoparietal hypometabolism (AD)[143] but also because of a significantly *higher* parietal-cerebellar rCMRgl ratio in the vascular dementias.[144] More recently, Duara and associates failed to find any significant differences in metabolic ratios between MID and AD patients on FDG PET scans.[135] They speculated that multiple subcortical vascular lesions may "deafferent" widespread cortical regions, leading to a more diffuse pattern of cerebral hypometabolism indistinguishable from that seen in more advanced stages of AD. This phenomenon of intracerebral deafferentation has been elegantly described in a CT-PET postmortem case report.[145]

Single photon emission tomographic scanning attained clinical research prominence at the same time that autopsy and anatomic imaging studies were emphasizing the difficulties in diagnosing vascular dementia.[130,135] Recent years have therefore seen a number of studies evaluating the role of SPECT in the differential diagnosis of dementia, especially in distinguishing MID from AD (Fig. 10-24). Since SPECT can theoretically detect areas of decreased CBF before abnormalities are seen on anatomic scans, SPECT may be an important clinical tool in diagnosing specific dementing disorders even in the face of normal or minimally abnormal MRIs. In addition, SPECT may be useful in determining if there is an underlying "AD pattern" in patients who also have MID, thus aiding the diagnosis of mixed degenerative-vascular dementia. The results of these studies, unfortunately, have been conflicting. Some investigators have found the sensitivity and specificity of SPECT in differentiating MID from AD to be as high

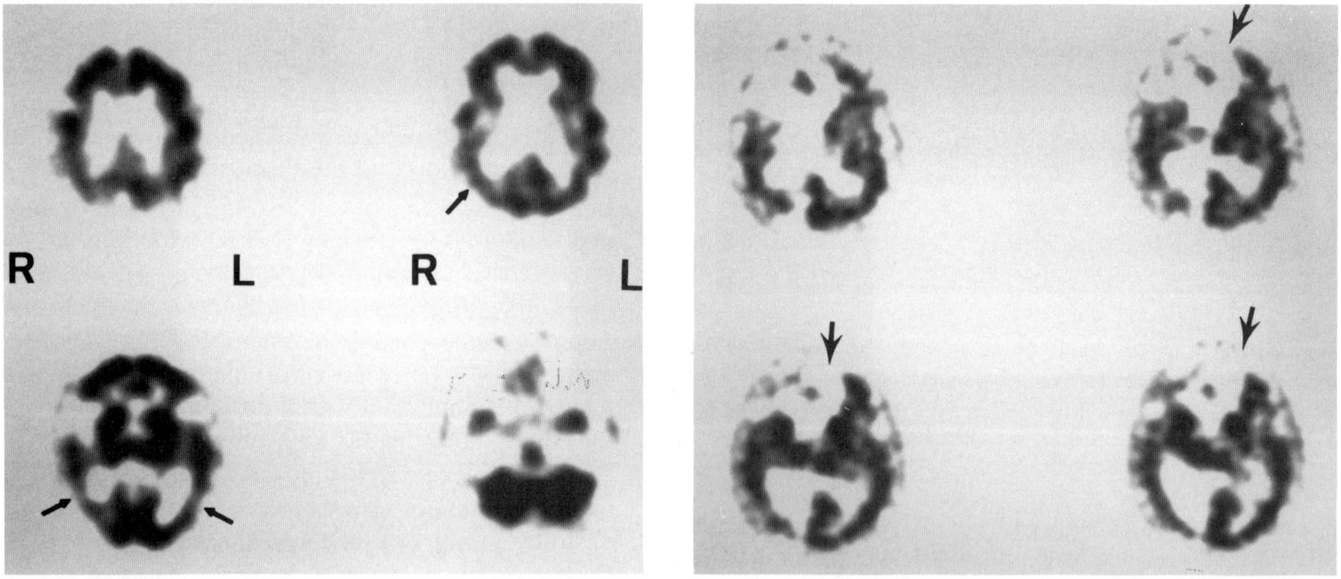

A B

Figure 10-24
HMPAO SPECT studies contrasting AD with MID. **(A)** *Patient with moderately severe AD shows bilateral temporoparietal hypoperfusion (arrows), greater on the right. Perisylvian atrophy is also greater on the right.* **(B)** *Patient with recurrent strokes and cognitive deterioration. SPECT scan shows marked perfusion deficits in the right frontal lobe and the right temporo-occipital region, and a lesser defect in the anterior left frontal lobe (arrows).*

as 80 percent.[146] Weinstein et al found that HMPAO SPECT was unable to differentiate AD from MID in a relatively small sample of 27 demented patients. Moreover there were no correlations between decreased tracer uptake and level of cognitive impairment.[147] Launes and associates studied 21 patients with psychiatric disorders (e.g., depression and anxiety) that may interfere with cognitive processes but who were not clinically demented.[107] Ten of the patients had one large or several small areas of hypoperfusion on HMPAO SPECT and were therefore classified as having MID, while three patients exhibited the "AD pattern" of bilateral temporoparietal hypoperfusion. Distinguishing MID and AD from various nondementing psychiatric disorders might not be possible using SPECT patterns of CBF.

Another form of vascular dementia, Binswanger disease (BD, also known as progressive subcortical arteriosclerotic encephalopathy), is suspected clinically when patients with vascular risk factors (especially hypertension and diabetes) demonstrate dementia, gait disorder, urinary incontinence, focal motor and/or sensory deficits, and pseudobulbar affect and/or signs in an either gradually progressive or stepwise fashion. Both CT and MRI demonstrate extensive periventricular ischemic damage, with ventricular enlargement and often discrete ischemic lesions in other subcortical zones. At times it may be difficult to distinguish BD from normal pressure hydrocephalus (NPH) on the basis of clinical criteria alone. The diagnosis of NPH is supported when MRI scans show prominent (low-signal-intensity) CSF flow voids involving the third ventricle, aqueduct of Sylvius, and fourth ventricle; marked thinning of the corpus callosum; and decreased CSF space over the vertex of the brain on sagittal views. The SPECT studies of BD characteristically demonstrate periventricular and supraventricular white matter hypoperfusion.[148] Toghi et al compared ^{123}I-IMP SPECT images in 18 patients with BD to scans from 25 AD patients and 14 age-matched control subjects.[149] Patients with BD of moderate severity exhibited a relative CBF decrement in the basal ganglia and frontal lobes. More severely affected BD patients suffered a more widespread cerebral hypoperfusion. The AD subjects displayed the typical bilateral temporoparietal pattern; more severely demented AD patients also had frontal lobe hypoperfusion. In the BD cohort, dementia severity correlated significantly with the decline in CBF.

The Neuroimaging of Other Dementias

Dementia is a cardinal feature of NPH, AIDS, and many movement disorders. The neuroimaging of these conditions is reviewed in the chapters specifically devoted to these disease processes (see Chaps. 1, 2, 11, and 14). The following sections briefly discuss neuroimaging findings in two degenerative disorders (Pick disease and primary progressive aphasia) and a slow virus encephalopathy (Creutzfeldt-Jakob disease, or CJD).

Pick Disease

Also called Pick lobar atrophy, Pick disease is characterized pathologically by prominent atrophy predominantly affecting the temporal and/or frontal lobes. Histologically there is neuronal loss that is mostly seen in the first three cortical layers. The swollen, degenerating neurons contain intracytoplasmic argentophilic Pick bodies, composed of straight fibrils as opposed to the paired helical filaments seen in the plaques and tangles of AD.[150] The diagnosis of Pick disease is difficult to establish antemortem, since patients display many of the features characteristic of AD and other dementias (memory loss, confusion, language disturbance, disintegration of social skills, etc.). The age of onset more often corresponds to the presenile form of AD (i.e., before age 60); the disease is somewhat more common in women. Clinical clues to the diagnosis are a prominent language disturbance at the onset of the dementia and early behavioral changes (e.g., apathy, agitation, and hypersexuality).

Both CT and MRI may show anterior sulcal prominence, marked widening of the sylvian fissures, and preferential enlargement of the frontal or temporal horns of the lateral ventricles, which suggest the diagnosis of Pick disease in the appropriate clinical context[151] (Fig. 10-25). Little is known about parenchymal signal abnormalities on MRI scans of Pick patients. Studies of Pick disease using FDG PET have shown much greater hypometabolism in frontal regions than in temporal or parietal regions, distinguishing Pick disease from AD[152,153] (Fig. 10-26). Both ^{123}I-IMP and ^{99m}Tc-HMPAO SPECT have shown bilateral frontal and temporal hypoperfusion in patients with Pick disease.[111,154–156] In the early stages of presumed degenerative presenile dementia, anatomic and functional brain imaging may therefore provide valuable information supporting a diagnosis of Pick disease.

Primary Progressive Aphasia

In 1982, Mesulam reported the clinical features of an entity he called "slowly progressive aphasia without generalized dementia."[157] The six patients described in his seminal report suffered from aphasia of insidious onset and gradually progressive course, without evidence of a more generalized cognitive or behavioral disorder. In four patients, aphasia remained the only neuropsychologic deficit 5 to 11 years into the illness. The other two patients did develop a mild decline in nonlanguage cognitive skills, but only 7 or more years after disease onset, at a time when the aphasic distur-

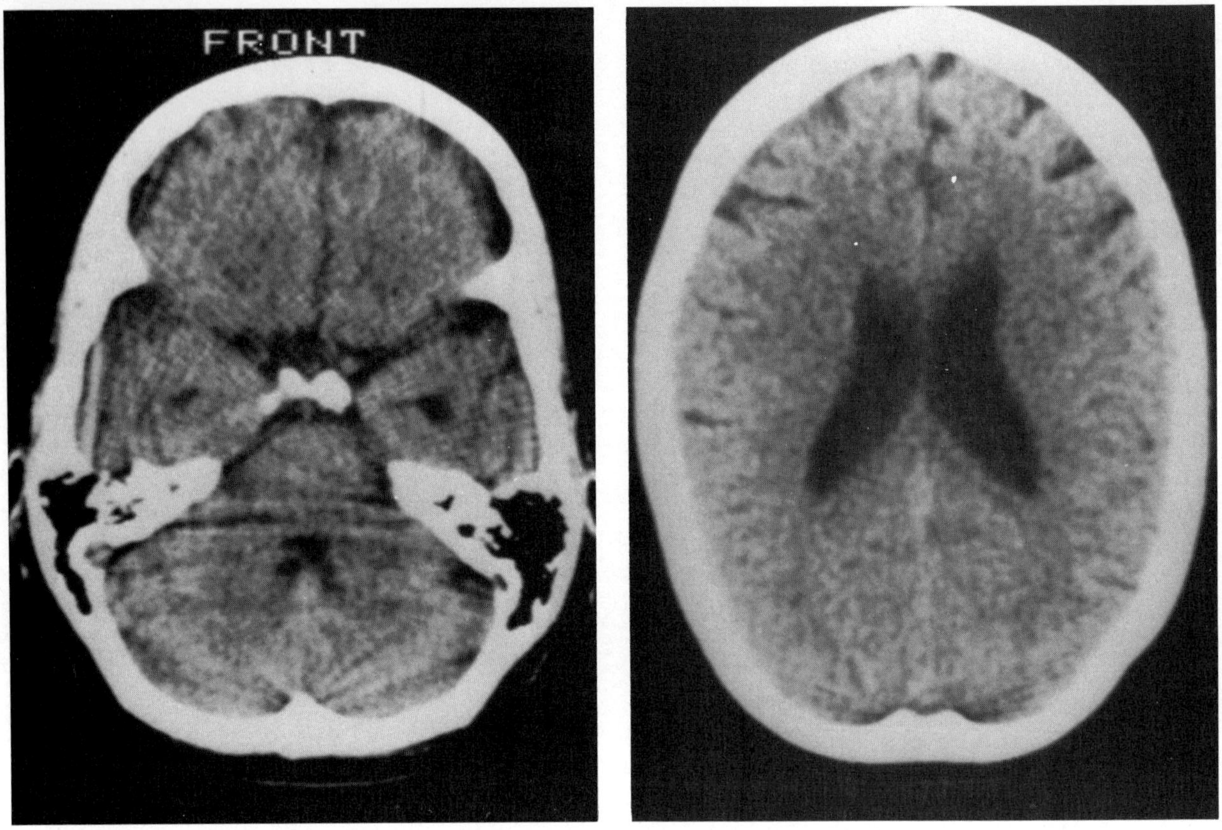

A B

Figure 10-25
CT scan of a 53-year-old woman with a clinical diagnosis of presumed Pick disease. **(A)** *Bilateral temporal horn enlargement, left greater than right.* **(B)** *Bilateral anterior sulcal prominence.*

bance was profound. Other reports soon followed supporting the existence of primary progressive aphasia, or PPA (a more widely appellation subsequently applied to the condition), as a distinct clinical syndrome.[158–160]

We reported FDG PET findings in two patients with PPA.[161] One patient had mild widening of the left sylvian fissure on CT scan. The other subject's CT scan was normal. Neither patient underwent MRI. Both patients

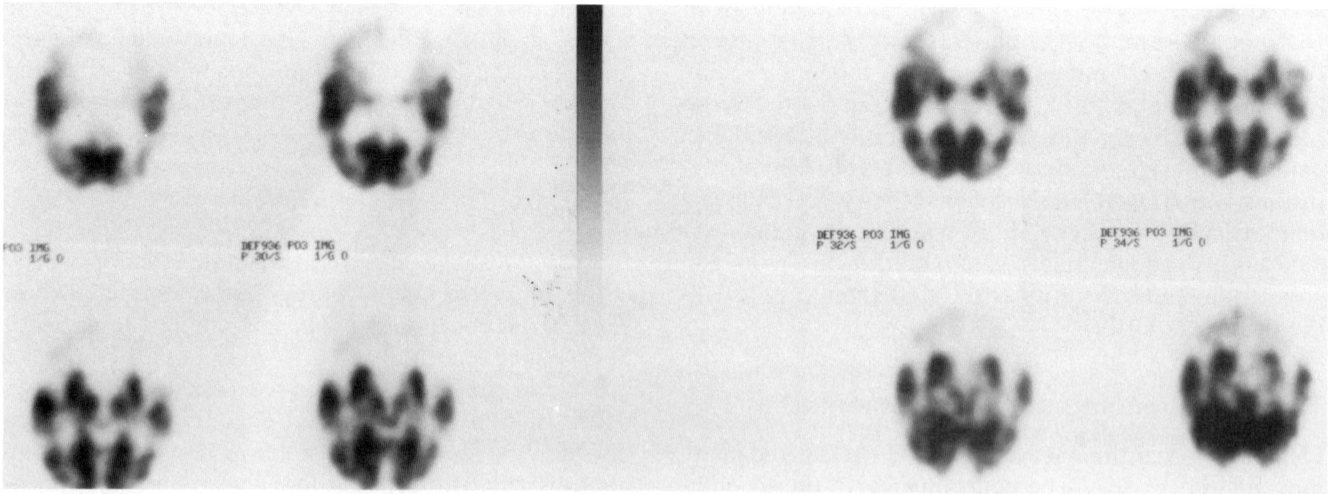

Figure 10-26
FDG PET scan of the patient in Fig. 10-25 (Pick disease). Note the profound bifrontal hypometabolism with relatively preserved metabolic activity elsehwere.

had striking focal left (dominant)-hemisphere hypometabolism on FDG PET scans, with normal right-hemisphere CMRgl, supporting the clinical impression that no nonlanguage cortical areas were involved. Other investigators have noted left sylvian fissure and temporal horn enlargement on CT and MRI scans in some PPA patients.[162,163] Further PET studies of PPA have also demonstrated focal left-hemisphere hypometabolism.[163–165] ^{99m}Tc-HMPAO SPECT scans have shown left-hemisphere hypoperfusion in PPA patients, even those with nondiagnostic anatomic scans[166] (Fig. 10-27).

The notion that PPA is nosologically distinct from AD or Pick disease has been debated since Mesulam's original report.[167] The two more common degenerative dementias (AD and Pick disease) can rarely present with an isolated progressive aphasia, preceding the onset of a more generalized cognitive decline by a year or more.[168–170] Progressive aphasia is also the salient feature of a familial dementia described by Morris et al, in which neuropathologic findings include aspects of Pick disease (focal lobar atrophy), AD (neuritic plaques), and Parkinson disease (substantia nigra degeneration).[172] Several independent autopsy examinations in PPA suggest a pathologic condition that is also distinct from other dementing illnesses.[157,173,174] One of Mesulam's original patients underwent a left superior temporal gyrus biopsy. The tissue showed mild neuronal loss and lipofuscin accumulation, with no findings suggesting one of the more common degenerative dementias.[157] Mehler and associates performed neurochemical and neuropathologic studies on one of two reported PPA patients.[174] They found asymmetrical cerebral atrophy and nonspecific histopathologic conditions, similar to Mesulam's biopsied case. Their neurochemical results were considerably more interesting. Choline acetyltransferase (CAT) activity, which is virtually always reduced in AD, was normal, whereas somatostatin levels were reduced throughout the neocortex and hippocampus. Although reduced somatostatin levels are frequently seen in AD,[175] the dissociation between CAT and somatostatin levels reported by Mehler et al is more typical of Pick disease. Given the absence of Pick bodies or other histopathologic features suggesting Pick disease, they refer to PPA as a non-Pick lobar atrophy.

Kirshner and colleagues, performing postmortem examinations on two PPA patients, also found highly focal histopathologic degeneration without Pick or Alzheimer features.[173] Both patients exhibited focal spongiform changes with neuronal loss and gliosis, primarily in layer 2 of the involved neocortex. In one patient, these findings were restricted to the left inferior frontal and superior temporal gyri. In the other, degeneration was seen in the left inferior frontal gyrus, the superior temporal gyrus not having been sectioned. Kirschner concluded that, although the histopathologic alterations were nonspecific, the extreme focality of the degenerative changes, coupled with the distinctive clinical presentation, supports the contention that PPA is not only a clinical syndrome but a discrete nosologic entity. Neuroimaging studies, especially emission tomographic scans, clearly serve a valuable role in detecting this uncommon but fascinating condition antemortem.

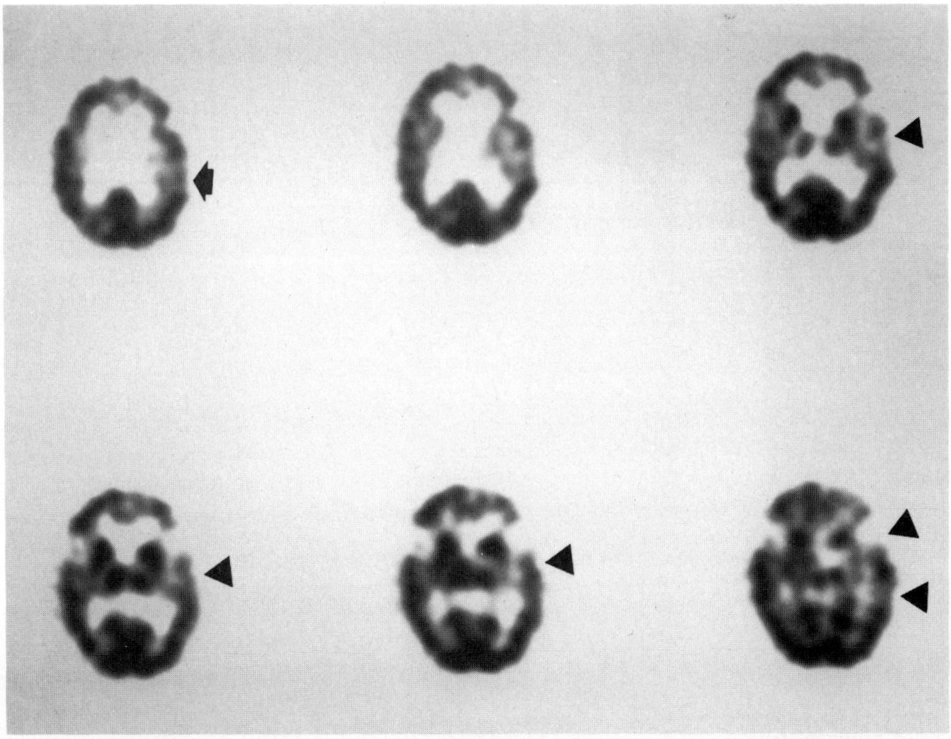

Figure 10-27
HMPAO SPECT scan of a patient with PPA. Note the left frontal, frontoparietal (arrow), and frontotemporal (arrowheads) hypoperfusion.

Creutzfeldt-Jakob Disease

Creutzfeldt-Jakob disease is a slow virus disease characterized clinically by a severe, rapidly progressive dementia, often with prominent spontaneous and reflex ("startle") myoclonus, and cerebellar ataxia. We have seen a pathologically proven case, however, with a clinical course indistinguishable from AD! The pathologic hallmark of CJD is widespread neuronal loss and gliosis with vacuolation, or spongiform change, in affected brain regions, hence the term *subacute spongiform encephalopathy.* Anatomic scans generally show diffuse, nonspecific cerebral atrophy with ventricular enlargement and sulcal widening,[176] although one MRI case study suggests that bilateral basal ganglia high-signal abnormalities may be seen.[177]

The FDG-PET scans of three reported CJD cases demonstrated scattered areas of reduced metabolism[178] or bitemporal hypometabolism differing little from that seen in AD.[179] In our unreported autopsy-proven case mentioned above, the PET rCMRgl pattern was similar to that seen in severe AD patients (profound frontal, temporal, and parietal hypometabolism, with relative sparing of the primary sensorimotor and visual cortices). In fact, the diagnosis of CJD at autopsy came as a complete surprise!

An ^{99m}Tc-HMPAO SPECT study performed in a patient with biopsy-proven CJD demonstrated focal perfusion defects in the left frontal and right temporoparietal areas despite a normal CT scan.[180] We also scanned one patient with biopsy-proven CJD using HMPAO SPECT, finding mild bilateral parietal and anterior temporal hypoperfusion (Fig. 10-28).

Based on the investigations reviewed above, it would appear that the neuroimaging findings in CJD are rather nonspecific. Anatomic scan features generally cannot be distinguished from AD or other diffuse atrophic conditions, while functional images may mimic those seen in AD or MID.

CONCLUSION

Neuroimaging of the human brain from birth to senescence has provided us with valuable insights into the processes of normal brain development, maturation, and aging, as well as diagnostic assistance in distinguishing among a variety of dementing illnesses. For example, the observation that "incomplete infarction" is commonly present in older AD patients would most likely have remained buried in the neuropathology literature were it not for the surprising frequency of WMHs on MRI scans of those suffering from AD. Despite the incredible technologic advancements in brain imaging over the past 25 years, however, the neurologic clinician has not been replaced by machines. In their study, Mattman and coworkers found that the accuracy of an AD diagnosis using only CT and SPECT was below that achieved using standard clinical criteria.[181] The CT, MRI, PET, or SPECT scans of a normal elderly individual may look like those of an early Alzheimer patient at a point in time when the experienced neurologist can establish the correct diagnosis with a careful history, physical examination, and longitudinal follow-up care. Patients with MID may resemble nondemented individ-

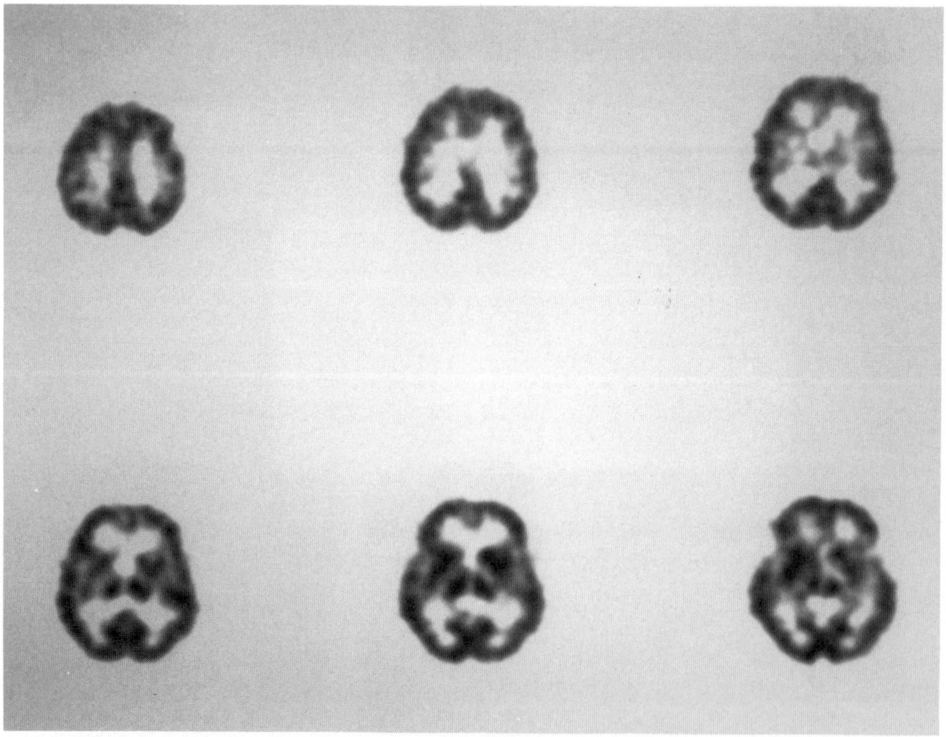

Figure 10-28
HMPAO SPECT study of a patient with biopsy-proven CJD. There is mild bilateral parietal and anterior temporal hypoperfusion.

uals with severe atherosclerotic vascular disease on the basis of MRIs. Patients with CJD may be identical to patients with AD or MID on the basis of CT, MRI, or emission tomographic scans.

Common to many of the studies reviewed in this chapter is the emphasis on the increased sensitivity of the newer tomographic modalities (MRI, PET, and SPECT). Careful observation and investigation have improved the specificity of these techniques as well, but not enough. Future clinical research will undoubtedly lead to even greater accuracy as specific diagnostic imaging criteria are established for the various dementias.

Newer MRI techniques are in their infancy as applied to the study of brain aging and dementia. Preliminary investigations using functional MRI (fMRI) correlate well with emission tomographic results.[182,183] If this early promise is fulfilled, the relative ease of implementing the fMRI technique, the absence of harmful ionizing radiation, and the superior spatial resolution may lead to the replacement of PET and SPECT with fMRI in CBF and metabolic studies. However, PET and SPECT will remain important modalities for in vivo neurotransmitter and neuroreceptor investigations.

In the future, phosphorous (^{31}P) magnetic resonance spectroscopy (MRS) may provide valuable information regarding membrane integrity (phospholipids) in AD.[184] Proton (^{1}H) MRS should eventually reveal regional bioenergetic and membrane structural abnormalities in AD. Early results using MRS in the study of dementia have been contradictory, however.[185–187]

The imaging modalities discussed here represent important adjuncts to the evaluation of dementia patients but are not alone capable of proving the presence of a given disease process. Nevertheless, the use of CT or MRI has become an essential part of the dementia evaluation, given the importance of detecting treatable structural disease. Setting aside economic issues, MRI is clearly the anatomic imaging modality of choice. The superior sensitivity of MRI facilitates the uncovering of treatable lesions, such as tumors, hematomas, and infections. Moreover, MRI can demonstrate temporal lobe atrophy, supporting a diagnosis of AD, and may reveal ischemic damage in MID that is not as conspicuous on CT images. In the late 1990s, emission tomography is not a necessary part of most dementia workups. However, PET or SPECT studies may be quite useful in discriminating Pick disease or PPA from AD. The current state of neurologic therapeutics limits the utility of this degree of diagnostic specificity. As pharmacologic advances in the treatment of degenerative and ischemic brain disorders occur, however, functional imaging may serve a more important neurodiagnostic purpose. The development of novel radiolabeled tracers, especially those capable of imaging the specific neurotransmitter systems affected in dementing illnesses (e.g., the cholinergic pathways in AD), will also broaden the role of emission tomography in diagnosing disorders of cerebral senescence.

REFERENCES

1. Adams RD, Victor M: *Principles of Neurology,* 5th ed. New York, McGraw-Hill, 1993, p 106.
2. Chawluk J, Alavi A, Hurtig H, et al: Altered patterns of regional cerebral glucose metabolism in aging and dementia. *J Cereb Blood Flow Metab* 5(suppl 1):121, 1985.
3. Chugani HT, Phelps ME: Maturational changes in cerebral function in infants determined by 18-FDG positron emission tomography. *Science* 231:840, 1986.
4. Brooks RA, DiChiro G: Beam hardening in x-ray reconstructive tomography. *Physiol Med Biol* 21:390, 1976.
5. Flechsig P: Developmental (myelogenetic) localisation of the cerebral cortex in the human subject. *Lancet* 2: 1027, 1901.
6. Barkovich AJ, Kjos BO, Jackson DE Jr, Norman D: Normal maturation of the neonatal and infant brain: MR imaging at 1.5 T. *Radiology* 166:173, 1988.
7. Dietrich RB, Bradley WG Jr: Normal and abnormal white matter maturation. *Semin Ultrasound CT MR* 9: 192, 1988.
8. van der Knaap MS, Valk J, Bakker CJ, et al: Myelination as an expression of the functional maturity of the brain. *Dev Med Child Neurol* 33:849, 1991.
9. Martin E, Krassnitzer S, Kaelin P, Boesch Ch: MR imaging of the brainstem: Normal postnatal development. *Neuroradiology* 33:391, 1991.
10. Freyhan FA, Woodford RB, Kety SS: Cerebral blood flow and metabolism in psychoses of senility. *J Nerv Ment Dis* 113:449, 1951.
11. Chugani HT, Phelps ME, Mazziotta JC: Positron emission tomography study of human brain functional development. *Ann Neurol* 22:487, 1987.
12. Chugani HT: Functional brain imaging in pediatrics. *Pediatr Clin North Am* 39:777, 1992.
13. Jernigan TL, Trauner DA, Hesselink JR, Tallal PA: Maturation of human cerebrum observed *in vivo* during adolescence. *Brain* 114:2037, 1991.
14. Tomlinson BE, Blessed G, Roth M: Observations on the brains of demented old people. *J Neurol Sci* 11:205, 1970.
15. Miller AKH, Alston RL, Corsellis JAN: Variation with age in the volumes of grey and white matter in the cerebral hemispheres of man: Measurements with an image analyser. *Neuropathol Appl Neurol* 6:119, 1980.
16. Paxton R, Ambrose J: The EMI scanner: A brief review of the first 650 patients. *Br J Radiol* 47:530, 1974.
17. Haug G: Age and sex dependence of the size of normal ventricles on computed tomography. *Neuroradiology* 14: 201, 1977.
18. Glydensted C, Kosteljanetz M: Measurements of the normal ventricular system with computer tomography. *Neuroradiology* 10:205, 1976.
19. Glydensted C: Measurements of the normal ventricular system and hemispheric sulci of 100 adults with computed tomography. *Neuroradiology* 14:183, 1977.
20. Earnest MP, Heaton RK, Wilkinson WE, Manke WR:

Cortical atrophy, ventricular enlargement and intellectual impairment in the aged. *Neurology* 29:1138, 1979.

21. Glydensted C, Kosteljanetz M: Measurements of the normal hemispheric sulci with computed tomography: A preliminary study of 44 adults. *Neuroradiology* 10:147, 1975.
22. George AE, de Leon MJ, Stylopoulos LA, et al: CT diagnostic features of Alzheimer disease: Importance of the choroidal/hippocampal fissure complex. *Am J Neuroradiol* 11:283, 1990.
23. Kido DK, Caine ED, LeMay M, et al: Temporal lobe atrophy in patients with Alzheimer disease: A CT study. *Am J Neuroradiol* 10:551, 1989.
24. Jobst KA, Smith AD, Szatmari M, et al: Detection in life of confirmed Alzheimer's disease using a simple measurement of medial temporal lobe atrophy by computed tomography. *Lancet* 340:1179, 1992.
25. DeLeon MJ, George AE, Golomb J, et al: Frequency of hippocampal atrophy in normal aging and Alzheimer's disease. *Neurobiol Aging* 18:1, 1997.
26. Chawluk J, Alavi A, Dann R, et al: PET measurements of cerebral metabolism corrected for CSF contributions. *J Nucl Med* 25(suppl 1):56, 1984.
27. Yue NC, Arnold AM, Longstreth WT Jr, et al: Sulcal, ventricular, and white matter changes at MR imaging in the aging brain: Data from the Cardiovascular Health Study. *Radiology* 202:33, 1997.
28. Wahlund LO, Almkvist O, Basun H, Julin P: MRI in successful aging: A 5-year follow-up study from the eighth to ninth decade of life. *Magn Reson Imaging* 14: 601, 1996.
29. Bradley WG Jr, Waluch V, Brant-Zawadzki M, et al: Patchy, periventricular white matter lesions in the elderly: A common observation during NMR imaging. *Noninv Med Imaging* 1:35, 1984.
30. Fazekas F, Chawluk JB, Alavi A, et al: Magnetic resonance signal abnormalities at 1.5T in Alzheimer's dementia and normal aging. *Am J Neuroradiol* 8:421, 1987.
31. Fazekas F, Schmidt R, Offenbacher H, et al: Prevalence of white matter and periventricular magnetic resonance hyperintensities in asymptomatic volunteers. *J Neuroimag* 1:27, 1991.

31a. Longstreth WJ Jr, Manolio TA, Arnold A, et al: Clinical correlates of white matter findings on cranial magnetic resonance imaging of 3301 elderly people: The Cardiovascular Health Study. *Stroke* 27:1274, 1996.

32. Awad IA, Spetzler RF, Hodak JA, et al: Incidental subcortical lesions identified on magnetic resonance imaging in the elderly: I. Correlation with age and cerebrovascular risk factors. *Stroke* 17:1084, 1986.
33. Austrom MG, Thompson RF Jr, Hendrie HC, et al: Foci of increased T2 signal intensity in MR images of healthy elderly subjects: A follow-up study. *J Am Geriatr Soc* 38:1133, 1990.
34. Junque C, Pujol J, Vendrell P, et al: Leuko-araiosis on magnetic resonance imaging in dementia. *Arch Neurol* 47:151, 1990.
35. Kozachuk WE, DeCarli C, Schapiro M, et al: White matter hyperintensities in dementia of Alzheimer's type and in healthy subjects without cerebrovascular risk factors: A magnetic resonance imaging study. *Arch Neurol* 47: 1306, 1990.
36. Brant-Zawadski M, Fein G, Van Dyke C, et al: MR imaging of the aging brain: Patchy white-matter lesions and dementia. *Am J Neuroradiol* 6:675, 1985.
37. Rao SM, Mittenberg W, Bernadin L, et al: Neuropsychological test findings in subjects with leukoaraiosis. *Arch Neurol* 46:40, 1989.
38. O'Brien JT, Desmond P, Ames D, et al: Magnetic resonance correlates of memory impairment in the healthy elderly: Association with medial temporal lobe atrophy but not white matter lesions. *Int J Geriatr Psychiatry* 12:369, 1997.
39. Kirkpatrick JB, Hayman LA: White-matter lesions in MR imaging of clinically healthy brains of elderly subjects: Possible pathologic basis. *Radiology* 162:509, 1987.
40. Cervos-Navarro J, Rozas IJ: The arteriole as a site of metabolic exchange. *Adv Neurol* 20:17, 1978.
41. Braffman BH, Zimmerman RA, Trojanowski JQ, et al: Brain MR: Pathologic correlation with gross and histopathology: 1. Lacunar infarction and Virchow-Robin spaces. *Am J Neuroradiol* 9:621, 1988.
42. Awad IA, Johnson PC, Spetzler RF, Hodak JA: Incidental subcortical lesions identified on magnetic resonance imaging in the elderly: II. Postmortem pathological correlations. *Stroke* 17:1090, 1986.
43. Braffman BH, Zimmerman RA, Trojanowski JQ, et al: Brain MR: Pathologic correlation with gross and histopathology: 2. Hyperintense white-matter foci in the elderly. *Am J Neuroradiol* 9:629, 1988.
44. Fazekas F, Kleinert R, Offenbacher H, et al: The morphologic correlate of incidental punctate white matter hyperintensities on MR images. *Am J Neuroradiol* 12: 915, 1991.
45. Grafton ST, Sumi SM, Stimac GK, et al: Comparison of postmortem magnetic resonance imaging and neuropathologic findings in the cerebral white matter. *Arch Neurol* 48:293, 1991.
46. van Swieten JC, van den Hout HW, van Ketel BA, et al: Periventricular lesions in the white matter on magnetic resonance imaging in the elderly: A morphometric correlation with arteriosclerosis and dilated perivascular spaces. *Brain* 114:761, 1991.
47. Munoz DG, Hastak SM, Harper B, et al: Pathologic correlates of increased signals of the centrum ovale on magnetic resonance imaging. *Arch Neurol* 50:492, 1993.
48. Leys D, Pruvo JP, Parent M, et al: Could wallerian degeneration contribute to "leuko-araiosis" in subjects free of any vascular disorder? *J Neurol Neurosurg Psychiatry* 54:46, 1991.
49. Wong KT, Grossman RI, Boorstein JM, et al: Magnetization transfer imaging of periventricular hyperintense white matter in the elderly. *Am J Neuroradiol* 16:253, 1995.
50. Rowe JW, Kahn RL: Human aging: Usual and successful. *Science* 237:143, 1987.
51. Kety SS, Schmidt CF: The nitrous oxide method for the quantitative determination of cerebral blood flow in man: Theory, procedure, and normal values. *J Clin Invest* 27:476, 1948.
52. Dastur DK, Lane MH, Hansen DB, et al: Effects of aging on cerebral circulation and metabolism in man, in Birren JE, Butler RN, Greenhouse SW, et al (eds): *Human Aging: A Biological and Behavioral Study*. NIH, DHEW

pub no 986. Bethesda, MD, U.S. Department of Health, Education and Welfare, 1963, pp 59–76.
53. Frackowiak RSJ, Wise RJS, Gibbs JM, et al: Positron emission tomographic studies in aging and cerebrovascular disease at the Hammersmith Hospital. *Ann Neurol* 15(suppl):S112, 1984.
54. Duara R, Margolin RA, Robertson-Tchabo EA, et al: Cerebral glucose utilization as measured with positron emission tomography in 21 resting healthy men between the ages of 21 and 83 years. *Brain* 106:761, 1983.
55. Rapoport SI, Horwitz B, Duara R: PET scanning demonstrates that aging in man is accompanied by loss of integration of regional brain activity without concurrent reduction in absolute regional cerebral metabolic rates for glucose. *J Cerebr Blood Flow Metab* 5(suppl 1):S119, 1985.
56. Chawluk JB, Alavi A, Jamieson DG, et al: Changes in local cerebral glucose metabolism with normal aging: The effects of cardiovascular and systemic health factors. *J Cerebr Blood Flow Metab* 7(suppl 1):S411, 1987.
57. Kuhl DE, Metter EF, Riege WH, Phelps ME: Effect of human aging on patterns of local cerebral glucose utilization determined by the [^{18}F]fluorodeoxyglucose method. *J Cerebr Blood Flow Metab* 2:163, 1982.
58. Yoshii F, Barker WW, Chang JY, et al: Sensitivity of cerebral glucose metabolism to age, gender, brain volume, brain atrophy, and cerebrovascular risk factors. *J Cerebr Blood Flow Metab* 8:654, 1988.
59. Chawluk JB, Alavi A, Dann R, et al: Positron emission tomography in aging and dementia: The effect of cerebral atrophy. *J Nucl Med* 28:431, 1987.
60. Herscovitch P, Archus AP, Gado M, et al: Correction of positron emission tomography data for cerebral atrophy. *J Cerebr Blood Flow Metab* 6:120, 1986.
61. Chawluk JB, Dann R, Alavi A, et al: The effect of focal cerebral atrophy in positron emission tomographic studies of aging and dementia. *Nucl Med Biol* 17:797, 1990.
62. Birren JE, Schaie KW (eds): *Handbook of the Psychology of Aging.* New York, Van Nostrand Reinhold, 1977.
63. Erkinjuntti T, Haltia M, Palo J, et al: Accuracy of the clinical diagnosis of vascular dementia: A prospective clinical and post-mortem neuropathological study. *J Neurol Neurosurg Psychiatry* 51:1037, 1988.
64. Lopez OL, Becker JT, Jungreis CA, et al: Computed tomography—but not magnetic resonance imaging—identified periventricular white-matter lesions predict symptomatic cerebrovascular disease in probable Alzheimer's disease. *Arch Neurol* 52:659, 1995.
65. Hyman BT, Van Hoesen GW, Damasio AR, Barnes CL: Alzheimer's disease: Cell-specific pathology isolates the hippocampal formation. *Science* 225:1168, 1984.
66. Kesslak JP, Nalcioglu O, Cotman CW: Quantification of magnetic resonance scans for hippocampal and parahippocampal atrophy in Alzheimer's disease. *Neurology* 41:51, 1991.
67. Folstein MF, Folstein SE, McHugh PR: Mini-mental state: A practical method for grading the cognitive state of patients for the clinician. *J Psychiatr Res* 12:189, 1975.
68. Barclay LL, Linden C, Murtagh R: Medial temporal atrophy as a magnetic resonance imaging marker for Alzheimer's disease. *J Neuroimag* 2:131, 1992.
69. Scheltens Ph, Leys D, Barkof F, et al: Atrophy of medial temporal lobes on MRI in "probable" Alzheimer's disease and normal aging: Diagnostic value and neuropsychological correlates. *J Neurol Neurosurg Psychiatry* 55:967, 1992.
70. Frisoni GB, Beltramello A, Weiss C, et al: Linear measures of atrophy in mild Alzheimer disease. *Am J Neuroradiol* 17:913, 1996.
71. Jack CR Jr, Petersen RC, Xu YC, et al: Medial temporal atrophy on MRI in normal aging and very mild Alzheimer's disease. *Neurology* 49:786, 1997.
72. Fox NC, Warrington EK, Freeborough PA, et al: Presymptomatic hippocampal volume reductions in individuals at risk for Alzheimer's disease. *Neurobiol Aging* 18:131, 1997.
73. Convit A, DeLeon MJ, Yarshish C, et al: Specific hippocampal volume reductions in individuals at risk for Alzheimer's disease. *Neurobiol Aging* 18:131, 1997.
74. Kaye JA, Swihart T, Howieson D, et al: Volume loss of the hippocampus and temporal lobe in healthy elderly persons destined to develop dementia. *Neurology* 48:1297, 1997.
75. Robakis NK, Oangalos MN: Involvement of amyloid as a central step in the development of Alzheimer's disease. *Neurobiol Aging* 15(suppl 2):S127, 1994.
76. Schroder J, Pantel J, Ida N, et al: Cerebral changes and cerebrospinal fluid beta-amyloid in Alzheimer's disease: A study with quantitative magnetic resonance imaging. *Mol Psychiatry* 2:505, 1997.
77. Saunders AM, Hulette O, Welsh-Bohmer KA, et al: Specificity, sensitivity, and predictive value of apolipoprotein-E genotyping for sporadic Alzheimer's disease. *Lancet* 348:90, 1996.
78. Lehtovirta M, Soininen H, Laasko MP, et al: SPECT and MRI analysis in Alzheimer's disease: Relation to apolipoprotein E epsilon 4 allele. *J Neurol Neurosurg Psychiatry* 60:644, 1996.
79. Alavi A, Reivich M, Ferris S, et al: Regional cerebral glucose metabolism in aging and senile dementia as determined by ^{18}F-deoxyglucose and positron emission tomography, in Hoyer S (ed): *The Aging Brain: Physiological and Pathophysiological Aspects.* Berlin, Springer-Verlag, 1982, pp 87–195.
80. Ferris S, DeLeon M, Wolf A, et al: Regional metabolism and cognitive deficits in aging and senile dementia, in Samuel D, Algeri S, Gershon S, et al (eds): *Aging of the Brain.* New York, Raven Press, 1983.
81. Frackowiak R, Pozzillic C, Legg N, et al: Regional cerebral oxygen supply and utilization in dementia: A clinical and physiological study with oxygen-15 and positron tomography. *Brain* 104:752, 1981.
82. DeLeon M, Ferris S, George A, et al: Computed tomography and positron emission transaxial tomography evaluations of normal aging and Alzheimer's disease. *J Cerebr Blood Flow Metab* 3:391, 1983.
83. Cutler N, Haxby J, Duara R, et al: Clinical history, brain metabolism and neuropsychological function in Alzheimer's disease. *Ann Neurol* 18:298, 1985.
84. Alavi A, Dann R, Chawluk J, et al: Positron emission tomography of regional cerebral glucose metabolism. *Semin Nucl Med* 16:2, 1986.

85. Duara R, Grady C, Haxby J, et al: Postron emission tomography in Alzheimer's disease. *Neurology* 36:879, 1986.
86. Haxby J, Duara R, Grady C, et al: Relations between neuropsychological and cerebral metabolic asymmetries in early Alzheimer's disease. *J Cerebr Blood Flow Metab* 5:193, 1985.
87. McGeer P, Kamo H, Harrop R, et al: Postron emission tomography in patients with clinically diagnosed Alzheimer's disease. *Can Med Assoc J* 134:597, 1986.
88. McGeer P, Kamo H, Harrop R, et al: Comparison of PET, MRI, and CT with pathology in a proven case of Alzheimer's disease. *Neurology* 36:1569, 1986.
89. Jamieson DG, Chawluk JB, Alavi A, et al: The effect of disease severity on local cerebral glucose metabolism in Alzheimer's disease. *J Cerebr Blood Flow Metab* 7(suppl 1):S410, 1987.
90. Lowenstein D, Yoshii F, Barker WW, et al: Predominant left hemisphere metabolic dysfunction in dementia. *Arch Neurol* 46:146, 1989.
91. Friedland R, Budinger T, Koss E, Ober B: Alzheimer's disease: Anterior-posterior and lateral hemispheric alterations in cortical glucose utilization. *Neurosci Lett* 53: 235, 1985.
92. Haxby JV, Grady C, Duara R, et al: Neocortical metabolic abnormalities precede nonmemory cognitive defects in early Alzheimer's-type dementia. *Arch Neurol* 43:882, 1986.
93. Benson D, Kuhl D, Hawkins R, et al: The fluorodeoxyglucose ^{18}F scan in Alzheimer's disease and multiinfarct dementia. *Arch Neurol* 40:711, 1983.
94. Chawluk JB, Alavi A, Hurtig H, et al: Altered patterns of regional cerebral glucose metabolism in aging and dementia. *J Cerebr Blood Flow Metab* 5(suppl 1):S121, 1985.
95. Friedland S, Brun A, Budinger T: Pathological and positron emission tomographic correlations in Alzheimer's disease. *Lancet* 1:228, 1985.
96. Yamaguchi S, Meguro K, Itoh M, et al: Decreased cortical glucose metabolism correlates with hippocampal atrophy in Alzheimer's disease as shown by MRI and PET. *J Neurol Neuorsurg Psychiatry* 62:596, 1997.
97. Jagust WJ, Friedland RP, Budinger TF, et al: Longitudinal studies of regional cerebral metabolism in Alzheimer's disease. *Neurology* 38:909, 1988.
98. Cutler N, Haxby J, Durara R, et al: Brain metabolism as measured with positron emission tomography: Serial assessment in a patient with familial Alzheimer's disease. *Neurology* 35:1556, 1985.
99. Small GW, Mazziotta JC, Collins MT, et al: Apolipoprotein E type 4 allele and cerebral glucose metabolism in relatives at risk for familial Alzheimer's disease. *JAMA* 273:942, 1995.
100. Polinsky R, Noble H, DiChiro G, et al: Dominantly inherited Alzheimer's disease: Cerebral glucose metabolism. *J Neurosurg Psychiatry* 50:752, 1987.
101. Luxenberg J, May C, Haxby J, et al: Cerebral metabolism, anatomy, and cognition in monozygotic twins discordant for dementia of the Alzheimer's type. *J Neurol Neurosurg Psychiatry* 50:333, 1987.
102. Bonte FJ, Ross ED, Chehabi HH, et al: SPECT study of regional cerebral blood flow in Alzheimer disease. *J Comput Assist Tomogr* 10:579, 1986.
103. Derouesne C, Rancurel G, Le Poncin H, et al: Variability of cerebral blood flow defects in Alzheimer's disease on 123-iodo-isopropyl-amphetamine and single photon emission tomography (letter). *Lancet* 1:1282, 1985.
104. Bartenstein P, Minoshima S, Hirsch C, et al: Quantitative assessment of cerebral blood flow in patients with Alzheimer's disease by SPECT. *J Nucl Med* 38:1095, 1997.
105. Nagel JS, Ichise M, Holman BL: The scintigraphic evaluation of Huntington's disease and other movement disorders using single photon emission computed tomography perfusion brain scans. *Semin Nucl Med* 21:11, 1991.
106. Pizzolato G, Dam M, Borsato N, et al: Tc-99m-HM-PAO SPECT in Parkinson's disease. *J Cerebr Blood Flow Metab* 8:S101, 1988.
107. Launes J, Sulkava R, Erkinjuntti T, et al: 99Tcm-HMPAO SPECT in suspected dementia. *Nucl Med Commun* 12:757, 1991.
108. Kuwabara Y, Ichiya Y, Otsuka M, et al: Differential diagnosis of bilateral parietal abnormalities in I-123 IMP SPECT imaging. *Clin Nucl Med* 15:893, 1990.
109. Grunwald F, Zierz S, Broich K, et al: HMPAO-SPECT imaging resembling Alzheimer-type dementia in mitochondrial encephalopathy with lactic acidosis and strokelike episodes (MELAS). *J Nucl Med* 31:1740, 1990.
110. Masterman DL, Mendez MF, Fairbanks LA, et al: Sensitivity, specificity, and positive predictive value of technetium 99-HMPAO SPECT in discriminating Alzheimer's disease from other dementias. *J Geriatr Psychiatry Neurol* 10:15, 1997.
111. Kuwabara Y, Ichiya Y, Otsuka M, et al: Comparison of I-123 and Tc-99m HMPAO SPECT studies with PET in dementia. *Ann Nucl Med* 4:75, 1990.
112. Gemmell HG, Evans NT, Besson JA, et al: Regional cerebral blood flow imaging: A quantitative comparison of technetium-99m-HMPAO SPECT with C15-02 PET. *J Nucl Med* 31:1595, 1990.
113. Jagust WJ, Budinger TF, Reed BR, et al: The diagnosis of dementia with single photon emission computed tomography. *Arch Neurol* 44:258, 1987.
114. Johnson KA, Holman BL, Rosen TJ, et al: Iofetamine I-123 single photon emission computed tomography is accurate in the diagnosis of Alzheimer's disease. *Arch Intern Med* 150:752, 1990.
115. Neary D, Snowden JS, Shields TA, et al: Single photon emission tomography using Tc-99m-HM-PAO in the investigation of dementia. *J Neurol Neurosurg Psychiatry* 50:1101, 1987.
116. Perani D, DiPiero V, Vallar G, et al: Technetium-99m HM-PAO SPECT study of regional cerebral perfusion in early Alzheimer's disease. *J Nucl Med* 29:1507, 1988.
117. Sharp P, Gemmell H, Cherryman G, et al: Application of iodine-123-labeled isopropylamphetamine imaging to the study of dementia. *J Nucl Med* 27:761, 1986.
118. Testa HJ, Snowden JS, Neary D, et al: The use of Tc-99m HM-PAO in the diagnosis of primary degenerative dementia. *J Cerebr Blood Flow Metab* 8:S123, 1988.
119. Holman BL, Johnson KA, Garada B, et al: The scintigraphic appearance of Alzheimer's disease: A prospec-

tive study using technetium-99m-HMPAO SPECT. *J Nucl Med* 33:181, 1992.

120. Agnoli A, Fabbrini G, Fioravanti M, et al: CBF and cognitive evaluation of Alzheimer type patients before and after IMAO-B treatment: A pilot study. *Eur Neuropsychoparmacol* 2:31, 1992.
121. Holman BL, Hellman RS, Goldsmith SJ, et al: Biodistribution, dosimetry, and clinical evaluation of technetium-99m ethyl cysteinate dimer in normal subjects and in patients with chronic cerebral infarction. *J Nucl Med* 30:1018, 1989.
122. Weinberger DR, Gibson R, Coppola R, et al: The distribution of cerebral muscarinic acetylcholine receptors *in vivo* in patients with dementia: A controlled study with ^{123}I-QNB and single photon emission computed tomography. *Arch Neurol* 48:169, 1991.
123. Weinberger DR, Jones D, Reba RC, et al: A comparison of FDG PET and IQNB SPECT in normal subjects and in patients with dementia. *J Neuropsychiatry Clin Neurosci* 4:239, 1992.
124. Kuhl DE, Minoshima S, Fessler JA, et al: In vivo mapping of cholinergic terminals in normal aging, Alzheimer's disease, and Parkinson's disease. *Ann Neurol* 40:399, 1996.
125. Davies P, Maloney AJF: Selective loss of central cholinergic neurons in Alzheimer's disease. *Lancet* 2:1403, 1976.
126. Perry EK, Perry RH, Blessed G, Tomlinson BE: Necropsy evidence of central cholinergic deficits in senile dementia. *Lancet* 1:189, 1977.
127. Hachinski VC, Zilhka E, DuBoulay GH, et al: Cerebral blood flow in dementia. *Arch Neurol* 32:632, 1975.
128. Rosen W, Terry RD, Fuld PA, et al: Pathological verification of ischemic score in differentiation of dementias. *Ann Neurol* 7:486, 1980.
129. Molsa PK, Paljarvi L, Rinne JO, et al: Validity of clinical diagnosis in dementia: A prospective clinicopathological study. *J Neurol Neurosurg Psychiatry* 48:1085, 1985.
130. Wade JPH, Mirsen TR, Hachinski VC, et al: The clinical diagnosis of Alzheimer's disease. *Arch Neurol* 44:24, 1987.
131. Ladurner G, Iliff LD, Lechner H: Clinical factors associated with dementia in ischemic stroke. *J Neurol Neurosurg Psychiatry* 45:97, 1982.
132. Ladurner G, Sager MD, Iliff LD, Lechner H: A correlation of clinical findings and CT in ischaemic cerebrovascular disease. *Eur Neurol* 18:281, 1978.
133. Goto K, Ishii N, Fukasawa H: Diffuse white matter disease in the geriatric population: A clinical, neuropathological, and CT study. *Radiology* 141:687, 1981.
134. Radue E-W, duBoulay GH, Harrison MJG, Thomas DJ: Comparison of angiographic and CT findings between patients with multi-infarct dementia and those with dementia due to primary neuronal degeneration. *Neuroradiology* 16:113, 1978.
135. Duara R, Barker W, Loewenstein D, et al: Sensitivity and specificity of positron emission tomography and magnetic resonance imaging studies in Alzheimer's disease and multi-infarct dementia. *Eur Neurol* 29(suppl 3):9, 1989.
136. Bowen BC, Barker WW, Loewenstein DA, et al: MR signal abnormalities in memory disorder and dementia. *Am J Neuroradiol* 11:283, 1990.
137. Leys D, Soetaert G, Petit H, et al: Periventricular and white matter magnetic resonance imaging hyperintensities do not differ between Alzheimer's disease and normal aging. *Arch Neurol* 47:524, 1990.
138. Mantyla R, Erkinjuntti T, Salonen O, et al: Variable agreement between visual rating scales for white matter hyperintensities on MRI: Comparison of 13 rating scales in a poststroke cohort. *Stroke* 28:1614, 1997.
139. Erkinjuntti T, Ketonen L, Sulkava R, et al: Do white matter changes on MRI and CT differentiate vascular dementia from Alzheimer's disease? *J Neurol Neurosurg Psychiatry* 50:37, 1987.
140. Scheltens PP, Barkhof F, Valk J, et al: White matter lesions on magnetic resonance imaging in clinically diagnosed Alzheimer's disease: Evidence for heterogeneity. *Brain* 115:735, 1992.
141. Pullicino P, Benedict RHB, Capruso DX, et al: Neuroimaging criteria for vascular dementia. *Arch Neurol* 53: 723, 1996.
142. Stout JC, Jernigan TL, Archibald SL, Salmon DP: Association of dementia severity with cortical gray matter and abnormal white matter volumes in dementia of the Alzheimer type. *Arch Neurol* 53:742, 1996.
143. Kuhl DE, Metter EJ, Riege WH, et al: Local cerebral glucose utilization in elderly patients with depression, multiple infarct dementia, and Alzheimer's disease. *J Cerebr Blood Flow Metab* 3(suppl 1):S494, 1983.
144. Kuhl D, Metter E, Benson F, et al: Similarities of cerebral glucose metabolism in Alzheimer's and Parkinson's dementia. *J Cerebr Blood Flow Metab* 5(suppl 1):S169, 1985.
145. Metter EJ, Mazziotta JC, Itabashi HH, et al: Comparison of glucose metabolism, x-ray CT, and postmortem data in a patient with multiple cerebral infarcts. *Neurology* 35:1695, 1985.
146. Dewan MJ, Gupta S: Toward a definite diagnosis of Alzheimer's disease. *Compr Psychiatry* 33:282, 1992.
147. Weinstein HC, Hean J, van Royen EA, et al: SPECT in the diagnosis of Alzheimer's disease and multi-infarct dementia. *Clin Neurol Neurosurg* 93:39, 1991.
148. De Cristofaro MT, Masclachi M, Pupi A, et al: Subcortical arteriosclerotic encephalopathy: Single photon emission computed tomography–magnetic resonance imaging correlation. *Am J Physiol Imaging* 5:68, 1990.
149. Toghi H, Chiba K, Sasaki K, et al: Cerebral perfusion patterns in vascular dementia of Binswanger type compared with senile dementia of the Alzheimer type: A SPECT study. *J Neurol* 238:365, 1991.
150. Adams RD, Victor M: *Principles of Neurology,* 5th ed. New York, McGraw-Hill, 1993, pp 966–968.
151. Davis DO, Pressman BD: Computerized tomography of the brain. *Radiol Clin North Am* 12:297, 1974.
152. Friedland RP, Jagust WJ, Ober BA, et al: The pathophysiology of Pick's disease: A comprehensive case study. *Neurology* 36(suppl 1):268, 1986.
153. Kamo H, McGeer PL, Harrop R, et al: Positron emission tomography and histopathology in Pick's disease. *Neurology* 37:439, 1987.
154. Bonte FJ, Hom J, Tintner R, et al: Single photon tomog-

raphy in Alzheimer's disease and the dementias. *Semin Nucl Med* 20:342, 1990.
155. Momose T, Kosaka N, Nishikawa J, et al: *N*-isopropyl I-123 *p*-iodoamphetamine (IMP) brain SPECT in dementia. *J Nucl Med* 25:1311, 1988.
156. Weinstein HC, Hijdra A, van Royen EA, et al: Determination of cerebral blood flow by SPECT: A valuable tool in the investigation of dementia? *Clin Neurol Neurosurg* 91:13, 1989.
157. Mesulam M-M: Slowly progressive aphasia without generalized dementia. *Ann Neurol* 11:592, 1982.
158. Heath PD, Kennedy P, Kapur N: Slowly progressive aphasia without generalized dementia. *Neurology* 13: 687, 1983.
159. Kirschner HS, Webb WG, Kelly MP, Wells CE: Language disturbance: An initial symptom of cortical degenerations and dementia. *Arch Neurol* 41:491, 1984.
160. Assal G, Favre C, Regli F: Aphasie dégénérative. *Rev Neurol (Paris)* 141:245, 1985.
161. Chawluk JB, Mesulam M-M, Hurtig H, et al: Slowly progressive aphasia without generalized dementia: Studies with positron emission tomography. *Ann Neurol* 19: 68, 1986.
162. Sapin LR, Anderson FH, Pulaski PD: Progressive aphasia without dementia: Further documentation. *Ann Neurol* 25:411, 1989.
163. Tyrell PJ, Warrington EK, Frackowiak RSJ, et al: Heterogeneity in progressive aphasia due to focal cortical atrophy. *Brain* 113:1321, 1990.
164. Kempler D, Metter EJ, Riege WH, et al: Slowly progressive aphasia: Three cases with language, memory, CT and PET data. *J Neurol Neurosurg Psychiatry* 53:987, 1990.
165. Newberg A, Alavi A, Souder E, et al: Quantitative PET and MRI analysis in patients with primary progressive aphasia (PPA). *J Nucl Med* 33:857, 1992.
166. Lee H, Kramer JH: Brain SPECT imaging in progressive aphasia. *Clin Nucl Med* 17:800, 1992.
167. Foster NL, Chase TN: Diffuse involvement in progressive aphasia. *Ann Neurol* 13:224, 1983.
168. Wechsler AF: Presenile dementia presenting as aphasia. *J Neurol Neurosurg Psychiatry* 40:303, 1977.
169. Pogacar S, Williams RS: Alzheimer's disease presenting as slowly progressive aphasia. *RI Med J* 67:181, 1984.
170. Holland AL, McBurney DH, Moossy J, Reinmuth OM: The dissolution of language in Pick's disease with neurofibrillary tangles: A case study. *Brain Lang* 24:36, 1985.
171. Greene JDW, Patterson K, Xuereb J, Hodges JR: Alzheimer disease and nonfluent progressive aphasia. *Arch Neurol* 53:1072, 1996.
172. Morris C, Cole M, Banker BG, Wright D: Hereditary dysphasic dementia and the Pick-Alzheimer spectrum. *Ann Neurol* 16:455, 1984.
173. Kirschner HS, Tanridag O, Thurman L, Whetsell WO Jr: Progressive aphasia without dementia: Two cases with focal spongiform degeneration. *Ann Neurol* 22:527, 1987.
174. Mehler MF, Horoupian DS, Dickson DW: Reduced somatostatin-like immunoreactivity in cerebral cortex in nonfamilial dysphasic dementia. *Neurology* 37:1448, 1987.
175. Beal MF, Mazurek MF, Svendsen CN, et al: Widespread reduction of somatostatin-like immunoreactivity in the cerebral cortex in Alzheimer's disease. *Ann Neurol* 20: 489, 1986.
176. Schneck SA, Hedley-White ET: Case records of the Massachusetts General Hospital: Case 49. *N Engl J Med* 309:1440, 1983.
177. Milton WJ, Atlas SW, Lavi E, Mollman JE: Magnetic resonance imaging of Creutzfeldt-Jakob disease. *Ann Neurol* 29:438, 1991.
178. Horowitz S, Benson DF, Kuhl DE: FDG scan to confirm Creutzfeldt-Jakob diagnosis. *Neurology* 32:2, 1982.
179. Friedland RP, Prusiner SB, Jagust WJ: Bitemporal hypometabolism in Creutzfeldt-Jakob disease measured by positron emission tomography with [^{18}F]-2-fluoro-deoxyglucose. *J Comput Assist Tomogr* 8:978, 1984.
180. Cohen D, Krausz Y, Lossos A, et al: Brain SPECT imaging with Tc-99m HM-PAO in Creutzfeldt-Jakob disease. *Clin Nucl Med* 14:808, 1989.
181. Mattman A, Feldman H, Forster B, et al: Regional HmPAO SPECT and CT measurements in the diagnosis of Alzheimer's disease. *Can J Neurol Sci* 24:22, 1997.
182. Gonzalez RG, Fischman AJ, Guimaraes AR, et al: Functional MR in the evaluation of dementia: Correlation of abnormal dynamic cerebral blood volume measurements with changes in cerebral metabolism on positron emission tomography with fluorodeoxyglucose F 18. *Am J Neuroradiol* 16:1763, 1995.
183. Sandson TA, O'Connor M, Sperling RA, et al: Noninvasive perfusion MRI in Alzheimer's disease: A preliminary report. *Neurology* 47:1339, 1996.
184. Gonzalez RG, Guimaraes AR, Moore GJ, et al: Quantitative in vivo ^{31}P magnetic resonance spectroscopy of Alzheimer disease. *Alzheimer Dis Assoc Disord* 10:46, 1996.
185. Tedeschi G, Bertolino A, Lundblom N, et al: Cortical and subcortical chemical pathology in Alzheimer's disease as assessed by multislice proton magnetic resonance spectroscopic imaging. *Neurology* 47:696, 1996.
186. Constans JM, Meyerhoff DJ, Gerson J, et al: H-1 MR spectroscopic imaging of white matter signal hyperintensities: Alzheimer disease and ischemic vascular dementia. *Radiology* 197:517, 1995.
187. Heun R, Schlegel S, Graf-Morgenstern M, et al: Proton magnetic resonance spectroscopy in dementia of Alzheimer type. *Int J Geriatr Psychiatry* 12:349, 1997.

PART THREE

THE MAJOR CATEGORIES OF NEUROLOGIC DISEASE

DISTURBANCES OF CEREBROSPINAL FLUID CIRCULATION, INCLUDING HYDROCEPHALUS AND MENINGEAL REACTIONS

Suzan Khoromi
Leon D. Prockop

INTRODUCTION

CSF Dynamics

Cerebrospinal fluid (CSF) is produced at the rate of 20 mL/h, or approximately 500 mL/day, in adults. Of this volume only 100 to 150 mL is retained, 25 mL of which is contained in the ventricular system. Most of this fluid is produced by the choroid plexus of the third, fourth, and especially the lateral ventricles.[1] Smaller amounts enter the CSF compartment from the ependymal and arachnoidal lining and perivascular spaces.[1] CSF flows from the lateral ventricles via the foramen of Monro to the third ventricle and through the aqueduct of Sylvius to the fourth ventricle, entering the cisterna magna via the foramen of Magendie, then passing superiorly into the subarachnoid space (SAS) over the cerebellar hemispheres, caudally into the spinal SAS, and cephalad into the prepontine and interpeduncular cisterns. CSF exiting the foramina of Luschka bathes the brainstem, the cerebellopontine angle, and the prepontine cisterns. From the basal cisterns, CSF travels superiorly, ultimately reaching the cerebral convexities and the dural sinuses. By bulk flow, CSF is absorbed in the arachnoid villi, which allow direct communication between CSF and the venous blood. The arachnoid villi consist of arachnoid granulations or pacchionian bodies. These villi are concentrated along the parasagittal regions of the cerebral cortex. Hydrostatic pressure differences between CSF and the venous sinus are the driving force for absorption of CSF into the arachnoid villi, along with diffusion into the brain and brain capillaries. The capacity for CSF absorption is 2 to 4 times greater than normal CSF synthesis.[2] The functions of CSF are many: providing protection and buoyancy to the central nervous system (CNS), transporting nutrients and metabolites, minimizing fluctuations in intracranial pressure, and accommodating rapid shifts in CSF volume.

Imaging Techniques

Historically, pneumoencephalography was used to study the ventricular system. This technique was abandoned in favor of computed tomography (CT) and magnetic resonance imaging (MRI) and their derivatives, such as cine MR, which is particularly helpful in investigating CSF flow dynamics. This technique is based on cardiac-gated, low-flip-angle, gradient-echo MRI in the mid-sagittal plane. Cardiac gating can be performed in a retrospective or a prospective manner. In the prospective form, the "cine frame rate" equals the repetition time (TR), which depends on the patient's RR interval. Acquisition starts immediately after the R wave and continues at approximately 50- to 75-ms intervals to within 200 ms of the next R wave. This information then is displayed in a closed-loop cine format.[3] Quantitative and qualitative assessments of CSF flow can be based on this technique. Qualitative cine MRI allows a rapid evaluation of CSF motion. Phase-contrast evaluation of CSF flow gives more quantitative information about CSF velocity and information about areas of slow CSF flow.[4] Figures 11-1A and B and 11-2A and B illustrate normal flow of CSF during the cardiac cycle. In cases where the basis of ventricular enlargement is unclear, that is, atrophic versus obstructive, cine MRI is a particularly valuable tool.

Clinicoanatomic correlations have been greatly facilitated by new techniques such as three-dimensional reconstruction. This method is based on information derived from T1-weighted, T2-weighted, and proton-density weighted images. "Feature vectors" are thus formed in which each pixel has attributes of all three sequences. These compiled data are then subjected to segmentation through pattern recognition which can be performed in a supervised, that is, operator-dependent, or unsupervised fashion. The disadvantage of the operator-dependent method is lack of reproducibility, and

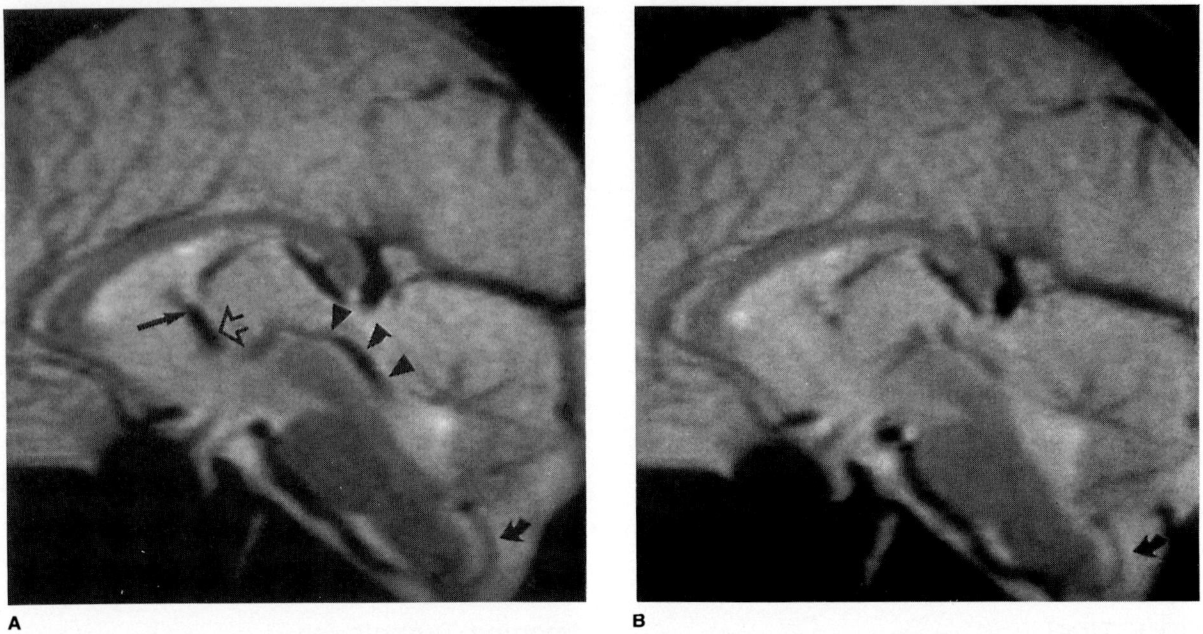

Figure 11-1

(A *and* **B)** *Normal CSF flow. Variation in the normal CSF flow pattern throughout the cardiac cycle is seen. Shortly after the peak of the R wave* **(A),** *marked hypointensity related to rapidly flowing CSF is seen starting at the level of the foramen of Monro (straight arrow), into the third ventricle (open arrow), and continuing throughout the length of the aqueduct of Sylvius (arrowheads). Later* **(B)** *in the cardiac cycle (during diastole), a greatly diminished flow void is identified in these regions, indicating a lessened velocity of CSF flow. The small curved arrows in* **A** *and* **B** *indicate the posterior inferior cerebellar artery, not flow out of the fourth ventricle. Evaluation of the multiframe sequence in a cine format disclosed a normal "to-and-fro" movement of CSF through the aqueduct. (Quencer RM: Intracranial CSF flow in pediatric hydrocephalus: Evaluation with cine-MR imaging.* AJNR *13:602–607, 1992.)*

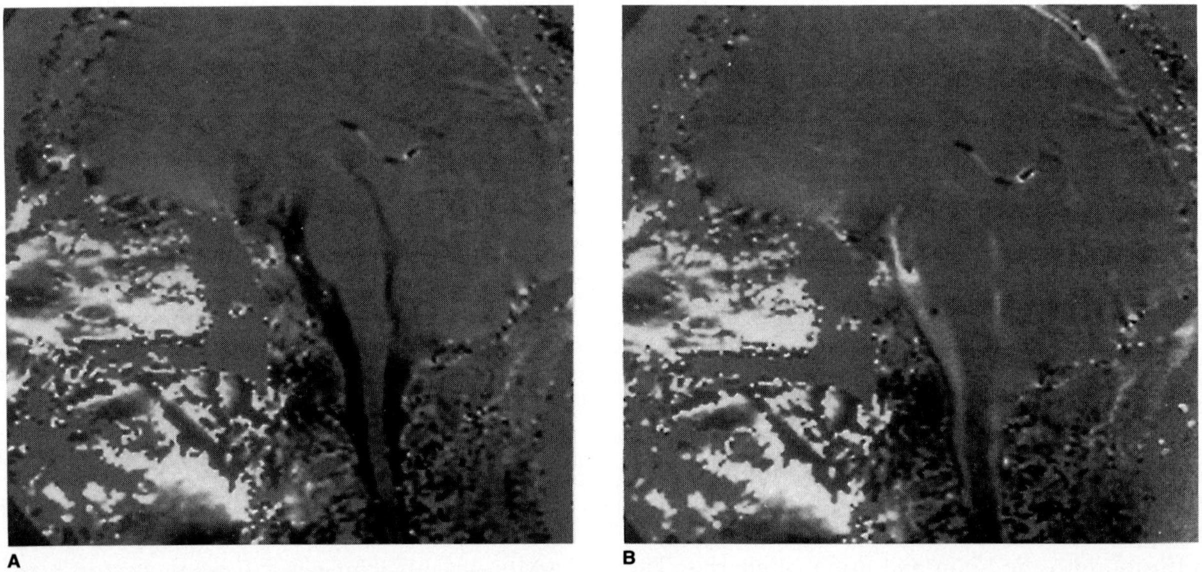

Figure 11-2

Normal CSF-phase imaging. With flow sensitization along the cranial to caudal axis, phase imaging in systole is hypointense **(A),** *indicating caudal flow of CSF within the cisterns, aqueduct, fourth ventricle, foramen of Magendie, and cervical subarachnoid space. This situation reverses in* **B,** *where cranial (retrograde) flow is identified as signal hyperintensity in the same structures. Whenever phase contrast imaging is performed and compared with magnitude imaging (e.g.,* **A** *and* **B***), phase imaging is seen to have greater sensitivity to areas of slower flow. (Quencer RM: Intracranial CSF flow in pediatric hydrocephalus: Evaluation with cine-MR imaging,* AJNR *13:602–607, 1992.)*

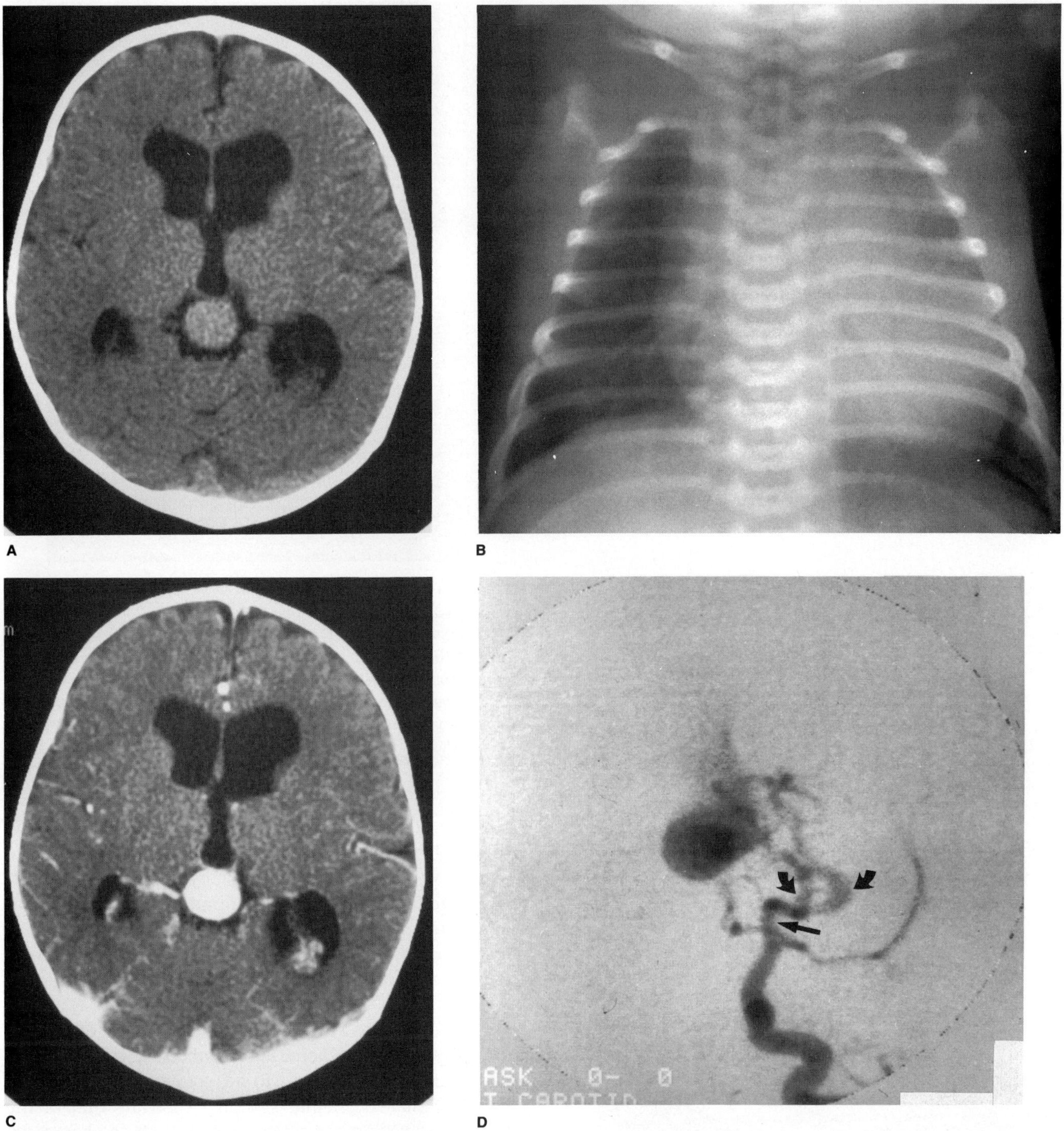

Figure 11-13

Vein of Galen aneurysm (galenic AVM). A 5-month-old presenting with increased head size and cranial bruit. **(A)** *Nonenhanced CT scan of the brain demonstrates a rounded, well-circumscribed lesion in the area of the vein of Galen. This is causing obstruction at the level of the cerebral aqueduct and dilatation of the third and lateral ventricles.* **(B)** *Chest x-ray shows predominantly right-sided cardiomegaly. The superior mediastinum is widened. The pulmonary vasculature is normal. There is no evidence of increased pulmonary perfusion to suggest a left-to-right shunt, nor is there any sign of pulmonary edema.* **(C)** *In the same patient, contrast-enhanced CT scan of the brain shows intense homogeneous enhancement, along with vessels feeding and/or draining the AVM. (Courtesy of Dr. J.C. Barnes, Department of Radiology, All Children's Hospital, St. Petersburg, Fla.)* **(D)** *digital subtraction angiography reveals a dilated posterior cerebral artery (straight arrow) with choroidal branches (curved arrows) supplying a vascular malformation. There was a rapid arteriovenous shunting into the dilated sac-like vein of Galen and straight sinus.*

ing hydrocephalus by compressing the cerebral aqueduct. These tumors include germinomas, pineocytomas, pineoblastomas, and teratomas. Pineocytomas and pineoblastomas originate from parenchymal cells. Lesions usually are well delineated on MRI and cranial CT. On contrasted CT, pineocytomas are iso- or hyperdense, occasionally associated with calcification. There is homogeneous enhancement with contrast. MRI abnormalities are profound but nonspecific.[10] Teratomas typically show calcifications on CT (Fig. 11-14).

Other common causes of CSF obstruction include intraventricular neoplasms occluding the foramen of Monro, the aqueduct of Sylvius, and the foramina of Luschka and Magendie.

Giant-cell astrocytomas, which are thought to arise from malignant transformation of subspendymal hamartomas, typically occur within the lateral ventricles. They are commonly associated with tuberous sclerosis and may or may not be calcified. CT without contrast will show an isodense or slightly hyperdense mass lesion, with enhancement after intravenous administration of contrast. The MRI appearance of a giant-cell astrocytoma is hypointense or isointense to normal brain tissue on T1-weighted images and hyperintense on T2-weighted images. With gadolinium, there is uniform enhancement of the tumor (Fig. 11-15). Because of their location in the proximity of the foramina of Monro, they often cause obstruction at this level, as is illustrated in Fig. 11-15.

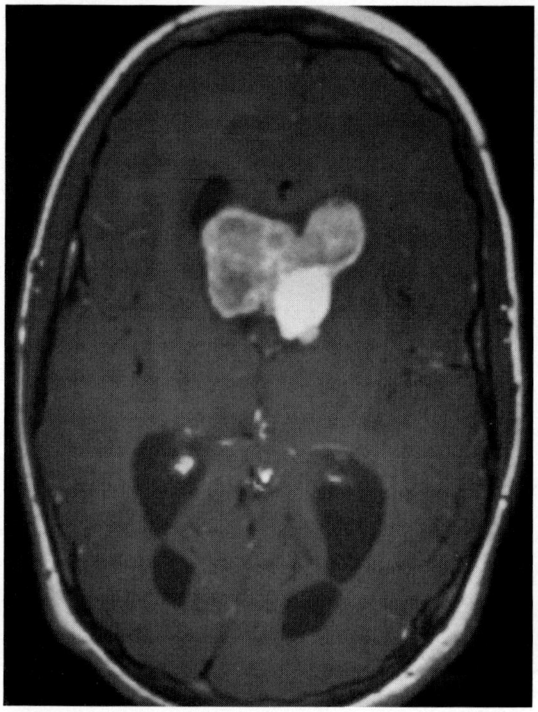

Figure 11-15
Tuberous sclerosis with giant-cell astrocytoma. Contrast-enhanced T1-weighted axial MRI of the brain demonstrates a large inhomogeneously enhancing tumor centered at the foramen of Monro and causing obstructive hydrocephalus. A subependymal nodule is visualized in the left lateral ventricle. The diagnosis was made at the time of surgery. (Courtesy of Dr. J.C. Barnes, Department of Radiology, All Children's Hospital, St. Petersburg, Fla.)

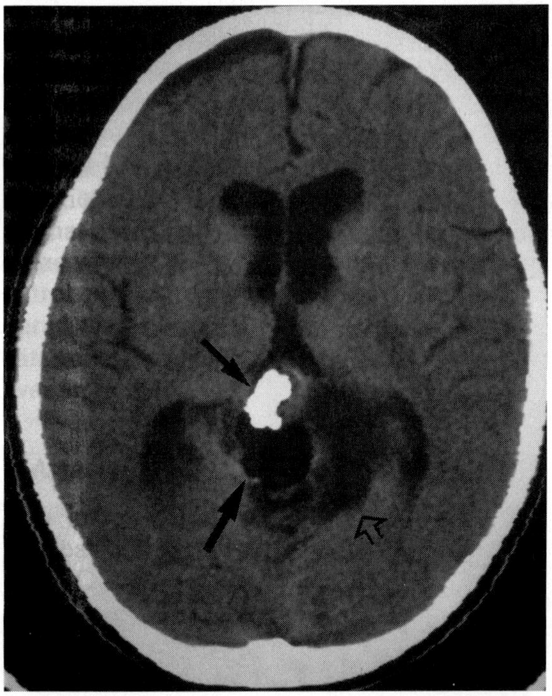

Figure 11-14
Teratoma of the pineal gland. Brain CT without contrast shows the presence of an inhomogeneous mass lesion posterior to the third ventricle and thalamus. It is predominantly inferior to the posterior aspect of the corpus callosum, mostly in the area of the pineal gland. Calcification is visualized within this lesion (short black arrow). The fatty portion of the tumor (long black arrow) is mostly seen extending behind the pineal gland, whereas the cystic component of the lesion bulges into the atrium of the left lateral ventricle (open arrow). Dilatation of the lateral and third ventricles most likely is due to obstruction at the level of the aqueduct of Sylvius. At surgery this mass proved to be a pineal gland teratoma. (Courtesy of Dr. J.C. Barnes, Department of Radiology, All Children's Hospital, St. Petersburg, Fla.)

Ependymomas (Fig. 11-16) typically have decreased intensity on T1 and increased signal on T2. In the pediatric population, they tend to arise from the ependymal lining of the ventricular system, especially that of the fourth and lateral ventricles. MRI reflects the heterogeneity of these tumors, which consist of cystic, calcified, and hemorrhagic regions.[10] Enhancement is speckled with gadolinium, as opposed to choroid plexus papillomas, which typically show diffuse enhancement.

Meningiomas also occur in the ventricular system on occasion. The glomus of the lateral ventricle is the most common site of occurrence of intraventricular meningiomas.[10] On CT, a reliable feature is homogeneously increased density.[11] On T1-weighted sequences, meningiomas may appear slightly hypo- to isointense with cerebral cortex. On T2-weighted images, they appear slightly hyper- to isointense. Intravenous contrast leads

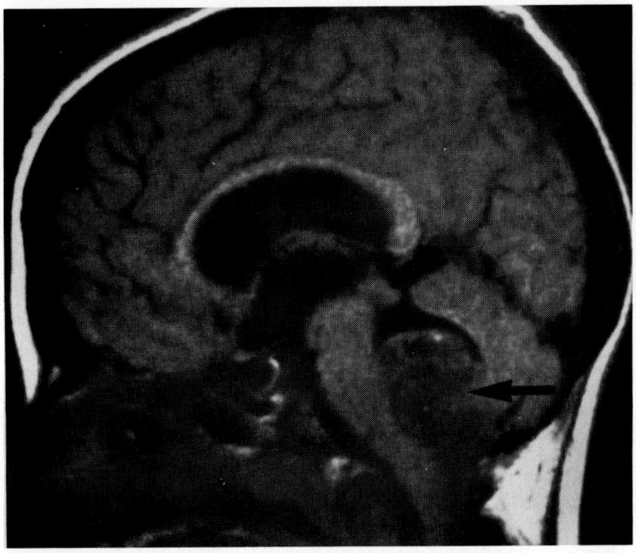

Figure 11-16
Ependymoma. A 12-year-old white male presenting with nausea, vomiting, and headaches. T1-weighted sagittal MRI shows a lobulated, mostly hypointense mass (arrow) occupying most of the fourth ventricle and causing hydrocephalic dilatation of the third and lateral ventricles. Biopsy obtained at time of surgery was consistent with an ependymoma. (Courtesy of Dr. J.C. Barnes, Department of Radiology, All Children's Hospital, St. Petersburg, Fla.)

to a marked signal increase in T1-weighted sequences (Fig. 11-17). The presence of hydrocephalus is less common than is the case with choroid plexus papillomas.

Colloid cysts commonly occur at the level of the third ventricle, yielding a characteristic MRI presentation (Fig. 11-18). They account for 0.5 to 2 percent of all intracranial tumors.[9] The cyst usually contains break-

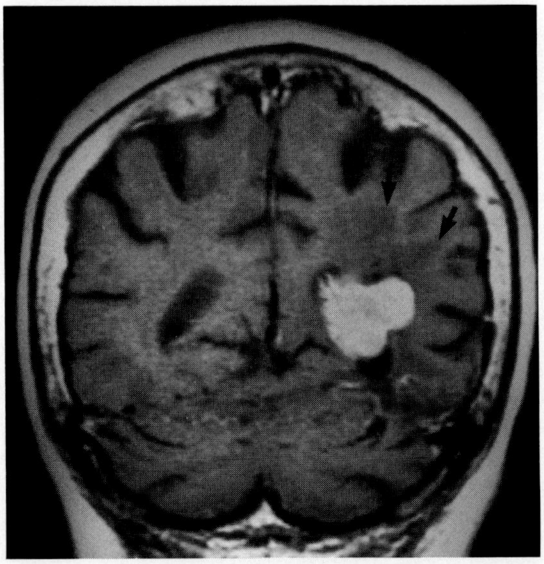

Figure 11-17
Intraventricular meningioma. T1-weighted coronal MRI of the brain with gadolinium shows the presence of a diffusely hyperintense mass in the atrium of the left lateral ventricle causing dilatation of the left lateral ventricle. Periventricular edema is noted (arrows).

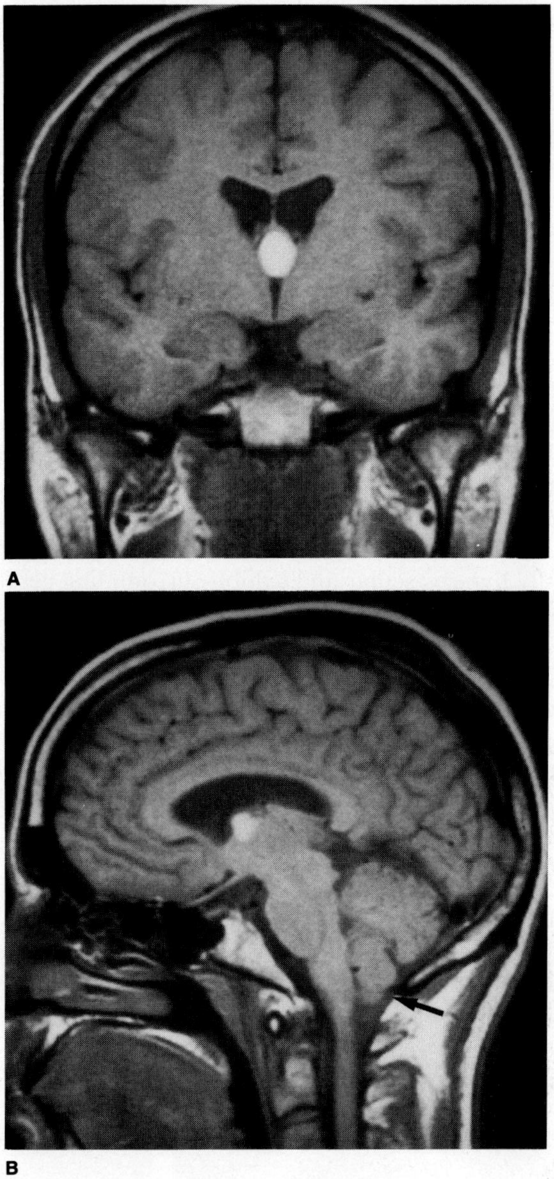

Figure 11-18
Colloid cyst and Arnold-Chiari I malformation. **(A)** *Coronal T1-weighted MRI of the brain demonstrates a well-circumscribed mass situated within the third ventricle with partial compression of the foramina of Monro bilaterally; mild dilatation of the lateral ventricles is noted. The homogeneously hyperintense nature of this lesion on T1-is characteristic of a colloid cyst.* **(B)** *Sagittal T1-weighted MRI also shows the presence of tonsillar ectopia consistent with a type I Chiari malformation (arrow).*

down products of the epithelial lining of the cyst, old blood, hemosiderin-laden macrophages, cholesterol, and CSF. Variation in the contents of the cyst account for various densities on MRI. On CT colloid cysts usually show hyperdensity, and on MRI signal intensity varies according to content. Contrasted CT may or may not show enhancement. When obstructive hydrocephalus is present, periventricular interstitial edema may be visualized on CT.

Mass Lesions with Increased CSF Production

Choroid plexus papilloma and carcinoma account for 0.5 to 0.6 percent of all intracranial tumors.[9] These tumors share with normal choroid plexus the property of CSF production and thus can cause hydrocephalus through excess CSF synthesis. CT without contrast usually shows a lobulated mass of increased density, which enhances markedly with contrast (Fig. 11-19A,B,C).[11] Calcification and hemorrhage may be present and detectable on CT. MRI signal characteristics of choroid plexus papilloma are intermediate signal on T1-weighted images and intermediate to increased signal on T2 W sequences. Communicating hydrocephalus is another characteristic feature. Choroid plexus carcinomas are found mainly in infants and children, typically originating in one of the lateral ventricles.[8] They are usually hypervascular and exhibit surrounding cerebral edema and midline shift. Hydrocephalus is present but is not always as pronounced as it is with choroid plexus papilloma. This can result not only from CSF overproduction but from obstruction of the CSF pathways. Spread through the CSF pathway is also common; MRI with gadolinium will show characteristic enhancement.

Congenital Abnormalities

Congenital syndromes such as Arnold-Chiari (A-C) malformation also are associated with particular abnormalities of the ventricular system and hydrocephalus. A-C malformation can present with obstruction of the aqueduct of Sylvius. The MRI may show absence of flow void in the cerebral aqueduct, but flow can be seen in the inferior portion of the fourth ventricle.[4] Aqueductal stenosis may cause only partial obstruction if there is forking or membrane formation.

However, if complete, it can cause enlargment of the lateral and third ventricles. Arnold-Chiari malformation (A-C MF) is classified into four groups, mostly according to the severity of tonsillar herniation. In A-C MF type I the hydrocephalus is usually not present, whereas in A-C MF type II midsagittal MRI (Fig. 11-20A and B) characteristically shows elongation and caudal displacement of the cerebellar vermis, cerebellar tonsils, and caudal fourth ventricle through the foramen magnum into the cervical canal. The dorsal part of the medulla is also displaced caudally, producing a "kink" at the cervicomedullary junction.[12] The diagnosis can be made if cerebellar tonsils extend more than 5 mm below the foramen magnum. Other parameters include a sagittal diameter of the foramen magnum greater than 42 mm. In an MRI study comparing normal controls with patients with A-C MF, the tip of the cerebellar tonsils in the latter group was found to be on average 10.3 mm below the foramen magnum versus 2.9 mm above the foramen in the normal controls.[12] Up to 2 mm of protrusion below the foramen magnum is considered insignificant.[13] Types II and III A-C malformations are commonly associated with obstructive hydrocephalus as a result of elongation or stenosis of the cerebral aqueduct or as a result of narrowing, stretching, and compression of the fourth ventricle. Cine MR is helpful in answering several questions about CSF flow in A-C MF, including (1) patency of the cerebral aqueduct and the fourth ventricular foramina to CSF flow, (2) the significance

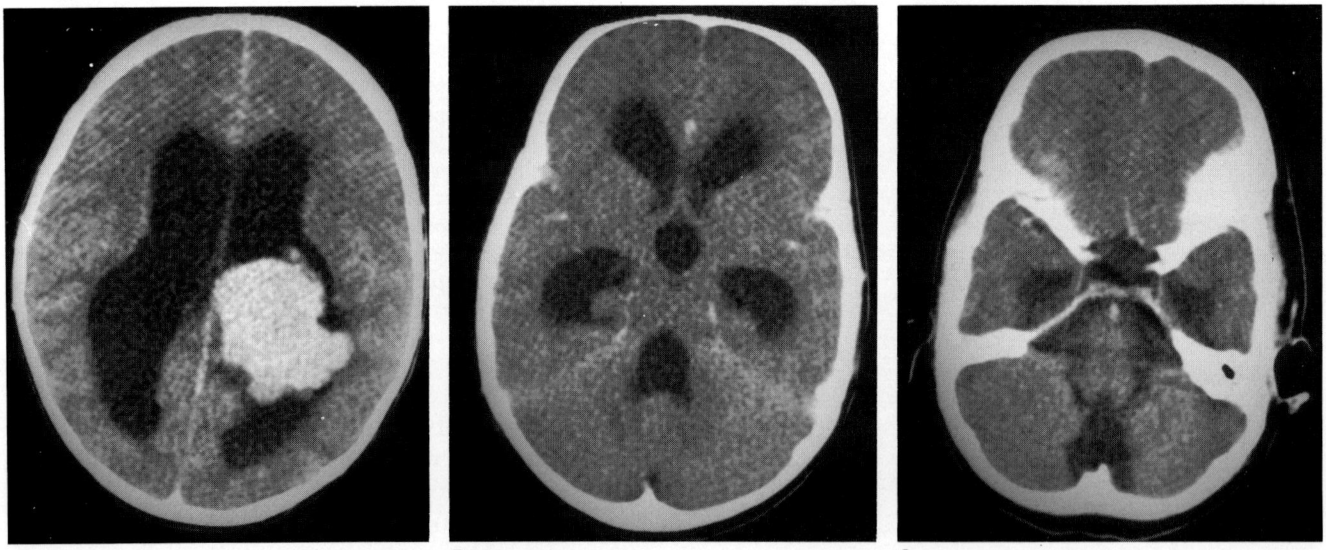

A B C

Figure 11-19

Choroid plexus carcinoma. CT with contrast shows **(A)** *marked enhancement of a lobulated mass within the atrium of the left lateral ventricle.* **(B)** *Diffuse ventricular enlargement involving the lateral, third, and fourth ventricles.* **(C)** *Prominence of the basilar cisterns. At surgery, the tissue diagnosis was choroid plexus carcinoma.*

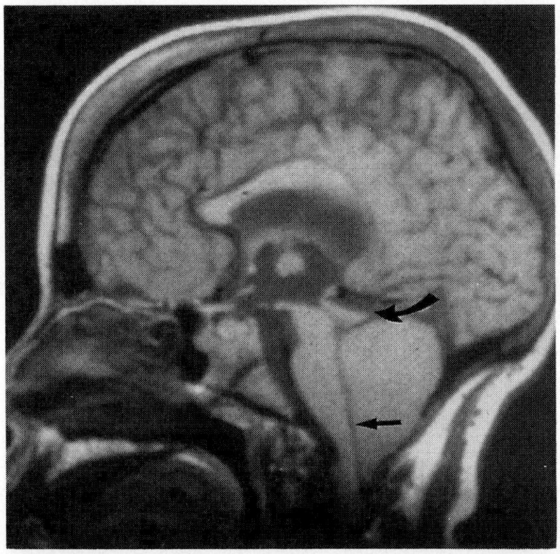

A

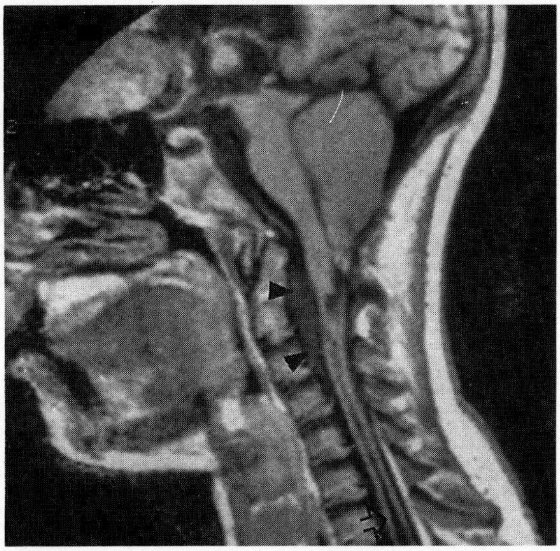

B

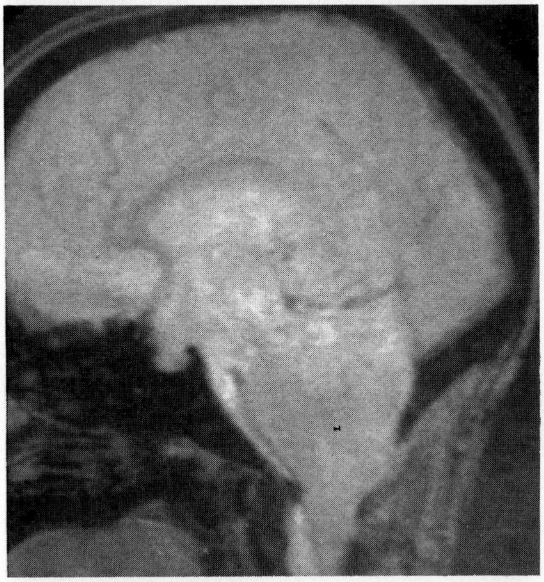

C

Figure 11-20

(A–E) *Chiari II malformation with syringohydromyelia. The classic findings of the Chiari II malformation are shown in* **A** *and* **B***; these include an elongated (closed arrow) and an inferiorly displaced fourth ventricle, a featureless and caudally displaced cerebellum, a beaked tectum (curved arrow), a kinked and displaced medulla, partial absence of the corpus callosum, and a syringohydromyelic cavity. Closed arrowheads in* **B** *indicate the CSF collection anterior to the cord at* C_2. *An open arrow indicates the syrinx. In* **C** *no flow is noted at the level of the foramen of Magendie or in the dorsal cervical subarachnoid space (SAS). In* **D,** *the low-lying cerebellar tissue impacted at the foramen magnum and* C_1 *level directs the bulk of CSF flow inferiorly in the anterior SAS (solid arrows). The anterior arachnoid cyst at* C_2 *appears isolated from the adjacent CSF flow within the syringohydromyelic cavity in* **D** *(open arrows). In* **E** *(later in the cardiac cycle), flow in the anterior SAS at* C_2 *and* C_3 *is not seen (compare* **D** *with* **E***) (and there is a diminished flow void in the syrinx cavity). This was more convincingly demonstrated on the cine display, where to-and-fro movement of CSF was clearly seen. (Quencer RM: Intracranial CSF flow in pediatric hydrocephalus: Evaluation with cine-MR imaging.* AJNR *13:602–607, 1992.)*

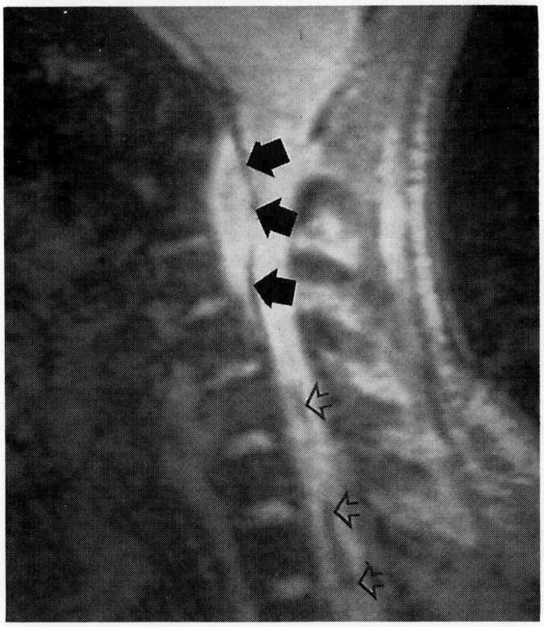

D

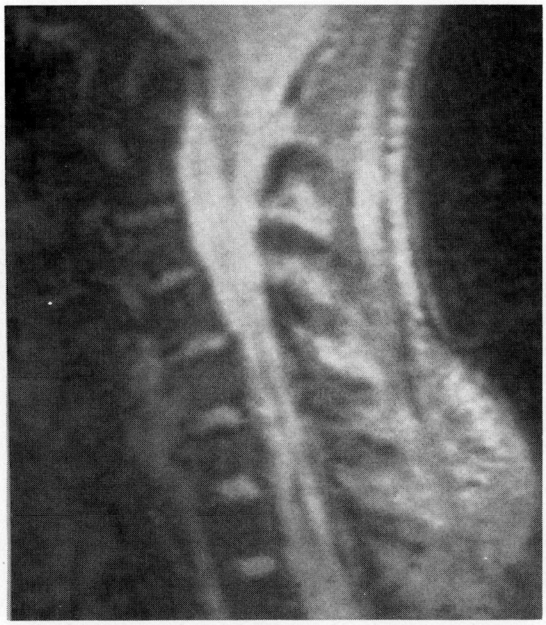

E

of CSF flow in the syrinx, if present, and (3) whether CSF collection anterior to the cervical cord communicates with the adjacent subarachnoid space (Fig. 11-20C to E). Type IV consists of a single abnormality, hypoplasia of the cerebellum.

Other developmental anomalies associated with A-C MF include meningomyelocele, heterotopias, polymicrogyria, agenesis of the corpus callosum, platybasia, syringomyelia, and Klippel-Feil syndrome.

The degree of herniation of the brainstem into the cervical canal and the associated hydrocephalus are critical parameters for surgical intervention. However, aqueductal stenosis may occur without other abnormalities. Cine MR is particularly helpful in cases in which enlarged lateral ventricles coexist with a normal fourth ventricle (Fig. 11-21).

The Dandy-Walker (D-W) complex is another syndrome with associated ventricular malformation and hydrocephalus. Here the abnormality consists of marked cystic dilatation of the fourth ventricle communicating with an enlarged posterior fossa and partial or complete agenesis of the cerebellar vermis with anterosuperior displacement of a small cerebellum (Fig. 11-22). In addition, the cerebral aqueduct and the supratentorial ventricles may be dilated, the brainstem hypoplastic, and the corpus callosum partially or completely absent (Fig. 11-22). The fourth ventricular foramina may be patent or occluded.[14] D-W complex is probably a developmental anomaly of rhombencephalic midline structures that occurs before the sixth or seventh week of gestation as a result of in utero insult to the cerebellum and the fourth ventricle.[15] Proposed etiologies include chromosomal abnormalities[16] and infectious agents such as cytomegalovirus, rubella, and toxoplasma as well as chemical factors. Over 80 percent of patients with D-W present with hydrocephalus at a young age, in 75 percent by 3 months.[14]

The site of obstruction varies. In a series by Carmel and associates[17] obstruction was due to aqueductal stenosis in 28 percent of cases, to communication between the third ventricle and the cyst in 72 percent, to obstruction of the incisure in 11 percent, and to obstruction distal to the fourth ventricular foramina in 39 percent. If the lateral ventricles are shunted in the presence of aqueductal stenosis, upward herniation of the fourth ventricular cyst may occur. However, hydrocephalus is not always present.[18] Other CNS abnormalities include cerebral gyral malformations, occipital encephaloceles, aqueductal stenosis, and malformation of the inferior olives. Figure 11-23 shows a classical D-W cyst. MRI also may show absence of the inferior vermis, superior displacement of the cerebellar vermis between the tentorial incisure and the quadrigeminal region, downward displacement of the floor of the fourth ventricle, absence

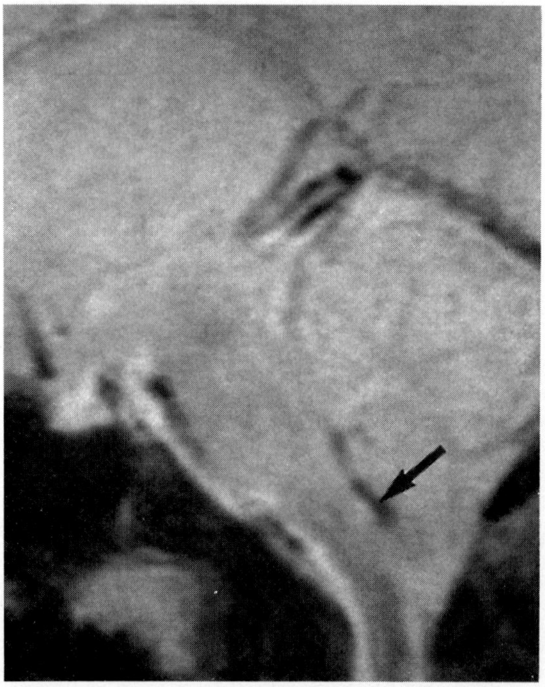
A

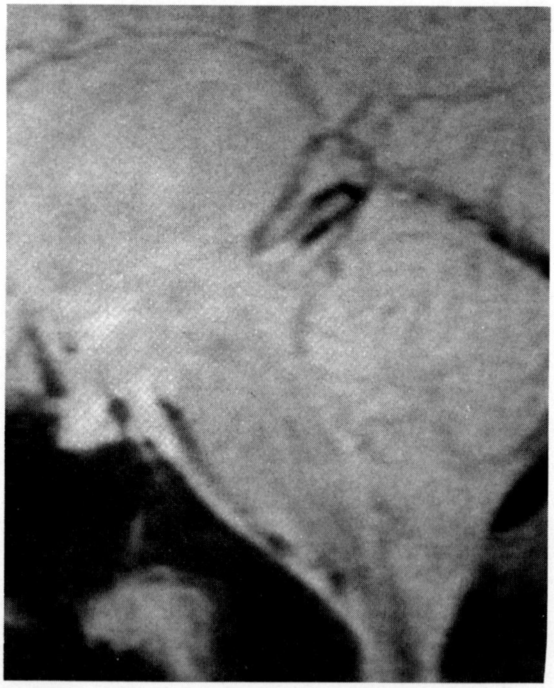
B

Figure 11-21

(A *and* **B)** *Aqueductal stenosis. Here frames from a 12-frame cine study in systole* **(A)** *and diastole* **(B)** *show no evidence of aqueductal flow. Nonetheless, flow out of the fourth ventricle (arrows in* **A***) is seen. This is consistent with aqueductal stenosis. (Figure reprinted from* Neuroradiology *32:371–391, 1990.) (Quencer RM: Intracranial CSF flow in pediatric hydrocephalus: Evaluation with cine-MR imaging.* AJNR *13:602–607, 1992.)*

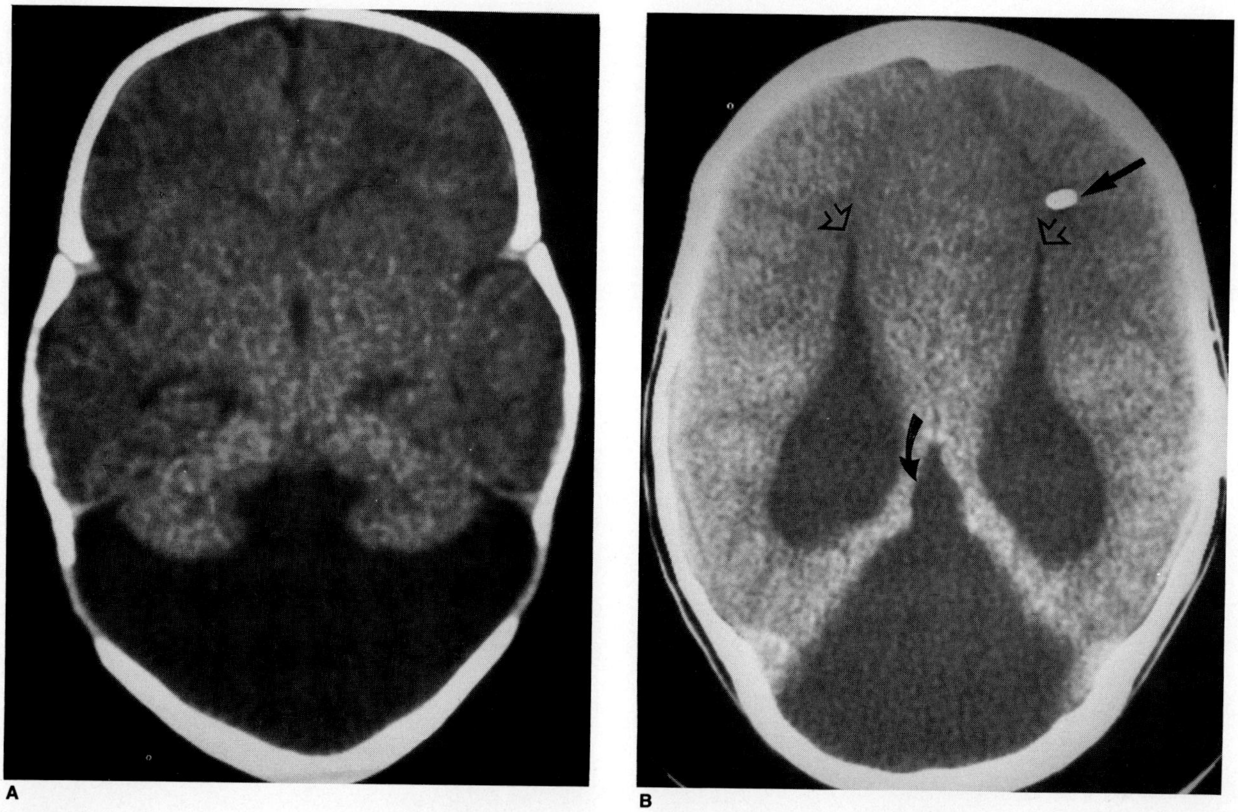

A B

Figure 11-22

Dandy-Walker syndrome. **(A)** *Head CT without contrast shows a very large low-density extra-axial fluid collection in the posterior fossa. There is no identifiable fourth ventricle separate from this fluid collection. The cerebellar hemispheres are hypoplastic, and the vermis is absent.* **(B)** *Agenesis of the corpus callosum, a common abnormality associated with Dandy-Walker syndrome, is present in this patient, who has a ventriculopleural shunt (arrow). The agenesis is demonstrated by the wide separation of the lateral ventricles with beaking of the frontal horns (open arrows) and the interposition of the third ventricle (curved arrow) between the lateral ventricles. In this case, the third ventricle appears to communicate with the cyst. (Courtesy of Dr. J.C. Barnes, Department of Radiology, All Children's Hospital, St. Petersburg, Fla.)*

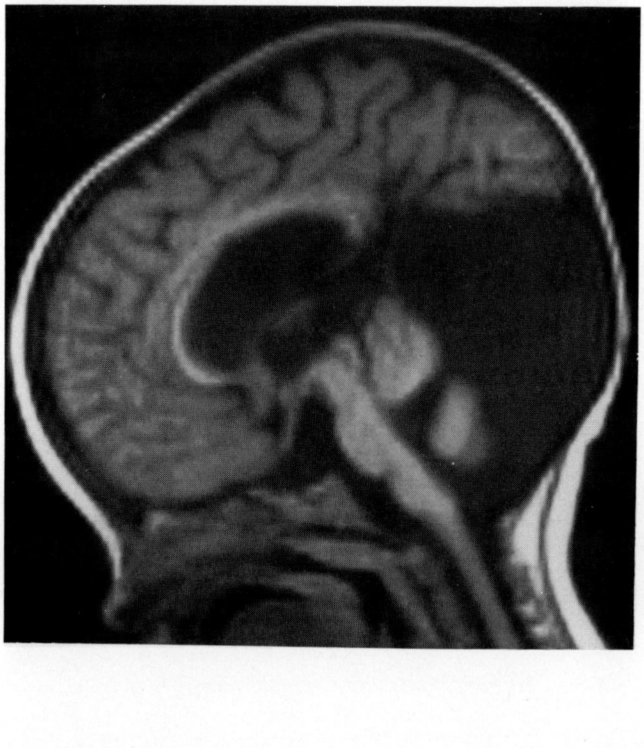

Figure 11-23

Dandy-Walker cyst. Sagittal T1-weighted MRI of the brain demonstrates an enlarged ventricular system with a thin cortical mantle. The posterior fossa contains a large cyst communicating with the fourth ventricle, diagnostic of a Dandy-Walker cyst. (Courtesy of Dr. J.C. Barnes, Department of Radiology, All Children's Hospital, St. Petersburg, Fla.)

of torcular-lambdoid inversion, and elevation of the straight sinus.[19] Sonography may detect the D-W syndrome prenatally.[20] Transverse planes show a posterior fossa cyst and splaying of the cerebellar hemispheres.

A D-W variant has an expanded fourth ventricular roof that communicates with a cisterna magna of variable size. These cysts tend to be of a smaller size than are standard D-W cysts.[21] Furthermore, hypoplasia of the inferior cerebellar vermis is often present, and the fourth ventricle is smaller and better formed than it is in standard cases.[18] The variant also may be accompanied by hydrocephalus. Cine MR may help establish whether obstruction is present at the level of the aqueduct or that of the cyst and/or fourth ventricular outlets (Fig. 11-24A to C). The D-W complex should be distinguished from other cystic anomalies of the posterior fossa, such as a posterior fossa arachnoid cyst and a giant cisterna magna. In the case of an arachnoid cyst, a normally sized but displaced fourth ventricle does not communicate with the cyst. Likewise, the cerebellar vermis is normal but may be displaced.[8] The cyst is unilocular, round, oval, or crescentic. The cyst fluid has

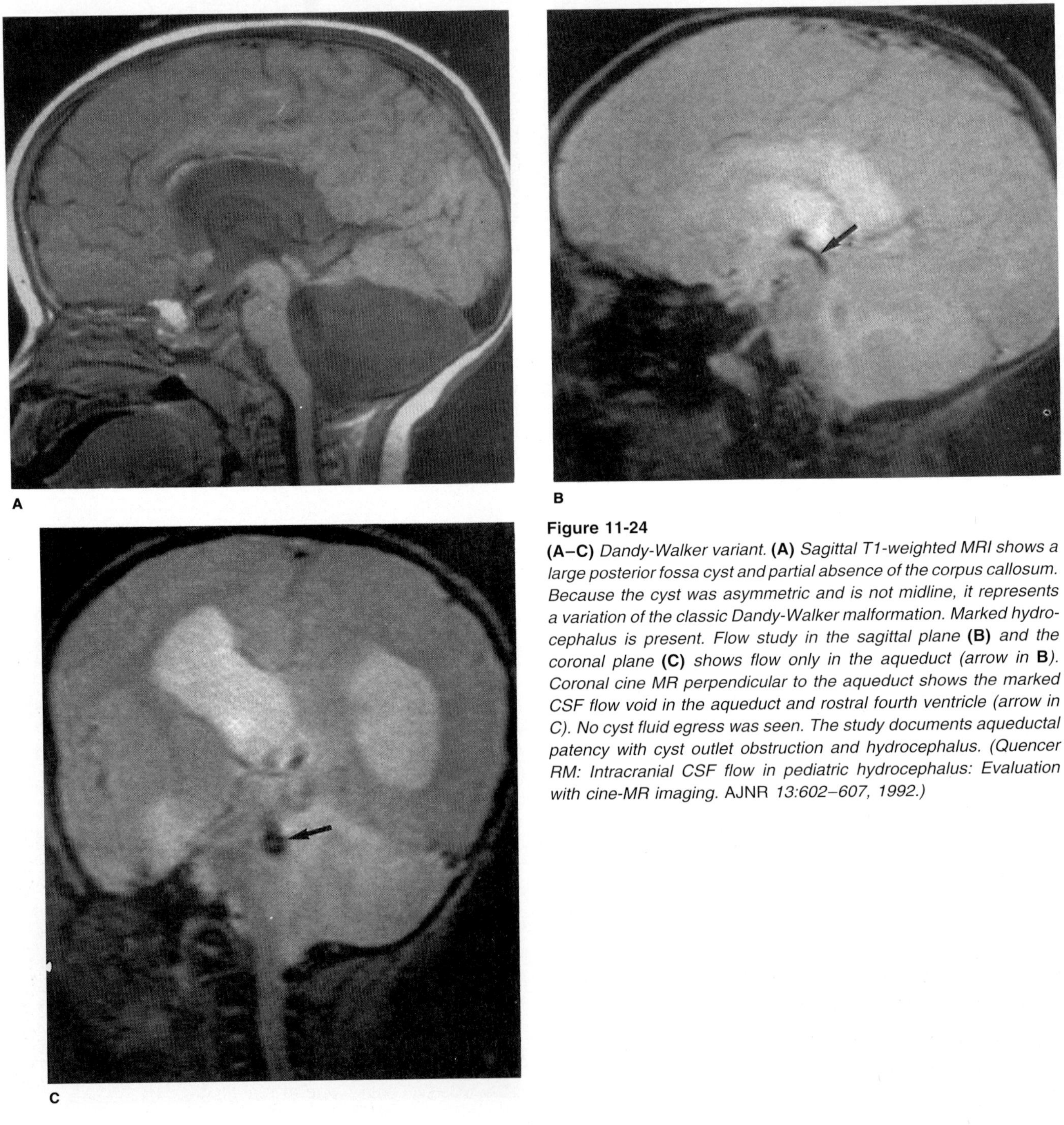

A

B

C

Figure 11-24

(A–C) *Dandy-Walker variant.* **(A)** *Sagittal T1-weighted MRI shows a large posterior fossa cyst and partial absence of the corpus callosum. Because the cyst was asymmetric and is not midline, it represents a variation of the classic Dandy-Walker malformation. Marked hydrocephalus is present. Flow study in the sagittal plane* **(B)** *and the coronal plane* **(C)** *shows flow only in the aqueduct (arrow in* **B***). Coronal cine MR perpendicular to the aqueduct shows the marked CSF flow void in the aqueduct and rostral fourth ventricle (arrow in C). No cyst fluid egress was seen. The study documents aqueductal patency with cyst outlet obstruction and hydrocephalus. (Quencer RM: Intracranial CSF flow in pediatric hydrocephalus: Evaluation with cine-MR imaging.* AJNR *13:602–607, 1992.)*

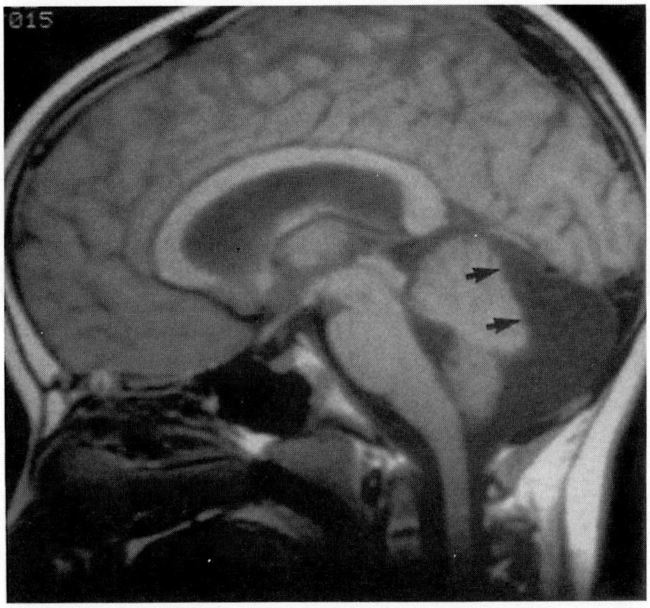

A

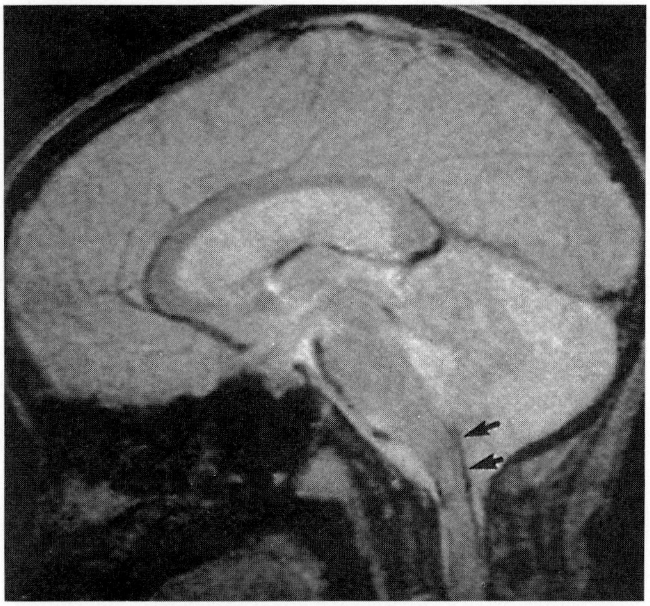

B

Figure 11-25
(A *and* **B)** *giant cisterna magna vs. arachnoid cyst. Despite absence of mass effect on the fourth ventricle or brainstem, the flattening of the posterior surface of the cerebellum (arrowheads in* **A***) suggested the presence of an arachnoid cyst and possible fourth ventricular outlet obstruction. Sagittal cine MR* **(B)** *clearly shows flow out of the fourth ventricle into the cisterna magna (arrows in* **B***). (Quencer RM: Intracranial CSF flow in pediatric hydrocephalus: Evaluation with cine-MR imaging.* AJNR *13:602–607, 1992.)*

nearly CSF intensity by MRI (Fig. 11-25A). The mega cisterna magna is characterized by an enlarged cisterna magna and an enlarged bony posterior fossa. The fourth ventricle communicates with the SAS, but unlike the D-W malformation, the brainstem and the cerebellum are usually normal and hydrocephalus is absent.[21]

Cine MR may distinguish between giant cisterna magna and posterior fossa arachnoid cyst (Fig. 11-25B).

Infectious and Inflammatory Processes

Inflammatory and infectious processes also may cause impairment of CSF flow. Among parasitic infections, cysticercosis has varied appearances. Neurocysticercosis is classified into four types: parenchymal, meningeal (subarachnoid), intraventricular, and mixed.[10] MRI is more sensitive than CT in detecting parenchymal and subarachnoid lesions. Intraventricular cysts may be present in the absence of parenchymal cysts (Fig. 11-26A,B,C). Typically, these cysts are 10 to 20 mm in diameter and are iso- to hyperintense to CSF. The presence of proteinaceous material within the degenerating cysts may appear hyperintense on both short and long TR images.[10] Enhancement of the basal cisterns and of the ependymal lining as a result of granulomatous meningitis also can be demonstrated on MRI with contrast as represented by an ependymal rim of hyperintensity (Fig. 11-26C). Cysticercus lesions also may be present in the basal subarachnoid cisterns (Fig. 11-26B), appearing as large "grape-like clusters" also known as racemose cysts.[10] They usually are located at the cerebellopontine angle or in the suprasellar cisterns. MRI also can demonstrate extraventricular hydrocephalus that is present as a result of parasitic infestation of the subarachnoid space.

Tuberculosis (TB), a granulomatous infection, may present with hydrocephalus. Granulomatous meningitis has a predilection for the basal cisterns. Unenhanced CT scans may demonstrate obliteration of the basal cisterns secondary to meningeal hyperemia or subarachnoid exudate. Blockage of the basal cisterns by this inflammatory exudate can cause EVOH. Purulent exudate causes obstructive hydrocephalus as a result of granulomatous ependymitis.[8] In partially treated meningitis, cellular debris blocks the ventricular outlets or CSF flow through the basal cisterns,[22] with resultant hydrocephalus. Postcontrast leptomeningeal enhancement reflects the inflammatory reaction to bacteria and the granulation tissue caused by cell-mediated response (Fig. 11-27). Cine MR may further elucidate EVOH in TB meningitis (Fig. 11-28A to D).

Neonatal purulent meningitis also may present with ventriculitis. The bacterial inflammatory response of ependymal lining causes obstruction of the aqueduct of Sylvius, increased intracranial pressure, and brainstem herniation. Viral encephalitis secondary to toxoplasma, rubella, cytomegalovirus (CMV), and herpes (TORCH) may also cause hydrocephalus. CMV commonly causes congenital microcephaly.[23] However, hydrocephalus is also one of many CNS sequelae of CMV

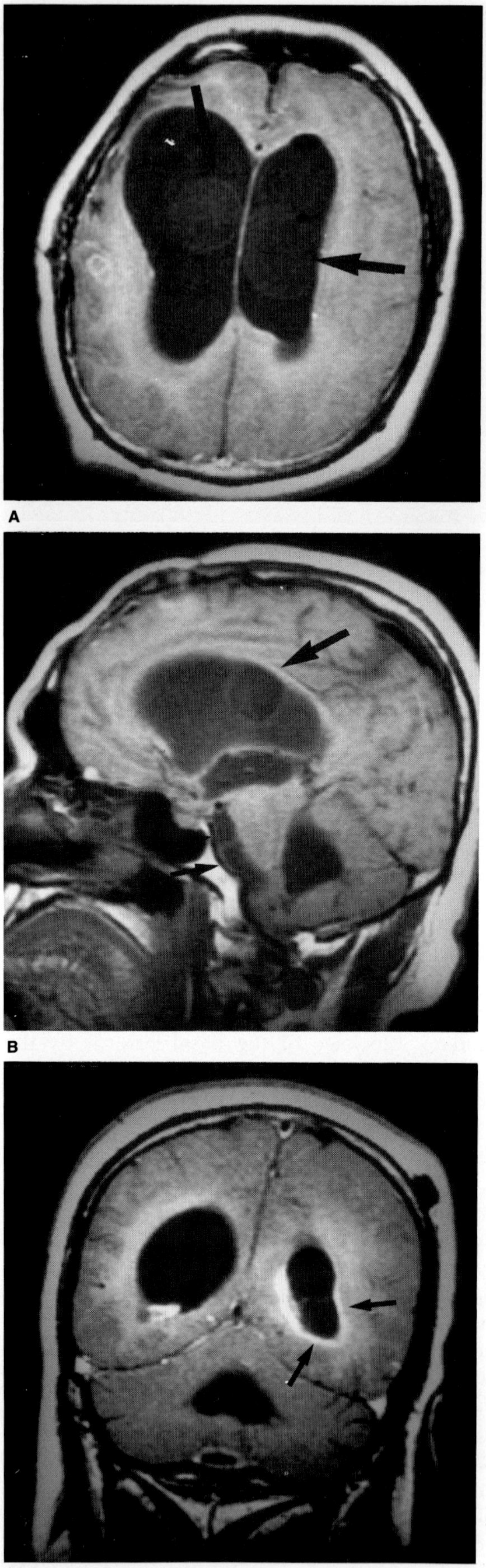

A

B

C

Figure 11-26
Intraventricular cysticercus. T1-weighted axial **(A)** *image with T1-weighted sagittal* **(B)** *image without gadolinium in a patient with several episodes of cysticercus meningitis demonstrating several distinct intraventricular cysts, two in the left lateral ventricle and one in the right lateral ventricle (long black arrows). Additional cysts are seen in the prepontine cistern extending into both cerebellopontine angles (short black arrows).* **(C)** *After contrast injection, T1-weighted coronal image shows mild ependymal enhancement (black arrows) and synechia within the ventricles. Marked dilatation of the lateral, third, and fourth ventricles is also noted. Hyperintensity in the periventricular white matter is suggestive of the interstitial edema frequently associated with obstructive hydrocephalus. (Tip of ventriculoperitoneal shunt is also noted.) (Courtesy of Dr. C. Martinez, Department of Radiology, USF, Tampa, Fla.)*

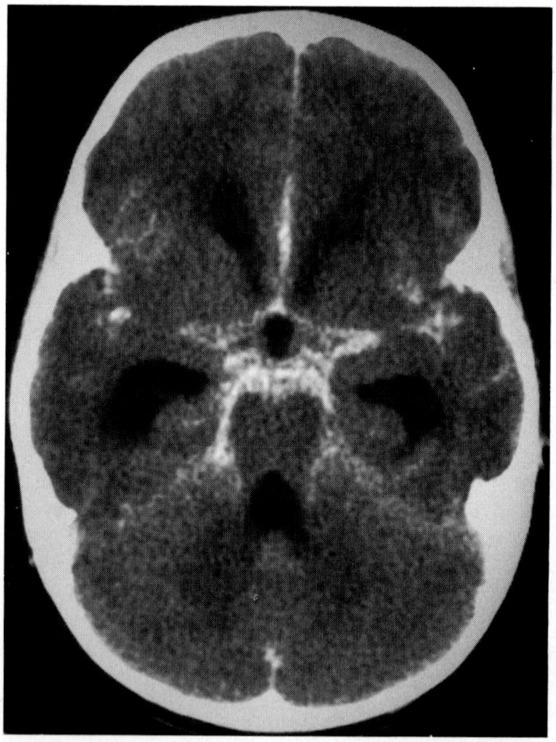

Figure 11-27
Tuberculous meningitis with obstructive hydrocephalus: A 3-year-old child previously treated for tuberculous meningitis presented with recurrent meningeal symptoms and signs. Brain CT with contrast shows prominent enhancement of the prepontine cisterns with dilated lateral, third, and fourth ventricles consistent with EVOH. (Courtesy of Dr. J.C. Barnes, Department of Radiology, All Children's Hospital, St. Petersburg, Fla.)

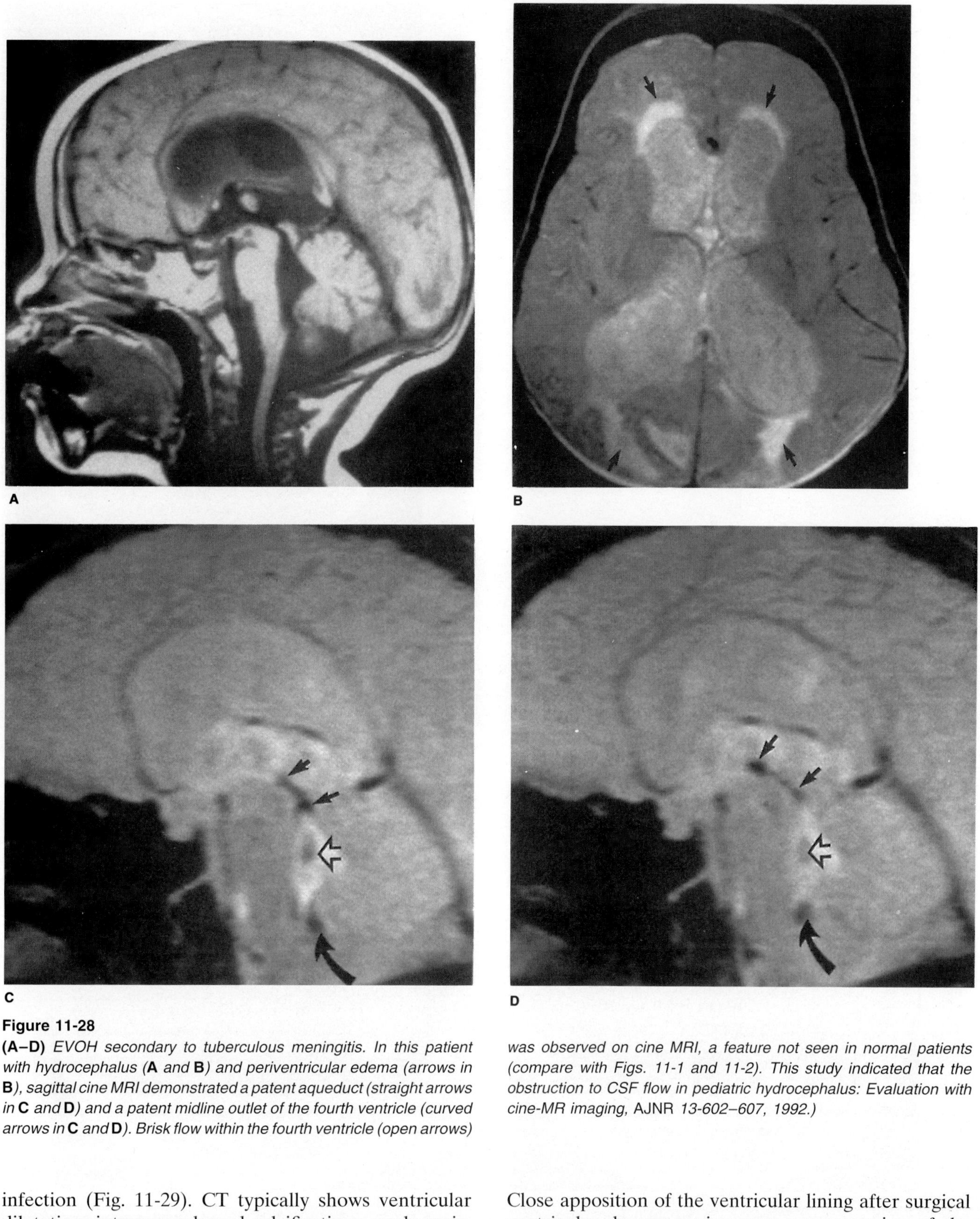

Figure 11-28

(A–D) *EVOH secondary to tuberculous meningitis. In this patient with hydrocephalus (***A** *and* **B***) and periventricular edema (arrows in* **B***), sagittal cine MRI demonstrated a patent aqueduct (straight arrows in* **C** *and* **D***) and a patent midline outlet of the fourth ventricle (curved arrows in* **C** *and* **D***). Brisk flow within the fourth ventricle (open arrows) was observed on cine MRI, a feature not seen in normal patients (compare with Figs. 11-1 and 11-2). This study indicated that the obstruction to CSF flow in pediatric hydrocephalus: Evaluation with cine-MR imaging,* AJNR *13-602–607, 1992.)*

infection (Fig. 11-29). CT typically shows ventricular dilatation, intraparenchymal calcifications, pachygyria, and cerebral or cerebellar atrophy. Ventriculitis occasionally causes entrapment of part of the ventricular system (Fig. 11-30). Chemical reactions and inflammation may be associated with foreign bodies or blood. Close apposition of the ventricular lining after surgical ventricular decompression may cause scarring of the ependymal linings and adhesions that lead to ventricular distortion (Fig. 11-31).

Subdural effusion, another complication of meningitis, rarely occurs if meningitis is responsive to antibiotics.

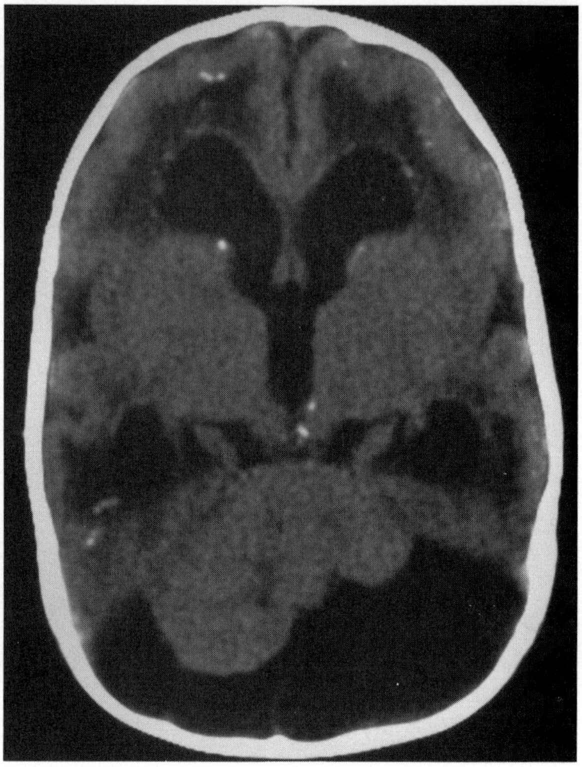

Figure 11-29

Congenital CMV encephalitis. In a 1-month-old infant with congenital CMV and intrauterine growth retardation, nonenhanced brain CT demonstrates ventricular dilatation with areas of low attenuation surrounding the ventricles. These areas represent encephalomalacia. Multiple calcifications are visualized throughout the brain, including the periventricular area and the corticomedullary junction. Hypoplasia of the left cerebellar hemisphere is also present. (Courtesy of Dr. J.C. Barnes, Department of Radiology, All Children's Hospital, St. Petersburg, Fla.)

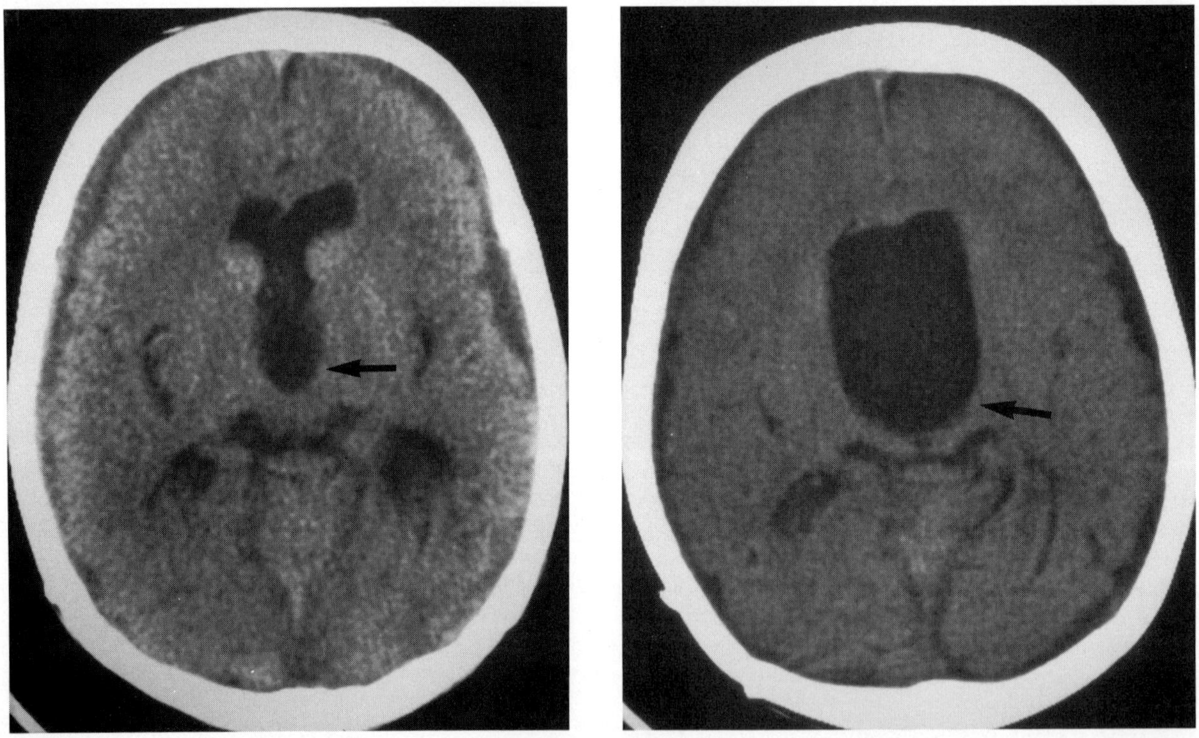

A

B

Figure 11-30

Ventriculitis with a trapped third ventricle. **(A)** *A brain CT in a 4-year-old boy treated by ventriculoperitoneal (VP) shunt at birth for hydrocephalus of unknown etiology shows dilatation of the third (arrow) and lateral ventricles. Shortly after this CT, another VP shunt decompressed the obstructed ventricles.* **(B)** *Brain CT in the same patient at age 6 shows marked dilatation of the third ventricle only (arrow), representing a trapped third ventricle. This child required another shunt.*

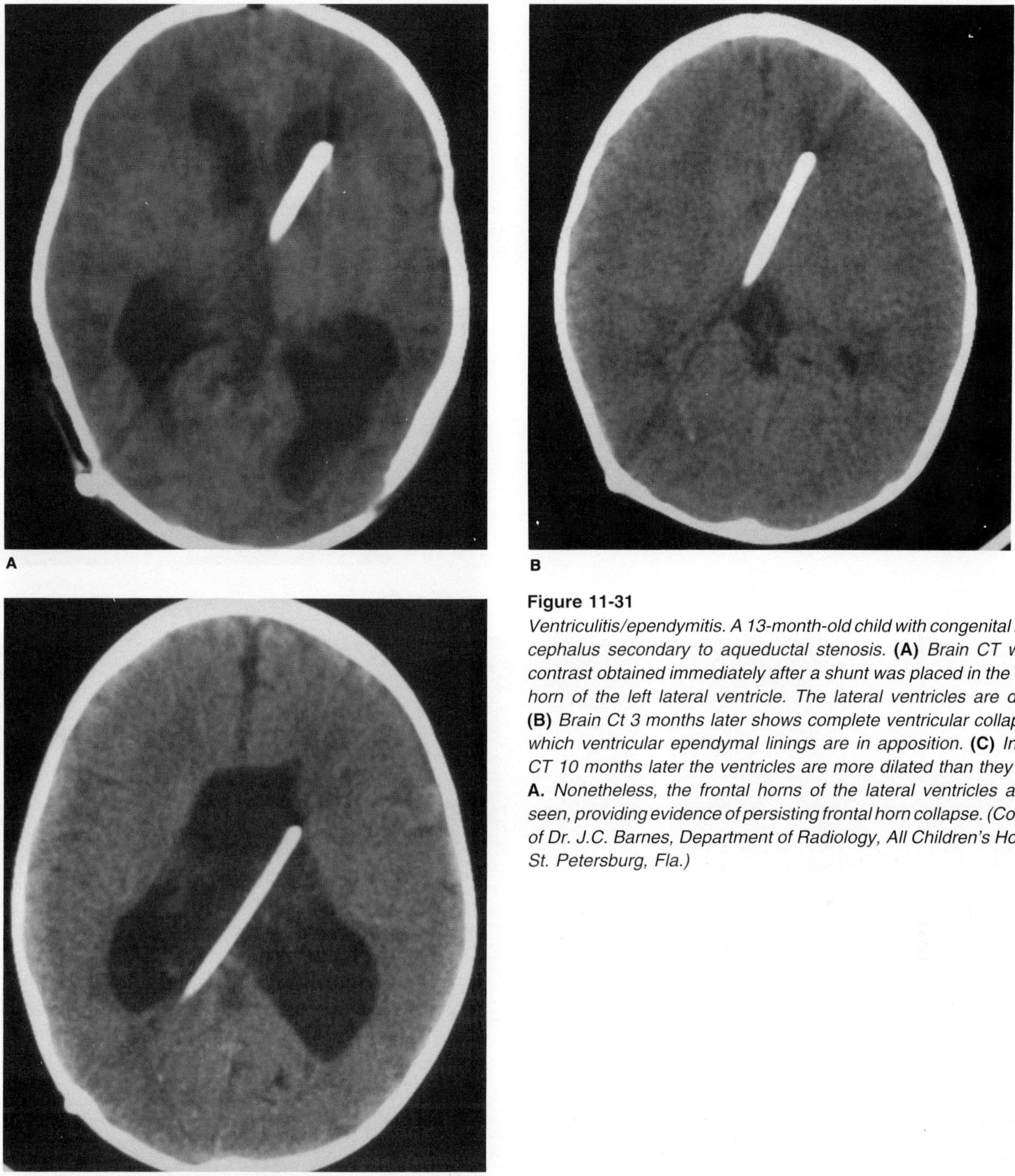

A B C

Figure 11-31
Ventriculitis/ependymitis. A 13-month-old child with congenital hydrocephalus secondary to aqueductal stenosis. **(A)** *Brain CT without contrast obtained immediately after a shunt was placed in the frontal horn of the left lateral ventricle. The lateral ventricles are dilated.* **(B)** *Brain Ct 3 months later shows complete ventricular collapse by which ventricular ependymal linings are in apposition.* **(C)** *In brain CT 10 months later the ventricles are more dilated than they are in* **A.** *Nonetheless, the frontal horns of the lateral ventricles are not seen, providing evidence of persisting frontal horn collapse. (Courtesy of Dr. J.C. Barnes, Department of Radiology, All Children's Hospital, St. Petersburg, Fla.)*

In chronic or complicated meningitis, contrast enhancement of the brain-meningeal surface is seen initially. Meningeal inflammation subsequently may produce sterile subdural effusion (Fig. 11-32) or a subdural empyema. Other complications of meningitis include hydrocephalus and ventriculitis. Bacteria that commonly produce subdural effusions include *Haemophilus influenzae,* pneumococcus, and meningococcus, in decreasing order of frequency.[23] Subdural effusions, although rare, can cause increased intracranial pressure.

Arachnoiditis, or scarring of the arachnoid and pial membranes, is another common inflammatory process.

Vascular damage to the dura mater is accompanied by an inflammatory response that is mainly a fibrinous exudate containing only a few phagocytic cells with fibrinolytic enzymes. The enzyme sparsity yields insufficient lysis of fibrous bands deposited by proliferating fibroblasts that invade the arachnoid mater, deposit collagen, and coat the nerve roots and the arachnoid membrane.[24] This leads to scarring and adhesions. In addi-

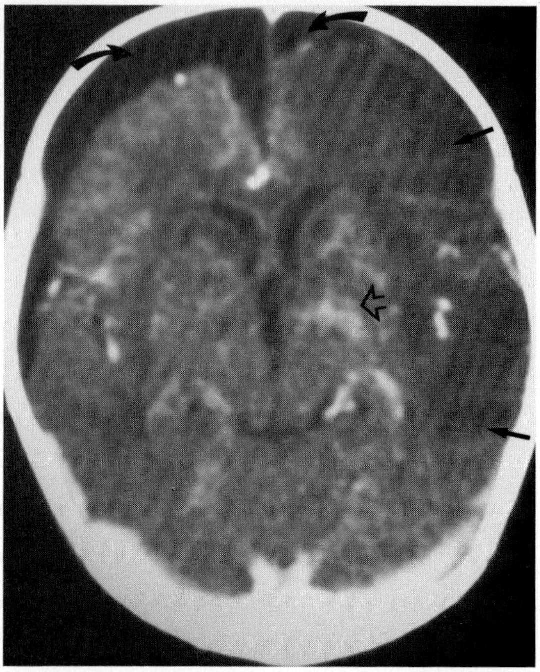

Figure 11-32
Subdural effusion in meningitis. Head CT with contrast in a 3-month-old boy with meningitis. Bilateral hypodense lesions, greater on the right than on the left, consistent with subdural effusions are visualized (curved arrows). Decreased attenuation seen in the distribution of the left middle cerebral artery represents encephalomalacia (short arrows), most likely caused by vascular occlusion associated with meningitis. Areas of decreased attenuation visualized in the deep white matter on the right side represent ischemia. An area of increased attenuation in the region of the left basal ganglia represents luxury perfusion and/or hemorrhagic focus (open arrow). (Courtesy of Dr. J.C. Barnes, Department of Radiology, All Children's Hospital, St. Petersburg, Fla.)

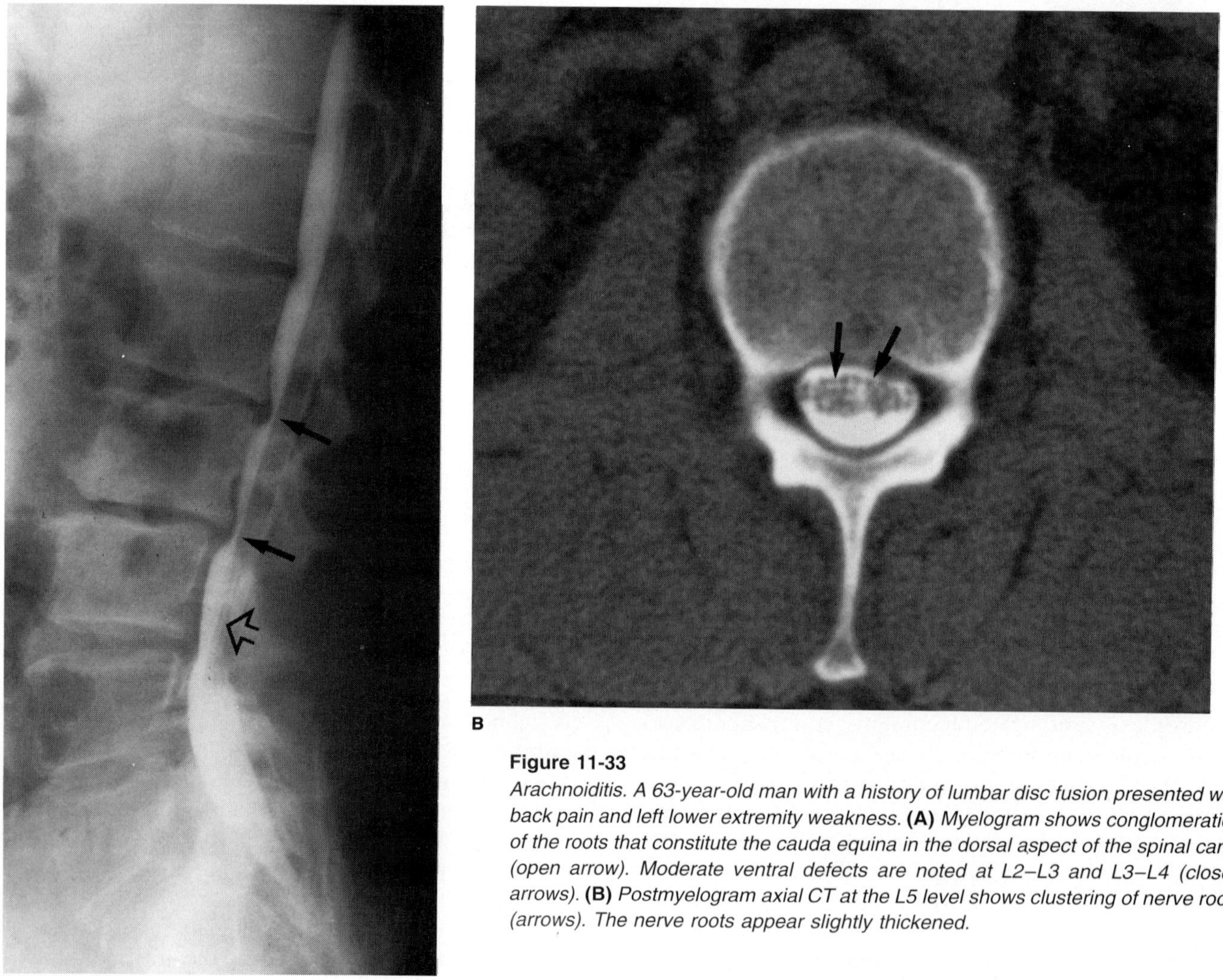

A

B

Figure 11-33
Arachnoiditis. A 63-year-old man with a history of lumbar disc fusion presented with back pain and left lower extremity weakness. **(A)** *Myelogram shows conglomeration of the roots that constitute the cauda equina in the dorsal aspect of the spinal canal (open arrow). Moderate ventral defects are noted at L2–L3 and L3–L4 (closed arrows).* **(B)** *Postmyelogram axial CT at the L5 level shows clustering of nerve roots (arrows). The nerve roots appear slightly thickened.*

tion, serum enzymatic defects have been reported in patients with arachnoiditis.[25]

Arachnoiditis is of a known cause in 94 percent of cases.[26] Disc herniation, postsurgical changes, infection, trauma, and the injection of nonsoluble contrast material, anesthetic agents, and steroids into the subarachnoid space (SAS) are the most common causes of arachnoiditis. Patients present with radicular symptoms of pain and motor or sensory loss. Most cases evolve over years.

Although plain CT is not diagnostic of arachnoiditis, calcifications noted within the linings of the thecal sac by CT are almost pathognomonic of chronic adhesive arachnoiditis.[27] Because arachnoiditis is an avascular process, CT with intravenous contrast is not helpful. Therefore, CT diagnosis of arachnoiditis requires the administration of intrathecal contrast. Two distinct types of arachnoiditis have been described on CT and myelography.[10] In the first type, cases show thickened, "sleeveless" nerve roots caused by adhesions of the roots to the inside of the meninges. In the second group, myelographic filling defects, narrowing of the thecal sac (Fig. 11-33A), or myelographic block may be present. On postmyelography CT, the clumping of the roots is seen (Fig. 11-33B).[10] Intradural adhesions may lead to fixation of the cord and occasionally cause syrinx formation. Extradural fibrosis secondary to trauma or surgery can cause displacement of the thecal sac, a process that may be diffuse or chronic.[27] Adhesion of roots to the thecal sac may appear as a featureless "empty sac" in the second group.[10] In these patients, the subarachnoid space is filled by dense fibrous tissue and scarred nerve roots that may compress the spinal cord and interfere with CSF flow. If the cord is compressed, these patients usually present with pyramidal tract findings.

As in CT and myelography, MRI without contrast also detects arachnoiditis. MRI demonstrates the roots that constitute the cauda equina in 78 percent of cases.[10]

Delamarter and associates[28] performed MRI studies of previously demonstrated cases of arachnoiditis. In all, MRI abnormalities were well defined.[28] Three groups were described on the basis of MRI findings: One group showed root conglomeration in the center of the sac; another showed flattening of the agglomerated roots against the sac wall (Fig. 11-34A and B), producing an "empty sac" appearance; in the third, the sac was filled with granulation tissue (Fig. 11-35A,B,C.).

On myelography, the third group showed complete block. Axial T1- and T2-weighted sequence images were most helpful. However, segmental root fusion in mild arachnoiditis may be difficult to detect on MRI and may require myelography to demonstrate lack of filling in one or more nerve root sleeves or lack of subtle indentations in the column of dye.

In a group of patients with benign arachnoiditis established by a previous myelogram or noncontrast MRI, gadopentetate dimeglumine MRI showed moderate enhancement in only a few cases.[29] Therefore, MRI

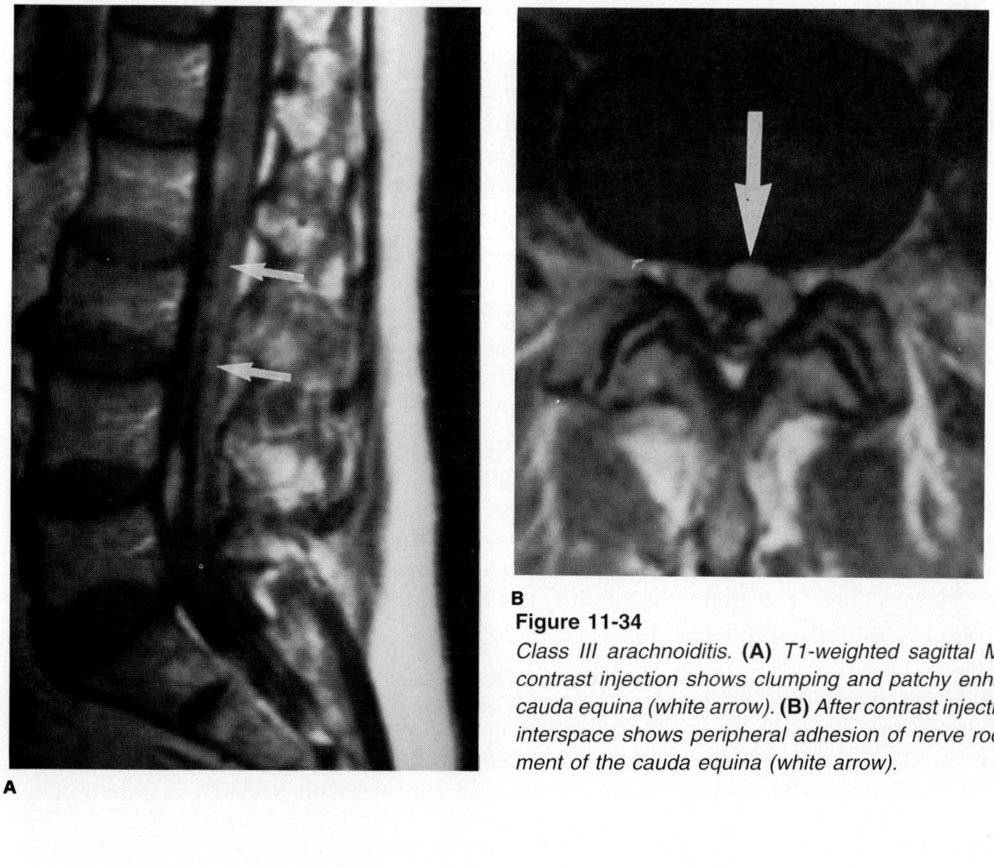

A

B

Figure 11-34

Class III arachnoiditis. **(A)** *T1-weighted sagittal MRI of the lumbosacral spine after contrast injection shows clumping and patchy enhancement of the nerve roots of the cauda equina (white arrow).* **(B)** *After contrast injection, T1-weighted axial MRI at L4–L5 interspace shows peripheral adhesion of nerve roots to the thecal sac and enhancement of the cauda equina (white arrow).*

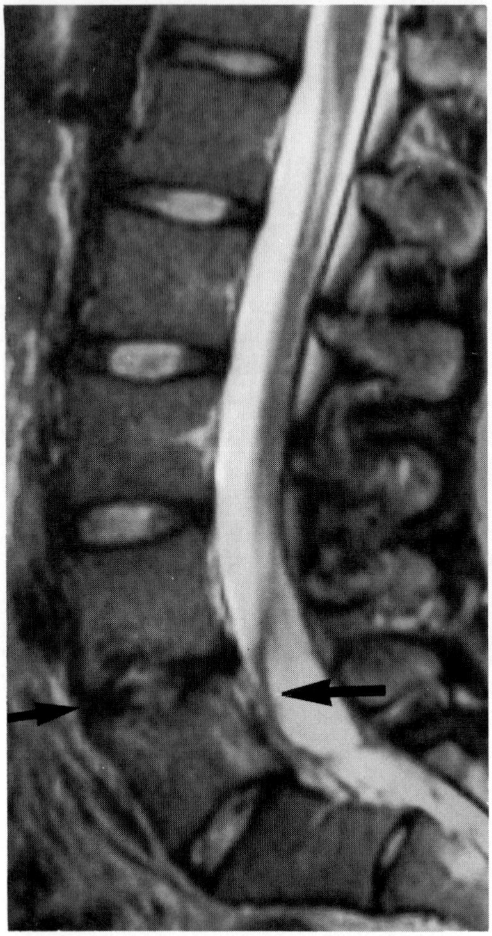

A

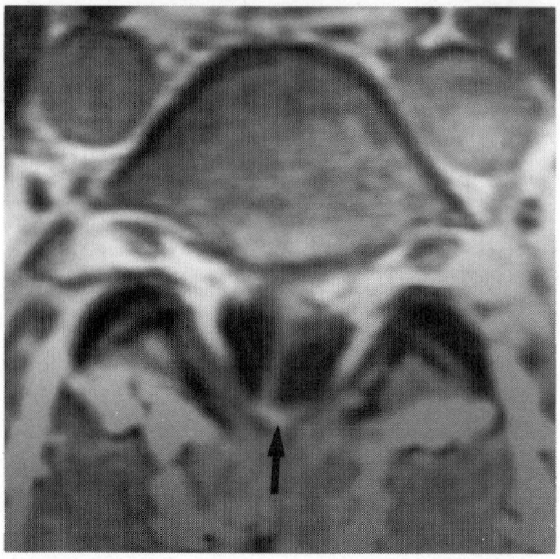

B

Figure 11-35

Arachnoiditis. A 16-year-old male presenting with a gunshot wound to the back. **(A)** *Fast spin echo T2-weighted sagittal image of the lumbar spine shows decreased height of the L4–L5 intervertebral disc (short black arrow). The area of low signal in the inferior portion of the body of the fourth lumbar vertebrae is consistent with the bullet itself. A bundle of nerve roots displaced anteriorly toward the fifth lumbar body and then taking a more tortuous course inferiorly is consistent with tethering as a result of severe arachnoiditis (long black arrow).* **(B)** *T1-weighted axial MRI with gadolinium at the level of body of L4 shows abnormal enhancement and clumping of nerve roots to the posterior aspect of the thecal sac consistent with arachnoiditis (black arrow). (Courtesy of Dr. C. Martinez, Department of Radiology, USF, Tampa, Fla.)*

contrast seems to have little additional value in the diagnosis of lumbar arachnoiditis. Enhancement on MRI may be based on the development of a vascular matrix within the fibrous meshwork. Supporting evidence for this hypothesis comes from histologic examination that has shown proliferation of blood vessels in arachnoiditis lesions.[30] However, dural thickening is better visualized on CT and myelography than it is on MRI.[27] Therefore, strong enhancement of the thecal sac on CT and myelography can be used as a marker of arachnoiditis.

Vascular Abnormalities

Impaired drainage of CSF into the cerebral venous system also occurs in venous sinus thrombosis as a result of diseases such as congenital and acquired hypercoagulable states or as an idiopathic abnormality. The first category includes protein C, protein S, antithrombin III deficiency, and homocysteinuria.

Acquired hypercoagulopathies are associated with trauma, surgery, infection, inflammatory diseases, and pregnancy. Increased superior sagittal sinus venous pressure (SSVP) may be associated with increased intracranial pressure (ICP) and hydrocephalus.[31] It can result from structural lesions causing narrowing of the venous sinuses, such as achondroplasia, craniosynostosis, and Arnold-Chiari malformation with chronically increased ICP.[32,33] Unenhanced CT shows the intraluminal clot as high signal intensity. Within several days the thrombus usually becomes isodense to brain. The thrombosed vein does not enhance with contrast but is indicated by the absence of contrast opacification and intense enhancement of dural walls and collateral veins. MRI shows greater detail: MRI features of a subacute thrombus are hyperintensity on T1-weighted (Fig. 11-36A,B,C) and moderate intensity on T2-weighted sequences.

Cerebral angiography (Fig. 11-36C) may show the extent of the venous thrombosis with delineation of superficial venous collaterals.

Intraventricular hemorrhage also may cause hydrocephalus, IVOH acutely, or EVOH chronically.

Acquired Diseases of Infancy and Childhood

Intraventricular hemorrhage (IVH) is especially common in premature infants. In adults, it may be a result from aneurysmal rupture with SAH or intraparenchy-

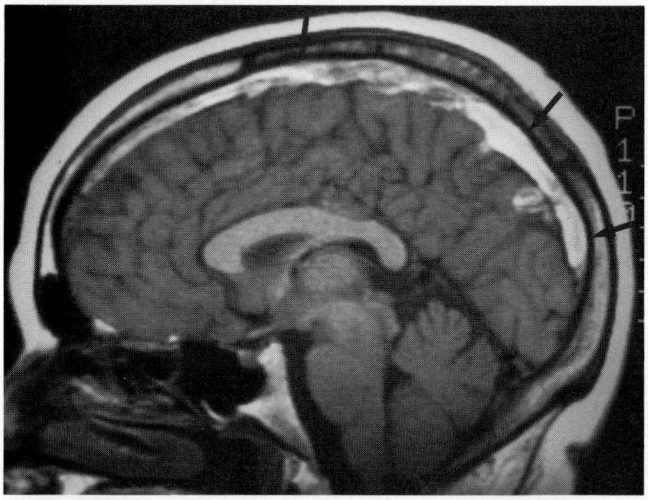

A

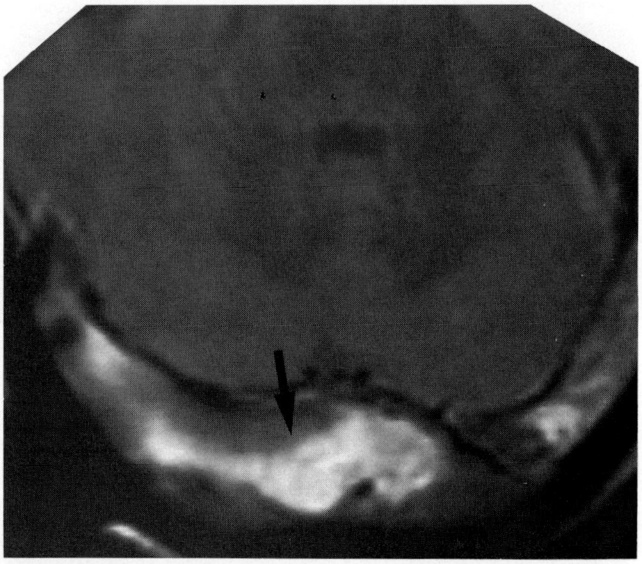

B

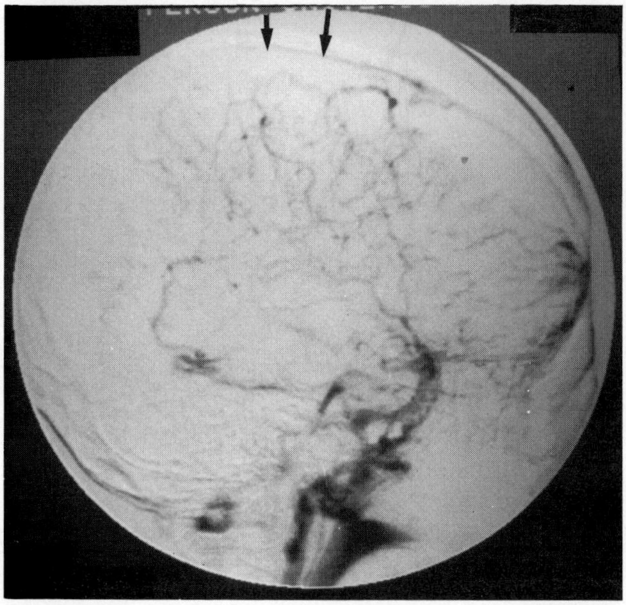

C

Figure 11-36

Sagittal sinus thrombosis. **(A)** *T1-weighted sagittal image demonstrates a large region of high signal intensity in the sagittal sinus consistent with sagittal sinus thrombosis (black arrow).* **(B)** *Magnified axial T1-weighted image shows high intensity in the right transverse sinus consistent with venous thrombosis (black arrow).* **(C)** *Lateral cerebral angiogram in the venous phase shows absence of sagittal sinus opacification (black arrow). (Courtesy of Dr. J.C. Barnes, Department of Radiology, All Children's Hospital, St. Petersburg, Fla.)*

mal bleed with extension into the ventricular system, usually after trauma, hypertensive bleed, or rarely, hemorrhagic infarction.

IVH occurs in 34 to 49 percent of premature infants.[34] The subependymal germinal matrix, which contains thin-walled vessels that are highly susceptible to hypoxia, is the source of bleeding. A grading system related to the severity of bleeding has been devised for sonographic classification of IVH: Grade I indicates germinal matrix hemorrhage with minimal or no IVH ($<$10 percent of the ventricular area on parasagittal view); grade II is characterized by IVH (10 to 50 percent of the ventricular area on parasagittal view); grade III is associated with IVH of $>$50 percent of the ventricular area on parasagittal view, associated with ventricular distention; and grade IV is characterized by periventricular echogenicity (Fig. 11-37A).

Hydrocephalus is the third most common complication of IVH.[34] In patients with grade III and IV IVH (Fig. 11-37B), it occurs in nearly all cases.

Blood in the ventricular system may lead to arachnoiditis and obstruction of CSF flow (Fig. 11-38). Blood clots also may hinder CSF circulation at the aqueduct of Sylvius and the arachnoid villi. Acoustic interfaces resulting from fibrin within the blood clot form the physical basis for detecting hemorrhage by ultrasound.[35] CT and MRI are also excellent tools to demonstrate IVH; in the chronic state, however, the distinction between ventricular dilatation secondary to impaired CSF flow and that from compensatory ventricular dilation re-

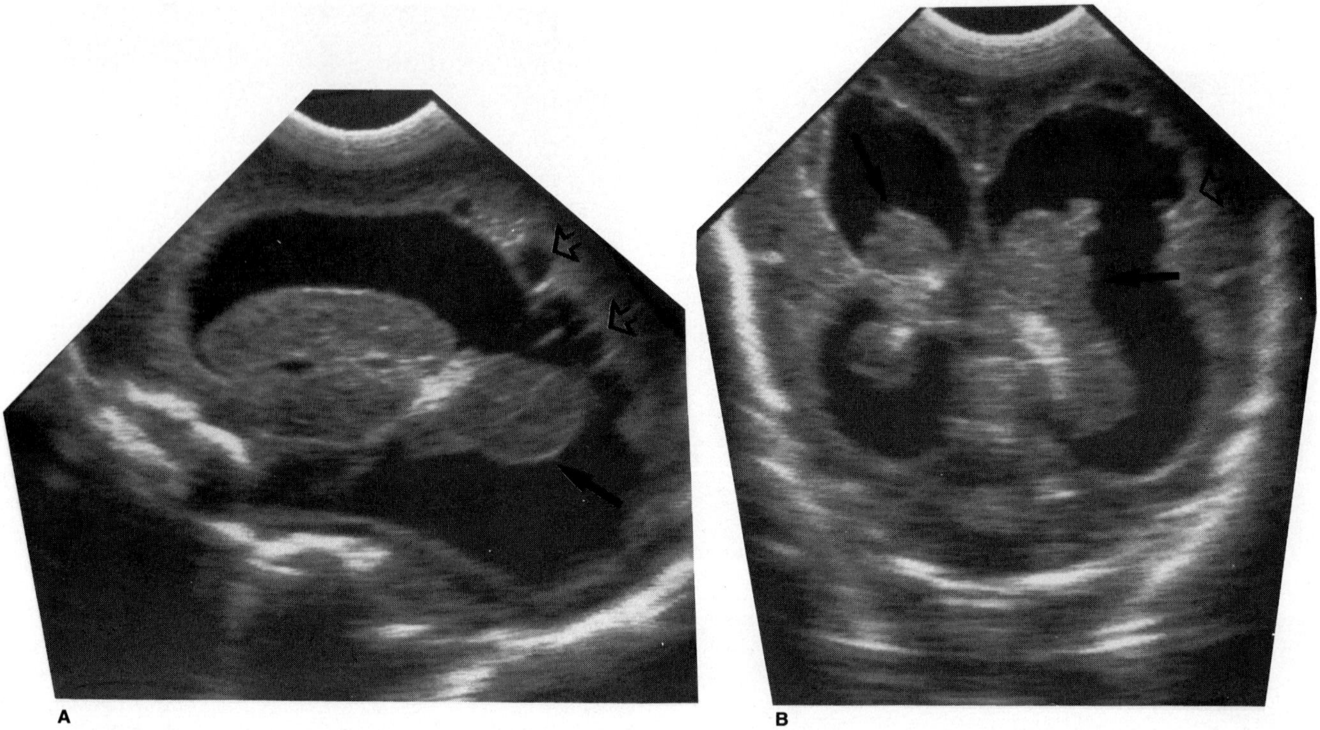

Figure 11-37

Grade IV intraventricular hemorrhage. Cerebral ultrasound of a 23-day-old infant born at 28 weeks of gestation, weighing 1200 g. **(A** *and* **B)** *the ventricular dilatation is caused by intraventricular hemorrhage. The lateral ventricles and the third ventricle are distended. Large clots are noted in both lateral ventricles around the choroid plexus (black arrows). The clots are moderately echogenic. Intraventricular clots become less echogenic over time and may liquefy. Periventricular porencephaly is caused by periventricular leukomalacia secondary to ischemia (short open arrows). This patient underwent ventriculoperitoneal shunting shortly after this sonogram. (Courtesy of Dr. J.C. Barnes, Department of Radiology, All Children's Hospital, St. Petersburg, Fla.)*

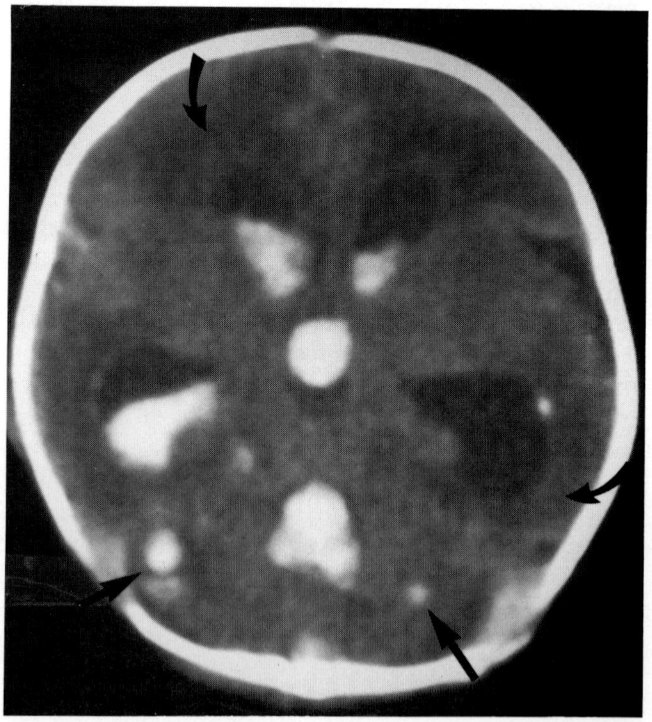

Figure 11-38

Intraventricular hemorrhage (grade IV) with bilateral cerebellar hemorrhage. Brain CT without contrast shows areas of increased attenuation within the lateral, third, and fourth ventricles, which are consistent with hemorrhage. Global ventricular dilatation consistent with extraventricular hydrocephalus also is noted. This results from the decreased ability of subarachnoid granulation to reabsorb CSF in the presence of blood, which is thus disrupting the fine balance between CSF synthesis and reabsorption. Two punctate areas of hemorrhage (straight arrows) are noted within the cerebellar hemispheres, the one on the right being slightly larger than the one on the left. In addition, areas of low density are seen in the periventricular white matter (curved arrows). These findings are consistent with grade IV IVH. (Courtesy of Dr. J.C. Barnes, Department of Radiology, All Children's Hospital, St. Petersburg, Fla.)

sulting from periventricular leukomalacia or infarct can be difficult. Bleeding into the subarachnoid space may lead to the syndrome of normal-pressure hydrocephalus as well.

Meningeal Carcinomatosis

Beerman introduced the term *leptomeningeal carcinomatosis* in 1912.[36] In 1904, malignant cells were first detected in the CSF,[37] and hypoglycorrhachia was reported.[38] Leptomeningeal carcinomatosis is diffuse or focal involvement of the subarachnoid space by spread from a primary CNS tumor or by metastasis from a distant systemic malignancy. Primary CNS tumors with a predilection for CSF invasion include medulloblastomas, glioblastomas, and ependymomas. Extraneural malignancies with a similar propensity include adenocarcinomas, especially from the lung, the breast, the stomach, and the ovary.[10] Leukemia and lymphoma also can be associated with carcinomatosis. Tumor cells enter the CSF in several ways: (1) hematogenous invasion via the superficial meningeal arteries, (2) contiguous penetration from superficial parenchymal metastases, (3) spread from dural metastasis, and (4) extension along nerve roots via cranial and spinal foramina via lymphatics.[39]

Once in the CSF, tumor cells may spread in sheetlike fashion, causing either regional or diffuse meningeal involvement. These malignant cells are associated with an inflammatory process that results in a reactive meningeal fibrosis.[9] Frequently, tumor deposits also are found along the ependymal lining of the ventricles and may be responsible for diffuse subarachnoid extension of malignant cells.[9] In cranial carcinomatosis, contrast-enhanced CT may show EVOH with abnormal enhancement of the tentorium cerebelli, sylvian fissures, basal cisterns, and cortical subarachnoid spaces. Contrasted CT is usually insensitive to leptomeningeal metastatic disease (Fig. 11-39A), particularly when associated with leukemia or lymphoma.[40] This technique had a 44 percent false negativity in one series.[41] MRI without contrast also has been reported to be insensitive to meningeal metastases from primary CNS and distant neoplasms.[42] In a series comparing contrasted CT and myelography with MRI of the cranium and spine, respectively, Krol and associate[41] found abnormalities in only 56 percent of the cases. Contrasted cranial CT abnormalities consisted of abnormal enhancement of the subarachnoid spaces and ventricular walls, obliteration of the cortical sulci, and enhancing nodules within the subarachnoid cisterns and the lateral ventricles. These features were equally well seen on unenhanced cranial MRI. However, involvement of the ventricular linings, tentorium, and subarachnoid cisterns was better demonstrated on contrasted CT than it was on routine T1- and T2-weighted spin echo sequences. CT and MRI were found to be associated with 44 percent and 65 percent false negativity, respectively.[41] The nonspecific MRI features included poor definition of structures within the subarachnoid space, such as the distal spinal cord and the CSF, and a ground-glass appearance of the subarachnoid spaces.[41]

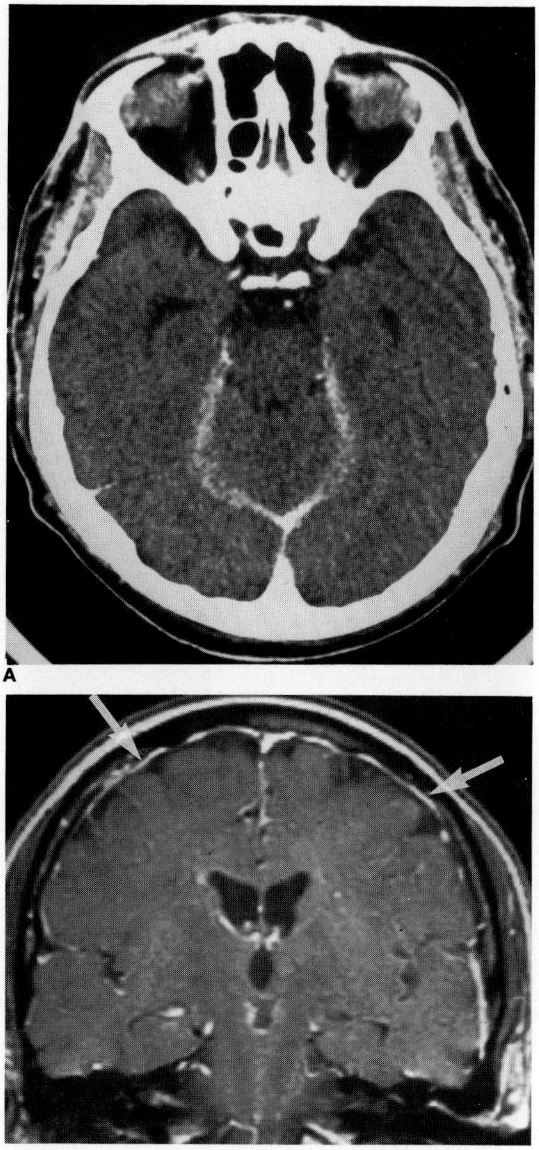

A

B

Figure 11-39
Carcinomatous meningitis in a 65-year-old man with history of metastatic melanoma. **(A)** *Contrasted CT without abnormal enhancement.* **(B)** *T1-weighted coronal MRI of the brain with gadolinium shows evidence of diffuse enhancement consistent with leptomeningeal carcinomatosis (arrows). This process is mostly noticeable over the cerebral convexities.*

In meningeal carcinomatosis of the spine, contrasted CT has no value. Myelographic abnormalities include nodular filling defects within the subarachnoid space; thickening, crowding, and irregularities of the roots of the cauda equina; longitudinal striations; and scalloping of the subarachnoid space.[41] In one study,[41] only 27 percent of patients with positive myelograms exhibited a positive unenhanced MRI (Fig. 11-40A and B). The uncontrasted spinal MRI did not visualize lesions

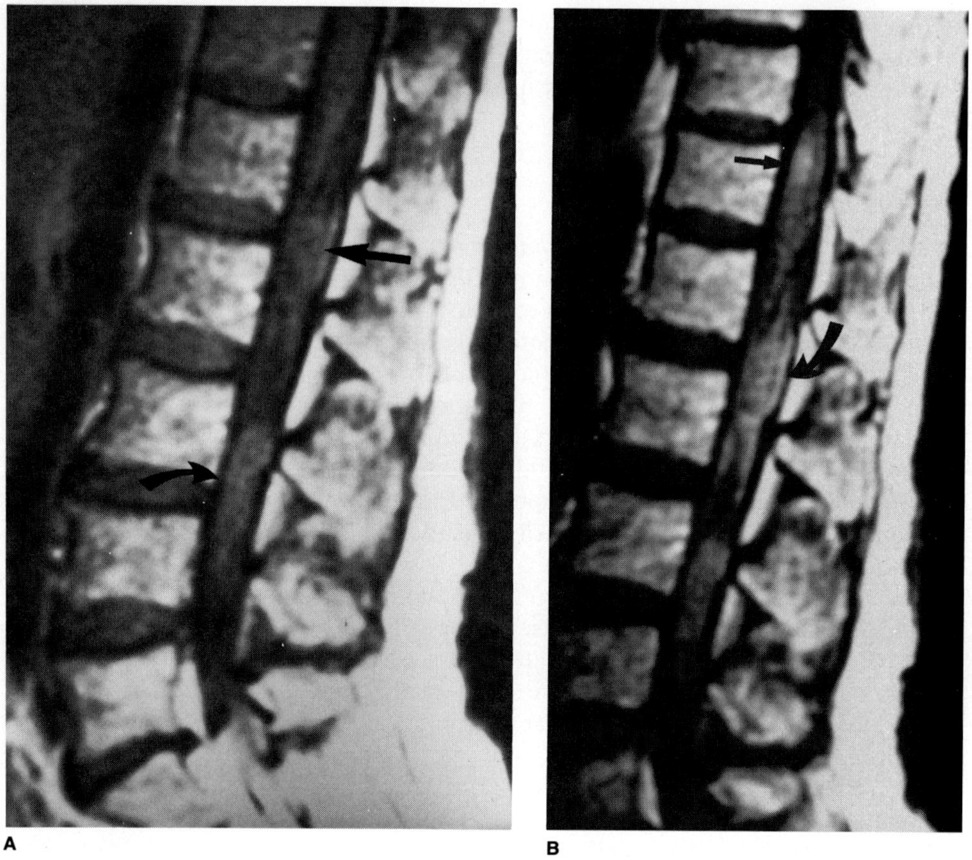

Figure 11-40
Leptomeningeal carcinomatosis. A 67-year-old woman with lung cancer and brain metastases who presented with back pain and progressive left leg weakness. **(A)** *Sagittal T1-weighted MRI without gadolinium demonstrates the spinal column from T11 to the upper aspect of S1. The vertebral bodies are normal. There is no evidence of metastasis to the vertebral bodies. Abnormal signals consistent with mass lesions are noted at L1–L2 (straight arrow) and L3–L4 (curved arrow).* **(B)** *After contrast injection, T1-weighted sagittal MRI shows focal enhancement of a 12-mm mass in the anterior portion of the spinal canal at T12–L1 at the level of the conus medullaris (short arrow). Areas of patchy enhancement also are seen along with dural lining (curved arrow) and the cauda equina.*

(Fig. 11-41A to C) in 65 percent of patients, in whom myelography delineated all lesions. Common features on MRI with gadolinium (Fig. 11-40B) include inhomogeneous, patchy, or nodular enhancement of the dura and the subarachnoid space. However, contrasted MRI is very sensitive to leptomeningeal disease.[10] In a series by Sze and associates,[39] 22 of 30 clinically suspicious cases were found to have abnormal meningeal enhancement on MRI. In this prospective study, MRI with gadolinium demonstrated abnormal meningeal enhancement in 15 of 21 patients with positive CSF cytology. Only one case with negative cytology showed abnormal enhancement on MRI. CT with contrast showed abnormality in only 18 of the 22 cases that were found to be abnormal on MRI.

When abnormal, both CT and MRI show prominent leptomeningeal enhancement. Subependymal and ependymal seeding do not always enhance.

In cranial carcinomatosis, coronal and axial MRI studies may be more sensitive than sagittal MRI to abnormality (Fig. 11-39B). The normal enhancement of the dural reflections around the superior sagittal sinus makes the sagittal planes unreliable in establishing abnormal meningeal enhancement. MRI appearance varies from diffuse enhancement encasing the entire brain to nodular foci involving patchy areas of the leptomeninges and leptomeningeal tumor with parenchymal invasion. Nodular or invasive lesions usually are detected by CT, whereas diffuse leptomeningeal involvement along the inner aspect of the skull usually is undetectable on CT because of bony skull artifact.[39]

In focal subdural collections, enhancement on MRI with gadolinium is usually more prominent along the skull, that is, the outer edge of the effusion, than along the brain parenchyma. Thus far there is no correlation between the degree of increased CSF protein in suspicious cases and meningeal enhancement.

Despite its high degree of sensitivity, MRI with gadolinium is not specific for leptomeningeal carcinomatosis. The differential diagnosis includes fungal or granulomatous meningitis and complications of trauma, subdural hematoma, intrathecal radiation, chemotherapy, and subacute infarction.[39] Idiopathic enhancement of the pachymeninges does not penetrate into the sulci, a characteristic that distinguishes it from the conditions mentioned above.

In conclusion, although CSF cytology provides a definitive diagnosis of leptomeningeal carcinomatosis, with abnormal CSF noted in up to 55 percent of cases after the first spinal tap and in up to 90 percent after the third,[43,44] MRI with gadolinium is a useful ancillary diagnostic tool, especially when lumbar puncture is contraindicated or CSF cytology is equivocal.

"Hydrocephalus Ex Vacuo"

Historically, hydrocephalus ex vacuo refers to ventricular enlargement in the presence of cerebral atrophy or

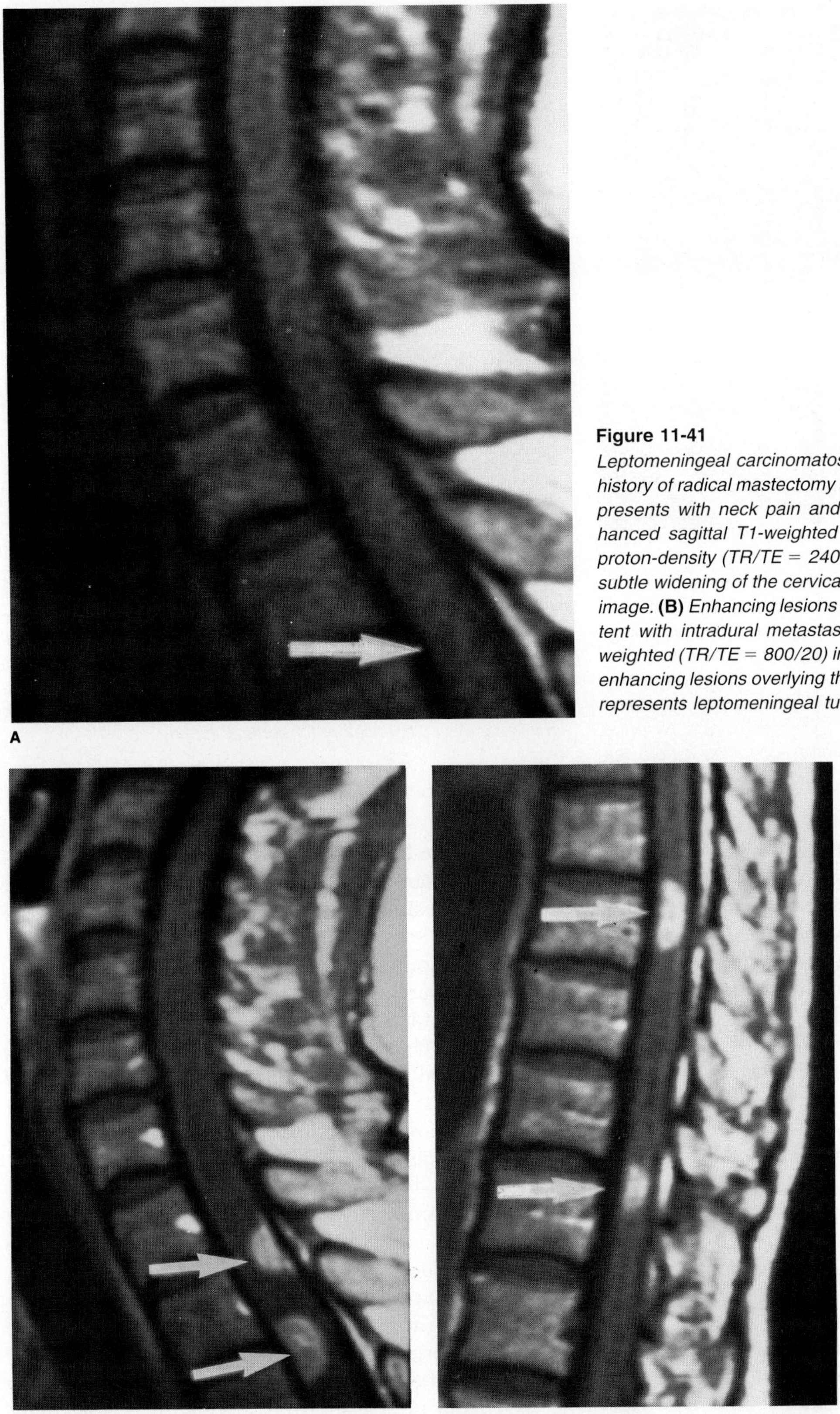

Figure 11-41

Leptomeningeal carcinomatosis. A 38-year-old woman with a 1-year history of radical mastectomy and lymphadenectomy for breast cancer presents with neck pain and upper extremity weakness. **(A)** *Unenhanced sagittal T1-weighted (TR/TE = 800/20) and cardiac-gated proton-density (TR/TE = 2400/30) images of the cervical spine show subtle widening of the cervical spinal cord (arrow) on the T1-weighted image.* **(B)** *Enhancing lesions are also seen in the cervical cord consistent with intradural metastasis (arrows).* **(C)** *Enhanced sagittal T1-weighted (TR/TE = 800/20) images of the thoracic spine demonstrate enhancing lesions overlying the spinal cord (arrows). This appearance represents leptomeningeal tumor seeding with invasion of the cord.*

A

B

C

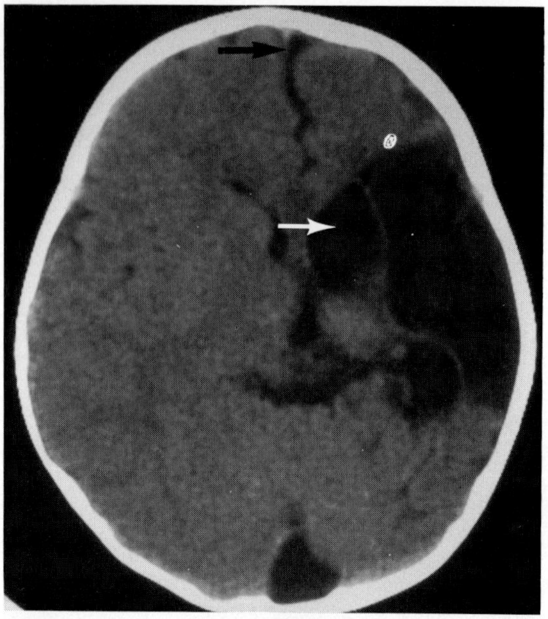

A

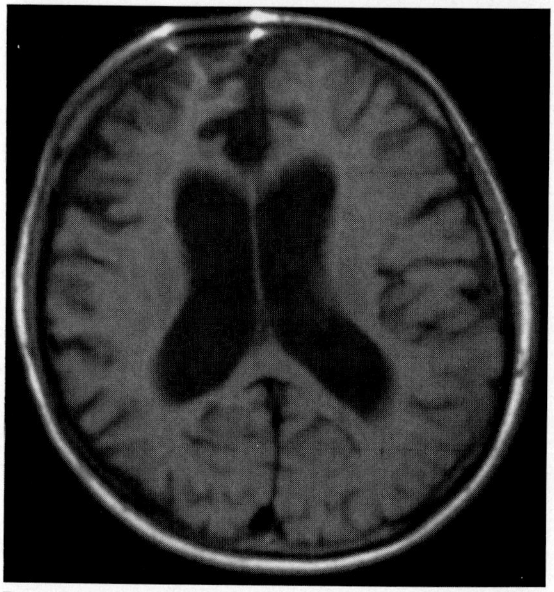

B

Figure 11-42

(A) *Left middle cerebral artery infarct with hydrocephalus ex vacuo. Brain CT without contrast shows a hypodense area in the territory of the left middle cerebral artery, indicating encephalomalacia with density similar to that of CSF. Note the shift of the anterior falx toward the lesion (arrow). The frontal horn and the body of the left lateral ventricle are dilated in response to the encephalomalacia. Note the lateral wall (curved arrow) of the ventricle separating it from the encephalomalacia. (Courtesy of Dr. J.C. Barnes, Department of Radiology, All Children's Hospital, St. Petersburg, Fla.)* **(B)** *MRI. Sagittal brain MRI without contrast in a patient with Alzheimer disease shows marked enlargement of the lateral ventricles along with diffuse cerebral atrophy as indicated by widening of the sulci. Ventricular dilatation in this case is compensatory for cortical atrophy.*

irreversible loss of brain parenchyma. The most common causes of this CT or MRI finding include infarction (Fig. 11-42A), demyelination, infection, hypoxia, and degenerative diseases such as Alzheimer disease. (Fig. 11-42B). Enlargement of the cortical sulci allows distinction of atrophy from hydrocephalus. When both the ventricular system and the cortical sulci are enlarged, sulcal widening out of proportion to ventricular dilatation suggests cortical atrophy. However, this pattern is associated with diffuse cortical atrophy as opposed to disease states, such as advanced multiple sclerosis, that may resemble hydrocephalus on CT.[45]

IDIOPATHIC ENTITIES

Normal-Pressure Hydrocephalus

In 1956, Hakim and Adams established the clinical importance of normal-pressure hydrocephalus (NPH). This syndrome consists of a triad of cognitive impairment, gait disturbance, and urinary incontinence with normal CSF opening pressure and enlarged ventricles that are out of proportion to the degree of cerebral atrophy[46] on CT or MRI. Although in some cases no cause can be determined, subarachnoid hemorrhage, trauma, or infection precedes NPH in many patients.

Because it is a potentially treatable cause of dementia, this syndrome has stimulated investigation and controversy. Some but not all patients with the triad improve after surgical shunting.

It has been suggested that NPH results from deficient CSF absorption into the dural sinuses[47,48] leading to increased pressure and reflux of CSF within the ventricular system and transependymal flow of CSF into the periventricular white matter. Transverse shearing forces on the mesial fibers of the frontal lobes may cause the symptoms.

Cisternography sometimes is used to evaluate NPH. It allows visualization of the reversed CSF flow in NPH. Although 131-I serum albumin was first used as a tracer, 111-In-DTPA and ^{99m}Tc-DTPA are used now. Between 500 μCi and 1 mCi of In-DTPA is administered into the subarachnoid space via lumbar puncture. Images are recorded at 6, 24, 48, and 72 h. At 6 h, tracer activity extends along the spine and reaches the basal cisterns, the interhemispheric fissure, and the sylvian cisterns. At 24 h, it reaches the cerebral convexities and then is cleared from the basal cisterns. By 48 h, radioactivity should be mainly present at the vertex while being reabsorbed in the sagittal sinus. Normally, the tracer does not enter the lateral ventricles. In a group of patients with NPH, there is preferential and persistent activity in the lateral ventricles, which disappears after successful surgical shunting. However, NPH patients display a wide range of cisternographic patterns. Often a "mixed pattern" is present (Fig. 11-43A to C). Furthermore, these radionuclide findings are not diagnostic for NPH. Patients with compensated ventricular enlargement secondary to cerebral atrophy and with entities such as Binswanger disease[49,50] may present with ventricular penetration, as do occasional normal controls.

In one study using quantitative contrast, resolution of the symptoms of NPH was found to be independent of total CSF clearance in shunted patients.[50]

MRI has largely replaced cisternography in the diagnostic evaluation of NPH. As was stated above, MRI and cine MR visualize CSF flow dynamics. CSF flows anterograde, that is, toward the fourth ventricle, in systole and flows retrograde, that is, toward the third ventricle, during diastole (Figs. 11-1 and 11-2). Cardiac pulsations and CSF volume affect the velocity of CSF through the ventricular system. Based on Bernoulli's principle, the highest velocity of CSF is through the aqueduct of Sylvius. Bernoulli's principle states that for constant volumetric flow, tubes with smaller cross-sectional areas have higher linear velocities than do those with larger cross-sectional areas.[45] Quantitative information about CSF velocity and aqueductal CSF stroke volume during each cardiac cycle may be obtained through the use of high-resolution axial MRI sequences by integrating the velocity measurement of 30 0.3-mm pixels in the cerebral aqueduct over time.[45] Despite normal opening pressure, elevated CSF pulse pressure with values 6 to 8 times higher than normal have been documented in NPH.[45]

Hyperdynamic CSF flow in NPH causes an excessive to-and-fro motion of CSF through the ventricular system, giving rise to a marked flow void in the cerebral aqueduct, the third ventricle, and part of the fourth ventricle on MRI (Fig. 11-44A to C). This is best visualized on sagittal and axial MRI planes[51] and on proton-density weighted images.[52] In a study of 20 patients with the clinical criteria for NPH, patients with larger flow void from the third ventricle responded well to VP shunting, whereas patients with a minimal degree of flow void had only a fair to poor response.[53] Therefore, MRI flow void abnormality was suggested as a predictor of surgical outcome. The same authors reported similar

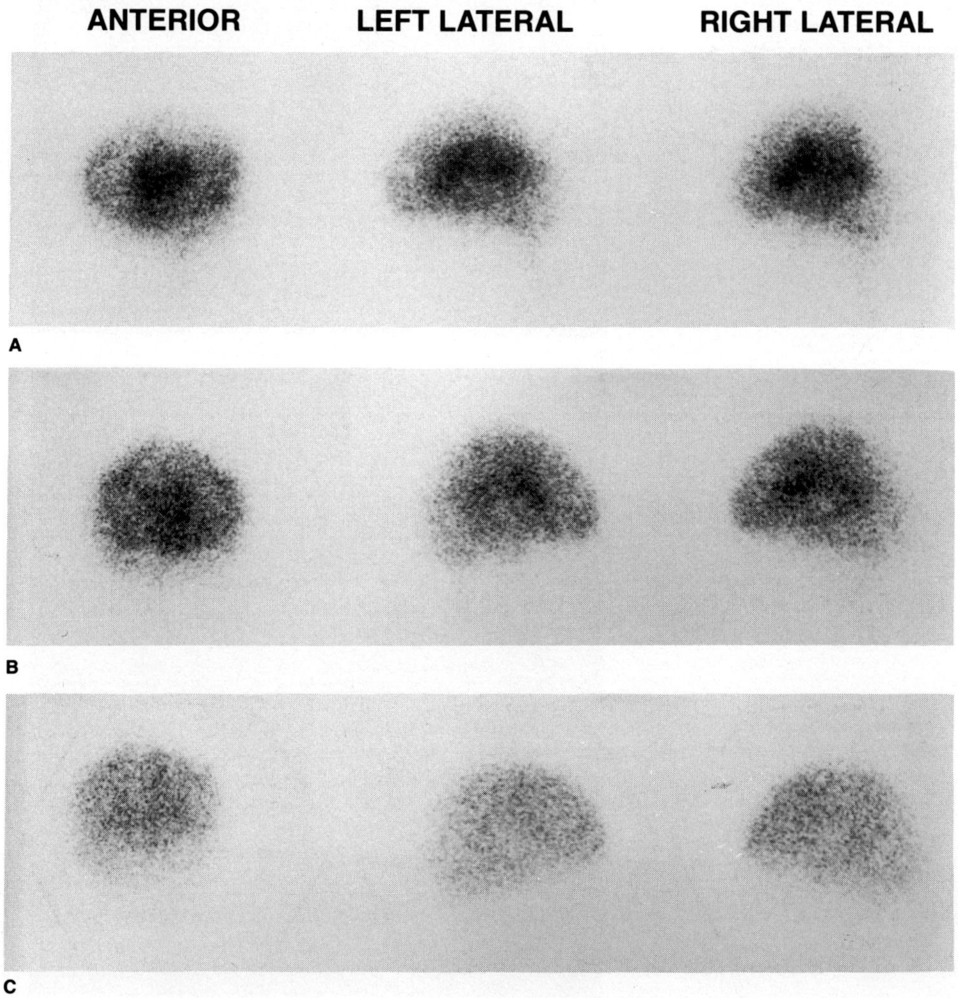

Figure 11-43
NPH. Cisternogram in a 40-year-old white man with a history of a motor vehicle accident 20 years earlier presenting with ataxia, dementia, and urinary incontinence. **(A)** *111-In-DTPA CSF flow study showing anterior and lateral images at 24 h. Activity is quite prominent in the lateral ventricles, with only minimal activity over the cerebral convexities.* **(B)** *At 48 h, activity ascends over the cerebral convexities with partial clearance from the lateral ventricles. This represents the "mixed" pattern of CSF ascent.* **(C)** *At 72 h after injection, most of the activity has cleared from the lateral ventricles.*

Figure 11-44

A 66-year-old man with NPH. **(A)** *T1-weighted sagittal MRI shows that the ventricles are significantly enlarged, including the lateral, third, and fourth ventricles. The pituitary gland is normal in size. The aqueduct is patent. There is no periventricular lucency.* **(B** *and* **C)** *Spin echo axial T1-weighted MRI shows very prominent flow void at the upper portion of the fourth ventricle (arrow)* **(B)** *and third ventricle (arrow)* **(C).**

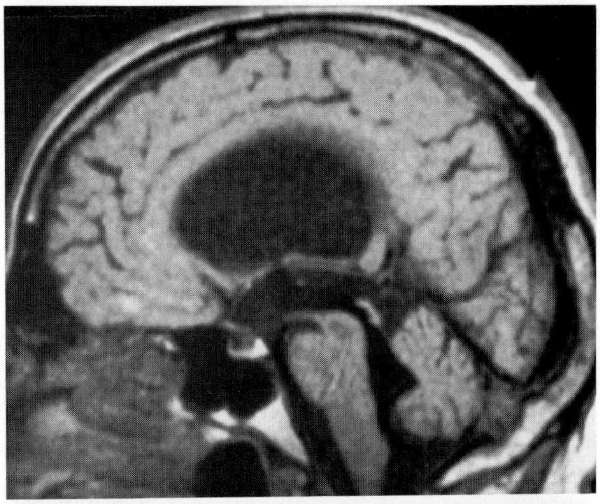

A

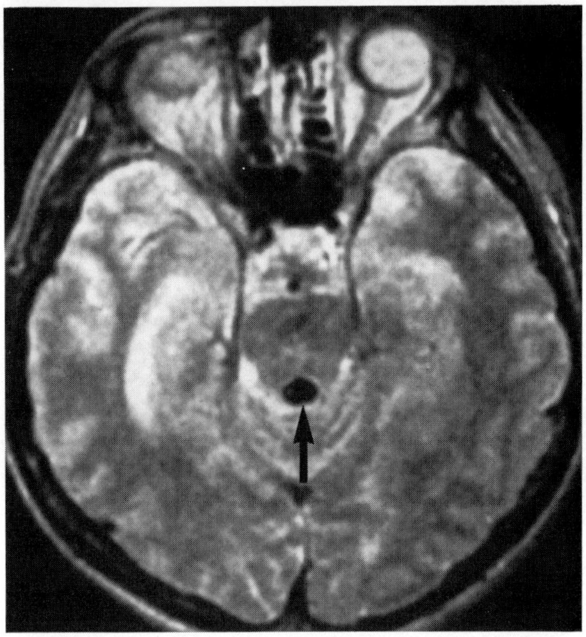

B

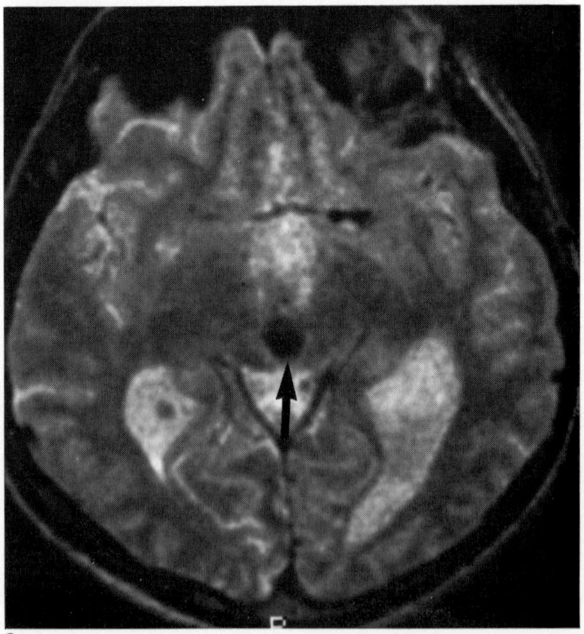

C

CHAPTER 12

INTRACRANIAL NEOPLASMS

Jack O. Greenberg
Ilydio Polachini, Jr.

Approximately 35,000 Americans develop new intracranial neoplasms each year.[1] The annual incidence has been estimated at 17,000 for primary neoplasms and 17,400 for secondary neoplasms, corresponding to 8.2 and 8.3 per 100,000 U.S. population respectively.[1] Intracranial neoplasm ranks as the second most common cause of death from intracranial disease and is surpassed only by stroke.[2] The advent of computed tomography (CT) in the 1970s and magnetic resonance imaging (MRI) in the 1980s dramatically improved the ability to diagnose brain tumors, completely replacing pneumoencephalograms and radioactive brain scans and relegating diagnostic contrast angiography to an occasional secondary role. Positron emission tomography (PET) is useful in identifying hypermetabolic, aggressive astrocytomas and differentiating radiation necrosis from recurrent tumor, but the expense, general unavailability, and poor resolution associated with this technique have limited its applications. Single photon emission computed tomography (SPECT) can provide similar information, although with poorer resolution and sensitivity. Among all the imaging modalities utilized in the investigation of intracranial neoplasms, MRI has become the method of choice. Its inherent multiplanar capability permits accurate localization of tumors and their relationship to landmark anatomic structures. The technique has superb sensitivity, and the "low" specificity cited in the initial results has been largely corrected by accumulated experience and the use of paramagnetic contrast agents. There is now wide recognition of MRI features of common tumors as well as an appreciation of the specific MRI appearance of uncommon tumors.

GENERAL IMAGING CONSIDERATIONS OF INTRACRANIAL NEOPLASMS

Once a tumor has been detected in MRI or CT, ascertaining the following parameters will help characterize it further, with the main objective of establishing a specific diagnosis or a differential diagnosis.

Tumor Location and Size

Establishing whether an intracranial neoplasm is situated in the extra-axial (extraparenchymal) or intra-axial (intraparenchymal) compartment narrows the differential diagnosis. For instance, meningiomas are extra-axial, whereas astrocytomas are intra-axial. A sharp border with a cleft composed of cerebrospinal fluid (CSF) between brain parenchyma and tumor is presumptive of an extra-axial mass such as a meningioma.[3] Inward displacement of the brain surface and focal deviation of the white matter, the "buckled white matter sign," when present, is also consistent with an extra-axial mass.[4] Whenever possible, tumor size should be estimated in three dimensions.

Signal Intensity and Absorption Coefficient

While absorption coefficient numbers on CT are relatively easy to measure and interpret, allowing for quick identification of calcification, acute hemorrhage, and fat, signal intensity and contrast in MRI are complex phenomena that are dependent on several factors. Neoplastic tissue in general has prolonged T1 and T2 relaxation times, so that most tumors are hypointense in T1-weighted images (T1 WI) and hyperintense in proton-density weighted images (PD WI) and T2-weighted images (T2 WI). Quantitative analysis of T1 and T2 is of limited value and does little to increase specificity.[5] Signal intensity within the same tumor can be quite variable, depending on the presence of cystic changes, necrosis, hemorrhage, calcification, fat, and vascularity. The qualitative analysis of signal intensity requires several pulse sequences, which should include precontrast T1 WI, PD WI, and T2 WI. T2*-weighted gradient echo sequences are more sensitive to magnetic susceptibility artifacts and better in detecting calcification and acute hemorrhage, especially at midfield operation. Tables 12-1 through 12-4 summarize the etiology of focal changes in T1 and T2 relaxation times.[6–8] Tables 12-5 and 12-6 provide a summary of contrast mechanisms on spin echo and gradient echo images.

Contrast Enhancement

The use of iodinated and paramagnetic intravenous contrast in CT and MRI, respectively, is an essential step in the imaging evaluation of brain tumors. When enhancement occurs in intra-axial tumors, it reflects breakdown of the blood-brain barrier. Most extra-axial

Table 12-1
Focal changes in T1—etiology
Long (hypo in T1 WI)

Increased water
Edema
Tumor
Infarction
Demyelinating disease
Abscess
Chronic hemorrhage
Calcification
Flow void

Table 12-2
Focal changes in T1—etiology
Short (hyper in T1 WI)

Methemoglobin
Subacute, chronic hemorrhage
Melanin
Fat
High protein
Slow-flowing blood
Paramagnetic agents
Gadolinium
Manganese
Copper
Calcium phosphate crystals (nonheme T1 shortening)
Laminar necrosis of cerebral infarction

Table 12-3
Focal changes in T2—etiology
Long (hyper in T2 WI)

Increased water
Edema
Tumor
Infarction
Abscess
Subdural
Demyelinating disease
Extracellular methemoglobin
Subacute hemorrhage

Table 12-4
Focal changes in T2—etiology
Short (hypo in T2 WI)

Low proton density
Calcification
High nuclear and cytoplasmic ratio
Fibrotic stroma
Paramagnetic substances
Deoxyhemoglobin
Intracellular methemoglobin
Iron
Ferritin
Hemosiderin
Melanin
Macromolecular content
Very high protein
Concentration
Signal void

Table 12-5
Spin echo contrast*

	TR: Short	TR: Long
TE: Short	T1 WI	PD
TE: Long		T2 WI

** Also valid for fast spin echo contrast.*

Table 12-6
Gradient echo contrast*

	TR: Short (> 100 ms)	TR: Long
Flip angle: Small	PD	PD T2*W with long TE
Flip angle: Large	T1 WI T1/T2 with TR <50 ms	T1 WI

** No RF spoiling of transverse magnetization, no inversion pulse.*

neoplasms enhance intensely because of an absent endothelial barrier. Also, with contrast enhancement it is possible to differentiate gross tumor margins from edema. One may infer the degree of malignancy, as tumors with a high malignancy grade tend to show more enhancement and certain patterns. The atomic numbers of gadolinium (64) and iodine (53) are close, and the patterns of enhancement with these two completely different contrast media are similar. However, unlike iodine, which is visualized directly by attenuating an x-ray beam, paramagnetic contrast agents of MRI are visualized indirectly by diffusing to the extracellular space, where they enhance the relaxation rates of nearby water protons. Both T1 and T2 relaxation times decrease, but the effect is primarily in T1 with the usual dose of 0.1 m*M*/kg for gadopentetate dimeglumine (Gd-DTPA), an ionic paramagnetic contrast agent, and up to 0.2 m*M*/kg for the nonionic forms, gadoteridol and gadodiomide.

Peritumoral Edema—Mass Effect

Peritumoral edema is the vasogenic type, in which there is increased permeability of brain-capillary endothelial cells to macromolecules (blood-brain barrier breakdown) such as albumin and various other molecules.[9] It is more prominent in the white matter, where it may extend along its tracts like fingers or pseudopods. Vasogenic edema is hypodense in CT, hypointense in T1 WI relative to normal white matter or gray matter, and hyperintense in T2 WI relative to normal white matter. When a brain tumor obstructs CSF pathways, causing hydrocephalus, interstitial edema in the periventricular white matter may occur from movement of CSF across ventricular walls.[10] Brain tumor and the associated edema raise intracranial pressure, and this may result in internal brain herniation. Subfalcine, transtentorial, and cerebellar tonsillar herniations are the three main types, as illustrated in Figs. 12-1 to 12-3.

This chapter reviews the MRI and CT features and relevant neuropathology of intracranial neoplasms according to their dominant mode of clinical presentation as described in Adams and Victor's *Textbook of Neurology*.

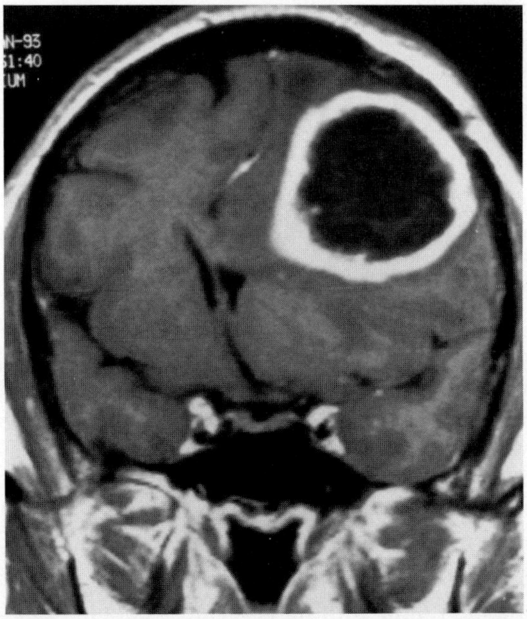

Figure 12-1
Postcontrast T1 WI. Subfalcine herniation in large left frontal glioblastoma multiforme.

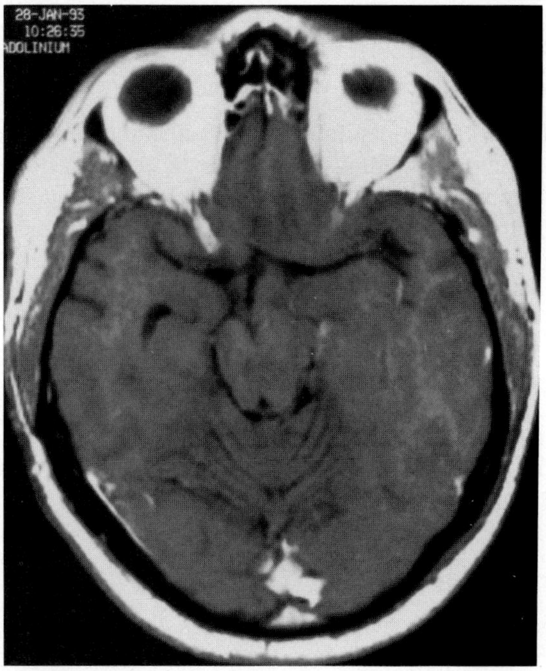

Figure 12-2
Postcontrast T1 WI. Left uncal herniation in same patient.

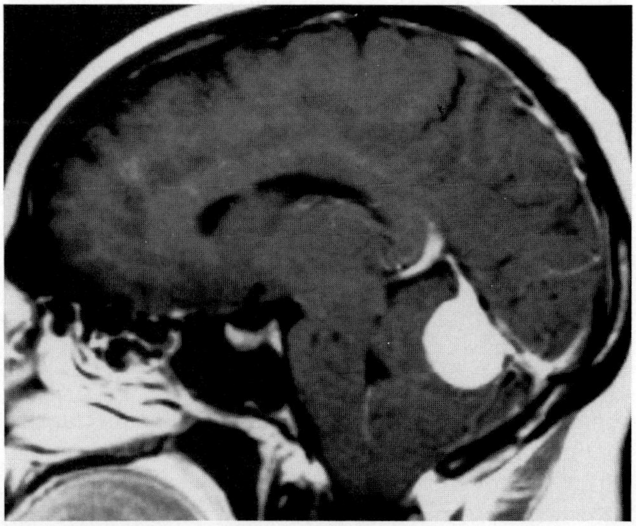

Figure 12-3
Postcontrast T1 WI. Cerebellar tonsil herniation from tentorial meningioma with dural tail sign.

PATIENTS PRESENTING WITH GENERAL IMPAIRMENT OF CEREBRAL FUNCTION, HEADACHES, OR SEIZURES

Virtually any hemispheric neoplasm can give rise to the above clinical findings, singly or in combination. The most common hemispheric neoplasms will be described in groups, according to their histopathologic classification, as follows.

Hemispheric Astrocytoma

Definition

Astrocytoma is a type of glioma derived from and composed of astrocytes that show varying degrees of maturity.

Epidemiology

In general, astrocytoma constitutes about 30 percent of all hemispheric gliomas, excluding glioblastoma multiforme. This number varies widely with the source reviewed.[11,12] Diffuse, low-grade hemispheric astrocytoma occurs more commonly in adults in the third and fourth decades.[12–14] Anaplastic astrocytoma tends to be diagnosed a decade later than is low-grade astrocytoma.[13]

In the pediatric age group astrocytoma accounts for 30 percent of supratentorial brain tumors when visual pathway gliomas are included.[15] Hemispheric astrocytoma represents half of these tumors and is more frequently of the well-circumscribed, pilocytic type rather than diffuse, as is seen in the adult population.[16] The peak incidence is in the second half of the first decade of life.[16]

Pathology

Most hemispheric low-grade astrocytomas in adults are generally solid, poorly defined gray-white infiltrative tumors.[12–14] The frequency of location in any lobe is proportional to its content of white matter from where it extends to involve the cortex or deep structures.[11,13] When it arises from the corpus callosum, spread to both hemispheres is common.[12] Macroscopically, anaplastic astrocytoma is often indistinguishable from low-grade astrocytoma.[12] Histologically, diffuse low-grade astrocytoma is composed of well-differentiated astrocytes that show infiltrative growth, mild uneven hypercellularity, scant mitotic figures, mild nuclear abnormalities, absent vascular endothelial proliferation, and no necrosis.[12–14] Anaplastic astrocytoma results from malignant transformation of low-grade astrocytoma featuring greater infiltrative growth, anaplasia, hypercellularity, higher mitotic activity, minimal endothelial proliferation, and absent necrosis.[12–14] CSF-borne metastases may occur with anaplastic astrocytoma.[12] Areas of low-grade and high-grade malignant changes frequently coexist in anaplastic astrocytoma, and this may lead to erroneously low estimates of tumor grade in limited surgical biopsy sampling.[14] In low-grade astrocytoma, the 5-year and 10-year survival rates are 65 percent and 25 percent, respectively.[14] In anaplastic astrocytoma, median survival is 24 to 36 months.[12]

Hemispheric pilocytic astrocytoma in children and young adolescents is well circumscribed, cystic with a mural nodule or solid tumor of lobar location (most frequently in the temporal lobe), or arising in the walls and floor of the third ventricle or thalamus.[11,12,16] Histologically, these tumors are composed of well-differentiated, strongly fibrillated fusiform-shaped or polar astrocytes, among which are prominent Rosenthal fibers.[11] Vascular endothelial proliferation is present in pilocytic astrocytoma, but in the absence of other anaplastic changes, it does not have a poor prognosis.[11] The prognosis is excellent in this type of astrocytoma, with virtually no tendency for anaplastic transformation and infrequent recurrence after surgical removal.[12]

Imaging Findings

In general, imaging studies (CT and MRI) display typical diffuse low-grade astrocytoma as a well-defined, intraparenchymal homogeneous lesion involving the white matter, corticomedullary junction, or gray matter regions with minimal or no enhancement after contrast infusion and minimal mass effect (Fig. 12-4).[17–21] On noncontrast CT, low-grade astrocytoma is homogeneous, hypodense, and occasionally calcified and exhibits minimal or no surrounding edema. Low-grade astrocytoma is better demonstrated by MRI, especially PD WI and T2 WI, as a homogeneously hyperintense intraparenchymal lesion with minimal mass effect and surrounding edema.[19–21] Corresponding hypointensity in T1 WI is less conspicuous.

Anaplastic astrocytomas usually exhibit a more heterogeneous appearance, more edema, and greater mass effect on both CT and MRI studies (Figs. 12-5 to 12-7).[17,18,20,21] Noncontrast CT displays anaplastic astrocytoma more typically as a heterogeneous, hypodense, or mixed high-density and low-density lesion with variable enhancement that includes ring-like or nodular patterns.[18,21] Compared with low-grade gliomas on MRI studies, anaplastic astrocytoma is more heterogeneous, hypointense in T1 WI and hyperintense in PD WI and T2 WI, and less well defined and has more mass effect and vasogenic edema. There is a greater tendency for enhancement in anaplastic astrocytoma, and the pattern on MRI is the same as that observed on CT.

Pilocytic astrocytoma appears on CT and MRI as sharply demarcated, round, and cystic with a mural nodule or solid tumor without associated edema in the temporal lobe or around the third ventricle (Fig. 12-8).[116,221] Solid tumor and the mural nodule show marked enhancement with contrast. Solid tumor and mural nodule

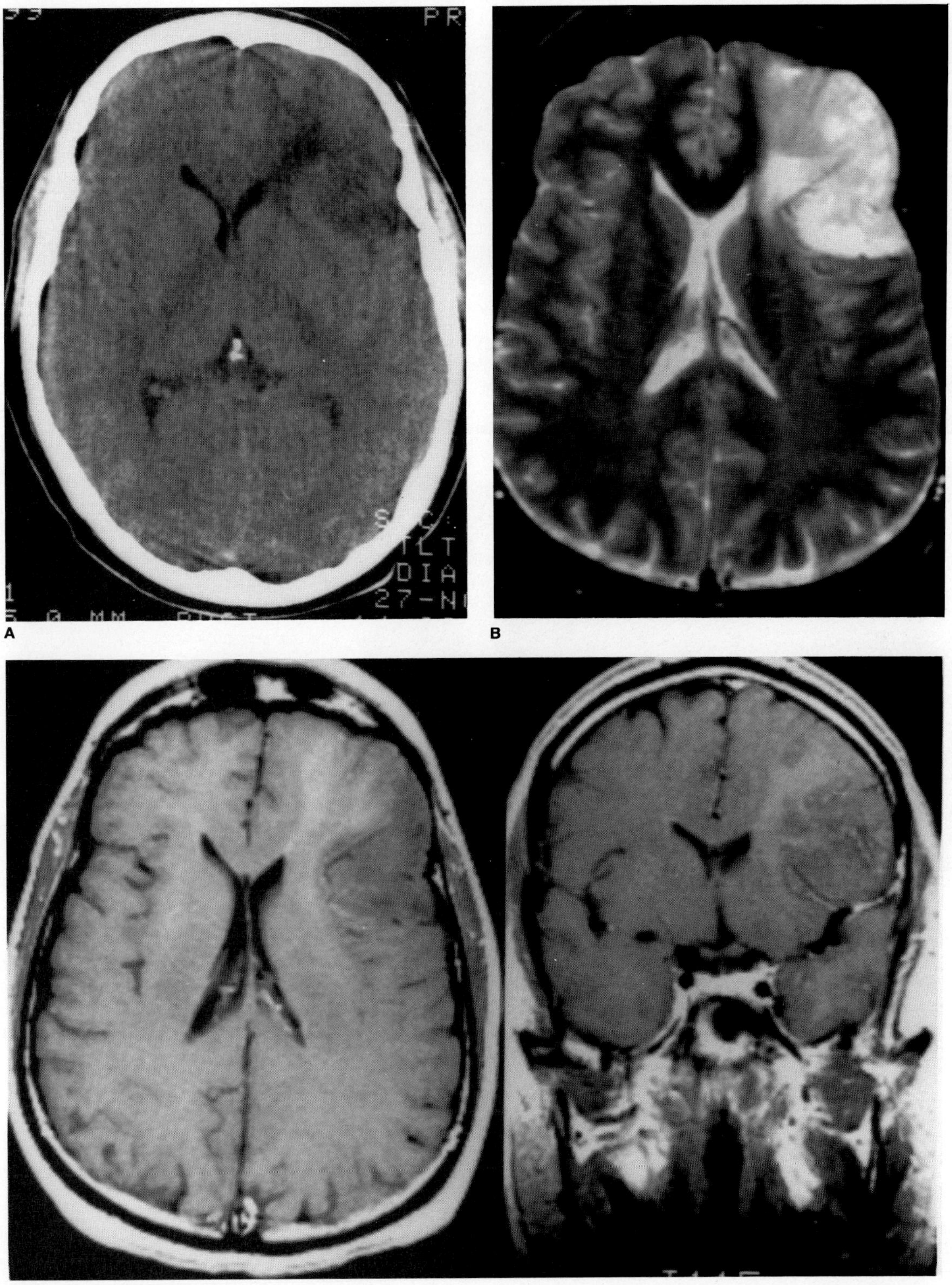

Figure 12-4
Low-grade astrocytoma, left frontal lobe, in a 36-year-old man presenting with 2-week history of headaches. **(A)** *Noncontrast CT. Tumor is ill-defined hypodensity on the left.* **(B)** *T2 WI. Tumor is well delineated; homogeneous hyperintensity in left midfrontal lobe without significant edema and minimal mass effect.* **(C)** *Transverse and coronal postcontrast T1 WI. Tumor is nonenhancing; inconspicuous hypointensity involving the left inferior frontal gyri with associated effacement of cortical sulci and mild shift of midline.*

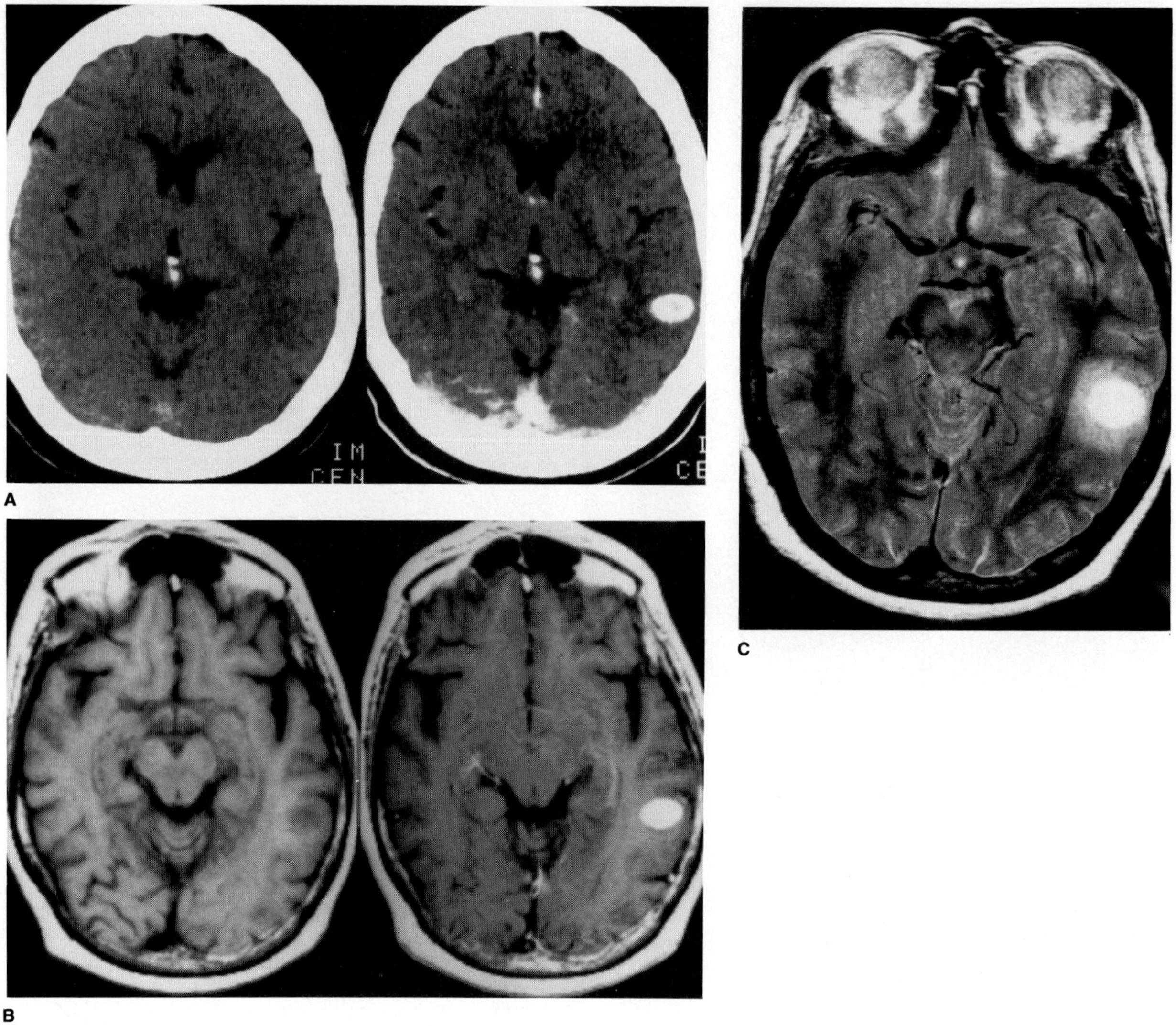

Figure 12-5

Anaplastic astrocytoma, left temporal lobe, in a 67-year-old woman presenting with a spell of speech arrest. **(A)** *Pre- and postcontrast CT. Precontrast study shows minimal hypodensity in the left posterior temporal lobe. Contrast study reveals tumor as cortical nodule of marked enhancement.* **(B)** *Pre- and postcontrast T1 WI. Tumor is inconspicuous, roundish, hypointense intra-axial lesion in posterior temporal cortex that markedly enhances in a nodular pattern. Marked enhancement is more characteristic of high-grade than low-grade astrocytomas.* **(C)** *PD WI. Tumor is roundish, homogeneous area of hyperintensity with minimal surrounding edema in the left posterior temporal lobe. The main differential diagnosis in this case would be single metastasis.*

are isodense to hypodense in noncontrast CT, isointense to hypointense on T1 WI relative to gray matter, and hyperintense on PD WI and T2 WI relative to CSF.[22]

Glioblastoma Multiforme

Definition

Glioblastoma multiforme is the most anaplastic form of glioma arising from extreme dedifferentiation of a preexisting astrocytoma or "de novo."[11,12] Positive staining for glial fibrillary acidic protein in most glioblastomas attests to their astrocytic origin.

Epidemiology

Glioblastoma multiforme represents about 15 to 20 percent of primary intracranial neoplasms and 50 percent of cerebral gliomas.[12] It is rare under age 30, and its peak incidence occurs in the fifth and sixth decades, with a slight predominance in males.[12,13]

Pathology

Macroscopically, glioblastoma multiforme has a variegated cut surface appearance with ill-defined margins, areas of solid growth alternating with zones of necrosis,

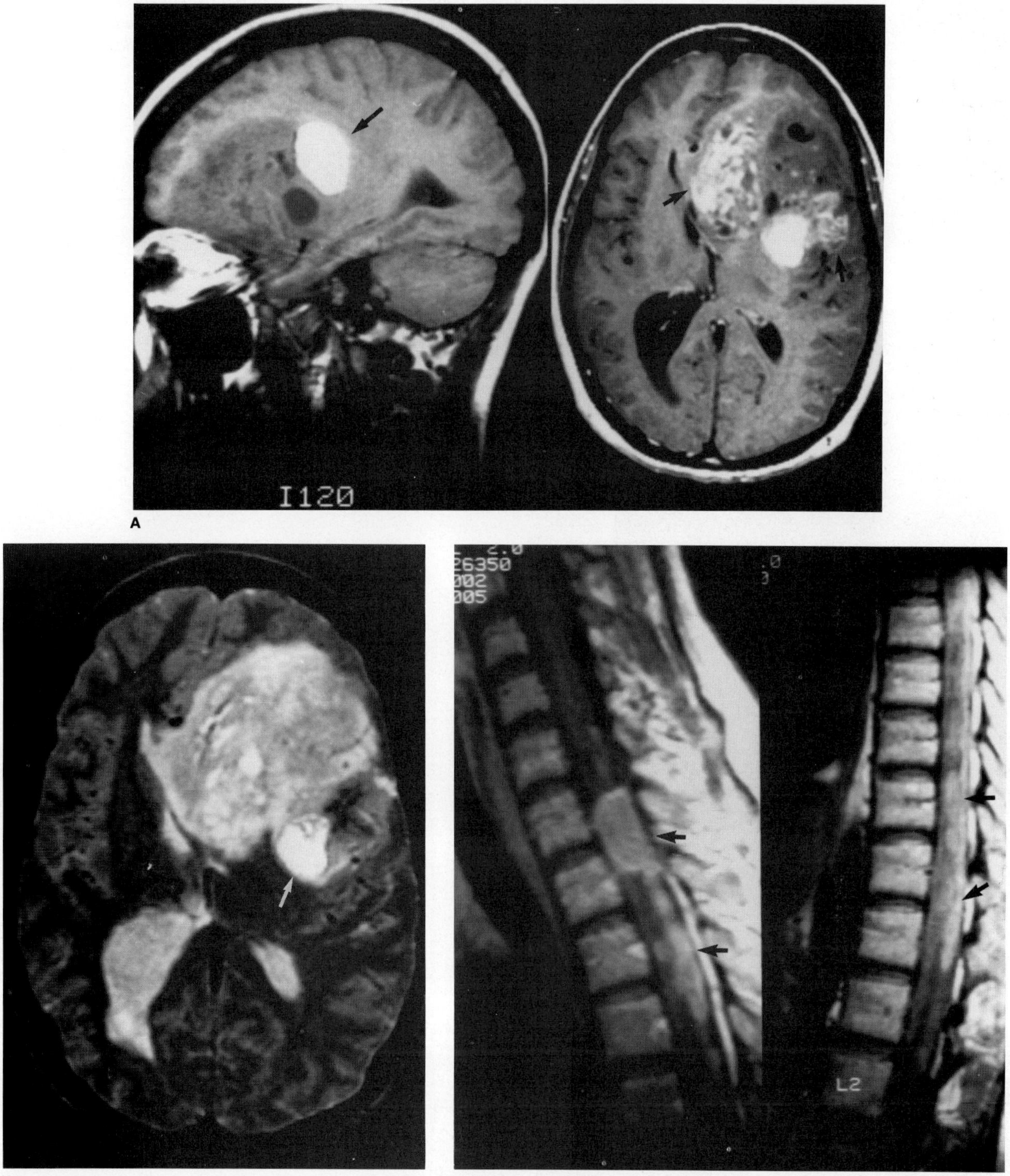

A

B

C

Figure 12-6

Anaplastic astrocytoma, left frontal lobe, in a 23-year-old woman with a 2-month history of headaches and seizures. **(A)** *Precontrast sagittal and postcontrast transverse T1 WI. In sagittal view, tumor appears as a large area of inhomogeneous hypointensity with cystic changes and focal area of hyperintensity representative of subacute hemorrhage (arrow). In transverse views enhancement is seen medially and laterally to hemorrhage (arrows) with nonenhancing cystic and solid tumor. Tumor infiltrates corpus callosum and causes marked shift of midline.* **(B)** *T2 WI. Large tumor exhibits inhomogeneous hyperintensity. Posterior hemorrhagic focus appears hyperintense, denoting extracellular methemoglobin (arrows).* **(C)** *Postcontrast sagittal cervical and thoracic T1 WI. There are multiple nodular enhancing drop metastases in intradural, extramedullary space (arrows).*

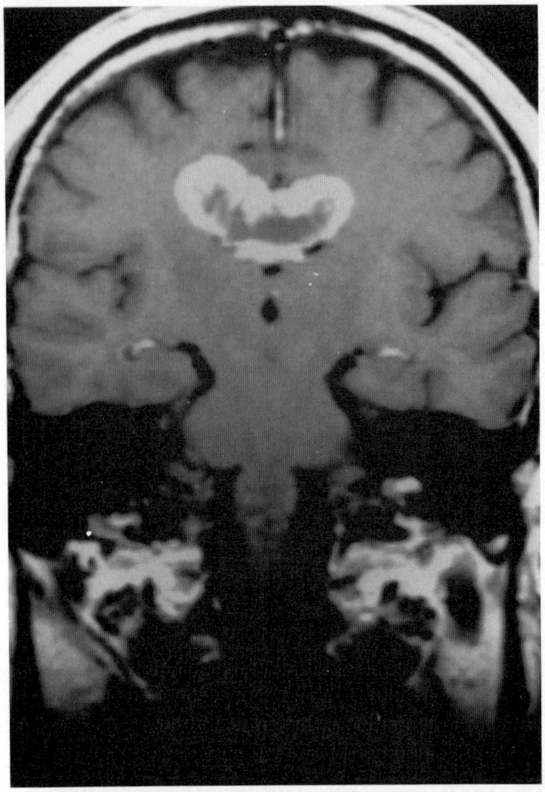

Figure 12-7

Anaplastic astrocytoma, corpus callosum in a 68-year-old man presenting with weakness of right leg, coronal postcontrast T1 WI. Ring of enhancement has wall width of varying thickness typical of high-grade malignant changes in astrocytoma. Tumor center is in the corpus callosum, extending to both sides (butterfly pattern).

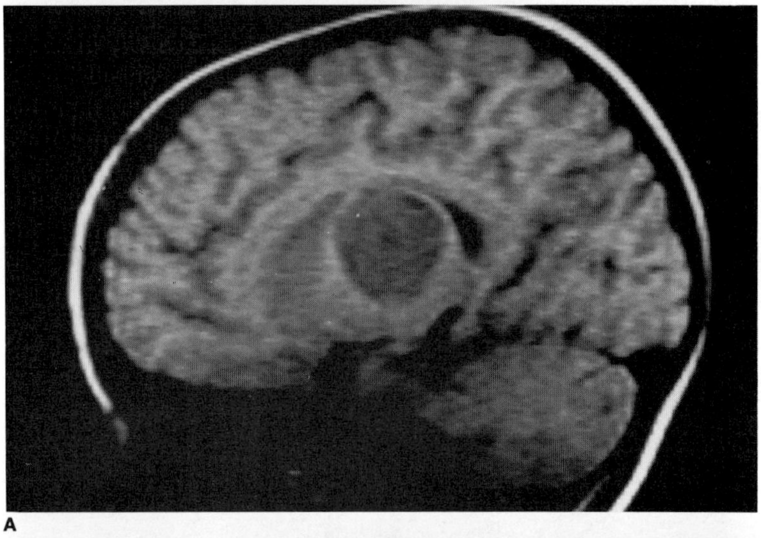

A

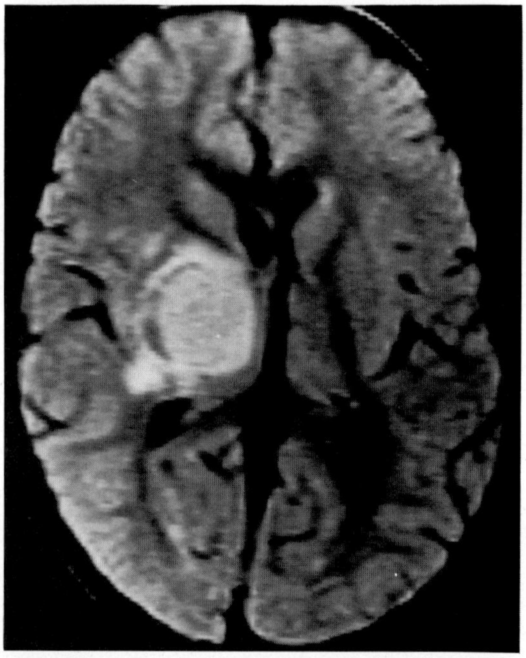

B

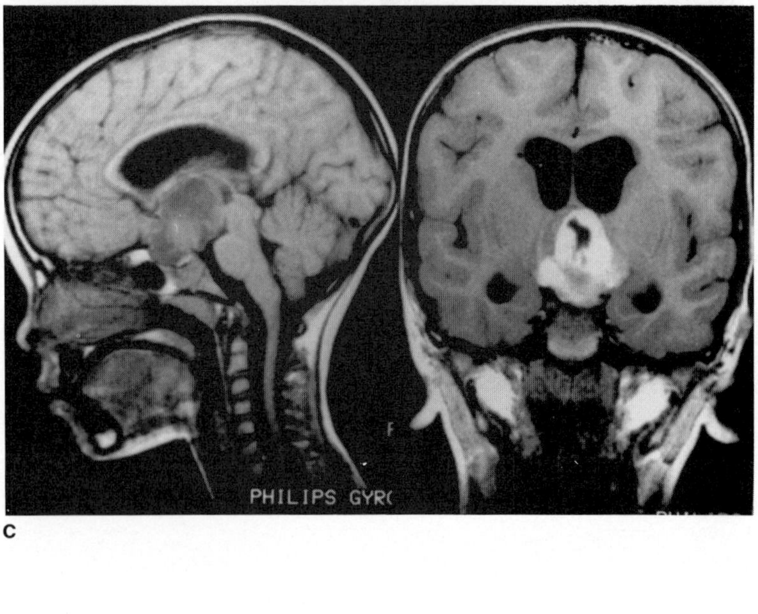

C

Figure 12-8

Pilocytic astrocytoma. **(A)** *A 4-year-old girl presenting with left hemiparesis, sagittal T1 WI. Tumor is well demarcated, solid, hypointense mass in thalamus.* **(B)** *Same patient, PD WI. Tumor appears homogeneous, hyperintense, with minimal surrounding edema in right thalamus.* **(C)** *A 5-year-old girl with a 3-week history of headaches and vomiting, precontrast sagittal and postcontrast coronal T1 WI. Large mixed iso- and hypointense tumor fills the third ventricle and extends into the sella turcica. Note marked enhancement which is typical of pilocytic astrocytoma despite its benign histology. The main differential diagnosis in this case is craniopharyngioma.*

and frequently old or recent hemorrhagic foci.[11,12] Cystic changes are common and may be multiple.[11] Common sites are the lobar white matter extending to gray matter (anterior greater than posterior); corpus callosum, from where it may grow to both sides of the centrum semiovale (butterfly glioblastoma); basal ganglia; and thalamus.[11,12] Six percent of glioblastomas have a multicentric origin.[12] Histologically, glioblastoma multiforme shows marked cellularity, nuclear pleomorphism, hyperchromatism, and many mitotic figures. Marked proliferation and hypertrophy of endothelial cells and zones of necrosis with or without a perimeter of neoplastic cells (pseudopallisading) are hallmarks of glioblastoma multiforme.[11–14] With multimodality therapy (surgery plus radiation plus chemotherapy), median survival time is 1 year or more, and 25 to 30 percent of patients survive for 18 months.[23]

Imaging Studies

On noncontrast CT studies, glioblastoma multiforme exhibits more frequently a heterogeneous mixed pattern of a slight hyperdense zone, ring-like, surrounding a hypodense center (Fig. 12-9).[24] A homogeneous hypodense lesion without clear separation of peripheral and central zones is the next most common appearance on noncontrast CT. Ninety to 100 percent of glioblastomas enhance by CT, more frequently in a ring-like or annular pattern corresponding to the hypercellular gross margins of the tumor that surround a central hypointense area of necrosis or cystic change.[17,24] The walls of the ring are usually thick and of irregular width. The other patterns on contrast CT are the mixed type, in which variable zones of enhancement are seen corresponding to a mixture of solid and cystic tumor and are nodular without cystic changes.[17,21,24] Hemorrhagic changes are more common in glioblastoma multiforme and can be recent or chronic in the form of hemosiderin.[20,21] Peritumoral vasogenic edema that may follow and expand the nearby white matter tracts in a "pseudopod" fashion is seen in up to 88 percent of glioblastomas.[17,24]

On MRI studies, glioblastoma usually exhibits heterogeneous hypointensity in T1 and hyperintensity in T2 WI (Figs. 12-9 and 12-10). The appearance of glioblastoma multiforme on contrast MRI is similar to the appearance on CT, and the most common pattern is ring-like enhancement of irregular and varying wall thickness surrounding a central area of hypointensity on T1 WI. Peritumoral pseudopod-like edema may appear more extensive in MRI studies. In both imaging methods the zones of enhancement correspond to tumor itself, whereas edematous regions include edema only or edema plus microscopic tumor.[25] Although MRI is considered more sensitive in demonstrating tumor extent and spread of malignant astrocytomas, microscopic tumor beyond the zone of hyperintensity depicted in T2 WI still occurs, as demonstrated in stereotactic biopsy specimens and postmortem studies.[25–27] Despite these

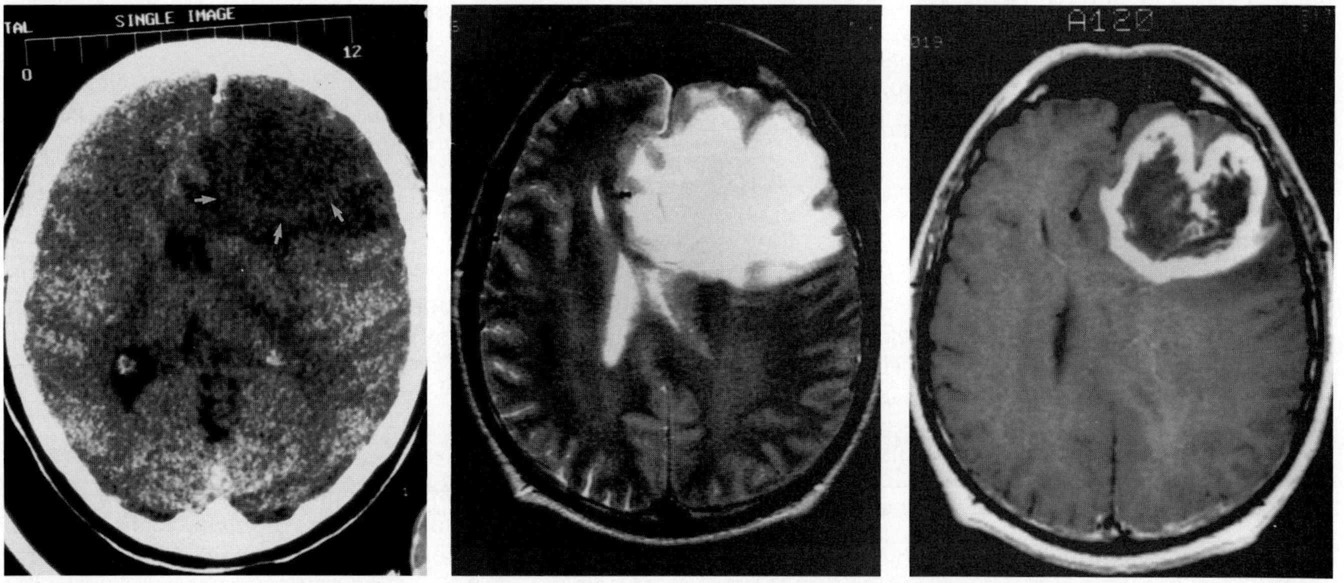

A B C

Figure 12-9
Glioblastoma multiforme, left frontal lobe, in a 53-year-old with a several-week history of headaches and personality changes. **(A)** *Noncontrast CT. Tumor has hypodense center with peripheral, slightly hyperdense zone (arrows) and surrounding edema.* **(B)** *T2 WI. Gross tumor margins and edema blend without distinction and appear as large hyperintense area.* **(C)** *Postcontrast T1 WI. Enhancement clearly depicts gross margin of tumor as rim of irregular, variable wall thickness. Center contains solid enhancing and nonenhancing necrotic and/or cystic tumor. Note subfalcine herniation.*

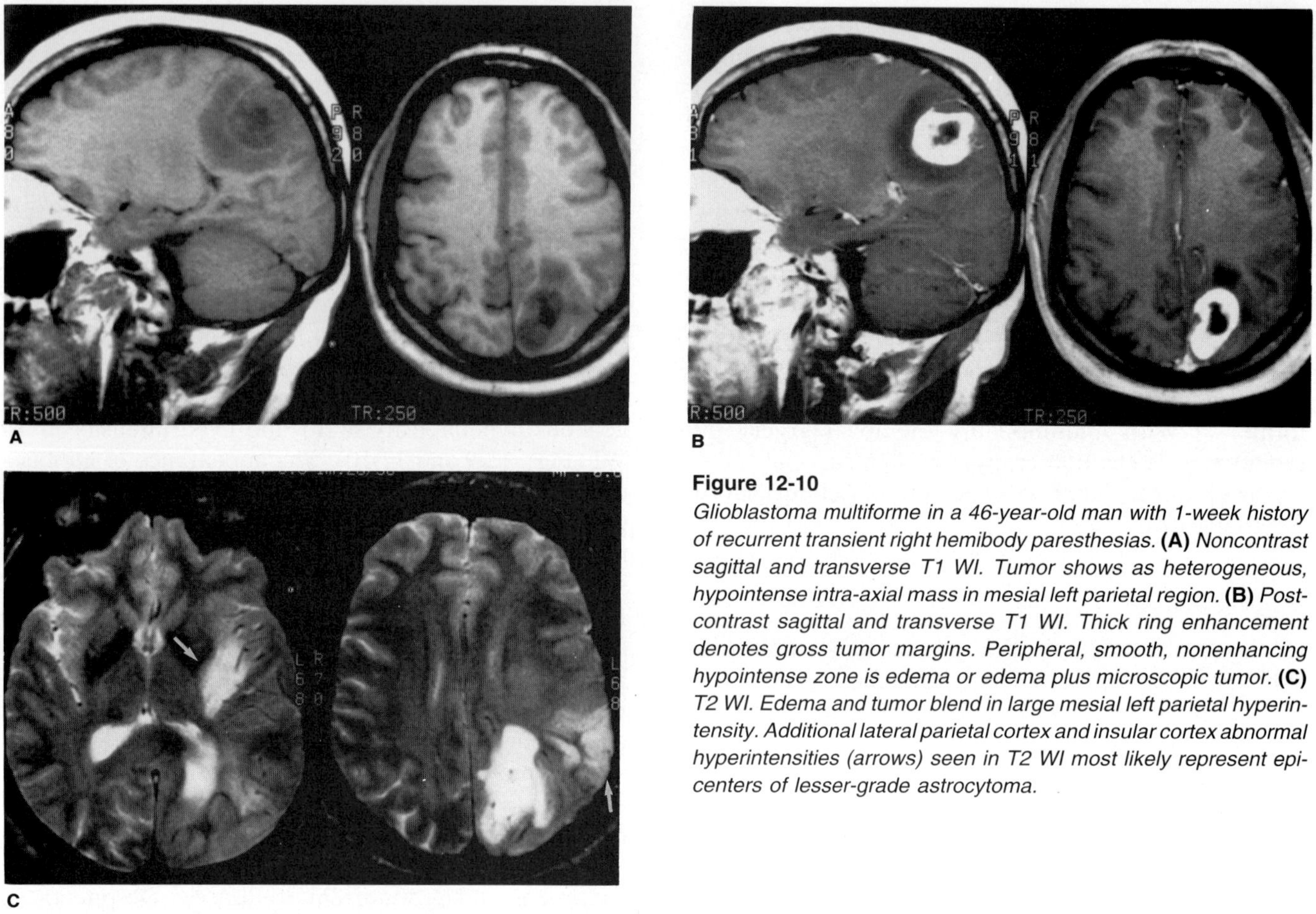

Figure 12-10
Glioblastoma multiforme in a 46-year-old man with 1-week history of recurrent transient right hemibody paresthesias. **(A)** *Noncontrast sagittal and transverse T1 WI. Tumor shows as heterogeneous, hypointense intra-axial mass in mesial left parietal region.* **(B)** *Postcontrast sagittal and transverse T1 WI. Thick ring enhancement denotes gross tumor margins. Peripheral, smooth, nonenhancing hypointense zone is edema or edema plus microscopic tumor.* **(C)** *T2 WI. Edema and tumor blend in large mesial left parietal hyperintensity. Additional lateral parietal cortex and insular cortex abnormal hyperintensities (arrows) seen in T2 WI most likely represent epicenters of lesser-grade astrocytoma.*

limitations, multiplanar MRI utilizing pre- and postcontrast T1 WI and T2 WI offers the best gross total assessment of tumor size, location, and follow-up in glioblastoma multiforme and less malignant hemispheric astrocytomas.[25]

Gliomatosis Cerebri

Definition

Gliomatosis cerebri is a diffusely infiltrative, variably differentiated astrocytic neoplasm without a necrotic glioblastomatous center. It occurs over geographically wide areas of the central nervous system (CNS).[13,14,28]

Epidemiology

The age of onset of gliomatosis cerebri varies from 6 to 60 years, with most cases reported in the first and second decades of life. Its true incidence is not known, but the condition is considered quite rare. The most common clinical findings are personality changes and a decline in mental status, followed by hemiparesis, ataxia, papilledema, headaches, seizures, and brainstem findings.[29]

Pathology

As it infiltrates diffuse portions of the brain, gliomatosis cerebri enlarges the cerebral hemispheres, cerebellum, or brainstem without causing focal tumefaction.[13,14] Microscopically, gliomatosis cerebri consists of extensive gray and white matter infiltration by undifferentiated cells with foci of better-differentiated neoplastic astrocytes arranged in a perineuronal, perivascular, and subpial distribution.[13] The prognosis is variable, with survival measured in months to years.[29]

Imaging Studies

The CT appearance of gliomatosis cerebri is that of inconspicuous, homogeneous, nonenhancing hypodensity spreading over large areas of white and gray matter, loss of gray-white matter differentiation, or a swollen hemisphere (Fig. 12-11).[30]

MRI displays gliomatosis cerebri as homogeneous hypointensity in T1 WI and hyperintensity in PD WI and T2 WI, invariably involving diffuse areas of gray and white matter of supratentorial and infratentorial compartments (Fig. 12-12).[31] The involvement may be unilat-

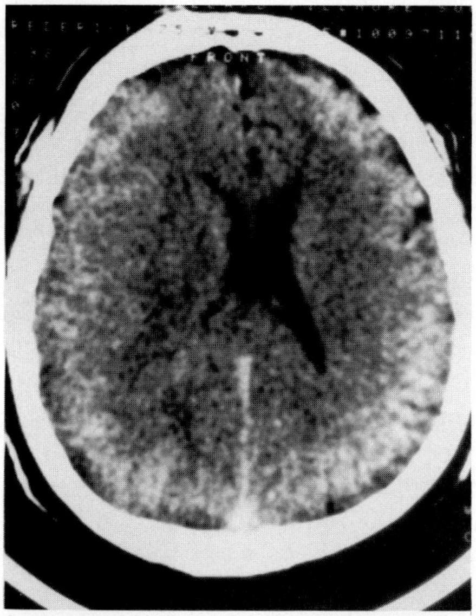

A

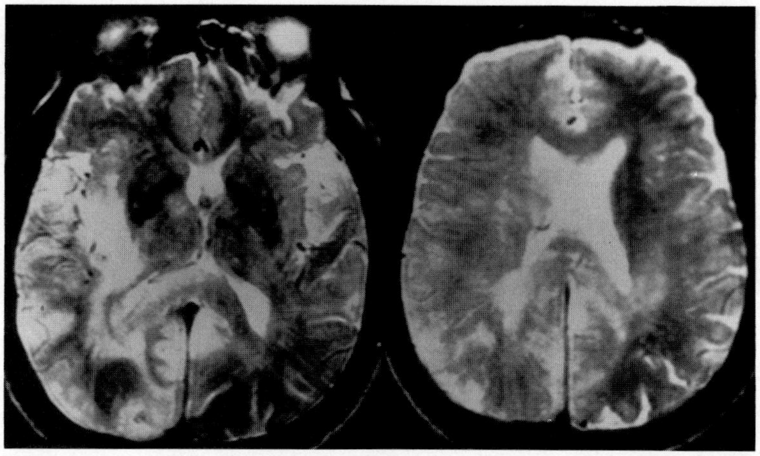

B

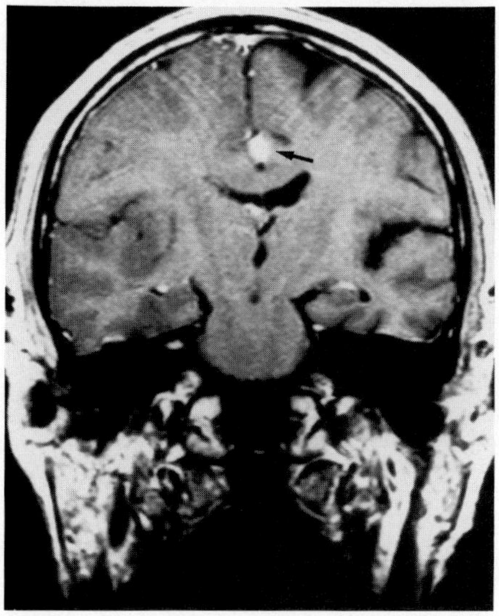

C

Figure 12-11
Gliomatosis cerebri in a 73-year-old man presenting with seizures and dementia. **(A)** *Noncontrast CT. Appearance is that of a swollen right hemisphere with slight shift of midline.* **(B)** *T2 WI. Gliomatosis appears as abnormal hyperintensity involving wide areas of temporal, occipital, and parietal gray and white matter and left mesioparietal gray matter.* **(C)** *Coronal postcontrast T1 WI. Right hemisphere appears swollen as denoted by effacement of cortical sulci, sylvian fissure. Note hypointensity of temporal and insular cortex and focal abnormal enhancement of left cingulate gyrus (arrow).*

eral or bilateral, and enhancement with contrast infusion is usually minimal or absent.

Oligodendroglioma

Definition

Oligodendroglioma is an intraparenchymal CNS tumor arising from oligodendrocytes, the supportive cells of the central nervous system that make up the central myelin.[13,14]

Epidemiology

Oligodendroglioma represents 5 to 15 percent of gliomas and is as common as low-grade astrocytoma, according to some authors.[13,14] Typically, oligodendroglioma is a tumor of the adult population, with a peak incidence in the fourth to fifth decades, although it may rarely occur in children.[13,14]

Pathology

Macroscopically, oligodendroglioma appears as a moderately well-circumscribed gray mass, often with cysts, focal hemorrhage, and calcification.[13,14] The most common location is the white matter of the frontal lobe, followed by the parietal, temporal, and occipital lobes.[13] From the hemispheric white matter the tumor extends outwardly, causing expansion of the overlying cortex.[13,14] Prominent in oligodendroglioma is the presence of calcifications in calcific grains or calcospherites, which are found microscopically in up to 90 percent of these tumors.[12–14] Microscopically, these are densely cellular tumors composed in most cases of patternless sheets

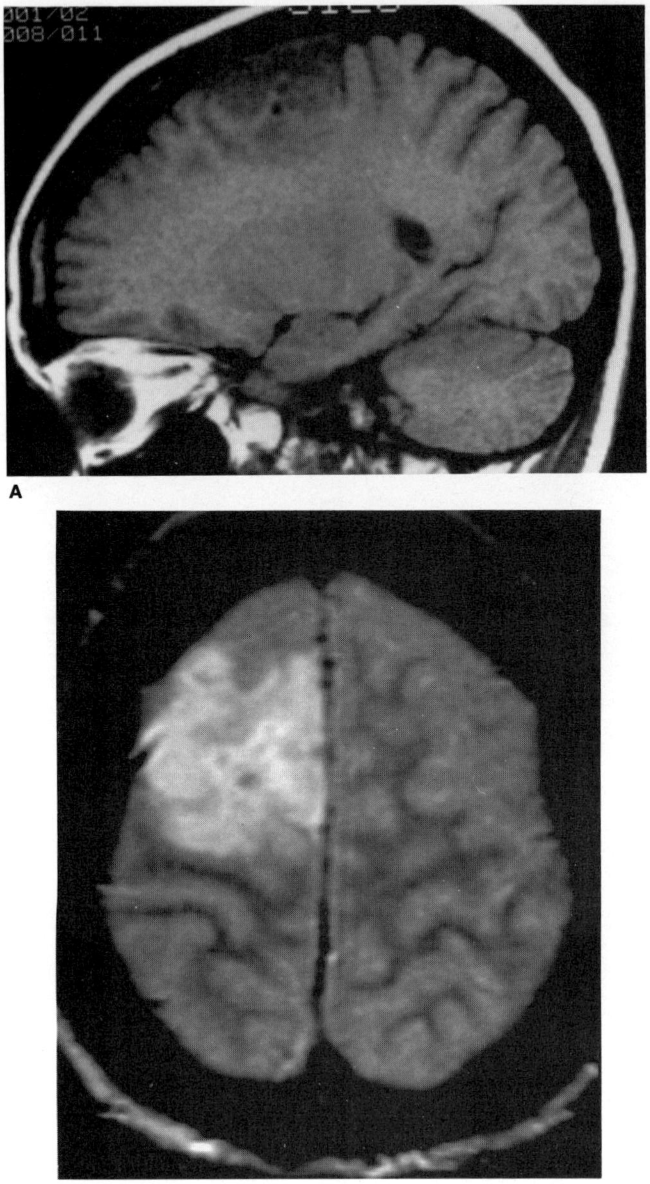

A

B

Figure 12-12
Oligodendroglioma, right posterior mesial frontal lobe, in a 38-year-old woman with a history of focal motor epilepsy. **(A)** *T1 WI. Tumor shows as intra-axial hypointense inhomogeneous cortical lesion.* **(B)** *PD WI. Tumor appears as homogeneous hyperintense cortical intra-axial lesion.*

of well-differentiated oligodendrocytes with perinuclear halos. The halos are considered an artifact of delayed fixation that gives the cells an appearance of "fried eggs" in permanent sections of nonfrozen tissue.[13] In some oligodendrogliomas there may be a component of neoplastic astrocytes, in which case the tumor is called a mixed glioma or oligoastrocytoma. A small proportion of oligodendrogliomas undergo malignant transformation featuring abundant mitotic activity, nuclear pleomorphism, vascular proliferation, and necrosis. The most common clinical presentation is a long-standing history of seizures.

Imaging Studies

Noncontrast CT studies display oligodendroglioma as a hypodense, homogeneous, or heterogeneous hemispheric mass lesion involving white matter and extending to the overlying gray matter, with calcification in 50 to 90 percent of cases (Fig. 12-13). Oligodendroglioma without anaplastic transformation usually shows little edema and minimal enhancement.[32]

MRI studies display oligodendroglioma as a homogeneous or heterogeneous hypointense lesion in T1 WI and hyperintense in PD WI and T2 WI, with minimal edema and enhancement unless there is anaplastic transformation (Figs. 12-12 and 12-13).[33] Calcification may not be well visualized in routine spin echo sequences, and its detection may require the use of T2*-weighted gradient echo sequences.

Dysembryoplastic Neuroepithelial Tumor

Definition

Dysembryoplastic neuroepithelial tumors (DNETS) constitute a supratentorial, morphologically unique, and surgically curable group of neuroepithelial tumors of heterogeneous cellular components that include astrocytes, oligodendrocytes, and neurons.[34]

Epidemiology

The age at the onset of symptoms ranges from 1 to 19 years (mean, 9 years). Chronic seizure is the typical mode of presentation in the large majority of these patients. These lesions are associated with a good prognosis and are potentially curable by surgical resection.[34]

Pathology

DNETs are primarily cortical in location, involving the temporal, frontal, and parieto-occipital lobes in decreasing order of frequency. As many as one-third of these patients have an overlying focal calvarial deformity, indicating the early onset and long-standing evolution.[34,35] The pathologic features are multinodularity and cellular heterogeneity characterized by neurons floating within pools of oligodendrocytes and, to a lesser extent, astrocytes.[34,35] Unlike oligodendrogliomas, which predominantly involve white matter and secondarily involve gray matter, a DNET is primarily intracortical in location. The term *dysembryoplastic neuroepithelial tumor* was proposed because the clinicopathologic features suggest a dysembryoplastic origin.[34]

Imaging Findings

The imaging findings in DNET are essential in the prebiopsy diagnosis and are characterized in CT studies as typically pseudocystic (Fig. 12-14), predominantly cortical, well-demarcated, low-density intraparenchymal le-

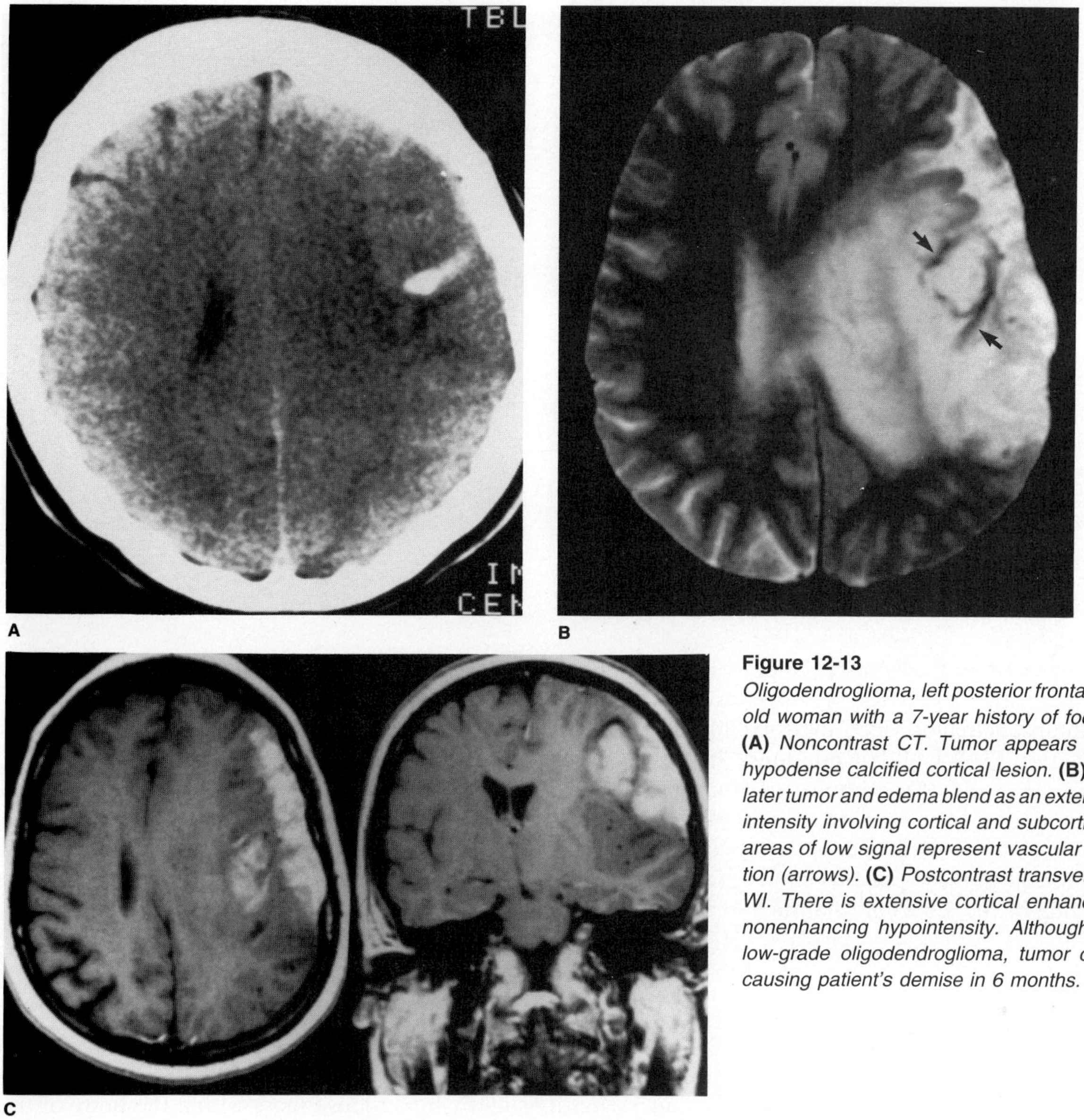

Figure 12-13
Oligodendroglioma, left posterior frontal lobe, in a 37-year-old woman with a 7-year history of focal motor seizures. **(A)** *Noncontrast CT. Tumor appears as mixed iso- and hypodense calcified cortical lesion.* **(B)** *T2 WI. Five years later tumor and edema blend as an extensive area of hyperintensity involving cortical and subcortical regions. Linear areas of low signal represent vascular supply or calcification (arrows).* **(C)** *Postcontrast transverse and coronal T1 WI. There is extensive cortical enhancement mixed with nonenhancing hypointensity. Although surgery revealed low-grade oligodendroglioma, tumor continued to grow, causing patient's demise in 6 months.*

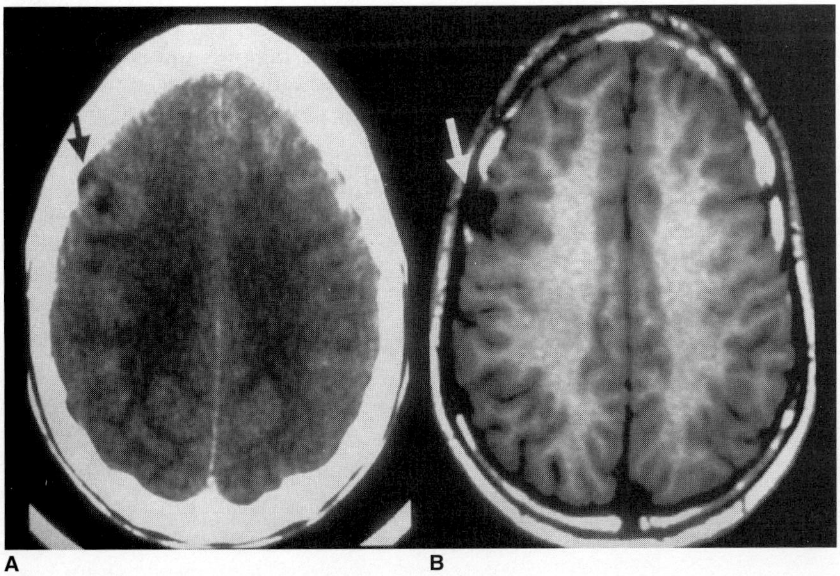

Figure 12-14
Dysembryoplastic neuroepithelial tumor in the right frontal lobe in a 17-year-old male presenting with seizures. Noncontrast CT **(A)** *shows the tumor as a pseudocystic cortical hypodense lesion (black arrow), and noncontrast T1 WI* **(B)** *shows it as a cortical hypointense lesion (white arrow). There was no enhancement with contrast.*

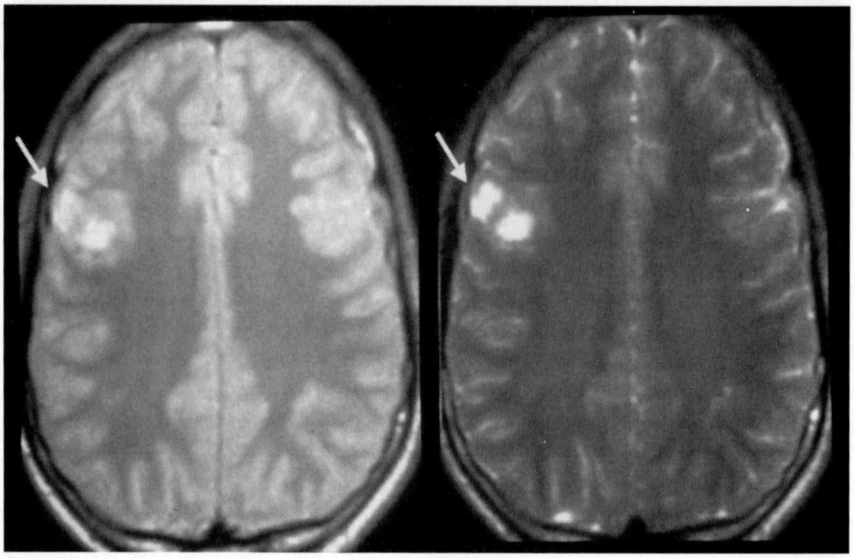

Figure 12-15
Dysembryoplastic neuroepithelial tumor in the same patient shown in Fig. 12-14. Both PD WI **(A)** *and T2 WI* **(B)** *show the tumor as a well-circumscribed cortical hyperintense lesion without peritumoral edema (white arrows).*

sions, in some cases with enhancement (18 percent) or calcification (23 percent).[34] On MRI, the appearance is that of a hyperintense, circumscribed gyriform-like lesion on PD WI and T2 WI and hypointense in T1-weighted images (Fig. 12-15) without peritumoral edema.[36,37] The temporal lobe is most commonly involved, followed by the frontal and parieto-occipital lobes. Over 50 percent of these patients show evidence of bone remodeling of the adjacent calvaria.[37]

Central Neurocytoma

Definition

Central neurocytomas are rare, usually benign, intraventricular tumors of neuronal origin that occur in young adults.[35,38]

Epidemiology

Usually these tumors have a favorable prognosis, although there have been some reports of malignant transformation.[39] With total or nearly complete excision, the prognosis is quite favorable.

Pathology

Neurocytomas occur typically in the lateral and third ventricles near the foramen of Monro, with the septum pellucidum being a common site of origin. They appear sharply demarcated and lobulated and usually fill the ventricular space but usually do not infiltrate the surrounding parenchyma. Microscopic features are characterized by monotonous hypercellularity. The cells are strikingly uniform in nuclear contour, with rare mitosis.[35] Neurocytomas originally were classified as intraventricular oligodendrogliomas because of their similar cellular appearance, but this tumor is now considered a well-differentiated neuronal neoplasm, based on ultrastructural findings of neuritic processes with neurotubules, occasional synapses and neurosecretory vesicles, and immunohistochemical reactivity for synaptophysin and neuron-specific enolase, both of which are neuronal markers.[35] Complete removal of the tumor mass without radiotherapy is the treatment of choice. The prognosis is usually favorable, without recurrence.[40]

Imaging Findings

On CT, central neurocytoma usually presents as a primarily slightly hyperdense mass within the body of the lateral ventricle or third ventricle with moderate contrast enhancement.[38] The majority of these tumors contain small multiple cysts and calcifications and exhibit a characteristic broad-based attachment to the superior-lateral ventricular wall.[38] On MRI, the tumors frequently appear isointense relative to the cortex in T1- and T2-weighted images or slightly hyperintense relative to cortex in T2 WI (Fig. 12-16). Calcifications are not well visualized by MRI. Intratumoral hemorrhage may be present occasionally on MRI but usually is not seen on CT.[41] Contrast enhancement is variable in degree and pattern in both MRI and CT images.[38,41]

Ependymoma

Definition

Ependymoma is a glioma that arises from neoplastic transformation of ependymal cells that line the ventricular system surfaces.

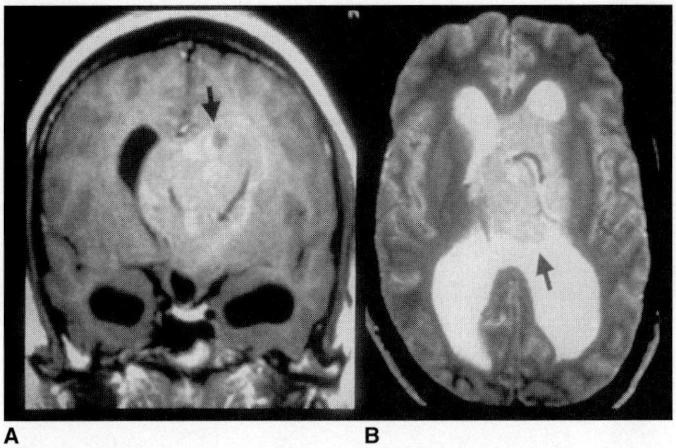

Figure 12-16
Central neurocytoma in a 23-year-old male presenting with headaches and papilledema. Postcontrast T1 WI **(A)** *shows the tumor as a large, solid, hypointense, minimally enhancing mass with cyst formation (black arrow) filling the ventricular system. In T2 WI* **(B)** *the tumor appears as relatively hypointense intraventricular mass (black arrow). Note that there is no apparent invasion of neighboring brain parenchyma. Curvilinear low-signal-intensity structures within the tumor represent vessels.*

Epidemiology

Ependymoma accounts for 2 to 6 percent of all gliomas. Primarily a tumor of children and adolescents, it has its peak incidence in the 10- to 15-year-old age group.[12,13] In classic neuropathology teaching, ependymoma is listed as the most common hemispheric glioma tumor in children.[14] Sixty percent of ependymomas are infratentorial, and 40 percent are supratentorial.

Pathology

Macroscopically, ependymoma is usually well circumscribed, with a homogeneous and occasionally hemorrhagic cut surface. Large tumors, especially those situated above the tentorium, may be cystic with small gritty foci of calcification.[12] The most common site of occurrence is the fourth ventricle, which accounts for 70 percent of cases, followed by the lateral ventricular region and the third ventricle. In cerebral ependymoma, the origin is in the lateral ventricular surface or ependymal rests near the ventricular surface.[12] The tumor extends from the lateral ventricle toward the hemisphere. Microscopically, ependymoma consists of a monotonous proliferation of neoplastic ependymal cells that often are engaged in the formation of perivascular pseudorosettes and true ependymal rosettes.[12,13] In perivascular pseudo rosettes delicate cytoplasmic processes converge toward a blood vessel, and true ependymal rosette cells are arranged to form a gland or canal-like structure.[13] Most ependymomas are benign, featuring infrequent mitosis and mild cell pleomorphism only. Anaplastic transformation in which the ependymal features are lost may occur, but this is uncommon. Because of their close relationship to the ventricles, CSF-borne metastases may occur.[12]

Imaging Studies

Supratentorial hemispheric ependymoma is periventricular and intraparenchymal in about 75 percent of cases rather than purely intraventricular, a feature that is most commonly seen in the posterior fossa ependymoma. Cerebral ependymoma is usually a large, cystic lesion, hypodense on noncontrast CT, with moderate to intense homogeneous or ring enhancement after contrast infusion.[42] Tumor calcification is present in one-third of cases, and peritumoral edema in 50 percent. Hemorrhages are difficult to detect on CT.[42] On MRI studies, the appearance of cerebral ependymoma is that of a solid or cystic hypointense mass lesion in T1 WI and hyperintense in PD WI and T2 WI (Fig. 12-17). Foci of signal heterogeneity usually denote hemorrhage in different stages, necrosis, calcification, and vascularity.[43] The pattern of enhancement with MRI contrast agents has not been documented in large series.

The appearance of posterior fossa ependymoma is outlined in the next section.

Ganglioglioma

Definition

Ganglioglioma is an intraparenchymal CNS tumor composed of neoplastic mature neurons and neoplastic astrocytes.[12]

Epidemiology

Ganglioglioma represents 3 percent of brain tumors in children with a peak incidence between 9 and 18 years of age.[16] Eighty percent of gangliogliomas present in patients under the age of 30.[12]

Pathology

The macroscopic appearance of ganglioglioma varies from small solid to large cystic, with mural nodule intraparenchymal tumor most often located in the cerebrum, typically in the temporal lobe.[12] Other locations include the floor of the third ventricle, other ventricles, basal ganglia, and cerebellum.[12] Microscopically, ganglioglioma is composed of neoplastic astrocytes and abnormal bizarre neurons of varying size and shape, including giant and binucleated forms with anomalous, irregularly oriented processes.[12,14] Mitotic figures are not seen in neuronal forms. Cytologically, ganglioglioma is con-

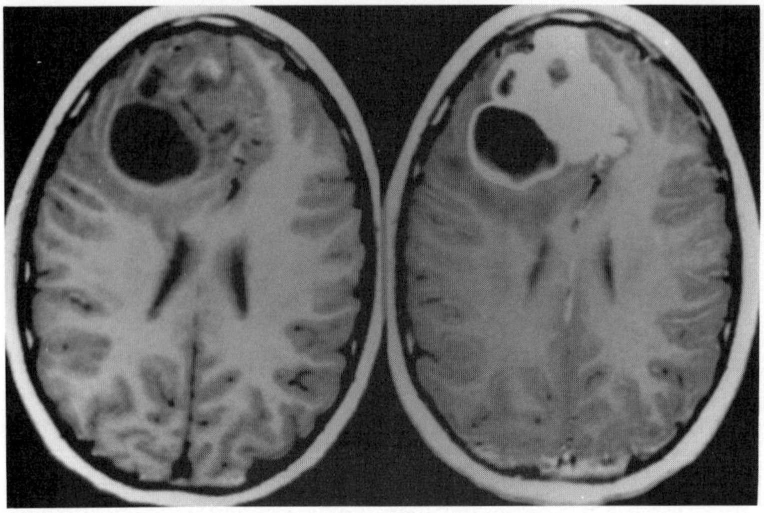

A

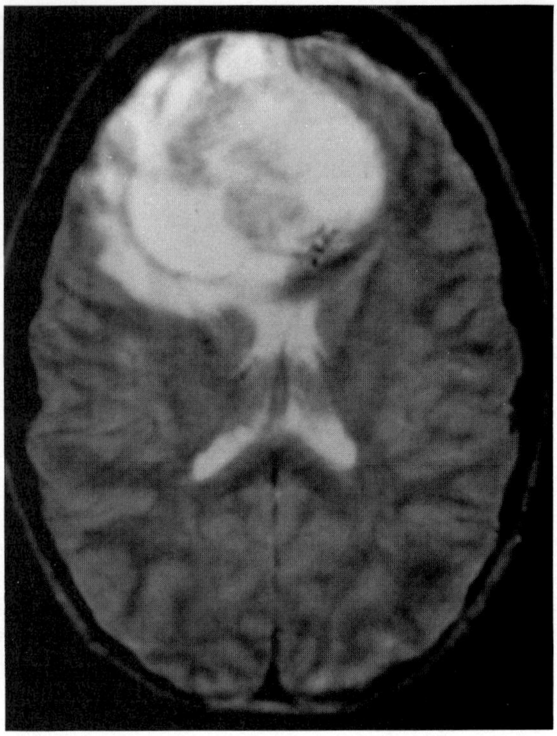

B

Figure 12-17

Supratentorial ependymoma in an 11-year-old boy. **(A)** *Pre- and postcontrast T1 WI. Tumor appears as large, intra-axial, heterogeneous, solid, and cystic tumor in the right frontal lobe. Solid portions of the tumor markedly enhance with gadolinium. Note marked mass effect from right to left.* **(B)** *T2 WI. Tumor is not as well delineated as in T1 WI, appearing as an iso- and hyperintense mass with surrounding edema.*

sidered a slow-growing benign tumor, a feature that translates into a stable clinical course. Most patients present with long-standing clinical findings that depend on the tumor location, such as partial epilepsy with cerebral lesions.

Imaging Studies

The appearance of ganglioglioma in imaging studies (CT and MRI) is that of a variably circumscribed, small to large, solid with cystic changes, and largely cystic intraparenchymal mass located by decreasing order of frequency in the temporal, frontal, and parieto-occipital regions with little or no surrounding edema.[44,45]

On noncontrast CT, the density of ganglioglioma varies from homogeneously isodense in small solid lesions to hypodense in cystic types. Calcification, which is present in 35 percent of gangliogliomas, occurs focally along the cyst wall or in solid portions of the tumor (Fig. 12-18).[44] Moderate enhancement on CT occurs in 50 percent of cases.

Cystic gangliogliomas are homogeneously or heterogeneously hypointense and solid tumors are iso- or hypointense relative to gray matter on T1 WI[45] (Figs. 12-18 and 12-19). On PD WI and T2 WI both solid and cystic varieties are usually homogeneously hyperintense relative to surrounding brain.[45] MRI contrast enhancement has not been evaluated in large series of gangliogliomas. Although cystic gangliogliomas with mural nodules have been described in pathology texts, this appearance has not been emphasized in the imaging literature.[12,44,45]

Meningioma

Definition

Meningioma is a common extra-axial intracranial neoplasm that originates from meningothelial or arachnoid cells. These cells are found clustered in arachnoid villae seen close to venous sinuses but also are scattered throughout the intracranial and spinal arachnoid membranes.[12,13] In patients with meningiomas, genetic analysis frequently demonstrates multiple lesions on chromosome 22, presumably leading to loss of regulation function and tumor cell proliferation.[12,13] Progesterone receptors are found in the majority of meningiomas, and this may explain tumor growth during pregnancy and in association with breast carcinoma in the same patient.[12,13]

Epidemiology

Meningioma is the most common benign brain tumor, accounting for 13 to 19 percent of intracranial neoplasms.[12,46] Its peak incidence is between the ages of 40 to 60, and women are affected twice as often as one men.[47] Meningioma is distinctly uncommon in children, in whom it constitutes 1 to 2 percent of intracranial tumors.[47]

Pathology

Meningioma arises from the inner surface of the dura, growing slowly to form a small or large, bulky, round,

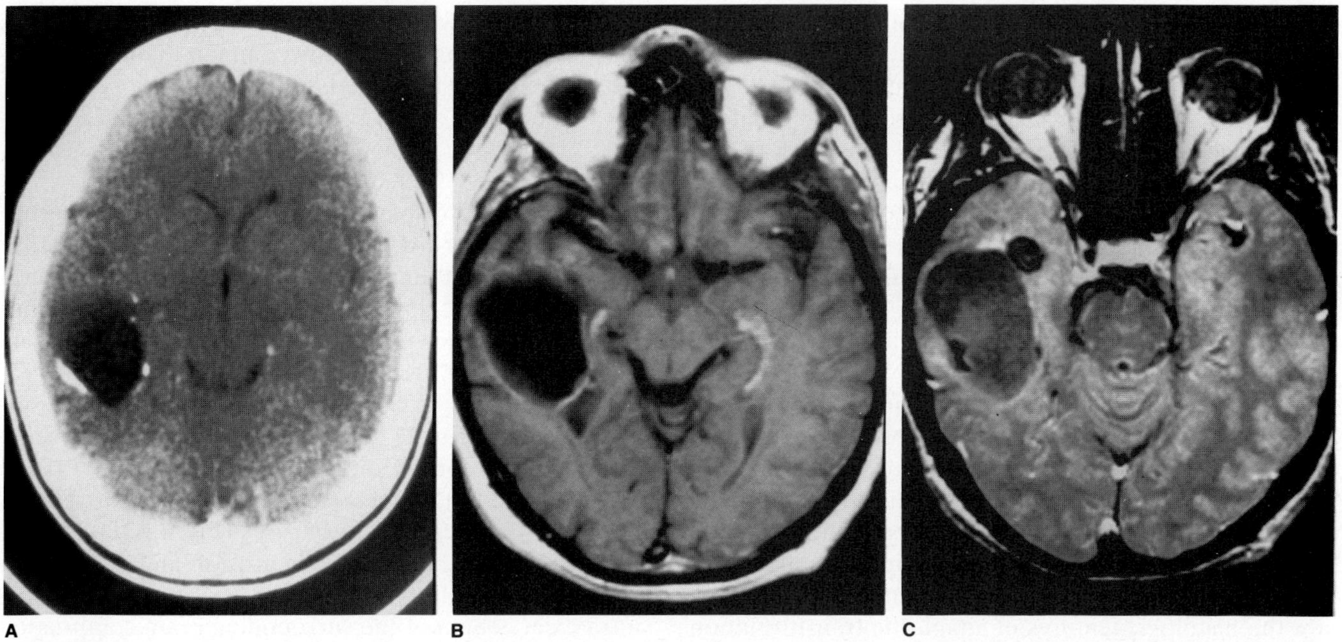

Figure 12-18
Cystic ganglioglioma, right temporal lobe, in a 36-year-old man with a lifelong history of psychomotor seizures. **(A)** *Noncontrast CT shows tumors as well demarcated, hypodense cystic lesion with foci of calcification along cyst wall.* **(B)** *Postcontrast T1 WI. Tumor appears as large, homogeneous, hypointense intraaxial temporal lobe cyst with minimal enhancement along its wall. Calcifications are not seen.* **(C)** *PD WI. Cyst exhibits mixed iso- and hypointensity that is different from CSF's. Calcifications are seen as marked hypointense foci along cyst wall.*

soft to tough, generally solid globoid tumor with a narrow or broad dural attachment that displaces rather than infiltrates the brain underneath.[12,13,47] When arranged in a thin, carpetlike, soft gelatinous pannus, meningioma is aptly termed "en plaque."[12,13,47,48] Globoid meningioma typically occurs in the convexity, suprasellar, and olfactory groove regions, whereas en plaque meningioma is more common in the region of the pterion and sphenoid ridge.[13] Thirty to 40 percent of meningiomas are encountered in the convexity (parasagittal and free convexity), followed in decreasing order of frequency by the sphenoid ridge, olfactory groove, suprasellar region, falx, posterior fossa, and temporal fossa.[47,48] When arising from the tela choroidea or velum interpositum, meningioma has no dural attachment and grows into the lateral, third, and fourth ventricles, where it usually remains confined without invading the brain. With dural invasion, meningiomas may grow in the extradural space, and in the case of bone erosion, extracranial extension may result. Examples are the convexity and olfactory groove meningiomas that erode the calvarium and cribriform plate, extending to the subgaleal and nasal fossa compartments, respectively.[48] Histologically, meningioma can be classified into four basic types: syncytial or meningothelial, transitional, fibroblastic, and angioblastic.[12,13] In syncytial meningioma, meningothelial cells with pale nuclei aggregated in whorls and lobules dominate the histologic picture.[13] The fibroblastic meningi-

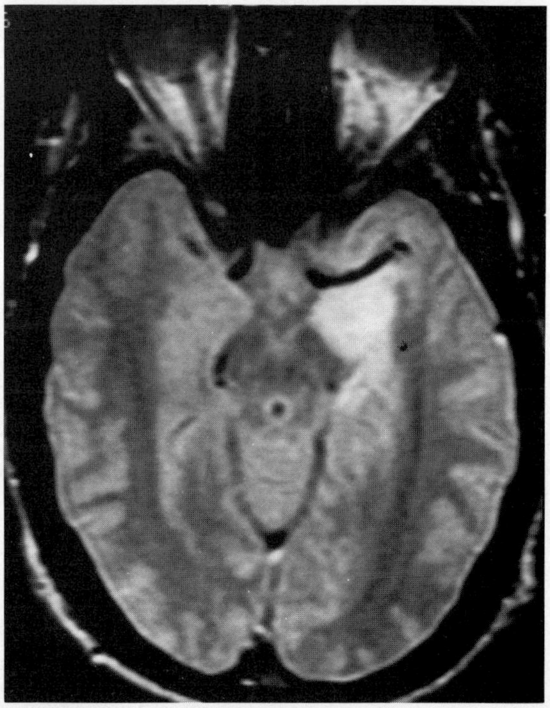

Figure 12-19
Solid ganglioglioma in a 28-year-old man with 5-year history of psychomotor seizures, PD WI. Tumor shows as well-delineated hyperintense lesion in left uncus.

oma is characterized by elongated, spindle-shaped cells in sheets and fascicles, often without whorls or lobularity.[13] Transitional meningioma contains features of both syncytial and fibroblastic types. Psammomatous bodies, which are calcified structures consisting of calcium apatite crystals admixed with concentrically arranged collagenous fibers, are more common in transitional meningioma but may be seen in the other two types described above and at times may dominate the histologic picture (psammmomatous meningioma).[12,13] The term *angioblastic* was used initially to describe a variety of meningioma characterized by hypercellularity, numerous thin-walled vascular channels, and aggressive growth.[47] Some neuropathologists consider them true hemangiopericytomas, malignant neoplasms derived from pericytes of periendothelial localization and of mesenchymal origin but distinct from meningothelial cells.[13] An increase in mitotic activity, infiltration of CNS parenchyma, microscopic necrosis, and cellular atypia are the histologic features of anaplastic transformation that may occur with all types of meningiomas.[12,13] Anaplastic transformation is more common in the hemangiopericytic or angioblastic type.

Imaging Findings

Noncontrast CT displays typical meningiomas as homogeneous, slightly hyperdense (70 percent) or isodense (25 percent), well-demarcated masses adjacent to dural surfaces (Figs. 12-20 to 12-24).[21,48,49] Their close proximity to dural sinuses may lead to invasion and ultimately obstruction of those structures. Hypodense meningiomas represent 1 to 6 percent of cases.[48] Calcifications are present in 15 to 27 percent of cases, appearing evenly distributed or focally throughout the tumor[21,48,50] (Figs. 12-21 and 12-24). Hyperostosis, either focal or diffuse, occurs in 15 to 20 percent of cases (Fig. 12-21).[48] Other osseous changes, such as bone erosion and destruction with extracranial growth, also may occur.[48] Vasogenic intra-axial edema of the surrounding brain compressed

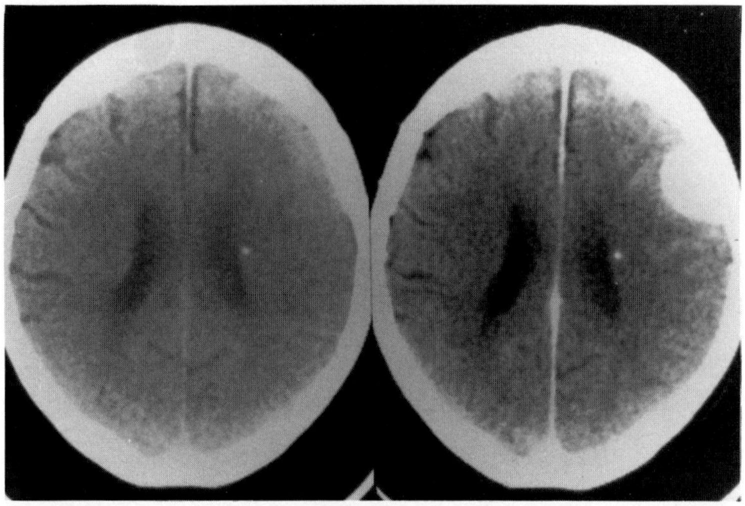

A

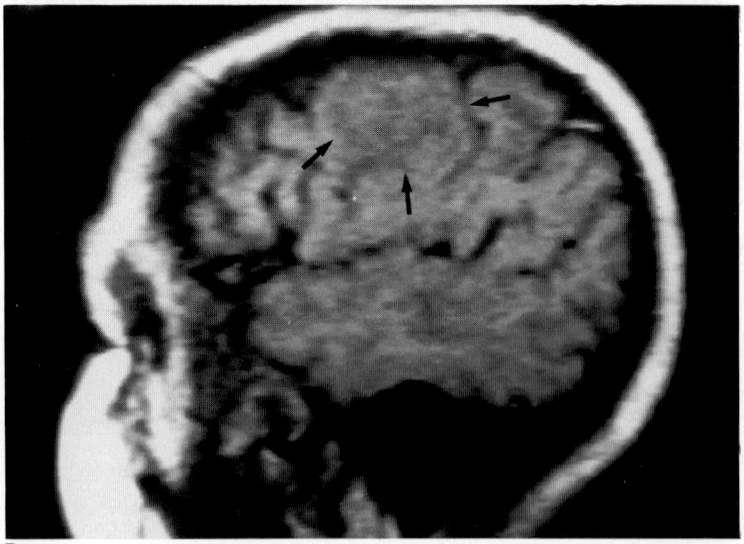

B

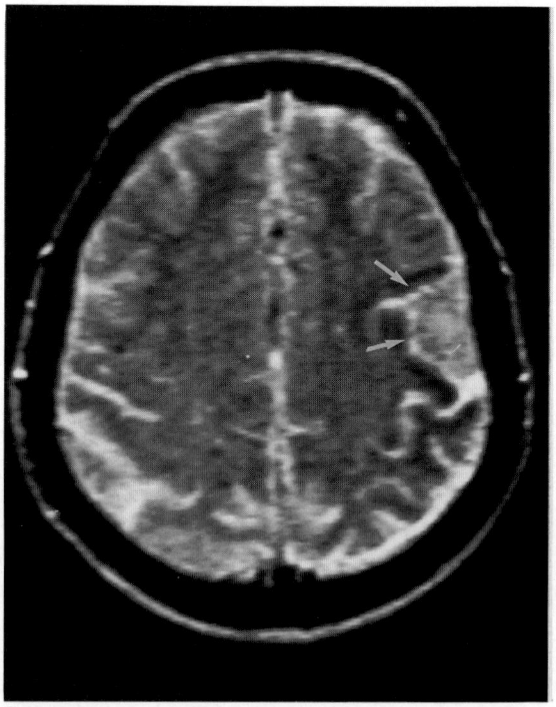

C

Figure 12-20

Syncytial meningioma, left frontal convexity, in a 79-year-old man with 3-year history of focal right-sided motor seizures. **(A)** *Pre- and postcontrast CT. In precontrast study isodense tumor is not seen, but it causes blurring of cortical sulci. Postcontrast image shows homogeneous, intense enhancement typical of meningioma.* **(B)** *T1 WI. Tumor is isointense and could be easily missed. Note blurring of cortical sulci by tumor (arrows).* **(C)** *T2 WI. Tumor is isointense relative to gray matter and could go unnoticed (arrows). This case illustrates the difficulty MRI had in identifying isointense meningiomas before gadolinium was available.*

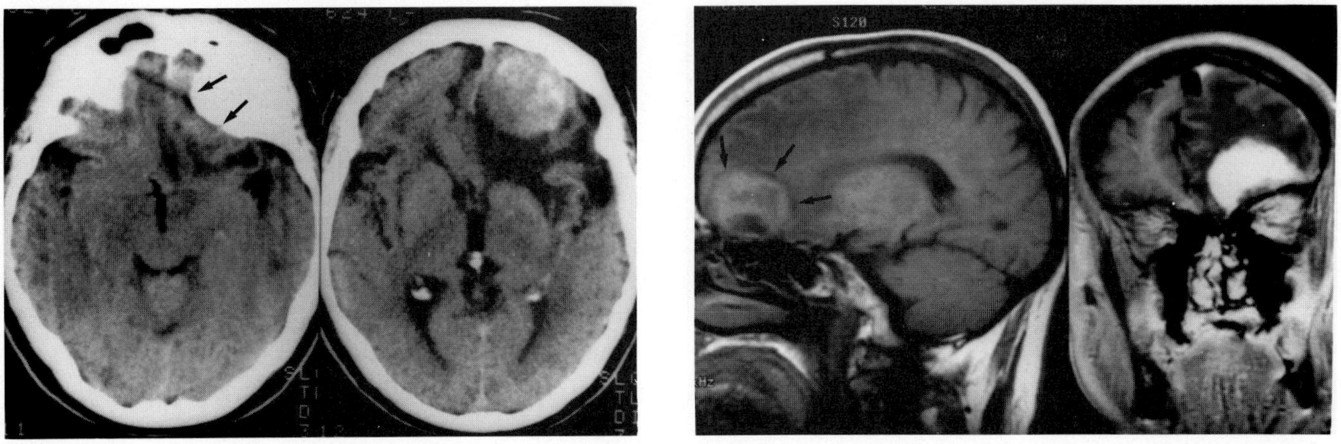

A B

Figure 12-21

Transitional meningioma, left anterior fossa, in an 80-year-old man presenting with headaches. **(A)** *Noncontrast CT. Meningioma appears hyperdense and well demarcated from edema. Note hyperostosis (arrows).* **(B)** *Precontrast sagittal and postcontrast coronal T1 WI. Note peritumoral halo in sagittal view (arrows) separating isointense tumor from brain. Coronal views show marked homogeneous enhancement and dural base inferiorly. Extensive edema disproportionate to tumor size as seen in this case may occur with subfrontal meningiomas.*

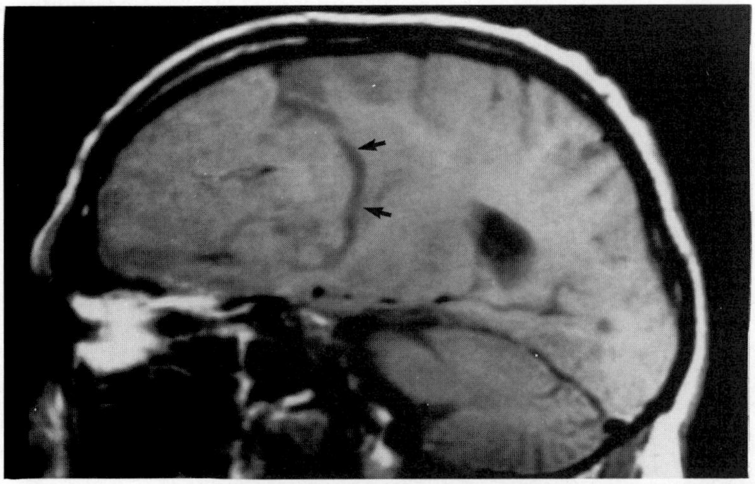

A

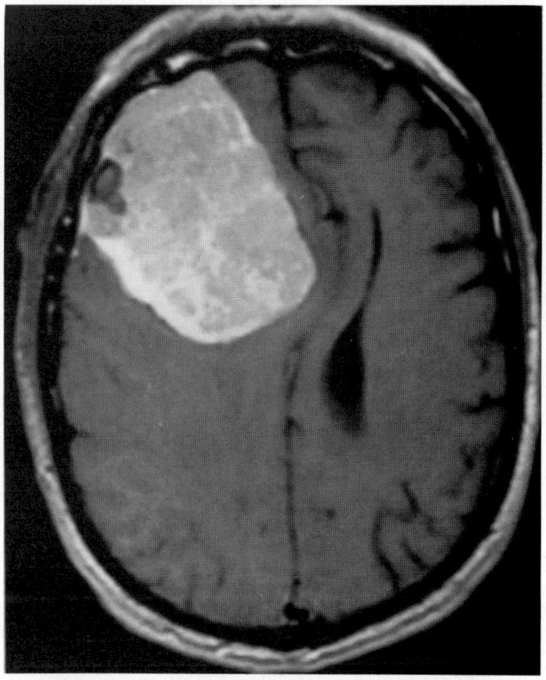

B

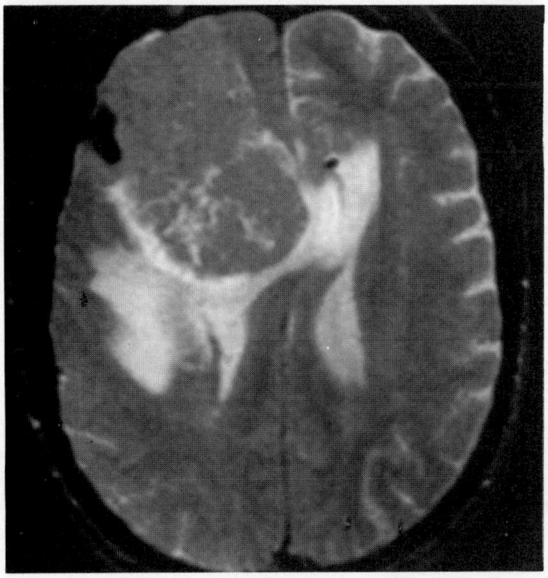

C

Figure 12-22

Transitional meningioma, right frontal convexity, in a 76-year-old man with several months' history of headaches and forgetfulness. **(A)** *T1 WI. Tumor is isointense but well demarcated at its periphery by hypointense halo (arrows).* **(B)** *Contrast T1 WI. Tumor enhances homogeneously. Mesial portion of tumor causes buckling of corpus callosum. Unenhanced nodule represents calcification.* **(C)** *T2 WI. Tumor is isointense relative to gray matter, as expected with transitional type; edema is moderate despite large tumor size. Calcification shows as marked hypointense nodule in this pulse sequence.*

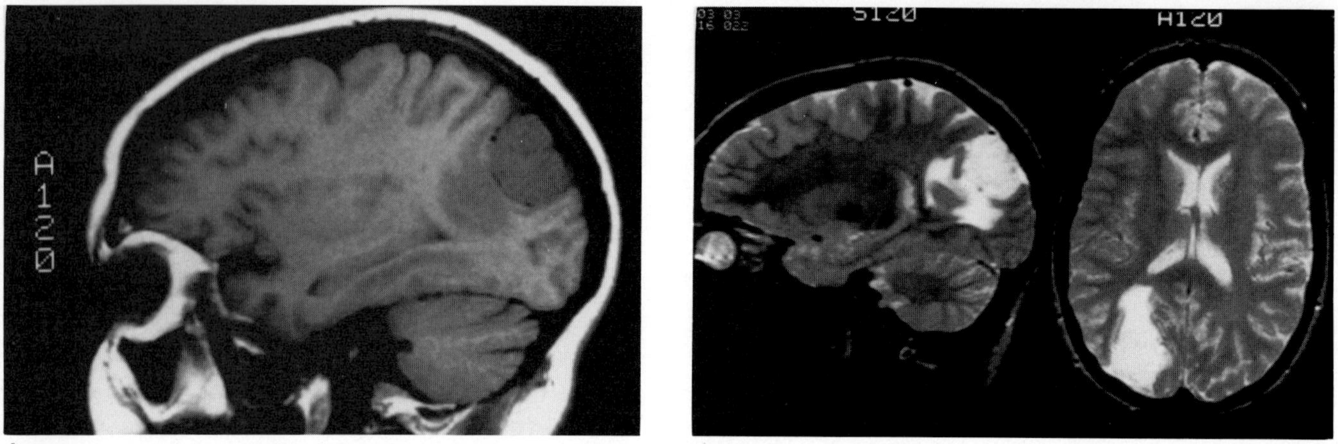

A B

Figure 12-23
Angioblastic meningioma in a 28-year-old woman with recent onset of episodic headaches. **(A)** *T1 WI. Tumor is homogeneously hypointense with a dural base and well demarcated by inner peritumoral halo. Vasogenic edema appears disproportionately large relative to tumor size, a feature that may be present in angioblastic meningioma.* **(B)** *T2 WI. Tumor and edema are hyperintense and cannot be easily separated. Angioblastic meningiomas are more often hyperintense in T2 WI than other types.*

by meningiomas occurs in 60 percent of cases, appearing as finger-like projections of low density that extend through white matter tracks.[48] Edema correlates poorly with tumor size and better with location (Figs. 12-21 and 12-22).[48] Thus, small subfrontal, frontal, and sphenoid wing meningiomas may elicit considerable edema that is disproportionate to tumor size. Atrophy of adjacent brain may result from chronic compression at the brain-tumor interface, giving rise to an arc-shaped CSF-filled cleft that appears in imaging studies as peritumoral halo.[3] Compression by a meningioma or another extra-axial mass lesion may cause inward displacement of the brain surface and focal deviation of the white matter, giving rise to the "buckled white matter sign."[4] Ninety-five percent of meningiomas show moderate to intense enhancement with contrast that is nodular homogeneous in 70 percent, mixed inhomogeneous in 24 percent, and ring-like in 2 percent of cases.[48] Densely

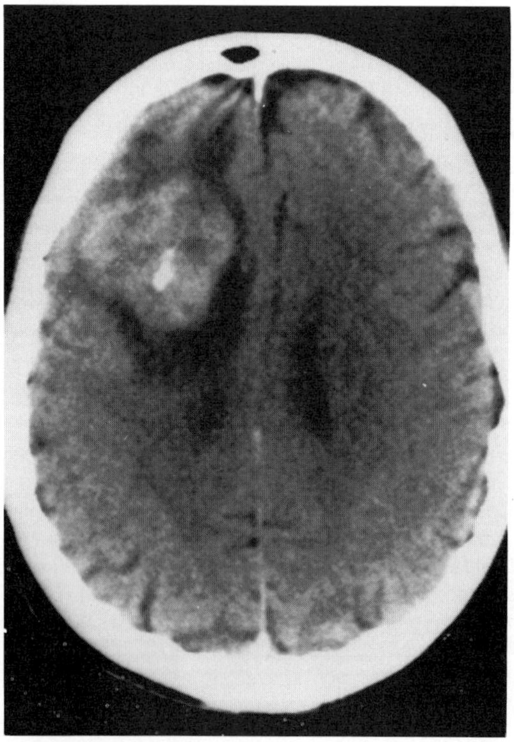

A

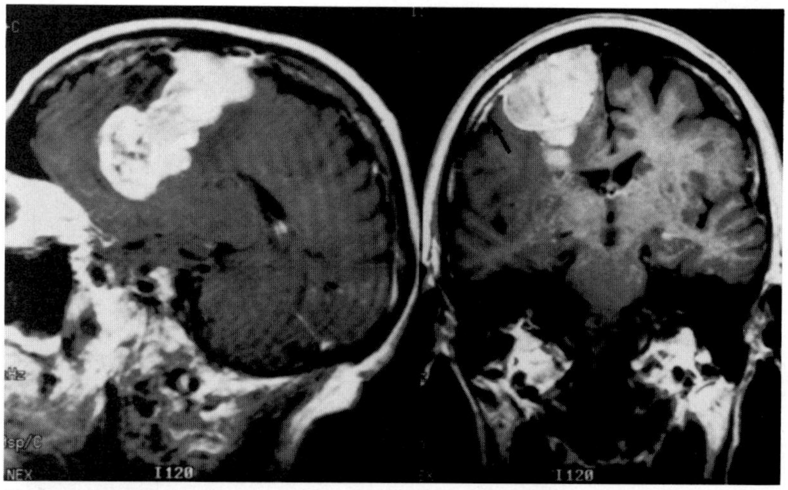

B

Figure 12-24
Parasagittal malignant meningioma in a 76-year-old man with a 2-month history of confusion. **(A)** *Noncontrast CT. Tumor is hyperdense with a focal central area of calcification and moderate surrounding edema. It cannot be easily classified as extra-axial by CT.* **(B)** *Contrast sagittal and coronal T1 WI. Parasagittal dural base, dural tail sign (arrows), homogeneous enhancement, and sharp borders characterize this tumor as meningioma. Lobulation and mushrooming (intracranial extension is larger than dural base) further characterize this tumor as malignant atypical meningioma.*

calcified meningiomas may not show enhancement. Attempts to project the histologic variety of meningiomas by CT have met with some success.[49] The presence of calcium, well-defined margins, and homogeneous enhancement are more common in fibroblastic and transitional types. Angioblastic and syncytial variants exhibit a greater tendency to show low-density, nonenhancing cystic areas and poorly defined irregular tumor margins or fringes. However, in typical benign meningiomas, little prognostic value is attached to microscopic characterization. Marked surrounding edema, absent calcifications, heterogeneous enhancement, cystic changes, poorly defined borders, and a multilobulated, mushrooming appearance are features of atypical meningioma and indicate a greater likelihood of anaplastic transformation.[21,48,49]

Benign typical meningiomas are isotense (60 percent) to slightly hypointense (30 percent) in noncontrast T1-weighted images and isotense (50 percent) to hyperintense (40 percent) in T2-weighted images relative to gray matter (Figs. 12-18 to 12-24).[21,51–53] In densely calcified tumors hypointensity prevails in both T1- and T2-weighted sequences. Minimal calcification is best demonstrated with T2*-weighted gradient echo sequences. The local effects of meningioma, such as peritumoral halo of low signal intensity, vasogenic intra-axial edema, and the buckled white matter sign, are also well seen in MRI and were greatly relied on for its diagnosis before paramagnetic contrast agents became available (Figs. 12-21 to 12-23). Almost all meningiomas enhance with paramagnetic contrast infusion, showing basically the same pattern as that described in CT studies. Sixty percent of meningiomas exhibit meningeal enhancement adjacent to their dural-based attachment on contrast-enhanced T1 WI, the so-called dural tail sign (Figs. 12-3 and 12-24).[54] However, this finding is nonspecific and can be found in other conditions, such as postsurgical changes, radiation, sarcoidosis, lymphoma, chordoma, aspergillosis, metastasis, and schwannomas.[55] In T2 WI the signal intensity of meningiomas may help predict histology.[51,56] Syncytial and angioblastic types tend to display high signal intensity in T2 WI, whereas fibroblastic and transitional types more frequently exhibit lower signal intensity in T2 WI. There is poor correlation if one utilizes T1 WI.[51] The features of atypical meningioma described for CT also apply to MRI studies.

Primary Cerebral Lymphomas

Definition

Primary cerebral lymphomas are malignant intra-axial neoplasms that are similar histologically to non-Hodgkin systemic lymphomas derived from B lymphocytes but occurring in the absence of recognized systemic disease. In the past these tumors were called reticulum cell sarcomas or microgliomas, implying an origin from microglia. This concept, however, has been questioned, and these terms have fallen into disuse.[12,13] CNS lymphomas also may occur secondarily as metastatic lesions from systemic lymphoma.

Epidemiology

Primary CNS lymphoma is considered a rare intracranial neoplasm accounting for 0.8 to 1.5 percent of intracranial tumors.[12,13] It may occur at any age, but in sporadic cases without associated conditions the peak incidence occurs between the ages of 50 and 60, with a male-to-female ratio of 3:2.[12] Individuals with congenital immunodeficiency disorders such as Wiskott-Aldrich syndrome or acquired disorders such as therapeutic immunosuppression in organ transplantation are particularly at risk for developing primary CNS lymphoma. In patients with AIDS the incidence of primary CNS lymphoma is estimated at 6 percent in those with neurologic manifestations.[12] The common denominator present in CNS lymphomas in immunocompromised patients seems to be a dysfunction of the suppressor T-cell system that permits proliferation and eventual neoplastic transformation of B lymphocytes.

Pathology

Macroscopically, primary CNS lymphomas range from well-demarcated or ill-defined, solid, partially necrotic tumors to multifocal infiltrates.[12–14] Multicentricity occurs in 25 percent of cases, and the hemispheres, cerebellum, and brainstem may be affected.[12] In the hemispheres, deep-seated lesions predominantly involve basal ganglia and periventricular regions with subependymal extension.[12] Leptomeningeal involvement is more common in secondary lymphomas.[14] Histologically, primary CNS lymphomas are diffuse rather than nodular and display a range of cytologic differentiation from small cell to mixed forms and large cell types.[14] The vast majority have B-cell surface markers.[14] Perivascular arrangement of tumor cells, reactive lymphocytes, perivascular deposition of reticulin, and monotypic immunostaining are common features of primary CNS lymphomas regardless of the cell subtype.[12–14]

Clinically, hemispheric primary CNS lymphomas cause behavior disturbances, personality changes, and focal findings rather than headaches or signs of increased intracranial pressure.[2] The prognosis is poor, with an expected median survival of 1 year or less in patients treated with radiation therapy.[57]

Imaging Findings

In noncontrast CT, primary CNS lymphomas typically appear as deep-seated, slightly hyperdense, poorly defined lesions that often are in contact with ventricular

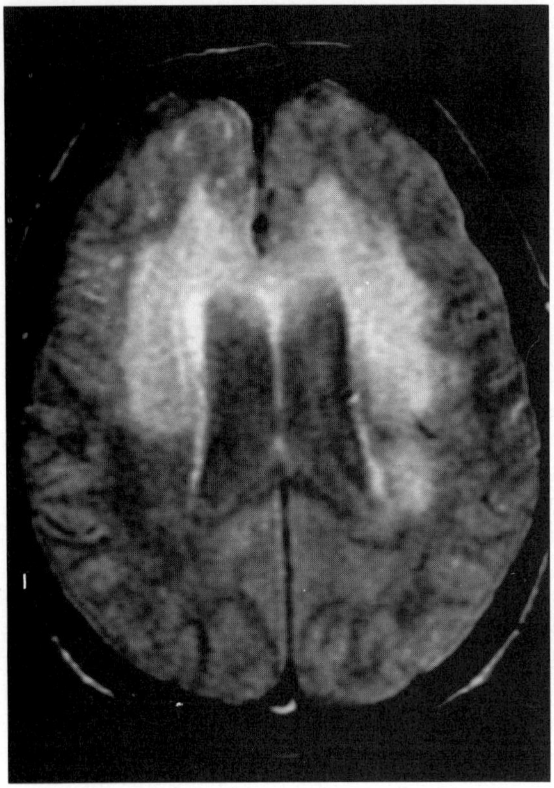

Figure 12-25
Primary CNS lymphoma, small cell type, in a 67-year-old woman presenting with dementia, PD WI. Tumor appears as bilateral, symmetrical, abnormal hyperintensity infiltrating anterior periventricular white matter. The patient had a negative CT and contrast T1 WI.

ependyma.[58,59] Noncontrast MRI shows primary CNS lymphomas as poorly defined, hypointense, or isointense lesions in T1 WI and hypointense to slightly hyperintense lesions in PD WI and T2 WI relative to gray matter (Fig. 12-25).[60] Enhancement in both MRI and CT studies is the rule, and it is more commonly homogeneous (Fig. 12-26). Edema and mass effect may be inconspicuous. Bilateral lesions occur in approximately 25 percent of cases from neuropathologic studies.[12]

In AIDS patients, the lesions are more often multiple and usually are less than 2 cm in diameter.[60] The main differential diagnosis in these patients is toxoplasmosis. Toxoplasmosis features more numerous lesions, a ring-enhancing pattern, more edema, and a predilection for basal ganglia and corticomedullary involvement.[61]

Metastatic Neoplasms

Definition

In its more general use, metastatic disease of the brain and its coverings (skull and meninges) refers to malignant tumor growths that arise more commonly from hematogenous spread of primary neoplasms situated at a distant site. Alternatively, metastatic disease may occur by extension through the basal skull foramina of head and neck tumors. Some primary brain tumors, notably medulloblastomas and ependymomas, may seed via CSF pathways to distant sites of the neuraxis, giving rise to so-called drop metastases.

Epidemiology

Metastatic disease of the brain is a common occurrence, accounting for 25 percent of intracranial tumors in the adult population.[62] In decreasing order of frequency, the most common primary sources of metastatic disease in adults are bronchogenic carcinoma, breast carcinoma, malignant melanoma, kidney, gastrointestinal tract, lymphoma, and leukemia.[12,13,63] The incidence of metastatic brain disease in cases of bronchogenic carcinoma, breast carcinoma, and malignant melanoma is 30 percent, 30 percent, and 22 percent, respectively.[12,63] The incidence of metastatic brain disease increases with age from the fifth decade through the seventh decade, and this disease is rare in childhood.[64]

Leptomeningeal carcinomatosis occurs in 5 to 8 percent of patients with solid tumors, 5 to 29 percent of those with non-Hodgkin lymphoma, and 11 to 70 per-

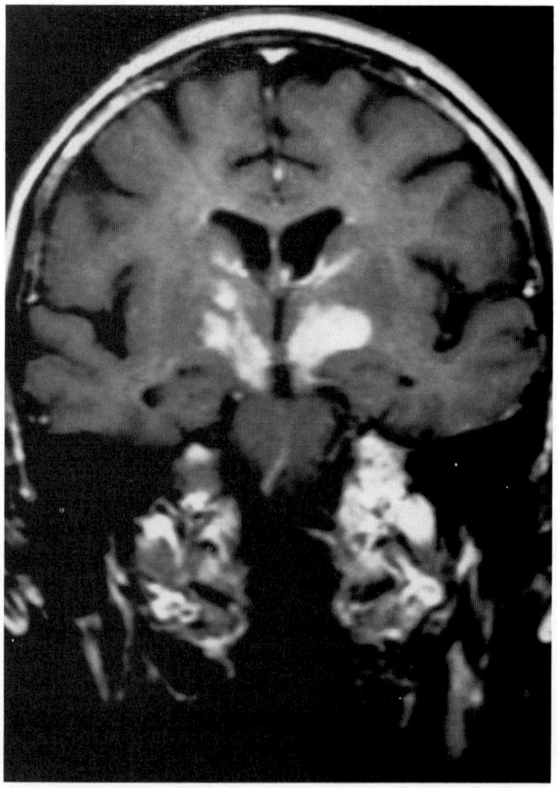

Figure 12-26
Primary CNS lymphoma, large cell type, in a 78-year-old woman with subacute onset of dementia, coronal postcontrast T1 WI. Note intensely enhancing tumor involving hypothalamic, thalamic, and subependymal regions.

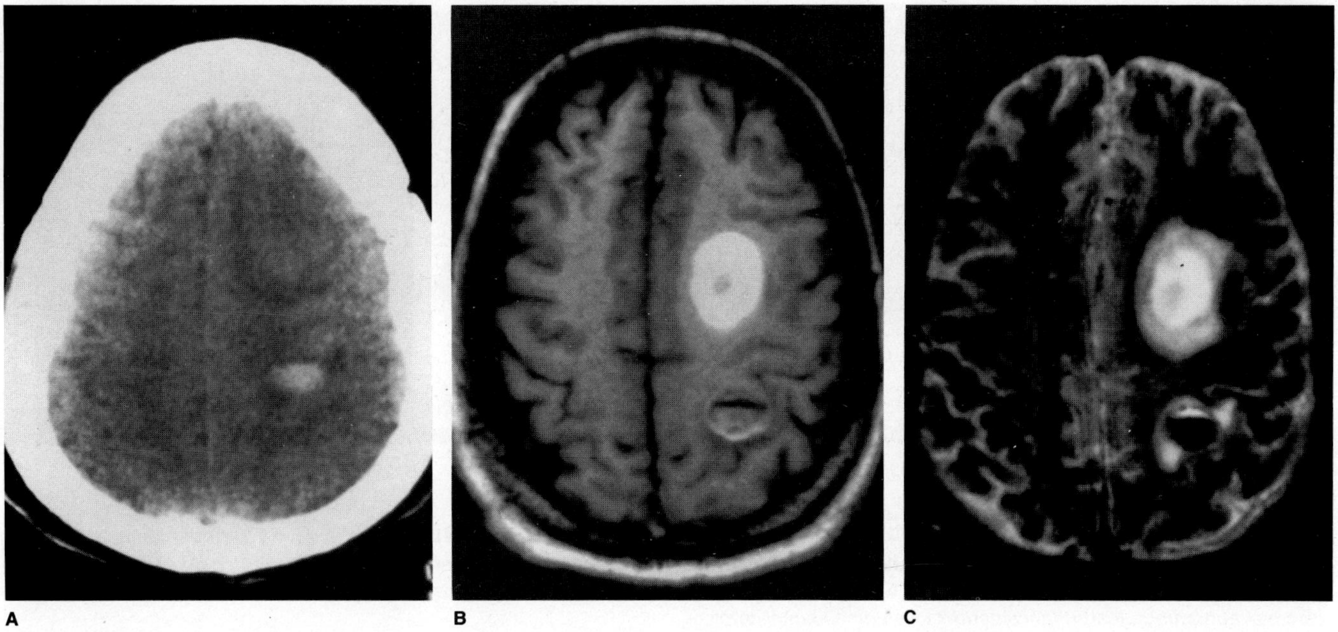

Figure 12-32

Hemorrhagic metastatic lung carcinoma, left hemisphere, in a 57-year-old man. **(A)** *Noncontrast CT. Lesion in the left parietal corticomedullary junction shows a hemorrhage; edema surrounds an inconspicuous, slightly hyperdense second lesion more anteriorly.* **(B)** *Noncontrast T1 WI shows subacute hemorrhagic lesion in left centrum semiovale and acute isointense hemorrhage with fluid level more posteriorly.* **(C)** *Heavily T2 WI. It characterizes extracellular methemoglobin of subacute hemorrhage in centrum semiovale metastasis and deoxyhemoglobin of acute hemorrhage in posterior metastasis. Edema surrounding both lesions is demonstrated better with this sequence. High signal intensity in T2 WI and low signal intensity in T1 WI of supernatant in posterior lesion indicates non-hemorrhagic tumor tissue. This case study documents the classical appearance of tumor hemorrhage, i.e., multiple hemorrhagic lesions in different stages.*

have an aggressive and fatal history with increased mitotic figures, necrosis, and spread to other areas.[12,78] A benign melanocytoma may recur locally.

Leptomeningeal carcinomatosis is seen in contrast CT and contrast MRI as nodular or diffuse, cistern, convexity, or subependymal enhancement with or without hydrocephalus (Figs. 12-34 and 12-35).[79,80] PD WI and T2 WI may show leptomeningeal carcinomatosis as diffusely increased signal intensity along convexity meninges (Fig. 12-34). Contrast MRI is more sensitive than CT in the detection of leptomeningeal enhancement of carcinomatosis.[80] Other conditions, such as meningitis, prior intracranial surgery, intrathecal chemotherapy, and radiotherapy, also can cause leptomeningeal enhancement and should be considered in the differential diagnosis.

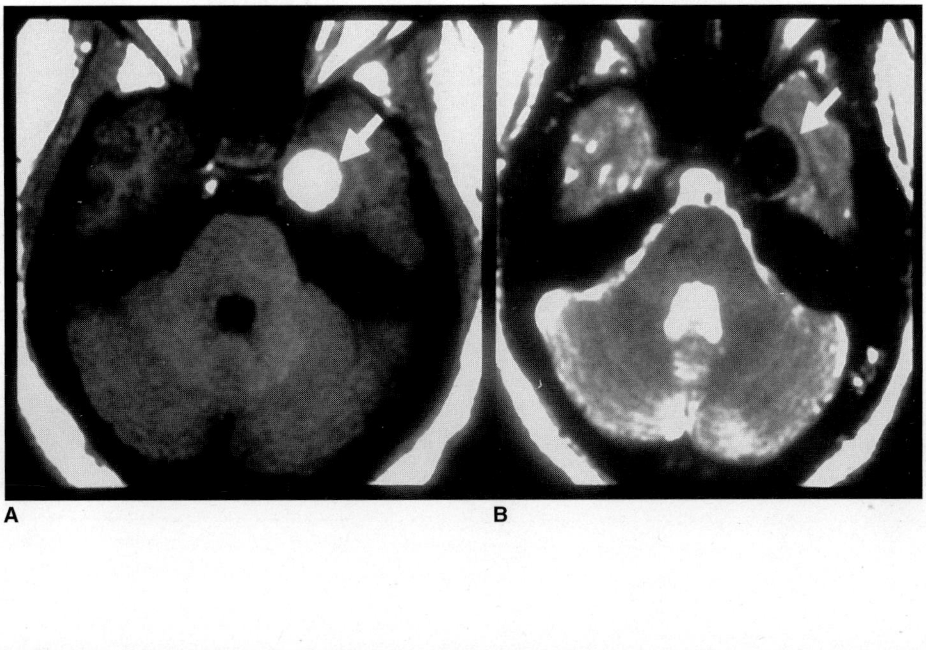

Figure 12-33

Meningeal melanocytoma in the left cavernous sinus region in a 30-year-old woman presenting with headaches. The tumor is extra-axial and well demarcated (white arrows) and shows in noncontrast T1 WI **(A)** *and T2 WI* **(B)** as hyperintense and hypointense, respectively, reflecting T1 and shortening caused by free radicals in melanin. With MRI it is not possible to distinguish it from malignant meningeal melanoma or a hemorrhagic lesion in the subacute stage (intracellular methemoglobin).

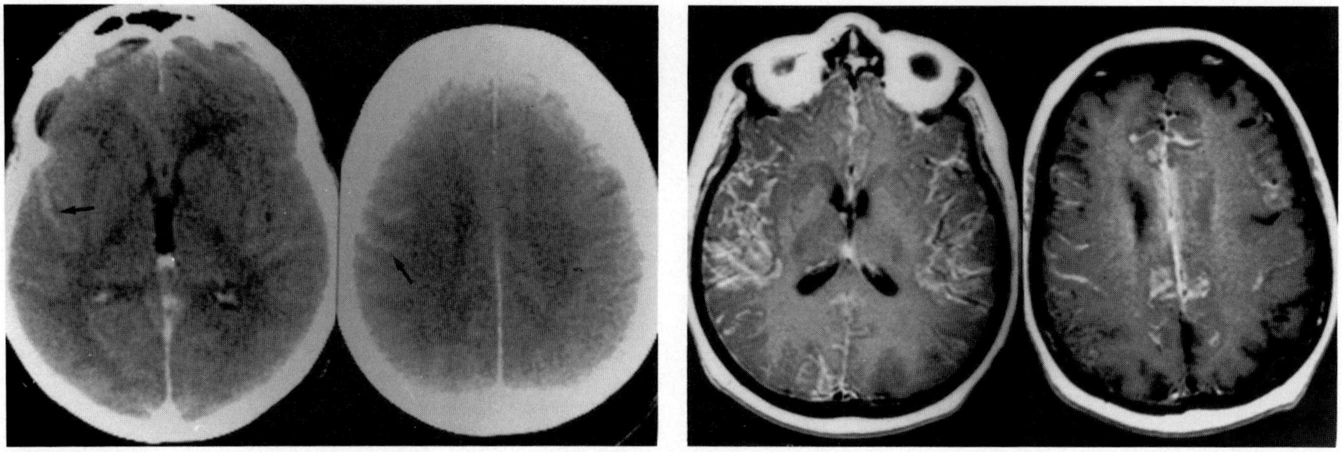

A B

Figure 12-34

Leptomeningeal carcinomatosis from systemic lymphoma in a 69-year-old woman presenting with a 2-week history of generalized weakness and decline in mental function. **(A)** *Contrast CT. Note discrete, abnormal sulcal enhancement from leptomeningeal carcinomatosis (arrows).* **(B)** *Postcontrast T1 WI. Note markedly abnormal pial enhancement in sylvian cistern and convexity sulci from leptomeningeal carcinomatosis.*

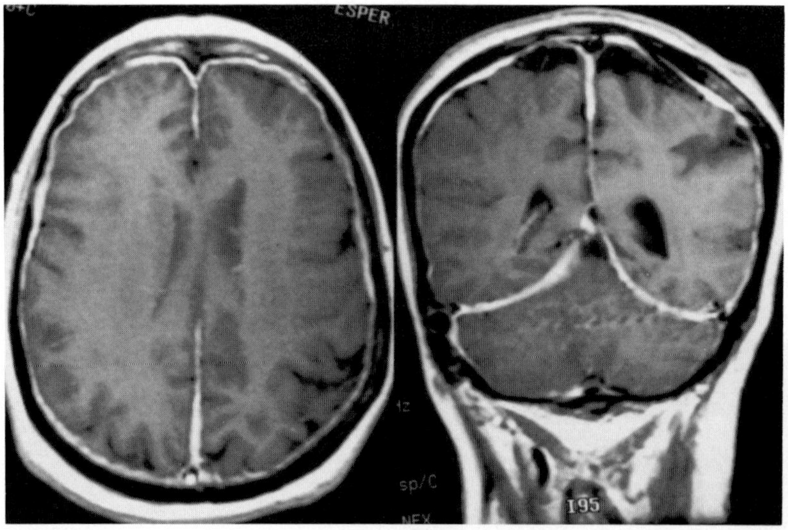

A

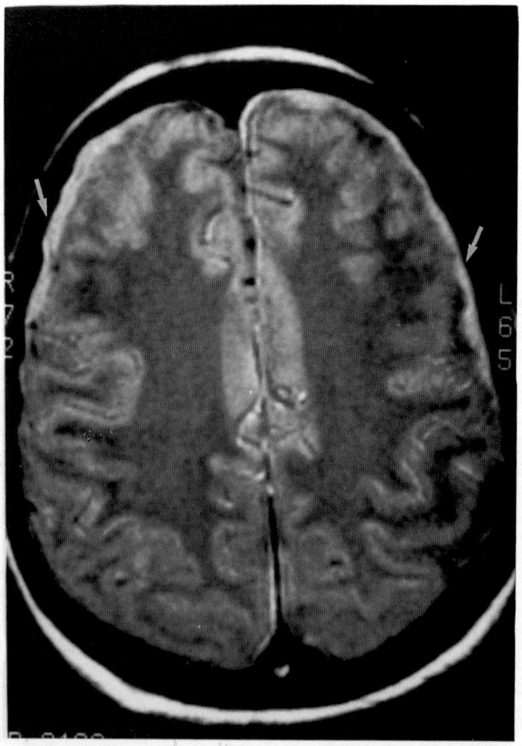

B

Figure 12-35

Leptomeningeal carcinomatosis from breast carcinoma in a 67-year-old woman presenting with a several-week history of headaches and confusion. **(A)** *Transverse and coronal postcontrast T1 WI. There is abnormal, marked, contiguous enhancement of dura mater.* **(B)** *PD WI. Note discrete, abnormal hyperintensity and thickening of frontal convexity leptomeninges (arrows).*

PATIENTS PRESENTING WITH SIGNS OF INCREASED INTRACRANIAL PRESSURE

Brain tumors cause increased intracranial pressure by virtue of mass effect from their size and associated edema, hydrocephalus from their location obstructing CSF pathways, or a combination of these mechanisms. The following tumors have a tendency to produce the syndrome of increased intracranial pressure while causing inconspicuous focal or lateralizing findings.

Medulloblastoma

Definition

Medulloblastoma is a malignant intraparenchymal cerebellar tumor composed of neoplastic primitive embryonal cells originating from germinal matrix zones in the posterior medullary vellum.[12,14] During embryonic development these germinal matrix cells migrate upward and laterally to form the external granular layer of the cerebellum, which gradually regresses during the first year of life. Medulloblastomas may occur anywhere along this migratory path, either medially or laterally.

Epidemiology

Medulloblastoma accounts for 7 to 8 percent of all intracranial tumors of neuroepithelial origin, but in childhood this proportion rises to 10 to 20 percent.[12,16,81] It is slightly less common than cerebellar astrocytomas, accounting for slightly less than 30 percent of posterior fossa neoplasms in children.[16] Males are affected twice as often as are females, and the peak incidence is from 1 to 10 years of age.[16] Forty percent of patients present within the first 5 years of life, and 75 percent within the first decade.[81] The 5-year survival rate is 60 percent for patients without leptomeningeal metastases treated with craniospinal radiotherapy.[82]

Pathology

Microscopically, medulloblastomas are densely cellular tumors composed of small oval to carrot-shaped cells with hyperchromatic nuclei, scarce cytoplasm, and variable mitotic figures.[14,82] Cell arrangement is patternless and may show Homer-Wright rosettes. In the latter case, cells surround small stellate areas of fibrillarity without a central lumen or blood vessel and indicate neuroblastic differentiation.[13] Glial differentiation in medulloblastoma is rare.[13,14] Seventy-five percent of medulloblastomas occur in the vermis, and 25 percent in the lateral cerebellar hemispheres.[14] Midline vermian medulloblastomas predominate in the young, appearing variably demarcated and soft, gray-red with variable foci of necrosis.[12,14] Laterally placed medulloblastomas are more common in adults, appearing well demarcated with a woody, tough consistency that reflects their nodular, desmoplastic histologic pattern.[12,14] Tumor dissemination by subarachnoid seeding occurs in the majority of patients with medulloblastoma.[16] Tumor cells may accumulate in the basilar cisterns, the sylvian fissure, the ependymal surfaces, and the intradural extramedullary space, from where it may extend to the intramedullary space.[14,16] Distant metastases outside the CNS may occur in bones, peritoneum (via shunt), lung, and liver.[16] The most common symptoms—nausea, vomiting, and headaches—are those of increased intracranial pressure from obstructive hydrocephalus. Symptomatology is usually of short duration, averaging 1 month in 50 percent of patients before the diagnosis is established.[81]

Imaging Findings

Imaging studies (CT and MRI) show typical medulloblastoma as a round, moderately well-demarcated, solid midline cerebellar mass arising in the vermis that compresses and obstructs the fourth ventricle.[16,81,83] Hy-

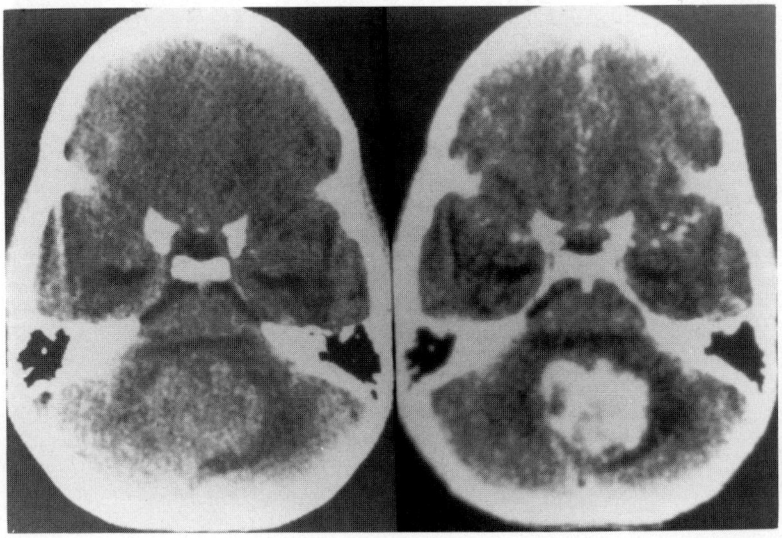

Figure 12-36
Medulloblastoma, midline cerebellum in a 6-year-old girl. Pre- and postcontrast CT. Precontrast CT shows classical appearance of medulloblastoma as solid, slightly hyperdense intra-axial tumor that enhances with contrast infusion.

drocephalus is present in 80 to 90 percent of patients at the time of diagnosis.[81] Cystic and necrotic areas may be seen occasionally. Small foci of calcification occur in 10 to 15 percent of cases.[84] Laterally placed medulloblastomas are more common in adults.[81] Edema is usually not prominent.

On noncontrast CT, typical medulloblastoma is isodense to hyperdense and homogeneous (Figs. 12-36 and 12-37).[83] On MRI, the appearance is that of a homogeneous, hypointense mass in the precontrast T1 WI and iso- or hyperintense mass in PD WI and T2 WI (Fig. 12-37).[84] Contrast enhancement is usually moderate and homogeneous in both CT and MRI studies. The hypointensity observed in T2-weighted images of medulloblastoma may reflect a high nuclear-cytoplasmic ratio of the tumor cells, its hypercellularity and the consequent little free water.[81] Cystic changes and necrosis may give rise to a heterogeneous appearance in both CT and MRI studies. The presence of leptomeningeal metastasis is best evaluated by craniospinal postcontrast T1 WI (Fig. 12-38). This should be done at the time of diagnosis, since it is present in 20 to 30 percent of patients.[82]

Primitive Neuroectodermal Tumors

There are other tumors of the CNS that like the medulloblastoma, arise from embryonal, uncommitted germinal matrix cells. The term *primitive neuroectodermal*

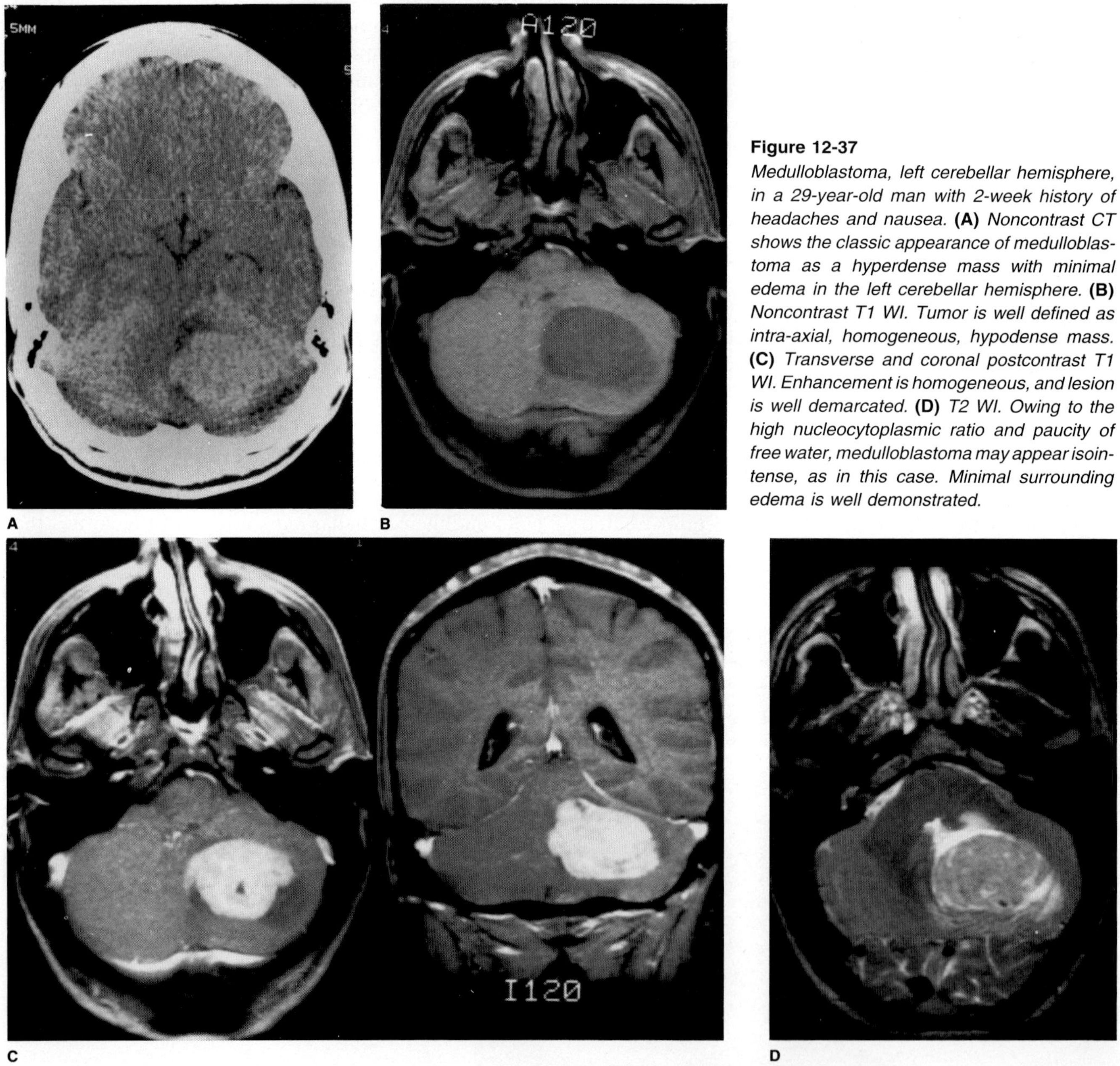

Figure 12-37
Medulloblastoma, left cerebellar hemisphere, in a 29-year-old man with 2-week history of headaches and nausea. **(A)** *Noncontrast CT shows the classic appearance of medulloblastoma as a hyperdense mass with minimal edema in the left cerebellar hemisphere.* **(B)** *Noncontrast T1 WI. Tumor is well defined as intra-axial, homogeneous, hypodense mass.* **(C)** *Transverse and coronal postcontrast T1 WI. Enhancement is homogeneous, and lesion is well demarcated.* **(D)** *T2 WI. Owing to the high nucleocytoplasmic ratio and paucity of free water, medulloblastoma may appear isointense, as in this case. Minimal surrounding edema is well demonstrated.*

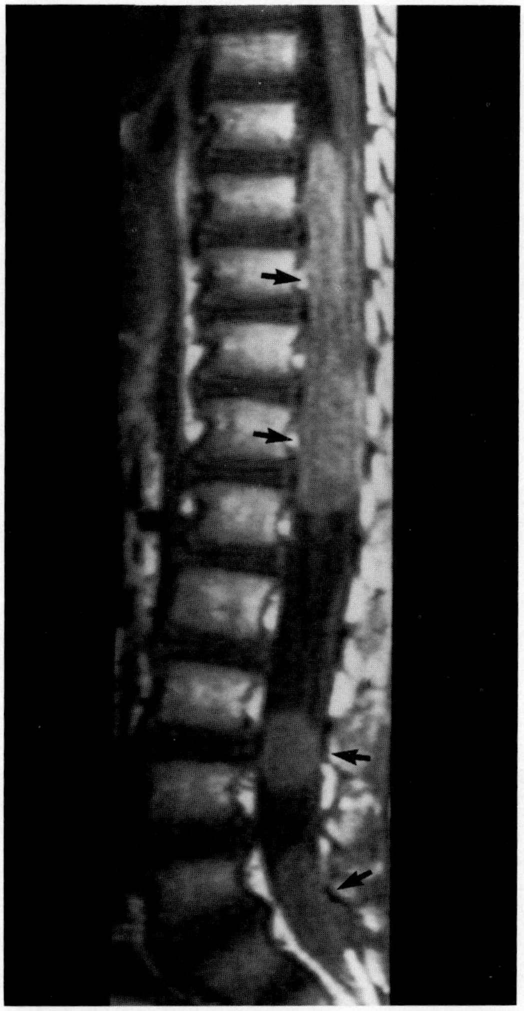

Figure 12-38

Drop metastases from medulloblastoma in a 2-year-old boy. Postcontrast sagittal T1 WI. Metastases are bulky, slightly enhancing, intra- and extramedullary masses between T9 and L1, at L3–L4, and in the sacral region (arrows).

tumor (PNET) was coined by Hart and Earle to describe a highly malignant and uncommon childhood cerebral neoplasm composed of neoplastic embryonal, mostly undifferentiated cells but capable of glioneuronal differentiation.[85]

Traditionally known by the term *cerebral neuroblastoma,* this rare tumor has a peak incidence in the 1- to 5-year age group, no sex predominance, and a short duration of symptoms (usually less than 6 months) that are usually those of increased intracranial pressure: nausea, vomiting, and headaches.[86]

On gross pathology the tumor is a gray-white, usually well-circumscribed mass measuring an average of 7 cm at the time of diagnosis and located more frequently in the deep white matter of the frontoparietal regions.[86] Cystic areas, necrosis, hemorrhage, and calcifications are common.

On imaging studies, cerebral neuroblastoma or supratentorial PNET typically shows as a bulky, large, well-circumscribed, heterogeneous intraparenchymal hemispheric mass with inconspicuous edema in the frontoparietal white matter (Fig. 12-39). The heterogeneous appearance in imaging studies (high and low density in CT and variable signal intensity in T1 WI, PD WI, and T2 WI) denotes a combination of cystic changes, necrosis, hemorrhage, and calcification. Contrast enhancement is also heterogeneous. Leptomeningeal dissemination is common, and metastases outside the CNS also occur as they do with medulloblastoma.[14,86]

The concept of PNET was later applied by some authors to describe all tumors that might share a common origin from neuroepithelial precursors not only in the cerebral hemisphere (neuroblastoma) but also in the cerebellum (medulloblastoma), olfactory region (esthesioneuroblastoma), retina (retinoblastoma), and pineal region (pineoblastoma). However, classic neuropathology texts still prefer to clearly distinguish traditional neoplasms such as medulloblastoma and pineoblastoma with their characteristic histology, predictable regional localization, and clinical course separately from the all-encompassing term *PNET.*[13,14]

Cerebellar Astrocytoma

Definition

Cerebellar astrocytoma in its most typical form is a relatively well-circumscribed, low-grade astrocytic glioma composed of bipolar fibrous astrocytes, hence the term *juvenile pilocytic astrocytoma* (JPA).[12–14]

Epidemiology

Cerebellar astrocytoma is the most common posterior fossa neoplasm in children, accounting for approximately 30 percent of tumors in that location and approximately 40 percent of all astrocytomas in the pediatric age group.[16] JPA represents 75 percent of all cerebellar astrocytomas and the diffuse type, which is indistinguishable from the adult type, represents the remaining 25 percent.[16] It affects male and females equally and has a peak incidence from birth to 9 years, while the diffuse type peaks between 10 and 14 years of age.[16,87]

Pathology

Macroscopically, juvenile pilocytic astrocytoma is a solid (50 percent) or cystic (25 percent) mass usually greater than 5 cm with discrete borders that arise in the midline or cerebellar hemisphere.[13,14] One form of cystic JPA consists of a unilocular cyst with a wall of nonneoplastic compressed glial cerebellar tissue and a mural nodule of tumor.[16] Other juvenile pilocytic astrocytomas contain multiple small tumor-lined cysts or a large necrotic center surrounded by tumor.[13,16] Microcystic degenera-

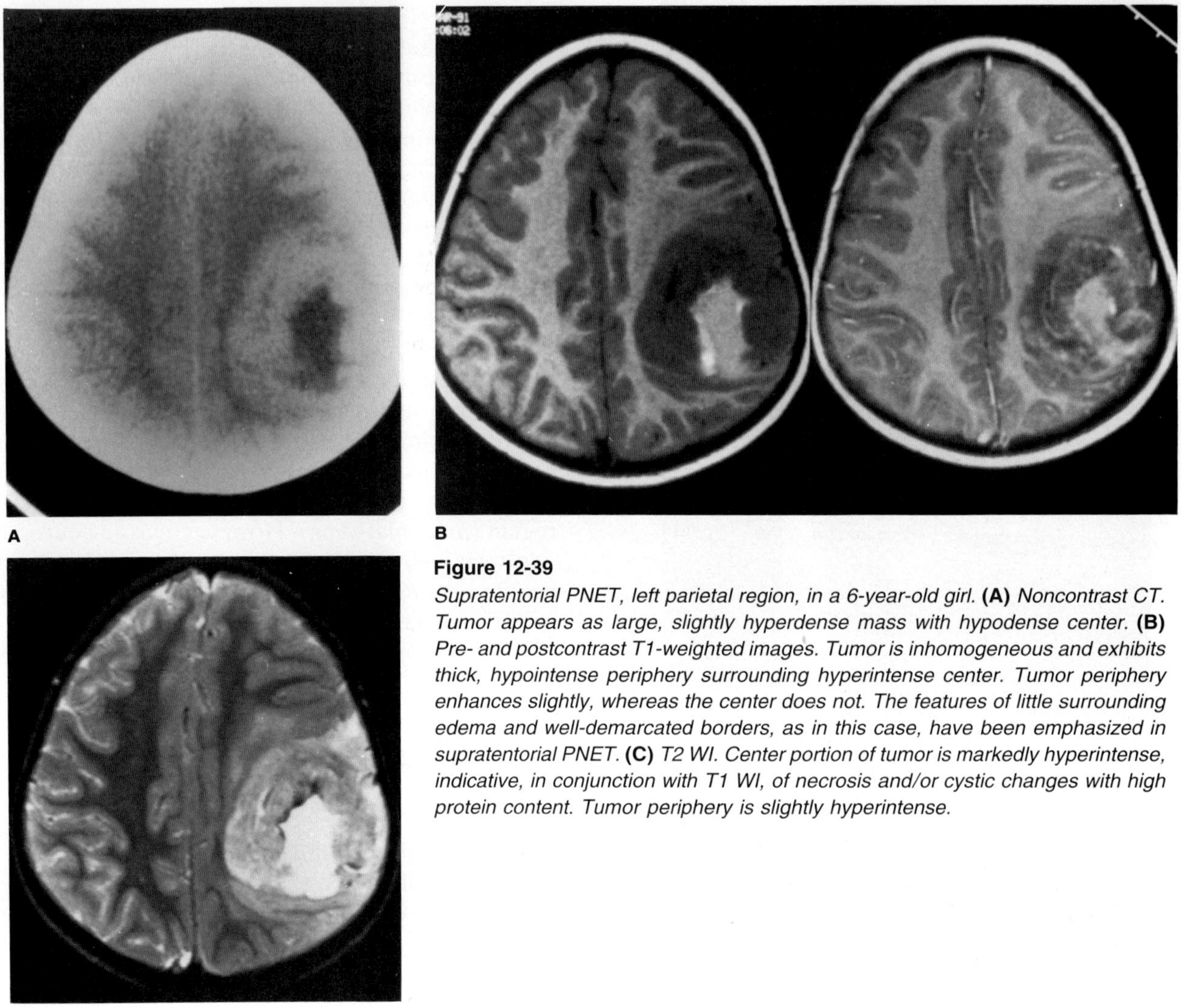

Figure 12-39

Supratentorial PNET, left parietal region, in a 6-year-old girl. **(A)** *Noncontrast CT. Tumor appears as large, slightly hyperdense mass with hypodense center.* **(B)** *Pre- and postcontrast T1-weighted images. Tumor is inhomogeneous and exhibits thick, hypointense periphery surrounding hyperintense center. Tumor periphery enhances slightly, whereas the center does not. The features of little surrounding edema and well-demarcated borders, as in this case, have been emphasized in supratentorial PNET.* **(C)** *T2 WI. Center portion of tumor is markedly hyperintense, indicative, in conjunction with T1 WI, of necrosis and/or cystic changes with high protein content. Tumor periphery is slightly hyperintense.*

tion is also the rule in apparent solid tumors when examined microscopically. Microscopically, cerebellar astrocytomas are composed primarily of bipolar, fibrous astrocytes that are often are arranged in intersecting bundles with Rosenthal fibers situated among tumor cells.[16] Occasional cellular atypia may be seen but mitotic figures are rare.[13,14] Histologically, they are identical to supratentorial pilocytic astocytoma. Clinical findings are those of increased intracranial pressure from structural hydrocephalus as the tumor grows and compresses the fourth ventricle and signs of cerebellar dysfunction.[88] The prognosis is excellent in juvenile pilocytic astrocytoma with a 25-year survival rate of 94 percent. That rate drops to 38 percent for the diffuse type.[87]

Imaging Studies

In imaging studies the appearance that most easily identifies a cerebellar pilocytic astrocytoma is a well-circumscribed vermian or hemispheric intra-axial cerebellar cystic mass with a well-defined, rounded, or plaque-like mural nodule attached to the wall (Fig. 12-40).[15,88] Alternatively, cyst formation may be multiple amid portions of solid tumor with no discrete mural nodule.[88] A large central cyst surrounded by tumor also may result from necrosis. On CT studies, 70 percent of cerebellar astrocytomas are cystic and 30 percent are solid.[16] Obstructive hydrocephalus from compression of the fourth ventricle is usually present at the time of diagnosis.[15] Intense homogeneous enhancement of the mural nodule is the rule, but the cyst wall typically shows little or no enhancement.[15] On noncontrast CT, cyst fluid is usually hyperdense relative to CSF and the tumor nodule may be hypo-, iso-, or hyperdense relative to cerebellum.[16] Calcification occurs in up to 20 percent of cases.[15] On MRI studies both cystic and solid components appear homogeneously or heterogeneously hypointense in T1 WI and hyperintense in PD WI and T2 WI.[15] Hemosiderin-laden areas denoting previous hemorrhage may be seen along the cyst walls.[15]

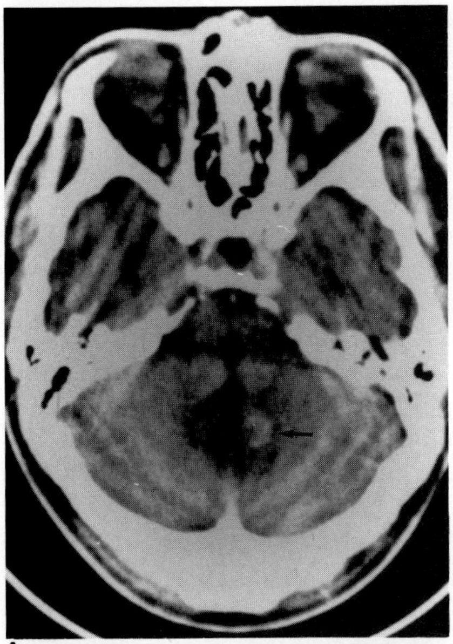

A

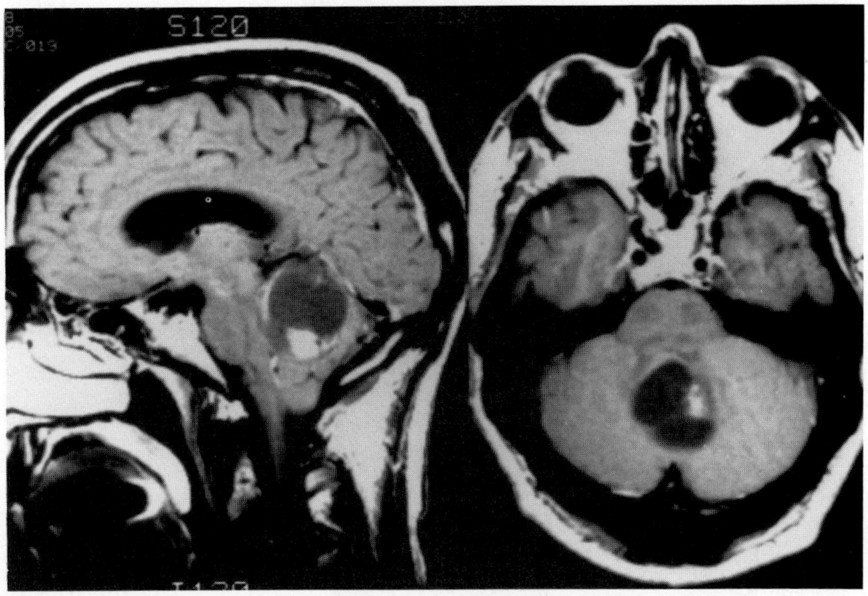

B

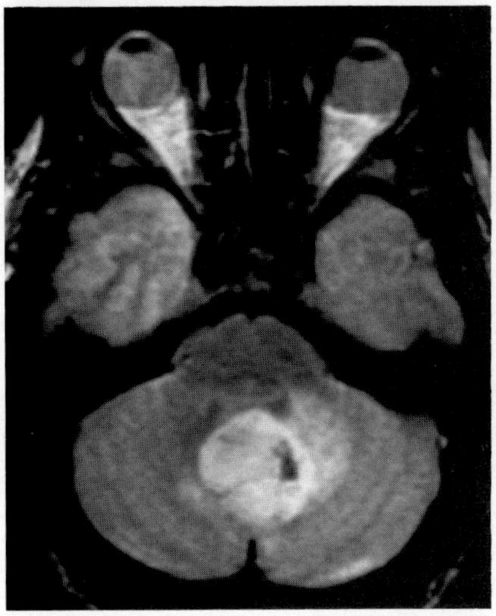

C

Figure 12-40
Cystic cerebellar astrocytoma in a 49-year-old man with a 4-month history of imbalance. **(A)** *Noncontrast CT. Tumor is midline cyst with hyperdense, slightly calcified mural nodule (arrow).* **(B)** *Sagittal and transverse postcontrast T1 WI. Tumor is composed of a large midline hypointense cyst with enhancing mural nodule. Cyst wall shows minimal enhancement of its anterior segment.* **(C)** *PD WI. Cyst content is hyperintense and mural nodule is hypointense, reflecting calcification. The main differential diagnosis of this case in this age group is hemangioblastoma.*

Ependymomas of the Fourth Ventricle

The definition, epidemiology, and pathologic features of ependymomas were described in the previous section.

Infratentorial ependymoma has two peak incidences, the first within the first 5 years of life and the other during the fourth decade.[88]

The majority of posterior fossa ependymomas grow in the fourth ventricle, from where they may extend to the lateral recesses, the foramen of Lushka, and the cerebellar pontine angle.[89] Downward extension of tumor through the foramen of Magendie may surround the medulla and fill the cisterna magna (plastic ependymoma) (Fig. 12-41).[12]

On noncontrast CT posterior fossa ependymoma is most often isodense with flecks of calcification in 50 percent of cases (Fig. 12-42).[89]

On MRI studies posterior fossa ependymoma is usually solid, iso- to hypointense in T1 WI, and hyperintense in PD WI and T2 WI.[84] Signal heterogeneity, mixed high and low in both pulse sequences, results from calcification, previous hemorrhage, and vascularity.[15,43,84] Inhomogeneous enhancement occurs in most ependymomas.[88] CSF-borne metastases are common and are best demonstrated with postcontrast T1 WI. (Fig. 12-43).

Choroid Plexus Papilloma

Definition

Choroid plexus papilloma is a rare intracranial tumor that arises from the epithelium of the choroid plexus.

Epidemiology

Choroid plexus papilloma accounts for 3 to 5 percent of intracranial neoplasms in children[81] and rarely occurs in the adult years.[13] There is a marked male predomi-

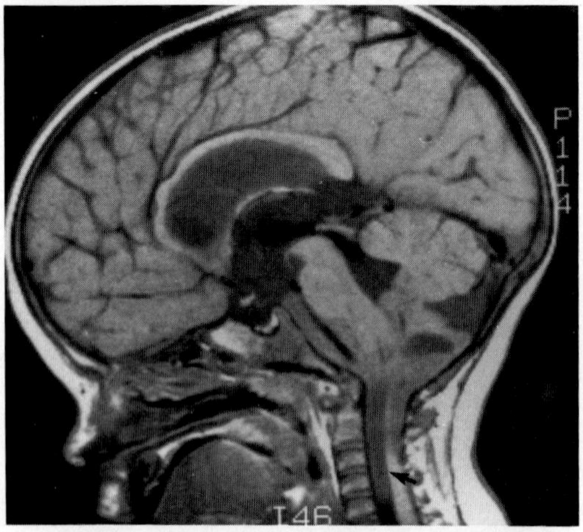

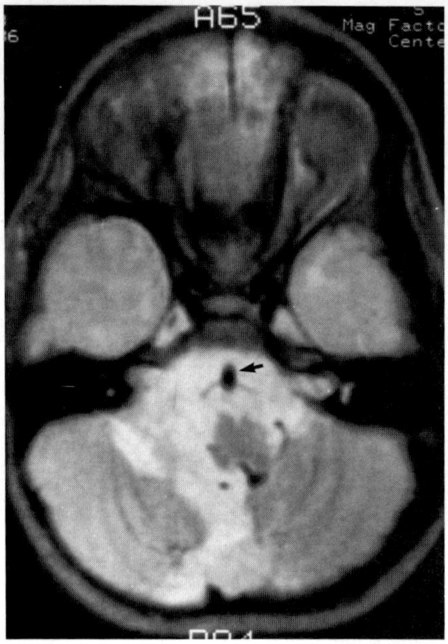

Figure 12-41
Plastic fourth ventricle ependymoma in a 19-month-old infant presenting with opisthotonos. **(A)** *Noncontrast sagittal T1 WI. Slightly hypointense tumor oozes out of the fourth ventricle, partially filling the cisterna magna and prepontine cistern where it girdles the basilar artery. It also projects like a tongue into anterior cervical subarachnoid space (arrow).* **(B)** *Transverse T2 WI. Homogeneous hyperintense tumor fills the right lateral recess, extends out to the right cerebellopontine angle, and encases the basilar artery in the prepontine cistern (arrow).*

nance for both choroid plexus papilloma and carcinoma.[81]

Pathology

Choroid plexus papilloma is an intraventricular tumor that occurs most commonly in the lateral ventricles of children, whereas the fourth ventricle is the usual site in adults.[11,13] Typically, a choroid plexus papilloma is a lobulated intraventricular mass with a rough surface architecture resembling cauliflower.[11,13,14] Microscopically, the picture is that of papillae composed of epithelial, cuboid, or columnar-like cells seated in a fibrovascular stroma. Other than some degree of disorganization and crowding, these cells are like regular choroid plexus cells.[13] Mitotic activity is typically absent. Calcifications are common. Loss of papillary architecture, pleomorphism, and invasiveness characterize the choroid plexus carcinoma, which tends to grow into neighboring brain, eliciting vasogenic edema.[11,13] Dissemination via CSF pathways also may occur in choroid plexus carcinoma. Choroid plexus papillomas usually present with hydrocephalus by obstructing CSF pathways or through overproduction of CSF. In choroid plexus carcinoma, a focal neurologic deficit may occur from invasion of neighboring structures.[81,88] Choroid plexus papillomas are benign tumors and are potentially curable with total resection.

Imaging Findings

In noncontrast CT the typical findings are those of an intraventricular isodense or hyperdense mass lesion with calcification in the region of the trigone or filling the fourth ventricle (Figs. 12-44 and 12-45).[81,90] When it is in the fourth ventricle, the tumor may extend to the lateral recess and the cerebellopontine angle.[90] Homogeneous enhancement usually occurs with contrast infusion.

In noncontrast MRI, T1 WI choroid plexus papillomas are isointense or hypointense lobulated masses relative to surrounding brain (Figs. 12-44 to 12-46). In T2 WI these tumors are usually hyperintense relative to brain. Inhomogeneous signal intensity in T1 WI and T2 WI denotes calcification and/or tumor vascularity.[81] Enhancement is common with MRI contrast agents. In choroid plexus carcinoma, CT and MRI usually demonstrate mixed density and inhomogeneous signal intensity, respectively, cystic changes, invasiveness, and edema of neighboring brain (Fig. 12-46).

Hemangioblastoma

Definition

Cerebellar hemangioblastoma is a benign intraparenchymal tumor of unknown histogenesis composed of vascular spaces lined by endothelial cells that are separated by lipid-rich larger cells called stromal cells.[12,14]

Epidemiology

Cerebellar hemangioblastoma represents approximately 7 percent of primary tumors in the posterior fossa.[12] Hemangioblastoma in general (including all CNS locations) accounts for 1 to 2.5 percent of all intracranial tumors.[12] Peak incidence is in the third through

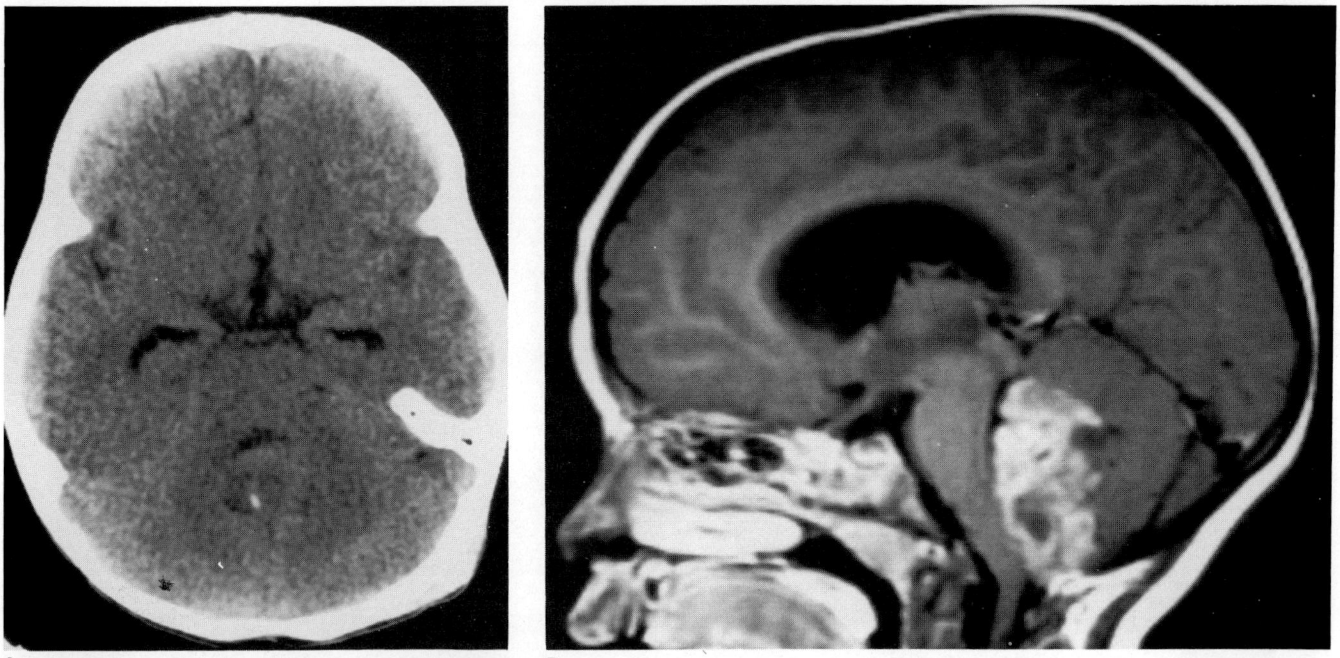

A B

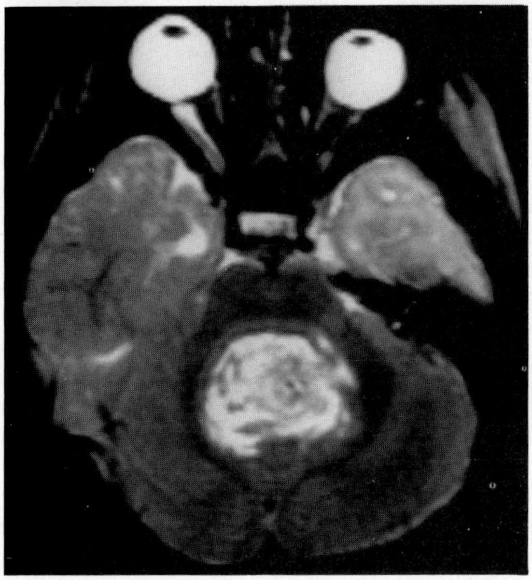

C

Figure 12-42

Fourth ventricle ependymoma in a 2½-year-old girl presenting with emesis and imbalance. **(A)** *Noncontrast CT. Fourth ventricle is obliterated by isodense mass with foci of calcification. Ependymoma is the tumor of the posterior fossa that most often calcifies.* **(B)** *Sagittal postcontrast T1 WI. Well-demarcated tumor fills the fourth ventricle extending out inferiorly and markedly enhances, although inhomogeneously.* **(C)** *T2 WI. Tumor mass exhibits mixed iso- and hyperintensity with no significant edema, completely filling the fourth ventricle in this section.*

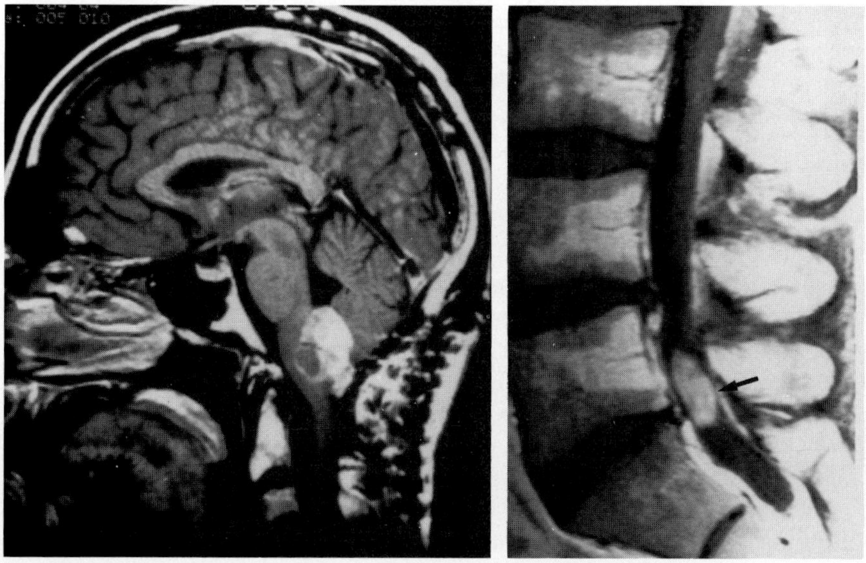

A B

Figure 12-43

Recurrent fourth ventricle ependymoma in a 42-year-old man complaining of back pain. **(A)** *Postcontrast sagittal T1 WI. Enhancing tumor has sharp borders invading the brainstem from inferior fourth ventricle.* **(B)** *Postcontrast sagittal T1 WI, lumbosacral region. Large intradural drop metastasis to lumbosacral region is present in the same patient (arrow).*

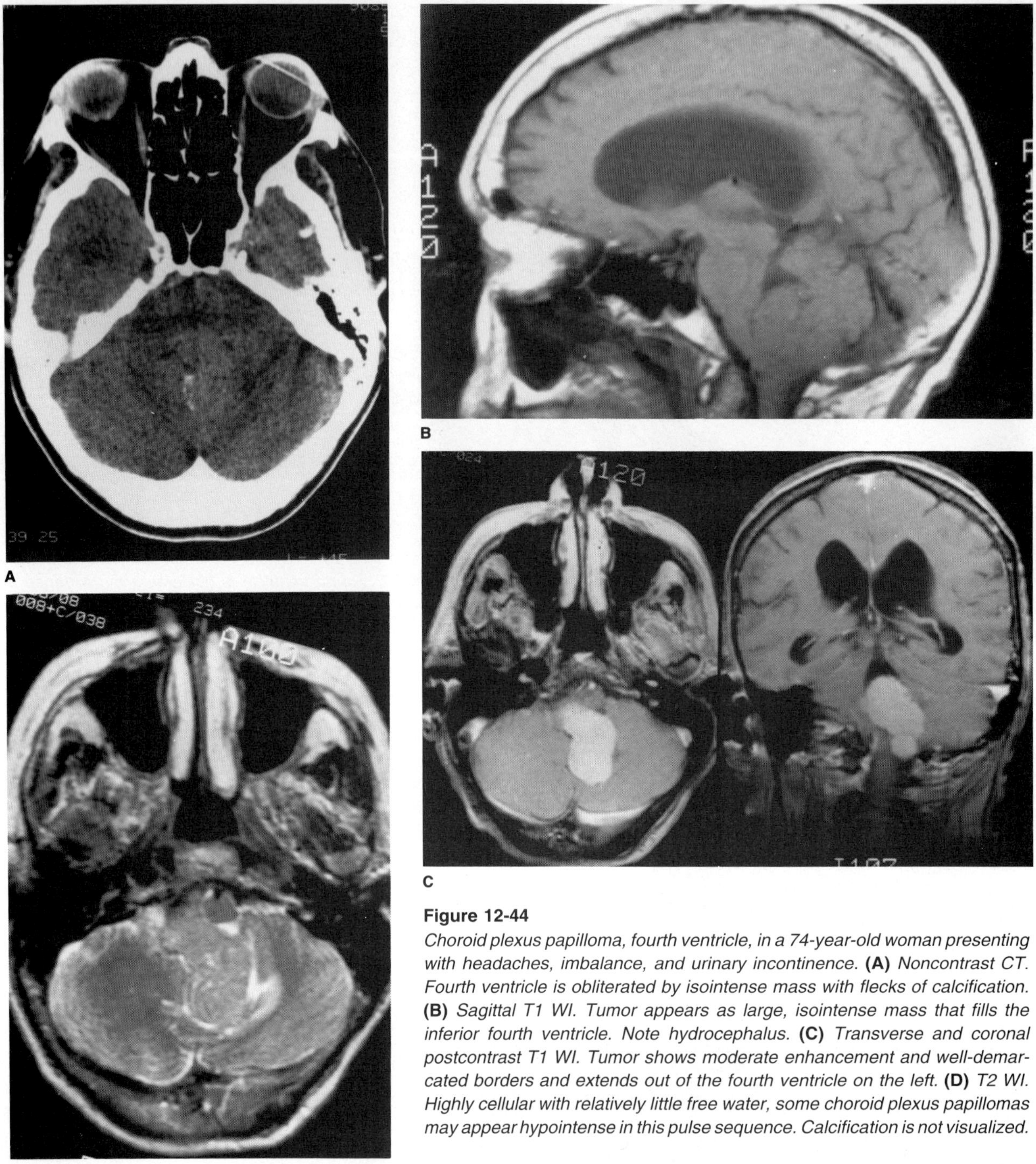

Figure 12-44

Choroid plexus papilloma, fourth ventricle, in a 74-year-old woman presenting with headaches, imbalance, and urinary incontinence. **(A)** *Noncontrast CT. Fourth ventricle is obliterated by isointense mass with flecks of calcification.* **(B)** *Sagittal T1 WI. Tumor appears as large, isointense mass that fills the inferior fourth ventricle. Note hydrocephalus.* **(C)** *Transverse and coronal postcontrast T1 WI. Tumor shows moderate enhancement and well-demarcated borders and extends out of the fourth ventricle on the left.* **(D)** *T2 WI. Highly cellular with relatively little free water, some choroid plexus papillomas may appear hypointense in this pulse sequence. Calcification is not visualized.*

fifth decades, with a slight male predilection. In about 20 percent of cases hemangioblastoma occurs as part of von Hippel–Lindau syndrome, an autosomal dominant inherited phakomatosis. Von Hippel–Lindau syndrome includes different combinations of single or multiple hemangioblastomas (cerebellum, eye, medulla, spinal cord, cerebrum), congenital nonneoplastic cysts of kidney and pancreas, and tumors of the adrenals, pancreas, and kidneys, among other abnormalities.[12,13,91] The symptoms and signs of cerebellar hemangioblastomas are mainly those of increased intracranial pressure (headache, nausea, vomiting) from obstructive hydrocephalus and cerebellar dysfunction, lasting an average of 6 to 10 months before prompting medical attention.[91] The prognosis for isolated cases of cerebellar hemangioblastoma is excellent, with 85 percent of patients surviving 5 to 20 years after surgical removal.[91]

Pathology

The cerebellum is the most common location of hemangioblastoma (83 to 85 percent), which also can be found

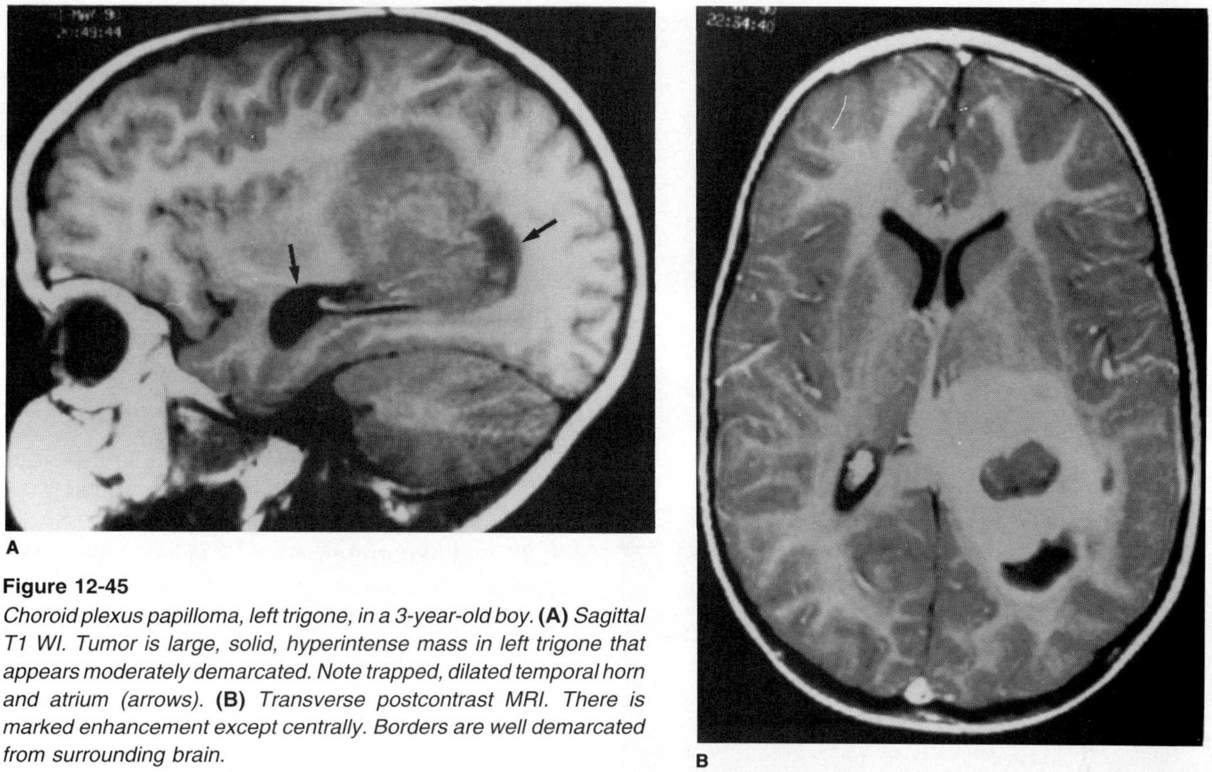

A

B

Figure 12-45
Choroid plexus papilloma, left trigone, in a 3-year-old boy. **(A)** *Sagittal T1 WI. Tumor is large, solid, hyperintense mass in left trigone that appears moderately demarcated. Note trapped, dilated temporal horn and atrium (arrows).* **(B)** *Transverse postcontrast MRI. There is marked enhancement except centrally. Borders are well demarcated from surrounding brain.*

by decreasing order of frequency in the spinal cord, medulla, and cerebrum.[12–14,91] The typical cerebellar hemangioblastoma is a paramedian or hemispheric well-circumscribed, unencapsulated large cystic mass (60 percent) with a variably sized mural nodule.[12–14] In 40 percent of the cases the tumor is solid without a surrounding cyst.[12,91] Microscopically, this highly cellular tumor consists of blood spaces and channels lined by plump endothelial cells that are separated by lipid-laden larger cells with pale nuclei termed stromal cells.[12–14] Focal cellular atypia may be present without prognostic importance, and mitotic figures are typically absent.[12,13] In cystic hemangioblastoma, the mural nodule represents the tumor whereas the cyst wall is usually devoid of neoplastic features consisting of fibrillary neuroglia.[12] Hemorrhage and necrosis are uncommon in hemangioblastomas.[12,91] Polycythemia, which results from the production of erythropoietin by the tumor, occurs in 10 percent of patients with hemangioblastoma.[13]

Imaging Findings

CT and MRI display hemangioblastoma most commonly as a cyst with a mural nodule (35 percent) or solid (33 percent) (Figs. 12-47 and 12-48).[91] Less frequently the appearance is solid with a cyst, purely cystic, or cystic nodule.[91] The mural nodule enhances intensely with contrast, and the cyst wall only occasionally. Obstructive hydrocephalus is common with cerebellar hemangioblastoma from compression of the fourth ventricle.

On noncontrast CT, the cyst is hypodense and the mural nodule is isodense relative to cerebellum.[21,91,92] Solid hemangioblastomas are usually isodense, are occasionally hyperdense on noncontrast CT, and enhance homogeneously with iodine infusion.[91] On precontrast T1 WI, the cystic component of cerebellar hemangioblastoma is typically hypointense and the mural nodule is hypointense or isointense relative to the cerebellum.[91,93] Solid cerebellar hemangioblastomas are hypointense to isointense relative to cerebellum in T1 WI.

In PD WI and T2 WI both cystic and solid cerebellar hemangioblastomas appear hyperintense relative to cerebellum and CSF.[91,93] Central or peripheral zones of serpentine signal void are common in cerebellar hemangioblastomas, denoting their rich vascular supply identified pathologically and angiographically.[91,93] The findings of serpentine signal void in a cystic paramedian cerebellar mass with a mural nodule are highly presumptive of the diagnosis of cerebellar hemangioblastoma.[93] Occasionally cerebellar hemangioblastomas exhibit hyperintense foci in precontrast T1-weighted images owing to lipid-laden stromal cells or hemorrhage.[21]

An unusual space-occupying cerebellar lesion that looks like but is not a tumor is referred to as Lhermitte-Duclos disease. It is also called dysplastic gangliocytoma of the cerebellum. It is a rare focally indolent growth of the cerebellar cortex in which folia enlarge as a result of a profusion of dysplastic cortical neurons and a thickening of the molecular layer. It presents with symptoms of increased intracranial pressure in young adults.[94]

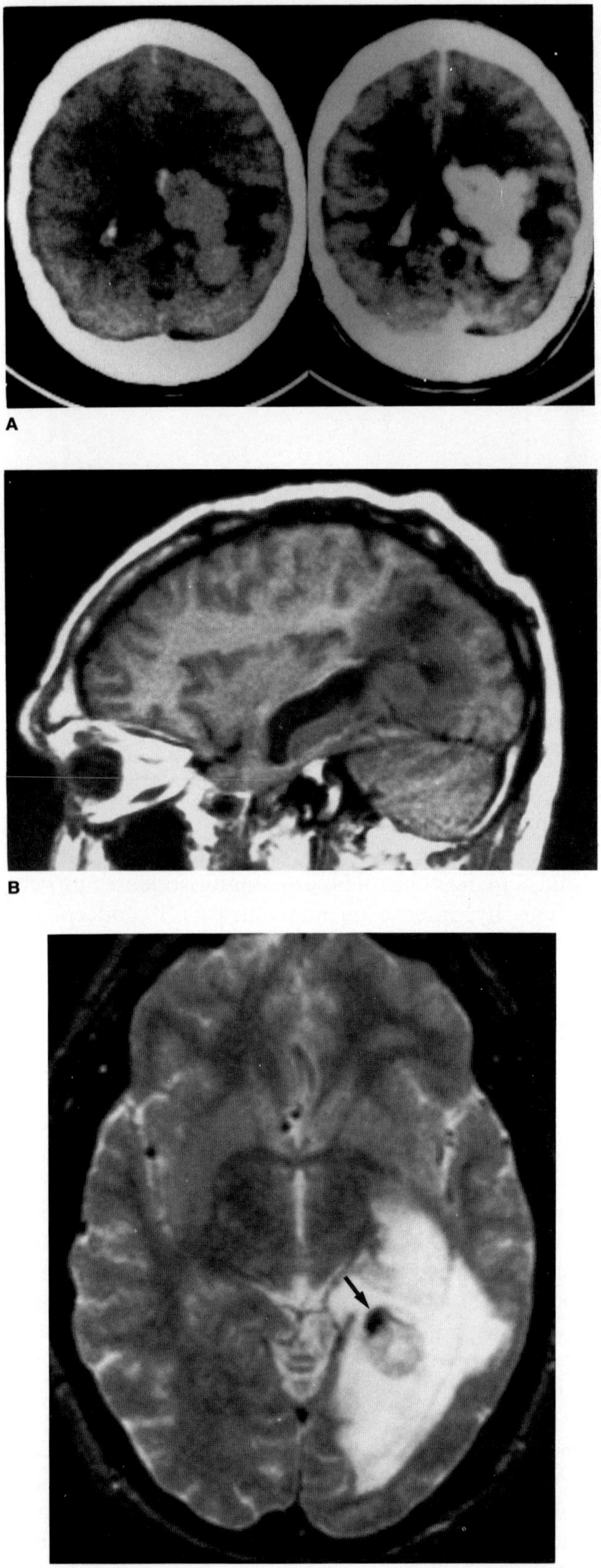

Figure 12-46
Choroid plexus papilloma, carcinoma, left lateral ventricle, in a 28-year-old man. **(A)** *Pre- and postcontrast CT. Tumor is lobulated and hyperdense and shows marked enhancement and well-defined borders with contrast. Pathology revealed choroid plexus papilloma.* **(B)** *Sagittal T1 WI. Tumor recurred 4 years after surgery, and it is shown here as an isointense (relative to gray matter) roundish mass in the left trigone.* **(C)** *T2 WI. Isointense, recurrent tumor nodule shows focus of acute hemorrhage (arrow). Note extensive hyperintense surrounding edema. Biopsy revealed malignant transformation to choroid plexus carcinoma with invasion of neighboring brain.*

There is a characteristic pattern on some CTs and all MRIs with laminated or striated patterns of cortical architecture with alternating layers that are hypointense on T1 and hyperintense on T2 (Fig. 12-49). The pathogenesis is unclear. It has been considered a developmental disorder, a hamartoma, or another type of low-grade neoplasm.[95]

Pineal Region Tumors

Neoplasms of the pineal region constitute a heterogeneous group that accounts for 0.4 to 1 percent of all intracranial neoplasms.[14] The two major groups are those originating from totipotential germ cells sequestered in this location during embryonic development and those derived from the pineal parenchyma.[13]

A simplified scheme listing neoplasms of the pineal region is shown in Table 12-8.[14,96,97]

Table 12-8
Neoplasms—pineal region

Germ cell origin
Germinoma
Embryonal carcinoma
Teratoma
Choriocarcinoma
Yolk sac tumor (endodermal sinus)
Mixed germ cell tumor
Pineal cell origin
Pineoblastoma
Pineocytoma
Other origin
Astrocytoma
Glioblastoma multiforme
Metastatic
Hemangiopericytoma
Meningioma
Ganglioneuroma
Ganglioglioma

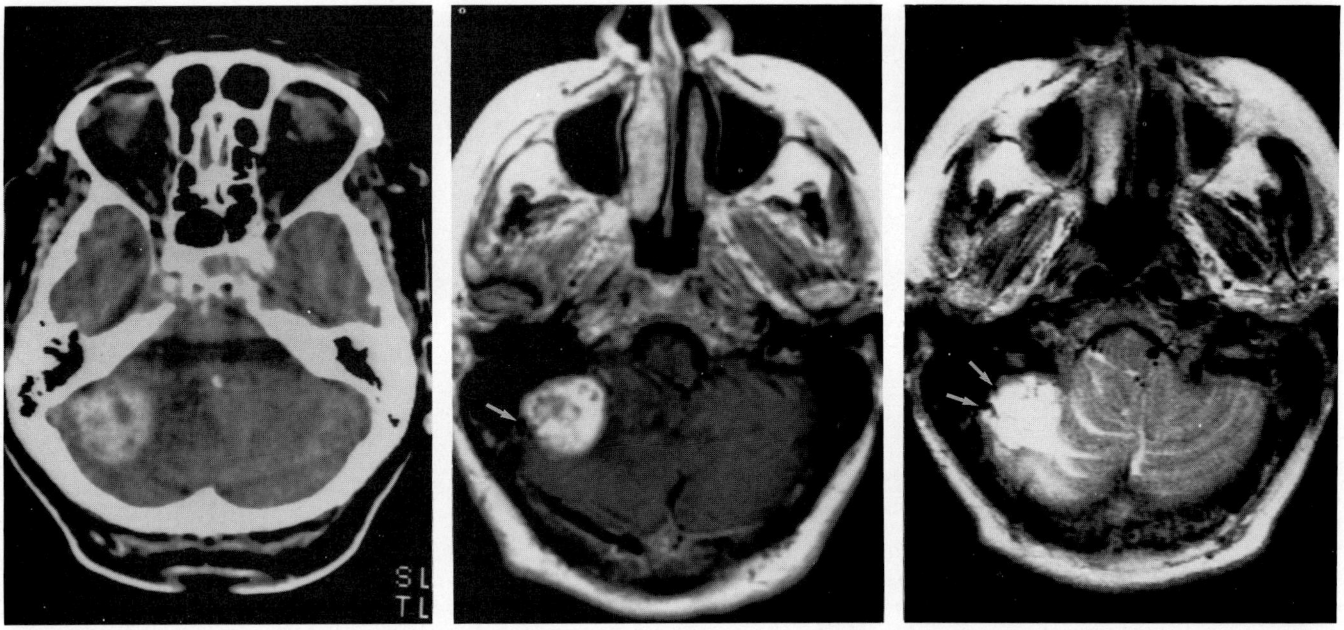

A B C

Figure 12-47
Solid cerebellar hemangioblastoma in a 74-year-old woman presenting with headaches and imbalance. **(A)** *Postcontrast CT. There is inhomogeneous, moderate enhancement of solid tumor situated in the lateral aspect of the right cerebellar hemisphere with inconspicuous surrounding edema.* **(B)** *Postcontrast transverse T1 WI. Solid tumor is well demarcated and shows marked enhancement with sharp borders. Note tubular flow void signal typical of hemangioblastoma indicating vascularity (arrow).* **(C)** *T2 WI. Tumor is hyperintense with surrounding edema, and again noted are serpiginous and tubular areas of flow void signal or vessels (arrows).*

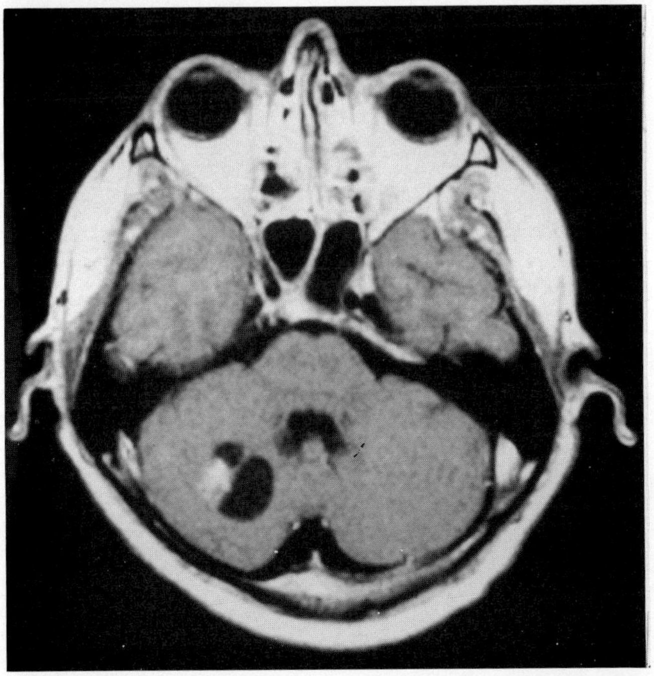

Figure 12-48
Cystic right cerebellar hemangioblastoma, postcontrast transverse T1 WI. Tumor has classical appearance of hypointense cyst with enhancing mural nodule. The main differential diagnosis in this case is with cystic astrocytoma.

Pineal Germinoma

Definition

Pineal germinoma is a tumor arising from neoplastic transformation of primitive germ cells that migrate to this region during embryonic development.[14]

Epidemiology

Pineal germinoma is the most common variant of germ cell neoplasm in this region, accounting for 50 percent of pineal neoplasms.[12] Peak incidence is in the middle of the second decade of life, with a marked male predominance.[88]

Pathology

Variably circumscribed or infiltrative, germinomas often are spread by discontinuous growth in the subarachnoid space, and CSFs borne metastases are common.[14] The majority occur in the pineal region, but in one-third of cases there is involvement of both the pineal and the hypothalamic-suprasellar regions.[14] Histologically, germinomas are identical to seminomas, consisting of neoplastic primitive germ cells, interspersed lymphocytes, and delicate septa of fibrous tissue.[13]

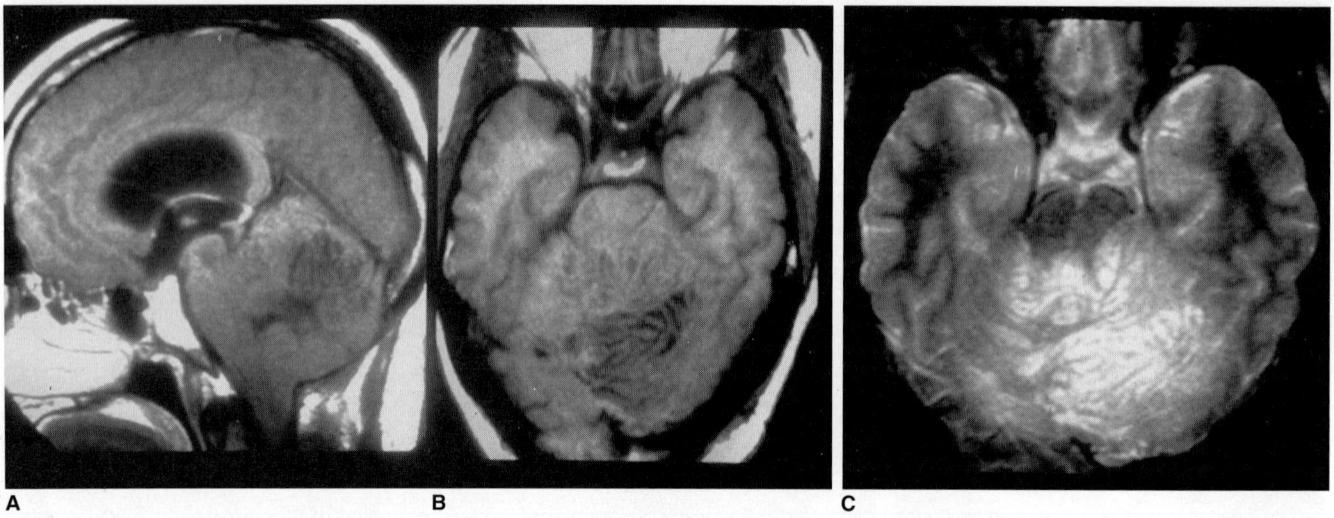

Figure 12-49
Lhermitte-Duclos disease in a 32-year-old man presenting with headaches and ataxia. The lesion is intraparenchymal in the left cerebellum and is characterized by a striated hypointense pattern in noncontrast sagittal T1 WI **(A)**, *transverse* **(B)** *and hyperintense in T2 WI* **(C)**, *representing the abnormally thickened folia. (Courtesy of Robert Quencer, M.D.)*

Imaging Findings

Noncontrast CT displays typical germinoma as a well-circumscribed, iso- to hyperdense mass in the pineal or suprasellar regions (Fig. 12-50).[88] Premature calcification of the pineal gland may be seen in germinomas in this region.[15,88]

MRI studies display a typical pineal germinoma as a rounded, well-circumscribed, or lobulated iso- to hypointense mass on precontrast T1 WI and iso- to hyperintense in PD WI and T2 WI (Fig. 12-50).[88,97,98] Homogeneous enhancement is common in both CT and MRI studies.[97,98]

Teratoma

Definition

Teratoma is a tumor composed of tissues derived from all three germ cell layers.[14] Intracranially, teratomas occur more commonly in the pineal and suprasellar regions.[14]

Epidemiology

Teratoma is the second most common pineal region tumor, with an incidence that is half that of germinoma. It shows a marked male predilection, and peak incidence is in children and adolescents.[14]

Pathology

Teratoma is usually well defined with a rounded or lobulated contour and heterogeneous cut surface denoting the presence of several tissue elements, such as bone, cartilage, and hair.[12] Microscopically, there is a wide range of histologic patterns related to the tissue types expressed by endodermal, mesodermal, and ectodermal layers.[12] Immature teratoma, the more aggressive type, contains embryonic or fetal-appearing elements, whereas the less aggressive mature teratoma shows components that resemble adult tissues.[14]

Imaging Findings

In imaging studies teratoma may exhibit marked heterogeneity owing to the presence of cysts, blood, fat, and calcification.[88] Thus, on CT a spectrum of densities from fat to bone attenuation values, cystic, and solid components may be observed (Fig. 12-51).[88,98]

On MRI studies teratoma can be quite heterogeneous, producing variable hypo- to hyperintense zones in T1 WI, PD WI, and T2 WI (Figs. 12-52 and 12-53).[88,98] Enhancement is variable in both imaging studies.

Pineocytoma and Pineoblastoma

Definition

Pineocytoma and pineoblastoma are tumors originating from neoplastic transformation of the pineocyte, the parenchymal pineal cell of neuroepithelial origin.[12] Discounting the transitional forms, pineocytoma represents the well-differentiated low-grade variant, and pineoblastoma the poorly differentiated high-grade variant of pineal parenchymal neoplasms.

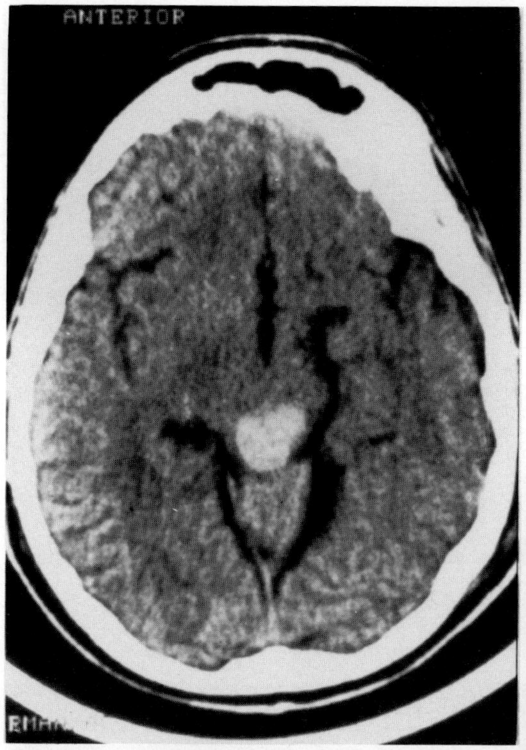

A

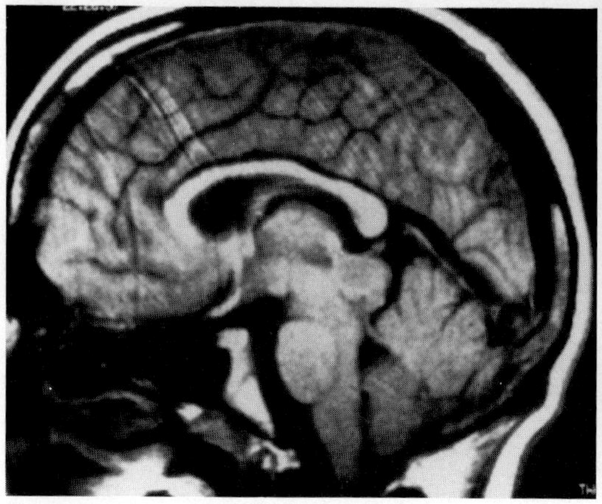

B

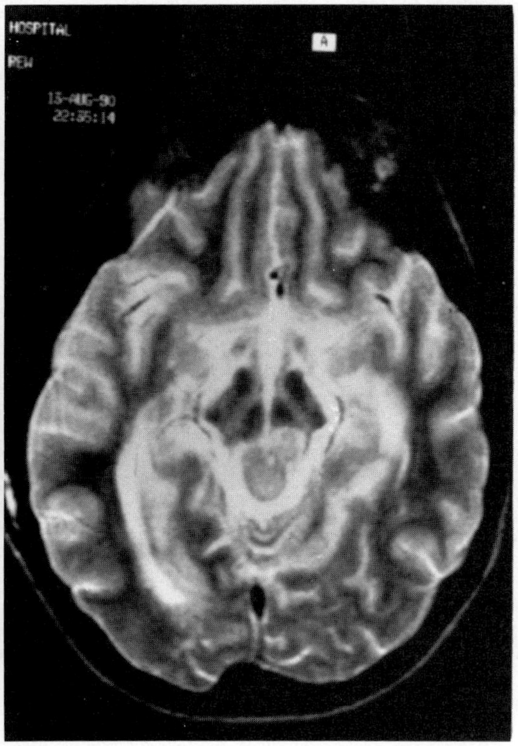

C

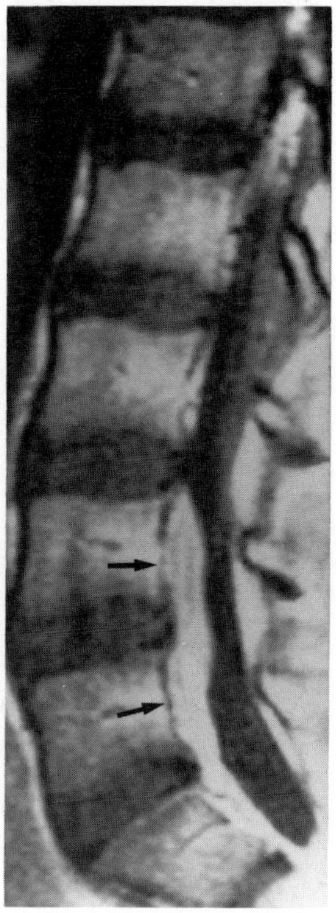

D

Figure 12-50
Pineal germinoma in a 14-year-old boy. **(A)** *Noncontrast CT. Tumor appears hyperdense.* **(B)** *Sagittal T1 WI. Tumor has slightly hypointense center. Note compression of aqueduct.* **(C)** *T2 WI. Tumor is well demarcated as isointense (relative to gray matter) mass in pineal region. Germinomas represent 50 percent of neoplasms in the pineal region.* **(D)** *Postcontrast sagittal T1 WI, LS spine. CSF-borne metastases are common in germinomas, as shown in this case as bulky sausage-shaped area of marked enhancement in the anterior spinal canal (arrows).*

Epidemiology

Pineocytoma and pineoblastoma are quite rare neoplasms and are less common than germ cell neoplasms of the pineal region.[12] Pineocytoma is more common in adolescents and adults without sex predominance; pineoblastoma has a peak incidence in the first decade with a 2:1 male predominance.[13,88]

Pathology

Pineocytoma is usually well circumscribed, slow-growing, moderately cellular, and well differentiated and exhibits an architectural pattern similar to that of a normal pineal gland.[14] Pineoblastoma, the anaplastic counterpart of pineocytoma, is composed of a dense population of primitive small cells often arranged to form Homer-Wright rosettes.[12] The histologic features, age of incidence, morphologic appearance, aggressive behavior, and tendency for CSF-borne metastases in pineoblastoma parallel those in medulloblastoma.[13]

Imaging Studies

On noncontrast CT both pineocytoma and pineoblastoma appear solid, hypo- to hyperdense, with prominent homogeneous enhancement after contrast infusion (Figs. 12-54 and 12-55).[88,98] A heterogeneous appearance occurs more frequently in pineoblastoma.

On MRI these tumors usually appear solid, well circumscribed, and hypointense to isointense in precontrast T1 WI. On PD WI and T2 WI pineocytoma tends

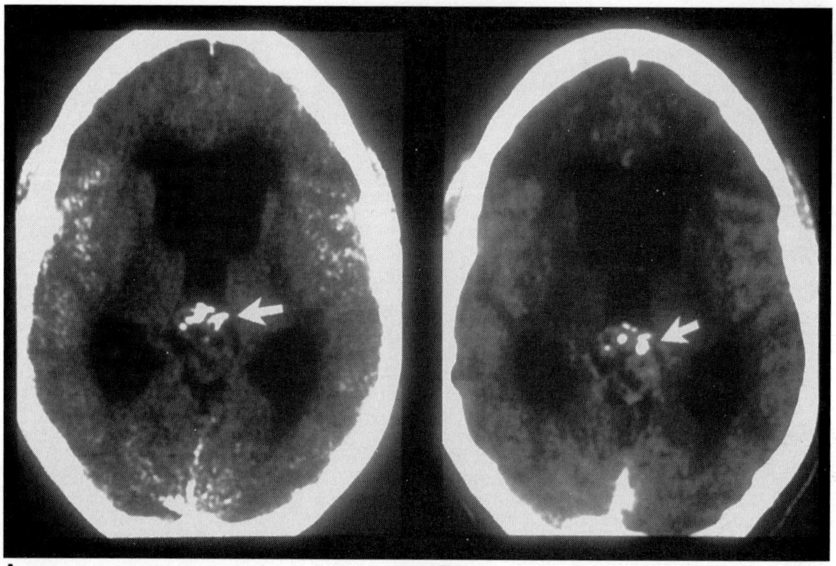

A B

Figure 12-51
Teratoma in the pineal region in an adolescent presenting with headaches. Precontrast **(A)** *and postcontrast* **(B)** *CT show the tumor as sizable heterogeneous, slightly hyperdense pineal mass with calcification (white arrows).*

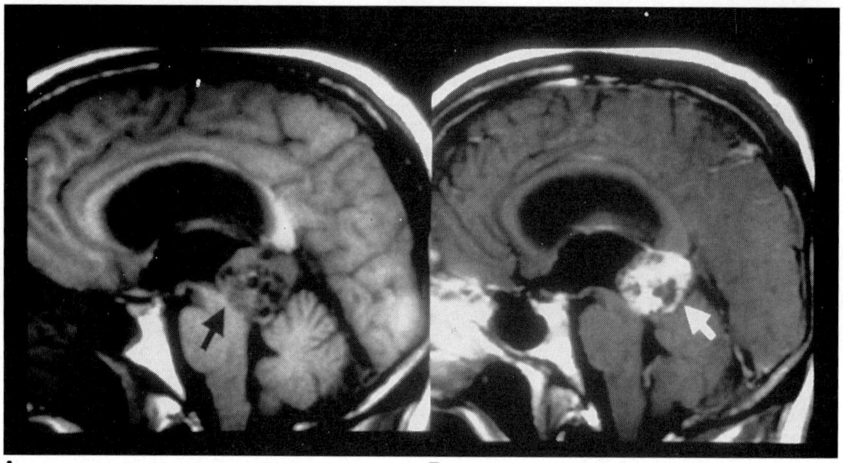

A B

Figure 12-52
Teratoma in the patient shown in Fig. 12-51. Precontrast **(A)** *and postcontrast* **(B)** *T1 WI shows the tumor as a large heterogeneous enhancing mass with central areas of fatty content (black arrow) and calcification (white arrow). Note compression of aqueduct and hydrocephalus.*

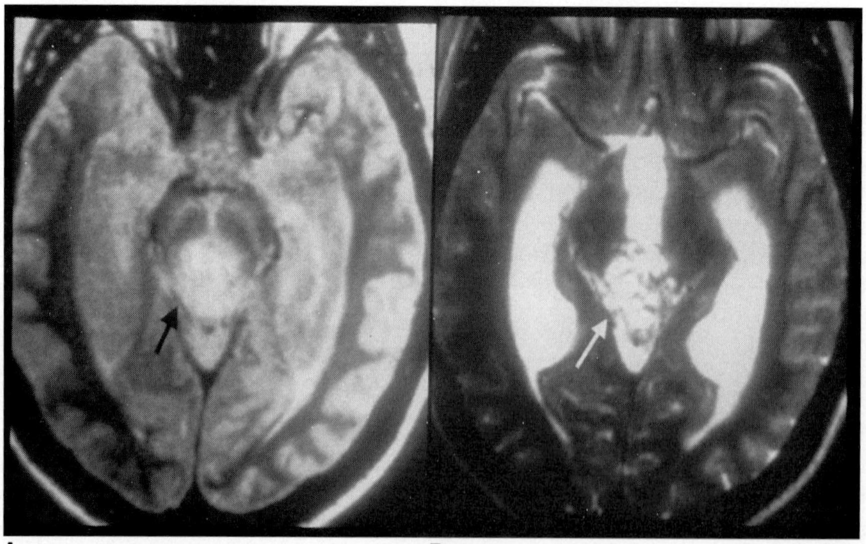

A B

Figure 12-53
Teratoma in the same patient shown in Fig. 12-52. In PD WI **(A)** *the tumor is homogeneously hyperintense (black arrow), but in T2 WI* **(B)** *there is heterogeneous mixed hypointensity and hyperintensity (white arrow), reflecting the complex pathology of these lesions, which may contain tissues from all three germ cell layers.*

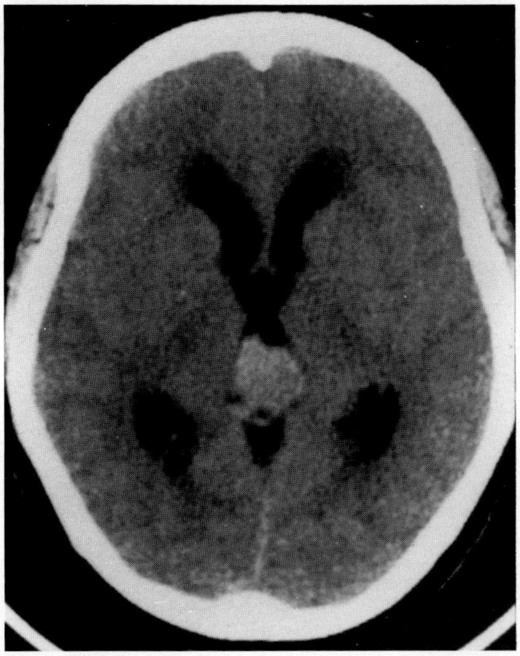

A

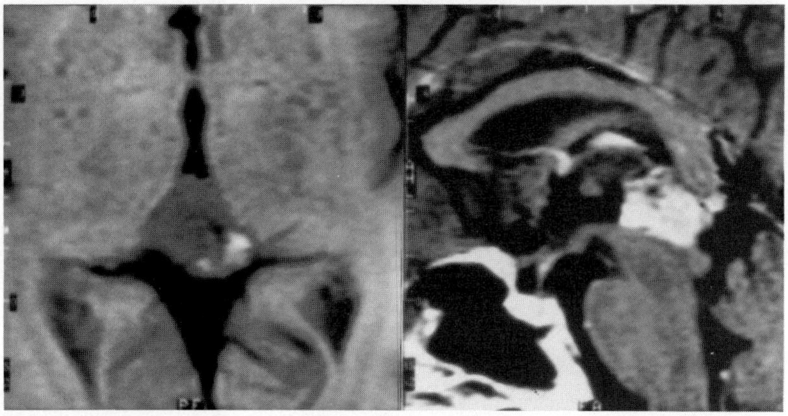

B

Figure 12-54
Pineocytoma in a 37-year-old woman presenting with headaches. **(A)** *Noncontrast CT. Tumor appears as lobulated, slightly hyperdense mass in the pineal region. Note associated enlargement of lateral ventricles.* **(B)** *Precontrast transverse and postcontrast sagittal T1 WI. Tumor is hypointense but has foci of slightly increased intensity denoting subacute hemorrhage. After contrast there is marked homogeneous enhancement of tumor in the pineal region.*

to be hyperintense. The appearance of pineoblastoma in PD WI and T2 WI is more variable, from hypo- to hyperintense or mixed high and low signal intensity.[97]

Pineal Cysts

A relatively common incidental finding in sagittal T1-weighted MRI examination is the presence of a well-circumscribed, centrally hypointense, round or ovoid enlargement of the pineal gland of pineal cyst (Fig. 12-56). In PD WI the cyst content may exhibit higher signal than CSF, and in T2-weighted images its signal is hyperintense.

Pineal cysts are usually smaller than 1 cm but occasionally expand to above 1 cm. Usually asymptomatic, a pineal cyst may very rarely give rise to clinical symptoms of obstructive hydrocephalus by compressing the region of the aqueduct.[88] Its origin is attributed to the degeneration of the central core of fibrillary glia in the pineal gland. On pathologic examination, the cyst contains thin, clear fluid and its lining consists of dense neuroglial fibers.[12] Pineal cysts can be differentiated from pineal tumors by their smooth, regular contour and shape, smaller size, and lack of internal structure.[88]

Colloid Cyst

Definition

Colloid cyst is a benign unilocular cyst of neuroepithelial origin that is consistently located in the anterior third ventricle.[14,99]

Epidemiology

When classified as a brain tumor of malformative neuroepithelial origin, colloid cyst represents 2 percent of intracranial tumors.[12] Colloid cyst is primarily a lesion of adults in the third to fifth decade, affecting males and females equally.[12,14]

Pathology

On gross pathology, colloid cyst has a spherical, globular shape with a smooth surface made up of a thin, fibrous capsule that encases gray, viscid, hyaline material.[12–14] Varying in size from 0.5 to 4 cm, colloid cyst consistently lies attached to the third ventricle roof, where it splays the column of the fornix. As it grows, the foramen of Monro is obstructed, leading to hydrocephalus. Some colloid cysts are mobile, and symptoms of hydrocephalus may be intermittent as the foramen of Monro is obstructed with changes in head position.[12] Microscopically, colloid cyst consists of an outer capsule of fibrous connective tissue and an inner epithelial layer composed of ciliated or mucin-producing columnar cells.[13,14] Growth in colloid cyst occurs by mucin production and desquamation of cells that become entrapped in the central amorphous material.[13] The content of a colloid cyst may show evidence of new or old hemorrhage.[12]

Imaging Findings

Noncontrast CT displays colloid cyst as a hypo-, iso-, or hyperdense, more frequently homogeneous, well-

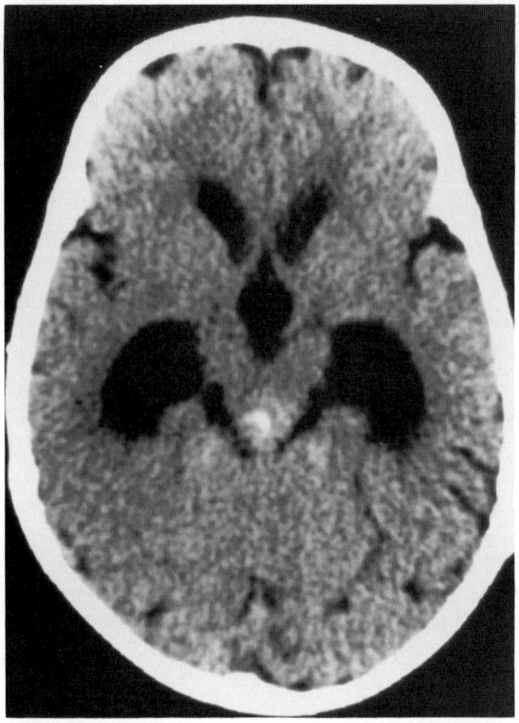

A

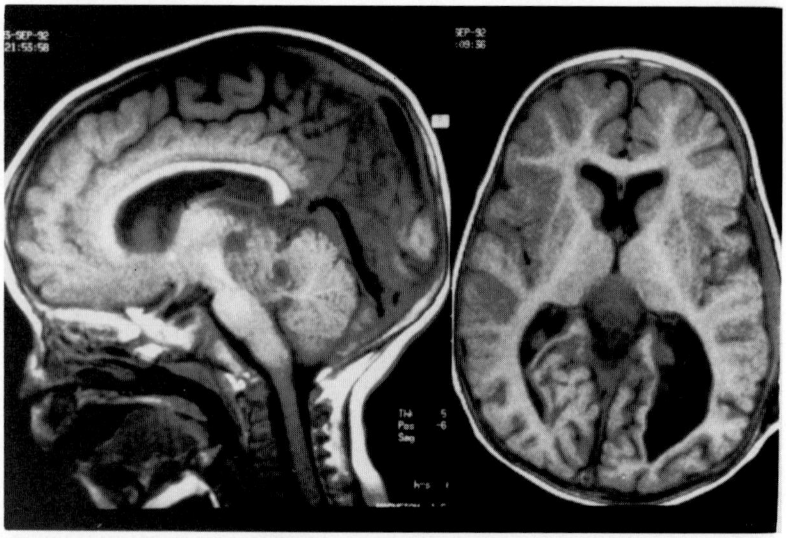

B

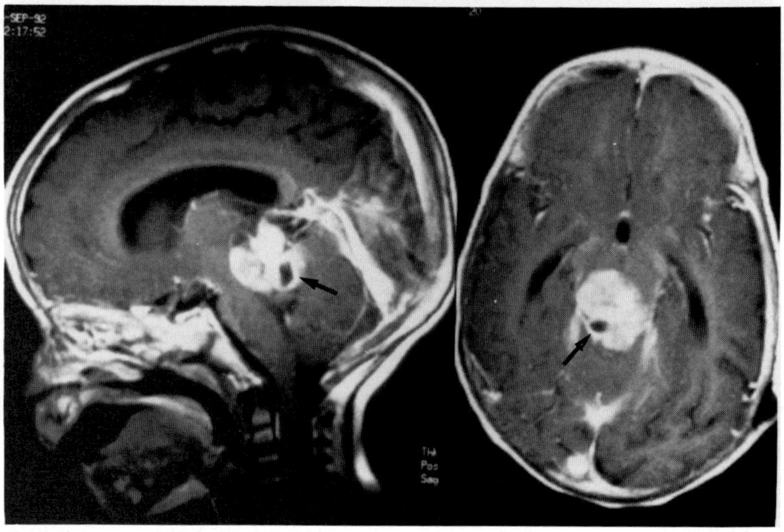

C

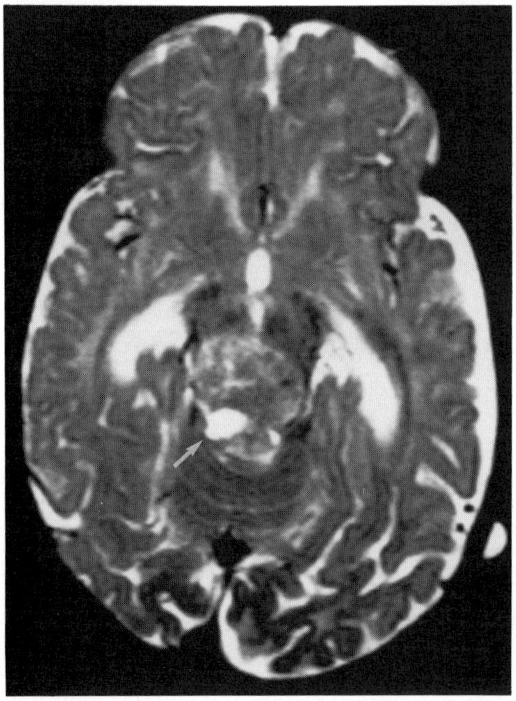

D

Figure 12-55

Pineoblastoma in a 7-month-old girl. **(A)** *Noncontrast CT. Tumor is identified as enlarged slightly hyperdense pineal gland that also exhibits premature calcification.* **(B)** *Precontrast sagittal and transverse T1 WI. Note marked enlargement of the pineal gland occupied by mixed iso- and hypointense tumor.* **(C)** *Postcontrast sagittal and transverse T1 WI. Note marked homogeneous enhancement except for cystic portion of tumor (arrow).* **(D)** *T2 WI. High cellularity, nuclear-cytoplasmic ratio in pineoblastoma leads to hypointensity except where there is cystic degeneration (arrow).*

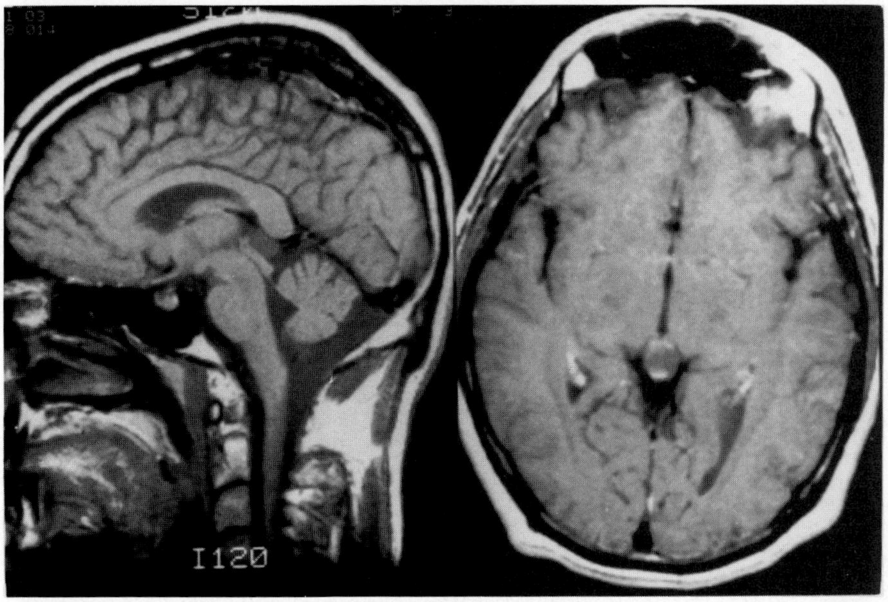

Figure 12-56
Pineal cyst in a 35-year-old man, precontrast sagittal and postcontrast transverse T1 WI. Note cyst as ovoid, slight hypointense enlargement of pineal gland; there is minimal enhancement of cyst wall with contrast in transverse images.

delineated, round or ovoid mass in the superior and anterior third ventricle, near or at the foramen of Monro.[100,101] Contrast enhancement is typically absent or minimal in some cases.[101]

Colloid cyst is better demonstrated in MRI owing to its multiplanar capability, (Figs. 12-57 and 12-58). There is no typical signal intensity pattern, and the pattern may vary from homogeneously or heterogeneously hypointense to hyperintense in T1-weighted images and T2-weighted images.[101] High signal intensity in T1-weighted images correlates with a high cholesterol content.[101] Rarely, a colloid cyst may become hemorrhagic.[12,102] The most helpful characteristic in MRI, as in CT, is the finding of a sharply demarcated round or ovoid mass in the anterior and superior third ventricle near or at the foramen of Monro. Obstructive hydrocephalus in the form of enlarged lateral ventricles is seen in most patients with colloid cyst.

Craniopharyngioma

Definition

Craniopharyngioma is a histologically benign CNS tumor arising from nests of squamous cells along the involuted pathway of the craniopharyngeal duct or Rathke's pouch.

Epidemiology

Craniopharyngioma represents to 3 percent of all intracranial tumors when all age groups are considered.[12,14] In children the incidence rises to 15 percent of supratentorial tumors and 50 percent of suprasellar tumors.[88] There is a bimodal age distribution, with one peak occurring in the first and second decades and the other between the fourth and sixth decades of life.[88]

Pathology

Craniopharyngioma typically occurs in the suprasellar region, from where it can extend superiorly to fill the third ventricle, inferiorly into the sellar region, laterally into the temporal lobes, or posteriorly along the clivus. Craniopharyngioma varies in size from small to large, and on gross examination the appearance is that of a well-circumscribed, round, or multilobulated, largely cystic or partly solid and cystic mass.[12–14] Its cut surface reveals a complex pattern of cyst, fibrous tissue, necrotic debris and calcification. Notable is the presence of encysted straw-colored or turbid brown oil with droplets of cholesterol crystals.[13] Microscopically, the histologic pattern is variable, consisting of neoplastic cells in a stratified squamous or columnar epithelial arrangement interspersed in the cyst, necrotic debris containing cholesterol clefts, and keratinized nodules.[12–14] Clinical findings include visual symptoms, endocrine dysfunction from compression of the visual tract and hypothalamus, and obstructive hydrocephalus. Recurrence is common in craniopharyngioma, as total excision is often difficult because of the location of the tumor.[14]

Imaging Findings

The classic findings are the presence of suprasellar calcification, expansion of the sella, and erosion of the dorsum sella. When encountered in a child, these radiographic findings are highly presumptive of the diagnosis of craniopharyngioma.

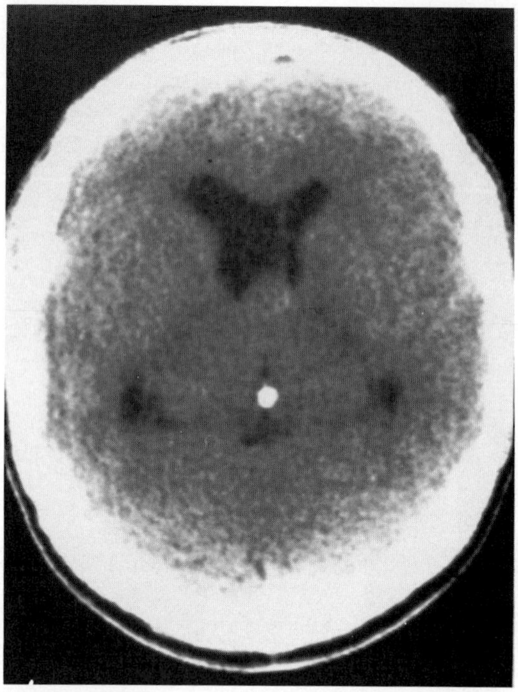

A

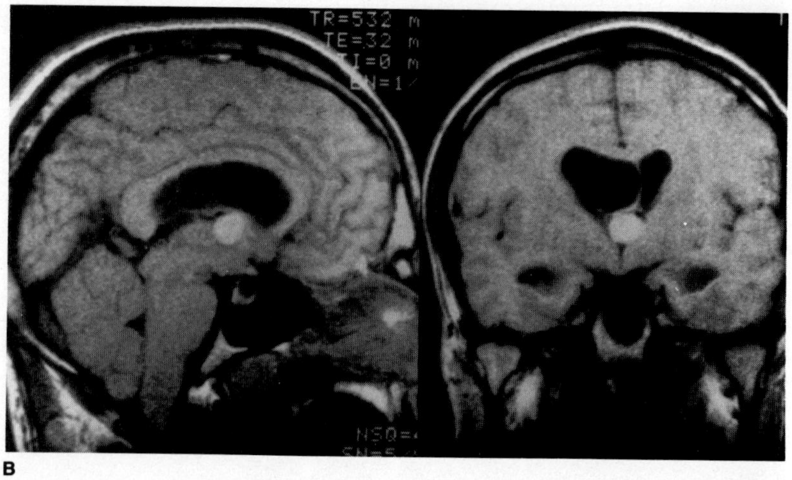

B

Figure 12-57
Colloid cyst in a 29-year-old man presenting with headaches. **(A)** *Noncontrast CT shows isodense roundish mass at the foramen of Monro.* **(B)** *Sagittal and coronal T1 WI. Diagnosis of colloid cyst is based on the location of round mass in superior and anterior third ventricle near or at the foramen of Monro. Cyst in this case is hyperintense relative to white matter. Note hydrocephalus.* **(C)** *PD WI. Colloid cyst is hyperintense.*

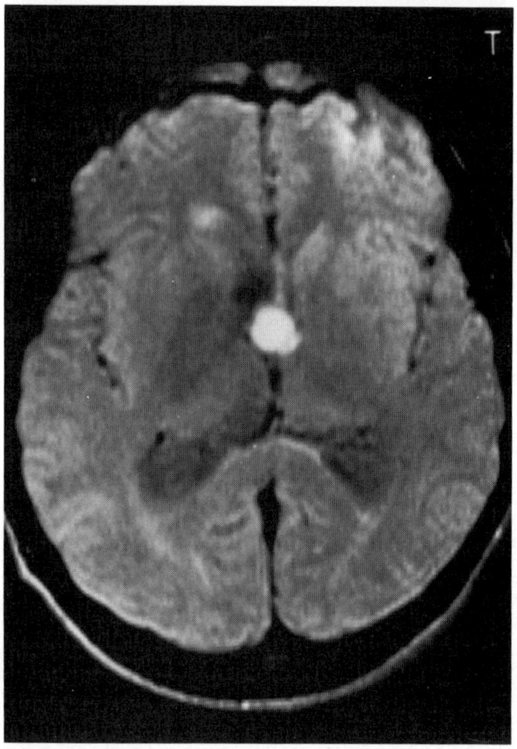

C

On noncontrast CT the classic appearance is that of a heterogeneous, partially calcified suprasellar mass with cystic and solid components (Fig. 12-59).[88] Calcification occurs along the wall of the cyst or in solid portions of the tumor.[103] The solid portion of the tumor and the cyst wall usually enhance (Fig. 12-60).

On MRI the characteristic finding is a round or lobulated largely cystic suprasellar mass that most often is heterogeneously hypointense but occasionally is hyperintense in T1 WI and homogeneously hyperintense in PD WI and T2 WI (Fig. 12-59).[88,104] Hyperintensity in T1 WI is attributed to the T1 shortening effect of cholesterol crystals.[104] Marked hypointensity in T2-weighted images may occur in heavily calcified craniopharyngiomas (Fig. 12-59). Enhancement is moderate to intense in solid portions of the tumor (Fig. 12-60).

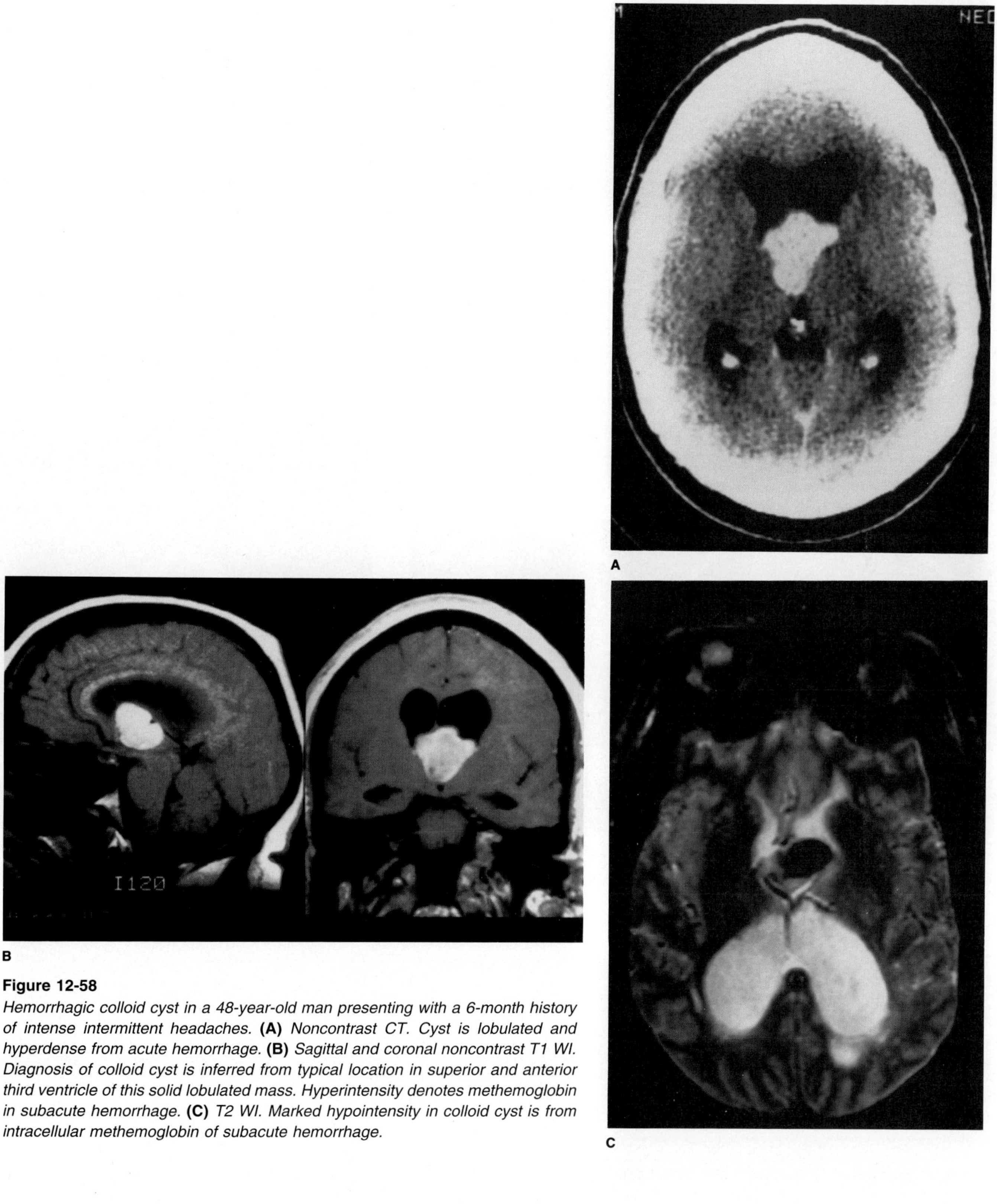

A

B

C

Figure 12-58

Hemorrhagic colloid cyst in a 48-year-old man presenting with a 6-month history of intense intermittent headaches. **(A)** *Noncontrast CT. Cyst is lobulated and hyperdense from acute hemorrhage.* **(B)** *Sagittal and coronal noncontrast T1 WI. Diagnosis of colloid cyst is inferred from typical location in superior and anterior third ventricle of this solid lobulated mass. Hyperintensity denotes methemoglobin in subacute hemorrhage.* **(C)** *T2 WI. Marked hypointensity in colloid cyst is from intracellular methemoglobin of subacute hemorrhage.*

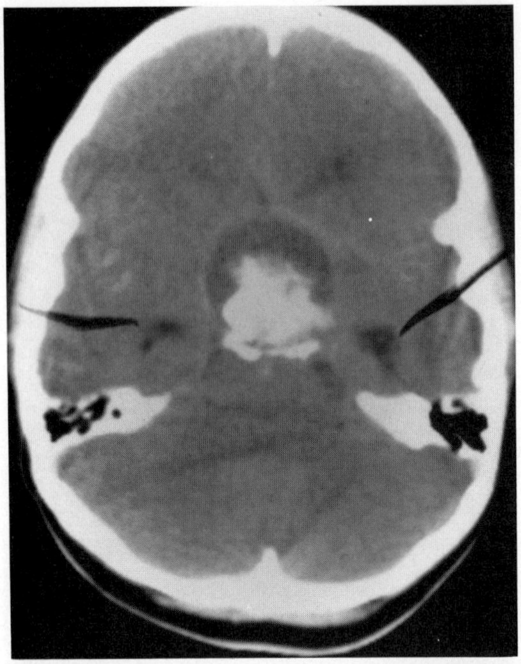

A

Figure 12-59

Cystic, calcified craniopharyngioma in a 7-year-old girl presenting with headaches. **(A)** *Noncontrast CT. Tumor consists of large hypodense cyst with heavily calcified solid center.* **(B)** *Sagittal and coronal noncontrast T1 WI. Tumor is well delineated, multilobulated, and markedly hyperintense owing to high protein or cholesterol content. Calcified center is hypointense. MRI defines large suprasellar component with downward sellar and upper third ventricular extension much better than does CT. Note enlargement of left lateral ventricle.* **(C)** *T2 WI. Tumor appears sharply demarcated with peripheral hyperintensity owing to high protein and hypointense calcified center.*

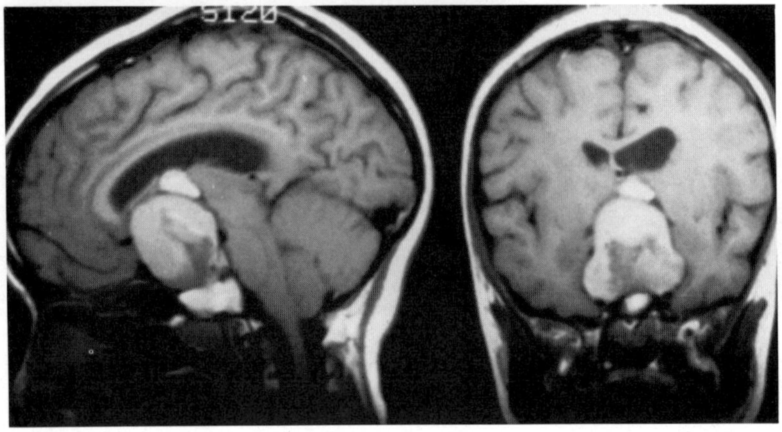

B

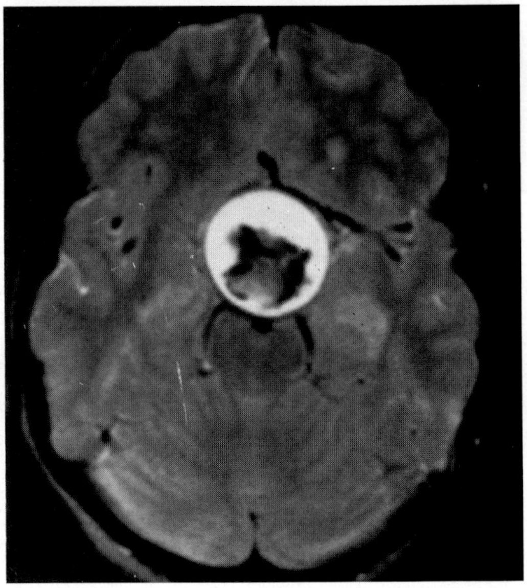

C

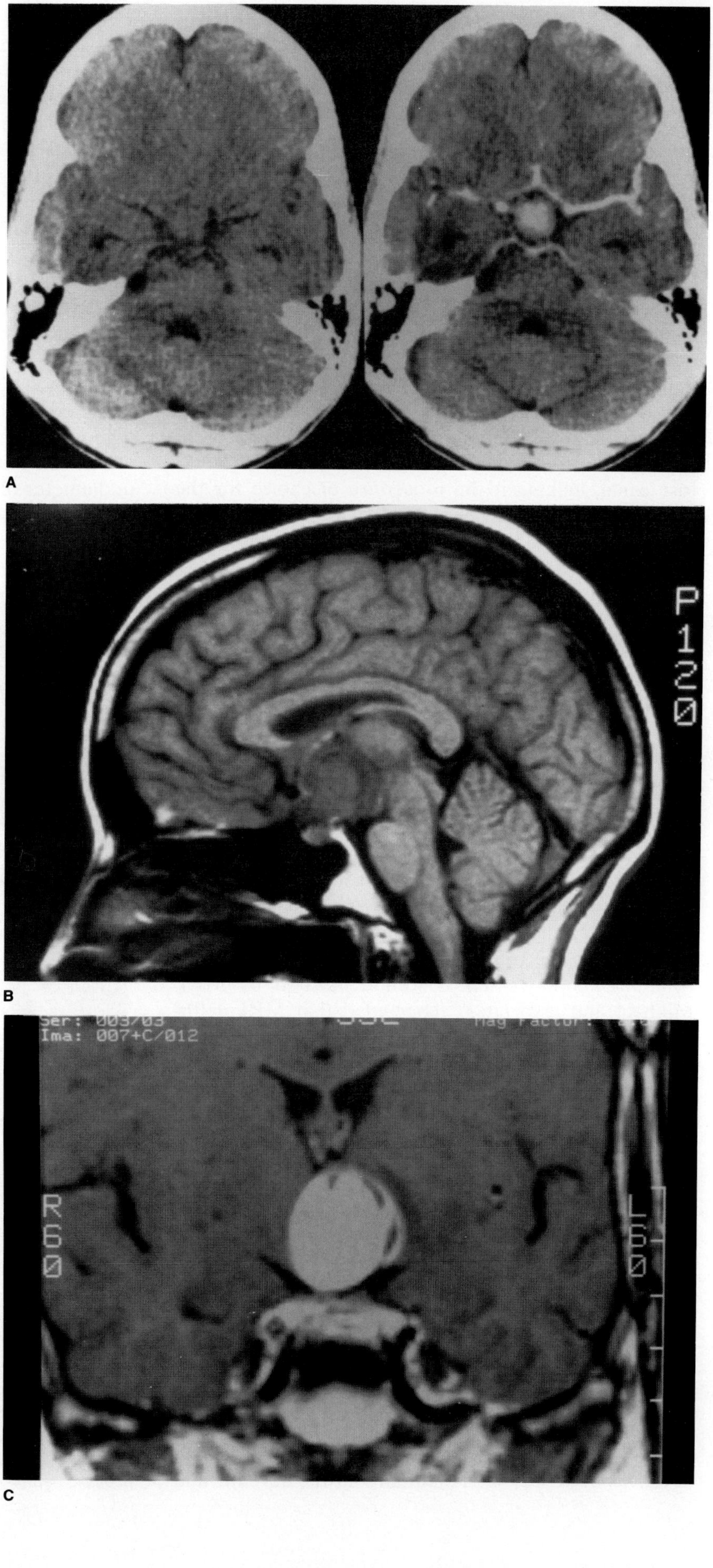

Figure 12-60
Solid craniopharyngioma in a 35-year-old woman with bitemporal visual field defect. **(A)** *Pre- and postcontrast CT. Tumor is isodense mass filling the suprasellar cistern; note marked enhancement with contrast.* **(B)** *Sagittal T1 WI. Large hypointense tumor fills suprasellar cistern and third ventricle. Optic track cannot be clearly visualized, but it may be draped over the tumor.* **(C)** *Coronal postcontrast T1 WI. Solid craniopharyngiomas tend to enhance homogeneously with sharp borders, as in this case. There is no sellar extension, but the third ventricle is filled with tumor. In adults craniopharyngiomas are more often solid.*

PATIENTS WHO PRESENT WITH SPECIFIC INTRACRANIAL TUMOR SYNDROMES

Acoustic Neuroma

The diagnosis of acoustic neuroma previously required conventional x-ray, tomography, and pantopaque cisternography. CT was excellent but small intracanalicular tumors were missed. Gas CT cysternography then became the procedure of choice. MRI has replaced all of the above.

CT visualizes the bony canal but not the nerves. Enlargement can be inferred only from secondary bone erosion. Beam hardening artifacts limit CT, especially in the posterior fossa. CT often requires iodinated contrast that increases the risks. The absence of beam hardening artifacts, multiplanar capability, and greater soft tissue contrast make MRI better than CT. MRI is able to demonstrate the normal contents of the internal auditory canal, making it the procedure of choice for the diagnosis of acoustic neuroma. It is cost-effective because most of the time no other studies are necessary. Unlike cysternography, it is an outpatient procedure. There are no known biologic health hazards.

Mikhael and associates[105] reported 51 acoustic neuromas. Thirty-six (70.5 percent) were large enough to be seen on routine CT. Fifteen were intracanalicular and missed on CT but diagnosed with cisternography and MRI. In another group of 23 acoustic neuromas, 15 were seen on CT and all by MRI. All studies so far show MRI to be better than CT in the diagnosis of posterior fossa tumors.[106,107] In 176 patients with sensorineural hearing loss, 65 had abnormal MRI.[108] CT was also done in 25 of these patients. In 18 (72 percent), MRI was superior to CT for lesion display. In 30 normal patients, MRI demonstrated the cochlea in all cases and the vestibulocochlear nerve in 77 percent. The relationship of the lesion to the brainstem, fourth ventricle, and surrounding blood vessels is well delineated by MRI. Mikhael and associates[105] concluded that MRI delineates the acoustic pathway more clearly than does CT.

Selection of protocols is most important for accurate imaging.[109,110] T1-weighted images most accurately demonstrate the seventh and eighth nerves in the internal auditory canal (IAC) and are most sensitive in detecting small tumors of the cerebellar pontine angle (CPA). On T1 images acoustic neuromas (ANS) are iso- or slightly hypointense to gray matter and on T2 are hyperintense. Usually the first sequence is a sagittal T1 study. The axial views use the pontomedullary junction as a center. These are 3-mm sections with short TR and TE. Thicker slices may decrease the potential for diagnosing these lesions. In the evaluation of the temporal bone for acoustic neuroma, both axial and coronal planes are necessary. Contrast agents such as gadolinium-DTPA will improve clarity and detail and indeed may diagnose a small tumor in the IAC not otherwise appreciated (Figs. 12-61 to 12-66). Potentially all the seventh and eighth cranial nerves will be seen in one scan plane as they course anteriorly from the brainstem and inferiorly in the coronal plane. The head must be straight in order to compare the two sides accurately. Flow compensation or motion-suppression techniques on T2 scans will minimize CSF pulsation artifacts. Short TR and TE images demonstrate greater contrast between CSF and tumor than do long TR and TE studies.

On normal thin-section T1-weighted images, cranial nerves VII and VIII can be seen as they exit the brainstem at the pontomedullary junction and course through the CPA cistern to the IAC. The IAC is a conical structure that tapers laterally at the cochlea and vestibule. The walls are cortical bone and have a low signal because the hydrogen protons are immobile. This allows for good contrast with the nerves. On T2 studies the nerves are partially obscured by CSF.

The size of the normal IAC may be as small as 2 mm in diameter or as wide as 12 mm. The average is 5 mm.

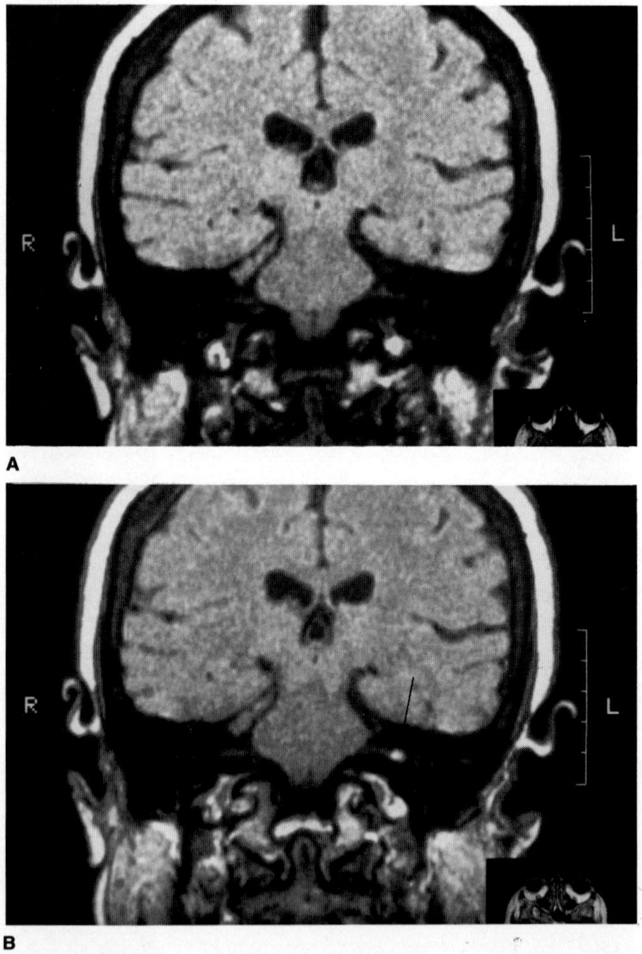

Figure 12-61
(A) *Short TR-short TE, 3-mm coronal through the eighth nerve complex in a patient with sensory neural hearing loss on the left. Study is normal.* **(B)** *After gadolinium, note enhancing 3-mm intracanalicular acoustic neuroma (arrow).*

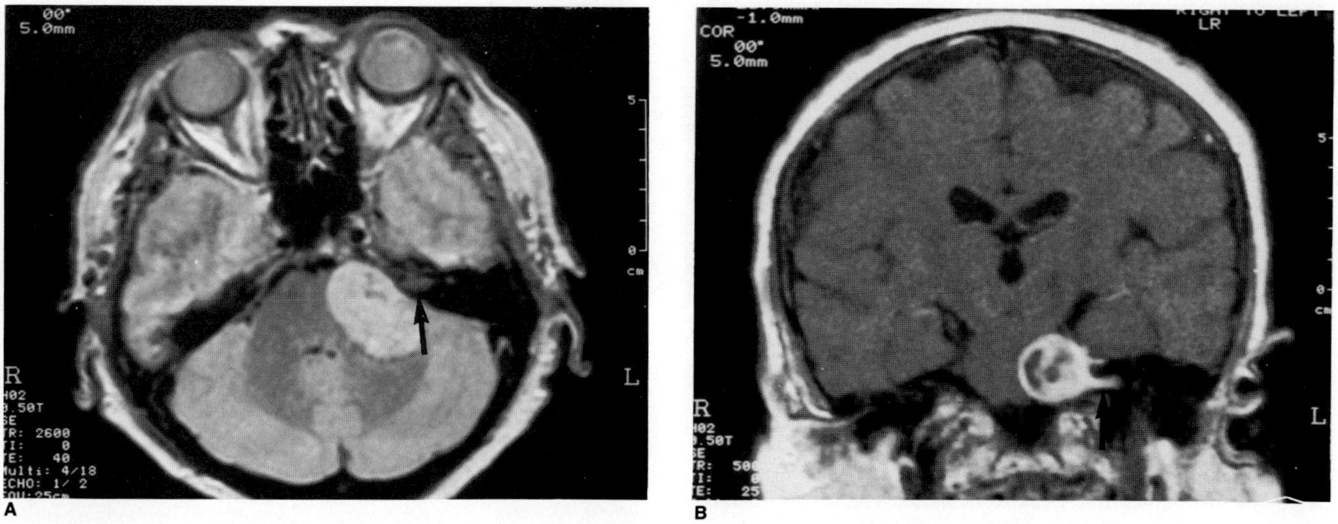

A B

Figure 12-62

(A) *Large tumor seen on long TR–short TE study could be acoustic neuroma or meningioma. The eighth nerve on the left is not bright (arrow).* **(B)** *Coronal view after gadolinium demonstrating enhancement of tumor and eighth nerve (arrow) proving an acoustic neuroma. Areas of low intensity represent cystic changes.*

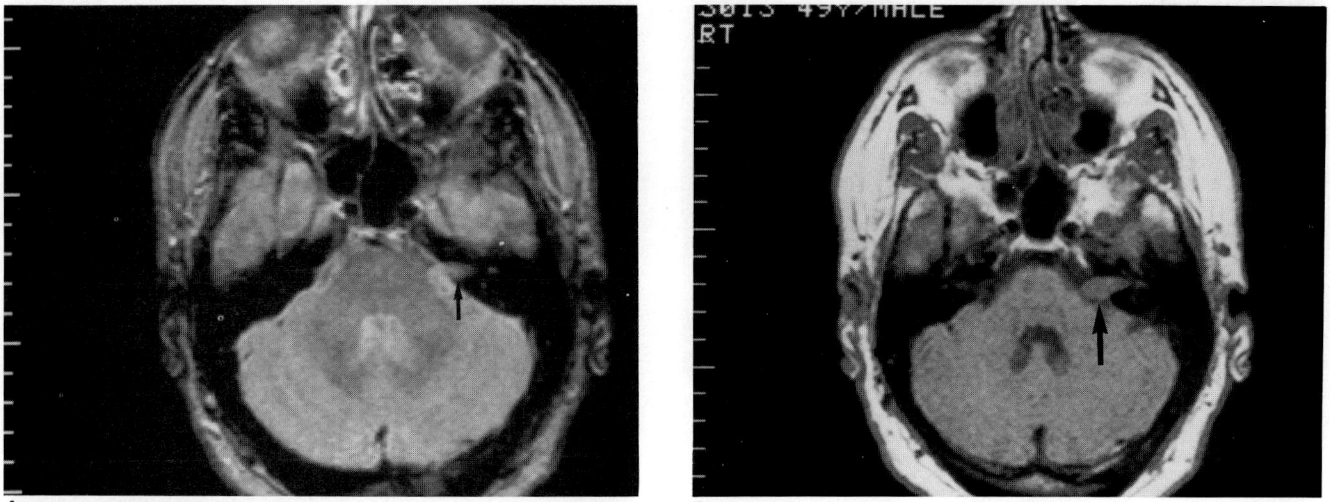

A B

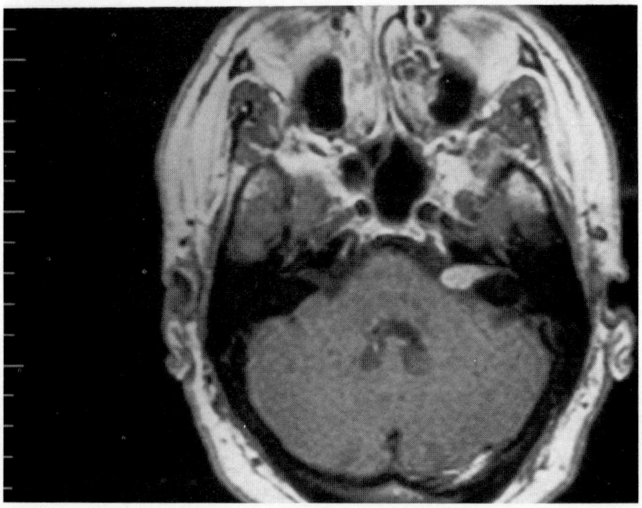

C

Figure 12-63

(A) *Axial long TR–long TE study. Right eighth nerve complex not seen. Left called normal (arrow).* **(B)** *Axial short TR–short TE left acoustic neuroma (arrow) shaped like ice cream cone.* **(C)** *Postgadolinium study demonstrates enhancement of tumor.*

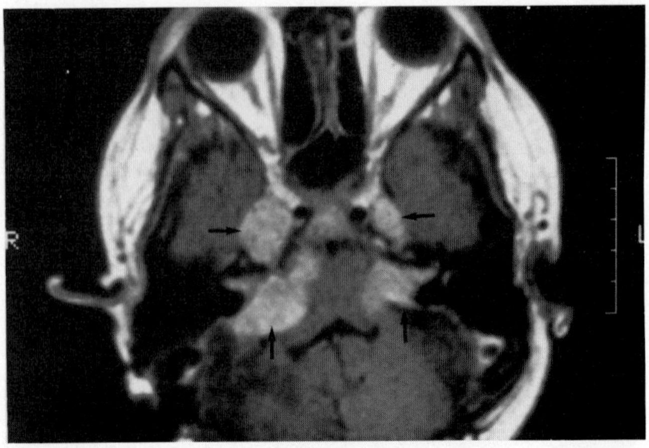

Figure 12-64
A 28-year-old female with neurofibromatosis type II demonstrating bilateral acoustic and trigeminal neuromas (T1 plus gadolinium) (arrows).

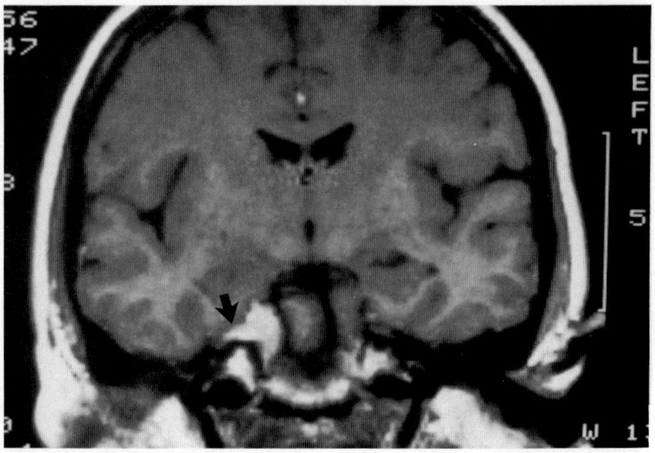

Figure 12-66
Short TR–short TE plus contrast demonstrating enhancing meningioma lateral to the pons originating from the tentorium. Arrow points to "dural tail."

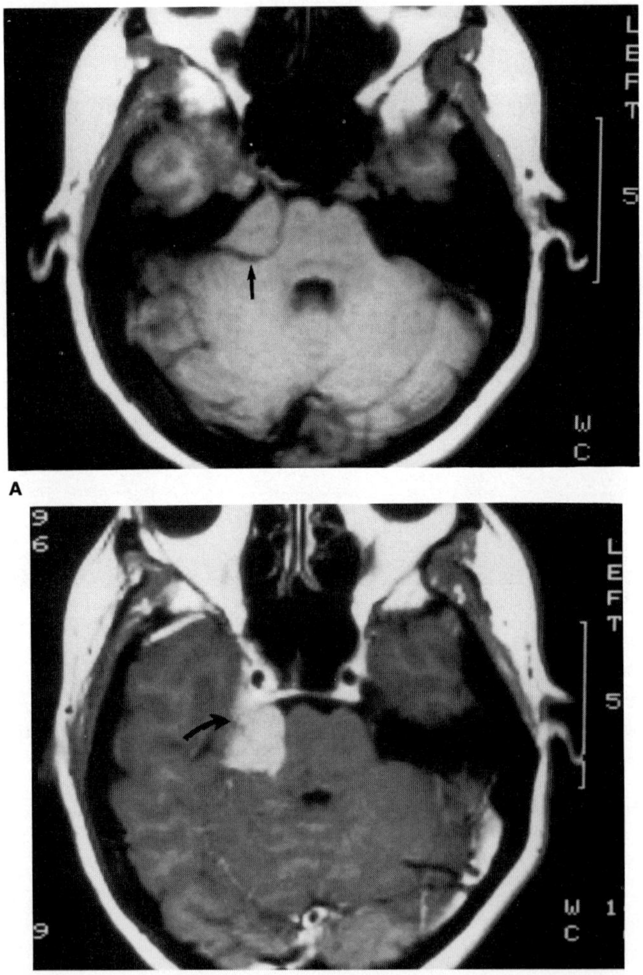

A

B

Figure 12-65
(A) *Short TR–short TE axial study demonstrating a meningioma in the left CPA with a flat base most likely originating from the tentorium (arrow).* **(B)** *Postcontrast study better demonstrating origin of tumor from the tentorium (arrow).*

The size of the neurovascular bundle is constant at 2 to 3 mm in diameter, and so the size of the subarachnoid space and the amount of CSF within the canal vary from almost nil to very conspicuous. The CPA cisterns may be asymmetrical and variable in size. Most acoustic neuromas arise within the IAC at the junction between two sheaths, the lateral myelinated sheath arising from the peripheral ganglia and the medial portion from neuroglial fibers extending from the brainstem. They arise at the glial-Schwann cell interface near the porus acousticus.

Press and Hesselink[111] reported 49 lesions of the CPA and IAC, of which 20 were acoustic neuromas. The ability to demonstrate the normal contents of the IAC by MRI facilitated the differentiation of acoustic neuromas from other lesions, especially meningiomas. Bilateral acoustic neuromas were seen in five patients, all with neurofibromatosis type 2 (Fig. 12-64). The T1 noncontrast study demonstrated 19 of 20 acoustic neuromas, while the proton-density and T2 sequences revealed 18 and 16, respectively. Long T2 sequences obscured the lesions because CSF and the tumor were equally bright. Erosion of the IAC was present in 15 tumors on noncontrast MRI. The smallest lesion seen on plain MRI was an intracanalicular lesion measuring 3 by 7 mm. The only lesion requiring contrast was the smallest, measuring 3 by 3 mm, located within the canal.

Noncontrast MRI findings of intracanalicular acoustic neuromas include erosion of the IAC, obscuration of margins of the seventh and eighth cranial nerves, and displacement of CSF from the canal. In all patients in whom the diagnosis of acoustic neuroma is suspected and the noncontrast study is normal, contrasted studies should be done to rule out a small lesion of the IAC (Fig. 12-61). The only exception to this is the elderly patient whose life expectancy is short and whose tumor will not grow enough to cause problems in such a time frame.

Other features of acoustic neuromas include cystic degeneration manifested on MR by hypointensity (Fig. 12-62B). There are two histologic types of tumors: Antoni A—small tumors that are densely packed—and Antoni B—larger tumors that are porous and less densely packed. Cystic degeneration is more likely in type B. Large tumors may compress and distort the brainstem and cerebellum. Rarely, calcification is present that is hypointense on MRI. At times the petrosal and capsular veins may form a hypointense ring around the tumor. The size of the mass will determine the amount of vascular displacement. The lesion is usually homogeneous, but heterogeneity of signal may be seen from volume averaging of normal CSF and the temporal bone surrounding the tumor.

Meningiomas of the CPA may be indistinguishable from acoustic neuromas. The ability to demonstrate normal contents of the IAC by MRI facilitates the differentiation of meningiomas from acoustic neuromas. Meningiomas are diagnosed by separation from the porus acousticus and cranial nerves VII and VIII. They may occur at the mouth of the IAC, the posterior aspect of the petrous ridge, the free edge of the tentorium, anterior to the foramen magnum, the superior aspect of the occipital bone, and within the jugular foramen. A widened IAC usually means an acoustic tumor, although occasionally a meningioma may do the same. Coronal views show the meningioma as a flat-based mass originating from the tentorium (Fig. 12-65). The shape of the acoustic lesion is more of an inverted ice cream cone (Fig. 12-63B). The meningioma spreads along the dura, causing the "tail" sign with contrast enhancement (Fig. 12-66). Rarely, even the acoustic tumor does the same.[112]

The signal of the meningioma is not predictable. At high field, most are hypointense on T1 and hyperintense on T2. On midfield magnets, only 10 percent show this pattern. They often are darker on T2 studies.[113] On T1 they are isointense and blend in with the brain. Small ones can be missed, and so contrast enhancement is absolutely necessary. The lack of eighth nerve enhancement in a CPA lesion should suggest a meningioma (Fig. 12-67B).

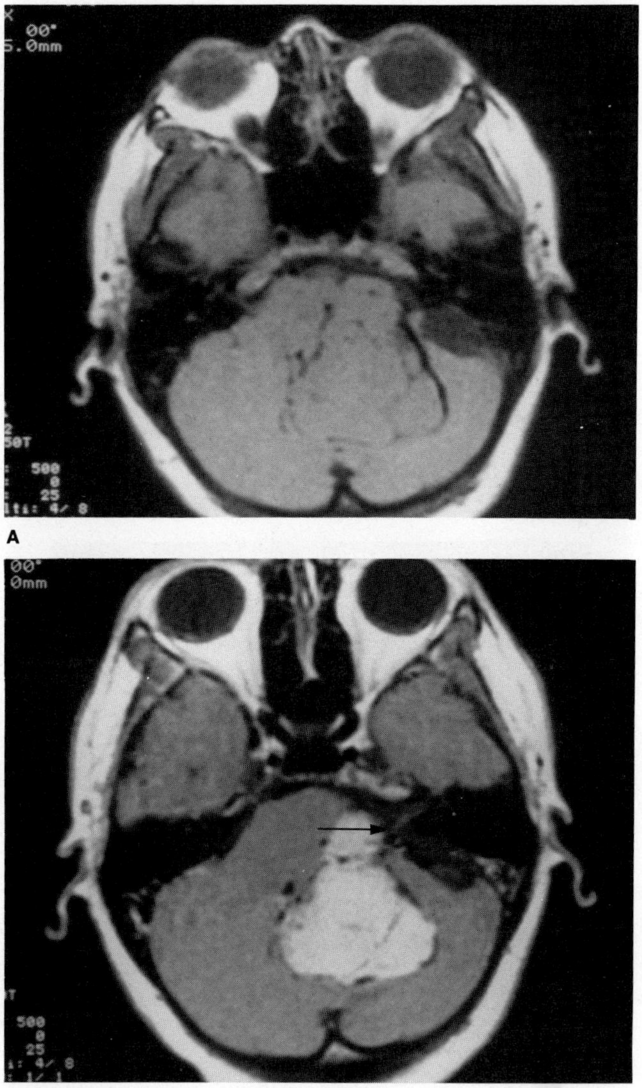
A
B

Figure 12-67
(A) *Short TR–short TE demonstrating large lesion isointense to brain outlined by a vascular capsule. Low signals within the tumor are either vessels or calcification.* **(B)** *After contrast, meningioma enhances but the eighth nerve complex (arrow) does not.*

Chen and associates[114] correlated MRI with the histopathology of meningiomas. They demonstrated that hyperintensity on the T2 study was correlated with microscopic increased vascularity, softness of the tumor, and more aggressive-type tumors. If a meningioma is bright on T2, it is more likely to be meningothelial, malignant, or angioblastic. If isointense, it is likely to be either fibroblastic-transitional or meningothelial. Malignant meningiomas often show marked edema, more so than do the other types. Contrast enhancement did not help the correlation of the histopathology, vascularity, or consistency of the tumor. A recent study[115] suggested that based on signal characteristics, a subgrouping of tumors as either fibroblastic-transitional or meningothelial-angioblastic was possible in 19 to 24 patients (80 percent). Utilizing other imaging features, such as mass effect, peritumoral edema, and intratumoral cyst formation, in conjunction with signal changes, permitted a correct histologic pattern in 96 percent (23 of 24). In the Chen and associates[114] study, there was no correlation between the degree of cerebral edema, mass effect, and histopathology of the tumor. The latter study[114] is twice as large as the former[115] and is statistically more valid.

Neurinoma or schwannoma of the trigeminal or gasserian ganglion may also be indistinguishable from an acoustic neuroma. Sevick[116] reported 5 trigeminal schwannomas, 2 of which had neurofibromatosis type 2. All

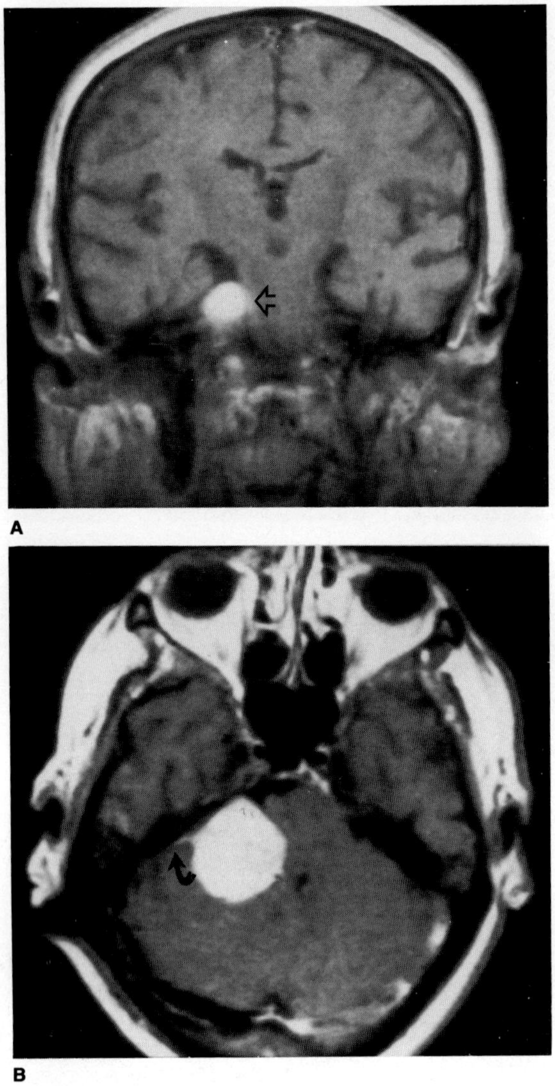

Figure 12-68
(A) *Short TR–short TE plus contrast demonstrates enhancing trigeminal neuroma (arrow) above nonenhancing eighth nerve complex.* **(B)** *Axial view of same patient demonstrating lesion growing toward Meckel's cave. Note the dural tail (arrow).*

enhanced with contrast (Fig. 12-68). In 17 patients with different types of tumors in this area (benign and malignant), Gd-DTPA improved lesion detection in 18 percent and conspicuity in 29 percent. Schwannomas were large, smooth-contoured, enhancing lesions at times with cyst formation. Smaller schwannomas occurred in patients with neurofibromatosis type 2 with its other multiple manifestations[117] (Fig. 12-64). They usually do not cause bone destruction but may expand Meckel's cave when the tumor is large. Facial neuromas may originate in the cisternal portion of the seventh nerve or more distally and are easily mistaken for an acoustic neuroma (Fig. 12-69). Schwannomas of other cranial nerves may be identified in the posterior fossa by MRI (Figs. 12-70 and 12-71).

A true cholesteatoma (epidermoid cyst) is a relatively rare tumor, 40 percent of which are found in the CPA. On CT these are well-defined lobulated masses with density similar to CSF because of high cholesterol and keratin. Twenty-five percent are calcified. Most do not enhance, although at times enhancement of tumor margin is present.[118,119] Occasionally they may be hyperdense on precontrast CT, possibly from (1) high protein, (2) bleeding, (3) excess leukocytes, (4) saponification of debris to calcium soaps, or (5) deposition of ferrocalcium or iron-containing pigments.[120]

With MRI they are hypointense on T1 but brighter than CSF and bright on protein density and T2 (Fig. 12-72). There is no enhancement with contrast. These characteristics depend on the relative composition of cholesterol and keratin within the cyst. The cholesterol is in a solid crystalline state and differs in signal from

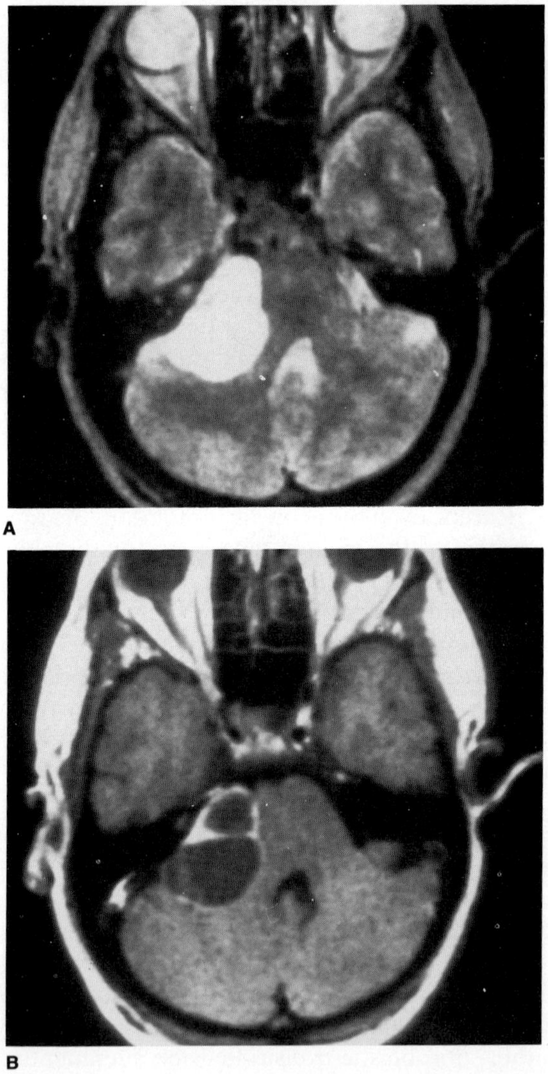

Figure 12-69
(A) *Long TR–long TE in a middle-aged woman with right facial weakness and numbness and normal hearing. Large high-intensity neuroma of seventh nerve is seen in the CPA.* **(B)** *Postcontrast demonstrates partially enhancing bilobed cystic neuroma of the seventh nerve.*

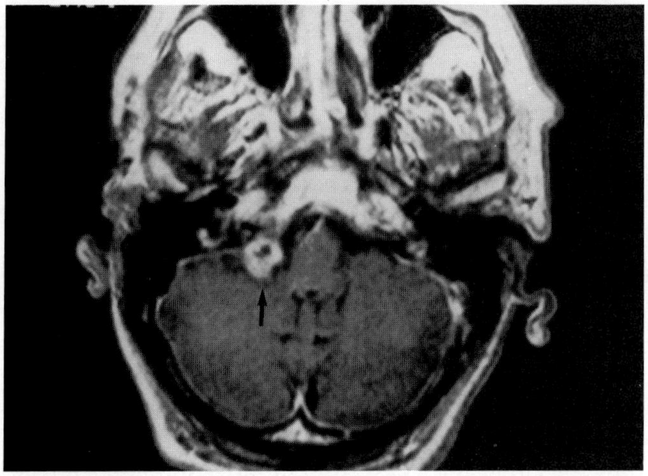

Figure 12-70
Short TR–short TE postcontrast demonstrating a schwannoma of the glossopharyngeal nerve lateral to the medulla (arrow).

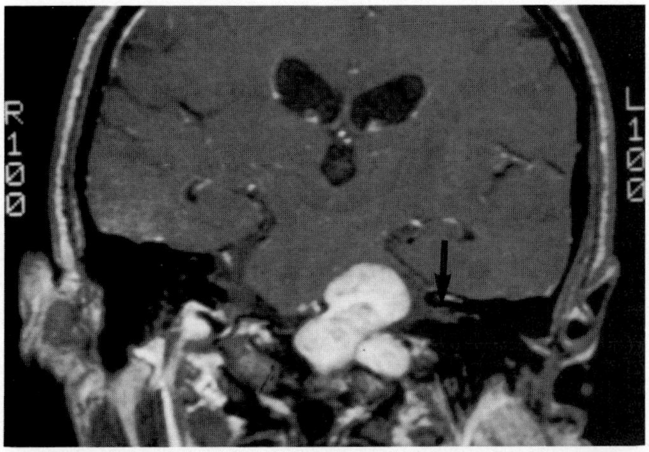

A

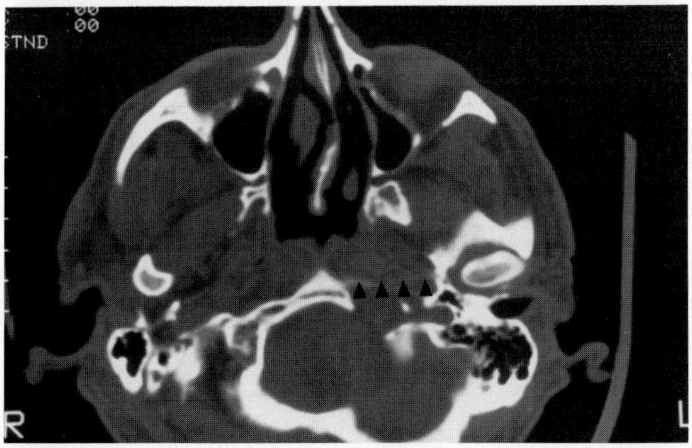

B

Figure 12-71
(A) *Short TR–short TE plus gadolinium demonstrating a large enhancing schwannoma of the hypoglossal nerve. Note that it is more inferior than other schwannomas presented (seventh, eighth, etc.). Also note sparing of seventh and eighth nerves complex on the left (arrow).* **(B)** *CAT scan demonstrating enlargement of hypoglossal canal on the left (arrowheads).*

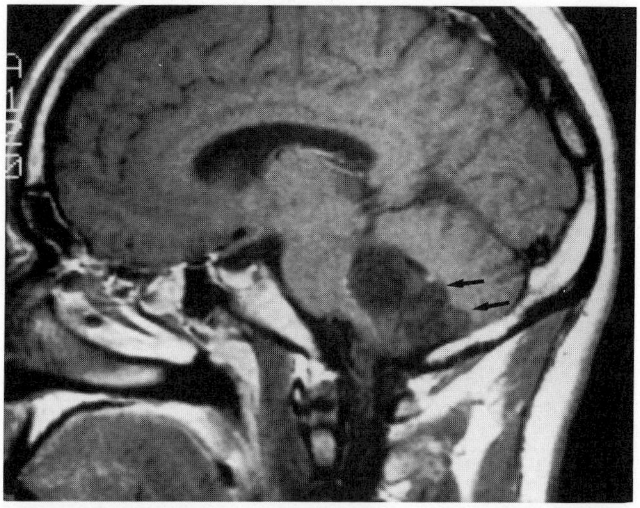

A

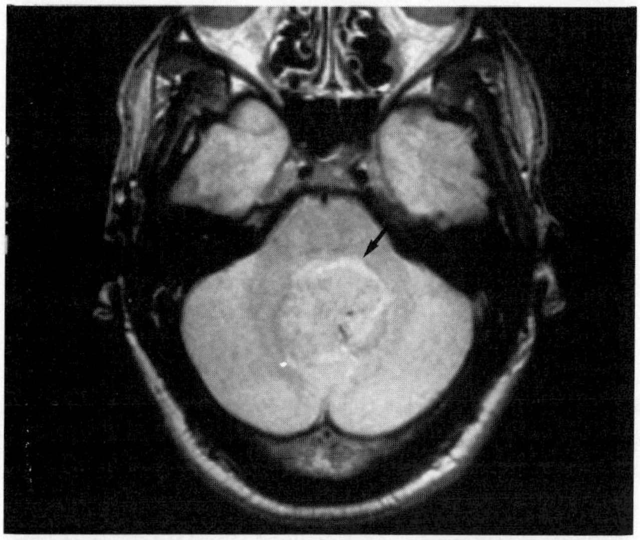

B

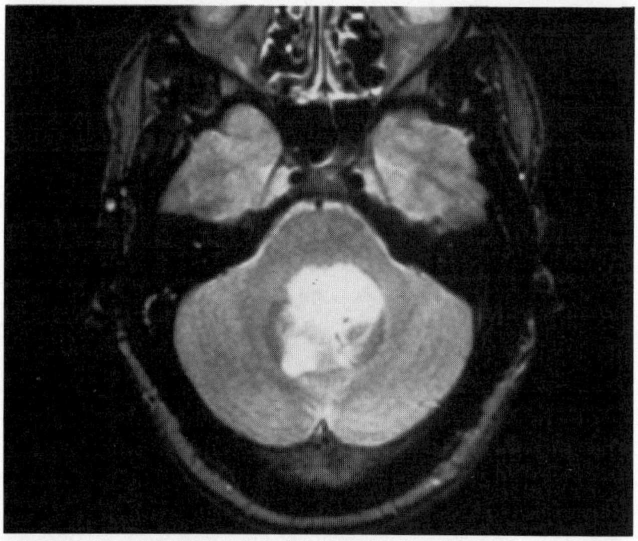

C

Figure 12-72
(A) *Short TR–short TE sagittal demonstrating a low-intensity epidermoid tumor in the fourth ventricle. See scalloped borders (arrow).* **(B)** *Long TR–short TE; see rim of high signal around the epidermoid (arrow). This possibly represents trapped CSF.* **(C)** *Long TR–long TE; the rim of CSF and tumor blend, and all is bright.*

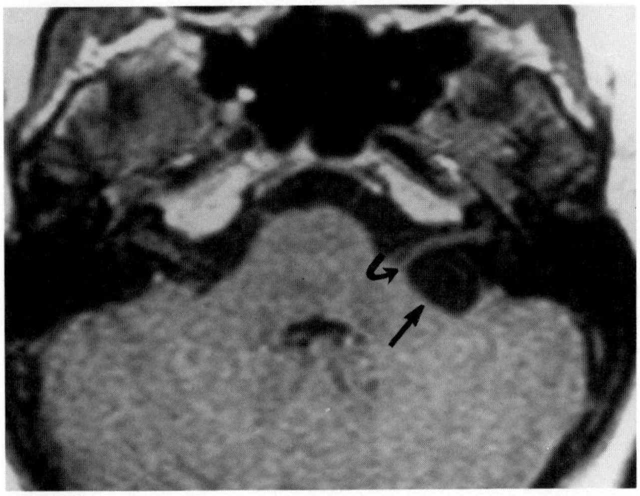

Figure 12-73
Short TR–short TE demonstrating an arachnoid cyst of the CPA (straight arrow). Note the eighth nerve as it curves around the cyst (curved arrow).

liquid cholesterol. (Craniopharyngiomas have liquid cholesterol and, like fat, are bright on T1.) On proton density there is a hyperintense rim representing CSF trapped around the extra-axial mass as it invaginates deeply into adjacent brain (Fig. 12-72B). There may be focal hypointensities due to calcium. Rarely they are so calcified that they are hypointense on T1 and T2. The tumors may be huge yet produce no edema. On MRI they may have a heterogeneous signal but on CT are homogeneous.[120] The heterogeneous signal is due to the mobile water protons of the complex proteinacious tumor and sometimes CSF-filled interstices with the tumor. MRI can differentiate CSF from tumor, but CT cannot. Subarachnoid cysts may pose a diagnostic problem in this area. The proton density is very helpful, because the cholesteatoma is bright on this sequence and the CSF in the subarachnoid cyst is isointense (Fig. 12-73). Fast gradient echo pulse sequences may demonstrate pulsatile fluid motion in subarachnoid cysts not seen in the more solid epidermoid.[121] The superior delineation of MRI provides better definition of the irregular margins than any other modality.

The cholesterol granuloma (giant cholesterol cyst) shares some morphologic similarities with epidermoids but is developmentally and histologically quite distinct.[122] Both contain keratin and cholesterol debris, but only the cholesterol cyst contains large amounts of iron-containing blood products (methemoglobin). Unlike cholesteatomas, these are bright on T1. They often occur in the petrous apex but can extend down into the CPA (Fig. 12-74).

Dermoids may present with cranial nerve signs and cerebellar dysfunction. Similar to epidermoids, their capsule is stratified squamous epithelium, but they also contain dermal elements and are firmer in texture. Dermoids remain along the midline. Calcification is more common and they are associated with dermal sinus tracts and skeletal anomalies. The MRI characteristics are more typical of fat. They are bright on T1 images and less so on T2 (Fig. 12-75).[123]

The MRI appearance of paragangliomas is quite characteristic, and they differ markedly from acoustic neuromas, meningiomas, and other lesions in this area. Hypervascularity is a prime feature of these lesions. Serpiginous areas of signal void representing high vascular flow are interspersed among areas of high signals

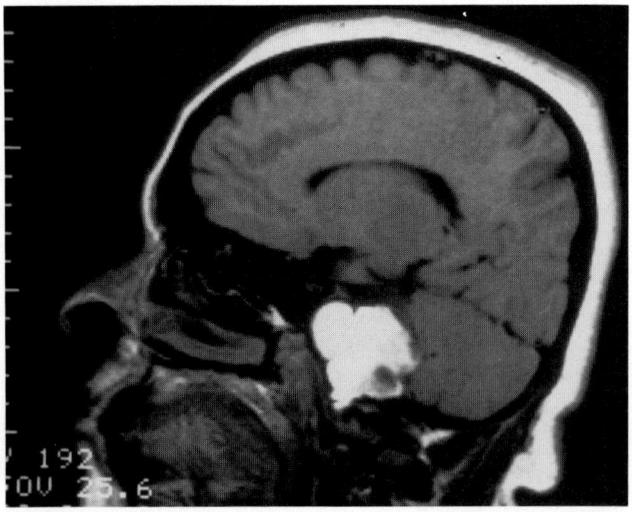

A

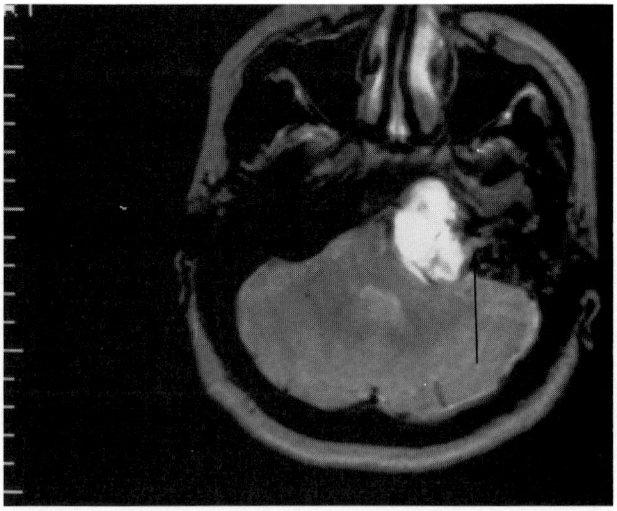

B

Figure 12-74
(A) *Short TR-short TE sagittal in a patient with vertigo, headaches, and hearing loss on the left. High-intensity lesion noted extending toward the foramen magnum.* **(B)** *Long TR–short TE axial with normal eighth nerve (arrow) on the left. This was a huge cholesterol granuloma originating in the petrous apex.*

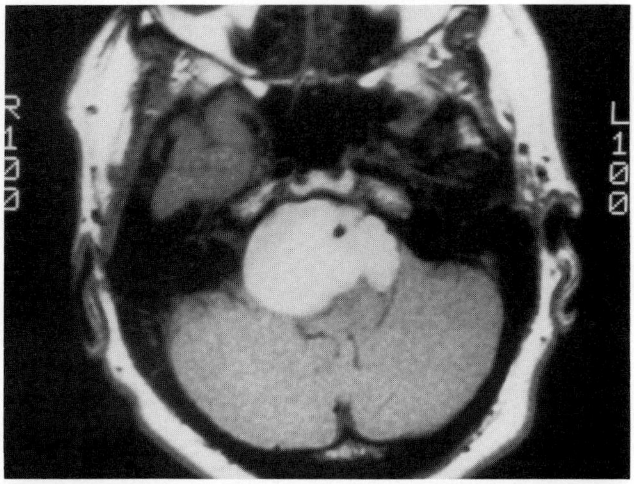
A

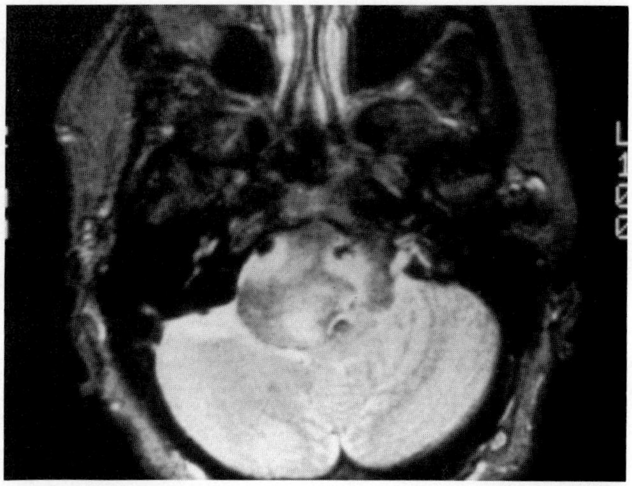
B

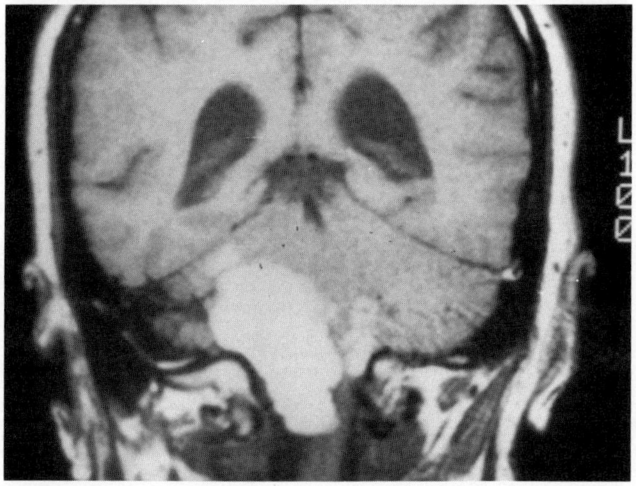
C

Figure 12-75
(A) *Short TR–short TE huge high signal lesion with low-intensity flow void or more likely calcification proved to be a dermoid.* **(B)** *Long TR–long TE lesion gets darker, proving that it is fat; more calcification and vessels seen on a lower slice than in* **A.** **(C)** *Short TR–short TE coronal demonstrating dermoid growing into foramen magnum.*

caused by tumor and slow-flowing blood. CT reveals bony changes of the skull and the relation of the middle ear better than does MRI. Angiography was necessary in the definitive diagnosis of these lesions previously, but now the location of the lesion at or extending into the jugular bulb, plus the vascularity and the "salt and pepper" appearance of MRI makes this an easy diagnosis for the experienced imager. Angiography will still be necessary to determine the vascular supply before surgical resection or for embolization. Coronal images localize these lesions easily and are best for evaluating intracranial extension (Fig. 12-76).[124,125]

Occasionally, brainstem tumors grow eccentrically and may present as a CPA syndrome. Gliomas usually originate in the pons and spread to the medulla and midbrain (Fig. 12-77). Posterior fossa beam hardening artifacts limit the success of CT in the diagnosis of these lesions. In a group of 18 patients with brainstem tumors Lee et al[126] found enlargement of the brainstem in all cases; exophytic growth was present in 8. Of 16 gliomas, MRI made a definite diagnosis of tumor in all, while CT was abnormal in 13. Decreased signal on T1 was

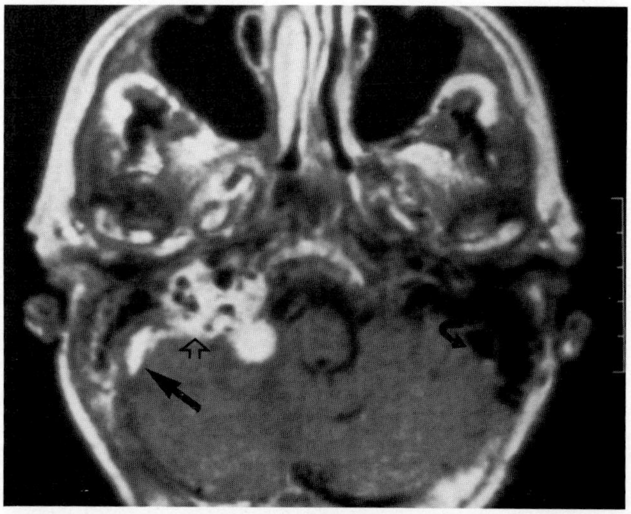

Figure 12-76
Short TR–short TE plus contrast demonstrates a paraganglioma in the region of the right jugular bulb (open arrow). Note multiple flow voids. See the normal sigmoid sinus flow void (curved arrow) on the left and probable thrombosis and/or tumor on the right (straight arrow).

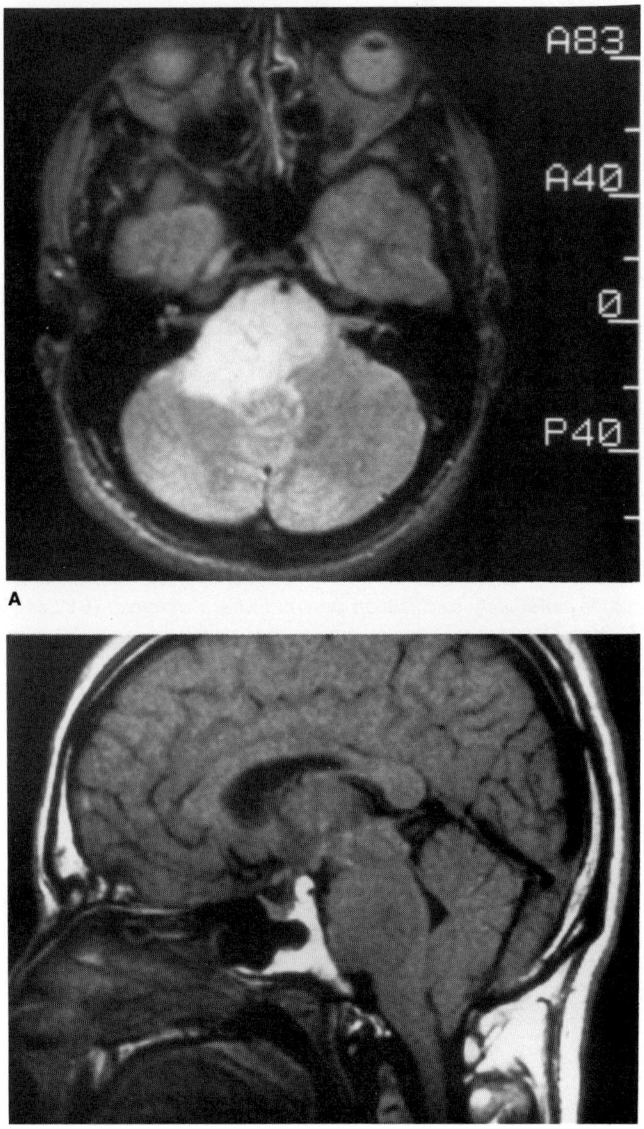

A

B

Figure 12-77
(A) *Long TR–long TE demonstrating a large high signal lesion in the brainstem. Note the eighth nerve complexes bilaterally are not involved.* **(B)** *Short TR–short TE demonstrates "fat" pons. Gadolinium is not necessary in this typical brainstem glioma.*

seen in six, and increased signal was present on the more T2-weighted studies in seven. Contrast enhancement was present in only two cases utilizing CT while contrast was not necessary for MRI. Two cases that enhanced were abnormal before enhancement. Rarely brainstem gliomas may be diffusely infiltrating, minimally destructive, nonexpanding, without gross hemorrhage, necrosis, or exophytic growth. These may appear with only subtle changes on MRI even with contrast enhancement. This is akin to gliomatosis cerebri.[127] Metastases to the brainstem may produce signal changes similar to primary tumors.

Vascular lesions usually have low signal intensities because of signal void caused by high flow velocity. At times high signal is due to flow-related enhancement.[128] These lesions include arteriovenous malformations (Fig. 12-78), vertebral basilar dolichoectasia, and aneurysms in the CPA (Fig. 12-79). Methemoglobin in a partially clotted aneurysm is at times responsible for high signal. Gentry and colleagues[129] reviewed 75 patients with CPA-petromastoid mass lesions. They suggest that the location, shape, contour, and internal architecture of the lesions were often of more value than signal characteristics. They found that CT demonstrated 95.8 percent and MRI 98.7 percent of the lesions. They used contrast in CT but not MRI. Its use in the latter would likely skew

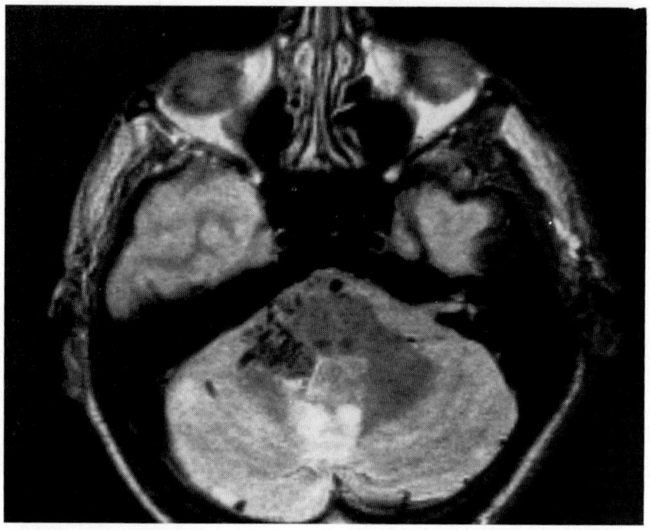

Figure 12-78
Long TR–long TE demonstrating multiple flow voids on the right. This was a proven arterial venous malformation that had bled 20 years previous to this study.

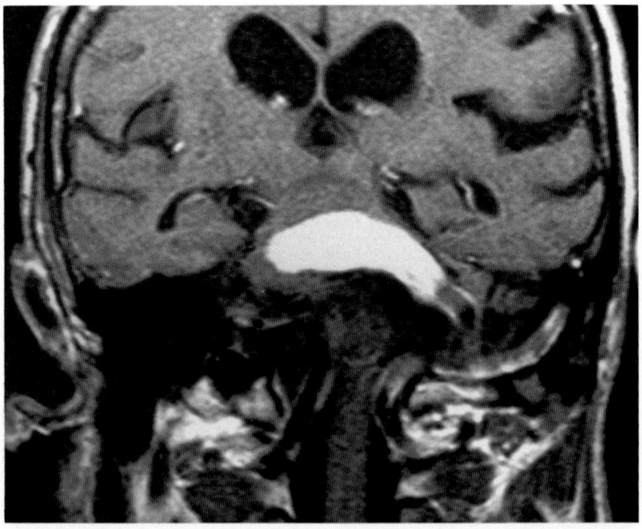

Figure 12-79
Short TR–short TE with contrast demonstrated dolichoectasia of both vertebral arteries leading into a fusiform aneurysm of the basilar artery. (With permission, Dr. T. Bloomberg.)

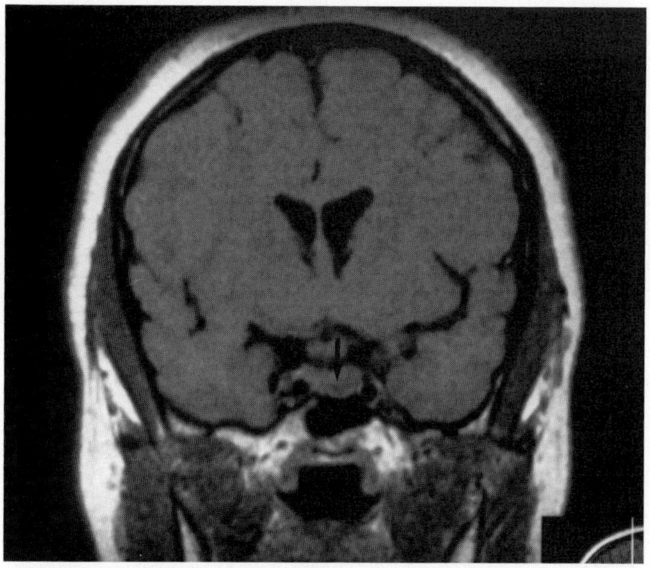

Figure 12-80
Short TR–short TE 3-mm coronal demonstrating low-signal microadenoma on the left (arrow) depression of the left sphenoid sinus and shift of the infundibulum to the right in a young female with amenorrhea, galactorrhea, and elevated prolactin.

the results even more favorably toward MRI except for the lesions involving bone.

Pituitary Adenomas

High-contrast, high-spatial-resolution MRI scanning with thin sections has become the procedure of choice in modern pituitary imaging. Three-millimeter T1 sagittal and coronal sections with a small field of view (16 to 20 mm) and four to six acquisitions all make the signal-to-noise ratio excellent enough to diagnose most lesions in this area (Figs. 12-80 and 12-81).

The normal pituitary gland has a variable size. The average height is 7 mm in females and 5 mm in males. The gland is adult size at puberty. The infundibular stalk should be present on all thin-section studies. The anterior and posterior lobes are seen but not the pars intermedia. The anterior lobe is homogeneous and has the same signal as normal white matter on T1 and T2 studies. The posterior lobe is bright on T1. This is thought to be due to the presence of antidiuretic hormone–neurophysin protein complex in the terminal axons of the neurohypophysis. Stress and dehydration may affect the size and signal intensity of the posterior lobe. The latter may also disappear in diabetes insipidus or traumatic stalk transection. In the latter the bright spot may be seen in the proximal end of the transected stalk.[130]

Pituitary adenomas are benign neoplasms of the adenohypophysis. They are micro (10 mm or less) or macro (>10 mm), functioning or nonfunctioning. The functioning lesions are usually microadenomas. They may secrete prolactin, growth hormone, or ACTH. MRI cannot discern among the latter three types. Macroadenomas are usually nonfunctioning and cause clinical symptoms by compression of structures such as the optic chiasm, cavernous sinus, or cranial nerves III to VI.

The imaging features of microadenomas are (1) focal hypointensity on T1 with iso- or hyperintensity on T2, (2) possible contour abnormality, especially a focal upward bulge that may or may not be associated with (3) stalk displacement (Fig. 12-80). Macroadenomas are usually iosintense on T1, but inhomogeneity is common

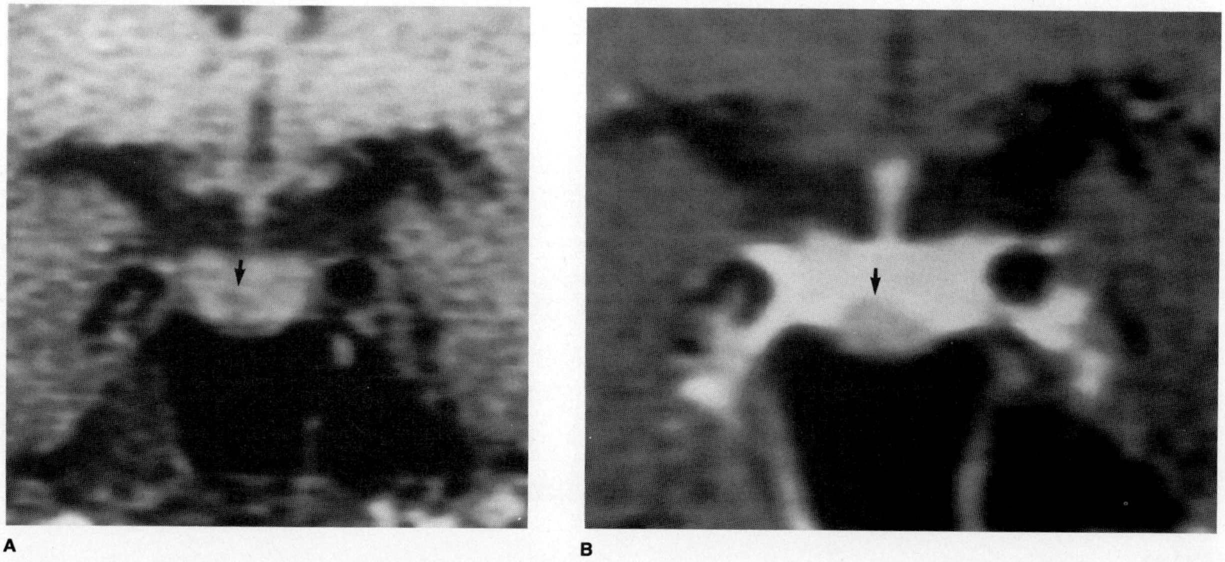

Figure 12-81
(A) *Short TR–short TE 3-mm noncontrast coronal demonstrating low-intensity microadenoma inferiorly and to the right (arrow).* **(B)** *After contrast the hypointense lesion is seen well (arrow); the normal pituitary enhances homogeneously. Floor of sella is depressed.*

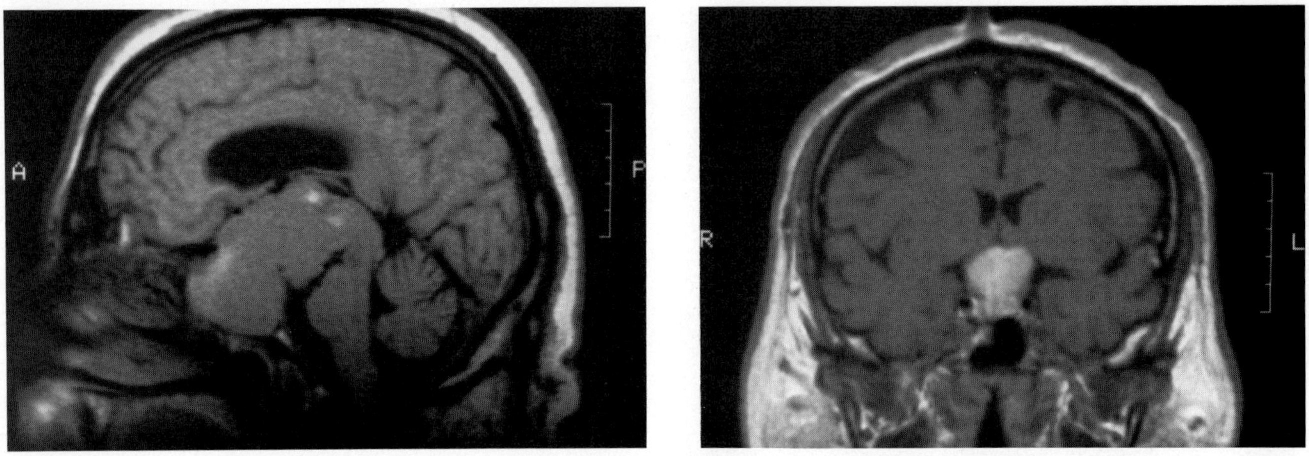

A B

Figure 12-82

(A) *Short TR–short TE noncontrast sagittal demonstrating a huge macroadenoma growing into the third ventricle, displacing midbrain posteriorly. High signals represent previous hemorrhage (methemoglobin).* **(B)** *Short TR-short TE plus contrast demonstrating another large macroadenoma that enhances homogeneously. Carotids appear not to be involved in the tumor. The chiasm is buried in the tumor.*

owing to necrosis, hemorrhage, or cyst formation (Fig. 12-82). MRI addresses important questions such as the determination of suprasellar extension and compression of the optic pathways, intrasellar extension into the sphenoid sinus, or lateral growth into the cavernous sinus. The sensitivity of MRI in differentiating between cavernous sinus invasion and compression is only 55 percent because of the inability to visualize the thin dura of the medial wall of the cavernous sinus.[130]

Dynamic scanning[131] with gadolinium caused the enhancement of the pituitary gland in 80 s and microadenomas in 60 to 200 s. Rapid scanning after bolus injection will allow for the visualization of a hypointense microadenoma with the bright gland for contrast. To differentiate a microadenoma from a cyst (Rathke's pouch), delayed scanning will enhance the tumor but not the cyst. Stadnik and associates[132] reviewed 27 microadenomas. Of 8 patients with false-negative MRIs on unenhanced studies, 3 were diagnosed with the use of contrast. Treatment with parlodal may lead to a false-negative MRI.[132] Macroadenomas usually enhance moderately with contrast. Hemorrhage is readily seen as a

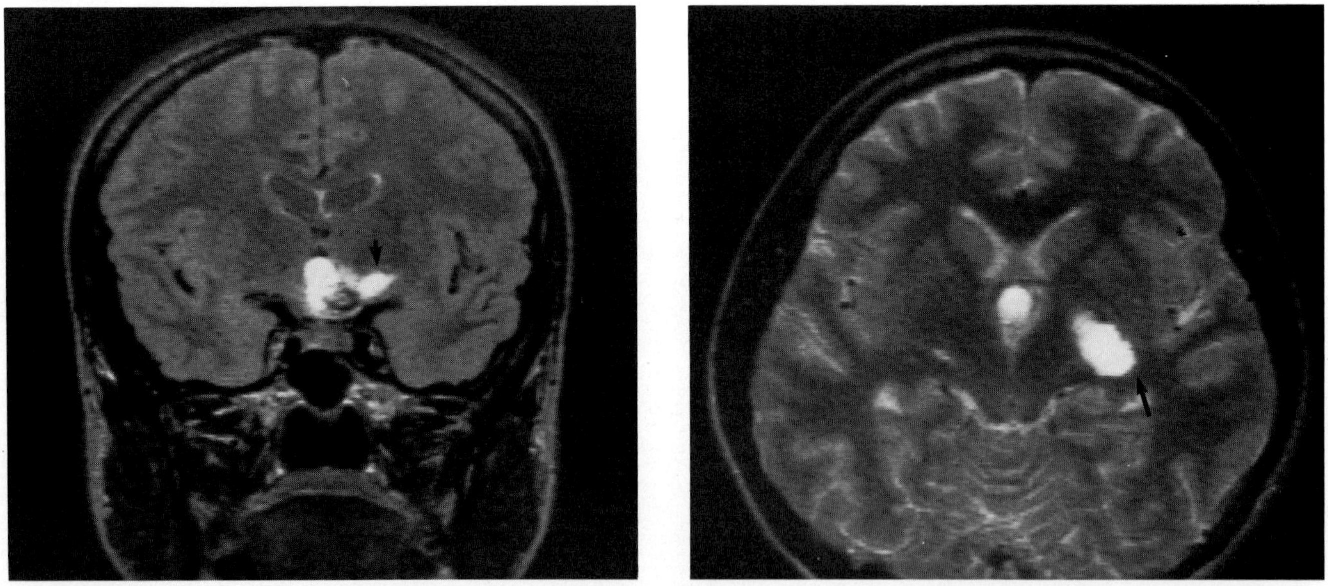

A B

Figure 12-83

(A) *Long TR–short TE coronal study demonstrating an optic glioma affecting the chiasm and growing to the left along the optic tract (arrow). Low-signal flow void representing a vessel is present.* **(B)** *Long TR–long TE axial in the same patient demonstrating optic glioma growing toward the lateral geniculate body (arrow).*

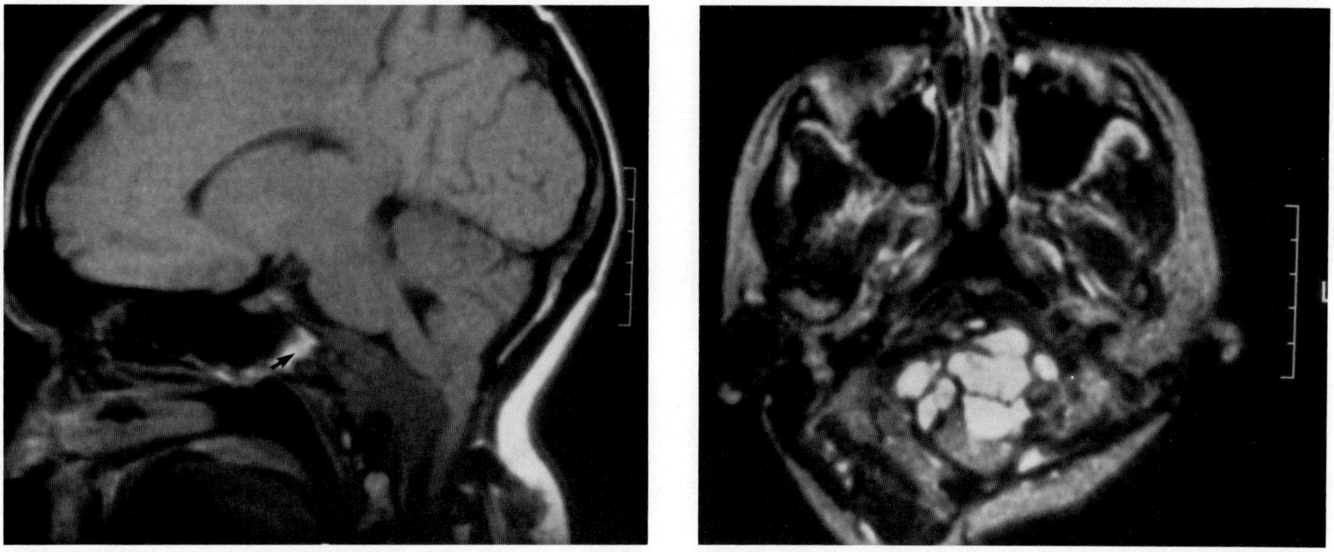

A B

Figure 12-84
(A) *Short TR–short TE noncontrast sagittal demonstrating a hypointense chordoma compressing and displacing the brainstem and destroying most of the clivus. High signal (arrow) is all that is left of the clivus. The lesion grows into the cervical canal.* **(B)** *Long TR–long TE axial demonstrating septations separating bright signal lobules in a chordoma.*

bright signal on T1. This is more common in prolactin-secreting lesions treated with bromocriptine. These may be silent but may occur with third nerve palsies, headache, and chiasmatic compression.

The differential diagnosis of macroadenomas includes meningiomas. The latter have a lower signal on T2 and more often surround carotid arteries. Craniopharyngiomas are separated by their anatomic location and have different signal characteristics already mentioned in this chapter. Optic gliomas occur in younger individuals and often infiltrate along the optic chiasm into the optic nerves. Aneurysms in the sella are easily diagnosed by their flow characteristics.

Optic nerve glioma is a low-grade astrocytoma that is often associated with neurofibromatosis (12 to 38 percent of cases). This is especially true in bilateral optic

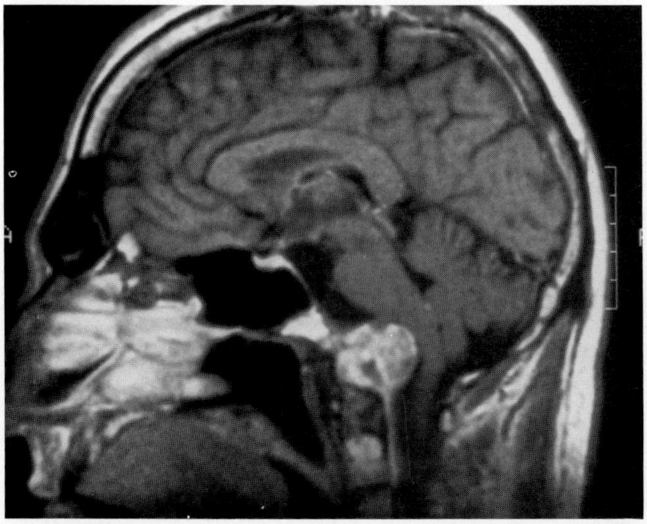

Figure 12-85
Short TR–short TE enhanced sagittal demonstrating another chordoma. Note "lollipop" configuration with round tumor indenting the medulla and "stick" extending down the cervical canal.

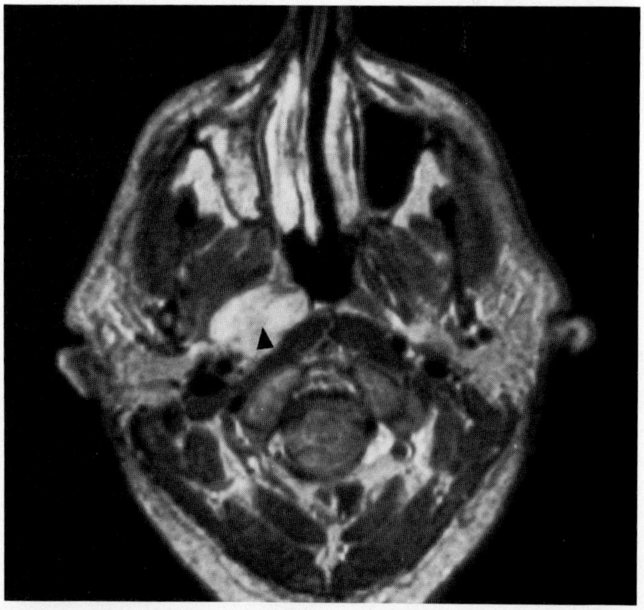

Figure 12-86
Long TR–short TE noncontrast axial demonstrating nasopharyngeal carcinoma in the right parapharyngeal space (arrowhead). There is distortion of the posterolateral aspect of the right nasopharyngeal wall.

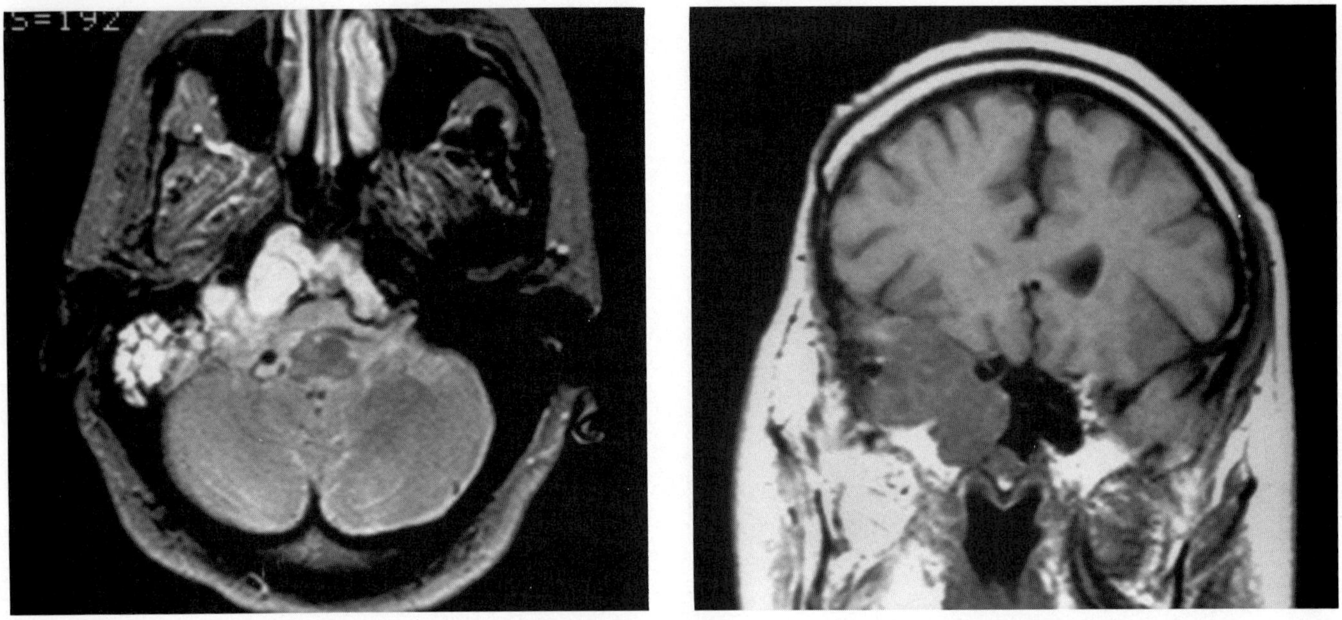

A B

Figure 12-87
(A) *Long TR–long TE noncontrast axial demonstrating a chondrosarcoma. It has the lobulated appearance of a chordoma. Chordomas, however, are usually closer to midline. High signals in the right mastoid could be tumor or inflammatory process from obstruction.* **(B)** *Short TR–short TE noncontrast coronal demonstrates large chondrosarcoma off the midline growing superiorly and displacing the right frontal lobe.*

gliomas.[12] MRI shows the optic nerve from its attachment to the globe through the optic canal and into the chiasm. At times a special orbital coil is helpful in demonstrating optic gliomas with exquisite detail. The glioma is isointense to normal white matter on short TR/TE and long TR/TE studies. This is true all the way along the tumor until the chiasm and beyond (optic tracts and lateral geniculates), when the tumor becomes bright on the T2 images. The low intensity on T2 in the prechiasmatic portion is thought to be due to fibrocollagenous reactive change (Fig. 12-83).[7]

The typical chordoma is a soft, jelly-like tumor that consists of cords of physaliphorous cells with a watery, gelatinous matrix. This type of consistency leads to an MRI signal of hypo- or isointensity on T1 and hyperintensity on T2. Septations of low signal separate lobulated areas of higher signal (Fig. 12-84). Chondroid chordomas have foci of cartilage-like tissue and are less intense on T2 than typical chordomas.

Sze et al[133] reported 20 chordomas—12 predominantly clival, 5 sellar or parasellar, and 3 vertebral. Fifteen of 20 were isointense on T1 and 5 were hypointense, while all were bright on T2. MRI and CT were equivalent in demonstrating the presence and site of the tumor. The boundaries of the tumor and its relationship to the vessels were better seen on MRI. A thin line of neoplastic tissue may extend down the anterior epidural space into the cervical spine with the appearance of a "lollipop" (Fig. 12-85). CT is better for demonstrating bone destruction and calcification. MRI is better to delineate the exact length of the lesion, the posterior margin of the tumor, and the nasopharyngeal extension.

Nasopharyngeal carcinoma is one of several tumors of the nasal cavity including squamous cell carcinoma, adenocarcinoma, and rare lesions such as melanoma and plasmocytoma. Signal characteristics alone will not differentiate these lesions. MRI will, however, demonstrate where the tumor arises in the nasal cavity or

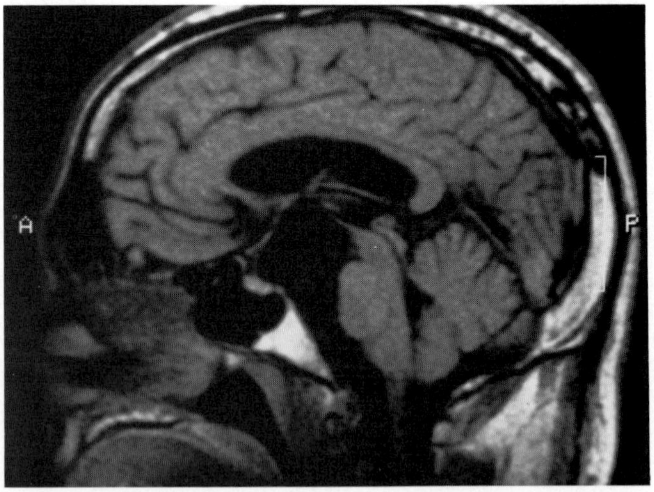

Figure 12-88
Short TR–short TE noncontrast sagittal demonstrating an arachnoid cyst in prepontine and suprasellar cisterns displacing the brainstem. It has the signal characteristics of CSF.

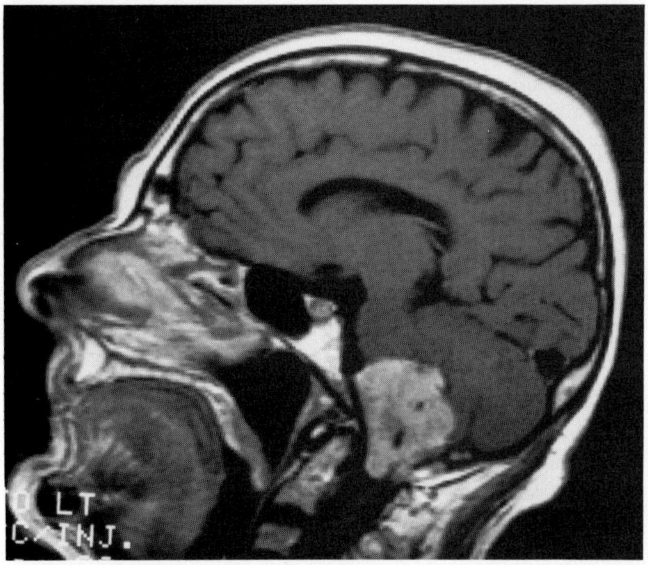

Figure 12-89
Short TR–short TE plus contrast demonstrating a large enhancing meningioma of the foramen magnum.

sinuses and extension, if any, through the skull base into the anterior or middle fossa (Fig. 12-86).

Other tumors of the base of the skull include osteomas, chondromas, lipomas, metastases, and chondrosarcomas. Chondrosarcomas look like chordomas, are more lateral, and often involve petroclival suture (Fig. 12-87).[7] Suprasellar arachnoid cysts also occur in this region (Fig. 12-88). They track CSF on all sequences, have no identifiable cyst wall on MRI, and do not enhance with gadolinium.

Tumors of the foramen magnum are readily visualized with MRI. Usually the first sequence on brain studies is a 5-mm T1 sagittal. The lesion will be seen immediately if it is large enough. The differential diagnosis includes multiple sclerosis, Chiari I malformation, syringomyelia, and bony abnormalities of the craniocervical junction. Tumors include neurofibromas, meningiomas, teratomas, dermoids, granulomas, cavernous hemangiomas, hemangioblastomas, lipomas, and epidural carcinomas (Fig. 12-89).[2]

REFERENCES

1. Walker AE, Robins M, Weinfield FD: Epidemiology of brain tumors: The national survey of intracranial neoplasms. *Neurology* 35:219–226, 1985.
2. Adams RD, Victor M: *Principles of Neurology,* 6th ed. New York, McGraw-Hill, 1997.
3. Sigel RM, Messina AV: Computer tomography: The anatomical basis of the zone of diminished density surrounding meningiomas. *J Neurosurg* 71:665–672, 1989.
4. George AE, Russell EJ, Kritcheff II: White matter buckling: CT signs of extra-axial intracranial mass. *AJN* 1:425–430, 1980.
5. Just M, Thelen M: Tissue characterization with T1, T2, and proton density values: Results in 1960 patients with brain tumors. *Radiology* 169:779–785, 1988.
6. Bydder GM, Kingsley PE, Brown W, et al: Clinical MR imaging of the brain. *AJR* 139:215–236, 1992.
7. Atlas SW: Intra-axial brain tumors, in Atlas SW, (ed): *Magnetic Resonance Imaging of the Brain and Spine.* New York, Raven Press, 1991, chap 10.
8. Boyko OB, Burger PC, Shelborne JD, et al: Non heme mechanism for T1 shortening: Pathologic, CT and MR elucidation. *AJNR* 13:1439–1444, 1992.
9. Klatzko I: Neuropathological aspects of brain edema. *J Neuropathol Exp Neurol* 26:1–14, 1967.
10. Fishman RA: Brain edema. *N Engl J Med* 273:706–711, 1975.
11. Rubinstein LJ: *Tumors of the Central Nervous System: Atlas of Tumor Pathology,* Washington DC, Armed Forces Institute of Pathology 1972.
12. Russell DS, Rubinstein LJ: *Pathology of Tumors of the Nervous System,* 5th ed. Baltimore, Williams & Wilkins, 1989.
13. Burger CP, Scheithauer BW, Vogel FS: *Surgical Pathology of the Nervous System and Its Coverings,* 3d ed. New York, Churchill Livingstone, 1991.
14. Okazaki H, Scheithauer BW: *Atlas of Neuropathology.* New York, Gower, 1988.
15. Zimmerman RA: Pediatric brain tumors, in Lee SH, Rao KCVZ, Zimmerman RA (eds): *Cranial MRI and CT,* 3d ed. New York, McGraw-Hill, 1992, chap 9.
16. Naidich TP, Zimmerman RA: Primary brain tumors in children. *Semin Roentgenol* 19:100–114, 1984.
17. Tchang S, Scotti G, Perbruge K, et al: Computerized tomography as a possible aid to histologic grading of supratentorial gliomas. *J Neurosurg* 45:735–739, 1997.
18. Tans JT, Jongh IE: Computed tomography of supratentorial astrocytoma. *Clin Neurol Neurosurg* 80:156–168, 1978.
19. Price AC, Runge VM, Allen JH, et al: Primary glioma: Diagnosis with magnetic resonance imaging. *CT* 10:325–334, 1986.
20. Dean BL, Drayer BP, Bird CR: Gliomas: Classification with MR imaging. *Radiology* 174:411–415, 1990.
21. Smirniotopoulos JG, Lee SH: Primary brain tumors in adults, in Lee SH, Rao KCVG, Zimmerman RA (eds): *Cranial MRI and CT,* 3d ed. New York, McGraw-Hill, 1992, chap 8.
22. Lee YY, Tassel PV, Bruner JM, et al: Juvenile pilocytic astrocytoma: CT and MR characteristics. *AJNR* 10:363–370, 1989.
23. Shapiro WR: Malignant neural tumors, in Johnson RT, Griffin JW (eds): *Current Therapy in Neurologic Disease,* 4th ed. St. Louis, Mosby Yearbook, 1993, pp 220–223.
24. Steinhoff H, Lanksch W, Kazner E, et al: Computed tomography in the diagnosis and differential diagnosis of glioblastomas. *Neuroradiology* 14:193–200, 1977.
25. Zimmerman RA: Imaging of adult central nervous system primary malignant gliomas: Staging and followup. *Cancer* 67:1278–1283, 1991.
26. Earnest F, Kelly PS, Scheithauer BW, et al: Cerebral astrocytomas: Histopathologic correlation of MR and CT contrast enhancement with stereotactic biopsy. *Radiology* 166:823–827, 1988.

27. Johnson PC, Hunt SJ, Drayer BP: Human cerebral gliomas: Correlation of post-mortem MR imaging and neuropathologic findings. *Radiology* 170:211–217, 1989.
28. Nevin S: Gliomatosis cerebri. *Brain* 61:170–191, 1938.
29. Couch JR, Wise SA: Gliomatosis cerebri. *Neurology* 24:504–511, 1974.
30. Geremia GK, Wellman R, Foust R: Computed tomography of gliomatosis cerebri. *J Comput Assist Tomogr* 12:698–701, 1988.
31. Spagnoli MV, Grossman RI, Packer RJ, et al: Magnetic resonance imaging determination of gliomatosis cerebri. *Neuroradiology* 29:15–18, 1987.
32. Vonofokos D, Marcu H, Hack H: Oligodendrogliomas: CT patterns with emphasis on features indicating malignancy. *J Comput Assist Tomogr* 3:733–788, 1979.
33. Lee YY, Tassell PV: Intracranial oligodendrogliomas: Imaging findings in 35 untreated cases. *AJNR* 10:119–127, 1989.
34. Daumas-Duport C, Scheithauer BW, Chodkiewicz JP, et al: Dysembryoplastic neuroepithelial tumor: A surgically curable tumor of young patients with intractable partial seizures: Report of thirty-nine cases. *Neurosurgery* 23(5):545–556, 1988.
35. Nelson JS, Parisi JE, Schochet SS Jr: *Principles and Practice of Neuropathology*. St. Louis, Mosby, 1993.
36. Koeller KK, Dillon WP: Dysembryoplastic neuroepithelial tumors: MR appearance. *Am J Neuroradiol* 13(5):1319–1325, 1992.
37. Kuroiwa T, Bergey GK, Rothman MI, et al: Radiologic appearance of the dysembryoplastic neuroepithelial tumor. *Radiology* 197(1):233–238, 1995.
38. Wichmann W, Schubiger O, von Deimling A, et al: Neuroradiology of central neurocytoma. *Neuroradiology* 33(2):143–148, 1991.
39. Sgouros S, Carey M, Aluwihare N, et al: Central neurocytoma: A correlative clinicopathologic and radiologic analysis. *Surg Neurol* 49(2):197–204, 1998.
40. Giangaspero F, Cenacchi G, Losi L, et al: Extraventricular neoplasms with neurocytoma features: A clinicopathological study of 11 cases. *Am J Surg Pathol* 21(2):206–212, 1997.
41. Chang KH, Han MH, Kim DG, et al: MR appearance of central neurocytoma. *Acta Radiol* 34(5):520–526, 1993.
42. Armington WG, Osborn AG, Cubberly D, et al: Supratentorial ependymoma: CT appearance. *Radiology* 157:367–372, 1985.
43. Spoto GP, Press GA, Hesselink JR, et al: Intracranial ependymoma and subependymoma: MR manifestations. *AJNR* 11:83–91, 1990.
44. Dorne HL, O'Gorman AM, Melanson D: Computed tomography of intracranial gangliogliomas. *AJNR* 7:281–285, 1986.
45. Castillo M, Davis PC, Takei Y, et al: Intracranial ganglioglioma: MR, CT, and clinical findings in 18 patients. *AJNR* 11:109–114, 1990.
46. Kepes JJ: *Meningiomas: Biology, Pathology, and Differential Diagnosis.* New York, Masson, 1982.
47. Cushing H, Eisenhardt L: *Meningiomas: Their Classification, Regional Behavior, Life History, and Surgical End Results,* Springfield, IL, Charles C. Thomas, 1938.
48. Naidich TP: Imaging evaluation of meningiomas, in Categorical course: *Neoplasms of the Central Nervous System.* Chicago, American Society of Neuroradiology, 1990.
49. Vassilouthis J, Ambrose J: Computerized tomography scanning appearances of intracranial meningiomas: An attempt to predict the histological features. *J Neurosurg* 50:320–327, 1979.
50. Rohringer M, Sutherland GR, Louw DF, et al: Incidence and clinical pathological features of meningiomas. *J Neurosurg* 71:665–672, 1989.
51. Zee CS, Chin T, Segall HD, et al: Magnetic resonance imaging of meningiomas. *Semin Ultrasound CT MRI* 13:154–169, 1992.
52. Zimmerman RD, Fleming CA, St. Louis LA, et al: Magnetic resonance imaging of meningiomas. *AJNR* 6:149–157, 1985.
53. Spagnoli MV, Goldberg H, Grossman RI, et al: Intracranial meningiomas: High field MR imaging. *Radiology* 161:369–375, 1986.
54. Goldsher D, Litt AW, Pinto RS, et al: Dural tail associated with meningiomas on gadolinium-DTPA enhanced images. *Radiology* 176:447–450, 1990.
55. Tien RD, Yang PJ, Chu PK: "Dural tail sign": A specific MR sign for meningioma? *J Comput Assist Tomogr* 15:64–66, 1991.
56. Elster AD, Challa VR, Gilbert TH, et al: Meningiomas: MR and histopathologic features. *Radiology* 170:857–862, 1989.
57. Black PM: Brain tumors. *N Engl J Med* 324:1555–1564, 1991.
58. Holtas S, Nyman U, Cronquist S: CT of malignant lymphoma of the brain. *Neuroradiology* 26:33–38, 1984.
59. Jack CR, Reese DF, Scheithauer BW: Radiographic findings in 32 cases of primary CNS lymphomas. *AJNR* 11:567–574, 1985.
60. Schwaighofer BW, Hesselink JR, Press GA, et al: Primary intracranial CNS lymphoma: MR manifestations. *AJN* 10:725–729, 1989.
61. Rovira MJ, Donovan PMJ, Bowen BC: Central nervous system infection in HIV-positive persons. *Neuroimaging Clin North Am* 1:179–200, 1992.
62. Posner JB: Neurologic complications of systemic cancer. *Med Clin North Am* 63:783–800, 1979.
63. Johnson CE, Sze G: Intracranial metastatic disease, in Lee SH, Rao KCVG, Zimmerman RA (eds): Cranial MRI and CT, 3d ed. New York, McGraw-Hill, 1992, pp 417–439.
64. Vanucci RC, Bathen M: Central metastatic disease in childhood. *Neurology* 24:981–985, 1976.
65. Grossman SA, Timothy JM: Neoplastic meningitis. *Neurol Clin* 9:843–956, 1991.
66. Patchell RA, Tibbs PA, Walsh JW, et al: A randomized trial of surgery in the treatment of single metastasis to the brain. *N Engl J Med* 322:494–500, 1990.
67. Byrne T, Waxman SG: *Spinal Cord Compression,* 1st ed. Philadelphia, Davis, 1990.
68. Delattre JY, Krol G, Thaler HT, et al: Distribution of brain metastases. *Arch Neurol* 45:741–744, 1988.
69. Weisberg LA: Hemorrhagic metastatic intracranial neoplasms: Clinical computed tomographic correlations. *J Comput Assist Tomogr* 9:105–114, 1985.
70. Hayman LA, Hinck VC: Delayed high iodine dose con-

trast computed tomography: Cranial neoplasms. *Radiology* 136:677–681, 1980.
71. Sze G, Shin J, Krol G, et al: Intraparenchymal brain metastases: MR imaging versus contrast enhanced CT. *Radiology* 168:187–194, 1988.
72. Davis PC, Hudgins PA, Peterman SBL: Diagnosis of cerebral metastasis: Double dose delayed CT versus contrast enhanced MR imaging. *AJNR* 12:293–300, 1991.
73. Sze G, Milano E, Johnson C, et al: Detection of brain metastases: Comparison of contrast enhanced MR and enhanced CT. *AJNR* 11:785–791, 1990.
74. Yuh WTC, Engelken JD, Muhonen NG, et al: Experience with high dose gadolinium MR imaging in the evaluation of brain metastasis. *Am J Neuroradiol* 13:335–345, 1992.
75. Atlas SW: Intracranial hemorrhage, in Atlas SW (ed): *Magnetic Resonance Imaging of the Brain and Spine.* New York, Raven Press, 1991, chap 9.
76. Faro SH, Koenigsberg RA, Turtz AR, et al: Melanocytoma of the cavernous sinus: CT and MR findings. *AJNR* 17(6):1087–1090, 1996.
77. Armvig J, Christensen E: Primary benign Intracranial Melanocytoma. *Acta Chir Scand* 82:218, 1939.
78. Botticelli AR, Villani M, Angiari P, et al: Meningeal melanocytoma of Meckel's cave associated with ipsilateral Ota's nevus: Case report. *Cancer* 51:2304–2310, 1983.
79. Lee YY, Glass JP, Geoffrey A, et al: Cranial computed tomographic abnormalities in leptomeningeal metastases. *AJNR* 5:559–563, 1984.
80. Sze G, Soletsky S, Bronen R, et al: MR imaging of cranial meninges with emphasis on contrast enhancement in meningeal carcinomatosis. *ANJR* 10:964–975, 1989.
81. Barkovich AJ, Edwards MSB: Brain tumors of childhood, in Barkovich AJ (ed): *Pediatric Neuroimaging.* New York, Raven Press, 1990, chap 6.
82. Parker RJ: Childhood brain tumors, in Johnson RT, Griffin WJ (eds): *Current Therapy in Neurology,* 4th ed. St. Louis, Mosby Yearbook, 1993, pp 215–223.
83. Zimmerman RA, Bilaniuk LT, Pahlajani H: Spectrum of medulloblastomas demonstrated by computed tomography. *Radiology* 126:137–141, 1978.
84. Gusnard PA: Cerebellar neoplasms in children. *Semin Roentgenol* 25:263–278, 1990.
85. Hart MN, Earle KM: Primitive neuroectodermal tumors of the brain in children. *Cancer* 32:890–896, 1973.
86. Robles HA, Smirniotopoulos JG, Figuero RE: Understanding the radiology of intracranial neuroectodermal tumors from a pathological perspective: A review. *Semin Ultrasound, CT MRI* 13:170–181, 1992.
87. Gjerris F, Klinkein L: Long-term prognosis in children with benign cerebellar astrocytoma. *J Neurosurg* 49:179–184, 1978.
88. Maroldo TV, Barkovich AJ: Pediatric brain tumors. *Semin Ultrasound, CT MRI* 13:412–448, 1992.
89. Swartz JD, Zimmerman RA, Bilaniuk LT: Computed tomography of intracranial ependymomas. *Radiology* 143:97–102, 1982.
90. Zimmerman RA, Bilaniuk LT: Computed tomography of choroid plexus lesions. *J Comput Assist Tomog* 3(2): 93–103, 1979.
91. Ho VB, Smirniotopoulos JG, Murphy FM, et al: Radiologic–pathologic correlations: Hemangioblastoma. *AJNR* 13:1343–1352, 1992.
92. Adair LD, Ropper HH, Davis KR: Cerebellar hemangioblastoma: CT, angiographic, and clinical condition in seven cases. *J Comput Assist Tomogr* 2:281–294, 1978.
93. Lee SR, Sanches J, Mark AS, et al: Posterior fossa hemangioblastomas: MR imaging. *Radiology* 171:463–468, 1989.
94. Kulkantrakorn K, Awwad EE, Levy B, et al: MRI in Lhermitte-Duclos disease. *Neurology* 48:725–731, 1997.
95. Meltzer CC, Smirniotopoulos JG, Jones RV: The striated cerebellum: An MR imaging sign in Lhermitte-Duclos disease (dysplastic gangliocytoma). *Radiology* 194(3): 699–703, 1995.
96. Scheithauer BW: Neuropathology of pineal region tumors. *Clin Neurosurg* 32:351–383, 1985.
97. Zee CS, Segal H, Apuzzo M, et al: MR imaging of pineal region neoplasms. *J Comput Assist Tomogr* 15:56–63, 1991.
98. Zimmerman RA, Bilaniuk LT, Wood JH, et al: Computed tomography of pineal, parapineal, and histologically related tumors. *Radiology* 137:669–677, 1980.
99. Shuangshotti S, Netsky MG: Neuroepithelial (colloid) cysts of the nervous system: Further observations in pathogenesis, location, incidence, and histochemistry. *Neurology* 16:887–903, 1966.
100. Ganti SR, Antunes JL, Lewis KM, et al: CT in the diagnosis of colloid cysts of the third ventricle. *Radiology* 138:385–391, 1981.
101. Maeder PP, Holtas SL, Basibuyuk LN, et al: Colloid cysts of the third ventricle: Correlation of MR and CT findings with histology and chemical analysis. *AJNR* 11:575–581, 1990.
102. Malik GM: Colloid cysts. *Neurology* 13:73–77, 1980.
103. Rao KCVG, Fitz CR, Harwood-Nash DC: Craniopharyngiomas in children: Neuroradiological evaluation. *Rev Int Radiol* 2:149–157, 1977.
104. Pusey E, Kortman KE, Flannigan BD, et al: MR of craniopharyngiomas: Tumor delineation and characterization. *AJNR* 8:439–447, 1987.
105. Mikhael MA, Ciric IS, Wolff AP: MR diagnosis of acoustic neuromas. *J Comput Assist Tomogr* 11:232–235, 1987.
106. Young IR, Burl M, Clarke GJ, et al: Magnetic resonance properties of hydrogen: Imaging the posterior fossa. *AJR* 137:895–901, 1981.
107. Kingsley DPR, Brooks GB, Leung AW, et al: Acoustic neuroma: Evaluation by magnetic resonance imaging. *AJNR* 6:1–5, 1985.
108. Armington WG, Harnsberger HR, Smoker WR, et al: Normal and diseased acoustic pathway: Evaluation with MR imaging. *Radiology* 167:509–515, 1988.
109. Pykett IL, Newhouse JH, Buonanno FS: Principles of NMR imaging. *Radiology* 143:157–168, 1982.
110. Enzmann DR, O'Donhue J: Optimizing MR imaging for detecting small tumors in the cerebellopontine angle and internal auditory canal. *AJNR* 8:99–106, 1987.
111. Press GA, Hesselink JR: MR imaging of cerebellopontine angle and internal auditory canal lesions at 1.5 T. *AJNR* 9:241–151, 1988.
112. Kutcher TJ, Brown DC, Maurer PK, et al: Dural tail

adjacent to acoustic neuroma: MR features. *J Comput Assist Tomogr* 15:669–670, 1991.
113. Price AC, Runge VM, Nelson ICL, et al: MR of meningiomas. *MRI Decisions* 2:1–11, 1988.
114. Chen TC, Zee CS, Miller CA, et al: Magnetic resonance imaging and pathological correlates of meningiomas. *Neurosurgery* 31:1015–1022, 1992.
115. Kaplan RD, Coons SC, Drayer BP, et al: MR characteristics of meningioma subtypes at 1.5 tesla. *J. Comput Assist Tomogr* 16:366–367, 1992.
116. Sevick RJ, Dillon WP, Engstrom J, et al: Trigeminal neuropathy: GD-DTPA enhanced MR imaging. *J. Comput Assist Tomogr* 15:605–611, 1991.
117. Aoki S, Barkovich AJ, Nishimura K, et al: Neurofibromatosis Types 1 and 2: Cranial MR findings. *Radiology* 172:527–534, 1989.
118. Gualdi GF, DiBiasi C: Unusual MR and CT appearance of an epidermoid tumor. *AJNR* 12:771–772, 1991.
119. Savader SJ, Murtaugh FR, Savader BL, et al: Magnetic resonance imaging of intracranial epidermoid tumors. *Clin Radiol* 40:282–285, 1989.
120. Gao P, Osborn AG, Smirniotopoulos JG, et al: Epidermoid tumor of the cerebellopontine angle. *AJNR* 13:863–872, 1992.
121. Brooks ML, Jolesz FA, Patz S: MRI of pulsatile CSF motion within arachnoid cysts. *Magn Reson Imaging* 6:575–584, 1988.
122. Lo WW, Solti-Bohman LG, Brackmann DE, et al: Cholesterol granuloma of the petrous apex: CT diagnosis. *Radiology* 153:705–711, 1984.
123. Yasargil ML, Abernathy CD, Sarioglu AC: Microneurosurgical treatment of intracranial dermoid and epidermoid tumors. *Neurosurgery* 24:561–567, 1989.
124. Olsen WL, Dillon WP, Kelly WM, et al: MR imaging of paragangliomas. *AJNR* 7:1039–1042, 1986.
125. Volg T, Bruning R, Schedel H, et al: Paragangliomas of the jugular bulb and carotid body. *AJNR* 10:823–827, 1989.
126. Lee BCP, Kneeland JB, Walker RW: MAR imaging of brainstem tumors. *AJNR* 6:159–163, 1985.
127. Wilson WB, Kosmorsky GS, deMasters BK: Diffusely infiltrating brainstem gliomas. *Neurology* 40:1237–1241, 1990.
128. Bradley WG, Waluch V: Blood flow: Magnetic resonance imaging. *Radiology* 154:443–450, 1985.
129. Gentry LR, Jacoby CG, Turski PA, et al: Cerebellopontine angle-petromastoid mass lesions: Comparative study of diagnosis with MR imaging and CT. *Radiology* 162:513–520, 1987.
130. Patel SC, Sanders WP: MRI of the pituitary gland: Adenomas. *MRI Decisions* January/February 12–20, 1990.
131. Sakomoto Y, Takahashi M, Korogi Y, et al: Normal and abnormal pituitary glands: Gadopentetate dimeglumine-enhanced MR imaging. *Radiology* 178:441–445, 1991.
132. Stadnik T, Stevenaevt A, Beckers A, et al: Pituitary microadenomas: Diagnosis with two- and three-dimensional MR imaging at 1.5 T before and after injection of gadolinium. *Radiology* 176:419–428, 1990.
133. Sze G, Vichanco LS, Brant-Zawadski M, et al: Chordomas: MR imaging. *Radiology* 166:187–191, 1988.

VIRAL AND NONVIRAL INFECTIONS OF THE NERVOUS SYSTEM

Álvaro C. de Almeida Magalhães
Luiz Alberto Bacheschi
Antonio Alci Barone

VIRAL INFECTIONS OF THE NERVOUS SYSTEM

The introduction of computed tomography (CT) in the mid-1970s remarkably improved the evaluation and diagnosis of central nervous system (CNS) infections. Since then, considerable experience has been gained in the CT appearance of intracranial infectious and inflammatory processes. The advent of magnetic resonance imaging (MRI) strikingly increased the diagnostic possibilities. The multiplanar capabilities and the high-contrast resolution of MRI far exceed those of CT. Further advantages of MRI include its capacity to study arterial or venous infectious lesions by means of MRI angiography and to study the cerebrospinal fluid (CSF) flow disturbances with cine-flow MRI. When available, MRI is now the screening procedure of choice to be used in patients suspected of harboring a CNS infection.[1]

Both CT and MRI image the gross neuropathologic aspects of several infectious processes that involve the brain and the meninges.[1] However, it must be stressed that routinely neither MRI nor CT is specific for a particular disease process.[2] For example, brain multiple ring-enhanced lesions may be due to bacterial or nonbacterial infections, metastasis, or certain demyelinating diseases. Careful correlation of clinical examination, imaging findings, CSF analysis, and other laboratory data is mandatory to reach the correct diagnosis.

VIRAL MENINGITIS

Viruses may infect the leptomeninges with little or no parenchymal involvement of the CNS. The clinical syndrome produced is that of an acute febrile illness with headache, photophobia, meningismus, and often vomiting. Analysis of the CSF reveals a predominantly lymphocytic pleocytosis with normal CSF glucose levels: no organisms can be demonstrated by smear or routine bacterial or fungal cultures. These clinical and laboratory features are usually considered to indicate aseptic meningitis.

The most common etiologic agents are enteroviruses, primarily coxsackie virus and echovirus. Next in order of frequency are mumps, herpes simplex type 2, lymphocytic choriomeningitis (LCM), and adenovirus infections. Other causative agents include Epstein-Barr virus (EBV) and HIV. Some nonviral organisms may produce a clinical syndrome indistinguishable from viral meningitis; this can be seen in Lyme disease (borreliosis), leptospirosis, and *Mycoplasma pneumoniae* infection.[3]

There may be associated findings of systemic viral infection, and these may help to identify the etiologic agent. Neurologic signs are sparse; gross pathologic findings range from none to some meningeal or brain congestion. The CT and MRI scans are usually normal.

VIRAL ENCEPHALITIS

Viral encephalitis is usually an acute febrile illness, often associated with meningismus and a variable mental status disturbance, such as delirium, confusion, stupor, or coma. There is evidence of parenchymal involvement of the CNS with seizures and focal deficits.

The mortality rate is significant during the acute illness (5 to 20 percent for all cases of viral encephalitis), and there is a high incidence of permanent disabling sequelae. The prognosis depends on the etiologic agent. Polymerase chain reaction (PCR) can determine the etiologic diagnosis through a search of the viral nucleic acid (RNA or DNA).

The most common etiologic agents identified in this disease are mumps, lymphocytic choriomeningitis (LCM), herpes simplex, arboviruses, and rabies.[3]

Encephalitis caused by mumps or LCM virus is benign except in rare instances. The CT and MRI scans are usually normal.

The other viruses cause an encephalitic process in which the gross pathologic findings range from minimal edema to diffuse brain congestion with hemorrhage and necrosis. Extensive cell damage sometimes occurs, associated with severe clinical functional impairment without significant blood-brain barrier disruption and with normal CT and MRI scans. In herpes simplex encephalitis, the lesions demonstrate intense hemorrhagic necrosis of brain parenchyma easily seen by CT and MRI. The introduction of effective antiviral drugs such as acyclovir has dramatically changed the prognosis of these patients.

Arborviruses Encephalitis

The arthropod-borne viruses (arborviruses) constitute more than 500 strains of viruses usually transmitted biologically by mosquitoes or ticks. The arborvirus that causes encephalitis usually belongs to the flavivirus, togavirus, or bunyavirus family.

While the characteristics of the encephalitis are similar for arborviruses, the severity of the encephalitis varies with the virus strain. Some viruses cause severe encephalitis with mortality rates as high as 40 percent, and up to 50 percent of survivors have permanent neurologic sequelae. Other viruses may cause a mild encephalitis with fever, headache, and slight obtundation followed by full recovery.[3] By MRI the pathologic changes range from none to diffuse brain lesions with hemorrhage and mass effect.

Eastern equine encephalitis is the most severe, with a 70 to 90 percent incidence of death or disabling sequelae. Japanese B encephalitis, Russian spring-summer encephalitis, and Murray Valley encephalitis (Australian X disease) are also associated with high mortality rates (20 to 40 percent), and up to 50 percent of survivors have permanent neurologic sequelae.[4,5]

Western equine encephalitis and St. Louis encephalitis have mortality rates of less than 10 percent, and the diseases are usually benign, although they may be severe in younger children. California and Venezuelan equine encephalitis generally cause benign infections; death and disability are unusual.[5]

Rabies

Rabies is a form of viral encephalitis. Human cases of this disease are rare in developed countries. Virtually all cases of rabies are transmitted to humans by animal bites, causing severe brainstem encephalitis with a high mortality rate. The usual incubation period in humans is 30 to 60 days for extremity bites, but periods as long as 6 months have been reported. Bites on the face and neck can have an incubation period as short as 2 weeks.

Rabies is a polioencephalomyelitis with inflammatory changes occurring predominantly in the gray matter. The pathognomonic histologic feature is the Negri body, an eosinophilic neuronal cytoplasmic inclusion. The largest bodies are seen in the pyramidal cells of the hippocampus, in the Purkinje cells, and in the motor neurons of spinal cord.[6]

The clinical disease usually begins with personality change and a period of excitement. Then focal signs, especially those referable to the brainstem, develop. The characteristic hydrophobia is caused by dysphagia and hyperirritability of pharynx. Death results from respiratory failure or cardiac arrythmia. The disease is fatal during the acute stage in 95 percent of cases, but complete recovery has been reported.[7]

Findings on CT have been found to be unremarkable in rabies. In one case in the terminal stage, the CT scan demonstrated rounded areas of decreased attenuation in the supratentorial white matter, mainly in the frontotemporal areas. In that case, a low-field MRI revealed hyperintensity in T2-weighted images in the same areas described on CT.[8]

HERPES VIRUS INFECTIONS

Herpes Simplex Encephalitis

Herpes simplex encephalitis is the most common cause of fatal endemic or sporadic encephalitis. It may occur in patients of any age, of either sex, or of any socioeconomic status and at any time of the year.[3] Herpes simplex encephalitis has been reported to have a 10 to 40 percent mortality rate, with a corresponding high incidence of sequelae.[8]

Herpes characteristically produces destructive lesions of the anterior temporal and inferior frontal lobes. In adults the encephalitis is almost always due to herpes simplex virus type 1.

Most patients have the classic findings of encephalitis, including fever, headache, and altered consciousness. Focal and generalized seizures are common. Hemiparesis, memory loss, personality disorders, dementia, and aphasia may occur. The type 2 virus may also cause encephalitis, usually in the neonate, acquired during vaginal delivery. It is usually a fulminate, generalized, and rapidly fatal disease.[3,8]

Pathologic changes include infiltration of leptomeninges by inflammatory cells with bilateral and usually asymmetrical hemorrhagic necrosis predominating in the temporal lobes, affecting particularly the anterior part of the parahippocampal, the fusiform, and the inferior and middle temporal gyri, and the posterior orbital cortex. The necrosis also involves the white matter, the hippocampus, the amygdaloid nucleus, and the putamen.[6]

The CSF analysis is not specific and frequently reveals a white cell count in the range of 50 to 500 cells/μl, elevated protein concentration, and usually a normal glucose level.

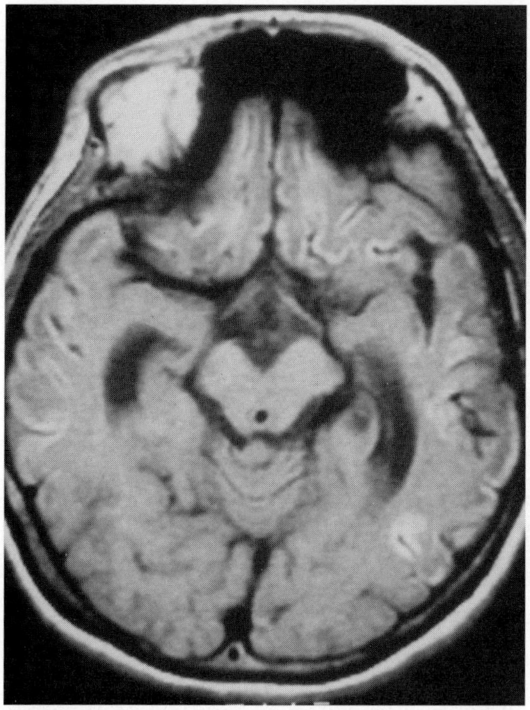

A

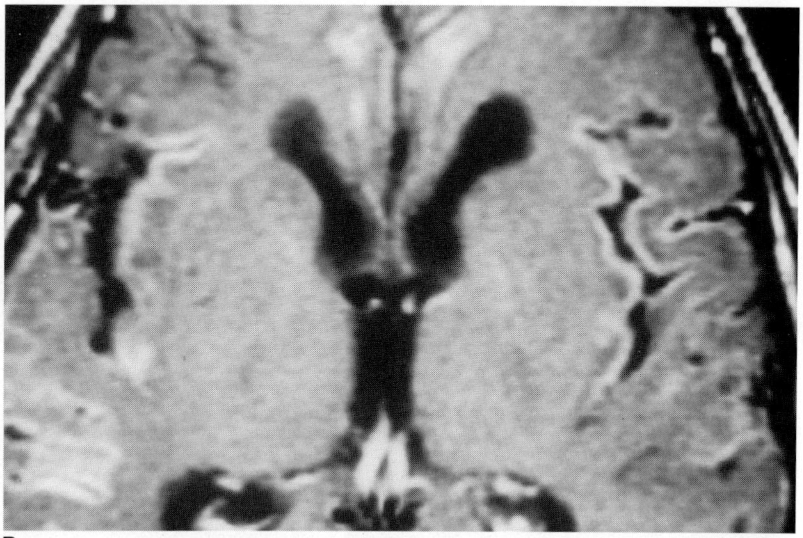

B

Figure 13-1
Subacute herpes simplex encephalitis presenting 4 weeks ago in a 28-year-old man with a history of fever. **(A)** *Axial T1-weighted image shows diffuse high signal in the cortex in the frontobasal and temporal regions.* **(B)** *Postcontrast axial T1-weighted image and* **(C)** *coronal T1-weighted image show enhancement of the cortex.*

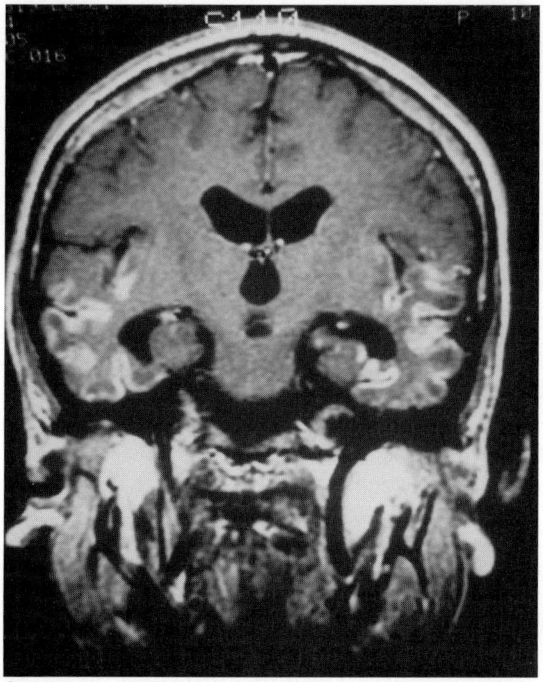

C

Neuroimaging is a very important diagnostic tool. Changes are usually seen on CT before the fifth day after the onset of symptoms.[9] In 50 to 60 percent of cases, the CT shows hypoattenuation involving the anterior and medial aspects of the temporal lobes and the inferior aspects of the frontal lobes. These usually are bilateral but asymmetrical. Hemorrhagic areas may be seen. However, MRI has greater sensitivity than CT in showing the temporal and frontal involvement. In the acute phase, MRI shows the temporal and inferior frontal lobes to be swollen, with low signal intensity on T1-weighted images and high signal intensity on T2-weighted images. T1-weighted images with gadolinium enhancement show cortical and pial abnormalities of the blood-brain barrier (Fig. 13-1). After the third week, the pathologic abnormalities are seen mainly in the gray matter. The temporal and frontobasal cortex and the hippocampi are especially affected. Cellular loss and atrophy occur. T1-weighted images reveal high signal intensity in the cortex that enhances after contrast administration (Fig. 13-1). In the chronic stage, MRI shows loss of substance, necrosis of the brain, enlargement of the sulci, and dilatation of the ventricles (Fig. 13-2).[8,10]

Varicella-Zoster Virus Infections

Varicella-zoster virus (VZV) is a human herpesvirus that causes both varicella and herpes zoster. Varicella (chickenpox) is a disease primarily of children, and reactivation causes herpes zoster (shingles), a disorder most common in the elderly.[11]

The most common neurologic complication associated with varicella is postinfectious encephalomyelitis, an acute demyelinating process that can assume features of an acute cerebellar ataxia or of an acute disseminated encephalomyelitis (ADEM). Another varicella complication is a syndrome of delayed vasculitis leading to infarction in the basal ganglia, internal capsule, and temporal lobe. Angiography reveals arterial irregular

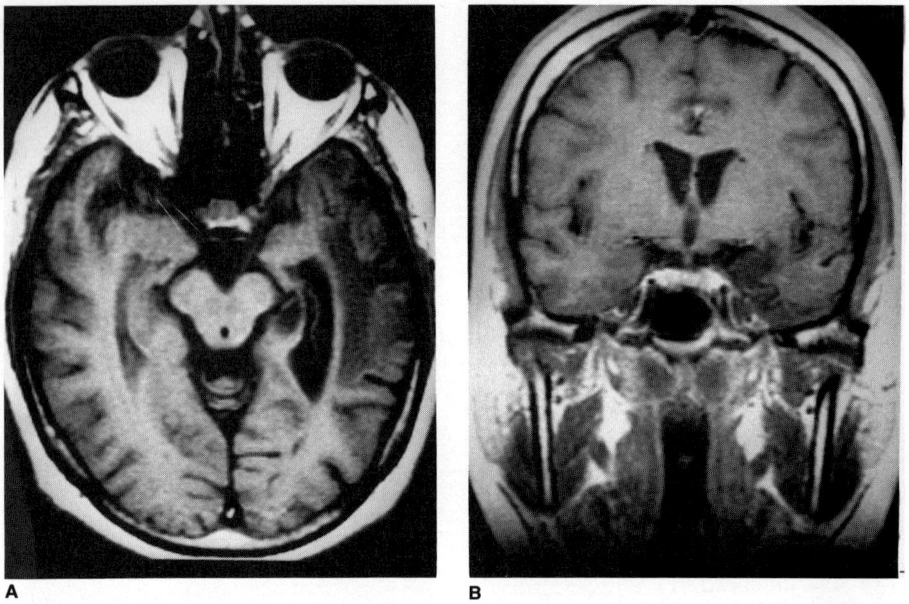

Figure 13-2
Chronic herpes simplex encephalitis. A 23-year-old woman presented 4 months ago with acute febrile illness with meningeal signs, seizures, and diminished consciousness. **(A and B)** *Axial T1-weighted image and postcontrast coronal T1-weighted image show diffuse hypointense area without enhancement, with volumetric reduction of the left temporal lobe and left ventricle temporal horn enlargement.*

narrowing and occlusion.[12] Reye's syndrome may develop after varicella infection.

Common neurologic complications of herpes zoster are acute and postherpetic neuralgia, segmental motor weakness (radiculitis), and cranial neuropathy. Myelitis and encephalomyelitis may occur in immunosuppressed patients, most frequently in AIDS.[11] A syndrome of postherpetic cerebral vasculopathy and infarction is well recognized. Cerebral infarction may occur after zoster in any location,[13] but most cases are due to zoster involvement of the ophthalmic division of the trigeminal nerve with vasculitis and occlusion of the ipsilateral middle cerebral artery.[11,14]

RETROVIRUS INFECTIONS

Acquired Immunodeficiency Syndrome

Imaging in CNS involvement by AIDS is presented in Chap. 14.

Tropical Spastic Paraparesis

Tropical spastic paraparesis (TSP), or HAM (HTLV-I associated myelopathy), is a chronic progressive demyelinating disease that predominantly affects the spinal cord.[15,16] The disease occurs in regions where the human T-cell lymphotropic virus type I (HTLV-1) is endemic: the Caribbean, Central and South America, southern Japan, and areas of Africa.[15,17,18]

The disease typically presents as symmetrical and slowly progressive weakness and stiffness of the lower extremities. On examination, the major finding is a spastic paraparesis with mild distal sensory loss.[19] The upper extremities may also be affected. Bladder as well as sexual function are impaired in some patients. The rate of progression varies and in most patients occurs over years.[15,19]

The pathology of TSP consists of myelin loss and some axonal degeneration in the white matter of the spinal cord. Some cases may show demyelination of optic and auditory nerves and demyelinated foci in the cerebral white matter.[6]

The CSF shows a mild pleocytosis and elevated oligoclonal IgG level, which are due to local synthesis. Spine MRI studies show only spinal cord atrophy in long-standing paresis; but brain MRI shows multiple foci of increased T2-weighted signal intensity in periventricular white matter in 50 to 75 percent of patients (Fig. 13-3).[20,21,22] Hyperintense foci have also been described in the pons and cerebellar white matter.[23] These findings can resemble those seen in multiple sclerosis.[22,23]

SLOW VIRUS DISEASES

Subacute Sclerosing Panencephalitis

Subacute sclerosing panencephalitis (SSPE) is a slow virus infection caused by the measles virus, although many questions remain as to how it produces slow infection and chronic disease. Pathologic findings include diffuse encephalitis of both gray and white matter affecting cerebral as well as brainstem structures. There is chronic inflammation, with perivascular cuffing, demyelination of cerebral white matter, and neuronal loss. Inclusion bodies are present in neurons, astrocytes, and oligodendrocytes.[24]

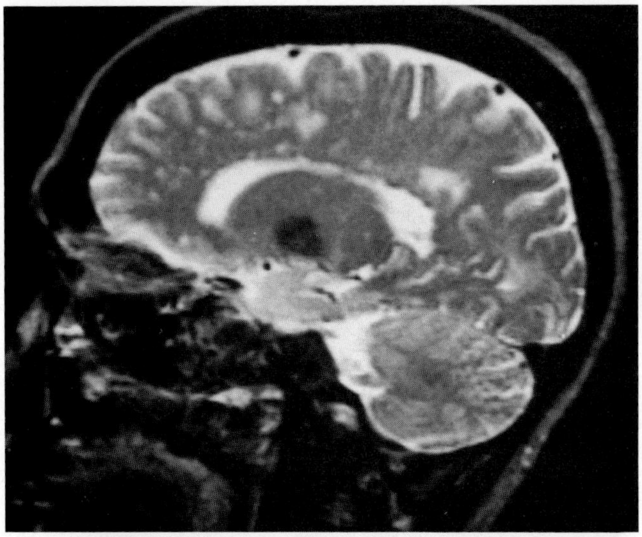

A

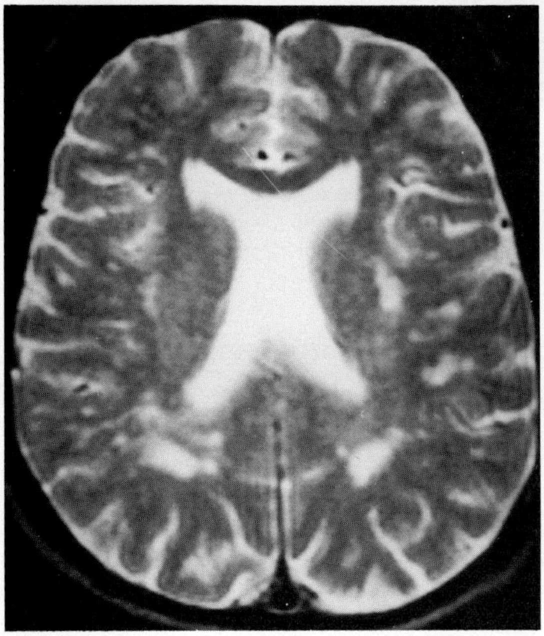

B

Figure 13-3
Tropical spastic paraparesis. This 41-year-old woman with progressive spastic crural paraparesis and HTLV-I positive. **(A and B)** *Sagittal and axial T2-weighted images show multiple bilateral nodular and punctate hyperintense foci in the periventricular and subcortical white matter.*

This infection is predominantly a disease of children and young adults. The first signs of SSPE are mental and behavioral changes. Focal neurologic signs appear and are followed by major, minor, myoclonic, and partial complex seizures. Periodic and generalized myoclonic jerks are frequent. The course is usually progressive, and the final stages are characterized by a vegetative state with decorticate or decerebrate posture and signs of autonomic dysfunction.[25] There is no effective treatment, and death occurs within 1 to 3 years. Spontaneous remission, partial or complete, occurs in about 4 percent of the cases.[24,25]

Early in the disease, the CT scan is usually normal, and then low-attenuation lesions may appear in the cerebral white matter and in the basal ganglia. Atrophy may be the only finding when the disease progresses.[26,27] The MRI usually shows a symmetrical diffuse involvement of the white matter, characterized by hyperintense areas in the T2-weighted images that become more evident with disease progression (Fig. 13-4).[27,28] Focal abnormalities of the white matter may also appear.[28]

Progressive Multifocal Leukoencephalopathy

Progressive multifocal leukoencephalopathy (PML) is a progressive demyelinating disease caused by an opportunistic papovavirus (JVC) that produces an infection in the oligodendrocytes of an immunodeficient host. This disease occurs principally in patients with AIDS, but it can occur in patients receiving immunosuppressive therapy, patients with lymphoma and leukemia, and patients with a generalized disorder, such as sarcoidosis associated with anergy.[29]

Pathologic study shows multifocal areas of demyelination, varying markedly in size, that originate in the subcortical hemispheric white matter, the cerebellum, and the brainstem. These areas may coalesce to form large atrophic regions. The parietal and occipital lobes are most commonly affected. Microscopic examination shows multiple, sometimes confluent, foci of demyelination. The most important pathologic finding is the presence of intranuclear inclusions, found mainly within large swollen oligodendrocytic nuclei, in the periphery of the demyelinated foci.[6]

Progressive dementia, hemiparesis, and hemianopsia are the most common clinical manifestations. Hemianesthesia, cerebellar, or brainstem symptoms and signs may occur. Seizures are infrequent and spinal cord involvement is rare.[29] Deterioration is usually rapid, leading to death within a few months, but there is much variation. Spontaneous remission has been reported.[24]

The CSF is usually normal. The CT scans demonstrate subcortical white matter hypointensity, and the lesions are often asymmetric and frequently begin in parietal-occipital areas. The MRIs in PML demonstrate T1 hypointensity and T2 hyperintensity of the lesions detected by CT. The T2-weighted images are more sensitive than CT and often show early white matter changes confirming the multifocal involvement.[30] There is less commonly cortical gray matter involvement. When the margin of the lesion reaches the cortex, a scalloped appearance results (Fig. 13-5).[31] Unusual MRI patterns include thalamic and basal ganglia involvement,[31] mass effect, and lesion enhancement.[32]

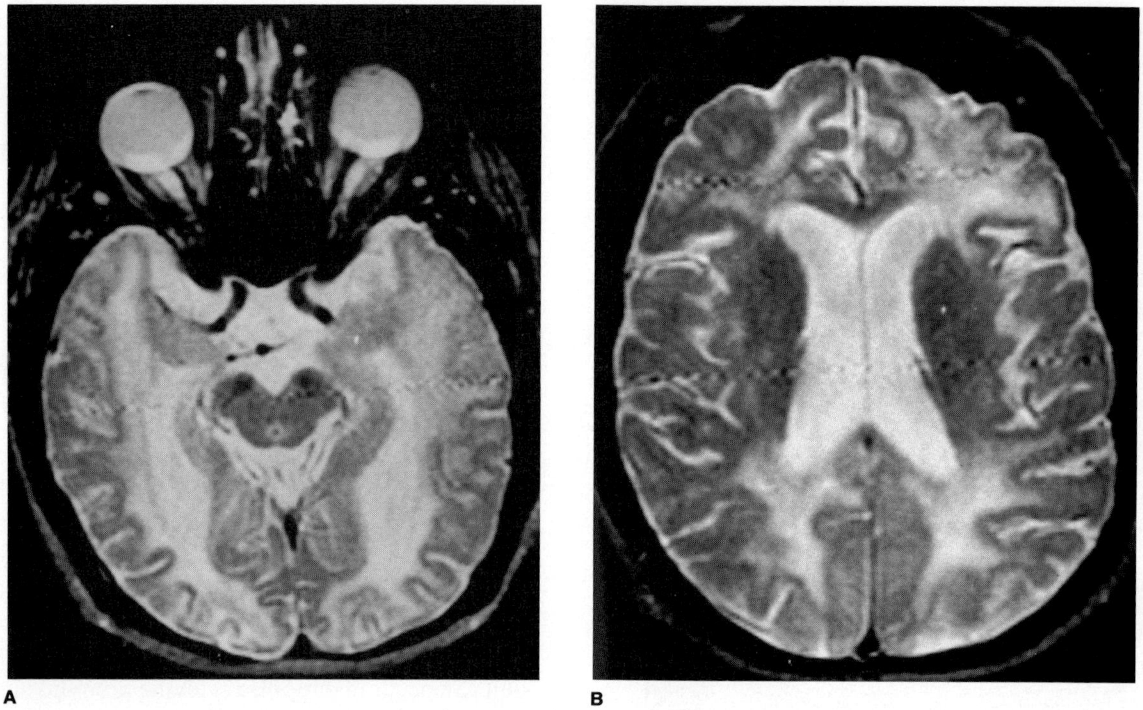

Figure 13-4
Subacute sclerosing panencephalitis (necropsy proven) in a 27-year-old woman with dementia, seizures, and myoclonus. Patient in clinical terminal stage. **(A and B)** *Axial T2-weighted image shows diffuse areas of hyperintensity in the white matter in both cerebral hemispheres, predominantly in the periventricular region. Ventricular and sulcul enlargement are also present.*

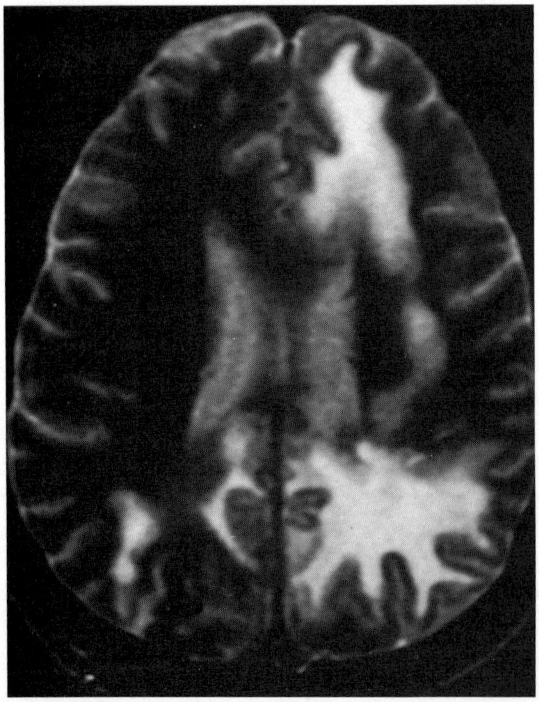

Figure 13-5
Progressive multifocal leukoencephalopathy. An HIV-positive 33-year-old man with cognitive dysfunction, right hemiparesis, and right hemianopsia. Axial T2-weighted image shows multifocal white matter lesions with hyperintensity in left frontal and bilateral parietal lobes.

Subacute Spongiform Encephalopathy

Subacute spongiform encephalitis (SSE) or Creutzfeldt-Jakob disease, is a transmissible slow virus infection of the group of human spongiform encephalopathies that includes the familiar Gerstmann-Straussler-Scheinker syndrome and kuru. These diseases, despite their rarity in humans, have attracted considerable interest because of the unique properties of the transmissible agent.[33,34] Prusiner coined the term *prion* to distinguish this transmissible agent from viruses.[34]

Pathologically, SSE is characterized by diffuse neuronal degeneration, mainly in cerebral and cerebellar gray matter, but also affecting the basal ganglia and spinal cord. There are widespread neuronal loss, cell vacuolation, and glial proliferation. No inflammatory reactions are seen.[6]

This disease occurs predominantly after the fifties with a peak incidence in the seventh decade. It is characterized by a rapidly progressive subacute dementia, sometimes accompanied by myoclonus, cerebellar signs, rigidity, and weakness. The course is invariably fatal, usually in the first year of the disease.[34,35]

The CT and MRI scans show progressive and diffuse cerebral atrophy with widened sulci and enlarged lateral ventricles. In a Japanese study, periventricular white matter hyperintensities in T2-weighted images were seen.[36]

POSSIBLE CNS VIRAL DISEASES

Rasmussen Encephalitis

Rasmussen encephalitis is a focal chronic encephalitis associated with severe intractable epilepsy and was first described and defined as a syndrome by Rasmussen et al. This entity usually has childhood onset, but adult onset has been described.[37]

The disease is characterized by intractable partial and secondary generalized seizures, often with epilepsia partialis continua and recurrent status epilepticus associated with progressive sensorimotor deficits, mainly hemiparesis, and cognitive decline.[37]

Studies with CT and MRI have revealed a nonspecific focal atrophy (Fig. 13-6), but the entire hemisphere may be affected.[38] The diagnosis was established at surgery for relief of epilepsy when there were noted to be features of encephalitis in the resected brain tissue.[6]

In some cases, the neurologic disease followed a febrile illness and had persisted up to 15 years. Recently, cytomegalovirus genome was found in brains of patients with this disease, suggesting a possible etiologic relationship.[39]

Behçet Disease

There is a group of obscure recurring disease with CSF findings of aseptic meningitis that includes Mollaret meningitis, Vogt-Koyanagi-Harada syndrome, and Behçet disease. No virus has been definitively established as the causative agent of these diseases.

Behçet disease most commonly presents as recurrent oral and genital aphthous ulcers accompanied by uveitis or iridocyclitis. Recurrent meningoencephalitis may occur, with sudden episodes of neurologic dysfunction resembling minor strokes. The CSF analysis shows pleocytosis and increased protein content. Usually there is spontaneous remission of the neurologic symptoms in a few weeks. Recurrent episodes of CNS dysfunction may leave permanent neurologic deficits.[40,41] The neuropathologic condition is characterized by multifocal inflammatory and necrotizing lesions and vasculitis that can occur in any part of nervous system.[41]

The MRI usually shows foci of high signal intensity on T2-weighted images within the brainstem, the diencephalon, and the basal ganglia.[40] All the CNS parts may be affected. Lesions in the brainstem and dienceph-

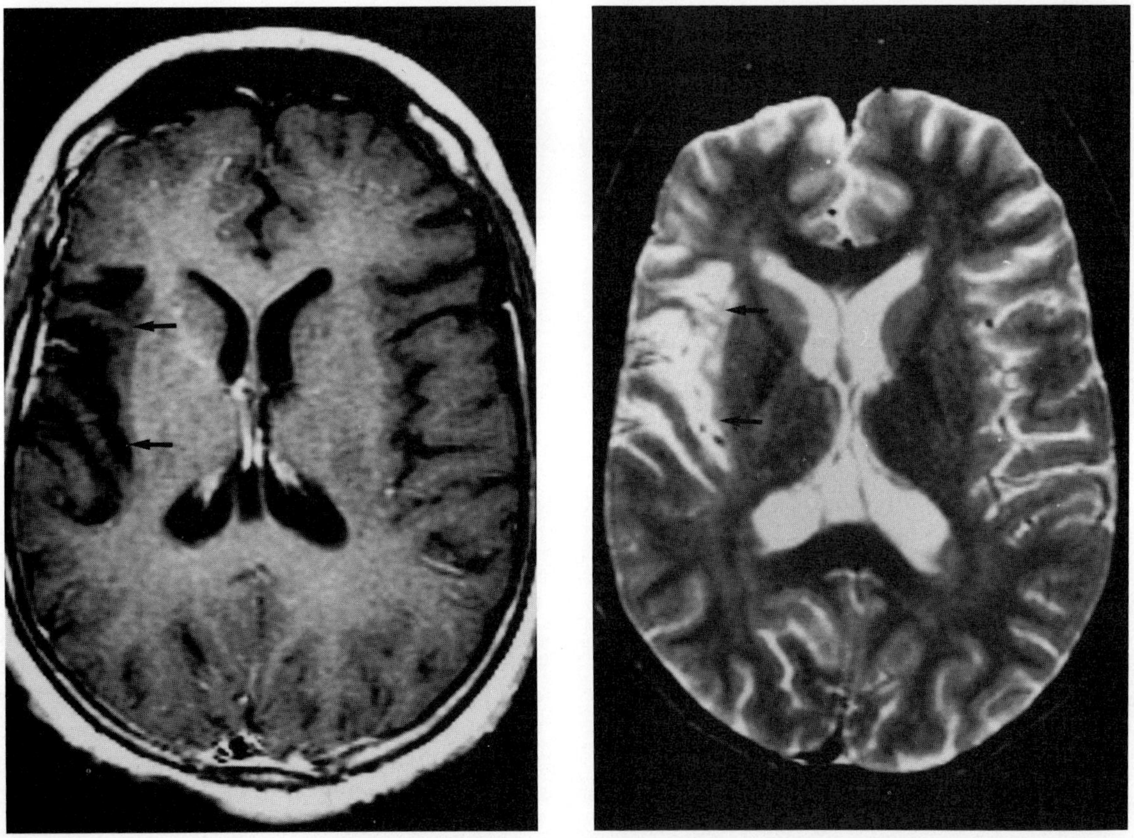

A B

Figure 13-6

Rasmussen encephalitis in a 21-year-old woman with intractable seizures and left hemiparesis. **(A and B)** *A T2-weighted image and postcontrast T1-weighted image also show right temporal atrophy with marked cortical shrinking without enhancement (arrows).*

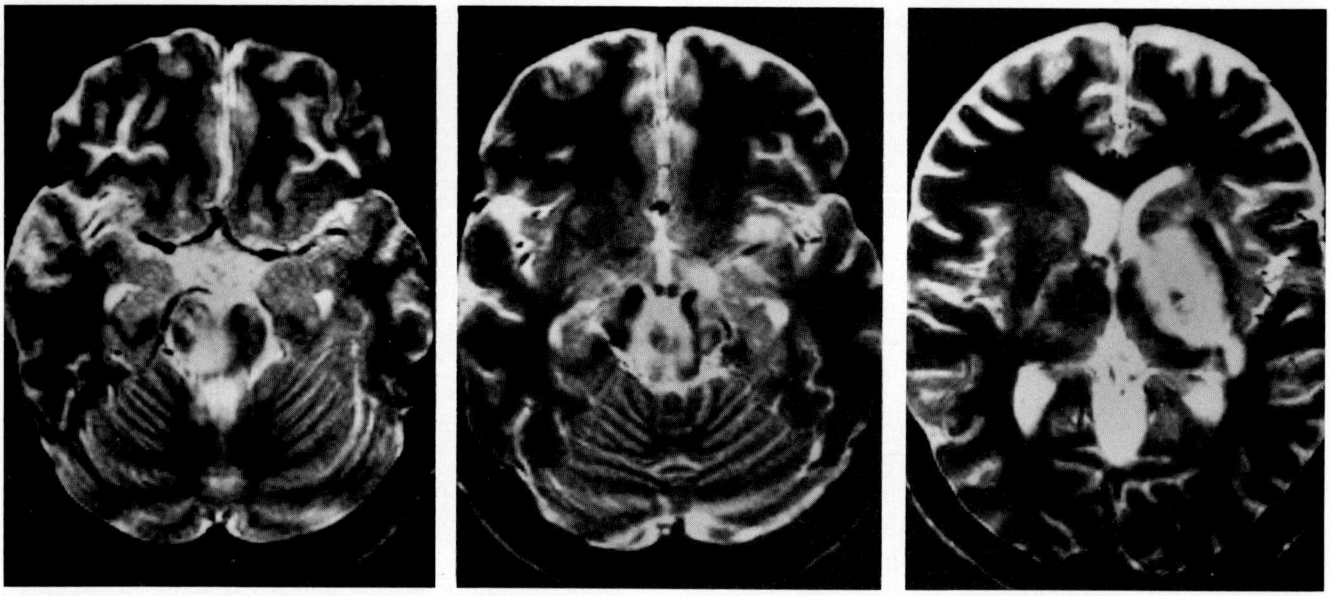

Figure 13-7
Behçet disease in a 33-year-old woman with recent complaint of diplopia and right hemiparesis, with spontaneous recovery within 2 months. **(A–C)** *Axial T2-weighted image shows hyperintense lesions in the midbrain, bilateral basal ganglia including internal capsule, more intense in the left side. These lesions are compatible with ischemic areas secondary to vasculitis.*

alon are sometimes perplexingly large despite few clinical signs (Fig. 13-7).[42] These lesions may show gadolinium enhancement that usually disappears with clinical improvement.[42]

VIRAL CONGENITAL INFECTIONS

Rubella, cytomegalovirus, herpes simplex, toxoplasmosis, and HIV infection represent the major causes of congenital CNS infections. These infections are usually acquired either transplacentally in utero or during the birth process itself when the fetus descends through the birth canal.[43] Manifestations depend on fetal age at time of insult. Infections during the first two trimesters generally lead to congenital malformations, whereas third-trimester infections result in destructive lesions. While MRI is more sensitive than CT in defining the extent of parenchymal lesions and in identifying delayed myelination, in congenital infections CT is also important because intracranial calcifications are better visualized with CT than with conventional MRI.[44] Congenital toxoplasmosis and HIV infection are discussed in Chap. 14.

Rubella

Rubella virus is transmitted to the fetus through the placenta during primary maternal infection. This devastating condition has dramatically diminished its frequency with rubella immunization.[43] The rubella syndrome is usually associated with infection during the first trimester and consists of a wide spectrum of multiorgan anomalies, including heart, eye, and CNS anomalies. Brain involvement results in microencephaly, hydrocephalus, deafness, and atrophy with calcification.[44]

The MRI examination can show malformations of the brain, delayed myelination, hydrocephalus, microcephaly, and microphthalmia. The intracranial calcification is better seen with CT.

Cytomegalovirus

Cytomegalovirus (CMV) is the most common and serious fetal congenital infection.[44] Congenital CMV infection not only occurs during primary maternal infection from transplacental transmission but can result from secondary infections as well.

Pathologically the entire brain may be involved with an encephalitic process. Chronically there are gliosis and calcification. The predilection for rapidly growing cells of germinal matrix leads to periventricular calcification. Cortical malformations such as oligopachygyria and polymicrogyria are identifiable and may be due to an insufficiency in cerebral blood supply.[45,46] Chorioretinitis, cerebellar hypoplasia, and microphthalmia may be seen. Clinically most patients infected congenitally with CMV have no external signs or symptoms.

The MRI findings of CMV include atrophy, hydrocephalus, infarction, and calcifications. Studies using MRI will delineate diffuse white matter abnormalities seen as high signal on T2-weighted sequences, indicative of abnormal myelination and gliosis secondary to the infective process. In addition, MRI demonstrates the neuronal migration anomalies resulting from these infections.

Herpes Simplex Virus

Most congenital infections are caused by herpes simplex virus (HSV) type 2. It may infect the fetus either hematogenously through the placenta or through the cervix prior to or during delivery. Infection during the first trimester commonly results in microcephaly, cerebral atrophy, hydranencephaly, cerebral and cerebellar necrosis, intracranial calcification, chorioretinitis, and multiple other cutaneous and systemic anomalies. Infection acquired through the birth canal during delivery may result in localized CNS involvement with or without infection of the skin and eyes.

The MRI findings of neonatal herpes encephalitis include hypointense signal in T1-weighted images and hyperintense signal on T2-weighted scans. All sequences may disclose loss of the gray-white matter interface. Hemorrhage may be seen. Gadolinium-enhanced images may demonstrate patchy and irregular enhancement of the parenchyma.[47]

NONVIRAL INFECTIONS OF THE NERVOUS SYSTEM

BACTERIAL INFECTIONS

Meningitis

Common causes of acute meningitis include viruses (mainly enteroviruses) and bacteria, such as *Haemophilus influenzae, Neisseria meningitides,* and *Streptococcus*

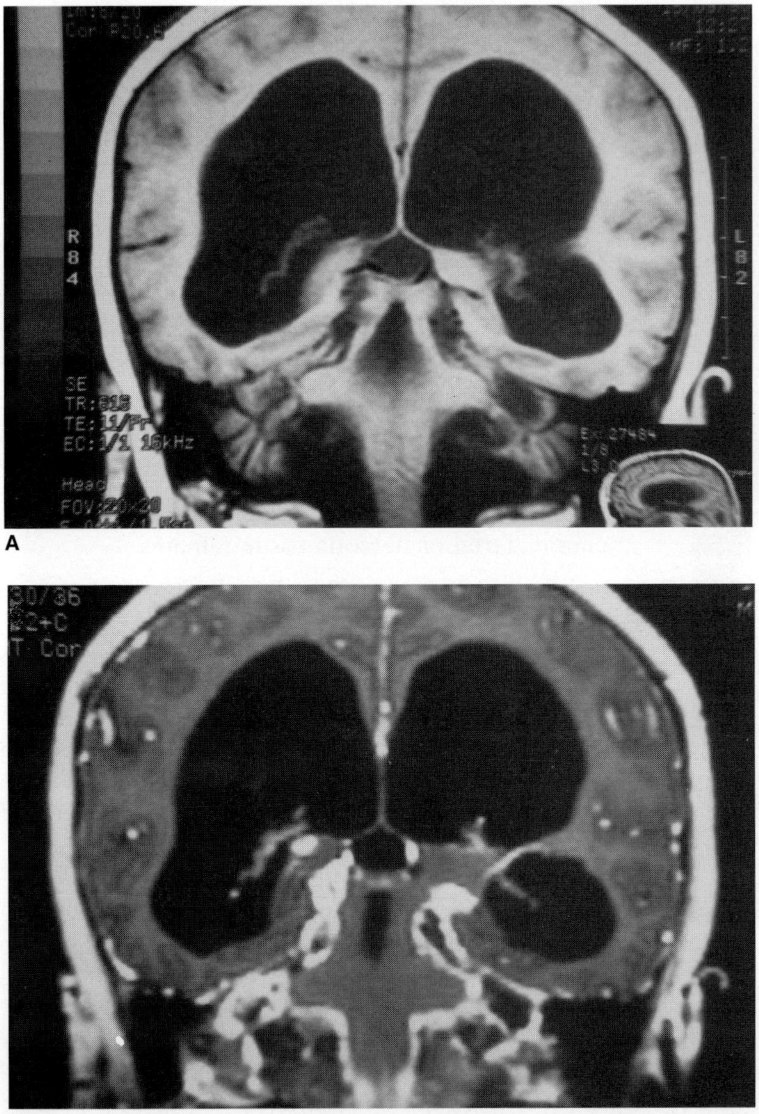

A

B

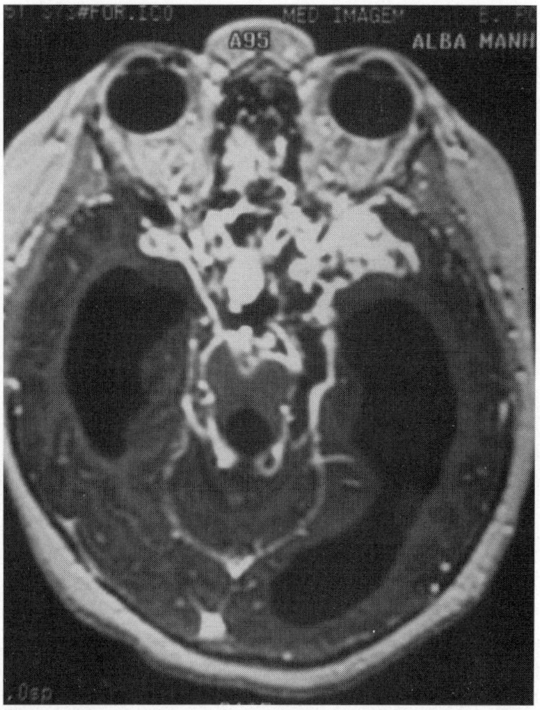

C

Figure 13-8

Bacterial meningitis in a 6-year-old boy with meningeal signs. **(A)** *Coronal T1-weighted image shows ventricular enlargement. Postcontrast* **(B)** *coronal and* **(C)** *axial T1-weighted image show diffuse leptomeningeal enhancement mainly in the basal meninges and around the upper cervical spinal cord, medulla, pons, and midbrain.*

species. In infants and weakened hosts, gram-negative bacteria and fungi are also important. Pathogens may enter hematogenously or, less commonly, by direct extension (temporal bone and sinuses). In the early stage, there is pial congestion, endothelial swelling, and inflammatory infiltrate of the vessel walls. In the midphase stage, there is vessel wall necrosis and thrombosis, which can lead to cortical infarction, cerebritis, and nidus for abscess development. In the later stage, exudate will be present in basal cisterns and sulci, and later thickened fibrotic leptomeninges develop. Hydrocephalus is a common complication of chronic fibrotic leptomeningitis (Fig. 13-8). Since the diagnosis of meningitis is almost always made clinically, imaging modalities assume a secondary role.

Enlarged sulci are usually the initial manifestation of bacterial meningitis and can be seen on CT and MRI. Contrast-enhanced CT is relatively less sensitive than enhanced MRI.[48]

The MRI scan could be normal in the early stages. Enhancement of the meninges may be seen after the administration of gadolinium. Magnetic resonance imaging is useful in assessing the possibility of complications. Hydrocephalus is a frequent concomitant condition. Ventricular enlargement has been found in up to 75 percent of symptomatic patients. Subdural effusions in meningitis constitute a special problem. Parenchymal changes include infarcts, diffuse cerebral edema, and abscess formation (Fig. 13-9). Magnetic resonance imaging is especially useful in determining dural sinus thrombosis, since moderate- to high-intensity signals will occupy the expected position of the sinus instead of the usual flow void (Fig. 13-10).[49]

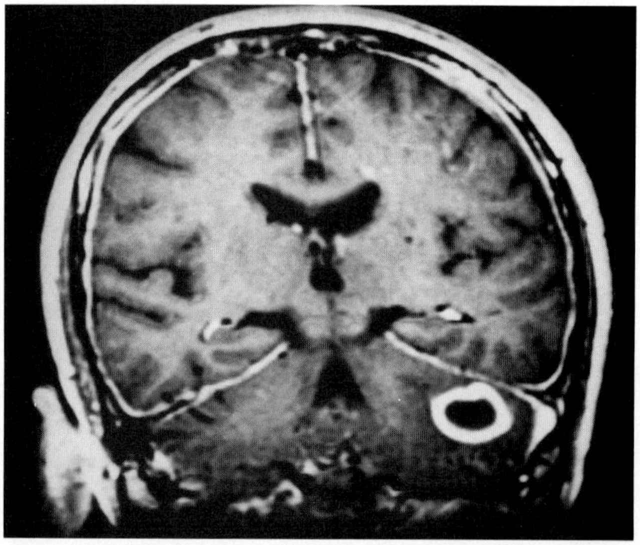

Figure 13-9
Bacterial meningitis and cerebellar abscess in a 58-year-old man with cerebellar ataxia, intracranial hypertension, and meningeal signs. Coronal postgadolinium T1-weighted image shows left cerebellar abscess with central hypointensity and thick ring enhancement. There is also enhancement of leptomeninges in the convexity, interhemispheric fissure, and tentorium.

Encephalitis

Encephalitis results from diffuse parenchymal infiltration, inflammatory cells that cause chromatolysis and pyknosis of neurons, and at times extensive necrosis. Although bacteria, rickettsia, fungi, and protozoa can invade brain tissue, the majority of diffuse infections are viral in origin.

Bacterial causes of meningoencephalitis are unusual but do occur in the first month of life. Most are gram negative. *Escherichia coli* and group B *Streptococcus* type 3 account for approximately 65 to 70 percent of cases in the newborn. Infection is usually a result of bacteremia from another focus, although a contiguous source, such as a middle ear infection, can result in meningoencephalitis. The infection tends to spread through the cerebrum rapidly and is often bilateral and symmetric.

Computed tomographic scans demonstrate large usually bilateral areas of low attenuation in the deep white matter. Contrast enhancement usually is peripheral. Multicystic encephalomalacia can be seen in the end stage.

Abscess

Cerebral abscesses are focal parenchymal infections characterized by a central zone of liquefaction necrosis surrounded by a unique fibrogliotic capsule that localizes the infection. The causes of focal abscesses include:

1. dissemination from infections elsewhere, from either bacteremia or septic emboli
2. direct extension from adjacent infections
3. trauma-related causes, especially if a nidus of foreign material or necrotic tissue remains

Common pathogens consist of both aerobic bacteria, especially *Streptococcus, Staphylococcus,* and gram-negative organisms, and anaerobic bacteria, such as *Bacteroides* and anaerobic *Streptococcus.* In debilitated patients, fungi, actinomycetes, mycobacteria, and protozoa can also lead to abscesses. With the increasing number of AIDS patients, toxoplasmosis has become one of the more frequently encountered causes of brain abscesses.

Acute cerebritis is the initial phase of abscess evolution and lasts 4 days. There is a focal or multifocal inflammatory process with edema, hyperemia, perivascular inflammatory infiltrate, petechial hemorrhage, and necrosis. On CT, the area of involvement needs to be relatively extensive so that the edema will create a low density or a mass effect that can be seen.[50] Magnetic resonance imaging shows well-defined regions of prolonged T1 and T2 relaxation times with mass effect;

ture into the subarachnoid space, producing a tuberculous meningitis. A thick, gelatinous exudate is formed within the basal cisterns (Fig. 13-14). Vessels and cranial nerves traversing the exudate may be compromised (Fig. 13-15).[55]

Magnetic resonance imaging is more sensitive than CT in making an early diagnosis of tuberculous meningitis. Hemorrhagic or ischemic infarcts, meningeal enhancement, ventriculitis, and granulomas are better visualized by MRI than by CT (Fig. 13-14). Intravenous gadolinium is essential to evaluate completely all the intracranial manifestations of tuberculosis. Small calcifications are better seen by CT than by MRI.[56,57]

Tuberculomas

Intracranial tuberculomas are more common in developing countries and occur more frequently in children and young adults. In developed countries, reports indicate a higher frequency in adults. Tuberculomas present as expanding intracranial lesions. The symptoms are related to the site of the lesion. Signs of increased intracranial pressure, headaches, fever, and seizures may be found. Tuberculomas are either solitary or multiple, situated in the cortical or subcortical regions. Most common sites are the cerebral hemisphere and basal ganglia in adults and the cerebellum in children. Intraventricular localization is rare.

Tuberculoma appears on CT most often as a discrete round lesion. It is usually found at the cortico-medullary junction, and it contrast-enhances. The typical size is 5 to 15 mm in diameter. Occasionally the lesion reaches such a size that it mimics a brain tumor. More often the lesion is multiple. Calcification, when present, is best seen on CT.[50,56]

Plain MRIs may not distinguish tuberculomas from surrounding brain and edema on both T1- and T2-weighted images. Sometimes a hypointense rim may separate the hyperintense center from the peripheral hyperintense edema on T2-weighted images. With gadolinium injection, T1-weighted images often show nodular ring enhancing lesions (Fig. 13-14).[57]

Tuberculous Abscess

Tuberculous brain abscess is a rare entity, even in areas where tuberculosis is abundant. It may be seen in the AIDS population.[58] It is defined as an encapsulated collection of pus-containing viable tubercle bacilli without evidence of the classic tubercular granuloma. It should be differentiated from granuloma with central caseation and liquefaction mimicking pus. Magnetic resonance imaging examination demonstrates a hypointense lesion on T1-weighted imaging, with a thick enhancing rim, difficult to differentiate from pyogenic abscess.[57] A case of tuberculous abscesses in a patient with AIDS is presented in Fig. 13-16.

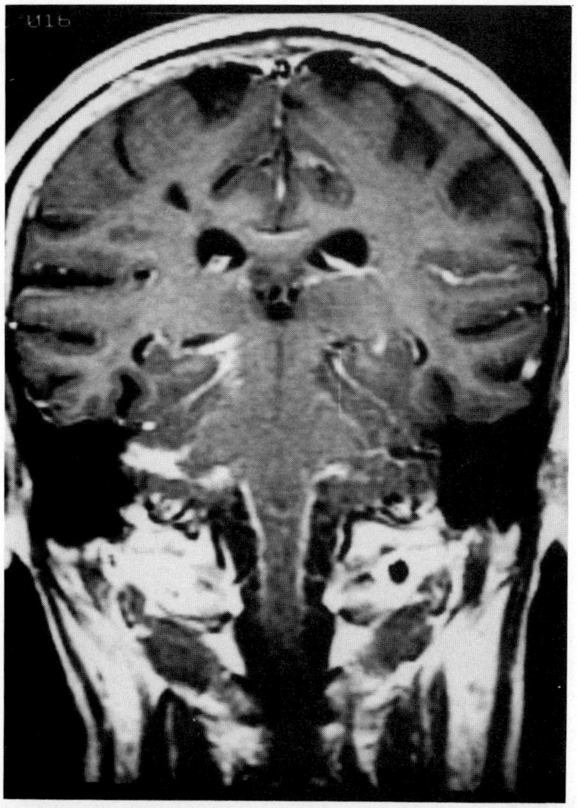

A

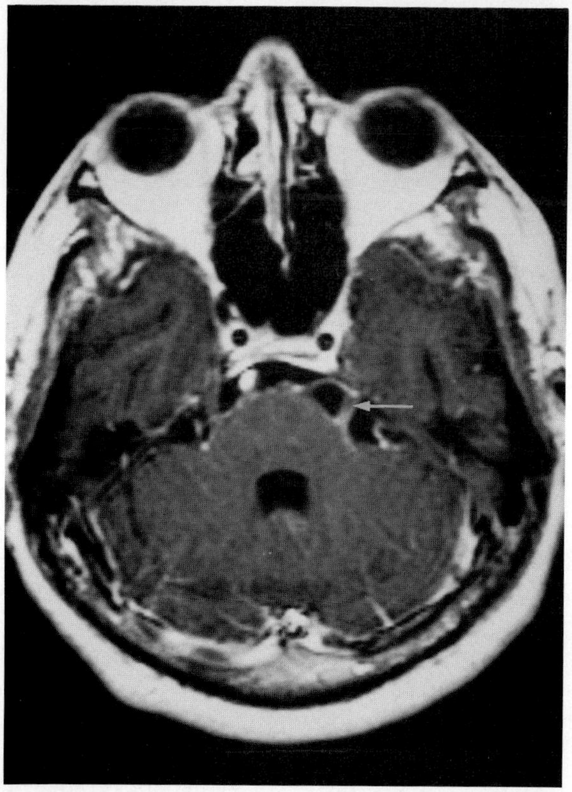

B

Figure 13-15
Tuberculous meningitis in a 44-year-old man with progressive headache, vomiting, vertigo, dysarthria, and sudden left hemiparesis. **(A and B)** *Postcontrast coronal and axial T1-weighted images show abnormal leptomeningeal enhancement mainly in the basal meninges around the upper cervical spinal cord, medulla, pons, and midbrain. The meningeal inflammation involves the left trigeminal nerve (arrow).*

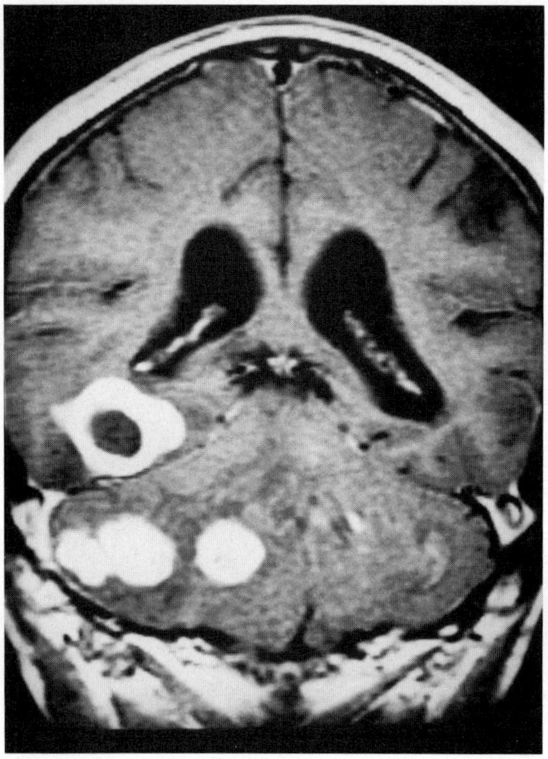

Figure 13-16

CNS tuberculosis in an HIV-positive 41-year-old man with cerebellar ataxia and intracranial hypertension. A coronal postcontrast T1-weighted image shows thick ring enhancement around the hypointense central area in the right temporoparietal region and the right cerebellar hemisphere. Ventricular enlargement can be seen.

SYPHILIS

Syphilis, caused by *Treponema pallidum,* is divided into primary, secondary, and tertiary states. Central nervous system involvement can occur in any of these states from weeks to decades after infection. The major symptomatic types of neurosyphilis are acute leptomeningitis in secondary syphilis and parenchymatous and meningovascular neurosyphilis in tertiary cases.

Chronic involvement of the meninges in the meningovascular type leads to frontal lobe atrophy, ependymitis, and ventricular dilatation. In the parenchymatous type, diffuse proliferative inflammatory changes are seen within the cerebral cortex, occasionally associated with either miliary, small, or large gummas.

Computed tomographic findings can closely resemble a demyelinating disease of the white matter or a cerebrovascular insult. Magnetic resonance imaging is not specific and shows the pattern of lesions related to vasculitis. The gumma should have the same appearance as a chronic inflammatory granuloma.

Tien et al[59] reported the MRI findings of neurosyphilis in six HIV-positive patients. Contrast-enhanced MRIs showed patchy enhancement involving the basal ganglia or middle cerebral artery territories in the first five patients and a convexity mass in the sixth patient, proved by biopsy to be a syphilitic gumma.

LYME DISEASE

Lyme disease is an infection (erythema chronicum migrans) caused by a tick-borne nonsyphilitic spirochete *(Borrelia burgdorferi).* Patients with neuroboreliosis show symptoms of meningoradiculoencephalomyelitis or lymphocytic meningoradiculitis. Computed tomography scans in patients with severe cerebral involvement have shown both enhancing and nonenhancing low-density lesions, mass effect, and cerebral demyelination.[50]

In the acute phase, MRI revealed edema and hypointense areas corresponding to ischemic lesions caused by vasculitis and multiple sclerosis–like lesions within the brain with vascular involvement.[60] Nelson et al[61] reported a case of cranial nerve involvement with Lyme borreliosis in which the inflammatory process was demonstrated only by using gadolinium.

SARCOIDOSIS

Sarcoidosis is a granulomatous disease of unknown cause characterized pathologically by the presence of noncaseating epithelioid granulomas. Central nervous system involvement occurs in approximately 5 percent of the cases of sarcoidosis. Most often, multisystem disease is present, but exclusive CNS involvement can occur. The main CNS manifestations of sarcoidosis include leptomeningitis and a meningovascular form with associated parenchymatous changes.

Sarcoidosis primarily involves the leptomeninges, causing leptomeningitis, which is well visualized on enhanced MRIs. Infiltration may occur along the surface of the brain or extend deep into the brain along the Virchow-Robin spaces. Enhancing linear and nodular areas from the pial surface in the white matter indicate infiltration along Virchow-Robin spaces, which may coalesce, producing parenchymal granuloma. Hydrocephalus may be caused by granulomatous compression of the aqueduct and fourth ventricle, by the granulomatous leptomeningitis, or by infiltration of the ependyma and choroid plexus.[62–64]

Any portion of the brain can be affected by sarcoidosis, but the basal portion is most commonly involved. This correlates with recent observations that CSF-filled Virchow-Robin spaces are routinely visualized in the basal areas of the brain. Anatomically, this area includes the anterior perforated substance, which is characterized by numerous penetrating, small blood vessels. In addition the blood-brain barrier is absent in the tuber cinereum, hypophysis, and preoptic region. Hypothalamic dysfunction is the most common manifestation of CNS sarcoidosis. Infiltrations of the chiasm, optic pathways, infundibulum, and hypophysis usually occur and are easily seen on enhanced MRIs (Fig. 13-17).[65–67]

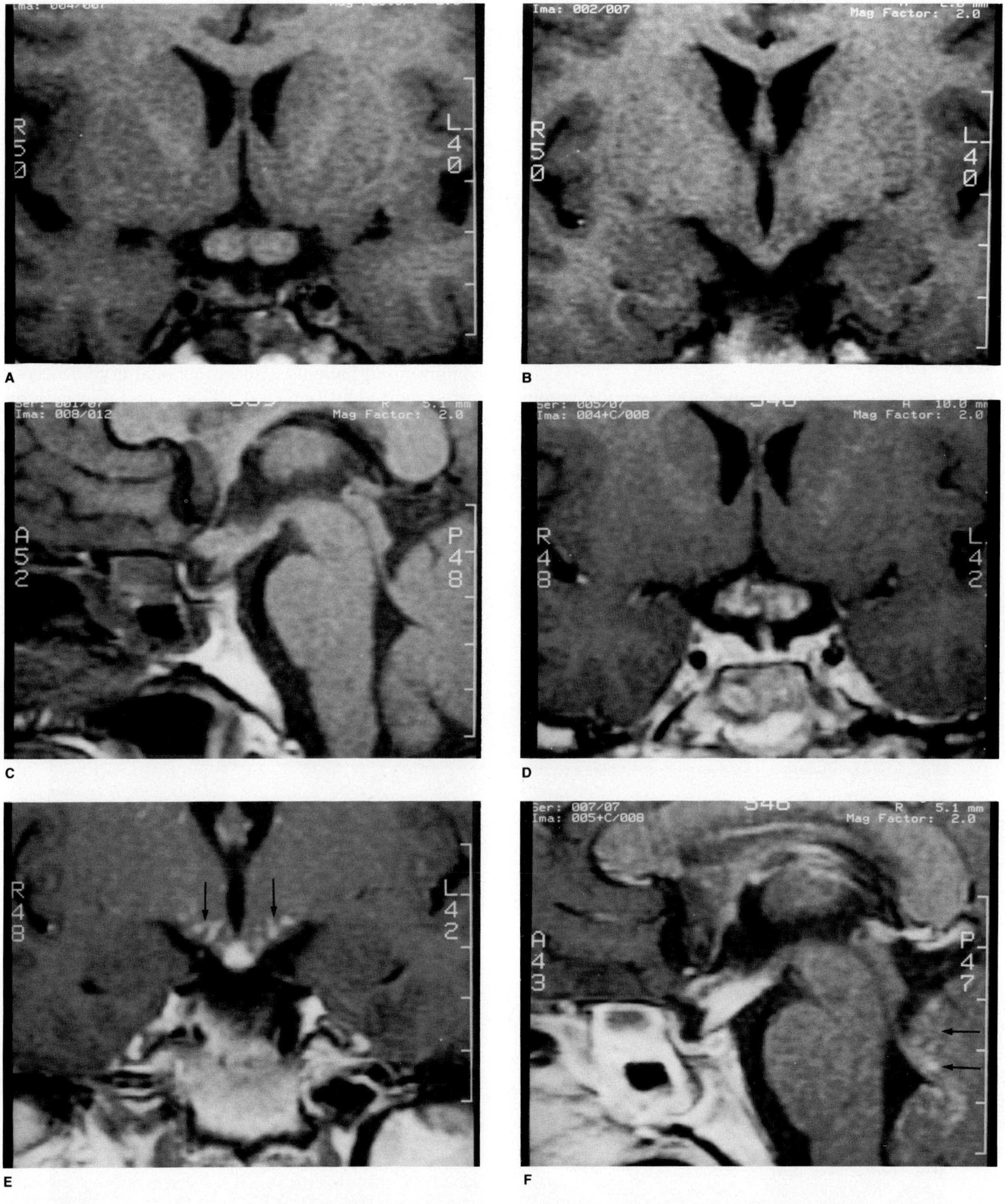

Figure 13-17

CNS sarcoidosis in a 22-year-old woman with panhypopituitarism and loss of vision. **(A–C)** *T1-weighted images show enlargement of the optic chiasm and optic nerves.* **(D)** *The postcontrast coronal T1-weighted image shows intense enhancement of the enlarged optic chiasm.* **(E)** *The postcontrast coronal T1-weighted images show infundibulum enhancement, with extension of the disease through anterior perforated substance into the hypothalamus (arrows).* **(F)** *The postcontrast sagittal T1-weighted image shows enhancement of the enlarged visual pathways and enhancement of the fourth ventricle ependymal lining with extension of the granulomatous process through the cerebellar parenchyma along the Virchow-Robin spaces (arrows).*

FUNGAL INFECTIONS

Fungal infections of the CNS can be classified in two groups:

1. infections caused by a true pathogenic fungus that is able to elicit a disease process in a host who is otherwise healthy, for example, *Paracoccidioides, Blastomyces, Coccidioides,* and *Histoplasma*
2. infections caused by fungus of low pathogenicity in a host whose resistance is impaired by an underlying debilitating condition, the most common opportunistic fungi being *Aspergillus, Candida,* Zygomycetes, *Nocardia,* and *Cryptococcus*

Cryptococcosis

Cryptococcus neoformans is the most common fungus to infect the CNS in the AIDS and non-AIDS population. The usual portal of entry is the lungs. The primary pulmonary infection in most cases seems to be asymptomatic. In terms of relative frequency, it is the third most common cause of CNS infection in AIDS patients, after HIV encephalitis and *Toxoplasma* encephalitis. Approximately 5 percent of AIDS patients develop CNS involvement by this fungus. It involves the CNS most commonly as a meningitis, less often as a focal cryptococcoma. Pathologically, the meningitis can be associated with meningeal thickening and widening of the subarachnoid space by a mucous exudate, but with minimal inflammatory reaction. Fungi can enter the Virchow-Robin spaces and give rise to small cysts or gelatinous pseudocysts within the parenchyma. The basal ganglia, thalami, and substantia nigra are the most frequent sites of these cysts. Both cryptococcoma and focal meningeal lesions can be secondary to hematogenous dissemination. The diagnosis of cryptococcosis is most often made by an India ink preparation of the CSF. Computed tomography scans of patients with intracranial cryptococcosis may show diffuse atrophy, mass lesions, hydrocephalus, and diffuse cerebral edema.[68]

Magnetic resonance imaging findings in 29 immunocompromised patients with intracranial cryptococcosis were reported by Tien et al.[69] They found four patterns of lesions: parenchymal masses, dilated Virchow-Robin spaces, miliary enhancing nodules, and mixed patterns. Within the perivascular space, fungi can proliferate, forming gelatinous masses. On T1-weighted images, the lesions are isointense to slightly hypointense, and hyperintense on T2-weighted images. The blood-brain barrier is not disrupted, so these lesions do not enhance (Fig. 13-18). Magnetic resonance imaging findings of dilated Virchow-Robin spaces are highly suggestive of crypto-

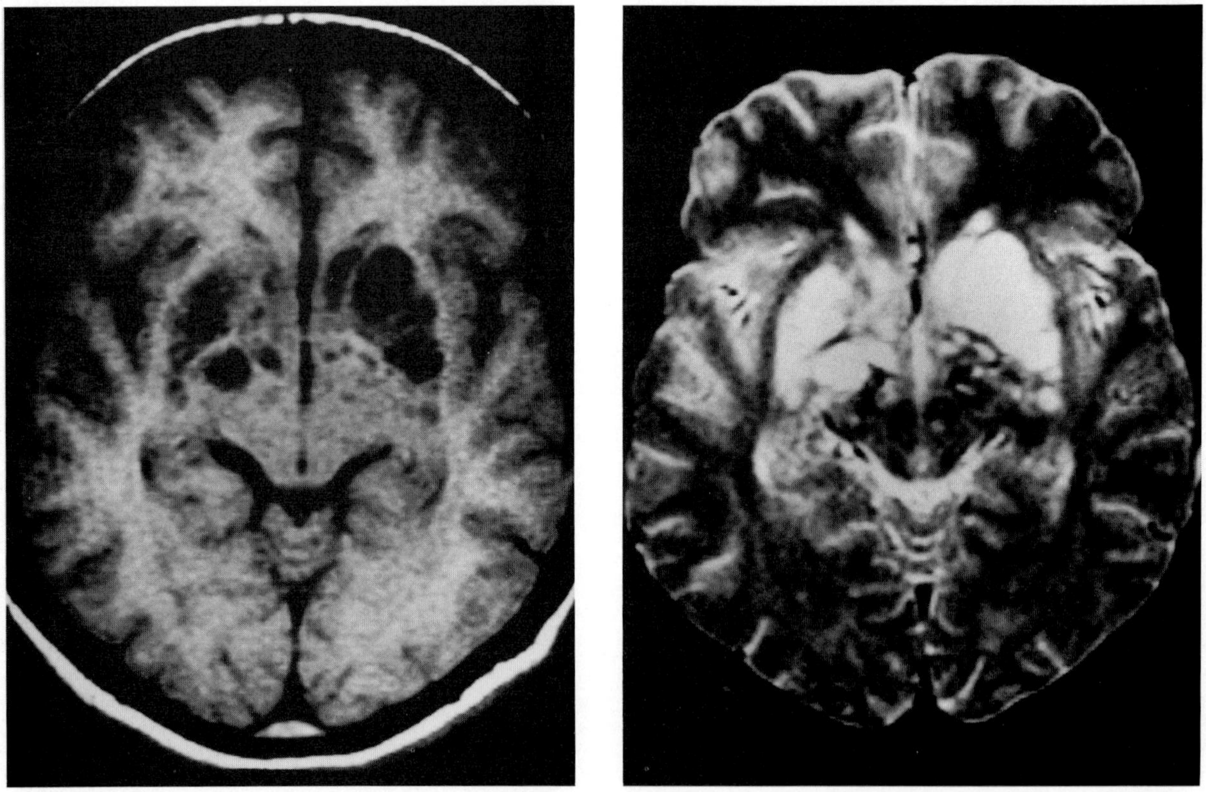

A B

Figure 13-18
Cryptococcosis in a 25-year-old man with meningeal symptoms who is HIV negative. **(A)** *The axial T1-weighted image shows multiple hypointense lesions in the basal ganglia. They did not enhance with gadolinium.* **(B)** *The axial T2-weighted image shows the hyperintense signal of the lesions, associated with perilesional edema.*

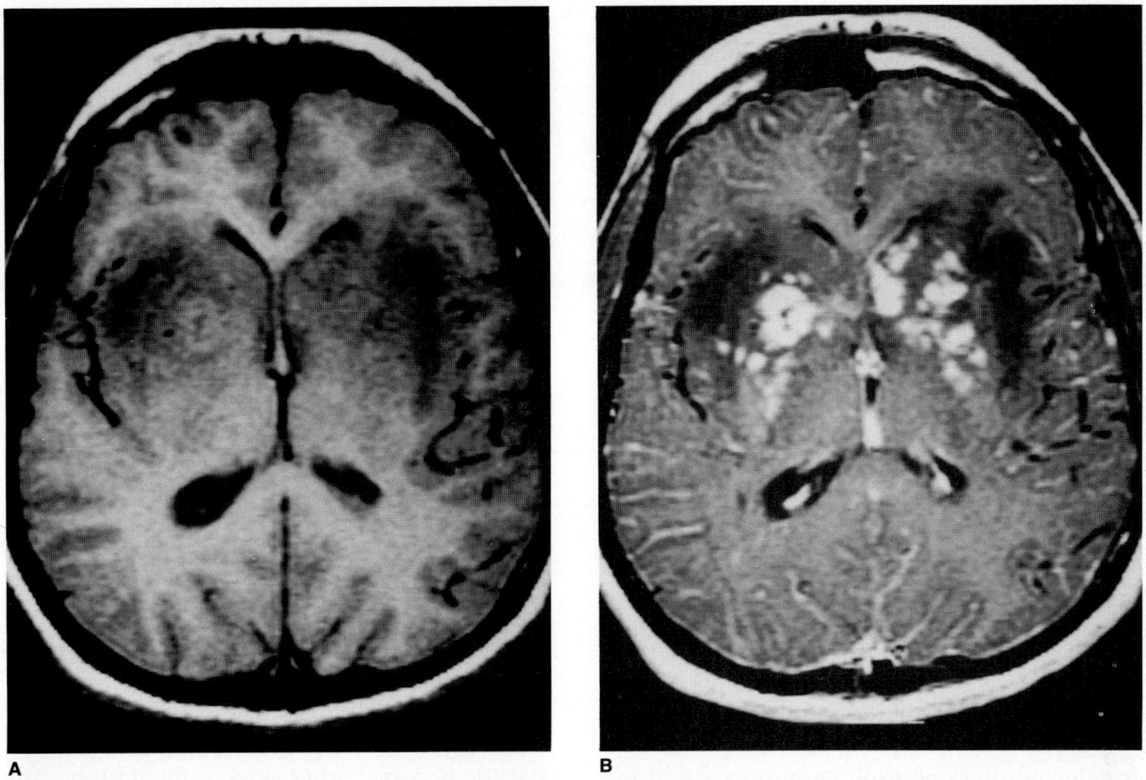

Figure 13-19
Cryptococcosis (the same case presented in Fig. 13-18), with clinical improvement after 4 months of treatment with amphotericin B. **(A)** *In the axial T1-weighted image, the cystic character of the lesion has disappeared, and only the edema is prominent.* **(B)** *The axial postcontrast T1-weighted image shows that the blood-brain barrier has been disrupted with multiple nodular enhancement of the lesions.*

coccosis. Sometimes the lesions can enhance after gadolinium when the blood-brain barrier is disrupted by an inflammatory process caused by treatment-induced lesion of the cryptococcus capsule (Fig. 13-19).[70]

Coccidioidomycosis

Coccidioidomycosis is caused by *Coccidioides immitis.* When inhaled into the lungs, it transforms itself into a spherule that may contain almost 100 endospores. Central nervous system infection results from hematogenous spread of endospores from a pulmonary lesion.

Meningeal involvement is the most common manifestation. Both CT and MRI show marked enhancement in the basal cisterns and meninges following administration of contrast material. Hydrocephalus is a common complication of coccidioidal meningitis. Less commonly, parenchymal enhancing lesions representing granulomas are identified. Infarcts may be seen in areas supplied by small penetrating arteries affected by endarteritis obliterans.[71,72]

Blastomycosis

Blastomycosis is caused by inhalation of *Blastomyces dermatitidis.* It begins as a pulmonary infection. Cutaneous lesions occur in 80 percent of patients. Bone and genitourinary tract are also involved. The CNS is involved in 3 to 10 percent of cases.

Meningitis is the most frequent CNS lesion, followed by intracranial granulomas and spinal epidural granulomas or abscesses. The CT scan and the MRI are described as nonspecific. Solitary granulomas usually present as ring enhancement and perifocal edema.[73]

Histoplasmosis

Histoplasmosis is caused by inhalation of the fungus *Histoplasma capsulatum.* Central nervous system involvement by histoplasmosis is rare except in the disseminated form seen in infants, the elderly, and immunocompromised patients.

There are four forms of CNS involvement: miliary granulomas, leptomeningitis, cerebritis, and spinal cord involvement. Both CT and MRI can show multiple cerebral ring-enhancing lesions associated with multiple spinal cord lesions.[74]

Aspergillosis

Aspergillosis refers to a large group of species only a few of which are pathogenic to humans. *Aspergillus fumigatus* is the species most often recovered from patients with invasive or disseminated infections.

The infection can enter the cranial cavity through the paranasal sinuses, ears, orbits, or hematogenously from the lungs. Disseminated aspergillosis occurs in patients with underlying predisposing conditions. Invasive aspergillosis usually affects the lungs. Erosion into small arteries results in fungal embolization.

The CNS manifestations of aspergillosis are meningitis, meningoencephalitis, abscesses, and granulomas. Computed tomography and MRI may show enhancement of the meninges, secondary hydrocephalus, solid nodules, or ring enhancement. The MRI of the abscess shows a hypointense lesion on T1-weighted images, hyperintense on T2-weighted images, with peripheral edema and ring enhancement.[75] Gupta et al[76] reported a case of an intracranial granuloma that presented as an isointense mass on both T1- and T2-weighted images with a pial vascular rim simulating a meningioma.

Candidiasis

Candida albicans is the species most frequently responsible for candidiasis in humans. This species is part of the normal flora of the gastrointestinal tract and mucocutaneous regions. Physiologic changes by pregnancy, diabetes, or steroid therapy result in an increase in the *Candida* population and predipose these individuals to potential infection. The prolonged administration of antibiotics reduces the normal inhibitory bacterial flora, allowing *Candida* to proliferate. Disruption of cutaneous barriers by burns and wounds, immunosuppression, and neoplasm can lead to candidiasis.

Brain involvement occurs by hematogenous spread late in the course of the generalized disease. The CT and MRI findings include hydrocephalus secondary to leptomeningeal involvement, enhancing nodules with perifocal edema, calcified or enhancing granulomas, signs of infarction and abscesses, hemorrhages, and enhancement of the basal cisterns.[77]

Zygomycosis

Zygomycosis refers to infections caused by a member of the class Zygomycetes. *Mucormycosis* was the term used to designate infections caused by members of the order Murales, which belong to the class Zygomycetes.

Infection is usually acquired by inhalation. Fungi can then invade the epithelial lining of the nasal passages, paranasal sinuses, and bronchi. Acute rhinocerebral zygomycosis is a rapidly progressive infection that has a predilection for diabetics. Reddish-black areas in the turbinate and nasal septum are characteristic. The infection spreads rapidly to the orbit, and intracranial extension may occur through the cribriform plate from the ethmoid sinuses, through the orbital apex, or along the ophthalmic vessels to the cavernous sinus. In the cavernous sinus the fungus may invade the internal carotid artery, producing a mycotic aneurysm and thrombosis. Meningeal or intracerebral infection may occur from direct extension of the orbital or sinus disease or from septic emboli following invasion of the carotid artery. Vascular occlusion leads to ischemia and infarcts.[78]

Computed tomographic manifestations of intracranial zygomycosis reflect the underlying pathologic condition. Nonenhancing hypodense lesions may represent areas of infarction or early abscess formation. Lesions have been reported to enhance homogeneously or peripherally.[79] Cavernous sinus involvement may be suspected by bulging of the lateral margin, and thrombosis of the cavernous sinus results in nonenhancement. Angiographic manifestations include arterial narrowing, mycotic aneurysm, intraluminal fungal thrombosis, and arterial occlusion.[80]

Nocardiosis

Nocardiosis was previously considered a fungal infection, but *Nocardia* is a filamentous bacteria of the order Actinomycetales. Most cases of nocardiosis are pulmonary and result from inhalation of spores. Cerebral involvement is reported in 25 to 33 percent of the cases. Hematogenous brain abscess can occur. Both CT and MRI demonstrate ring enhancement of the cerebral abscesses.[78]

Paracoccidioidomycosis

Paracoccidioidomycosis, also called South American blastomycosis, is a systemic mycosis caused by *Paracoccidioides brasiliensis,* endemic in many countries of South and Central America. The disease affects many organs, including the CNS. Central nervous system involvement is seen in almost 10 percent of the cases and is characterized by a meningeal form, with inflammation of the leptomeninges, predominantly in the skull base, and a pseudotumoral or granulomatous form.[81–83]

We studied five patients with intracranial paracoccidioidomycosis. All patients presented with multiple round or lobulated lesions, iso- or hyperintense in T1-weighted images and predominantly hypointense in T2-weighted images (Fig. 13-20). The lesions were distributed diffusely, with a slight predominance in the supratentorial compartment, although infratentorial lesions were also observed, mainly in the cerebellum. All lesions had ring or nodular contrast enhancement (Fig. 13-21). Three patients were reexamined after treatment, with disappearance of the lesions in two but with persistence of a hypointense area in T2-weighted images.

Magnetic resonance imaging is a good method of demonstrating intracranial granulomata of paracoccidioidomycosis, but a pathologic correlation of the lesions should be performed in order to better understand the multiple appearances of the signal intensity of lesions observed on T1- and T2-weighted images.

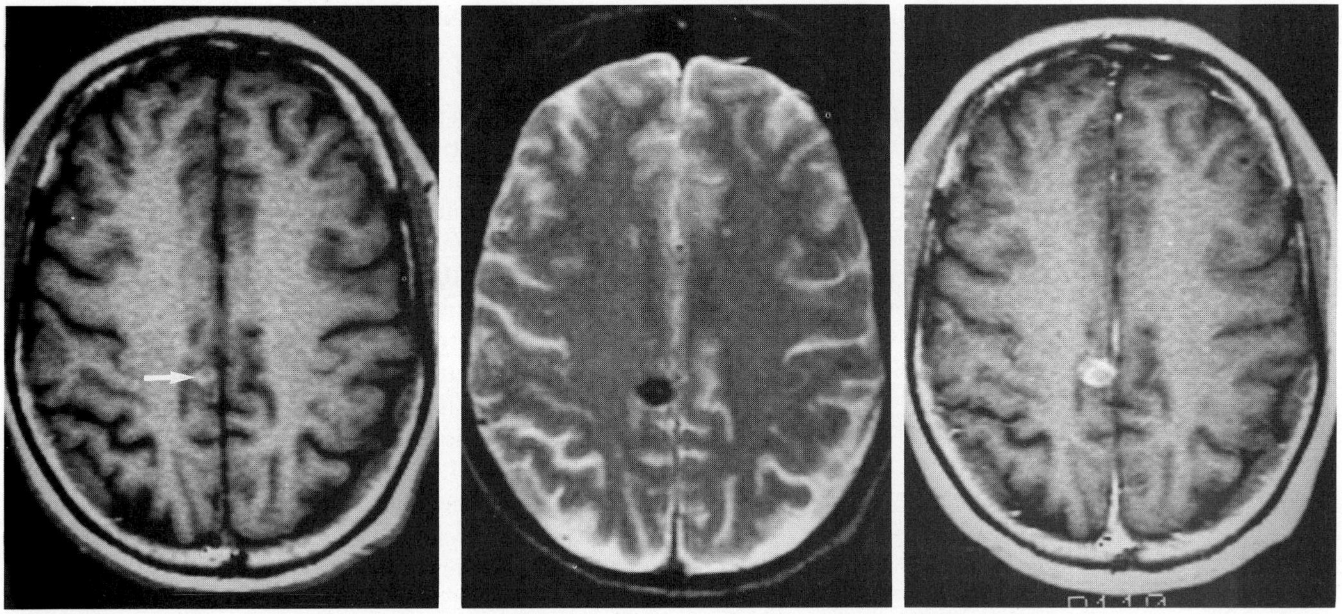

A B C

Figure 13-20

Paracoccidioidomycosis in a 46-year-old man with headache and seizures, and pulmonary paracoccidioidomycosis for 10 years. **(A)** *The axial T1-weighted image shows hyperintense lesions in the right mesial parietal lobe (arrow).* **(B)** *In the axial T2-weighted image, the parietal lesion is homogeneously hypointense. No peripheral edema is seen.* **(C)** *The postcontrast axial T1-weighted image shows irregular enhancement of the lesion.*

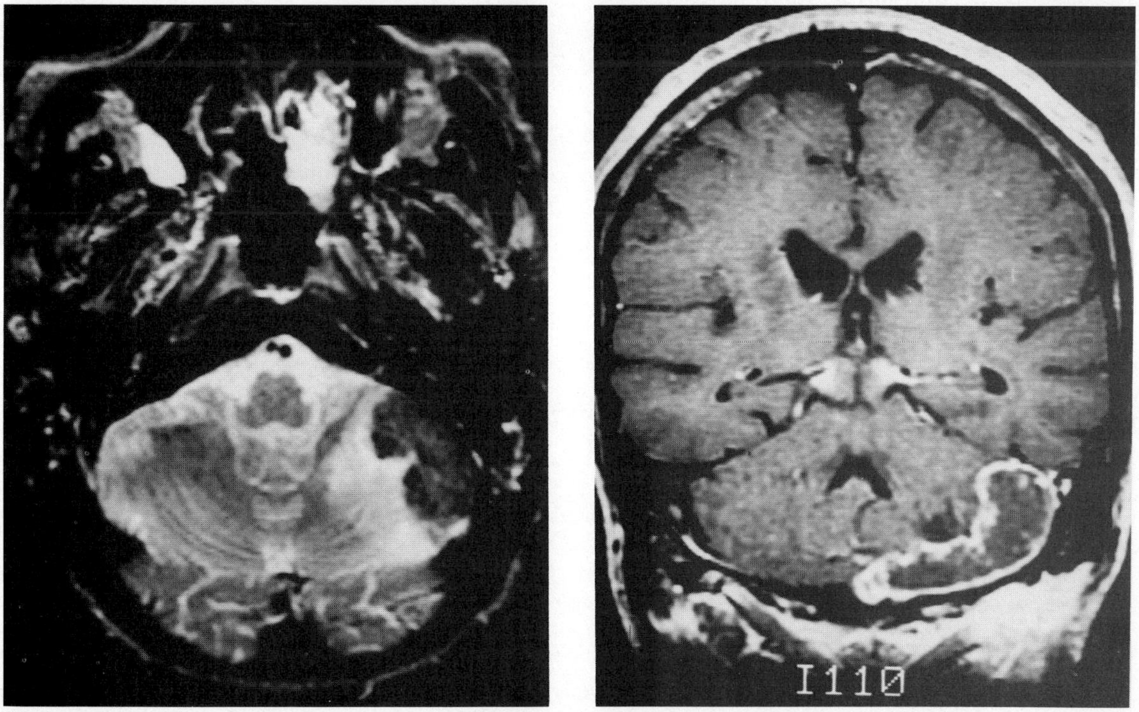

A B

Figure 13-21

Paracoccidioidomycosis in a 60-year-old with cerebellar ataxia. **(A)** *The axial T2-weighted image shows a large hypointense lesion in the left cerebellum, with moderate perilesional edema.* **(B)** *The post-contrast coronal T1-weighted image shows periperipheral enhancement of the lesion.*

PROTOZOAL INFECTIONS

Amebiasis

Cerebral amebiasis includes two distinctive varieties. Primary amebic meningoencephalitis is caused by free-living *Naegleria fowleri* and is usually rapidly progressive and fatal. Secondary amebiasis is caused by hematogenous spread of *Entamoeba histolytica* from the colon, causing brain abscess.

Dietz et al[84] presented a patient with multiple abscesses in the infratentorial and supratentorial compartments, with perifocal edema and partial compression of the fourth ventricle and aqueduct. The MRI and CT scans are not specific and show marked enhancement of the lesions.

Malaria

Malaria is caused by the parasite *Plasmodium falciparum* and can lead to cerebral involvement, with brain edema, vascular congestion, and petechial hemorrhages. Hemorrhage into the white matter in the form of a disseminated vasculomyelopathy is especially common.

The severe stage of malaria develops most often in a patient who has been ill for several days. Cerebral malaria may follow this pattern, or it may occur suddenly with a generalized seizure followed by persistent coma. The differential diagnosis includes bacterial and viral meningitis, encephalitis, and intracranial mass, such as neoplasm, abscess, and tuberculoma.[50]

Trypanosomiasis

American trypanosomiasis, also known as Chagas disease, is caused by infection with *Trypanosoma cruzi,* which is transmitted by the genus *Triatoma.* Acute CNS disease is most commonly a complication of congenital infection. Parasites can be found in the CSF following acute infection at any age, but clinical or pathologic meningoencephalitis is rare. When it occurs, it is usually fatal.[85] Mass lesions of the brain and granulomatous encephalitis Chagas disease have been described.[86] Recently, a number of cases of Chagas disease compromising the CNS have been described in immunosuppressed patients who have undergone organ transplantation and in AIDS patients. In these cases, lesions of the CNS result in the reactivation of a latent infection consequent to the decay of the immunocellular response of the patient.[87,88]

Toxoplasmosis

Imaging in CNS toxoplasmosis is covered in Chap. 14 under AIDS.

METAZOAL INFECTIONS

Cysticercosis

Neurocysticercosis is a parasitic infestation of the CNS caused by the larval stage of the pork tapeworm *Taenia solium.* It is common in some parts of the world (Mexico, Central and South America, eastern Europe, Africa, and Asia). Increased travel to and from endemic areas has resulted in the diagnosis of an increasing number of cases in nonendemic areas.

Humans are the definitive host for *T. solium* and harbor the adult tapeworm in the small intestine (taeniasis). Cysticercosis is acquired when humans inadvertently become the intermediate host by ingesting food or water contaminated with *T. solium* eggs. Oncospheres released from the eggs bore into the bowel wall, enter the circulatory system, and spread systemically. The oncospheres preferentially lodge in neural (CNS), muscular, and ocular tissues, where they develop into cysticerci (bladder larvae).

The pathologic changes of parenchymal cysticercosis have been classified into four stages: vesicular, vesicular colloidal, granular nodular, and nodular calcified. The vesicular stage consists of thin-walled cysts containing CSF-like fluid and a mural nodule, the scolex. In this stage the parasite is alive and incites little or no inflammatory response from the host. The vesicle could be single or multiple, in any localization of the CNS. In a massive infestation, a disseminated form could be present (Fig. 13-22).

When the larva dies, the cyst enters the vesicular colloidal stage. In this stage the cyst begins to shrink, the cyst wall thickens, the cyst fluid becomes turbid and jelly-like, and the scolex begins to calcify. These cyst changes are associated with an increased host inflammatory response. At this time, cyst wall enhancement and surrounding edema can be seen on MRI (Fig. 13-23).[23] The cyst fluid may also appear hyperintense to CSF on MRI.

As the process continues, the cyst becomes contracted and the scolex more calcified. This is the granular nodular stage. The lesion appears isodense to brain on CT, with a hyperdense calcified scolex. On MRI the lesion may be iso- to hypointense with surrounding edema and gadolinium enhancement. The final stage, nodular calcified, occurs when the lesion is totally calcified. The lesion is now only a fraction of its original size, and the inflammatory response has subsided. Surrounding edema and lesion enhancement have disappeared. On CT, calcified foci remain as evidence of the parasitic infestation. The calcified lesions are difficult to detect on MRI and are easily confused with the signal void of vascular structures.[89,90]

The racemose form of cysticercosis, grapelike clusters of cysts or very large cysts with multiple septations,

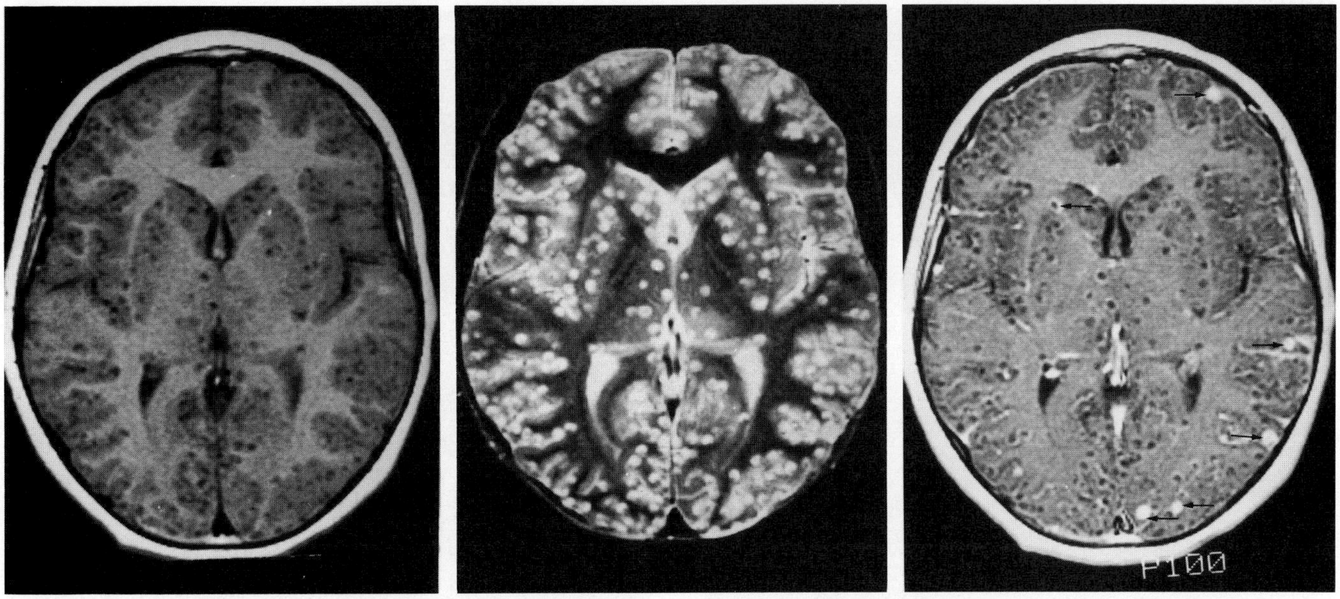

A B C

Figure 13-22

Cysticercosis. Massive recent infestation is seen in a 10-year-old girl. **(A)** *The T1-weighted image shows multiple round low-intensity lesions distributed mainly in the gray matter, including the cerebral cortex, basal ganglia, and thalami.* **(B)** *The T2-weighted image shows hyperintensity of the lesions.* **(C)** *Postgadolinium scans show that only a few lesions enhance with a ring or nodular pattern (arrows).*

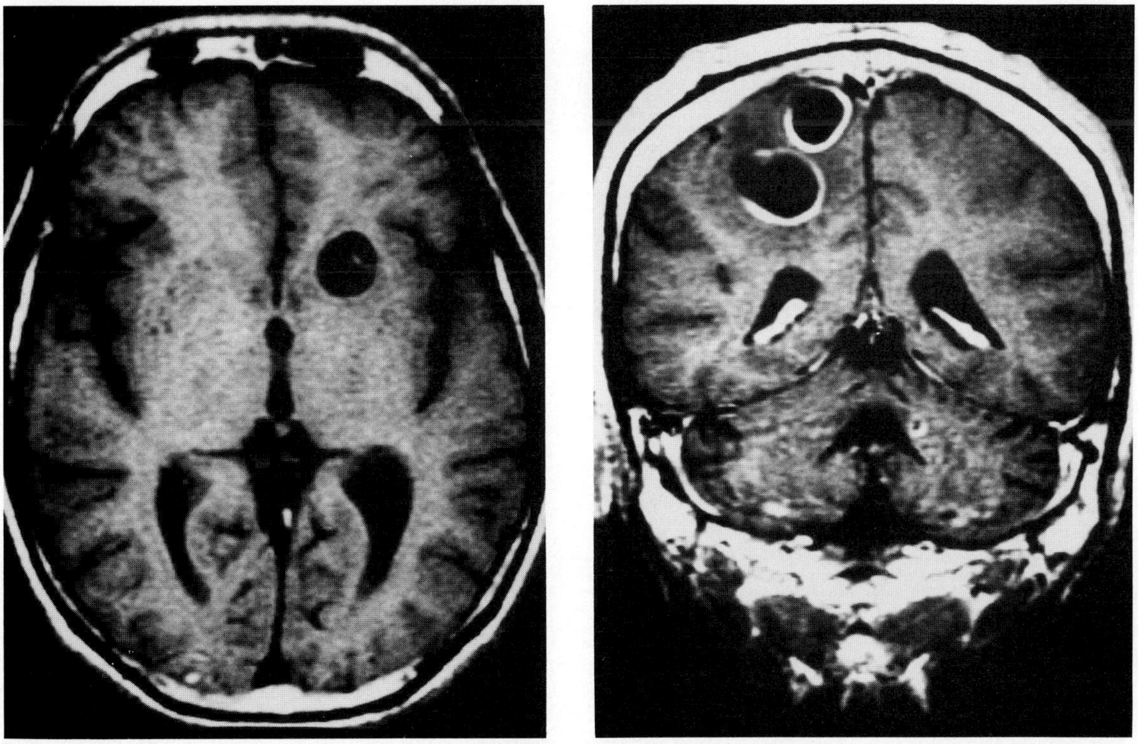

A B

Figure 13-23

Cysticercosis in a 57-year-old man with headache and seizures. **(A)** *The axial T1-weighted image shows a large cystic lesion in the left frontal lobe where the scolex can be seen.* **(B)** *The postcontrast coronal T1-weighted image shows ring enhancement of other lesions in the right parietal area.*

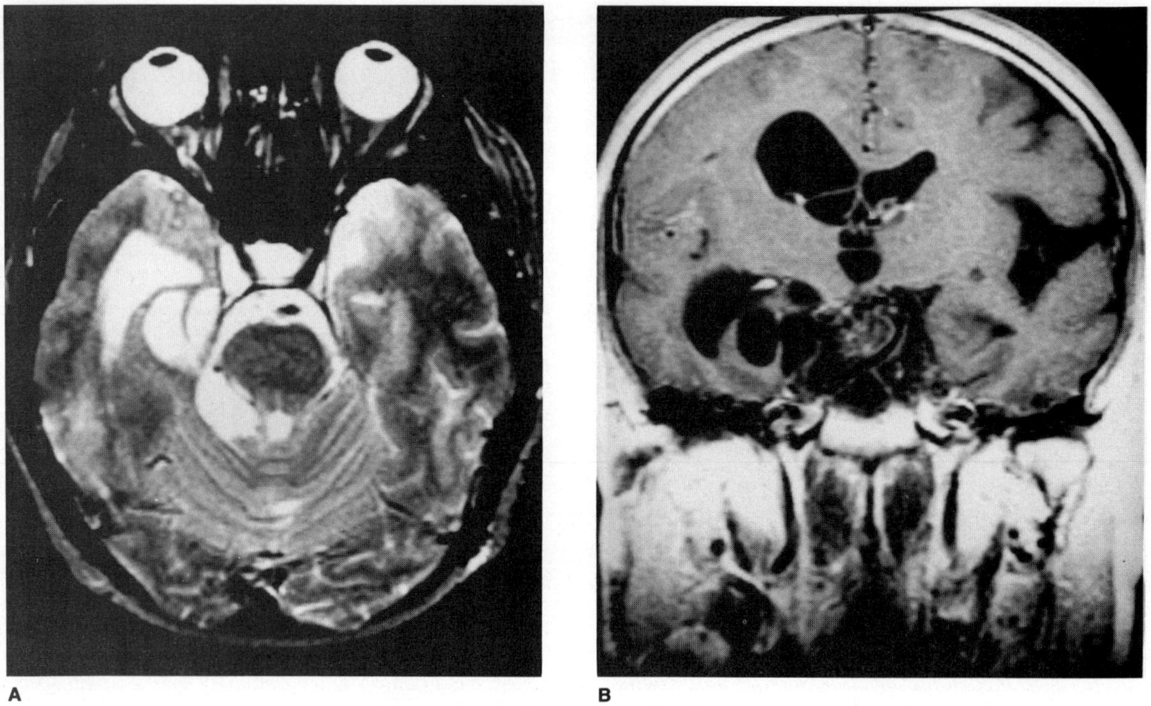

Figure 13-24
Neurocysticercosis, racematous ("malignant") form, in a 52-year-old man with intracranial hypertension. **(A and B)** *Axial T2-weighted and coronal postcontrast T1-weighted images show multiple cystic lesions invading the cisterns, with loculation of the third and lateral ventricles.*

occurs when the parasites lodge in the subarachnoid space or within the ventricles (Fig. 13-24). In these locations the parasites are able to grow larger, since they are not as confined as within the brain parenchyma. Within the ventricles, cysts may be free floating or attached to the ependyma. Racemose cysts often lack scolices and generally are much larger than parenchymal lesions (Fig. 13-25).[91,92]

Subarachnoid lesions are difficult to detect on routine CT examinations. Evidence of subarachnoid lesions includes distortion or enlargement of cisterns and fissures as well as excessive enhancement in these spaces. Computed tomographic ventriculography and cisternography can be used to better demonstrate racemose lesions. With its superior contrast resolution MRI can better detect lesions in the subarachnoid spaces and within the ventricles.[93,94]

Bazan et al[95] studied 40 patients with CT. In this study calcifications were the most frequent parenchymal lesions, followed by cysts, of which 66 percent had visible scolices, and then by enhancing lesions. Fourteen of these 40 patients also had MRI examinations that revealed 13 cysts, of which 46 percent had identifiable scolices, 11 enhancing lesions, and 9 calcifications. Comparing the utility of CT and MRI in the diagnosis of cysticercosis, CT was equivalent to MRI in 8 cases, superior to MR in 5 cases, and inferior to MRI in 1 case. However, MRI was superior to CT at detecting and demonstrating subarachnoid and intraventricular lesions without the need for contrast material. Also, MRI was more sensitive in detecting enhancing lesions. In 7 patients who were examined with both contrast CT and MRI, 10 enhancing lesions were revealed by MRI and 6 by CT. The researchers concluded that MRI was more sensitive in detecting subarachnoid, intraventricular, and enhancing lesions, while CT was superior in demonstrating calcified lesions. In their population of patients, calcifications were a prominent feature of neurocysticercosis. Computed tomography remains their modality of choice for initial imaging of patients with suspected neurocysticercosis.

When the cysticerci are viable, they do not induce an inflammatory response. However, when the cysticerci die, there is a immunologic response that incites an inflammatory reaction, resulting in high intensity in the adjacent brain tissue because of edema and peripheral enhancement of the cyst wall after gadolinium-DTPA (Fig. 13-23).

Echinococcosis

Echinococcosis, also known as hydatid cyst, is caused by *Echinococcus granulosus.* The definitive host is dog and the intermediate host usually sheep but occasionally

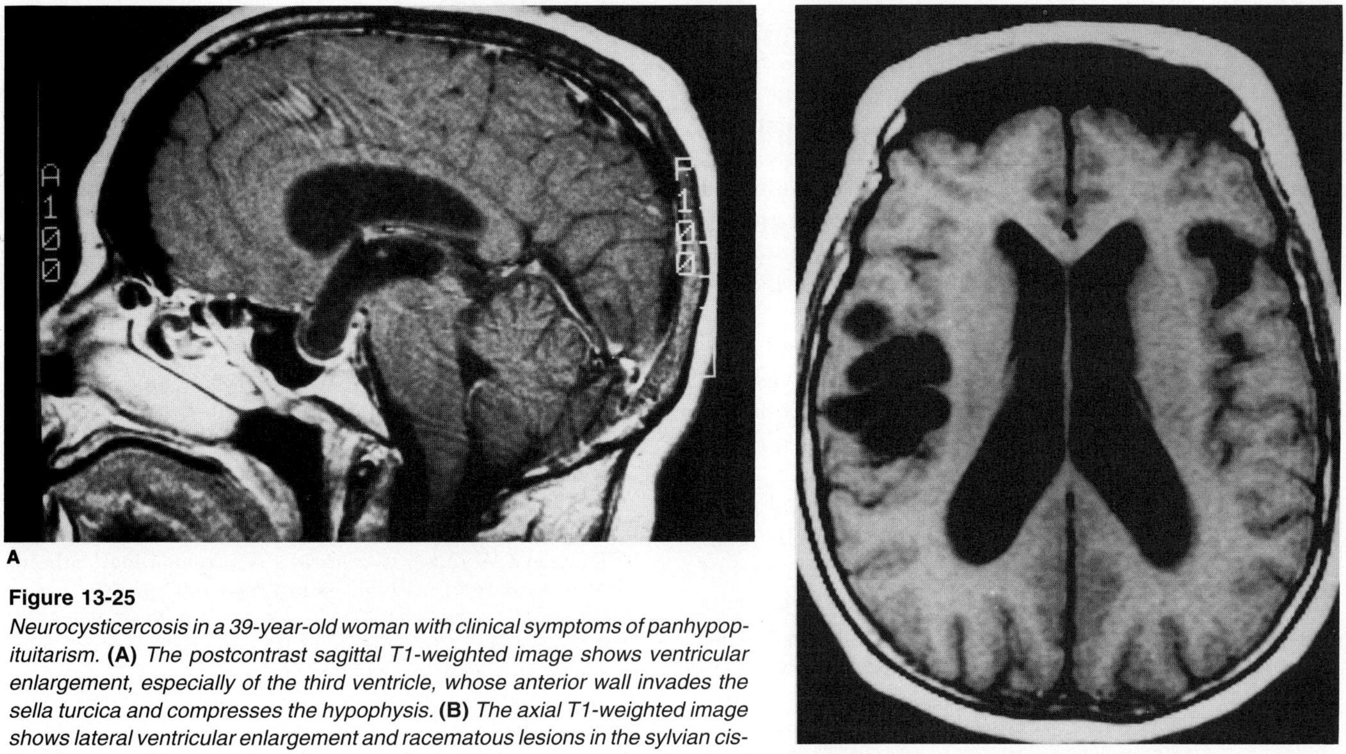

Figure 13-25
Neurocysticercosis in a 39-year-old woman with clinical symptoms of panhypopituitarism. **(A)** *The postcontrast sagittal T1-weighted image shows ventricular enlargement, especially of the third ventricle, whose anterior wall invades the sella turcica and compresses the hypophysis.* **(B)** *The axial T1-weighted image shows lateral ventricular enlargement and racematous lesions in the sylvian cisterns.*

human. The incidence of echinococcosis is highest in sheep-raising countries. The disease occurs by accidental ingestion of contaminated dog feces containing ova of a dog tapeworm. After ingestion, the ova hatch in the gastrointestinal tract, liberating embryos (oncospheres), which enter the circulatory system and are distributed throughout the body. The embryo develops into a cystic larva, which has been called echinococcal or hydatid cyst. Larvae settle in the liver preferentially, with involvement of the lungs, bone, and brain in decreasing order of frequency.

The cerebral infection usually occurs in the cerebral hemispheres, particularly in the parietal lobe. It is usually single and unilobular and may be quite large, up to 10 cm in size. When the cyst in the brain ruptures, it creates an extensive inflammatory reaction associated with eosinophilic leptomeningitis.

The CT features of cerebral hydatid cysts are classified in two groups. In the unilocular cases, the cyst is large, spherical in shape, with sharply defined boards. One side of the cyst wall is very close to the calvarium. The cyst may calcify and may have septa inside. There is no enhancement with contrast media and also no edema surrounding the cyst. In the second group are multiple and small multilocular cysts. The cysts are ovoid or polygonal, like a bunch of grapes, with perifocal edema. After contrast medium administration, there is enhancement in the cyst wall. On MRI, the spherical shape of the cyst is well demonstrated. The contents of the cyst have a signal intensity identical to that of CSF on T1- and T2-weighted images.[96]

Sparganosis

Cerebral sparganosis is a rare disease of the CNS caused by the larval tapeworm. These larvae originate from cestodes of the genus *Spirometra,* which are tapeworms of dogs and cats. The life cycle of these tapeworms is complex because two intermediate hosts are involved. After eggs are shed in the feces of dogs or cats into fresh water, they are infested by the first intermediate host, *Cyclops,* which are minute copepod crustaceans. In this host the proceroid larva develops. Certain vertebrates, including frogs, snakes, and mammals, can become the second intermediate host when they ingest *Cyclops.* In this stage the larvae, known as Spartan, develop. Humans can serve as accidental second intermediate hosts and also be infected by eating uncooked meat of intermediate host animals whose tissue contains Spartan. After reaching the human intestine, the worm's scolex can attach to and penetrate the intestinal wall. At this point, the worm can migrate into the tissues, where it grows back to full size, and produce chronic active granulomatous inflammation. The CT findings include hypodensity, with adjacent ventricular dilatation, irregular or nodular enhancing lesions, and small punctate calcification in the cerebral hemispheres, particularly in the frontal and parietal lobes.[97]

Schistosomiasis

Three species of blood flukes—*Schistosoma haematobium, Schistosoma japonicum,* and *Schistosoma mansoni*—cause human schistosomiasis. Focal granuloma of the brain develop around each egg, which is seeded hematogenously from blood vessels where adults are living. *Schistosoma mansoni* inhabits the inferior mesenteric vein, *S. haematobium* lives in the vein around the bladder, and *S. japonicum* inhabits the superior mesenteric vein.

Central nervous system schistosomiasis usually follows egg migration into the spinal cord or brain vasculature, leading to infarction or granuloma formation. The CT scan reveals many nonspecific enhancing nodules with surrounding edema.

Myelitis is a rare complication of *Schistosoma mansoni* and is characterized by a dramatic involvement of the lower part of the spinal cord. In most cases of transverse myelitis, the CT scan is normal. Magnetic resonance imaging may demonstrate a mild enlargement of the spinal cord, with a hyperintense signal on the midsagittal T1- and T2-weighted images. After intravenous injection of gadolinium, small and heterogeneous areas of intramedullary contrast uptake have been reported (Fig. 13-26).[98,99]

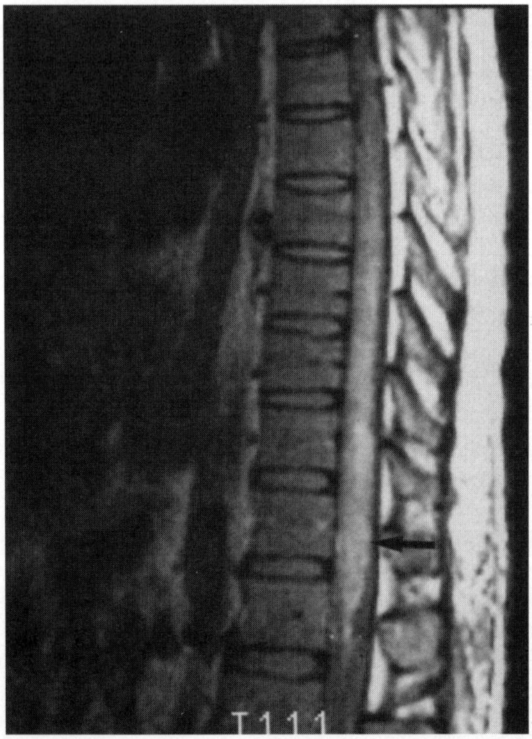

Figure 13-26

Schistosomal myelitis by S. mansoni. *A 35-year-old man with flaccid paraparesis. Postcontrast T1 W1 shows diffuse enhancement of the lower cord and proximal cauda equina, with conus medullaris enlargement (arrow).*

REFERENCES

1. Zimmerman RD: Imaging of intracranial infections, in Scheld WR, Witley RJ, Durack DT (eds): *Infections of the Central Nervous System.* New York, Raven Press, 1991, chap 37, p 442.
2. Bowen BC, Post MJD: Diagnostic imaging of CNS infection and inflammation, in Sclossberg D (ed): *Infections of the Nervous System.* New York, Springer-Verlag, 1990, p 315.
3. Davis LE: Acute viral meningitis and encephalitis, in Kennedy PGE, Johnson RT (eds): *Infections of the Nervous System.* London, Butterworths 1987, p 156.
4. Shoji H, Murakami T, Murai I: A follow-up study by CT and MRI in 3 cases of Japanese encephalitis. *Neuroradiology* 32:215, 1990.
5. Rennels MB: Arthropod-borne virus infections of the central nervous system. *Neurol Clin* 2:241, 1984.
6. Esiri MM, Kennedy PGE: Virus disease, in Adams JH, Duchen LW (eds): *Greenfield's Neuropathology,* 5th ed. New York, Oxford University Press, 1992, p 335.
7. Porras C, Barboza JJ, Fuenzalida E, et al: Recovery from rabies in man. *Ann Intern Med* 85:44, 1976.
8. Roine RO, Hillbom M, Jalle M, et al: Fatal encephalitis caused by a bat-borne rabies related virus. *Brain* 111: 1505–1516, 1988.
9. Whitley RJ, Soong S, Linneman C: Herpes simplex encephalitis. *JAMA* 247:317–320, 1982.
10. Zimmerman RD, Russell EJ, Leeds NE, Kaufman D: CT in the early diagnosis of herpes simplex encephalitis. *AJR* 134:61–66, 1980.
11. Schmidbauer M, Podreka I, Wimberger D: SPECT and MR imaging in herpes simplex encephalitis. *JCAT* 15: 811–815, 1991.
12. Kennedy PGE: Neurological complications of varicellazoster virus, in Kennedy PGE, Johnson RT: *Infections of the Nervous System.* London, Butterworths, 1987, pp 156–176.
13. Caekebeke J, Boudewyn Peters AC, et al: Cerebral vasculopathy associated with primary varicella infection. *Arch Neurol* 47:1033–1035, 1990.
14. Ross MH, Abend WK, Schwartz RB, Samuels MA: A case of herpes zoster with delayed bilateral pontine infarction. *Neurology* 41:1685–1686, 1991.
15. Hilt DC, Buchholtz D, Krumholz A, et al: Herpes zoster ophthalmicus and delayed contralateral hemiparesis caused by cerebral angitis: Diagnosis and management approaches. *Ann Neurol* 14:543–553, 1983.
16. Hollsberg P, Hafler DA: Pathogenesis of diseases induced by human lymphothropic virus type I infection. *N Engl J Med* 328:1173–1181, 1983.
17. Montgomery RD, Cruickshank EK, Robertson WB, McMenemey WH: Clinical and pathological observations on Jamaican neuropathy: A report on 206 cases. *Brain* 87:425–462, 1964.
18. Roman GC: The neuroepidemiology of tropical spastic paraparesis. *Ann Neurol* 23(suppl):S113–S120, 1988.
19. Shibasaki H, Endo C, Kuroda Y, et al: Clinical picture of HTLV-I-associated myelopathy. *J Neurol Sci* 87:15–24, 1988.
20. Roman GC, Vernant J-C, Osame M (eds): HTLV-I and

the nervous system, vol 51 of *Neurology and Neurobiology*. New York, Alan R Liss, 1980, pp 203–207.

21. Jacobson S, Gupta A, Mattson DH, et al: Immunological studies in tropical spastic paraparesis. *Ann Neurol* 27:149–156, 1990.
22. Miller DH, Newton MR, Rudge P, Cruickshank K: Magnetic resonance imaging in HTLV-I antibody positive patients. *Lancet* 2:514, 1987.
23. Rudge P, Ali A, Cruickshank K: Multiple sclerosis, tropical spastic paraparesis and HTLV-I infection in Afro-Caribbean patients in the United Kingdom. *J Neurol Neurosurg Psychiatry* 54:689–694, 1991.
24. Hara Y, Takahashi M, Ueno S, et al: MR imaging of the brain in myelopathy associated with human T-cell lymphotropic virus type I. *JCAT* 12:750–754, 1988.
25. Mattheus WB: Slow virus, in Kennedy PGE, Johnson RT (eds): *Infections of the Nervous System*. London, Butterworths, 1987, pp 227–247.
26. Haddad FS, Risk WS, Jabbour JT: Subacute sclerosing panencephalitis in the Middle East: Report of 99 cases. *Ann Neurol* 1:211–217, 1980.
27. Duda EE, Huttenlocker PR, Patronas NJ: CT of subacute sclerosing panencephalitis. *Am J Neuroradiol* 1:35–38, 1986.
28. Woodard KG, Weinberg PE, Lipton HL: Basal ganglia involvement in subacute sclerosing panencephalitis: CT and MR demonstration. *JCAT* 12:489–491, 1988.
29. Geller TJ, Vern BA, Sarwar M: Focal MRI findings in early SSPE. *Pediatric Neurol* 3:310–312, 1987.
30. Brooks BR, Walker DL: Progressive multifocal leukoencephalopathy. *Neurol Clin* 2:299–313, 1984.
31. Guilleux M-H, Steiner RE, Young IR: MR imaging in progressive multifocal leukoencephalopathy. *Am J Neuroradiol* 7: 1033–1035, 1986.
32. Mark AS, Atlas SW: Progressive multifocal leukoencephalopathy in patients with AIDS: Appearance on MR images. *Radiology* 173:517–520, 1989.
33. Bowen BC, Post MJD: Intracranial infection, in Atlas SW: *Magnetic Resonance Imaging of the Brain and Spine*. New York, Raven Press, 1991, pp 501–538.
34. Prusiner SB: Prions and neurodegenerative diseases. *N Engl J Med* 317:1571–1581, 1987.
35. Palmer MS, Collinge J: Human prion diseases. *Curr Opin Neurol Neurosurg* 5:895–901, 1992.
36. Uchino A, Yoshinaga M, Shiokawa O, et al: Serial MR imaging in Creutzfeldt-Jakob disease. *Neuroradiology* 33: 364–367, 1991.
37. Rasmussen T, Olszewski J, Lloyd-Smith D: Focal seizures due to chronic localized encephalitis. *Neurology* 8:435–445, 1958.
38. McLachlan RS, Girvin JP, Blume WT, Reichman H: Rasmussen's chronic encephalitis in adults. *Arch Neurol* 50: 269–274, 1993.
39. Tien RD, Ashdown BC, Lewis DV Jr, et al: Rasmussen encephalitis: Neuroimaging findings in four patients. *Am J Roentgenol* 158:1329–1332, 1992.
40. Power C, Poland SD, Blume WT, et al: Cytomegalovirus and Rasmussen's encephalitis. *Lancet* 1:1282–1284, 1990.
41. Banna M, El-Ramahi K: Neurologic involvement in Behçet disease: Imaging findings in 16 patients. *Am J Roentgenol* 157:867–872, 1991.
42. Nishimura M, Satoh K, Suga M, Oda M: Cerebral angio and neuro-Behçet syndrome: Neuroradiological and pathological study of one case. *J Neurol Sci* 106:19–24, 1991.
43. Erdem E, Carlier R, Idir ABC, et al: Gadolinium-enhanced MRI in central nervous system Behçet's disease. *Neuroradiology* 35:142–144, 1993.
44. Becker LE: Infections of the developing brain. *Am J Neuroradiol* 13:537–549, 1992.
45. Sugita K, Ando M, Makino M, et al: Magnetic resonance imaging of the brain in congenital rubella virus and cytomegalovirus infections. *Neuroradiology* 33:239–242, 1991.
46. Marques-Dias MJ, Harmant-van-Rijkevorsel G, Landrieu J, Lyon G: Prenatal cytomegalovirus disease and cerebral microgyria: Evidence for perfusion failure, not disturbance of histogenesis, as the major cause of cytomegalovirus encephalopathy. *Neuropaediatrics* 15:18–24, 1983.
47. Wolpert SM, Kaye EM: Intracranial inflammatory processes, in Wolpert SM, Barnes PD: *MRI in Pediatric Neuroradiology*. St Louis, Mosby Year-Book, 1992, pp 151–176.
48. Ogilvy CS, Chapman PH, McGrail K: Subdural empyema complicating bacterial meningitis in a child: Enhancement of membranes with gadolinium on magnetic resonance imaging in a patient without enhancement on computed tomography. *Surg Neurol* 32:138, 1992.
49. Chang KH, Han MH, Roh JK, et al: Gd-DTPA-enhanced MR imaging of the brain in patients with meningitis: Comparison with CT. *Am J Roentgenol* 154:809, 1990.
50. Zimmerman RA: Imaging of intracranial infections, in Scheld MW, Whitley RJ, Durack DT: *Infections of the Central Nervous System*. New York, Raven Press, 1991, pp 887–907.
51. Goldberg HI, Titelbaum DS, Grossman RI, et al: High field MR of brain abscess. *Am J Neuroradiol* 9:1036, 1988.
52. Haimes AB, Zimmerman RD, Morgello S, et al: MR imaging of brain abscesses. *Am J Neuroradiol* 10:279, 1989.
53. Barloon TJ, Yuh WTC, Knepper LE, et al: Cerebral ventriculitis: MR findings. *JCAT* 14:272, 1990.
54. Weingarten K, Zimmerman RD, Becker RD, et al: Subdural and epidural empyemas: MR imaging. *Am J Neuroradiol* 10: 81, 1989.
55. Wallace RC, Burton EM, Barrett FF, et al: Intracranial tuberculosis in children: CT appearance and clinical outcome. *Pediatr Radiol* 21:241, 1991.
56. Jinkins JR: Computed tomography of intracranial tuberculosis. *Neuroradiology* 33:126, 1991.
57. Chang KH, Han MH, Roh JR, et al: Gd-DTPA enhanced MR imaging in intracranial tuberculosis. *Neuroradiology* 32:19, 1990.
58. Villoria MF, de la Torre J, Fortea F, et al: Intracranial tuberculosis in AIDS: CT and MRI findings. *Neuroradiology* 34:11, 1992.
59. Tien RD, Gean-Marton AD, Mark AS: Neurosyphilis in HIV carriers: MR findings in six patients. *Am J Roentgenol* 158: 1325, 1992.
60. Reik L, Smith L, Khan A, Nelson W: Demyelinating encephalopathy in Lyme disease. *Neurology* 32:1302, 1985.
61. Nelson JA, Wolf MD, Yuh WT, Peeples ME: Cranial nerve involvement with Lyme borreliosis demonstrated by magnetic resonance imaging. *Neurology* 42:671, 1992.

62. Miller DH, Kendall BE, Barter S, et al: Magnetic resonance imaging in central nervous system sarcoidosis. *Neurology* 38:378, 1988.
63. Sherman JL, Stern BL: Sarcoidosis of CNS. *Am J Neuroradiol* 11: 915, 1990.
64. Seltzer S, Mark AS, Atlas SW: CNS sarcoidosis: Evaluation with contrast-enhanced MR imaging. *Am J Roentgenol* 158:391, 1992.
65. Liu DPC, Sze G: Intracranial sarcoidosis on gadolinium-enhanced MRI. *Neuroradiology* 33:189, 1991.
66. Engelken JD, Yuh WTC, Carter KD, et al: Optic nerve sarcoidosis: MR findings. *Am J Neuroradiol* 13:228, 1992.
67. Vogl TJ, Stelmmler J, Scriba PC, et al: Sarcoidosis of the hypothalamus and pituitary stalk. *Eur Radiol* 2:76, 1992.
68. Popovich MJ, Arthur RH, Helmer E: CT of intracranial cryptococcosis. *Am J Roentgenol* 154:603, 1990.
69. Tien RD, Chu PK, Hesselink JR, et al: Intracranial cryptococcosis in immunocompromised patients: CT and MR findings in 29 cases. *Am J Roentgenol* 156:1245, 1991.
70. Riccio IJ, Hesselink JR: Gd DTPA enhancement MR of multiple cryptococcal brain abscess. *Am J Neuroradiol* 10: 65, 1989.
71. McGahan JP, Graves DS, Palmer PES, et al: Classic and contemporary imaging of coccidioidomycosis. *Am J Roentgenol* 136: 393, 1981.
72. Wrobel CJ, Meyer S, Johnson RH, et al: MR findings in acute and chronic coccidioidomycosis meningitis. *Am J Neuroradiol* 13:241, 1992.
73. Roos KL, Bryan JP, Maggio WW, et al: Intracranial blastomycoma. *Medicine* 66:224, 1987.
74. Desai SP, Basan C III, Hummell W, et al: Disseminated CNS histoplasmosis. *Am J Neuroradiol* 12:290, 1991.
75. Mikhael MA, Ruschvitch AM, Ciric I: Magnetic resonance imaging of cerebral aspergillosis. *Comput Radiol* 9:85, 1985.
76. Gupta RK, Singh AK, Bishnu P, et al: Intracranial aspergillus granuloma simulating meningioma on MR imaging. *JCAT* 14:467, 1990.
77. Thron A, Wietholter H: Cerebral candidiasis: CT studies in a case of brain abscess and granuloma due to *Candida albicans. Neuroradiology* 23:223, 1982.
78. Bazan II C, Rinaldi MG, Rauch RR, Jinkins JR: Fungal infections of the brain, in Hesselink Jr: *Neuroimaging Clinics of North America.* Philadelphia, Saunders, 1991, pp 57–88.
79. Mikhael MA: Cerebral phycomycosis. *JCAT* 3:417, 1979.
80. Courey WR, New PFK, Price DL: Angiographic manifestations of craniofacial phycomycosis. *Radiology* 103:329, 1972.
81. Nobrega JPS: Micoses do sistema nervoso central. *Arq Bras Neurocirg* 1:157, 1982.
82. Minguetti G, Madalozzo LE: Paracoccidioidal granulomatosis of the brain. *Arch Neurol* 40:100, 1983.
83. Morato-Fernandez RN, Beraldo PPS, Masini M, Costa PHC: Paracoccidioidomicose de localização intramedular e cerebral. *Arq Neuropsiquiatr* 49:192, 1991.
84. Dietz R, Schanen G, Krammann B, et al: Intracranial amebic abscesses: CT and MR findings. *JCAT* 15:168, 1991.
85. Queiroz AC: Tumor-like lesion of the brain caused by *Trypanosoma cruzi. Am J Trop Med Hyg* 22:473, 1973.
86. Pittella JEH: Brain involvement in the chronic cardiac form of Chagas's disease. *J Trop Med Hyg* 88:313, 1985.
87. Monteverde DA, Taratuto AL, Lucatelli N et al: Meningoencefalitis chagasica aguda en pacientes imunossuprimidos. *Ver Neurol Arg* 2:260–266, 1976.
88. Sartori AMC, Shikanai-Yasuda MA, Amato Neto, V et al: Follow-up of 18 patients with HIV infection and chronic Chagas disease, with reactivation of Chagas disease causing cardiac disease in three patients. *CID* 26:177–179, 1998.
89. Lotz J, Hewlett R, Albert B, et al: Neurocysticercosis: Correlative pathomorphology and MR imaging. *Neuroradiology* 30:35, 1988.
90. Martinez HR, Rangel-Guerra R, Elizondo G, et al: MR imaging in neurocysticercosis: A study of 56 cases. *Am J Neuroradiol* 10:1011, 1989.
91. Rodacki MA, Detoni XA, Teixeira WR, et al: CT features of cellulosal and racemous neurocysticercosis. *JCAT* 13: 1013, 1989.
92. Ginier BL, Poirier VC: MR imaging of intraventricular cysticercosis. *Am J Neuroradiol* 13:1247, 1992.
93. Chang KH, Lee JH, Man MH, et al: The role of contrast enhanced MR imaging in the diagnosis of neurocysticercosis. *Am J Neuroradiol* 12:501, 1991.
94. Zee CS, Destian S, Coletti P, et al: Gadolinium-enhanced MR imaging in neurocysticercosis. *Radiology* 177:232, 1990.
95. Bazan C, Ripeckyj G, Kagen-Hallet: Neurocysticercosis CT and MR imaging. Paper presented at 76th Annual Meeting of the Radiological Society of North America, Chicago, December 1989.
96. Demir K, Karsli AF, Kaya T, et al: Cerebral hydatid cysts. *Neuroradiology* 33:22, 1991.
97. Chang KH, Chi JG, Cho SY, et al: Cerebral sparganosis: Analysis of 34 cases with emphasis on CT features. *Neuroradiology* 34:1, 1992.
98. Dupuis MJM, Atrouni S, Dooms GC, et al: MR imaging of schistosomal myelitis. *Am J Neuroradiol* 11:782, 1990.
99. Silbergleit R, Silbergleit R: Schistosomal granuloma of the spinal cord: Evaluation with MR imaging and intraoperative sonography. *Am J Roentgenol* 158:1351, 1992.

CHAPTER 14

THE ACQUIRED IMMUNODEFICIENCY SYNDROME

Joseph R. Berger
M. Judith Donovan Post
Robert M. Levy

SPECTRUM OF NEUROLOGIC DISEASES

The frequency with which neurologic disease complicates human immunodeficiency virus (HIV) infection probably exceeds 50 percent. In retrospective studies from San Francisco[1] and New York,[2] the incidence of neurologic complications occurring in association with AIDS was 39 and 41 percent, respectively. A study from south Florida detected neurologic illness in 63 percent of 132 patients with AIDS.[3] Autopsy studies reveal a substantially higher frequency of neurologic disease.[4] It is not uncommon to find that neurologic disease heralds HIV infection. The frequency with which neurologic disease is the harbinger of AIDS ranges from 10[5] to 20 percent.[3] Most commonly, neurologic disease occurs in the setting of advanced immunosuppression.

The spectrum of neurologic disease that complicates HIV is extremely broad. Any part of the neuraxis may be affected. These illnesses can be classified into those that are believed to be the direct result of involvement of the nervous system by HIV and those that result chiefly from the associated immunologic abnormalities.[6] The former include HIV-1-associated cognitive and/or motor disorders (AIDS dementia complex), HIV-associated myelopathy, HIV-associated peripheral neuropathy, and an HIV-related inflammatory myopathy. Although the latter category of disease is most often the consequence of HIV-induced cellular immunosuppression, it may arise in the absence of significant immunologic embarassment. As a general rule, the most common illnesses are infectious diseases, such as cerebral toxoplasmosis and cryptococcal meningitis. However, opportunistic infections are not the sole cause of neurologic disability in this category. Other causes of neurologic complications of HIV infection include primary and metastatic neoplasms, cerebrovascular disease, metabolic-nutritional disorders, and the neurotoxicity of drug therapy. A representative list of the more common neurologic complications may be found in Table 14-1.

The most important diagnostic utility of radiographic imaging with respect to the neurologic disease associated with AIDS, whether evaluating the brain or spine, is to determine whether there is a focal mass lesion. Distinguishing whether a mass lesion is present has significant implications both diagnostically and therapeutically.[7,8] Therefore, in discussing the neuroimaging of HIV infection, intracranial processes have been divided into those that are associated with focal mass effect versus those that are nonfocal and non-mass producing. Processes involving the spinal cord and nerve roots are considered separately but may also be classified similarly. A categorization by the typical nature of the lesions associated with some of the more commonly en-

Table 14-1
Neurological complications of HIV infection

Direct manifestations of HIV infection
HIV encephalopathy (AIDS dementia complex)
Vacuolar myelopathy
HIV-associated peripheral neuropathy
HIV-associated inflammatory myopathy
Indirect manifestations of HIV infection
Opportunistic infections
Toxoplasmosis encephalopathy
Cryptococcal meningitis
Tuberculous meningitis, brain abscess, and tuberculoma
Cytomegalovirus encephalitis
Progressive multifocal leukoencephalopathy
Neurosyphilis
Tumors
Primary CNS lymphoma
Gliomas*
Metastatic tumors
Kaposi's sarcoma
Cerebrovascular disease
Ischemic stroke
Hemorrhagic stroke
Transient ischemic attacks
Metabolic-nutritional disorders
Wernicke's encephalopathy
Vitamin B_{12} deficiency
Malnutrition
Drug neurotoxicity
Peripheral neuropathy secondary to didanosine (ddI)
Peripheral neuropathy secondary to zalcitabine (ddC)
Mitochondrial myopathy secondary to zidovudine

*Possible increased association with HIV infection.

Table 14-2
Intracranial lesions in HIV infection

I. Intracranial mass lesions
  A. Infections
    1. Toxoplasma encephalitis
    2. Tuberculous abscess
    3. Pyogenic abscess
    4. Syphilitic gumma
    5. *Candida* abscess
    6. *Nocardia* abscess
    7. Cryptococcoma
    8. Other
  B. Neoplasms
    1. Lymphoma
    2. Kaposi's sarcoma
  C. Cerebrovascular lesions
    1. Infarction
    2. Hemorrhage
II. Intracranial lesions usually without significant mass effect
  A. Infections
    1. Parenchymal
      a. PML
      b. HIV
      c. CMV
    2. Meningeal
      a. Fungal (e.g., *cryptococcus, candida*)
      b. Mycobacterial
      c. Bacterial (e.g., *Escherichia coli, T. pallidum*)
      d. Viral (e.g., HIV)
  B. Neoplasm
    1. Meningeal (e.g., lymphoma)

Source: Adapted from MJD Post, "Neuroimaging of HIV," 45th meeting of the American Academy of Neurology, New York, June 1993.

countered diseases of the brain and spine in patients with AIDS is provided in Tables 14-2 and 14-3.

IMAGING MODALITIES

Either magnetic resonance imaging (MRI) or computed tomography (CT) scanning is effective in determining the presence of a central nervous system (CNS) mass lesion. Both imaging modalities can detect focal mass lesions in the brain or spine, especially when aided by intravenous or intrathecal contrast material, respectively.[9] The use, following plain CT, of the double-dose delayed contrast-enhancement technique maximizes the detection of multiple enhancing lesions in the brain,[10] while the employment of intrathecal contrast material will aid in the display on CT of focal epidural and intramedullary spinal canal masses.[11] These findings on either CT or MRI are helpful in determining the patient's management, type of treatment, and response to therapy. When both imaging modalities are equally available, MRI is the preferred study to use in initiating the patient's evaluation for several reasons,[7,12–16] including (1) its noninvasive nature, (2) its superior contrast resolution, and (3) its multiplanar capabilities. Its sensitivity in detecting abnormal signal in intracranial or intraspinal soft tissue lesions, even in the absence of changes in size or configuration, renders it especially well suited for detecting non-mass-producing lesions. Furthermore, the sensitivity of MRI in detecting increased amounts of water make it ideal for ascertaining the edema caused by neoplasms, inflammatory lesions, or infarction and for detecting certain types of acute infection.[17,18] Increased water content results in a prolongation of T1 and T2 relaxation values and can readily be detected in either the brain or spine as areas of abnormal low-intensity signal on T1-weighted images and high-intensity signal on T2-weighted images.[9] Fluid-attenuated inversion-recovery (FLAIR) sequences appear to be superior to T2-weighted fast spin-echo images for detecting small lesions, lesions in the cortical and/or subcortical regions, and deep white matter lesions in AIDS-related brain diseases, particularly in patients with HIV encephalitis and progressive multifocal leukoencephalopathy.[19] Images obtained with FLAIR appear to be especially useful in detecting lesions adjacent to cerebrospinal fluid (CSF) spaces.[19] Potential pitfalls with FLAIR include CSF flow and misregistration artifacts, increased fat signal, decreased sensitivity to the detection of low-signal lesions, and lack of white matter tract detail.[20]

Table 14-3
Spinal lesions with HIV infection

I. Mass lesions
  A. Infection
    1. Epidural
      a. Pyogenic epidural abscess in parenteral drug abusers
      b. Tuberculous abscess
      c. Fungal abscess
      d. Miscellaneous
  B. Neoplasm
    1. Epidural
      a. Lymphoma
      b. Plasmacytoma
    2. Intramedullary
      a. Lymphoma
II. Spinal lesions usually without significant mass effect
  A. Infection
    1. Meningeal
    2. Intramedullary
      a. HIV
      b. PML
      c. CMV
      d. Others
  B. Neoplasm
    1. Meningeal
      a. Lymphoma

Source: Adapted from Post.[9]

The administration of intravenous paramagnetic contrast material, such as gadoliniumDTPA (gadopentate dimeglumine, MagnevistR, Berlex Pharmaceutical, Cedar Knolls, NJ)[12,21] increases the sensitivity of MRI in detecting intracranial and intraspinal lesions in HIV-infected patients. Similar to iodinated contrast material with CT scanning, the paramagnetic contrast material used with MRI accumulates in lesions that have an altered blood-brain-cord-barrier. Since paramagnetic contrast material shortens T1 relaxation values, parenchymal, subependymal, and meningeal lesions will appear bright on T1-weighted.[9] The lesions, whether mass producing or not, are more readily detected after paramagnetic contrast administration and distinguished with greater facility from adjacent edema and from normal structures.

In addition to providing anatomic information, MRI also provides both physiologic and biochemical information without resorting to invasive techniques. Examples of such techniques include (1) cardiac-gated cineflow MRI protocol, which employs gradient-recalled images in various portions of the patient's cardiac cycle, used to obtain physiologic information about obstruction to the ventricular and subarachnoid pathways;[12,22] (2) MRI angiography and MRI venography, which employ three-dimensional time-of-flight technique to detect vascular occlusions, aneurysms, and large vessel arteritis;[12] (3) diffusion-weighted MRI; and (4) MRI proton spectroscopy MRS), performed to detect biochemical abnormalities in HIV infection, such as decreased *N*-acetylaspartate (NAA) and changes in choline and creatine levels. A correlation exists between levels of NAA and neuronal integrity and between levels of choline and white matter disorders. In addition to its value in determining the pathogenetic abnormalities in HIV encephalitis,[23] proton MRS has been applied to the diagnosis of focal brain lesions in AIDS with some success.[24]

If contraindications to the performance of MRI exist (e.g., cardiac pacemaker, metallic clips, etc.), the procedure is not readily available, or additional complementary information is needed following a MRI study, other imaging modalities can be employed. A CT scan can also detect intacranial and intraspinal mass lesions and offers the advantage of depicting bony structures to excellent advantage because of its high spatial resolution. In this respect, it remains superior to MRI. Similarly, CT scanning is also better at detecting calcifications and acute hemorrhage, often indiscernible or difficult to appreciate on MRI.

While lacking the anatomic detail of MRI and CT, nuclear medicine studies have the advantage of being able to produce both physiologic and metabolic information. Single photon emission computed tomography (SPECT) using technetium 99m-hexamethylpropyleneamine oxime (HMPAO) allows for the identification of focal deficits in cerebral perfusion, and SPECT imaging with thallium201 (^{201}Th) may distinguish between intracranial neoplasm and infection, since intense focal uptake occurs on early and delayed images in lymphomas but not in inflammatory lesions.[25–27]

FOCAL INTRACRANIAL LESIONS

Focal neurologic disturbances, such as hemianopsia, hemiparesis, and hemianesthesia, occurring with HIV infection may result from a variety of lesions affecting the cerebrum. These lesions can be broadly classified, in order of frequency, as opportunistic infections, tumors, and cerebrovascular disease. The most common opportunistic infections in this category are toxoplasmosa encephalitis and progressive multifocal leukoencephalopathy (PML) lymphomas, although other primary CNS tumors and metastatic tumors have been reported. In the HIV-infected patient with focal neurologic signs, either a cranial MRI with gadolinium or a double-dose, delayed brain CT is mandated.

Lesions with Mass Effect

The most common causes of focal intracranial mass lesion in HIV infection are toxoplasma encephalitis followed in frequency by lymphoma.[2] The relative frequencies of these two causes of AIDS-associated intracranial mass lesions vary with the relative frequency of latent toxoplasmosis infection in the resident populations. Less common causes of intracranial lesions with mass effect are pyogenic abscess, syphilitic gumma, *candida* abscess, nocardia abscess, cryptococcoma and cryptococcal pseudocysts, and vascularocclusive lesions.[7] Cerebral aspergillosis[28] and mucormycosis[29] have also been reported with AIDS. Cysticercosis cysts,[30] *Trypanosoma cruzi* meningoencephalitis,[31] and granulomatous amebic encephalitis[32] have been observed in patients who had previously resided or currently reside in endemic areas. Whether these latter infections are coincidental or truly occur in increased relative numbers in association with HIV infection remains uncertain.

Toxoplasma Encephalitis

In most populations, *Toxoplasma gondii* is the most common cause of intracranial mass lesion occurring in association with HIV infection.[33,34] In a study from San Francisco, cerebral toxoplasmosis occurred in 28 percent of patients with AIDS[2] and, in a combined clinicopathologic series from Miami,[3] it accounted for 40 percent of all identified neurologic illnesses. At autopsy, between 10[35] and 30 percent[36] of AIDS patients have cerebral toxoplasmosis. Approximately 25 to 50 percent of AIDS patients who are seropositive for *T. gondii* will ultimately develop toxoplasmosis encephalopathy.

Toxoplasma gondii is an obligate intracellular parasite that is found worldwide in mammals. Humans typi-

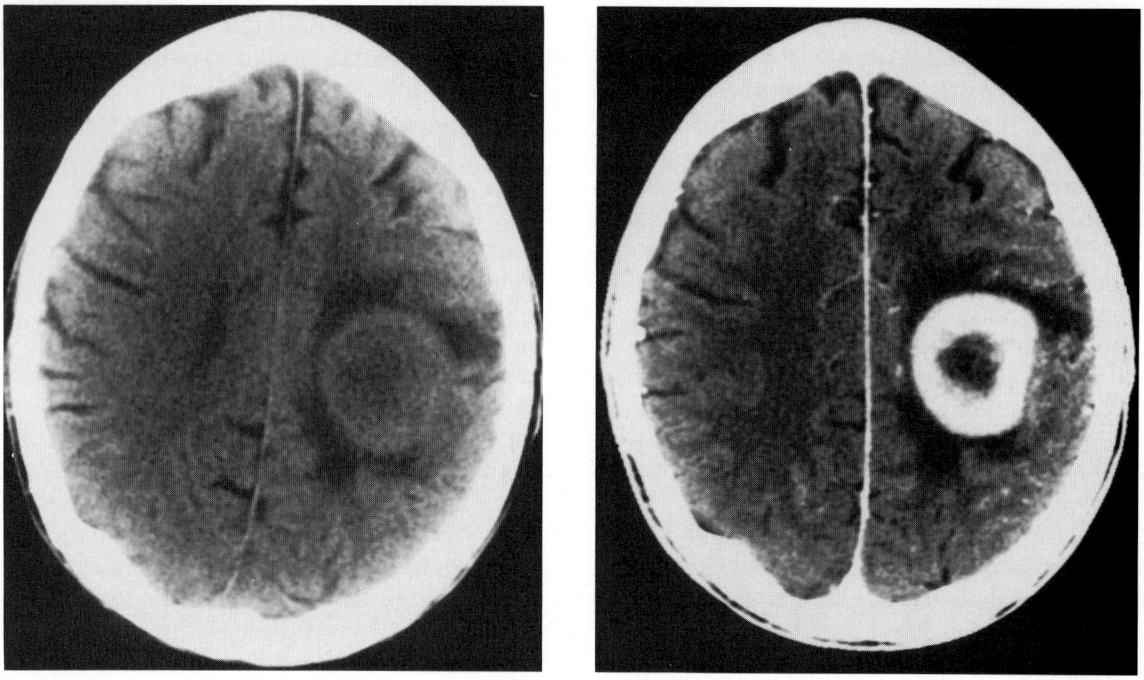

A B

Figure 14-1
Toxoplasmosis. **(A)** *Plain CT scan demonstrates a large lesion in the left frontoparietal lobe with surrounding edema.* **(B)** *CT scan with contrast demonstrates ring enhancement of the lesion.*

cally become infected after the ingestion of raw or undercooked meat that contains tissue cysts of the organisms or by the ingestion of oocysts released by infected cats, the normal host for this parasite.[37] Following the acute infection, the parasite assumes a latent form (tissue cysts containing bradyzoites). With a decline in cell-mediated immunity, these tissue cyts reactivate and rupture, resulting in the release of invasive trophozoites (tachyzoites). In almost all instances, toxoplasma encephalitis in AIDS patients represents a recrudence of infection rather than a newly acquired infection.[38] The presenting neurologic symptoms and signs in HIV-infected individuals with toxoplasma encephalitis are focal in nature, often superimposed on a global encephalopathy, and develop subacutely, usually over a period of 1 to 2 weeks. A prodrome of fever and malaise for several days to weeks before the onset of the neurologic illness is not uncommon.[39] Mild hemiparesis is the most common focal finding.[39] Brainstem and cerebellar involvement, seizures, confusion, and headache are also observed.[39] On rare occasion, cerebral toxoplasmosis may present as a global encephalopathy without significant focal findings.[40] The appearance of chorea in AIDS patients is believed to be virtually pathognomonic of toxoplasmosis.[41]

Pathologically, the lesions in toxoplasma encephalitis are unencapsulated and have three distinct zones.[42–45] A central zone composed of a solid and coagulated avascular necrotic center contains few organisms. The intermediate zone is characterized by an intense inflammatory reaction and numerous free extracellular and intracellular tachyzoites and few encysted forms. The peripheral zone contains more encysted forms and fewer free tachyzoites. The pathologic diagnosis can be

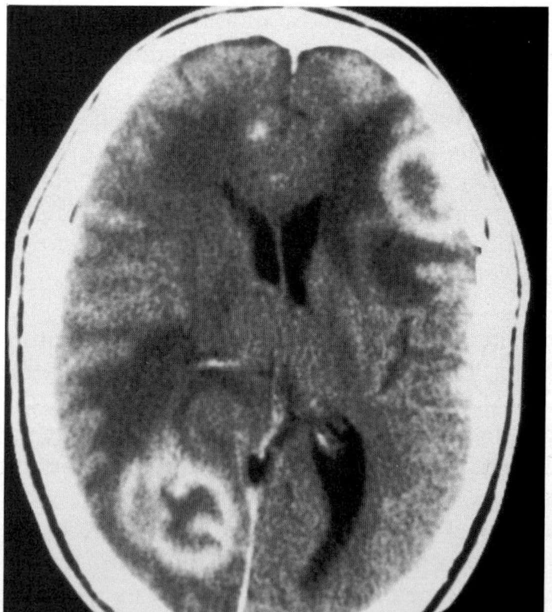

Figure 14-2
Toxoplasmosis. Double-dose delayed CT scan shows multiple ring enhancing lesions with accompanying edema.

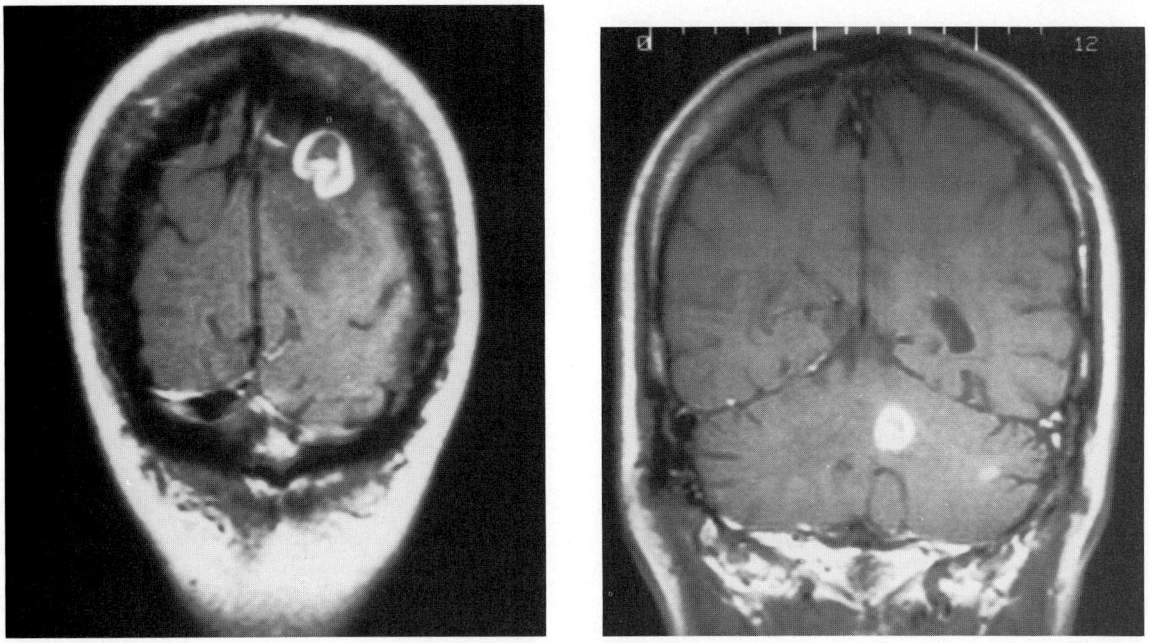

A B

Figure 14-3
Toxoplasmosis. **(A)** *MR with contrast showing ring enhancing lesion of the parietal lobe (From Post.[9] Used by permission.)* **(B)** *MR with contrast in the same patient as #3A showing nodular enhancement in the cerebellum (From Rovira et al.[8] Used by permission.)*

established by hematoxylin and eosin staining, but is best supplemented by Giemsa or immunoperoxidase stains.[42–45]

Cerebral lesions due to toxoplasma encephalitis appear as ring and/or nodular enhancing focal lesions with surrounding edema and mass effect[7,10,44] by both CT (Figs. 14-1 and 14-2) and MRI (Figs. 14-3 and 14-4). In our experience, single lesions are not infrequent with toxoplasmosis encephalopathy. Porter and Sande[46] observed isolated lesions in 27 percent of cases on CT scan and in 14 percent on MRI. However, toxoplasmosis encephalopathy more commonly affects multiple sites. The lesions are most frequently encountered at the corticomedullary junction and in the basal ganglia.[10] Next, in descending order of frequency, lesions are most commonly observed in the frontal lobe, basal ganglia, parietal lobe, occipital lobe, temporal lobe, cerebellum, centrum semiovale, and thalamus.[46] While typically over 1 cm in size, they can vary from under 5 mm to over 3 cm. On plain MRI, the lesions, especially those that are not large, may appear on T2-weighted images as nodular lesions isointense to gray matter silhouetted by the high-intensity signal of the surrounding edema.[9] On noncontrast MRI, large lesions may appear as an inhomogeneous signal.

Distinction of toxoplasma encephalitis from other focal mass lesions that occur in HIV-infected patients is not possible by either the clinical examination or by the MRI or CT scan, since neither imaging nor clinical findings are pathognomonic.[10] While the clinical symptoms may suggest an acute lesion with focal mass effect, they are nevertheless nonspecific. Serum titers for toxoplasma are not infrequently falsely negative.[46] A ^{201}Th SPECT scan may help in excluding alternative diagnostic possibilities, particulary lymphoma.[27,43,44] The resolution of lesions on serial MRI or CT scans following

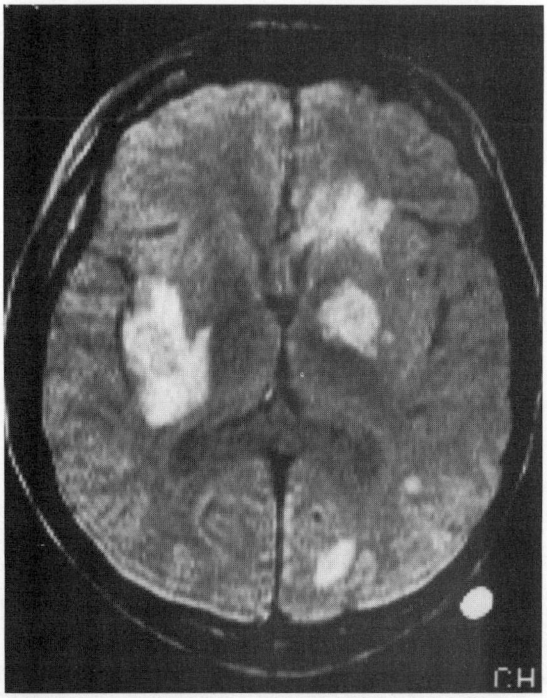

Figure 14-4
Toxoplasmosis. Proton density study showing multiple lesions.

the institution of antitoxoplasmosis therapy is extremely helpful in establishing the diagnosis of toxoplasma encephalitis. Alternatively, in the absence of substantial clinical and radiographic improvement with appropriate therapy, brain biopsy is required.

Establishing the diagnosis of toxoplasma encephalitis from an imaging standpoint requires a definite decrease in the number and size of the enhancing lesions[7,10] during 2 to 3 weeks of medical therapy (Fig. 14-5). A decrease in the amount of edema and mass is expected. Further time interval scans without and with contrast material will show a progressive decrease in the size and number of enhancing lesions and their eventual resolution. On long-term follow-up scans, calcifications, encephalomalacia, and focal atrophy may be seen at some of the sites of healed toxoplasma encephalitis, while at other sites there may be complete resolution of the lesions.

Essential to the interpretation of the radiographic images is determining whether the patient is on corticosteroid therapy.[7] Administration of corticosteroids may result in a seeming resolution of the lesions, whether due to toxoplasma encephalitis or some other pathologic process, due to their salutory effect on edema, mass effect, and contrast enhancement.

In addition, the proper interpretation of the interval images requires that similar scanning techniques are used and that similar amounts of contrast material are given on the follow-up studies. It is important to routinely obtain plain scans prior to the administration of the contrast material in order to distinguish enhancing lesions on CT from fresh hemorrhage or from calcifications. Hemorrhage has been infrequently observed in association with the lesions of toxoplasma encephalitis but in our experience is more common with lymphoma.

Interruption of medical therapy for toxoplasma encephalitis may result in its recurrence.[7,10,44] The latter can be diagnosed by obtaining plain and contrast MRI or CT scans and comparing the results to the initial pretreatment scans. In patients with recurrent disease, some of the enhancing lesions, edema, and mass effect that were seen on the initial study will reappear, and new sites of nodular or ring enhancement may also be visualized. Typically, reinstitution of antitoxoplasmosis therapy results in a progressive decrease in size and eventual resolution of the recurrent toxoplasma lesions. Coexistent pathologic conditions should always be considered in the face of new sites of contrast uptake. A progressive increase in the size of these lesions with resolution of the other lesions suggests a different pathologic process. A ^{201}Th SPECT scan may exclude a possible coexistent lymphoma.[9] Brain biopsy will be needed to determine the cause of the lesion not responding to medical therapy.

Cerebral Lymphoma

Primary lymphoma of the CNS (PCNSL) represents less than 1 percent of intracranial neoplasms and less than 1 percent of all non-Hodgkins lymphomas.[47,48] However, in the setting of immunodeficiency, the incidence in-

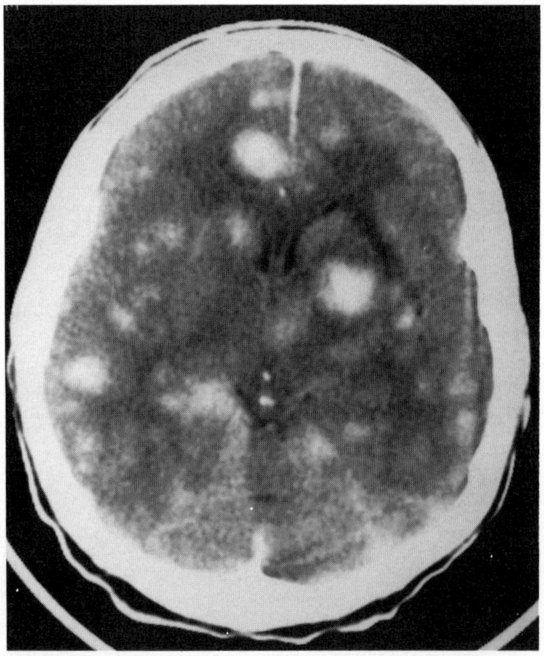

A

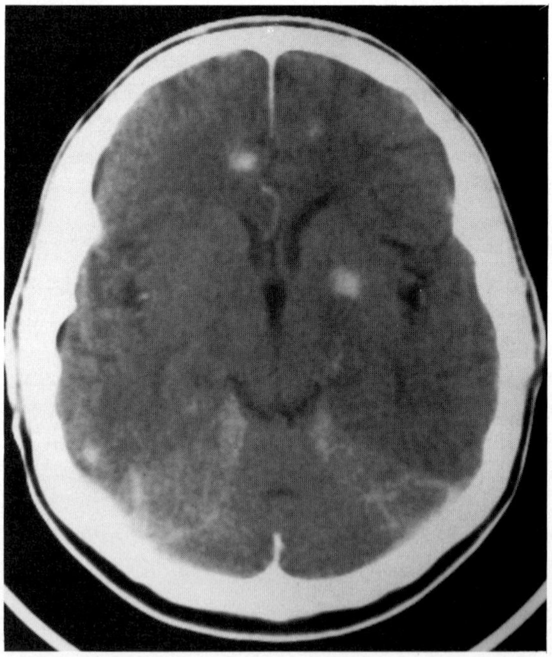

B

Figure 14-5

Toxoplasmosis. **(A)** *CT scan with multiple enhancing nodules and edema before the initiation of antitoxoplasmosis treatment. (From Rovira et al.[8] Used by permission.)* **(B)** *Dramatic but incomplete, resolution of lesions and edema during therapy. (From Post.[9] Used by permission.)*

creases substantially. For example, PCNSL is found in up to 0.6 percent of AIDS patients at the time of presentation and ultimately develops in up to 2.0 percent of all patients.[49] It is estimated that the incidence of AIDS-related PCNSL currently exceeds that of low-grade astrocytomas.[50] These tumors are mostly of B-cell origin, and both large-cell immunoblastic and small noncleaved lymphomas are seen.[51] Primary CNS lymphoma can present in several ways; focal neurologic deficits and impaired cognitive function are the most common presenting manifestations.

Hochberg and Miller[52] described four broad categories of PCNSL occurring with or without associated immunodeficiency: (1) solitary or multiple discrete intracranial nodules,(2) diffuse meningeal or periventricular lesions, (3) uveal or vitreous deposits (uveitis/vitreitis), (4) localized intradural spinal masses. These lymphomas usually present as single or multiple, multicentric focal mass lesions in brain parenchyma. Unlike other forms of lymphoma, PCNSL rarely involves the meninges. Curiously, PCNSL is more often necrotic in AIDS patients than in those patients with an intact immune system. The tumors are responsive to radiation therapy,[53] but median survival is 5.5 months,[54] with death often ensuing as a result of intercurrent illnesses. Epstein-Barr virus (EBV) expression is frequently, if not invariably, present in AIDS-related PCNSL,[54,55] suggesting that EBV plays a role in tumorigenesis.

On MRI or CT scan, cerebral lymphoma appears as solid or inhomogeneous enhancing focal lesions with surrounding edema and mass effect[2,7,8,56] (Figs. 14-6, 14-7, and 14-8). When ring enhancement occurs, it is typically thick, irregular, or nodular.[9] If not necrotic, lymphomas appear isointense to gray matter on T2-weighted plain MRIs. In necrotic lymphomas, there may be an isointense rim, but the necrotic center is hyperintense on T2-weighted images. Sites of predilection include the corpus callosum (Fig. 14-9), the subependymal-periventricular area, basal ganglia, and vermis. Other sites affected include cerebral cortex, thalamus, and brainstem.

There are no pathognomonic findings on MRI or CT for lymphoma. Toxoplasma encephalitis and other infectious disorders, such as tuberculoma and cryptococcoma, cannot be distinguished on the initial MRI or CT scan from cerebral lymphoma.[7,8] Helpful diagnostic features for the diagnosis of lymphoma include the following: (1) hyperdense mass on plain CT; (2) peripheral enhancement of thick, irregular, or nodular lesions; (4) involvement of the corpus callosum or subependymal and periventricular regions, (4) progression of disease during a short-interval follow-up scan during adequate medical therapy for toxoplasmosis; and (5) intense uptake on ^{201}Th SPECT.[27] The latter technique has evolved as the single most useful and cost-effective imaging study in the differentiation of PCNSL from infectious brain masses, particularly toxoplasma.[57] Its use has been

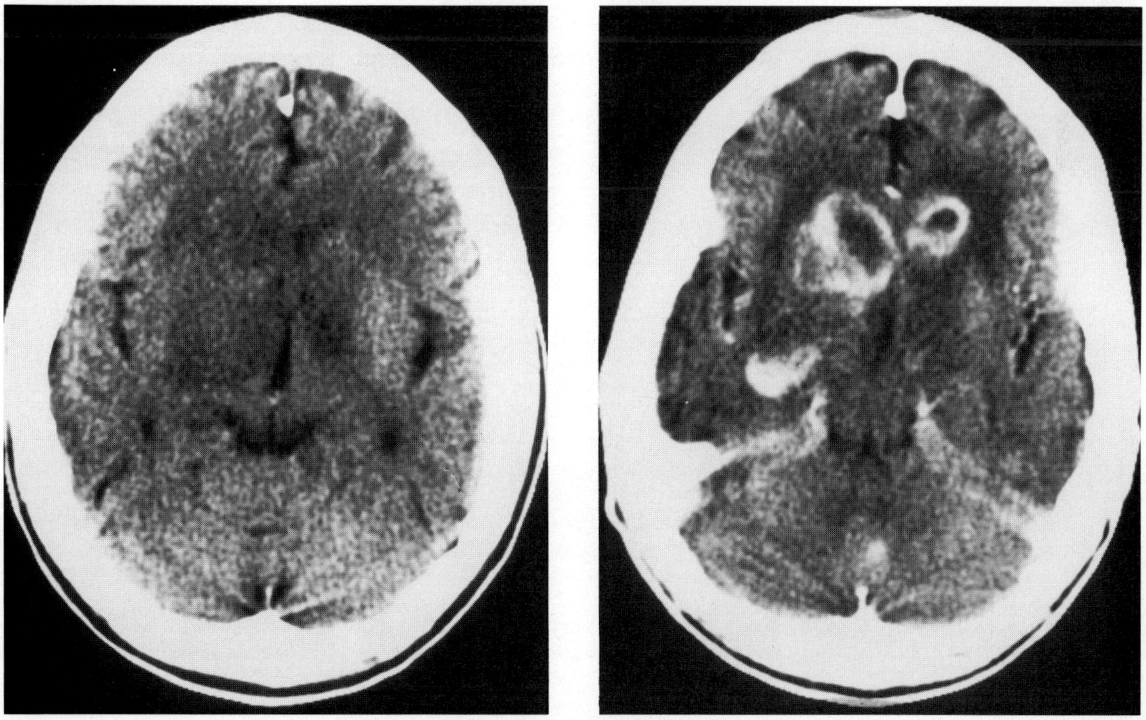

A B

Figure 14-6
Lymphoma. **(A)** *CT scan without contrast.* **(B)** *CT scan with contrast revealing irregular, thick, periventricular enhancement.*

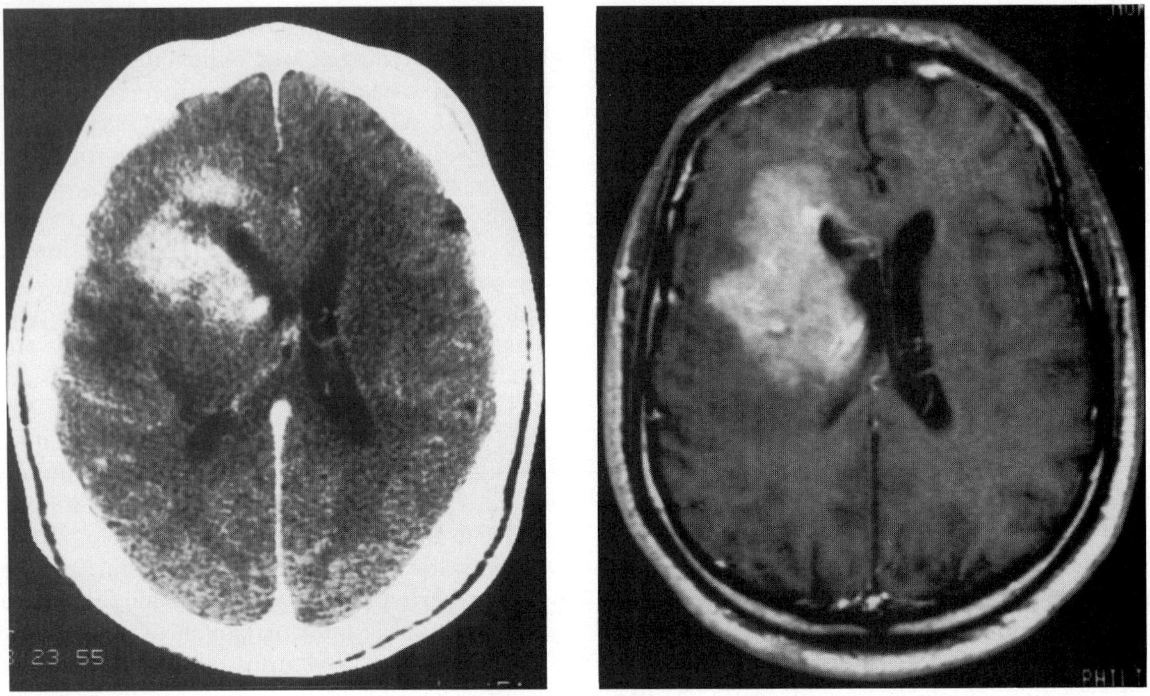

A B

Figure 14-7
Lymphoma. **(A)** *CT scan with contrast showing periventricular enhancement and an associated large parenchymal enhancing lesion with mass effect.* **(B)** *Axial MRI with contrast.*

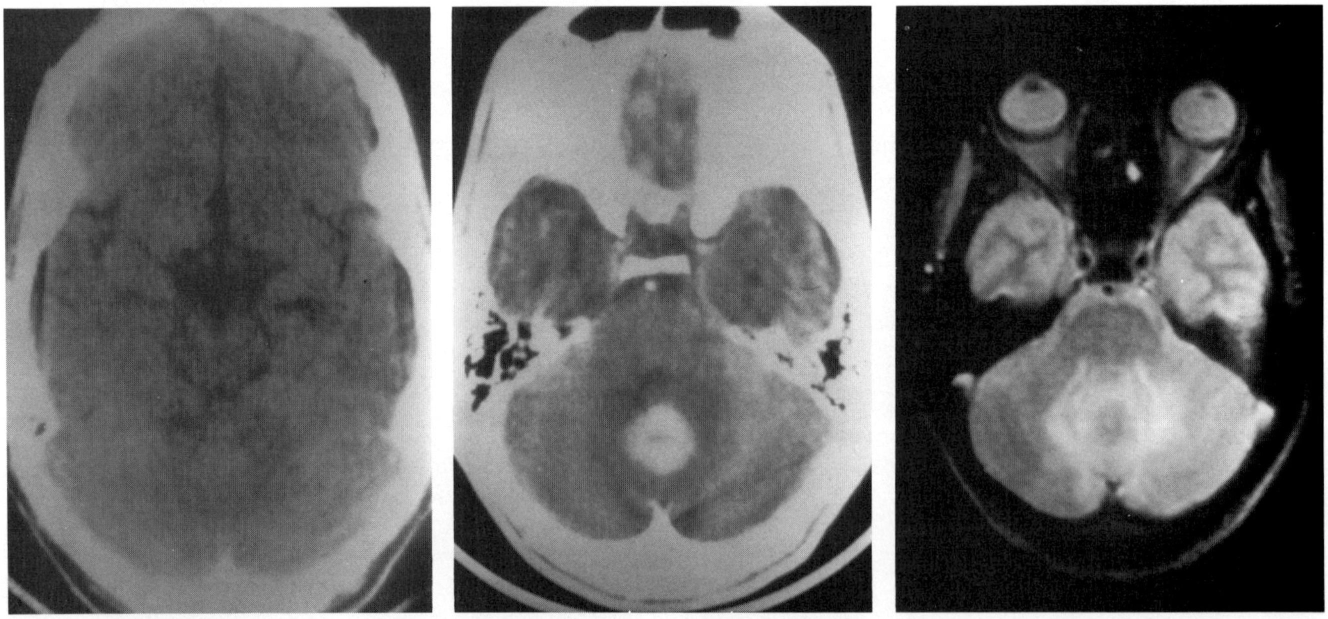

A B C

Figure 14-8
Lymphoma. **(A)** *On CT scan, vermian lesion is difficult to discern because of isointensity to gray matter.* **(B)** *Contrast MRI demonstrates nodular enhancement. (From Post.[9] Used by permission.)* **(C)** *In a T2-weighted MRI, the vermian lymphoma is isointense to gray matter, but surrounding edema is demonstrated.*

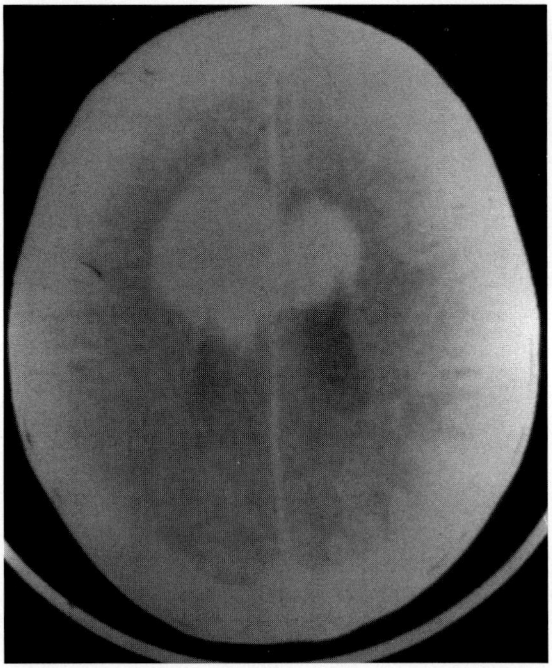

Figure 14-9
Lymphoma of the corpus callosum on contrast CT.

incorporated into the algorithm developed by the American Academy of Neurology Working Group for the evaluation of mass lesions of the brain in AIDS (Fig. 14-9B).[8] Further information on the radiographic manifestations of brain lymphoma and other tumors less commonly associated with HIV infection may be found in Chap. 12 (Fig. 14-10).

Tuberculous Abscess

Tuberculous meningitis remains the most common complication of mycobacterial infection in HIV-infected persons; however, other forms of CNS involvement include tuberculous abscess, tuberculoma, and subacute encephalitis.[7,58] Unlike *Mycobacterium tuberculosis,* which typically results in meningitis, *Mycobacterium avium-intracellularis* and other mycobacterial infections are more commonly associated with intracerebral mass lesions.

Tuberculous abscesses (Fig. 14-11) occur most often in association with immunocompromised states.[60] Tuberculous abscesses present as large focal mass lesions in the brain of AIDS patients.[10] Biopsy is required for definitive diagnosis, but there are some imaging clues that are suggestive of this disorder: (1) ring enhancement, a consequence of its resemblance to pyogenic abscesses and lack of typical giant cell and epitheloid cell granulomatous reaction:[7,8,59] (2) a multiloculated appearance; and (3) the presence of edema and mass effect. ^{201}Th SPECT may be helpful in distinguishing tuberculous abscesses from lymphoma.[27]

Pyogenic Abscess

Pyogenic abscess may also occur in the setting of HIV infection.[7,8] Parenteral drug abuse is a risk factor for both HIV infection and pyogenic abscess. In this population, the causative agent is often *Staphylococcus aureus.* These infections in the HIV-infected individual can cause either single or multiple lesions in the brain.

Pyogenic abscesses appear as ring enhancing lesions on contrast MRI and CT. Liquefactive necrosis is present in the center of a pyogenic abscess cavity, and the cavity fluid often has a signal intensity similar to that of CSF on MRI.[7,8,12,15,16,22] The abscess cavity appears bright on T2-weighted images unless the fluid is proteinaceous, since protein and other macromolecular components can shorten the T1 relaxation value.[12,61] On T1-weighted images, the rim of the pyogenic abscess will appear isointense to hyperintense, while on T2-weighted images the rim appears hypointense. On plain MRI, the characteristics of the signal of the abscess rim may be the consequence of collagen or paramagnetic free radicals within heterogeneously distributing macrophages in the abscess periphery.[12,14–16] If the abscess is mature, the enhancing ring is thin (Fig. 14-12). With medical or surgical therapy, the hypointense rim on T2-weighted images will resolve. The latter is a better indicator of therapeutic response than is resolution of a resolving ring or nodular enhancement on contrast MRI.[12,14]

Syphilitic Gummas and Infarcts

Neurosyphilis occurs in as many as 1.5 percent of some HIV-infected populations.[61] Neurosyphilis appears more aggressive in immunosuppressed HIV-infected individuals than in immunocompetent persons.[61–64] Involvement of the CNS by *Treponema pallidum* can cause a meningovasculitis with meningeal thickening, round cell infiltration of the meninges and small blood vessels, and luminal narrowing and ectasia of medium-sized to large vessels.[8] The vasculitis (see below) can result in cerebral ischemia and infarction. Gummas, on the other hand, result in focal circumscribed masses with granulation tissue that typically overlie the cerebral convexities and are adherent to the dura and brain.[65]

Among the imaging findings in neurosyphilis are nonspecific atrophy, infarctions, and gummas (peripherally enhancing nodules) over the cerebral convexities (Fig. 14-13).[65,66] Magnetic resonance imaging has a greater sensitivity than does CT scanning in displaying the detail of the affected blood vessels and in demonstrating small infarcts. The characteristic appearance of gummas include very peripheral nodular-enhancing lesions in the gray matter of the cerebral cortex, surrounded by edema and associated with an adjacent area of meningeal enhancement.[10] Resolution of the enhancing lesion during penicillin therapy is strongly suggestive of the diagnosis.

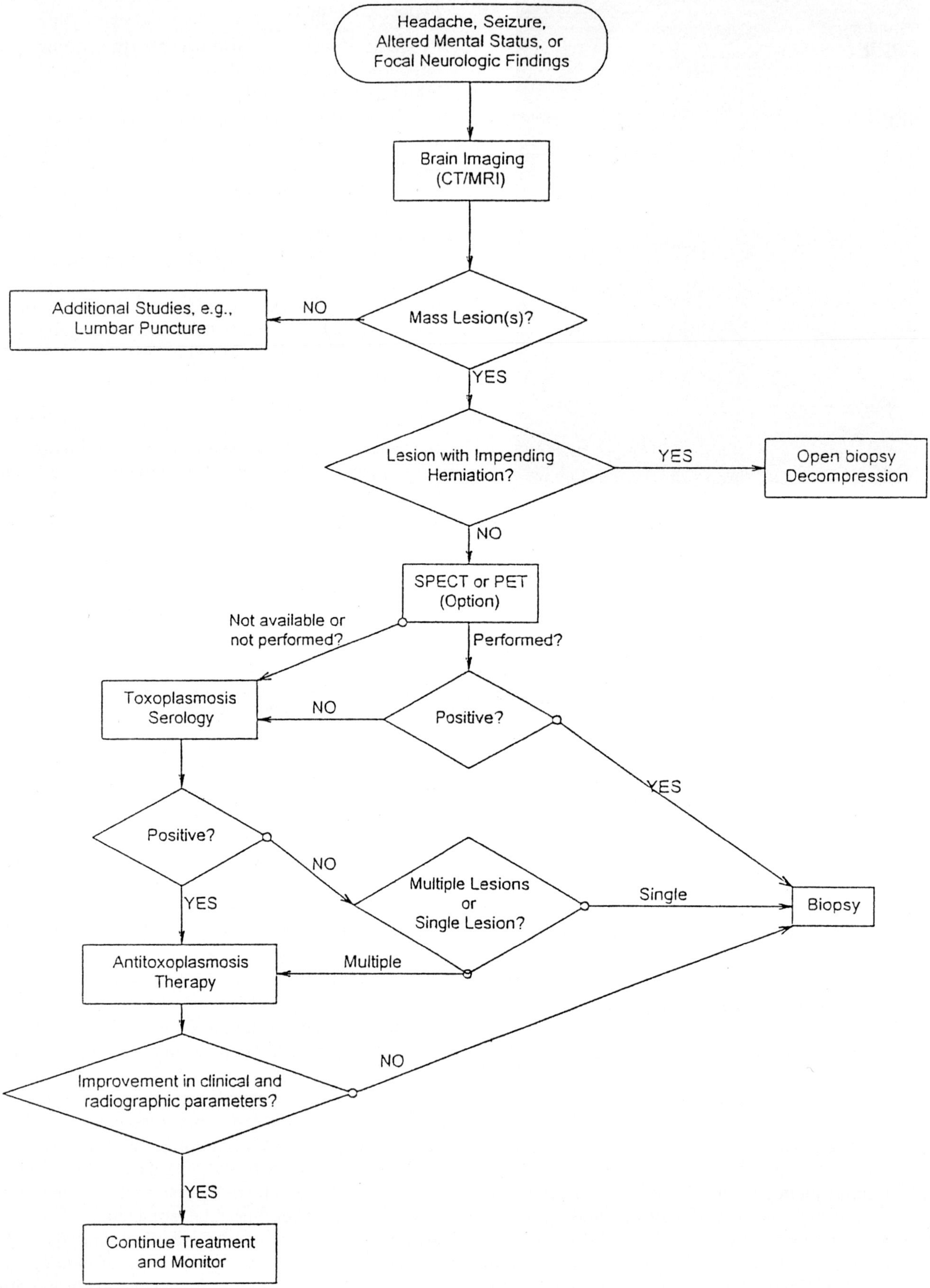

Figure 14-10
Algorithm for the evaluation of intracranial mass lesions in AIDS patients.

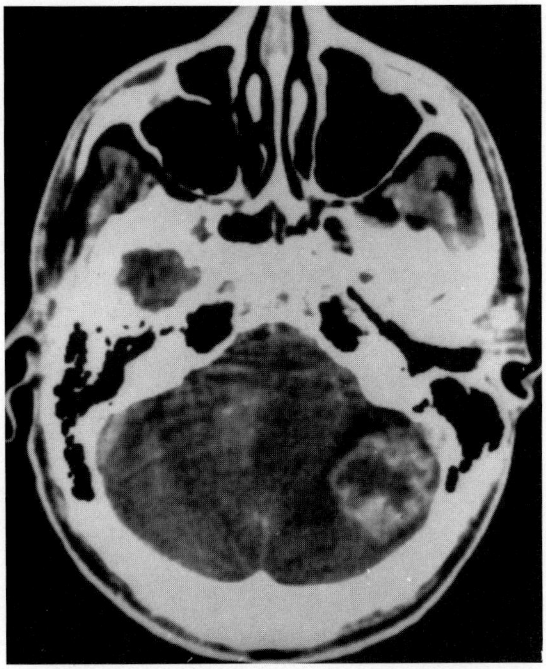

Figure 14-11
Tuberculosis. Tuberculous abscess of the cerebellum. (From Post.[9] Used by permission.)

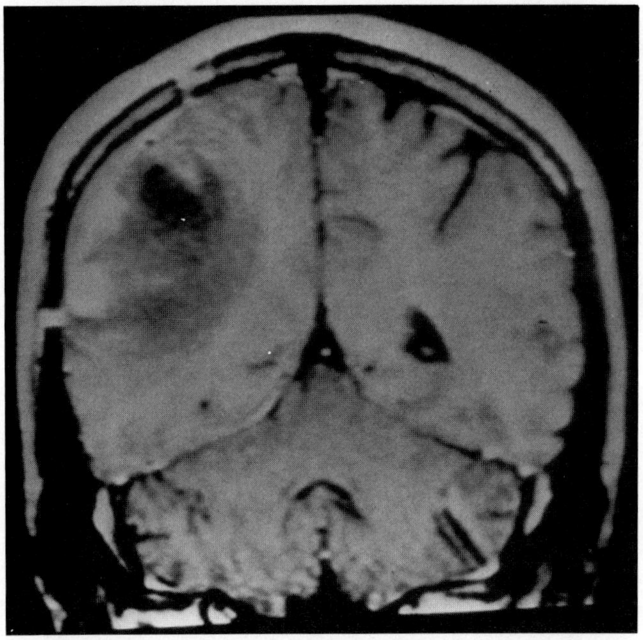

Figure 14-13
Neurosyphilis. Syphilitic cerebral gumma documented at biopsy. The lesion completely resolved following high-dose intravenous penicillin therapy.

Cryptococcoma and Cryptococcal Pseudocyst

In some series, *Cryptococcus neoformans* is the most common cause of CNS opportunistic infection in AIDS. Usually, *C. neoformans* presents as meningitis unaccompanied by other complications. The meningeal inflammatory response is often quite minimal, and therefore radiographic imaging studies are usually unremarkable. On rare occasions, cryptococcal meningitis may result in a focal mass lesion in the brain parenchyma, with imaging characteristics indistinguishable from pyogenic abscess. This lesion, referred to as a cryptococcoma, is the result of an extension of the organism from the perivascular space into the parenchyma, with an associated collection of inflammatory cells and gelatinous mucoid material. Ring enhancement on MRI or CT is characteristic.[67–69]

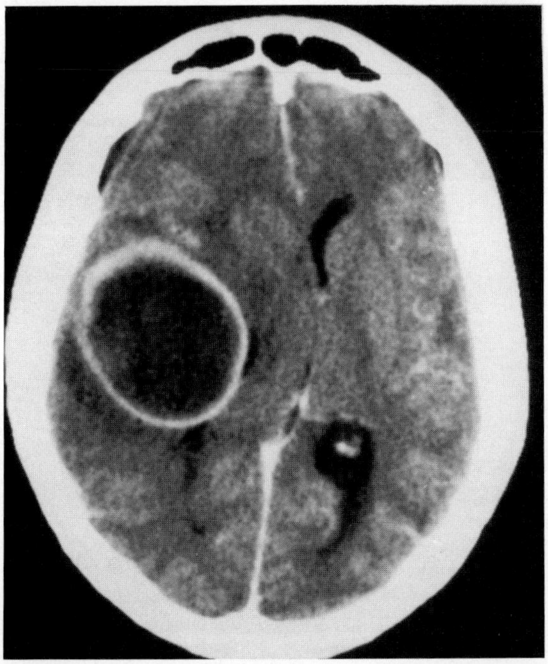

Figure 14-12
Pyogenic abscess. CT scan with contrast reveals ring enhancing lesion in a parenteral drug abuser (From Rovira et al.[8] Used by permission.)

Cryptococcal meningitis may also be associated with a secondary gelatinous pseudocyst formation that results from fungal invasion of dilated Virchow-Robin spaces. The cryptococcal pseudocyst is a CSF-equivalent lesion that does not contrast enhance and has a "soap bubble" appearance (Fig. 14-14).[67] These lesions have a predilection for the basal ganglia, presumably as a result of the large Virchow-Robin spaces in the territory of the branches of the middle cerebral arteries. While not pathognomonic, the appearance of lesions with the imaging characteristics of these pseudocysts is highly suggestive of cryptococcal infection. Another highly suggestive finding is the presence of choroid plexus granulomas.[70] Although CSF studies may not be readily obtainable because of the relative contraindication to lumbar puncture due to the presence of focal intracranial mass lesions, cryptococcus can frequently be cultured from the blood, and cryptococcal antigen is often de-

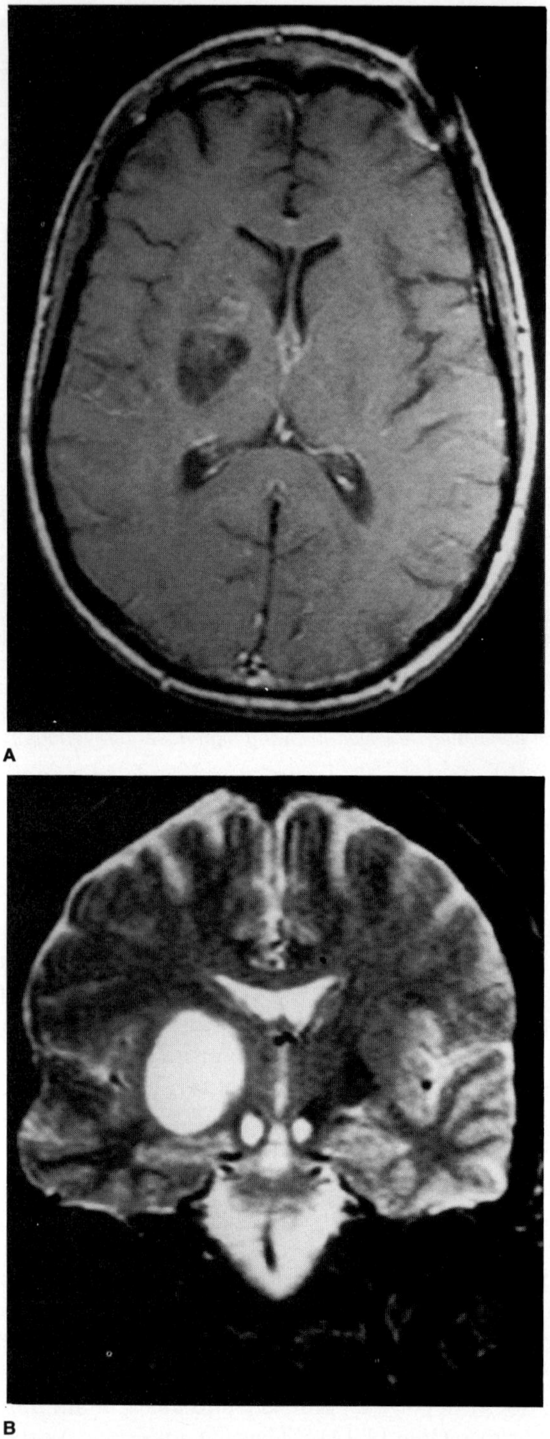

Figure 14-14
Cryptococcal pseudocyst. **(A)** *CSF-equivalent lesion on T1-weighted image in the basal ganglia in a patient with cryptococcal meningitis.* **(B)** *Hyperintense signal on a T2-weighted image.*

monstrable in the blood of patients with cryptococcal meningitis.

Other Focal Intracranial Lesions with Mass Effect

Other infections that may present as focal intracranial mass lesions in the HIV-infected patient include, *Candida albicans, Aspergillus fumigatus,* mucormycosis, *Histoplasma capsulatum, Coccidioides immitis, Blastomyces dermatitidis,* and cysticercosis.[2,7] Aspergillosis and mucormycosis germinate as hyphae and invade blood vessels, with consequent brain infarction. Herpes simplex encephalitis may also present as a focal lesion with mass effect (Fig. 14-15), occasionally displaying associated hemorrhage. A variety of neuroimaging abnormalities have been reported with some bacterial infections

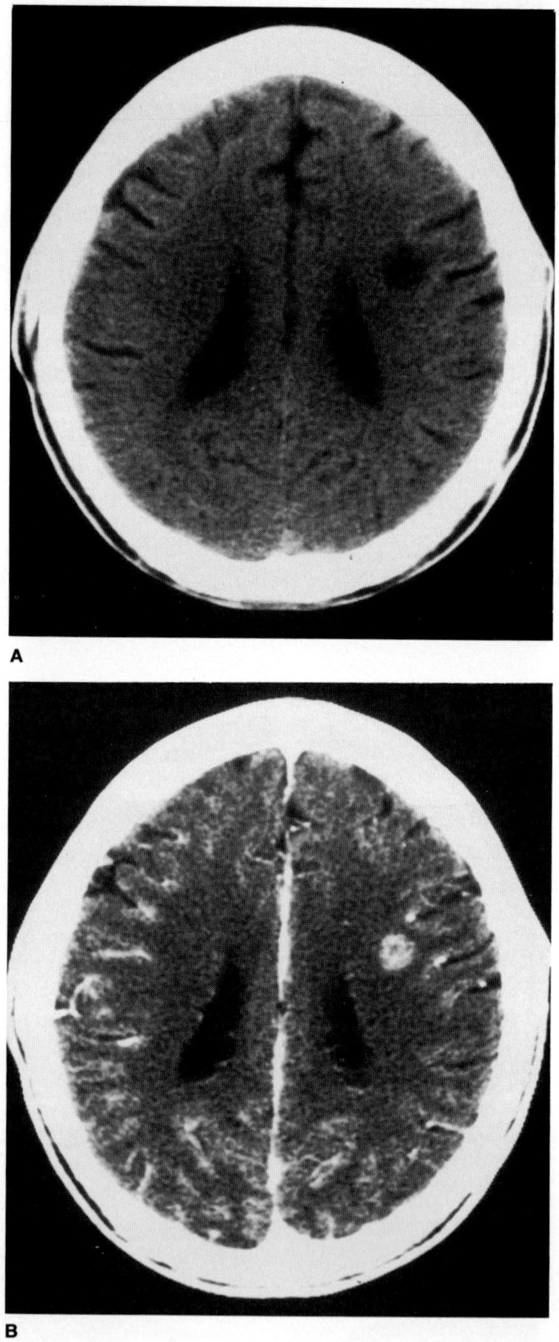

Figure 14-15
Herpes simplex encephalitis. **(A)** *CT scan without contrast revealing low-density left frontal lesion.* **(B)** *CT scan with contrast reveals contrast enhancement.*

(*Listeria monocytogenes, Nocardia asteroides, Bartonella henselae, Rhodococcus equi, Staphylococcus, Streptococcus,* and *Salmonella*) that are seen relatively rarely in association with AIDS.[71] Effective treatment for these disorders demands aggressive attempts to establish a diagnosis. Brain biopsy is required. All these lesions can appear on MRI or CT as ring or nodular enhancing lesions.

Cerebrovascular Lesions with or without Mass Effect

A wide variety of cerebrovascular lesions (Table 14-4) have been observed in the presence of HIV infection in both adults and children. Therefore, cerebrovascular disease must be included among the potential disorders that produce intracranial lesions with or without mass effect.[72] In one series of abnormal cranial MRI studies obtained over a 2-year period, 22 cerebral infarcts were observed in 13 (18 percent) of 71 HIV-infected patients.[73] This percentage is probably skewed and is significantly higher than that obtained from autopsy series.[72] Most infarcts appear to occur in the territory of the lenticulostriate arteries and affect the basal ganglia.[73] The cause of cerebral infarction in this population is multifactorial. Vasculitis may occur in the absence of an identifiable cause, presumably as the direct consequence of HIV infection (Fig. 14-16).[74] Established causes of vasculitis in HIV infection include such infections as herpes zoster and Treponema pallidum. A diagnosis of neurosyphilis should be strongly considered in any HIV-infected person presenting with a cerebral infarction (Fig. 14-17). Ruptured mycotic aneurysms need always be considered in the face of intracranial hemorrhage, particularly in parenteral drug abusers (Fig. 14-18). No radiographic appearances are specific for cerebrovascular disease complicating HIV infection. For a full discussion of these disorders, refer to Chap. 15.

Table 14-4
Potential causes of stroke occurring with HIV infection

- I. Ischemic stroke
  - A. Embolic
    - 1. Cardiac disease
      - a. Nonbacterial thrombotic endocarditis (marantic endocarditis)
      - b. Bacterial endocarditis
      - c. Other
  - B. Thrombotic
    - 1. Vasculitis
      - a. HIV-related
      - b. Non-HIV infectious etiologies
        - 1. Herpes zoster
        - 2. *T. pallidum*
        - 3. Tuberculous meningitis
    - 2. Cerebral vasospasm
    - 3. Hematologic conditions
      - a. Lupus anticoagulant
      - b. Disseminated intravascular coagulation
      - c. Hyperviscosity syndrome
    - 4. Cerebral venous thrombosis with cachexia and dehydration
- II. Intracranial hemorrhage
  - A. Thrombocytopenia
    - 1. Autoimmune
    - 2. Drug-induced
    - 3. Disseminated intravascular coagulation
    - 4. Other
  - B. Intracranial malignancy
    - 1. Kaposi's sarcoma
    - 2. Lymphoma
    - 3. Other
  - C. Vasculitis
  - D. Ruptured mycotic aneurysm

Source: Adapted from Berger et al.[73]

Without Mass Effect

The most common causes of non-mass-producing intracranial lesions in HIV-infected patients are PML, HIV encephalitis, and cytomegalovirus (CMV) encephalitis. Cerebrovascular disease frequently occurs in the absence of mass effect and is discussed in the previous section. Magnetic resonance imaging is the imaging study of choice due to its superior contrast resolution and marked sensitivity in detecting lesions that affect the white matter.

Progressive Multifocal Leukoencephalopathy

Progressive multifocal leukoencephalopathy is an opportunistic infection of the brain caused by the papovavirus JC virus. This infection ultimately develops in 4 to 5 percent of AIDS patients.[75] In as many as 25 percent of patients with PML complicating HIV infection, the neurologic deficit is the initial manifestation of AIDS.[75] The predominant clinical features of this illness are hemianopsia and motor impairment, but other neurologic signs include gait abnormalities, speech disturbances, ataxia, personality changes, and cognitive impairment. The illness is the consequence of a productive infection of oligodendrocytes by JC virus, with a resulting loss of myelin. Death typically ensues in less than 6 months, and no therapy has been demonstrated unequivocally to be effective.

Imaging findings include low-density lesions on CT and high-signal-intensity lesions on T2-weighted MRI (Figs. 14-19, 14-20, and 14-21).[75-78] The lesions are located in the white matter, usually do not enhance, and do not produce any mass effect. Involvement of the supratentorial white matter predominates. The parieto-occipital white matter and frontal white matter are most commonly affected. Involvement of the subcortical white matter U fibers often results in a scalloped appearance of the lesion. Internal and external capsules may

Figure 14-16
HIV vasculitis. **(A)** *CT scan with contrast revealing multiple superficial enhancing areas consistent with vasculitis.* **(B)** *Cerebral arteriogram (right internal carotid selective injection, anteroposterior view) reveals vasculitic changes with distal aneurysmal dilatation of vessels. Delayed clearance of contrast material was also observed.* **(C)** *Cerebral arteriogram (right internal carotid selective injection, lateral view) reveals vasculitic changes with distal aneurysmal dilatation of vessels.*

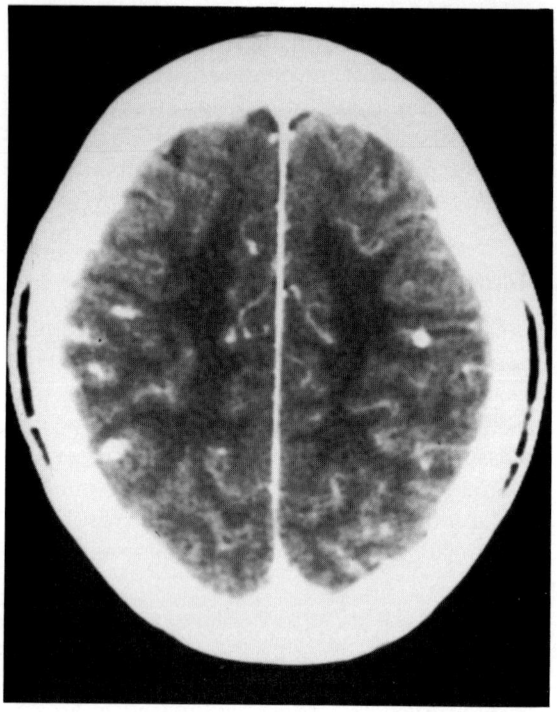
A

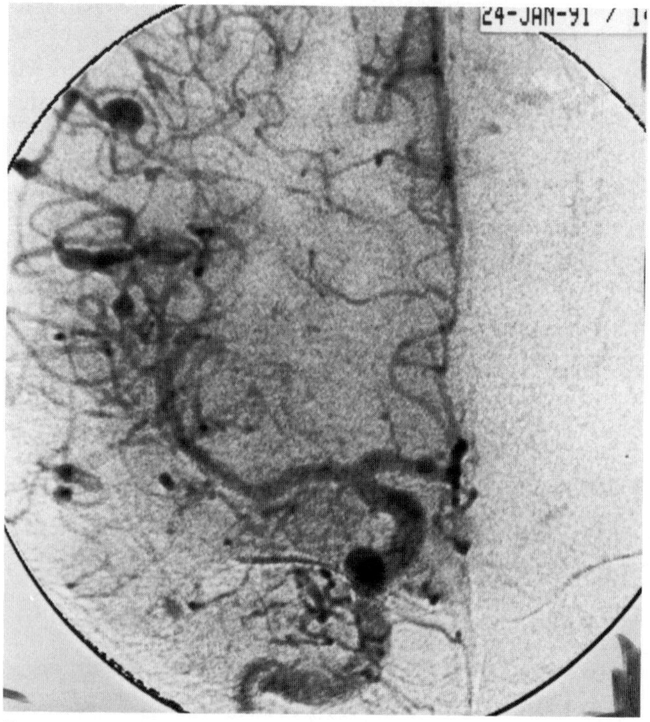

B

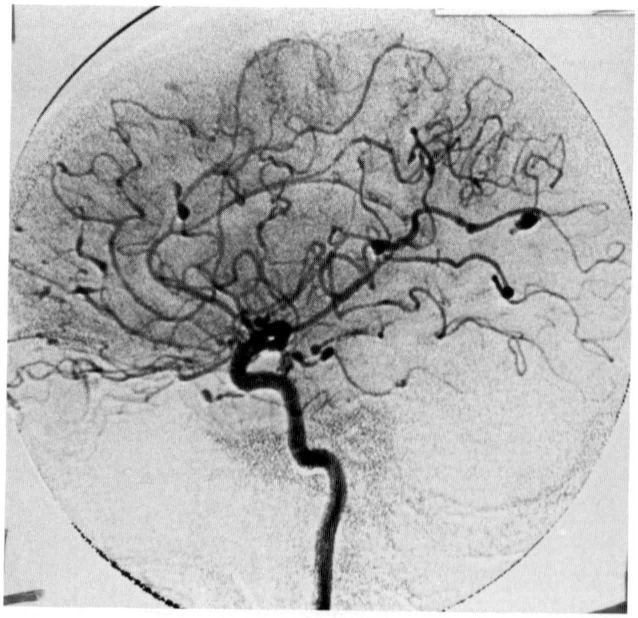
C

also appear demyelinated. The white matter lesions may be single and focal, but, as the name of the illness implies, multiple areas of white matter abnormality are the rule. When both cerebral hemispheres are affected, one side is usually more severely affected than the other. The brainstem and cerebellar white matter may also be involved (Fig. 14-22), and occasionally the posterior fossa may be the only site of disease. Radiographic imaging may reveal involvement of the deep gray matter, such as the basal ganglia and thalamus; however, this finding is generally a minor part of the disease. Corresponding pathologic studies indicate that this appearance is chiefly, if not exclusively, the result of involvement of the white matter tracts that course through the deep gray matter.[78] Serial MRI or CT scans in PML show a progressive increase in the size and number of the white matter lesions, with the focal lesions becoming diffuse and confluent. Rarely, the lesions may faintly contrast enhance in their periphery on either CT or MRI.

While the imaging findings of PML are not pathognomonic and while they may be impossible to distinguish from those of other infections that induce demyelination, such as HIV, some radiographic and clinical features are very suggestive of PML,[78] including (1) focal neurologic deficits, particularly visual field defects; (2) the absence of dementia; (3) white matter lesions in a parieto-occipital regions and subcortical white matter disease; and (4) a hypointense appearance on T1-weighted images. None of these features alone or in combination is unequivocally diagnostic. Furthermore, at the present time, no studies of the CSF for JC virus are sufficiently diagnostic to enable definitive diagnosis;

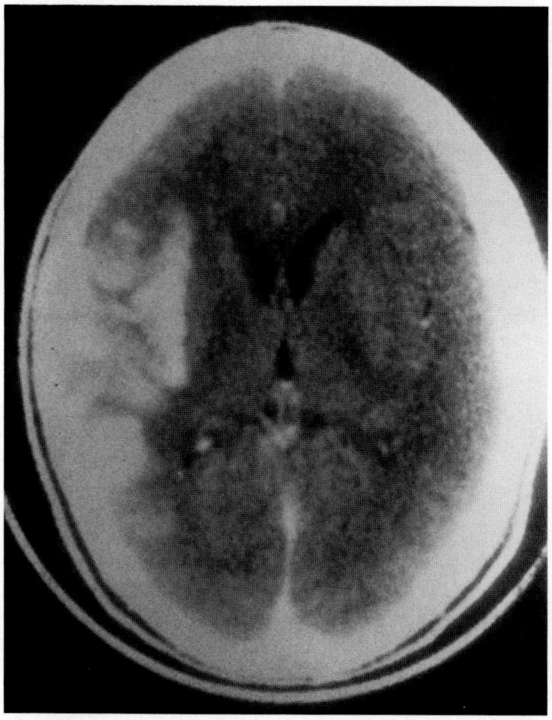

Figure 14-17
Meningovascular syphilis. CT with contrast reveals extensive middle cerebral artery distribution infarction accompanying meningovascular syphilis.

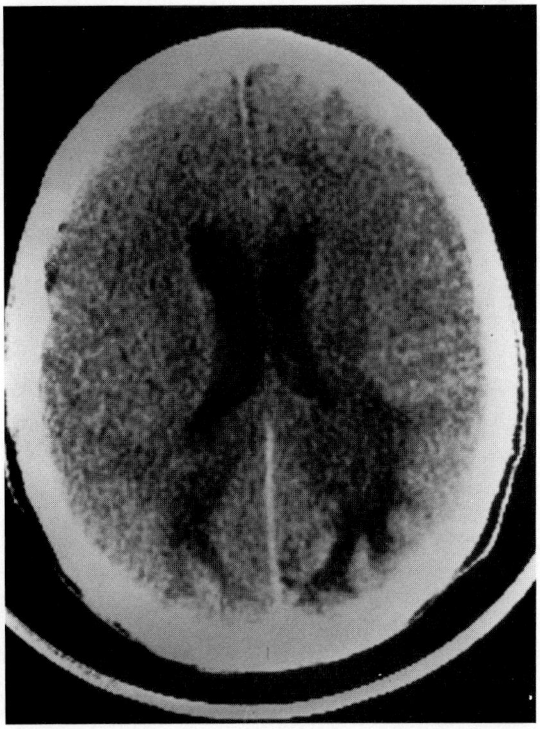

Figure 14-19
Progressive multifocal leukoencephalopathy. Typical hypointense lesions of the parieto-occipital white matter on plain CT scan.

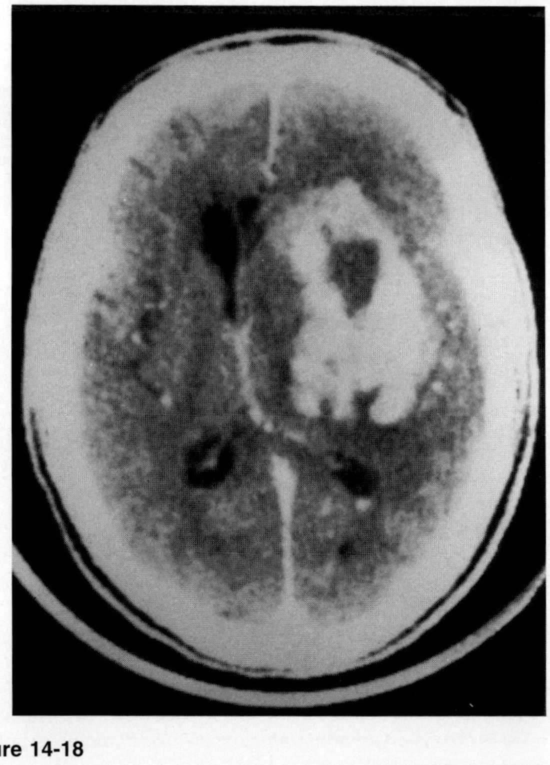

Figure 14-18
Ruptured mycotic aneurysm. CT scan reveals large, deep hemorrhage occurring as a consequence of a ruptured mycotic aneurysm.

hence, a tissue diagnosis is ultimately needed for confirmation.

HIV Infection

Infection by HIV may result in meningitis (both acute and chronic), subacute encephalitis, myelopathy, and peripheral neuropathy.[6] Animal experiments reveal that retroviruses cross the blood-brain barrier early in the course of infection. Anecdotally, HIV has been demonstrated in the brain within 2 weeks of infection. The virus can be cultured from the CSF,[79] and intra-blood-brain-barrier synthesis of antibody to HIV can be demonstrated in early stages of the infection.[80]

Although HIV encephalopathy is typically a disorder seen with advanced immunosuppression, estimates of its frequency as the initial AID-defining illness have ranged from 0.8[3] to 2.2 percent[49] of adult AIDS patients. In perinatally infected children, HIV encephalopathy developed in 16 percent of cases and was the initial manifestation of HIV infection in 77 percent of this group.[81] The illness is noted in approximately 7 percent of adults at the time the diagnosis of AIDS is established and develops at an annual rate between 7 and 14 percent once AIDS is diagnosed. In one series, more than two-thirds of AIDS patients had evidence of HIV encephalopathy in the terminal stages of their illness.[82] The gross

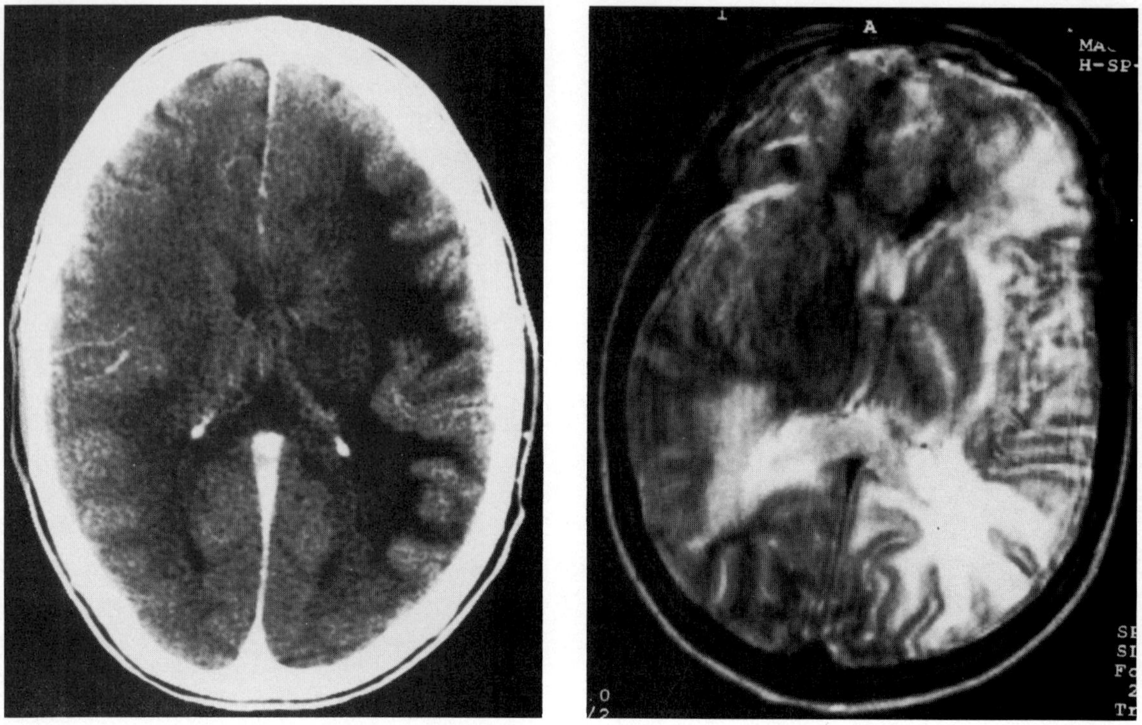

A B

Figure 14-20
Progressive multifocal leukoencephalopathy. **(A)** *CT scan reveals diffuse white matter involvement of the left hemisphere spreading across to the right parieto-occipital lobe white matter.* **(B)** *T2-weighted MRI shows hyperintense signals of the white matter in the same distribution.*

pathologic characteristics of HIV encephalopathy are brain atrophy with sulcal widening and ventricular dilatation. Meningeal fibrosis may occasionally be observed. Histologically, a common and distinctive feature of this illness is white matter pallor located chiefly in the periventricular and central white matter.[83] Multinucleate giant cells, the pathologic hallmark of the disease, appear to result from direct virus-induced cell fusion.[82] Clini-

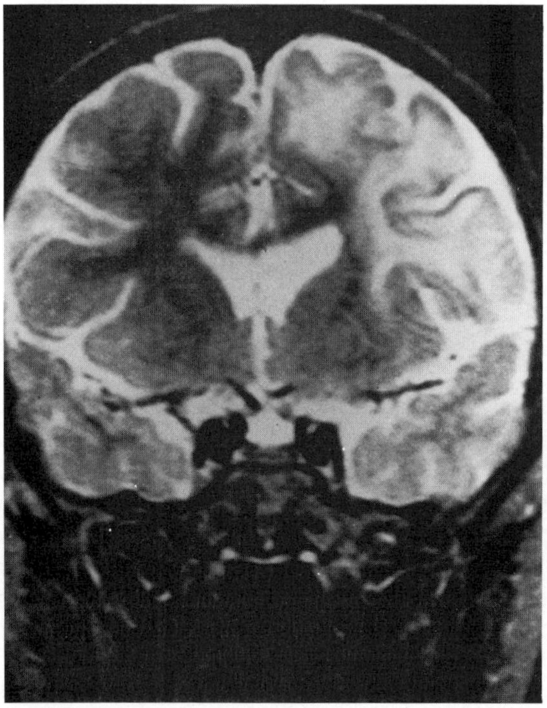

A

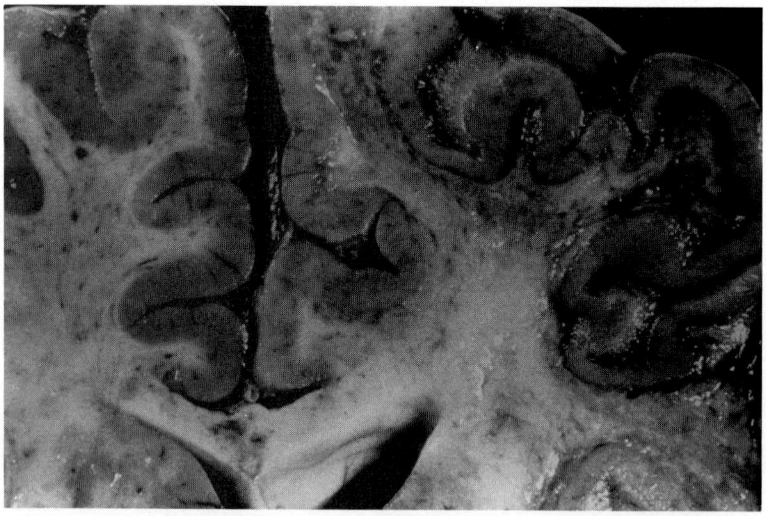

B

Figure 14-21
Progressive multifocal leukoencephalopathy. **(A)** *T2-weighted image shows extensive hyperintense white matter lesion of the left frontal lobe.* **(B)** *Section of the brain from the level of the lesion demonstrates excellent pathologic-radiologic correlation with respect to the extent of the lesion.*

PERIPHERAL NERVOUS SYSTEM

Infection with HIV-1 is associated with a diverse group of peripheral neuropathies. These neuropathies occur commonly, with prospective neurologic evaluation revealing evidence of peripheral neuropathy in up to 50 percent of patients with advanced HIV infection. The etiopathogenesis of these neuropathies is diverse. Imaging studies are particularly helpful in the polyradiculopathies that occur with HIV-associated lymphoma and progressive CMV polyradiculopathy.

Lymphoma may metastasize to the meninges and affect both cranial nerves and spinal roots. Imaging studies may reveal tumor nodules involving the meninges. Enhancing nodules may be evident on affected spinal nerve roots.

Cytomegalovirus progressive polyradiculomyelopathy[96,97] is typically characterized at onset by lower extremity and sacral paresthesias. Progressive paraparesis rapidly ensues, with concomitant areflexia, ascending sensory loss, and bowel and bladder incontinence. On occasion, MRI with gadolinium may reveal thickened clumped nerve roots of the cauda equina that contrast enhance (Fig. 14-27).

REFERENCES

1. Snider WD, Simpson DM, Nielsen S, et al: Neurological complications of acquired immunodeficiency syndrome: Analysis of 50 patients. *Ann Neurol* 14:403–418, 1983.
2. Levy RM, Bredesen DE, Rosenblum ML: Neurological manifestations of the immunodeficiency syndrome (AIDS): Experience at UCSF and review of the literature. *J Neurosurg* 62:475–495, 1985.
3. Berger JR, Moskowitz L, Fischl M, Kelley RE: Neurologic disease as the presenting manifestation of acquired immunodeficiency syndrome. *South Med J* 80:683–686, 1987.
4. Gray F, Gherardi R, Scaravilli F: The neuropathology of the acquired immune deficiency syndrome (AIDS). *Brain* 111:245–266, 1988.
5. Bredesen DE, Messing R: Neurological syndromes heralding the acquired immune deficiency syndrome (abstr). *Ann Neurol* 14:141, 1983.
6. Berger JR, Levy RM: The neurological complications of HIV-1 infection. *Med Clin North Am* 77:1–24, 1993.
7. Post MJD, Berger JR, Hensley CT: The radiology of central nervous system disease in acquired immunodeficiency syndrome, in Taveras JM, Ferucci JT (eds): *Radiology: Diagnosis, Imaging, Intervention,* vol. 3. Philadelphia, Lippincott, 1986, pp 1–26.
8. Quality Standards Subcommittee of the American Academy of Neurology (JR Berger, chair): Evaluation and management of intracranial mass lesions in AIDS. *Neurology* 50:21–26, 1998.
9. Post MJD: Neuroimaging of AIDS. *AIDS and the Nervous System,* course no. 140, Annual Meeting of the American Academy of Neurology, New York, April 25–May 1, 1993, pp 140–165.
10. Post MJD, Kursunoglu S, Hensley GT, et al: Cranial CT in acquired immunodeficiency syndrome: Spectrum of disease and optimal contrast enhancement technique. *Am J Neuroradiol* 6:743–754, 1985.
11. Post MJD, Sheldon JJ, Hensley GT, et al: Central nervous system disease in acquired immunodeficiency syndrome: prospective correlation using CT, MRI and pathologic studies. *Radiology* 158:141–148, 1986.
12. Bowen BC, Post MJD: Intracranial infections, in Atlas SW (ed): *Magnetic Resonance Imaging of the Brain and Spine.* New York, Raven Press, 1990, chap 16, pp 501–538.
13. Post MJD, Sze G, Quencer RM, et al: Gadolinium-enhanced MR in spinal infection. *J Comput Assist Tomogr* 14:721–729, 1990.
14. Sze G, Zimmerman RD: The magnetic resonance imaging of infections and inflammatory diseases. *Radiol Clin North Am* 26:839–859, 1985.
15. Zimmerman RD, Bilaniuk LT, Sze G: Intracranial infection, in Brant-Zawadzki M, Norman D (eds): *Magnetic Resonance Imaging of the Central Nervous System.* New York, Raven Press, 1987, pp 225–257.
16. Zimmerman RD, Becker RD, Devinsky O, et al: Magnetic resonance features: Cerebral abscesses and intracranial inflammatory lesions (abstr). *Acta Radiol* 369(suppl): 754, 1986.
17. Modic MT, Feiglin DH, Pirainio DW, et al: Vertebral osteomyelitis: Assessment using MR. *Radiology* 157:157–166, 1985.
18. Post MJD, Quencer RM, Montalvo BM, et al: Spinal infection: Evaluation with MR imaging and intraoperative US. *Radiology* 169:765–771, 1988.
19. Thurnher MM, Thurnher SA, Fleischmann D, et al: Comparison of T2-weighted and fluid-attenuated inversion-recovery fast spin-echo MR sequences in intracerebral AIDS-associated disease. *Am J Neuroradiol* 18:1601–1609, 1997.
20. Post MJD: Fluid-attenuated inversion-recovery fast spin-echo MR: A clinically useful tool in the evaluation of neurolgoically symptomatic HIV-positive patients. *Am J Neuroradiol* 18:1611–1616, 1997.
21. Haimes AB, Zimmerman RD, Morgello S, et al: MR imaging of brain abscesses. *Am J Radiol* 152:1073–1085, 1989.
22. Quencer RM, Post MJD, Hinks RS: Cine-MR in the evaluation of normal and abnormal CSF flow: Intracranial and intraspinal studies. *Neuroradiology* 32:371–391, 1990.
23. Navia BA, Gonzalez RG: Functional imaging of the AIDS dementia complex and the metabolic pathology of the HIV-1-infected brain. *Neuroimag Clin North Am* 7:431–445, 1997.
24. Chang L, Ernest T: MR spectroscopy and diffusion-weighted imaging in focal brain lesions in AIDS. *Neuroimag Clin North Am* 7:409–430, 1997.
25. Ganz WI, Serafini AN: The diagnostic role of nuclear medicine in the acquired immunodeficiency syndrome. *J Nucl Med* 30:1935–1945, 1989.
26. Vanarthos WJ, Ganz WI, Vanarthos JC, et al: Diagnostic uses of nuclear medicine in AIDS. *Radiographics* 12:731–749, 1992.
27. Ruiz A, Ganz WI, Post MJD: Use of thallium-201 brain SPECT to differentiate central lymphoma from toxoplasma encephalitis in AIDS patients. Annual Meeting

of the American Society of Neuroradiology, Vancouver, BC, 1993

28. Woods GL, Goldsmith JC: Aspergillus infection of the central nervous system in patients with acquired immunodeficiency syndrome. *Arch Neurol* 47:181–184, 1990.
29. Cuadrado LM, Gruerrero A, Garcia Asenjo JAL, et al:Cerebral mucormycosis in two cases of acquired immunodeficiency syndrome. *Arch Neurol* 45:109–111; 1988.
30. Thornton CA, Houston S, Latif AS: Neurocysticercosis and human immunodeficiency virus infection:Aa possible association. *Arch Neurol* 49:963–965, 1992.
31. Ferreira MS, Nishioka SA, Rocha A, et al: Acute fatal Trypanosoma cruzi meningoencephalitis in a human immunodeficiency virus-positive hemophiliac patient. *Am J Trop Med Hyg* 45:723–727, 1991.
32. Gardner HAR, Martinez AJ, Visvesvara GS, Sotrel A: Granulomatous amebic encephalitis in an AIDS patient. *Neurology* 41:1993–1995, 1991
33. McArthur JC: Neurologic manifestations of AIDS. *Medicine* 66:407–437, 1987.
34. Wanke C, Tuazon CU, Kovacs A, et al: Toxoplasma encephalitis in patients with acquired immunodeficiency syndrome: Diagnosis and response to therapy. *Am J Trop Med Hyg* 36:509–516, 1987.
35. Petito C, Cho E-S, Lemann W, et al: Neuropathology of acquired immunodeficiency syndrome (AIDS): An autopsy review. *J Neuropathol Exp Neurol* 45:635–646, 1986.
36. Moskowitz LB, Hensley GT, Chan JC, et al: The neuropathology of acquired immunodeficiency syndrome. *Arch Pathol Lab Med* 108:867–874, 1984.
37. Bia FJ, Barry M: Parasitic infections of the central nervous system. *Neurol Clin* 4:171–206, 1986.
38. Luft BJ, Remington JS: Toxoplasmic encephalitis. *J Infect Dis* 157:1–6, 1988.
39. Navia BA, Petito CK, Gold JW, et al: Cerebral toxoplasmosis complicating the acquired immune deficiency syndrome: clinical and neuropathological findings in 27 patients. *Ann Neurol* 19:224–238, 1986.
40. Gray F, Gherardi R, Wingate E, et al: Diffuse "encephalitic" cerebral toxoplasmosis in AIDS: Report of four cases. *J Neruol* 236:273–277, 1989.
41. Nath A, Jankovic J, Pettigrew LC: Movement disorders and AIDS. *Neurology* 37:37–41, 1987.
42. Frankel JK: Toxoplasmosis, in Minkler J (ed): *Pathology of the Nervous System.* New York, McGraw-Hill, pp 2521–2538, 1968.
43. Krick JA, Remington JS: Current concepts in parasitology: Toxoplasmosis in the adult—an overview. *N Engl J Med* 298:550–553, 1978.
44. Post MJD, Chan JC, Hensley GT, et al: Toxoplasma encephalitis in Haitian adults with acquired immunodeficiency syndrome: A clinical pathologic–CT correlation. *Am J Radiol* 140:861–868, 1983.
45. Moskowitz LB, Hensley GT, Chan KC, et al: Brain biopsies in patients with acquired immunodeficiency syndrome. *Arch Pathol Lab Med* 108:368–371, 1984.
46. Porter SB, Sande MA: Toxoplasmosis of the central nervous system in the acquired immunodeficiency syndrome. *N Engl J Med* 327:1643–1648, 1992.
47. Jellinger K, Radaskiewicz TH, Slowik F: Primary malignant lymphomas of the central nervous system in man. *Acta Neuropathol* Suppl (Berlin) 6:95–102, 1975.
48. Levitt LJ, Dawson DM, Rosenthal DS, Maloney WC: CNS involvement in the non-Hodgkin's lymphomas. *Cancer* 45:545–552, 1980.
49. Levy RM, Janssen RS, Bush TJ, et al: Neuroepidemiology of acquired immunodeficiency sydrome, in Rosenblum ML, Levy RM, Bredesen DE (eds): *AIDS and the Nervous System.* New York, Raven Press, 1988, pp 13–27.
50. Baumgartner JE, Rachlin JR, Beckstead JH, et al: Primary central nervous system lymphomas: Natural history and response to radiation therapy in 55 patients with acquired immunodeficiency syndrome. *J Neurosurg* 73:206–211, 1990.
51. So YT, Beckstead JH, Davis RL: Primary central nerous system lymphoma in acquired immune deficiency syndrome: A clincial and pathological study. *Ann Neurol* 20:566–572, 1986.
52. Hochberg FH, Miller DC: Primary central nervous system lymphoma. *J Neurosurg* 68:835–853, 1988.
53. Goldstein JS, Dickson DW, Moser FG, et al: Primary central nervous system lymphoma in acquired immune deficiency syndrome: A clinical and pathological study with results of treatment with radiation. *Cancer* 67:2756–2765, 1991.
54. Formenti SC, Gill PS, Lean E, Ranick M, Meyer PR, Boswell W, Petrovich Z, Chak I, Levine AM: Primary central nervous system lymphoma in AIDS; results of radiation therapy. *Cancer* 1989;63:1101–1107
55. MacMahon EME, Glass JD, Hayward SD, et al: Epstein-Barr virus (EBV) in AIDS-related primary central nervous system lymphoma. *Lancet* 1991;338:969–973.
56. Lee YY, Brunner JM, Tassel PV, et al: Primary and central nervous system lymphoma: CT and pathological correlation. *Am J Neuroradiol* 7:599–604, 1986.
57. Ruiz A, Post MJD, Bundschu C, et al: Primary central nervous system lymphoma in patients with AIDS. *Neuroimag Clin North Am* 7:281–296, 1997.
58. Bishburg E, Eng RHK, Jihad S, et al: Brain lesions in patients with acquired immunodeficiency syndrome. *Arch Intern Med* 149:941–943, 1989.
59. Whitener DR: Tuberculous brain abscess: Report of a case and review of the literature. *Arch Neurol* 35:148–155, 1978.
60. Som PM, Dillon WP, Fullerton GD, et al: Chronically obstructed sinonasal secretions: Observations on T1 and T2 shortening. *Radiology* 172:515–520, 1989.
61. Katz DA, Berger JR: Neurosyphilis in acquired immunodeficiency syndrome. *Arch Neurol* 46:895–898, 1989.
62. Katz DA, Berger JR, Duncan RC: Neurosyphilis: A comparative study of the effects of concomitant HIV-1 infection. *Arch Neurol* 50:243–249, 1993.
63. Hook EW: Syphilis and HIV infection. *J Infect Dis* 160:530–534, 1989.
64. Johns DR, Tierny M, Falsenstein D: Alteration in the natural history of neurosyphilis by concurrent infection with the human immunodeficiency virus. *N Engl J Med* 316:1587–1589, 1987.
65. Berger JR, Waskin H, Pall L, et al: Syphilitic cerebral gumma with HIV infection. *Neurology* 42:1282–1287, 1992.
66. Hollard BA, Perrett LV, Mills CM: Meningovascular syphilis: CT and MR findings. *Radiology* 158:439–442, 1986.

67. Tien RD, Chu PK, Hesselink J, et al: Intracranial cryptococcosis in immunocompromised patients: CT and MRI findings in 29 patients. *Am J Neuroradiol* 12:283–289, 1991.
68. Grafe MR, Press GA, Berthity DP, et al: Abnormalities of the brain in AIDS patients: Correlation of postmortem MR findings with neuropathology. *Am J Neuroradiol* 11:905–911, 1990
69. Popoyich MJ, Arthur RH, Helmer E: CT of intracranial cryptococcosis. *Am J Neuroradiol* 11:139–142, 1990.
70. Andreula CF, Burdi N, Carella A: CNS Cryptococcosis in AIDS: Spectrum of MR findings. *J Comput Assist Tomogr* 17:438–441, 1993.
71. Cohen WA: Intracranial bacterial infections in patients with AIDS. *Neuroimag Clin North Am* 7:223–229, 1997.
72. Berger JR, Harris JO, Gregorios J, Norenberg M: Cerebrovascular disease in AIDS: A case control study. *AIDS* 4:239–244, 1990.
73. Gilliams AR, Allen E, Hrieb K, et al: Cerebral infarction in patients with AIDS. *Am J Neuroradiol* 18:1581–1581, 1997.
74. Phillepet P, Blnache S, Sebag G, et al: Stroke and cerebral infarcts in children infected with human immunodeficiency virus. *Arch Pediatr Adolesc Med* 148:965–970, 1994.
75. Berger JR, Kaszowitz B, Dickinson G, Post MJD: Progressive multifocal leukoencephalopathy associated with human immunodeficiency virus infection: A review of the literature and report of 16 cases. *Ann Intern Med* 107:78–87, 1987.
76. Mark AS, Atlas SW: Progressive multifocal leukoencephalopathy in patients with AIDS: Appearance on MR images. *Radiology* 173:517–521, 1989.
77. Krup LB, Lipton RB, Swerdlow ML, et al: Progressive multifocal leukoencephalopathy: Clinical and radiographic features. *Ann Neurol* 17:344–349, 1985.
78. Whiteman MH, Post MJD, Berger JR, et al: PML in 47 HIV-seropositive patients: Neuroimaging with clinical and pathological correlations. *Radiology* 187:233–240, 1993.
79. Ho DD, Rota TR, Schooley RT: Isolation of HTVL-III from cerebrospinal fluid and neural tissue of patient with neurologic syndrome. *N Engl J Med* 313:1493–1497, 1985.
80. Resnick L, diMarzo-Veronese F, Schupbach J, et al: Intra-blood-brain-barrier synthesis of HTVL-III-specific IgG in patients with neurologic symptoms associated with AIDS or AIDS-related complex. *N Engl J Med* 313:1498–1504, 1985.
81. Scott G, Hutto C, Makuch RW, et al: Survival in children with perinatally acquired human immunodeficiency virus type infection. *N Engl J Med* 321:1791–1796, 1989.
82. Price RW, Brew B, Sidtis J, et al: The brain in AIDS: Central nervous system HIV-1 infection and AIDS dementia complex. *Science* 239:586–592, 1988.
83. Navia BA, Jordan BD, Price RW: The AIDS dementia complex: II. Neuropathology. *Ann Neurol* 19:525–535, 1986.
84. Navia BA, Jordan BD, Price RW: The AIDS dementia complex: I. Clinical features. *Ann Neurol* 19:517–524, 1986.
85. Chrysikopoulos HS, Press GA, Grafe MR, et al: Encephalitis caused by human immunodeficiency virus: CT and MR imaging manifestations with clinical and pathological correlation. *Radiology* 175:185–191, 1990.
86. Post MJD, Tate LG, Quencer RM, et al: CT, MR and pathology in HIV encephalitis and meningitis. *Am J Neuroradiol* 9:469–476, 1988.
87. Olsen WL, Longo FM, Mills CM, Normal D: White matter diseases in AIDS: Findings at MR imaging. *Radiology* 169:445–448, 1988.
88. Post MJD, Berger JR, Quencer RM: Asymptomatic and neurologically symptomatic HIV-seropositive individuals: Prospective evaluation with cranial MR imaging. *Radiology* 178:131–139, 1991.
89. Post MJD, Berger JR, Duncan R, et al: Long-term MR and clinical follow-up of HIV+ asymptomatic and neurologically symptomatic subjects. *Radiology* 188:173–179, 1993.
90. Post MJD, Levin BE, Berger JR, et al: Sequential cranial MR findings of asymptomatic and neurologically symptomatic HIV+ subjects. *Am J Neuroradiol* 13:359–370, 1992.
91. Reichert CM, O'Leary TJ, Levens DL, et al: Autopsy pathology in the acquired immune deficiency syndrome. *Am J Pathol* 112:357–382, 1983.
92. Kalayjian RC, Cohen ML, Bonomo RA, Flanigan TP: Cytomegalovirus ventriculoencephalitis in AIDS: A syndrome with distinct clinical and pathologic features. *Medicine* 72:67–77, 1993.
93. Post MJD, Hensley GT, Moskowitz LB, Fischl M: Cytomegalic inclusion virus encephalitis in patients with AIDS: CT, clinical and pathological correlation. *Am J Neuroradiol* 7:275–280, 1986.
94. Carne CA, Smith A, Elkington SG, et al: Acute encephalopathy coincident with seroconversion for anti-HTLV-III. *Lancet* 2:1206–1208, 1985.
95. Whiteman MLH: Neuroimaging of central nervous system tuberculosis in HIV-infected patients. *Neuroimag Clin North Am* 7:199–214, 1997.
96. Eidelberg D, Sotrel A, Vogel M, et al: Progressive polyradiculopathy in acquired immune deficiency syndrome. *Neurology*. 36:912–916, 1986.
97. Miller RG, Storey JR, Greco CM: Ganciclovir in the treatment of progressive AIDS-related polyradiculopathy. *Neurology* 1990;40:569–574.

CHAPTER 15

NEUROIMAGING IN PATIENTS WITH CEREBROVASCULAR DISEASE

Louis R. Caplan
L. Dana DeWitt
Joan C. Breen

Within two decades, the technological revolution in brain and vascular imaging and function tests has brought clinicians from famine to feast. A plethora of tests is now available, but the results are not always easy to interpret in relation to patients' symptoms and signs. For example, an early study of "normal prisoners" utilizing contrast cerebral angiography showed a high incidence of arterial occlusions and stenoses.[1] Similarly, brain imaging and vascular studies in a geriatric, stroke-prone population would undoubtedly contain a large number of clinically silent abnormalities, some of dubious clinical relevance. These observations belie the old adage, dear to many neurosurgeons, that an ounce of dye is worth all the neurologists in the room.

Clinicians have four basic goals when approaching stroke patients: (1) to identify the cause and mechanism of the stroke, (2) to localize the lesion or lesions within the brain and vascular system, (3) to quantify the severity of the brain damage sufficiently to guide prognosis and management decisions, and (4) to identify salient conditions and vascular lesions that might pose significant imminent or future risks of further strokes. Also, because most occlusive cerebrovascular lesions are due to atherosclerosis, a systemic disease, attention to risk factors and prevention of coronary-artery–related ischemia is very important. Clinicians must also keep the purse in mind; clearly, society cannot and will not be able to afford an unlimited array of expensive tests for all patients with vascular disease.

Given these goals and restraints, the following rules should guide the evaluation:

1. The clinical data should be acquired first before planning the laboratory and imaging evaluation.
2. At each stage of the evaluation—during and after the history, during and after the general and neurologic examinations, and during and after each important successive investigation—clinicians should generate and test hypotheses as to the *cause of the stroke* (*what?*) and the *location of the brain and vascular lesions* (*where?*).

Each evaluation should be hypothesis- and question-driven. This strategy for neurologic diagnosis is discussed elsewhere in more detail.[2,3] Succeeding chapters consider in detail the individual tests available. This chapter conveys the basic strategies and modus operandi for evaluating stroke patients and attempts to direct clinicians to the key questions that require answers. Once the important questions are recognized, the answers are not hard to obtain. Examples of specific patients are included to clarify the approach.

THE CLINICAL ENCOUNTER

The first important query in the mind of the clinician should be How ill is the patient? Is he or she a candidate for any form of specific therapy? Clearly, laboratory and imaging investigations are aimed at a specific diagnosis in order to guide prognosis and treatment. There are some patients in whom only symptomatic treatment is feasible and proper. In these patients, there is little reason to order needless tests.

The major guiding data in this decision should be the prior health and psychosocial state of the patient. A hopelessly demented nursing home resident of 91, a man 61 riddled with lung cancer and in constant pain, and a very depressed widower of 82 who had a prior disabling stroke are all clearly not candidates for aggressive treatment or testing.

More caution must be exercised in excluding patients from testing because of the acute stroke-related deficit. Although the initial deficit may be very severe when the patient is seen acutely, the *signs may be reversible later.* Most experienced clinicians have seen patients who entered the hospital in a coma, quadraplegic, or with severe hemiplegia and cognitive or aphasic deficits and who left the hospital with little or no permanent deficit. The term *spectacular shrinking deficit* was coined by Mohr to capture this turn of events. Also important is the notion that some lesions might be treatable, but others might not be. For example, the patient with a subdural hematoma, a drainable hemorrhage, acute hydrocephalus, and the like can be treated. In such a patient, some testing would be in order to exclude those treatable lesions. In many patients, time is a critical factor. If something can be done, it should be done quickly. If, under some circumstances, specific treatment is feasible, then the evaluation should proceed quickly to exclude those treatable conditions.

What Is the Cause (Mechanism) of the Stroke?

Table 15-1 lists the major stroke mechanisms that should be kept in mind as the clinician begins the history. The first branch point is separating *hemorrhage* from *ischemia*—too much blood in the head versus not enough. These are diametrically opposite problems that necessitate very different treatments and evaluations. Hemorrhage should be further divided into *subarachnoid hemorrhage (SAH)* and *intracerebral hemorrhage (ICH)*, since the causes and management strategies for these two types of hemorrhage are quite different. Subarachnoid hemorrhage is usually caused by an aneurysm at the base of the brain or a vascular malformation near the pial or ependymal surface. Bleeding is usually brisk, brief, and under arterial pressure. The bleeding quickly disseminates within the cerebrospinal fluid (CSF) and increases intracranial pressure abruptly. Bleeding is not usually into brain parenchyma. The common clinical symptoms are sudden severe headache, cessation of activity and recall, vomiting, and a change in the level of alertness (drowsiness or restlessness). Focal neurologic symptoms and signs are usually absent or minor or reflect pressure on adjacent cranial nerves by the aneurysm. In SAH, the clinical goal is to prevent the next bleed and to prevent vasoconstriction related to the blood already deposited around the brain. In ICH, the usual cause is hypertension, but vascular malformations, bleeding disorders, drugs, and other diverse causes are

Table 15-1
Stroke mechanisms

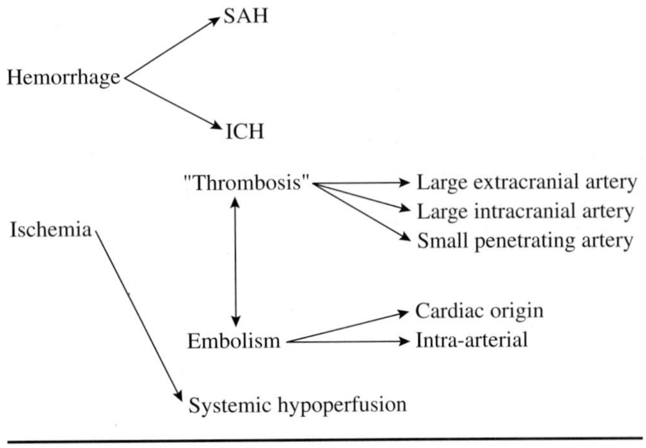

also important. Bleeding is usually under less pressure than in SAH and is directly into brain parenchyma. The initial symptoms and signs are related to dysfunction of the part of the brain harboring the hematoma. Hematomas often enlarge and extend gradually during minutes and sometimes hours. Rebleeding is less of a risk than in SAH. The clinician's goal is to minimize brain damage and pressure effects from the initial ICH.

Ischemic lesions are divided traditionally into "thrombotic," embolic, and pump failure with systemic hypoperfusion. The designation thrombotic is used when the vascular occlusive process originated within the vessel in situ. In embolism, vascular blockage is by a particle that came from somewhere else. In systemic hypoperfusion, there ordinarily is no focal vascular occlusion; the problem is failure of the heart to pump sufficient blood to the head. This could occur if blood volume or blood pressure were very low or if the pumping function of the heart failed because of arrythmia or cardiac arrest. Finding the mechanism of ischemia can be likened to the problem a plumber faces when you call him to your house because you have insufficient water flow and pressure in one of the third-floor showers. The plumber knows that the pipes to that third-floor bathroom might be blocked by rust or other local damage. Alternatively, there might be malfunction of the water tank or pump, or too little water in the system. Foreign material in the tank or pipes could have broken loose to block a pipe to the bathroom or to the shower. By testing a variety of pipes in that bathroom, the basement, and the first, second, and third floors, the plumber should be able to localize the problem as long as he knows where the pipes are. The plumber's repair strategy will vary considerably, depending on the cause—local pipe trouble, foreign material in the system, or pump or pressure trouble—as will the clinician's diagnostic and treatment plan, depending on the mechanism of the ischemia.

The key items of data that clinicians use to separate the conditions of thrombosis, embolism, and systemic hypoperfusion are listed in Table 15-2. Unfortunately, space does not permit an analysis of each of these items here, but they are discussed in detail elsewhere.[3]

Where Is the Lesion in the Brain? Where in the Vascular System?

The *where* question is very germane to the imaging and laboratory investigation. If the plumber has localized the problem to the large pipe supplying the third-floor shower and he knows exactly which pipes lead to that shower, he knows exactly where to look for mischief in the system. He would be greatly aided if he also knew which pipes were most likely to be injured, given the construction and physics of the system. Similarly, localization of the stroke to the anterior or posterior circulation and to the left or right side is an essential step. The data used to clinically judge location are quite different

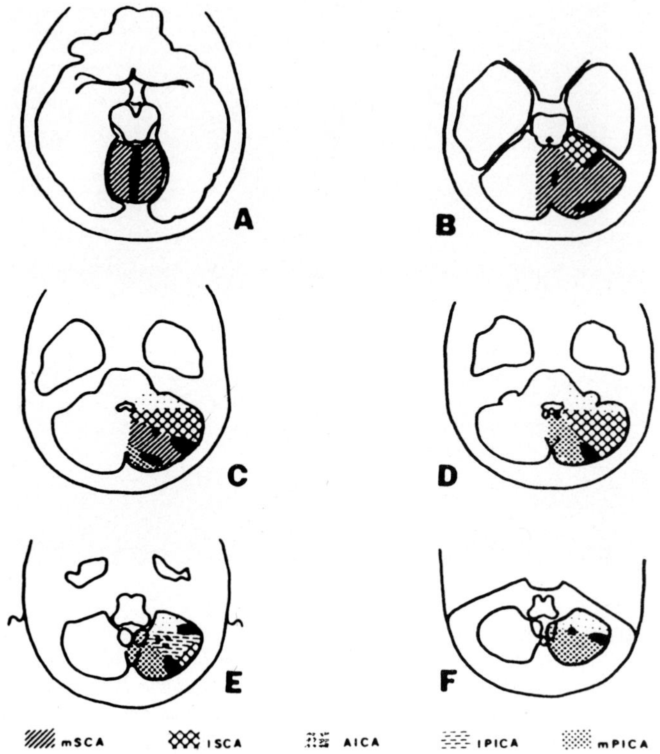

Figure 15-2
Arterial distribution of cerebellar infarcts. MSCA, medial superior cerebellar artery; ISCA, inferior superior cerebellar artery; AICA, anterior inferior cerebellar artery; IPCA, inferior posterior cerebellar artery; MPICA, medial posterior inferior cerebellar artery. (From Amarenco et al.[4])

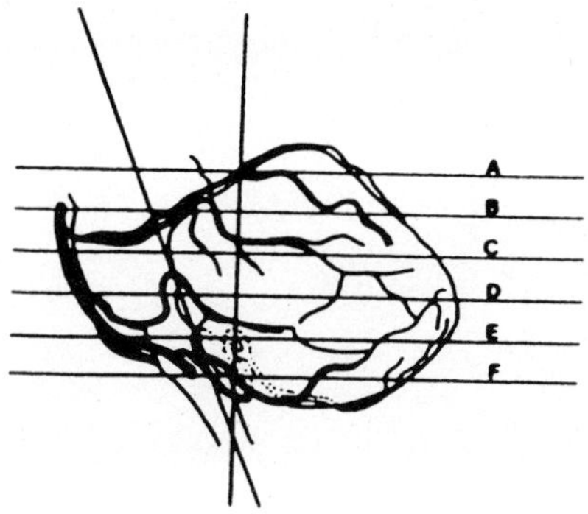

a known important complication of cocaine use. Moreover, we recalled that in individuals with cocaine-related ICH and SAH there was a higher incidence of underlying aneurysms and vascular malformations than in patients with hemorrhages related to amphetamines and other drugs.[18] An emergency CT scan was ordered. Magnetic resonance imaging was not as readily available early in the morning, and in ST, who was suspected of having a supratentorial hematoma, there was no clear superiority of MRI over CT. In fact, CT and MRI would probably have been equally able to show an acute hematoma.

The CT scan showed a very large hyperdense lesion in the right basal ganglia–internal capsule region (Figs. 15-4 and 15-5). The bleeding had dissected into the lateral ventricles, and some blood was also visible on the brain surface. There was some shift of the midline and dilatation of the contralateral lateral ventricle. The ipsilateral lateral ventricle was compressed.

Computed tomography had provided a variety of information concerning:

The stroke mechanism. Clearly, the hyperdense lesion represented a hematoma. Sometimes hyperdensity is admixed with hypodensity in hemorrhagic infarcts, but in this case the lesion was uniform and well circumscribed, and it spared the overlying cortex. There was no suggestion of infarcted tissue.

The vascular territory involved. In this case, the basal ganglionic hematoma was within the territory of the lateral lenticulostriate branches of the right MCA.

The size of the lesion. Using multiple sections, the maximal diameter of the hematoma on the slice showing the largest lesion can be measured, and the lesion volume can be estimated from the diameters on each slice and the number of slices involved. A useful method of measurement of hematoma volume on CT scans is to use the formula ABC/2, where A is the largest diameter, B is the diameter 90° to A, and C is the approximate number of slices that show hemorrhage multiplied by the thickness of each slice.[19] Newer scanners can calculate and print out the volume of circumscribed lesions. The prognosis of patients with hematomas depends heavily on the size of the lesion.[20,21]

Drainage patterns. Hematomas can remain entirely enclosed within brain parenchyma or can discharge (drain) contents into the CSF at either the pial surfaces or the ependymal surfaces of the ventricles. Spontaneous drainage allows for some egress of blood from within the brain and, with it, some decompression. The alternative is more bleeding into the brain.

The presence and amount of surrounding edema. Edema surrounding hematomas adds to the potential mass effect. The relative amount of hematoma versus edema may give information on the likely success of medical measures to reduce the mass effect of the lesion.

Mass effect. Displacement of midline structures and vertical displacement of the upper brainstem can be detected by both CT and MRI; the presence or absence of mass effects is useful in choosing medical or surgical decompression and in making a prognosis.

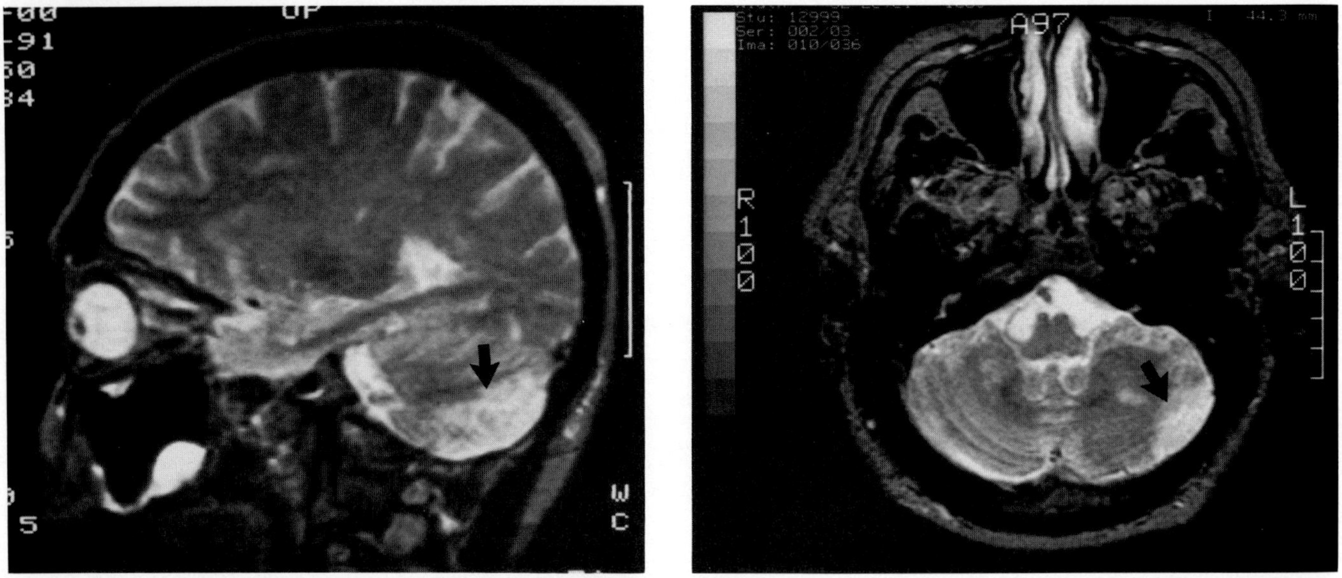

A

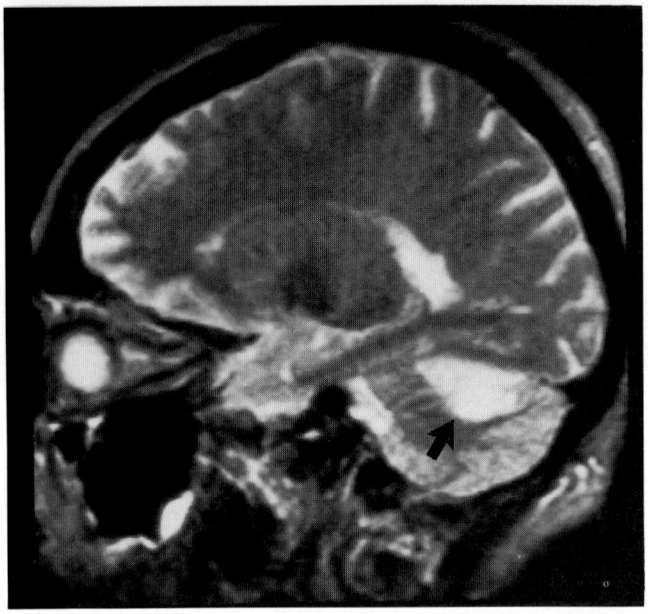

B

Figure 15-3

(A) *Sagittal (left) and axial (right) T2-weighted MRIs showing an infarct in the distribution of the lateral branch of the left posterior inferior cerebellar artery.* **(B)** *An infarct in the distribution of the right medial superior cerebellar artery is seen on this sagittal image.*

Blockage of CSF pathways causing hydrocephalus. Obstruction of the foramen of Monro (as in patient ST), the sylvian aqueduct, or the outflow foramina of the fourth ventricle is common in patients with hematomas. Computed tomography and MRI can readily define enlargement of one lateral ventricle, as in this case, and the pattern of general or localized ventricular enlargement. The presence of obstructive hydrocephalus raises the possibility of therapeutic ventricular drainage as a means of reducing intracranial pressure and decompressing the lesion.

The shape, homogeneity, and morphologic characteristics of the lesion. Hematomas that form within arteriovenous malformations (AVMs), cavernous angiomas, tumors, and infarcts often have different imaging characteristics from those found in spontaneous hematomas in which there is no preceding underlying structural lesion. The lesion in ST was homogeneous and well circumscribed and gave no hint of a prior process. Magnetic resonance imaging is superior to CT at suggesting underlying cavernous angiomas, AVMs, and tumors. Suspicion of one of these lesions would be an indication for MRI after CT.

The presence of additional brain lesions, especially old hematoma cavities. In ST, there were no other lesions. The presence of old slit cavities might have raised suspicion of amyloid angiopathy if the lesions were lobar and the patient were older. Prior hypertensive or cocaine-related bleeds were also possible. Alternatively, by showing other brain lesions that looked like cavernous angiomas (these lesions are often multiple) or tumors, suspicion of those disorders would be raised despite the

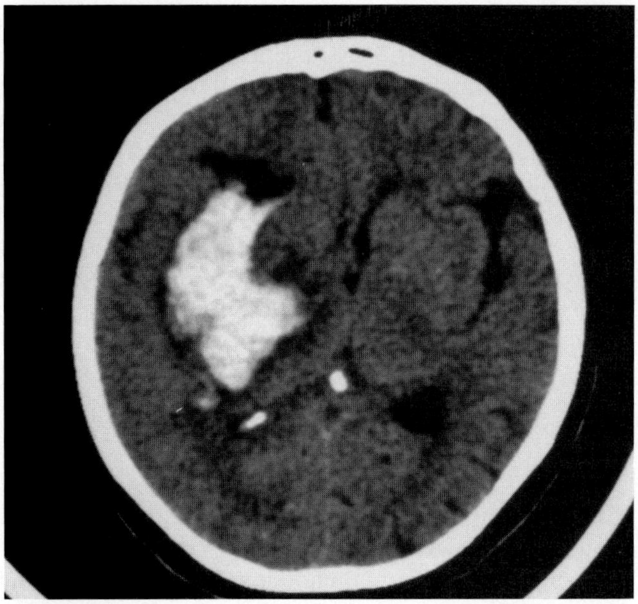

Figure 15-4
Noncontrast CT showing large intracerebral hemorrhage in the right basal ganglia.

fact that the symptomatic lesion did not suggest those disorders. Due to its ability to show hemosiderin, MRI, especially using gradient echo susceptibility images, is superior to CT in identifying old lesions as hemorrhagic foci.

In the patient ST, there seemed to be little additional benefit to ordering an MRI. Since he was restless and moving about, MRI would have required sedation, lending some risk to the procedure. We elected not to pursue brain imaging further at that time. If it had been important to define better the morphologic characteristics of the lesion because of a suspected infarct, AVM, angioma, or tumor or if it were important to establish the presence of old bleeds or acute contusions near the orbital and basal temporal surfaces of the brain, then MRI would have been potentially more fruitful.

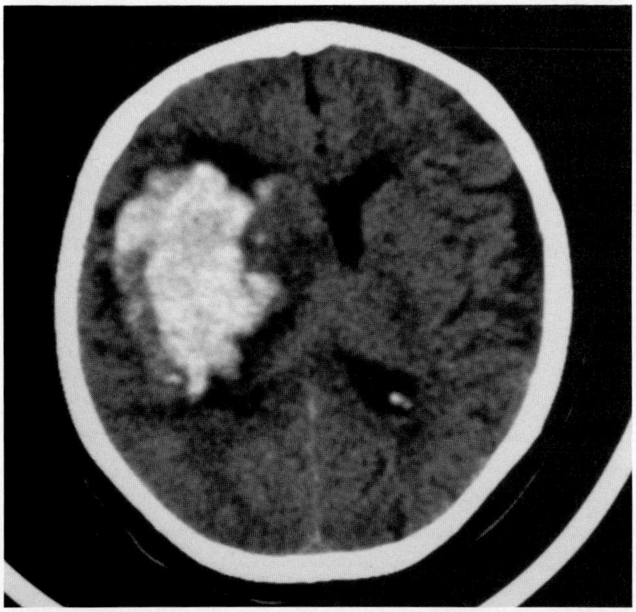

Figure 15-5
Higher cut shows hemorrhage plus dilatation of contralateral lateral ventricle.

What If the Lesion Is a SAH?

As discussed above, the two most common types of lesions are infarcts and hematomas. The other important intracranial vascular process is SAH, as illustrated by the following example:

A 23-year-old woman, RM, developed a very severe headache while having sex with her husband in the afternoon. She then became temporarily limp. Moments later she vomited, became restless and agitated, and seemed confused to her husband. On examination in the emergency room 1 h later, her blood pressure was 140/90 torr. She was quite restless and could not concentrate for cognitive testing. She did not recall the circumstance about the onset of the headache. Her neck was stiff, and she had a subhyaloid hemorrhage in the right optic fundus. There were no focal or lateralized neurologic signs. Both plantar responses were extensor.

In the patient RM, the diagnosis of SAH seemed straightforward. Her age, lack of stroke risk factors, and the onset during sex strongly favored SAH. In acute SAH, blood in the CSF is easier to detect and study with CT than with MRI. We ordered an urgent CT scan which confirmed the presence of a large quantity of blood within the subarachnoid space (Fig. 15-6). The *distribution of blood* can often yield clues to the location of the bleeding aneurysm. In patients with ruptured anterior communicating artery aneurysms, the blood often is centered near the anterior perforated substance on one side and may track into the basal frontal lobe, the septum pellucidum, and the lateral ventricles. In patients with MCA aneurysms, the blood is often laterally placed within the sylvian cistern and within the sulci on the convexal surface. In patients with hemorrhage from posterior communicating artery aneurysms, the blood may pool a bit more posteriorly, near the posterior perforated substance and the ICA on the side of the hemorrhage. When the bleeding aneurysm is within the posterior circulation, the blood may be more localized within the posterior fossa cisterns.

The thickness of the blood and the presence of thick clots can also yield information about the likelihood of development of delayed cerebral ischemia. Most observations indicate that local thick blood collection is more likely to be associated with vasoconstriction than are lesser degrees of diffusely disseminated blood.[22]

In some patients with SAH, the distribution of blood is primarily around the brainstem and the perimesencephalic and pontine cisterns. This distribution of SAH has been referred to by van Gijn and colleagues

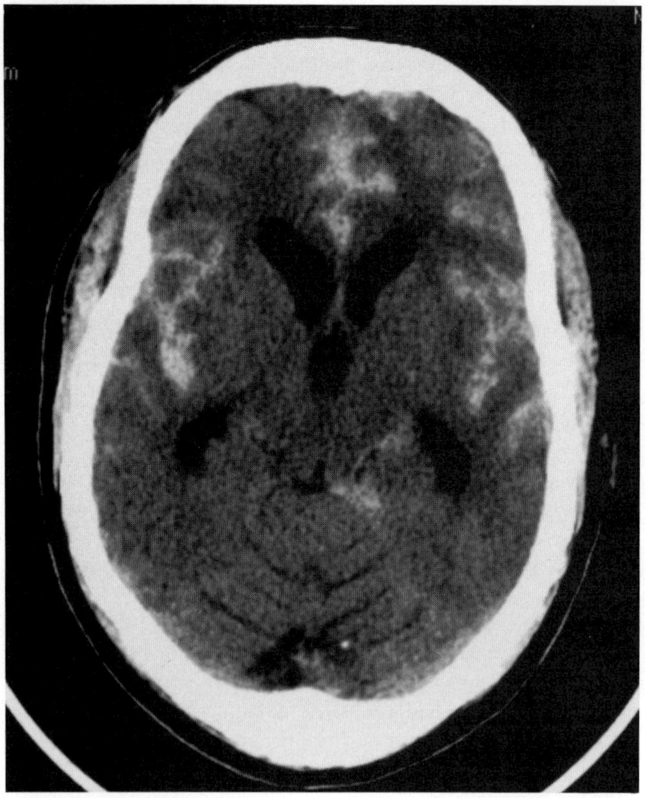

A

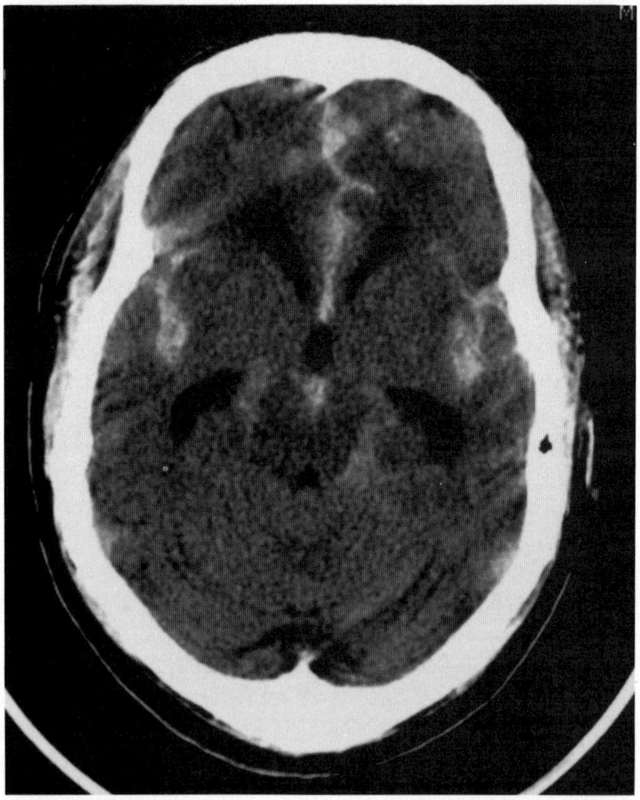

B

Figure 15-6
Noncontrast CT showing a large subarachnoid hemorrhage with subarachnoid blood located diffusely along the cortical surface. In this patient, subsequent angiography showed an anterior communicating artery aneurysm.

as perimesencephalic hemorrhage.[23,24] Figure 15-7 shows a CT scan from a patient with a perimesencephalic hemorrhage. Although the origin of the bleeding is not known, patients with this distribution of SAH have a better prognosis and have less probability of harboring aneurysms than do patients in whom SAH is more diffusely distributed within the CSF. The bleeding in patients with perimesencephalic hemorrhages may issue from venous structurers. In this patient and the vast majority of patients with SAH, there seemed to be little advantage to ordering an MRI.

What and Where Are the Vascular Lesions?

What If the Brain Lesion Is Ischemic?

The distribution and localization of infarcts within the brain on CT and MRI scans leads to preliminary hypotheses about the localization and nature of the underlying cardiovascular lesions. Of course, as mentioned earlier, the clinical signs must also be added to the imaging findings, since all ischemic brain lesions require an explanation. Figure 15-8 shows common infarct patterns

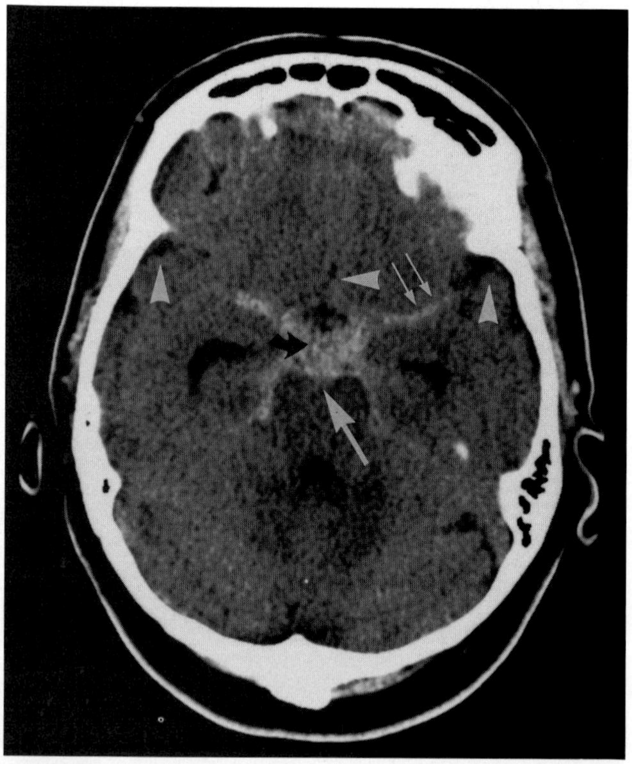

Figure 15-7
Noncontrast CT showing perimesencephalic subarachnoid hemorrhage. The center of the bleeding lies in the interpeduncular cistern (curved arrow). There is some extension to the central sylvian fissures and posterior part of the interhemispheric fissure (straight arrows) but not to the lateral part of the sylvian fissures or the anterior part of the interhemispheric fissure (arrowheads). There is no intraventricular blood. (Courtesy of Professors G.J.E. Rinkel and J. van Gijn, Department of Neurology, University of Utrecht, Utrecht, The Netherlands.)

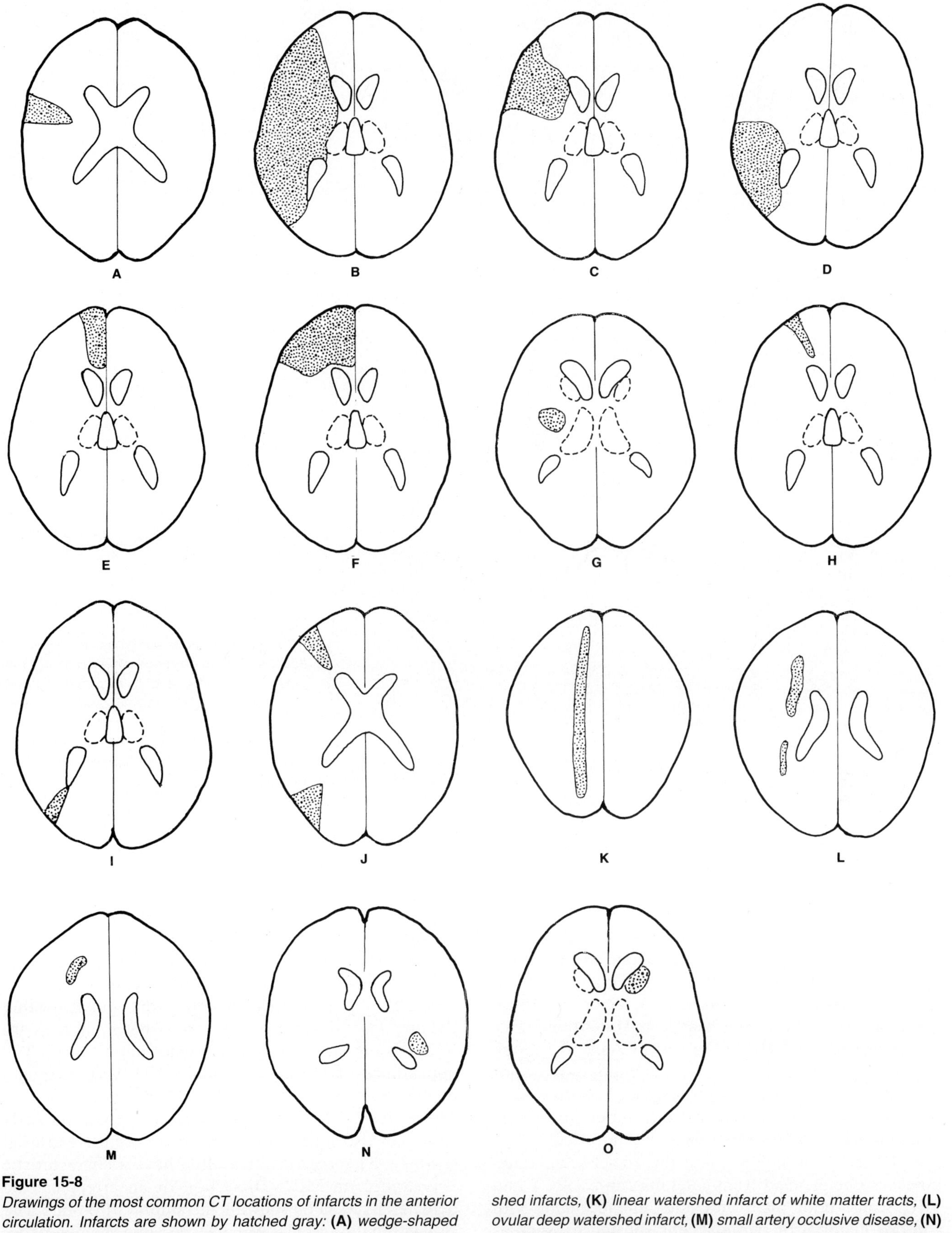

Figure 15-8

Drawings of the most common CT locations of infarcts in the anterior circulation. Infarcts are shown by hatched gray: **(A)** *wedge-shaped MCA infarct,* **(B)** *entire MCA territory,* **(C)** *superior division MCA,* **(D)** *inferior division MCA,* **(E)** *ACA,* **(F)** *ACA and MCA,* **(G)** *striatocapsular infarct,* **(H)** *wedge-shaped anterior watershed infarct,* **(I)** *wedge-shaped posterior watershed infarct,* **(J)** *anterior and posterior watershed infarcts,* **(K)** *linear watershed infarct of white matter tracts,* **(L)** *ovular deep watershed infarct,* **(M)** *small artery occlusive disease,* **(N)** *caudate infarct,* **(O)** *anterior choroidal artery territory infarct. (Modified from Caplan.[25] Used by permission. Artist, Harriet Greenfield, Boston.)*

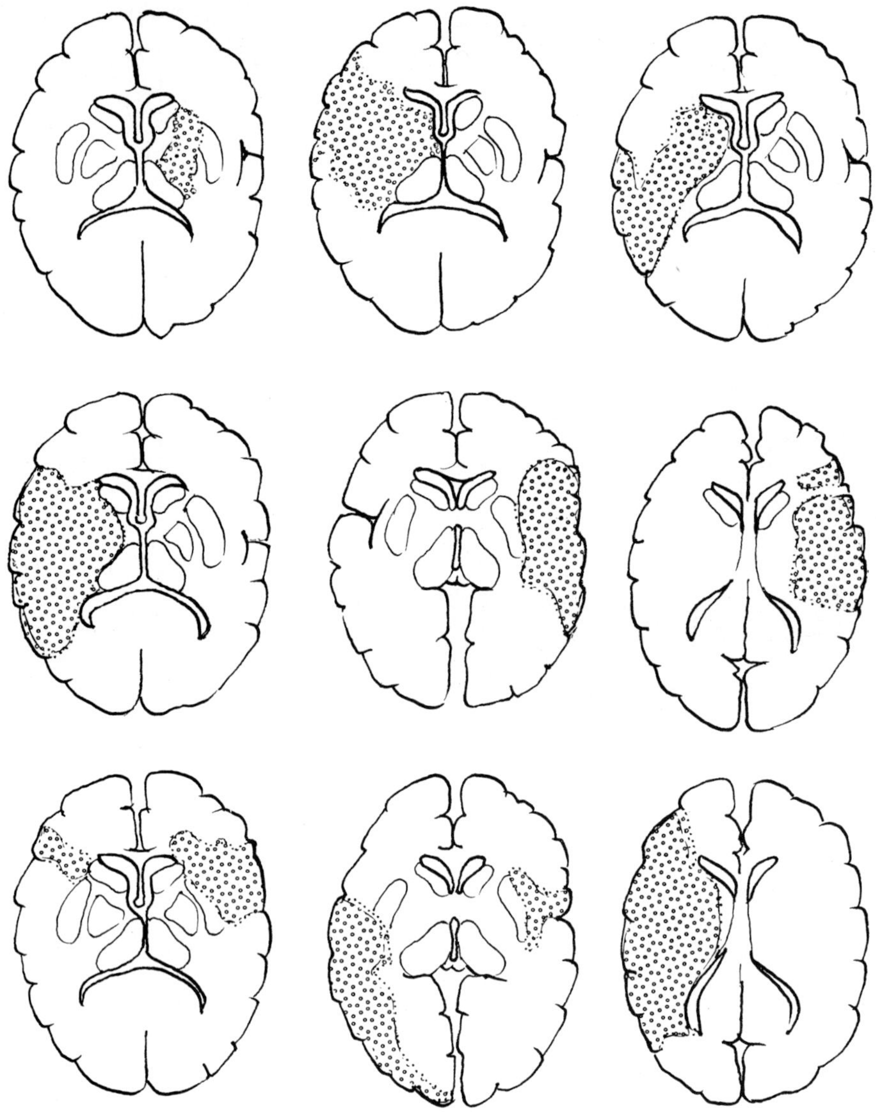

Figure 15-9

Drawings of common patterns of embolic brain infarcts. (Based on Ringelstein EB et al: Computer tomographic pattern of proven embolic infarctions. Ann Neurol *26:759–775, 1989. From Caplan.*[3] *Used by permission. Artist, Juan Sanchez-Ramos, Department of Neurology, University of Miami School of Medicine, Miami.)*

associated with occlusive lesions of the various anterior circulation arteries.[3,25] Figure 15-9 consists of an artist's drawings of CT scans taken from a series of patients with documented cardiac-origin brain embolism.[3,26] Our patient AH, however, had infarction within the posterior circulation. Studies of patients with posterior circulation embolism show that the most frequent recipient sites for emboli are the ICVA-PICA region, the distal basilar artery and its deep thalamic and midbrain perforating arteries, and the SCAs and PCAs.[17,27,28] Emboli sometimes go to the basilar artery. The sites of posterior circulation embolism are shown in Fig. 15-10.

The distribution of ischemia and infarction in the brain gives indirect information about the vascular process. Direct information about the vessels can sometimes also be gleaned from careful scrutiny of CT and MRI scans, both plain and after enhancement with contrast material or paramagnetic substances, such as gadolinium. Acute occlusive emboli may appear as cylindrical hyperdensities within the basal cisterns and subarachnoid space on plain unenhanced CT scans. Since the commonest artery involved is the MCA, the sign has been dubbed the hyperdense MCA sign.[29,30] Aneurysms, either dolichoectatic, fusiform expansions[31] or large berry-type aneurysms, can harbor clots and cause ischemia by embolization of clot material or blockage of branches by thrombus that remains within the aneurysm. Fusiform and large berry aneurysms are often visible on enhanced CT scans and on MRI. The appearance of the aneurysm on MRI with heterogeneous shadows can suggest the presence of thrombus. The absence of normal vascular flow voids on MRI scans can also suggest the presence of occlusive arterial lesions.[32] Dissected arteries often have a characteristic appearance on MRI. Dissection of an artery can be detected by MRI by showing intramural thrombus. The clot within the vascular wall has the same characteristics of hematomas as described earlier in this chapter. Typi-

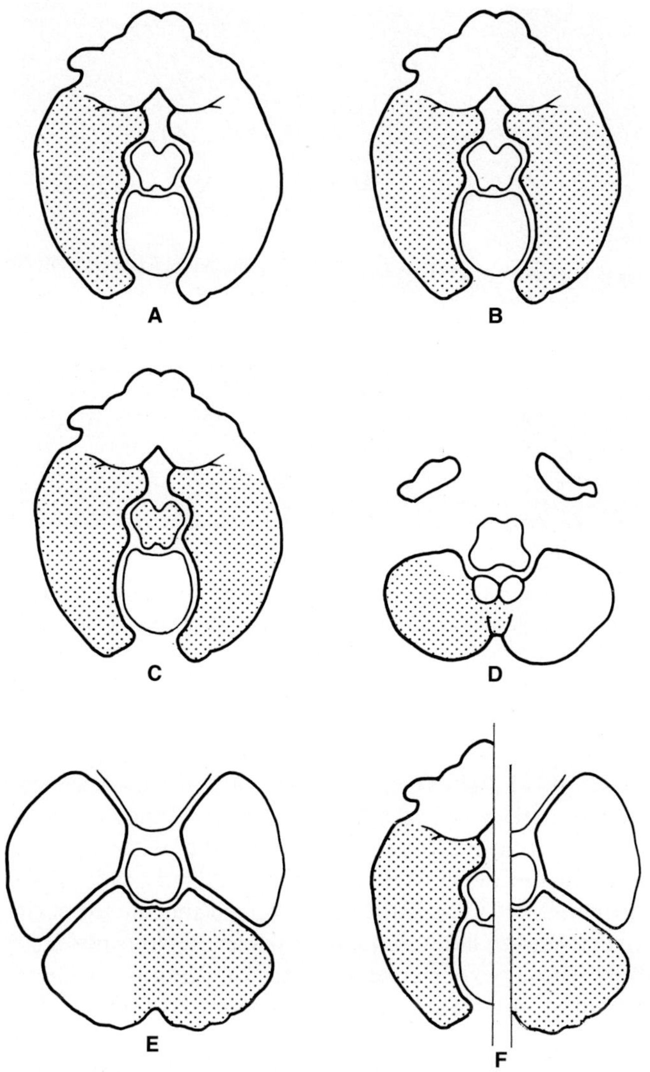

Figure 15-10
Drawings of the most common locations of infarcts in the posterior circulation. **(A)** *PCA territory infarct,* **(B)** *bilateral PCA territory infarcts,* **(C)** *top of the basilar territory infarct involving the PCAs and midbrain,* **(D)** *posterior ICA territory infarct,* **(E)** *SCA territory infarct,* **(F)** *tandem infarcts involving SCA (right half) and PCA (left half). (Artist, Harriet Greenfield, Boston.)*

cally, the intramural thrombus appears high intensity on an axial T1-weighted image and remains hyperintense on a T2-weighted image.[33] Often the lumen of the artery is eccentrically narrowed and may be thrombosed.

Magnetic resonance angiography is a very important investigation that promises to yield a great deal of information about vascular occlusive lesions. It has the additional positive feature of being able to be performed with and immediately after MRI. It is noninvasive and quite safe. Magnetic resonance angiography can be performed using a variety of techniques, including two-dimensional and three-dimensional time-of-flight and phase contrast imaging.[34–37] Magnetic resonance angiography is a functional technique that creates an image of flow in the artery. Unlike standard contrast injection angiograms, the images do not reflect anatomy. Within the anterior circulation, the ICA origins are usually well visualized, but at times MRA overestimates the degree of luminal narrowing.[38,39] The technique is quite accurate in patients with complete ICA occlusions and has a sensitivity and specificity comparable to that of duplex ultrasound in screening for the presence of severe ICA stenotic lesions.[39] The changing angles and curvature of the ICA in the siphon often make interpretation of this region more difficult than for the straight portions of the artery. The horizontal segment of the MCA is usually well shown. Figure 15-11 shows an MRA from a patient with severe stenosis of the MCA.

The MRA of the vertebral artery origins from the subclavian arteries is usually not adequate because of the overlapping of arteries. Similarly, arch injection contrast angiograms often do not show the vertebral artery origins (VAOs) very well unless special views are taken. The second portion of the vertebral artery (VA) within the intervertebral foramina is well shown on MRA. This region is poorly shown by color-flow Doppler studies. The third portion of the VA, the portion that curves around the rostral cervical vertebrae, is often not particularly well seen on MRA because of the sharp angulation and curvature of the artery. The ICVAs and the

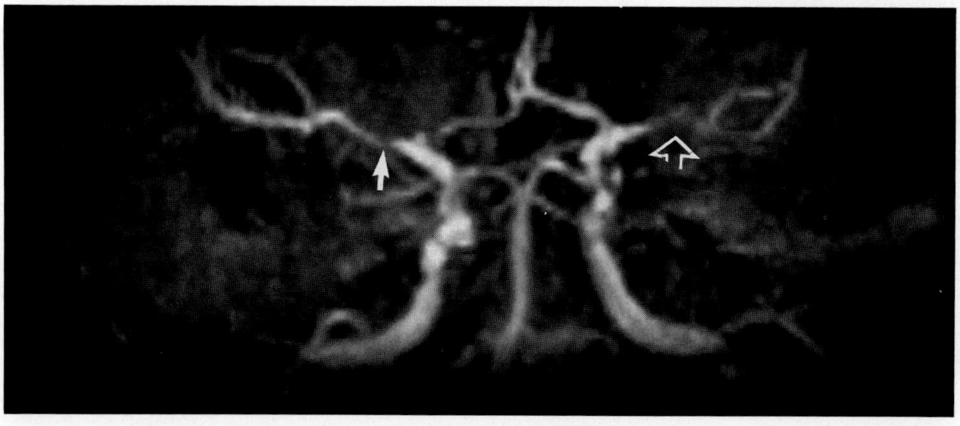

Figure 15-11
MRA showing severe stenosis of both left and right MCAs.

basilar artery are usually very well shown on intracranial MRA, especially the rostral bifurcation into the PCAs. Often the origins of PICAs, AICAs, and the SCAs are shown.

Quereshi and colleagues evaluated the ability of MRA to detect significant occlusive lesions among 118 patients with brain infarcts.[40] Among the 176 large arteries visualized by both MRA and conventional angiography, angiography confirmed 9 out of 10 (90 percent) extracranial and 32 out of 40 (80 percent) of intracranial abnormalities shown by MRA. There were few false-negative or -positive abnormalities.[40] In the patient AH, the MRA showed no definite abnormality in the neck. The ICVA on the left showed an area of stenosis (Fig. 15-12). The right SCA was not seen, but the left SCA and both PCAs were imaged and appeared normal. Our preliminary impression after the clinical encounter, brain imaging, and MRA was that there was an intrinsic lesion within the left ICVA upon which an occlusive thrombus had formed temporarily, and it embolized to the orifice of the right SCA.

Ultrasound is also an excellent technique for studying occlusive and embolic disease within the cervicocranial arteries. In the patient AH, we were particularly interested in the posterior circulation because of the known cerebellar infarcts and the abnormalities found on MRA. We began with a duplex scan of the region of the VAO; duplex scans include a combination of B-mode and pulsed-Doppler spectra. Figure 15-13 shows a B-mode image of the VA in the neck of a different patient. In patient AH, the probability of a VAO lesion was low, since he had no history of atherosclerosis elsewhere (no angina pectoris, myocardial infarction, claudication, or bruits) and he was of African-American descent. Blacks have a much lower incidence of extracranial occlusive disease involving the ICAs and the VAs in the neck. We have found duplex scans of the proximal VA to be quite sensitive and specific for occlusive disease when adequate scans are technically feasible.[17] In our experience, technical limitations are more common in the proximal subclavian/VAO region than at the ICA origin in the neck. The ICA begins higher in the neck, and the ICA is almost a 180° straight continuation of the common carotid artery; in contrast, the VAO begins very low in the neck quite near the clavicle, and the VA comes off at nearly a 90° angle from the subclavian artery. A color-flow Doppler study of the VAO region was also performed in patient AH; findings of both the duplex scan and the color-flow Doppler studies (Figure 15-14) were normal. Color-flow Doppler studies can usually show the subclavian artery and the proximal portion of the VA. When the VA enters the transverse foramina and courses cephalad, color-flow Doppler signals can still be obtained but the intervertebral regions show prominent artifacts that produce discontinuous images of the artery. This is usually not a problem because flow can be detected and velocities measured between the foramina.

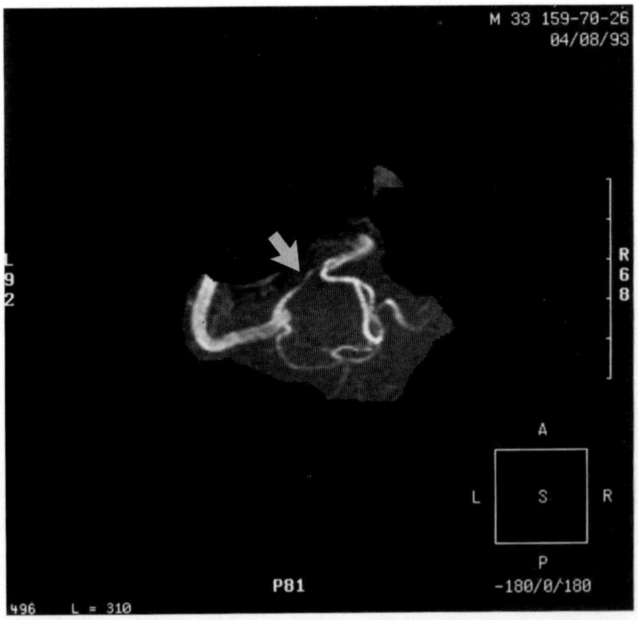

Figure 15-12
MRA showing left intracranial VA stenosis.

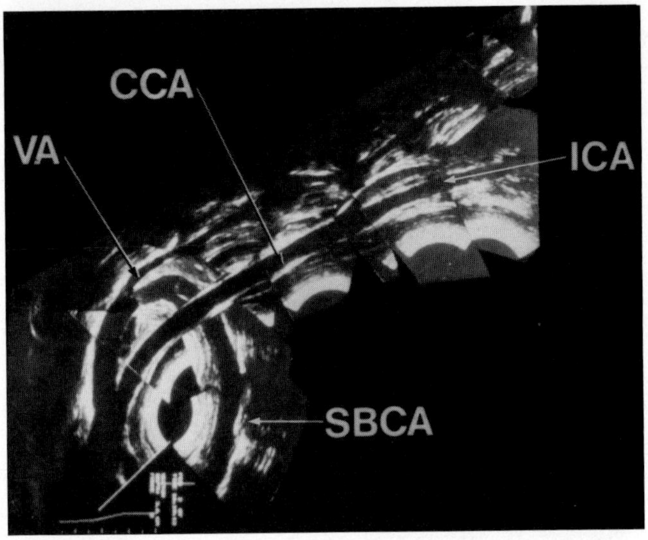

Figure 15-13
B-mode ultrasound image of major extracranial arteries. VA, vertebral artery; SBCA, subclavian artery; ICA, internal carotid artery; CCA, common carotid artery. (Courtesy of Professor Eikelboom, University of Utrecht, Utrecht, The Netherlands.)

In our vascular laboratory, we divide the extracranial VA into three portions: (1) the VAO region, (2) segment 1, between the VAO and where the artery enters the transverse foramina, and (3) segment 2, the intervertebral region. During 1 year, using color-flow Doppler, 565 extracranial VAs were studied (286 left VAs and 279 right VAs, fewer on the right due to intravenous line placement). We were unable to visualize the VA

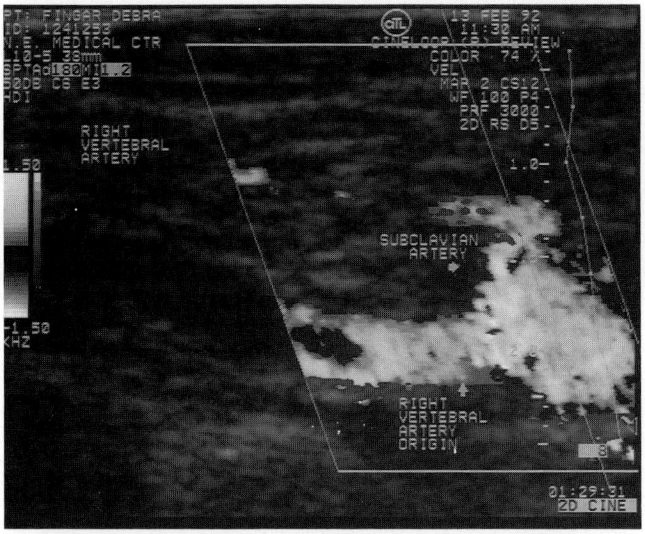

Figure 15-14 (Plate 28)
Color-flow Doppler ultrasound image showing normal VAO.

origins in 102 of 279 (37 percent) right VAs and in 129 of 286 (45 percent) left VAs. The first and second segments of the VAs were both seen and diagnostic of either normal or abnormal arteries in 260 of 279 (93 percent) right VAs and 232 of 286 (81 percent) left VAs. In a small number of patients (6 of 279 right VAs, 7 of 286 left VAs), the first segment was not seen, although the second segment was abnormal, with high velocities, suggesting stenosis, or damped flow, suggesting occlusion. In these patients, the difficulty in obtaining signals in the first segment of the VAs may have been due to disease in the second segment rather than to a technical limitation of the technique. In 7 right VAs and 6 left VAs, high velocity was detected at the origins, suggestive of stenosis at the origins. In 3 right VAs and 2 left VAs, the VAO and the first and second segments were seen and were diagnostic of VA occlusion.

We then continued the ultrasound examination of AH using a continuous-wave (C-W) Doppler probe and insonating along the posterior neck region and at the lateral border of the C2 vertebra. At this region, it is nearly always possible to define the direction of flow within the VA: purely cephalad, reversed, or to and fro. Dissections of the extracranial VA, which usually occur in the distal portion of the extracranial VA as it winds around the upper cervical vertebrae before piercing the dura mater to enter the cranium, can often be detected or suggested by Doppler ultrasound studies.[41,42] Touboul and colleagues described the ultrasound findings in 3 patients with bilateral extracranial VA dissections.[41] The diameter of the VA was often focally increased, and decreased pulsatility was found within these dilated segments. Abnormal intravascular echoes were also often present. Above the areas of dilatation, flow signals were often reduced in amplitude.[41] In patient AH, the C-W Doppler spectra showed normal antegrade flow and normal flow velocities.

We were now ready to perform transcranial Doppler ultrasound (TCD) evaluation of the intracranial posterior circulation arteries. Insonation is performed by placing the 2-mHz probe in the suboccipital window at the rim of the foramen magnum. Each VA can be insonated in turn by changing the direction of the probe. Flow velocities are then measured at 5-mm depth increments from the foramen magnum. In AH, the flow velocities in the left ICVA were increased sharply (Fig. 15-15). This finding indicated the high probability of a significant stenosing lesion of the left ICVA. The flow velocities in the right ICVA and the basilar artery were

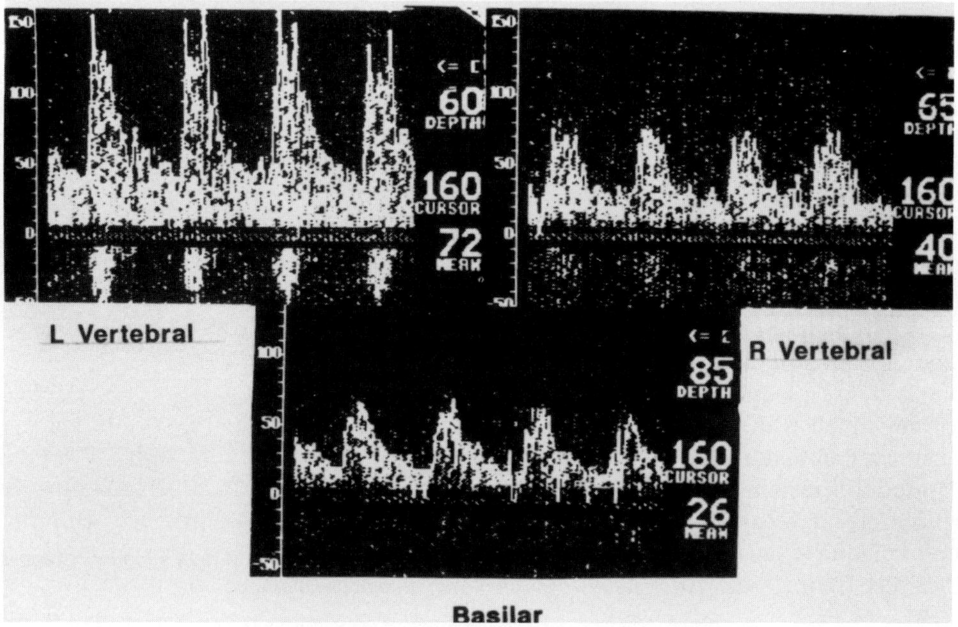

Figure 15-15
TCD of the left intracranial VA showing increased flow velocities consistent with stenosis.

within the normal range. Review of our own TCD studies in patients who also had posterior circulation angiography has shown that the sensitivity and specificity for detecting severely stenotic lesions of the ICVA are quite high.[43] The depth of the basilar artery origin and its cephalad curvature and course vary widely; thus, it is often difficult with TCD to be sure where the ICVA ends and where the basilar artery begins. In our experience, many stenotic and occlusive lesions of the middle and distal portions of the basilar artery have been missed by TCD because of the loss of signals at this depth from the foramen magnum.[43] The ability to insonate the distal basilar artery has improved significantly with technologic improvements in the ultrasound devices.

Magnetic resonance angiography and ultrasound are complementary in defining vascular lesions within the posterior circulation, and the combination of the two technologies is superior to either alone.[44] Magnetic resonance angiography is best in the intraosseous second portion of the extracranial VA and in the intracranial VA-basilar artery-PCAs region, while ultrasound is quite accurate at the VAO (a relatively blind spot for MRA) and the ICVA. In patient AH, we were quite confident, because of the concordance of the MRA and TCD findings, that a stenotic lesion was present in the left ICVA. This lesion could also explain both the PICA and SCA infarcts if we assumed that it provided a source for distal intra-arterial embolism to the right SCA.

In order to better define the ICVA lesion in AH, we elected to pursue standard contrast catheter angiography. Since we knew the region of interest, we could limit the angiography to a left VA injection. Findings of both ultrasound and MRA studies of the anterior circulation arteries had also been completely normal. The angiogram showed a long area of narrowing that appeared to represent an arterial dissection rather than an atherosclerotic occlusive process (Fig. 15-16). The remainder of the posterior circulation arteries were normal, except for a sharp amputation in the right SCA indicative of embolic blockage (Fig. 15-17).

Ultrasound has been even more intensely and thoroughly tested in its accuracy in detecting lesions within the anterior circulation. Duplex scans of the ICA origin region are nearly always technically possible. Usually, B-mode images can show the location, size, and contour of plaques. Often the sonographer can distinguish soft, irregular ulcerated plaques from firm fibrous or calcified plaques. Echolucent plaques are usually rich in cholesterol[45] and are susceptible to reduction in size as well as progression. Calcified, hard, echodense plaques, in contrast, usually do not change very much with time. Thrombi can often be detected using a combination of the Doppler flow spectra and B-mode ultrasound images. B-mode imaging is quite accurate at separating normal arteries and those with minor plaques from those arteries with severe stenosing lesions (more than 70

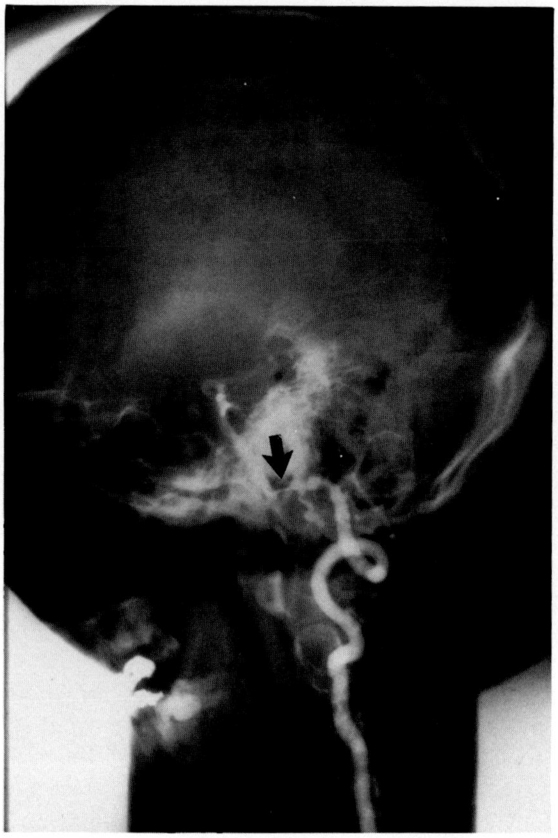

Figure 15-16
Angiogram showing left intracranial VA dissection.

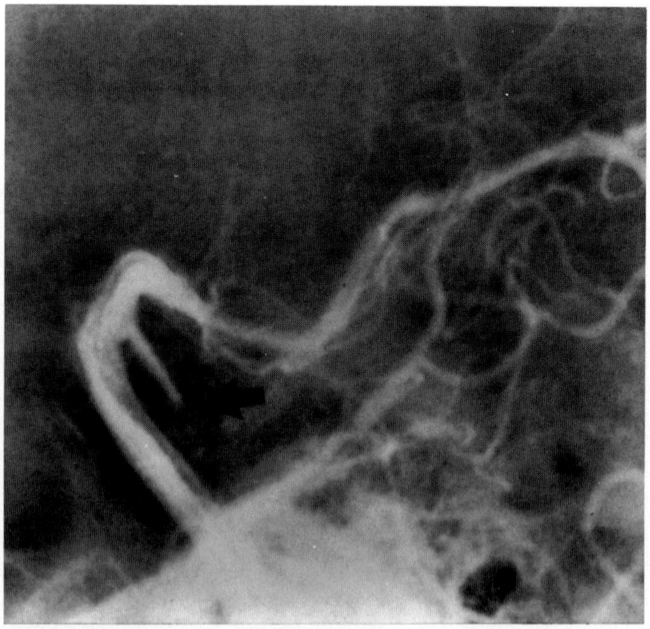

Figure 15-17
Angiogram showing abrupt lack of filling of right superior cerebellar artery consistent with an embolic blockage.

percent narrowed). More difficult is the separation of arteries with severe preocclusive stenosis from occluded arteries. Color-flow Doppler is very helpful in imaging flow and turbulence in the proximal ICA and occasionally can show some flow in vessels that appear occluded on MRA and standard angiography (so-called pseudo-occlusions).[46,47] However, color-flow Doppler does not always yield accurate reflections of the lumenal diameter when there is plaque calcification.[48]

The anterior neck region harboring the pharyngeal portion of the ICA can be explored using a hand-held continuous-wave Doppler probe. The most important and common lesion within the pharyngeal ICA above the bifurcation is dissection of the extracranial ICA. In ICA dissections, the Doppler spectral pattern usually shows a high-amplitude signal with very reduced systolic frequencies and alternating flow directions.[49] Duplex scans can show intimal flaps, regions of lumenal narrowing and dilatation, and false lumens and yield diagnostic information in addition to that shown by Doppler spectra.[50] These abnormalities are usually localized well above the bifurcation in the submandibular region in areas that angiography shows tapered narrowing of the pharyngeal ICA.

The TCD exploration of the anterior circulation intracranial arteries begins with the orbital windows. The probe is placed over the orbit. Usually, flow velocities in the ophthalmic artery, the ICA in the siphon, the distal ICA bifurcation (ICA-T portion), and the ACAs can be studied using this probe position by altering depth and angulation. At times, flow in the posterior communicating artery can also be well shown. Using a temporal, zygomatic window, flow velocities in the MCAs can be accessed at successive 5-mm depth intervals. Most useful is comparing the MCA velocities on the two sides. Flow in the PCAs can also usually be studied using the temporal window. Unfortunately, the temporal window depends on having a soft spot in the bone, and many patients do not have satisfactory temporal windows. Transcranial Doppler ultrasound is very useful in detecting severe occlusive lesions of the large basal intracranial arteries as well as reflecting the hemodynamic consequences of severe extracranial lesions.[51,52] Dolichoectatic dilated arteries also often give abnormal spectra on TCD. Reduced pulsatility and to-and-fro flow are common in this dilatative arteriopathy.

A recent new ultrasound technology, color-flow Doppler of the orbits, has also proved of great utility in patients with symptomatic transient or persistent retinal and optic nerve ischemia. Orbital ultrasound is also very helpful in assessing the hemodynamic consequences of proximal ICA occlusive disease. Figure 15-18 is a color-flow Doppler picture of the orbit showing a calcified particle within the central retinal artery, presumably arising from a calcified mitral anulus within the heart. This patient had the sudden onset of persistent monocular blindness, and her retina had the typical appearance of central retinal artery occlusion.[53]

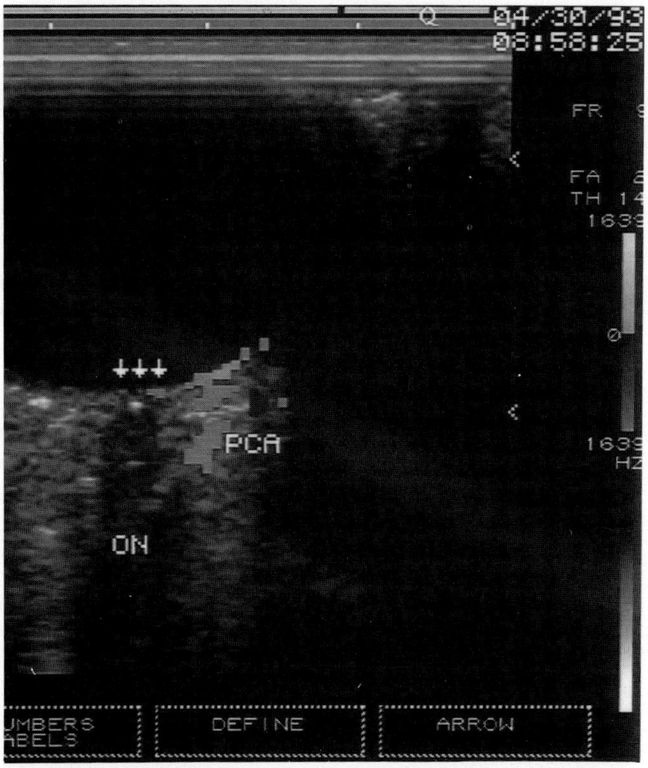

Figure 15-18 (Plate 29)
Color-flow Doppler ultrasound image of the orbit showing calcified particle obstructing the central retinal artery (arrows). ON, optic nerve; PCA, posterior choroidal artery. (Courtesy of Dr. Thomas Hedges III, New England Medical Center, Neuroophthalmology Department, Boston.)

Four recent applications of ultrasound technology have had an impact on the diagnosis of patients with brain ischemia: power Doppler imaging, TCD–color-coded sonography, the use of echo-enhancing contrast with TCD, and TCD emboli monitoring. Power Doppler is based on the display of the integrated power of the Doppler signal. Power Doppler imaging generates intravascular color signals based on the reflected echo amplitude, which depends mostly on the amount of erythrocytes within the sample volume.[54] The color display is independent of the angle of insonation and of the velocity and direction of moving red blood cells. Power Doppler images are not as confounded by plaque calcification as are color-flow Doppler images, and they provide somewhat more accurate visualization of the stenotic carotid artery vascular lumen than does color-flow Doppler.[54,55] Power Doppler technology can also be used transcranially.[55]

Transcranial color-coded sonography combines B-mode ultrasound with color-coded Doppler. The technique allows simultaneous visualization of brain parenchyma and basal cerebral artery blood flow using color-flow imaging.[56–61] Intracerebral hematomas can be diagnosed as hyperechoic regions within brain tissue.[61] Intracranial vascular occlusion can often be diagnosed using this method, which improves the localization of the intracranial vessels. However, failure to obtain a useful window is an important limitation of the method.[57]

Ultrasonographers have begun to use intravenous echo contrast agents in order to increase the intensity of Doppler signals. Increasing the signal-to-noise ratio increases the sensitivity of the ultrasound examination. A number of microparticles have been used, for example, a galactose/palmitic acid–based agent that on dissolution and agitation in sterile water generates air-filled microbubbles about 2 μm in diameter that are coated with palmitic acid.[62,63] These microbubbles can increase the signal by 10 to 30 dB.[62] Echo-enhancing contrast agents are particularly useful in transcranial Doppler examinations, especially in vessels that are difficult to insonate. Infusion of echo contrast agents during transcranial color-coded Duplex examinations often improves the B-mode images and promotes better identification of the various intracranial arteries and their branches.[62,63]

The most important advance in TCD has been the capability for emboli monitoring. In this technique, transcranial Doppler probes are positioned over brain arteries, most often the middle and posterior cerebral arteries on each side. Particles passing through the arteries being monitored produce an audible chirping noise and high-intensity transient signals (HITS) visible on an oscilloscope.[64–78] These signals are often referred to as microembolic signals (MES) because they are believed to represent the passage of small emboli through the vessel that is being monitored.

The microembolic signal character depends on the nature of the particles (gas, thrombus, calcium, cholesterol chrystal, etc.), particle size, and transit time. Monitoring probes can be placed on the neck and brain arteries. Emboli arising from the heart or aorta go equally to each side, proportionately to the anterior and posterior circulation arteries, and microembolic signals appear in the neck before appearing intracranially. In contrast, emboli that originate in a neck artery go only to the intracranial arterial branches on the side of the donor artery, and embolic signals do not appear in the neck. For example, emboli from the left ICA generate embolic signals detectable in the left MCA and not in the neck, posterior cerebral, or right-sided arteries. This technique allows better identification of the nature of embolic materials and their sources, quantification of the emboli load, and a means of monitoring the effect of various therapies on reducing that load.

Transcranial Doppler emboli monitoring has shown that embolism is a much more common cause of stroke than was thought in the past.[79] Physicians in the past thought that release of embolic materials was an unusual event with a high hit rate, that is, that emboli reaching intracranial arteries had a high likelihood of causing stroke and brain infarction. Recent data show that embolic particles are often found in the circulation but the hit rate is relatively very low.[64–78] Embolic particles can arise from a variety of donor sources, including the heart, aorta, and neck and intracranial arteries.

Many studies have detected HITS in the MCA distal to a carotid artery lesion and have studied the likelihood of their presence in carotid artery stenosis of various severity.[73–76] Orlandi et al found HITS on the same side as severe stenosis (70 to 99 percent narrowing) in 43.1 percent of patients monitored and on the same side as moderate stenosis (30 to 60 percent narrowing) in 13.5 percent of cases.[73] No HITS were detected on the side of normal control carotid arteries. They found that HITS were more prevalent on the same side as ulcerated plaques (60.9 percent) than on the same side as nonulcerated plaques (20 percent). All moderate stenoses that were associated with HITS had ulceration.[73] The same group of authors showed that no HITS were seen among 33 patients with severe carotid stenosis after carotid endarterectomy.[74] Other studies have shown an association among plaque ulceration, intraluminal thrombus, and cerebral microemboli but no definite correlation with plaque fissuring and intraplaque hemorrhage.[76,78] Babikian and colleagues found that microembolic signals were detected more often in symptomatic than in asymptomatic arteries (28.6 versus 12.4 percent).[70] They also found that microembolic signals were more frequent in arteries with lesions causing 70 percent or more stenosis or occlusion (26.3 percent) than in arteries with less than 70 percent stenosis (13.5 percent).[70] Siebler et al detected microembolic signals in 82 percent of 33 patients with symptomatic severe carotid stenosis (70 percent or greater luminal narrowing) and in only 16 percent of 56 neurologically asymptomatic patients with a comparable degree of stenosis.[75] Emboli were detected in the MCA distal to carotid artery dissection in 10 of 17 patients.[77] Patients with microemboli detected by TCD more often had strokes than did those who did not have microemboli.[77] Emboli monitoring with TCD after carotid endarterectomy showed that frequent signals (more than 50 microembolic signals/hour) occur in about 10 percent of patients during the early preoperative period and predict the development of ipsilateral cerebral ischemia.[72]

Microembolic signals are found more often in patients with carotid artery disease than in patients with potential cardiac sources of emboli.[68,69] Unilateral microembolic signals are associated with ipsilateral carotid artery disease, while bilateral signals predict cardiac disease.[69] Studies that compare the microembolic load in patients with stroke have found high loads in patients with large artery territory infarcts and no significant microembolic load in patients with lacunar infarcts.[68,71]

Emboli monitoring has also been used during cardiopulmonary bypass surgery. Monitoring of patients using TCD and transesophageal echocardiography shows that myriad microemboli are detected in the MCAs[80,81] and in the aortic lumen during and after cardiac surgery.[80–82] Most microembolic signals are recorded during clamping and unclamping of the aorta, but flurries of emboli are also detected during cannulation of the aorta and at the beginning and end of cardiac bypass.[80] Many more particles are detected in the aorta than in the MCAs. The total volume of embolic particles per heart operation within the aortic lumen is about 3.7 mL (range 0.57 to 11.2 mL), and the embolic load that reaches the brain is about 0.3 mL (range 0.06 to 0.5 mL).[80,82] The particles are of quite diverse composition and probably consist of air, atheromatous debris, lipid, and platelet-fibrin thrombi. Necropsy studies of patients and experimental animals that died after heart surgeries that included cardiopulmonary bypass show that the brains contain millions of small capillary and arteriolar dilatations thought to represent sites of microembolization.[83] Cardiac- and aortic-origin embolism undoubtedly contributes to the brain damage often noted after cardiac surgery.[84,85]

The development of more rapid spiral (helical) CT scanners has enabled the development of CT angiography (CTA) within the past 5 years. This technique involves intravenous injection of a bolus of dye followed by helical scanning. Volumetric data acquisition and improved computerized image manipulation have improved the CTA image display into three-dimensional reformations. The technique is based on anatomic imaging and has theoretical advantages over MRA, which is a functional imaging technique, when blood flow is greatly reduced. The ICAs are well seen in the neck, and the results of CTA for quantification of carotid stenosis are comparable to those obtained with MRA.[86–89] Compared with conventional angiography, there are few false-positive and -negative results.[86–89] In addition, CTA provides useful images of intracranial arteries and can show regions of intracranial stenosis, dolichoectasia, and aneurysms.[90–93] Intraobserver variability for both CTA and MRA is good, but different observers interpret CTA more variably than they do MRA.[93]

The new technology and improvements in older techniques provide clinicians with a menu of possible strategies for brain and vascular studies in patients with ischemia. All the investigations—MRI, fluid-attenuated inversion recovery (FLAIR) imaging, MRA, diffusion and perfusion MRI—can be performed using magnetic resonance technology within a relatively short period of time. Alternatively, especially if MRI is not readily available or cannot be used, spiral CT can be used to create brain images and CT angiography of the cervicocranial arteries. Computed tomography can also be used to quantify regional cerebral blood flow and blood volume.[94] Extracranial and transcranial ultrasound can be used as the diagnostic vascular tests in patients who have only had brain imaging or can be used to corroborate and quantify the blood flow effects of vascular lesions found by CTA and MRA. Ultrasound is also used effectively to monitor the progression and regression of vascular occlusive lesions once they are identified.

Cardiac imaging and rhythm monitoring are now also an integral part of the evaluation of patients with brain ischemia. Probably as many as 30 percent of ischemic lesions are cardioembolic, and a wide variety of cardiac lesions can give rise to embolism. We usually begin the cardiac evaluation with a routine electrocardiogram (ECG). Then a transthoracic echocardiogram (TTE) is ordered. When an intracardiac shunt is suggested, agitated saline solution should be introduced intravenously while the echocardiographer is listening over the cardiac septum with a Doppler probe. Air bubbles can be seen to pass through the septum and can be heard with the Doppler probe. We have found that a TCD probe placed over one of the MCAs is also very effective in detecting the rapid passage of air bubbles into the systemic circulation. Transthoracic echocardiography is not as effective as transesophageal echocardiography (TEE) in detecting many cardiac lesions. Since the esophagus lies just behind the left atrium, lesions of the atrial septum and the atria are much better imaged with TEE. Also, the ascending and thoracic portions of the aorta are well studied using TEE. Protruding aortic atheromas are especially important donor sites for brain embolism, particularly after angiography and cardiac surgery. Clamping of the aorta during surgery can provoke a flurry of cholesterol crystals and plaque emboli.

Atrial fibrillation and the sick-sinus syndrome are also important causes of cardiac-origin brain embolism. Each of these arrythmias becomes more common as patients age. In patients with known heart disease, in those with palpitations and irregular rhythms, and in those in whom preliminary vascular and cardiac evaluations have not revealed a cause of brain ischemia, cardiac rhythm monitoring is useful. Intermittent atrial fibrillation is often found. Recent studies have established the benefit of warfarin prophylaxis in patients with atrial fibrillation. Other cardiac tests, such as dipyridimole-thalium scanning and ultrafast CT, are useful in characterizing cardiac function in selected patients with known coronary and other heart disease.

In patients suspected of having extracranial large artery (ICA or VA in the neck) or intracranial large artery (intracranial VA, basilar artery, PCA, or MCA) disease, the combination of brain imaging (CT and/or MRI) and vascular tests (CTA, MRA, and/or extracranial and transcranial ultrasound) invariably show severe flow-reducing stenoses or occlusions. In patients with lacunar or branch artery disease, vascular investigations most often do not show severe occlusive arterial lesions that explain the clinical findings and acute infarcts found on brain imaging. In patients with suspected brain embolism, the investigations are directed toward both the recipient sites within the intracranial arteries and the potential donor sources in the heart, aorta, and the extracranial and proximal intracranial arteries. Nonstenosing plaques within the proximal arteries in both the anterior and posterior circulations can be the focus of white and red clot deposition, with subsequent intra-arterial embolism.

What If the Brain Lesion Is an ICH?

In ICH, the differential diagnosis is more limited than in brain ischemia. Furthermore, for a vascular lesion to cause bleeding within the brain, the bleeding lesion must be quite near the hematoma. Identification of the vessel suspected of harboring the causative vascular lesion is usually clear after neuroimagting with CT or MRI. Most often, the bleeding is from small arteries and arterioles not shown by MRA, CTA, or TCD, the most important noninvasive modalities for studying intracranial vascular lesions.

In hypertensive ICH, by far the commonest cause of bleeding into the brain, the responsible vascular lesion cannot be identified with any technique, including standard catheter-dye angiography. Similarly, in hematomas related to bleeding diatheses, amyloid angiopathy, and trauma, available vascular studies, including angiography, are not helpful except for excluding other causes. These disorders can be thought of as microangiopathies because the vascular lesion is usually visible only under the microscope. The two most important "macroangiopathies" that cause ICH and are usually visible grossly are aneurysms that send a jet of blood into the brain and vascular malformations within the brain substance. Among vascular malformations, cavernous and venous angiomas are usually well shown by MRI but are not easily detected by MRA or TCD. Only arteriovenous malformations (AVMs) are readily shown by angiography and can sometimes be identified using TCD and/or MRA.

In patient ST, the location of the hemorrhage in the right basal ganglionic region was typical for hypertensive ICH, and he was hypertensive when first examined. The only clinical feature that raised suspicion of another cause was the association in his case with the use of cocaine; patients with cocaine-related hemorrhages have a higher incidence of harboring aneurysms and AVMs than do hemorrhages complicating other drug use. As discussed previously, often the location, shape, and dissection patterns of the hemorrhage as imaged by CT or MRI can suggest the likelihood that the hemorrhage originated from rupture of a basal aneurysm. In patient ST, the lesion on CT did not suggest a pattern associated with an aneurysm. Both MRA and CTA probably have the capability of showing most bleeding aneurysms along the circle of Willis that cause ICH. Unfortunately, the quality and detail of the vascular images are not sufficient for surgeons to operate without a standard angiogram showing the aneurysm and its shape, the presence of a neck, and other morphologic details. If an AVM were suspected from the MRI, the large feeding arteries and draining veins would probably be shown by CTA or MRA. However, when an AVM is strongly suspected or known to be present, the detail of vascular filling and supply gained from MRA is usually not adequate, and catheter angiography with dye opacification is often needed. Therefore, CTA and MRA have little clinical use in patients with ICH at the present time.

Transcranial Doppler ultrasound is an effective technology for identifying large and medium-sized AVMs.[51,95] The TCD technique can show vascular flow patterns and the contribution of the various feeding arteries to the supply of the AVM. Arteries supplying high-flow malformations usually show increased flow volume, high velocity, and low resistance. Decreased resistance distally is due to venous runoff and leads to a decrease in arterial pulsatility. When multiple feeding arteries are present, the supply artery with the highest flow velocity usually also has the lowest pulsatility index.[51] Collateralization and "steal" effects are shown by reduction of mean and peak velocities below average normal values. While TCD is a useful adjunct to catheter angiography in patients with AVMs, it is seldom adequate by itself. It is very helpful in following patients after therapeutic embolization and radiation to show changes in blood supply and collateralization.

Contrast angiography is indicated in patients with ICH when aneurysms and AVMs are suspected from the clinical and neuroimaging data. The key clinical data derive from the demographic and risk factor profile. Youth and absence of risk factors for other causes of ICH make underlying vascular macroangiopathies more likely. A history of seizures, headaches, and prior bleeds favors an AVM. The location, shape, and dissection pattern of the hemorrhage on CT and MRI are also very important. In patients whose blood pressures are elevated at the time of the hemorrhage and who have a hematoma in a deep location typical of hypertensive ICH (putamen, caudate, thalamus, pons, or cerebellum), the yield of angiography is extremely low. In lobar hematomas and those near the basal and ventricular surface, the yield of angiography is higher, especially if the patient is not hypertensive. At times, serial MRIs after the acute hematoma has begun to resolve can give information about the presence of an underlying vascular malformation or tumor.

What If the Patient Has SAH?

The macroangiopathies that cause SAH (aneurysms and AVMs) are identical to those that cause ICH. In patients with SAH, just as in those with ICH, noninvasive testing with CTA, MRA, and TCD may have some utility in screening for causative vascular lesions near the brain surface. The comments about the utility of CTA, MRA, and TCD in identifying and following AVMs in patients with ICH hold equally well for patients with SAH. In patients with SAH, aneurysms are a more important and more urgent consideration than in patients with ICH. The ability to project image information at numerous angles and to view images from above and below has made CTA particularly advantageous in showing intracranial aneurysms. Standard catheter angiography with dye injection is still nearly always required for sufficient delineation of aneurysms when surgery is contemplated. In patient RM, an angiogram was performed on the second hospital day and showed an 8-mm aneurysm at the junction of the right PCA with the right ICA. Surgical clipping was performed on the same day.

Both MRA and CTA are useful screening tests for aneurysms in patients with known predisposing conditions (e.g., a strong family history of aneurysmal SAH or the known presence of polycystic kidneys or fibromuscular dysplasia). Either CTA or MRA might also be used if there is a rather recent history of a severe headache without a very high probability of SAH. These tests are also useful in follow-up studies of patients with surgically treated aneurysms.

Transcranial Doppler ultrasound is helpful in sequentially following the flow velocities in the basal brain arteries.[51,96,97] In patients with moderate- to large-volume SAH in whom no surgery is performed, flow velocities in the basal arteries are increased during days 3 to 10 after the onset of the bleeding. At times, the velocities continue to increase and reach a maximum between days 11 to 20. High velocities are rather well correlated with vasoconstriction as shown by catheter angiography. Velocities in the MCA over 200 cm/s predict the presence of severe vasoconstriction on angiography. Transcranial Doppler ultrasound can be used to monitor the effects of various treatments on the vasoconstriction. Systemic blood pressure, anemia, and intracranial pressure must be taken into consideration in evaluating blood flow velocities. Vasoconstriction is rare in patients with nonaneurysmal SAH; thus, TCD has less a role to play in evaluation of these patients.

Are Abnormalities in the Blood Causing or Adding to Brain Ischemia or Hemorrhage?

Hematologic abnormalities are important in causing and potentiating both brain ischemia and brain and subarachnoid hemorrhage. Screening of the cellular and serologic-coagulation functions of the blood should be a part of the evaluation of all patients with stroke.

In patients with brain ischemia, the key questions are, Could blood hypercoagulability have precipitated an occlusive thromboembolus? and Are there viscosity-related hemorrheologic factors present that might impede brain perfusion and so enhance ischemia? Increased red blood cell and platelet counts can precipitate thrombosis, especially in arteries already narrowed by atherosclerotic stenosis. Some qualitative disorders of erythrocytes, such as sickle cell disease and erythrocytosis, can also cause thrombosis and altered flow. Many of these hematologic disorders cause chronic anemia, and usually there are familial and genetic clues to their existence. Examination of a stained blood smear should give clues to the existence of these disorders in patients with anemia. Although qualitative disorders of platelets and their function do exist ("sticky platelets") and can enhance clotting in vivo, there are no generally accepted methods for studying platelet function in vitro that are widely available outside research laboratories. In most patients with hypercoagulable states, the prothrombin time (PT) and the activated partial thromboplastin time (aPTT) are abnormally accelerated. The battery of tests that we suggest for routine screening of patients with brain ischemia are hemoglobin level, hematocrit, white blood cell count, platelet count, PT, and aPTT. In patients with a personal or family history of hypercoagulability and in those whose early neuroimaging and cardiac and vascular testing has been unrevealing, we suggest also measuring antithrombin III, protein C, deficiency of activated protein C due to deficiency of Leiden factor, protein S, serine coagulation factor levels and activity (factors V, VII, VIII, IX, X, and XII), von Willebrand factor, and levels of tissue plasminogen activator and inhibitor. Antiphospholipid antibodies, including the lupus anticoagulant and anticardiolipin antibodies, should be measured in patients with lupus erythematosis; those with a history of frequent miscarriages, venous thromboembolism, and past myocardial ischemia and strokes; and those with thrombocytopenia and unexplained valvular cardiac lesions.

The two most important contributors to whole blood viscosity are the hematocrit and serum fibrinogen levels.[3,98] Cerebral blood flow at a hematocrit level of 45 is about half the flow in the same patient with a hematocrit of 33. Fibrinogen is an acute-phase reactant that contributes to coagulability as well as affecting blood viscosity and flow. We find it useful to measure fibrinogen levels, and at times whole blood and serum viscosity, in patients with brain ischemia, since reduction in viscosity might increase blood flow to the ischemic zone. Persistently high fibrinogen levels predict an important risk of coronary thrombosis and ischemic stroke.

In patients with intracranial hemorrhage, bleeding diatheses can cause both SAH and ICH. In other patients with localized intracerebral and subdural hematomas, particularly those due to head trauma, consumptive coagulopathies can develop secondary to the initial hemorrhage and augment bleeding. The commonest bleeding disorder that leads to intracranial hemorrhage is the iatrogenic prescription of anticoagulants. In patients who have been given anticoagulants because of prior brain ischemia, the occurrence of focal neurologic symptoms is often misinterpreted as being due to recurrent ischemia. Anticoagulant-related hemorrhages are particularly treacherous, since they may begin very insidiously and progress slowly. Inquiry as to the presence of past bleeding and familial bleeding disorders and the use of anticoagulants should be an important part of the evaluation of all patients with SAH and ICH. The skin and mucous membranes should be examined for purpura, and the urine and stool should be tested for blood. Usually, measurements of the platelet count, PT, and the aPTT are adequate to identify the vast majority of patients with bleeding disorders. If the results these tests are abnormal, further detailed testing is usually needed.

Are There Abnormalities of Brain Function, Metabolism, and Blood Flow Not Shown by CT, MRI, and Large Artery Vascular Studies That Are Important Clinically in Diagnosis and Treatment of Patients?

The standard testing described so far is available in many centers that treat stroke patients. These tests are adequate in the great majority of stroke patients to assist clinicians in making an accurate diagnosis and in planning appropriate treatment. In some patients, additional information gleaned from other tests of brain function, metabolism, and blood flow can be helpful in prognosticating and deciding on treatment options.

To treat stroke patients optimally, clinicians would like to know (1) the stroke mechanism (ischemia or hemorrhage); (2) the nature, location, and severity of the causative vascular lesion and the mechanism by which it causes ischemia (embolism and/or hypoperfusion) and/or hemorrhage; (3) the state of the blood; and (4) the state of the brain (normal, stunned—i.e., not functioning normally but not irreversibly damaged—or infarcted).

The standard neuroimaging tests do not give an accurate picture of the state of the brain. Computed tomography shows infarcted and edematous brain as hypodense lesions. Magnetic resonance imaging is more sensitive to water and electrolyte changes in cells and in the interstitial spaces. Ischemic changes are seen early because of water changes within cells that are usually the earliest morphologic signs of cell death. Neither test tells about tissue that is not functioning but is not yet infarcted.

The neurologic examination is a rather sensitive test of brain function. In a number of patients, sometimes during the early course, the neurologic examination shows abnormalities that are not matched by CT or MRI abnormalities. In these patients, there is a mismatch between the clinical and neuroimaging findings. The CT or MRI may show lesions without obvious corresponding signs of brain dysfunction (so-called silent infarcts), and the clinical examination may show signs related to brain regions that show no abnormality on neuroimaging tests. When the findings on examination exceed those found by neuroimaging, the most likely explanation is that there is viable brain tissue that is not functioning normally but has not yet been irreversibly infarcted.

The tests of vascular morphology and function discussed so far—CTA, MRA, ultrasound, and standard catheter angiography—are "macrovascular," that is, they give information about the large blood vessels and blood flow and velocities through these channels. These tests do not give detailed information about the microvasculature. The brain's network of tiny vessels within the microvasculature is many times the size and scope of the large arteries visible grossly on the surface. An embolus might block the MCA and pass, leaving the MCA widely patent by TCD and angiography, yet during the blockage, portions of the microvasculature supplied by the MCA may have become occluded, thus impeding perfusion of that region. Cerebral blood flow (CBF) and, more important, regional perfusion (rCBF) of specific regions can be measured and quantitated by other sophisticated technology.

Newer MRI techniques have the potential of yielding information about early brain infarction and brain perfusion in patients with ischemia.[12,13,99–102] For instance, MRI perfusion scans after the administration of contrast and paramagnetic agents have the potential of showing perfusion in various regions of interest. Echo-planar diffusion-weighted MRI (DWI) shows small early abnormalities of ion and water homeostasis very soon after the onset of brain ischemic events. The apparent diffusion coefficient (ADC) reflects a change in the self-diffusion of water in tissues, providing a quantitative means of assessing tissue status. Comparing the regions of abnormality shown on DWI scans with the area of decreased perfusion shown on perfusion scans gives information about the brain at risk for further ischemia: the so-called ischemic penumbra. When the perfusion defect exceeds the diffusion-weighted abnormality early after symptom onset, the volume of the abnormality on subsequent DWI scanning often expands.[102] The major practical advantage of the newer MRI techniques is that MRI offers the potential of being able to show infarction, blood flow, and the major arteries and veins (using MRA) during a brief single period of testing for the patient. Figure 15-19 shows the MRI studies of a single patient who had a cerebellar infarct related to occlusive disease of the intracranial vertebral arteries bilaterally. Figure 15-20 shows the MRI evaluation of a patient with an embolic PCA territory infarct.

The function of various brain regions can be assessed by electrophysiologic testing using standard electroencephalograms (EEGs), quantified electrophysiology (so-called brain mapping),[103,104] testing of evoked responses after sensory stimulation, and quantifying electrophysiologic reflexes.[105] Positron emission tomography

often referred to as diaschisis. Diaschisis is found in the thalamus ipsilateral to a cerebral lesion, the cerebral cortex ipsilateral to a thalamic lesion, portions of the cerebral hemisphere contralateral to a lesion of the other cerebral hemisphere, the cerebellar hemisphere contralateral to a cerebral lesion, and the cerebellar hemisphere ipsilateral to a pontine lesion.[3,116,117] In practice, identification of these regions of diaschisis helps explain some clinical findings but usually does not affect treatment in patients with hematomas.

In patients with SAH, TCD and SPECT are able to give information about vasoconstriction and regions of hypoperfusion. Increased blood flow velocities measured by TCD correlate well with vasoconstriction shown angiographically. Similarly, regions of reduced rCBF can be shown by SPECT scans and usually represent regions of underperfused brain in areas of vasoconstriction. These underperfused areas often become zones of delayed ischemic infarction unless vigorous treatment is pursued. The presence of vasoconstriction and zones of hypoperfusion is also used as a guide by some concerning the timing of surgery in patients with SAH. The use of TCD and SPECT can reduce the need for repeated angiography to assess the presence of vasoconstriction.

REFERENCES

1. Faris A, Poser C, Wilmore D et al: Radiologic visualization of neck vessels in health men. *Neurology* 13:386–396, 1963.
2. Caplan LR: *The Effective Clinical Neurologist* Boston, Blackwell, 1990.
3. Caplan LR: *Stroke: A clinical approach,* 2d ed. Boston, Butterworth-Heinemann, 1993.
4. Amarenco P, Hauw J-J, Caplan LR: Cerebellar infarctions, in Lechtenberg R (ed): *Handbook of Cerebellar Diseases.* New York, Marcel Dekker, 1993, pp 251–290.
5. Patel MR, Edelman RR, Warach S: Detection of hyperacute primary intraparenchymal hemorrhage by magnetic resonance imaging. *Stroke* 27:2321–2324, 1996.
6. Gomori JM, Grossman RI, Hackney DB, et al: Variable appearances of subacute intracranial hematomas on high-field spin echo MR. *Am J Neuroradiol* 8:1019–1026, 1987.
7. Dul K, Drayer BP: CT and MR imaging of intracerebral hemorrhage, in Kase CS, Caplan LR (eds): *Intracerebral Hemorrhage.* Boston, Butterworth-Heinemann, 1994, pp 73–93.
8. Bradley WG, Schmidt PG: Effect of methemoglobin formation on the MR appearance of subarachnoid hemorrhage. *Radiology* 156:99–103, 1985.
9. Kertesz A, Black SE, Nicholson L, Carr T: The sensitivity and specificity of MRI in stroke. *Neurology* 37:1580–1585, 1987.
10. Bell BA, Symon L, Branston NM: CBF and time threshold for the formation of ischemic cerebral edema, and effects of reperfusion in baboons. *J Neurosurg* 62:31–41, 1985.
11. Brant-Zawadzki M, Atkinson D, Detrick BS, et al: Fluid-attenuated inversion recovery (FLAIR) for assessment of cerebral infarction: initial clinical experience in 50 patients. *Stroke* 27:1187–1191, 1996.
12. Warach S, Chien D, Li W, et al: Fast magnetic resonance diffusion-weighted imaging of acute human stroke. *Neurology* 42:1719–1723, 1992.
13. Sorenson AG, Buonanno FS, Gonzales G, et al: Hyperacute stroke: Evaluation with combined multisection diffusion-weighted and hemodynamically weighted echo-planar MR imaging. *Radiology* 199:391–401, 1996.
14. Singer MB, Chong J, Lu D, et al: Diffusion-weighted MRI in acute subcortical infarction. *Stroke* 29:133–136, 1998.
15. Kistler JP, Buonanno FS, DeWitt LD, et al: Vertebral-basilar posterior cerebral territory stroke: Delineation by proton nuclear magnetic resonance imaging. *Stroke* 15:417–426, 1984.
16. Amarenco P: The spectrum of cerebellar infarctions. *Neurology* 41:973–979, 1991.
17. Caplan LR: *Posterior Circulation Disease: Clinical Findings, Diagnosis, and Management.* Boston, Blackwell Science, 1996.
18. Levine SR, Brust JCM, Futrell N, et al: Cerebrovascular complications of alkaloid cocaine. *N Engl J Med* 323:699–704, 1990.
19. Kothari RU, Brott T, Broderick JP, et al: The ABCs of measuring intracerebral hemorrhage volumes. *Stroke* 27:1304–1305, 1996.
20. Caplan LR, Kase CS: *Intracerebral Hemorrhage.* Boston, Butterworth-Heinemann, 1994.
21. Lampi Y, Gilad R, Esthel Y, Sarova-Pinhas I: Neurological and functional outcome in patients with supratentorial hemorrhages: A prospective study. *Stroke* 26:2249–2253, 1995.
22. Hijdra A, van Gijn J, Nagelkerke W, et al: Prediction of delayed cerebral ischemia, rebleeding, and outcome after aneurysmal subarachnoid hemorrhage. *Stroke* 19:1250–1256, 1988.
23. van Gijn J, van Dongen KJ, Vermeulen M, et al: Perimesencephalic hemorrhage: A nonaneurysmal and benign form of subarachnoid hemorrhage. *Neurology* 35:483–487, 1985.
24. Rinkel GJ, Wijdicks E, Vermeulen M, et al: Outcome in perimesencephalic (nonaneurysmal) subarachnoid hemorrhage: A follow up study in 37 patients. *Neurology* 40:1130–1132, 1990.
25. Caplan LR: Cerebrovascular disease: Large artery occlusive disease, in Appel S (ed): *Current Neurology,* vol 8. Chicago, Yearbook Medical, 1988, pp 179–226.
26. Ringelstein EB, Koschorke S, Holling A, et al: Computed tomographic patterns of proven embolic brain infarctions. *Ann Neurol* 26:759–765, 1989.
27. Caplan LR: The 1991 E Graeme Robertson lecture: Vertebrobasilar embolism. *Clin Exp Neurol* 28:1–23, 1991.
28. Caplan LR, Tettenborn B: Vertebrobasilar occlusive disease: Review of selected aspects: II. Posterior circulation embolism. *Cerebrovasc Dis* 2:320–326, 1992.
29. G'acs G, Fox A, Barnett HJM, et al: CT visualization of intracranial arterial thromboembolism. *Stroke* 15:756–762, 1983.
30. Yock D: CT appearance of cerebral emboli. *J Comput Assist Tomogr* 5:190–196, 1981.

31. Pessin MS, Chimowitz MI, Levine SR, et al: Stroke in patients with fusiform vertebrobasilar aneurysms. *Neurology* 39:16–21, 1989.
32. Levine R, Verro F, Korosec FR, et al: Magnetic resonance angiographic study of vertebrobasilar flow voids. *J Neuroimag* 2:175–180, 1992.
33. Goldberg HI, Grossman RI, Gomori JM, et al: Cervical internal carotid artery dissecting hemorrhage: Diagnosis using MR. *Radiology* 158:157–161, 1986.
34. Warach S, Li W, Ronthal M, Edelman R: Acute cerebral ischemia: Evaluation with dynamic contrast-enhanced MR imaging and MR angiography. *Radiology* 182:41–47, 1992.
35. Johnson BA, Heiserman JE, Drayer BP, Keller PJ: Intracranial MR angiography: Its role in the integrated approach to brain infarction. *Am J Neuroradiol* 15:901–908, 1994.
36. Gillard JH, Oliverio PJ, Barker PB, et al: MR angiography in acute cerebral ischemia of the anterior circulation: A preliminary report. *Am J Neuroradiol* 18:343–350, 1997.
37. Ruggieri PM, Masaryk T, Ross JS: Magnetic resonance angiography: Cerebrovascular applications. *Stroke* 23: 774–780, 1992.
38. Levi CR, Mitchell A, Fitt G, Donnan GA: The accuracy of magnetic resonance angiography in the assessment of extracranial carotid artery occlusive disease. *Cerebrovasc Dis* 6:231–236, 1996.
39. Mitti RL, Broderick M, Carpenter JP, et al: Blinded-reader comparison of magnetic resonance angiography and duplex ultrasonography for carotid artery bifurcation stenosis. *Stroke* 25:4–10, 1994.
40. Quereshi A, Isa A, Cinnamon J, et al: Magnetic resonance angiography in patients with brain infarction. *J Neuroimag* 8:65–70, 1998.
41. Touboul PJ, Mas JL, Bousser MG, Laplane D: Duplex scanning in extracranial vertebral artery dissection. *Stroke* 18:116–121, 1987.
42. Caplan LR, Tettenborn B: Vertebrobasilar occlusive disease: Review of selected aspects: I. Spontaneous dissection of extracranial and intracranial posterior circulation arteries. *Cerebrovasc Dis* 2:256–265, 1992.
43. Tettenborn B, Estol C, DeWitt LD, et al: Accuracy of transcranial Doppler in the vertebrobasilar circulation (abstract). *J Neurol* 237:159, 1990.
44. Rosengart A, DeWitt LD, Caplan LR, et al: Noninvasive tests in vertebro-basilar occlusive disease. *Ann Neurol* 32:265, 1992.
45. Gronholdt M-LM, Nordestgaard BG, Nielsen TG, Sillesen H: Echolucent carotid artery plaques are associated with elevated levels of fasting and postprandial triglyceride-rich lipoproteins. *Stroke* 27:2166–2172, 1996.
46. Steinke W, Kloetzsh C, Hennerici M: Carotid artery disease assessed by color Doppler flow imaging: Correlation with standard Doppler sonography and angiography. *Am J Neuroradiol* 11:259–266, 1990.
47. Berman SS, Devine JJ, Erdoes LS, Hunter GC: Distinguishing carotid artery pseudo-occlusion with color-flow Doppler. *Stroke* 26:434–438, 1995.
48. Steinke W, Hennerici M, Rautenberg W, Mohr JP: Symptomatic and asymptomatic high-grade carotid stenosis in Doppler color-flow imaging. *Neurology* 42:131–138, 1992.
49. Hennerici M, Steinke W, Rautenberg W: High resistance Doppler flow pattern in extracranial carotid dissection. *Arch Neurol* 46:670–672, 1989.
50. Sturznegger M: Ultrasound findings in spontaneous carotid artery dissection: The value of duplex sonography. *Arch Neurol* 48:1057–1063, 1991.
51. Caplan LR, Brass LM, DeWitt LD, et al: Transcranial Doppler ultrasound: Present status. *Neurology* 40:696–700, 1990.
52. Wilterdink JL, Feldmann E, Furie KL, et al: Transcranial Doppler ultrasound battery reliably identifies severe internal carotid artery stenosis. *Stroke* 28:133–136, 1997.
53. Wray SH: Occlusion of the central retinal artery, in Bernstein EF (ed): *Amaurosis Fugax.* New York, Springer-Verlag, 1988, pp 81–89.
54. Steinke W, Ries S, Artemis N, et al: Power Doppler imaging of carotid artery stenosis: Comparison with color Doppler flow imaging and angiography. *Stroke* 28:1981–1987, 1997.
55. Griewing B, Doherty C, Kessler Ch: Power Doppler ultrasound examination of the intracerebral and extracerebral vasculature. *J Neuroimag* 6:32–35, 1996.
56. Bogdahn U, Becker G, Winkler J, et al: Transcranial color-coded real-time sonography in adults. *Stroke* 21: 1680–1688, 1990.
57. Bartels E, Flugel KA: Quantitative measurements of blood flow velocities in basal cerebral arteries with transcranial duplex color-flow imaging. *J Neuroimag* 4:77–81, 1994.
58. Seidel G, Kaps M, Gerriets T: Potential and limitations of transcranial color-coded sonography in stroke patients. *Stroke* 26:2061–2066, 1995.
59. Kenton AR, Martin PJ, Abbott RJ, Moody AR: Comparison of transcranial color-coded sonography and magnetic resonance angiography in acute stroke. *Stroke* 28:1601–1606, 1997.
60. Klotzsch C, Popescu O, Berlit P: Assessment of the posterior communicating artery by transcranial color-coded duplex sonography. *Stroke* 27:486–489, 1996.
61. Seidel G, Kaps M, Dorndorf W: Transcranial color-coded duplex sonography of intracerebral hematomas in adults. *Stroke* 24:1519–1527, 1993.
62. Bogdahn U, Becker G, Schlief R, et al: Contrast-enhanced transcranial color-coded real-time sonography. *Stroke* 24:676–684, 1993.
63. Burns PN: Overview of echo-enhanced vascular ultrasound imaging for clinical diagnosis in neurosonology. *J Neuroimag* 7(suppl 1):S2–S14, 1997.
64. Markus HS: Transcranial Doppler detection of circulating cerebral emboli: A review. *Stroke* 24:1246–1250, 1993.
65. Markus HS, Harrison MJ: Microembolic signal detection using ultrasound. *Stroke* 26:1517–1519, 1995.
66. Tong DC, Albers GW: Transcranial Doppler-detected microemboli in patients with acute stroke. *Stroke* 26: 1588–1592, 1995.
67. Sliwka U, Job F-P, Wissuwa D, et al: Occurrence of transcranial Doppler high-intensity transient signals in patients with potential cardiac sources of embolism: A prospective study. *Stroke* 26:2067–2070, 1995.
68. Daffertshofer M, Ries S, Schminke U, Hennerici M: High-intensity transient signals in patients with cerebral ischemia. *Stroke* 27:1844–1849, 1996.

69. Sliwka U, Lingnau A, Stohlmann W-D, et al: Prevalence and time course of microembolic signals in patients with acute strokes: A prospective study. *Stroke* 28:358–363, 1997.
70. Babikian VL, Wijman CA, Hyde C, et al: Cerebral microembolism and early recurrent cerebral or retinal ischemic events. *Stroke* 28:1314–1318, 1997.
71. Grosset DG, Georgiadis D, Abdullah I, et al: Doppler embolic signals vary according to stroke subtype. *Stroke* 25:382–384, 1994.
72. Levi CR, O'Malley HM, Fell G, et al: Transcranial Doppler detected cerebral microembolism following carotid endarterectomy: High microembolic signal loads predict postoperative cerebral ischemia. *Brain* 120:621–629, 1997.
73. Orlandi G, Parenti G, Bertolucci A, et al: Carotid plaque features on angiography and asymptomatic cerebral microembolism. *Acta Neurol Scand* 96:183–186, 1997.
74. Orlandi G, Parenti G, Bertolucci A, Murri L: Silent cerebral microembolism in asymptomatic and symptomatic carotid artery stenoses of low and high degree. *Eur Neurol* 38:39–43, 1997.
75. Siebler M, Kleinschmidt A, Sitzer M, et al: Cerebral microembolism in symptomatic and asymptomatic high-grade internal carotid artery stenosis. *Neurology* 44:615–618, 1994.
76. Sitzer M, Muller W, Siebler M, et al: Plaque ulceration and lumen thrombosis are the main sources of cerebral microemboli in high-grade internal carotid artery stenosis. *Stroke* 26:1231–1233, 1995.
77. Srinivasian J, Newell DW, Sturznegger M, et al: Transcranial Doppler in the evaluation of internal carotid artery dissection. *Stroke* 27:1226–1230, 1996.
78. Valton L, Larrue V, Arrue P, et al: Asymptomatic cerebral embolic signals in patients with carotid stenosis. Correlation with appearance of plaque ulceration on angiography. *Stroke* 26:813–815, 1995.
79. Caplan LR: Brain embolism, revisited. *Neurology* 43: 1281–1287, 1993.
80. Barbut D, Caplan LR: Brain complications of cardiac surgery, in *Current Problems in Cardiology*. Mosby-Yearbook, 1997, pp 445–476.
81. Barbut D, Yao FS, Hager DN, et al: Comparison of transcranial Doppler ultrasonography and transesophageal echocardiography to monitor emboli during coronary artery bypass surgery. *Stroke* 27:87–90, 1996.
82. Barbut D, Yao FS, Lo Y, et al: Determination of size of aortic emboli and embolic load during coronary artery bypass grafting. *Ann Thor Surg* 63:1262–1267, 1997.
83. Moody DM, Bell MA, Johnston WE, et al: Brain microemboli during cardiac surgery or aortography. *Ann Neurol* 28:477–486, 1990.
84. Clark RE, Brillman J, Davis DA, et al: Microemboli during coronary artery bypass grafting: Genesis and effect on outcome. *J Thorac Cardiovasc Surg* 25:1393–1399, 1995.
85. Pugsley W, Klinger L, Paschalis C, et al: The impact of microemboli during cardiopulmonary bypass on neuropsychological functioning. *Stroke* 25:1393–1399, 1994.
86. Cumming MJ, Morrow IM: Carotid artery stenosis: A prospective comparison of CT angiography and conventional angiography. *Am J Roentgoenol* 163:517–523, 1994.
87. Dillon EH, van Leeuwen MS, Fernandez MA, et al: CT angiography: Applications to the evaluation of carotid artery stenosis. *Radiology* 189:211–219, 1993.
88. Marks MP, Napel S, Jordan JE, Enzmann DR: Diagnosis of carotid artery disease: Preliminary experience with maximum-intensity-projection spiral CT angiography. *Am J Radiol* 160:1267–1271, 1993.
89. Leclerc X, Godefroy O, Pruvo JP, Leys D: Computed tomographic angiography for the evaluation of carotid artery stenosis. *Stroke* 26:1577–1581, 1995.
90. Wong KS, Liang EY, Lam WWM, et al: Spiral computed tomography angiography in the assessment of middle cerebral artery occlusive disease. *J Neurol Neurosurg Psychiatry* 59:537–539, 1995.
91. von Kummer R, Weber J: Brain and vascular imaging in acute ischemic stroke: The potential of computed tomography. *Neurology* 49(suppl 4):S52–S55, 1997.
92. Alberico RA, Patel M, Casey S, et al: Evaluation of the circle of Willis with three-dimensional CT angiography in patients with suspected intracranial aneurysms. *Am J Neuroradiol* 16:1571–1578, 1995.
93. Wong KS, Lam WWM, Liang E, et al: Variability of magnetic resonance angiography and computed tomography angiography in grading middle cerebral artery stenosis. *Stroke* 27:1084–1087, 1996.
94. Steiger HJ, Aaslid R, Stooss R: Dynamic computed tomographic imaging of regional cerebral blood flow and blood volume. *Stroke* 24:591–597, 1993.
95. Schwartz A, Hennerici M: Non-invasive transcranial Doppler ultrasound in intracranial angiomas. *Neurology* 36:626–635, 1986.
96. Seklar L, Wechsler L, Yonas H, et al: Value of transcranial Doppler examination in the diagnosis of cerebral vasospasm after subarachnoid hemorrhage. *Neurosurgery* 22:813–821, 1988.
97. Sloan MA, Haley EC, Kassell NF, et al: Sensitivity and specificity of transcranial Doppler ultrasonography in the diagnosis of vasospasm following subarachnoid hemorrhage. *Neurology* 39:1514–1518, 1989.
98. Grotta J, Ackerman R, Correia J, et al: Whole blood viscosity in subjects with acute stroke, transient ischemic attacks, and risk factors for stroke. *Stroke* 22:162–168, 1991.
99. Fisher M, Sotak CH, Minematsu K, Li L: New magnetic resonance techniques for evaluating cerebrovascular disease. *Ann Neurol* 32:115–122, 1992.
100. Minematsu K, Fisher M, Li L, et al: Diffusion-weighted magnetic resonance imaging: Rapid quantitative detection of focal brain ischemia. *Neurology* 42:235–240, 1992.
101. Lutsep HL, Albert GW, DeCrespigny A, et al: Clinical utility of diffusion-weighted magnetic resonance imaging in the assessment of acute ischemic stroke. *Ann Neurol* 41: 574–580, 1997.
102. Baird AE, Benfield A, Schlaug G, et al: Enlargement of human cerebral ischemic lesion volumes measured by diffusion-weighted magnetic resonance imaging. *Ann Neurol* 41:581–589, 1997.
103. Duffy FH: Clinical value of topographic mapping and quantified neurophysiology. *Arch Neurol* 46:1133–1134, 1989.
104. Nuwer MR, Jordan SE, Ahn SS: Evaluation of stroke using EEG frequency analysis and topographic mapping. *Neurology* 37:1153–1159, 1987.

105. Tettenborn B, Caplan LR, Kramer G, Hopf HC: Electrophysiology in ischemic brain stem disease, in Bergeur R, Caplan LR (eds): *Vertebrobasilar Arterial Disease.* St. Louis, Quality Medical Publishing, 1992, pp 124–129.
106. Baron JC: Positron tomography in cerebral ischemia. *Neuroradiology* 27:509–516, 1985.
107. Powers W, Raichle ME: Positron emission tomography and its application to the study of cerebrovascular disease in man. *Stroke* 16:361–376, 1985.
108. Berkelbach JW, Luyten PR, van Rijen OC, et al: Cerebral lactate detected by regional proton magnetic resonance spectroscopy in a patient with cerebral infarction. *Stroke* 19:1556–1560, 1988.
109. Yonas H, Wolfson SK, Gur D, et al: Clinical experience with the use of xenon-enhanced CT blood flow imaging in cerebral vascular disease. *Stroke* 15:443–450, 1984.
110. Caplan LR: Question-driven technology assessment: SPECT as an example. *Neurology* 41:187–191, 1991.
111. Fayad P, Brass LM: Single photon emission tomography in cerebrovascular disease. *Stroke* 22:950–954, 1991.
112. Chimowitz M, Furlan AJ, Jones SC, et al: Transcranial Doppler assessment of cerebral perfusion reserve in patients with carotid occlusive disease and no evidence of cerebral infarction. *Neurology* 43:353–357, 1993.
113. Piepgras A, Schmiedek P, Leisinger G, et al: A simple test to assess cerebrovascular reserve capacity using transcranial Doppler and acetazolamide. *Stroke* 21:1306–1311, 1990.
114. Choksey MS, Costa DC, Ianotti F, et al: ^{99m}TC-HMPAO SPECT studies in traumatic intracerebral hematoma. *J Neurol Neurosurg Psychiatry* 54:6–11, 1991.
115. Metter EJ, Jackson C, Kempler D, et al: Left hemisphere intracerebral hemorrhages studied by (F-18) fluorodeoxyglucose PET. *Neurology* 36:1155–1162, 1986.
116. Martin W, Raichle M: Cerebellar blood flow and metabolism in cerebral hemisphere infarction. *Ann Neurol* 14: 168–176, 1983.
117. Bowler JV, Wade JP: Ipsilateral cerebellar diaschisis following pontine infarction. *Cerebrovasc Dis* 1:58–60, 1991.

CHAPTER 16

DISEASES OF THE SPINAL CORD

Franz Fazekas
Peter Kapeller

Magnetic resonance imaging (MRI) has become the imaging modality of choice for patients with suspected diseases of the spinal cord and therefore is the focus of this chapter.[1,2] The superiority of MRI to myelography and computed tomography (CT) for this indication results from (1) multiplanar imaging and reconstruction capabilities, including the sagittal plane, in a noninvasive manner, (2) exquisite tissue contrast, allowing separation of cerebrospinal fluid (CSF), spinal cord, bony structures, intervertebral disks, and other soft tissues, (3) high sensitivity for pathologic changes, (4) potential for tissue characterization by using different pulse sequences, and (5) the option of further diagnostic gain by intravenous application of contrast material in many instances. Consequently, spinal myelography has been almost abandoned, while the domain of CT in association with spinal cord syndromes remains primarily the delineation of osseous abnormalities of the spine following trauma. Angiography of the spinal arteries is reserved for the detection and interventional treatment of vascular anomalies or of unexplained ischemia to the cord.

MRI OF THE SPINAL CORD: NORMAL FINDINGS AND IMAGING STRATEGIES

For the evaluation of spinal cord abnormalities, both T1- and T2-weighted scans should be obtained. On T1-weighted images the cord looks grayish, and the surrounding CSF is dark. The bone-marrow–containing vertebral bodies appear of intermediate signal intensity and are separated by low-intensity intervertebral disks. Most often, alterations of the cord size and shape, distortions of the medulla, or a narrowing of the spinal canal can already be well appreciated on these images. T2-weighted scans serve to highlight intramedullary lesions and to better define the outer contours of the spinal cord against a bright CSF. Fast spin-echo techniques have become the preferred sequences at many institutions because they tend to reduce examination time and thus contribute to patients' tolerance. For subtle abnormalities, conventional spin-echo sequences with cardiac triggering may still be more sensitive, however.[3] Fluid-attenuated inversion recovery (FLAIR), a T2-weighted sequence with signal suppression of water, contributes significantly to the delineation of lesions in the brain, but its sensitivity for pathologic conditions of the spinal cord has been rather disappointing.[4] Following the application of contrast material, fat-suppression techniques are helpful with diseases preferentially involving the spinal column and paravertebral tissues.[5] These gadolinium chelates are given intravenously in a dosage of 0.1 mmol/kg body weight, and a minimum interval of 5 to 7 min should follow before the respective T1-weighted sequence is started in order to leave enough time for enhancement.[6] In general, slice thickness must not exceed 3 mm, and for many disorders it is wise to scan the entire cord, a procedure that has been greatly facilitated with the introduction of phased-array coils. Axial scans are needed to establish the relationship of the pathologic process to the various compartments of the spine and to delineate extradural extension, if present. They are also mandatory to confirm very small lesions suspected from sagittal images and to display their location in relation to the anatomy of the spinal cord.[7,8]

The normal shape of the spinal cord seen by MRI corresponds exactly to that known from anatomic studies, with a widening at the cervical and thoracolumbar region. Axial scans may be used to measure the anteroposterior (AP) and transverse cord diameters, and normative data have been accumulated for comparison with diseased states. In normal subjects, the average AP diameter of the cord at C3 to C5 is about 8.5 mm, and the transverse diameter ranges from 13 to 14 mm. At T3, an AP diameter of about 7 mm and a transverse diameter of about 10 mm were found.[9]

MYELOCOMPRESSIVE DISORDERS

There exist many causes for narrowing of the spinal canal and subsequent cord compression. The velocity of this process is crucial to the extent of associated clinical signs. Relatively minor but acute impingement upon the cord can result in a marked neurologic deficit, while chronically increasing compression may be associated with only minimal symptoms for years despite much higher grades of spinal canal stenosis. If patients with chronic compression suddenly start to deteriorate, it is probably a consequence of the development of compromise of blood supply to the spinal cord. Imaging is expected to identify and characterize the obstructive lesion and to display the extent of compression and intrinsic damage to the cord. In both respects, MRI is sensitive and rather specific. Therefore, MRI is a diagnostic emergency procedure for patients with rapidly developing spinal cord symptoms.[10] Immediate use of MRI not only increases the chance of helpful intervention for the individual patient but also appears to be of overall economic benefit.[11] Examination planning has to consider that misleading sensory levels as much as 5 to 12 segments below the actual lesion were found in 26 percent of patients with extra- or intramedullary spinal cord damage.[12] Additional levels of compression need not be apparent clinically but will significantly alter therapeutic approaches. Therefore, MRI of the whole spine should be performed in any patient with suspected malignant spinal cord compression.[13]

Neoplasms

The most frequent cause of cord compression is metastasis to the spine.[12] Tumors with the highest propensity to metastasize to vertebral bodies are lung, breast, and prostate carcinomas. Other tumors frequently affecting the spine are myeloma and lymphoma. Plain x-ray films can call attention to a destructive or lytic process, or metastases may be sclerotic, especially in prostate carcinoma, but in the early stage of infiltration they frequently go undetected. T1-weighted MRI shows metastases as hypointense lesions within the body or other parts of the vertebra and epidural extension in cases of cord compression (Fig. 16-1A). The areas of tumor infiltration are mostly hyperintense on T2-weighted images (Fig. 16-1B) but may also be isointense to hypointense with marked sclerosis. Signal abnormalities tend to involve the entire veretebral body or to be irregular and frequently extend into the pedicles and paravertebral tissue but spare the intervertebral spaces.[14,15] Multi-

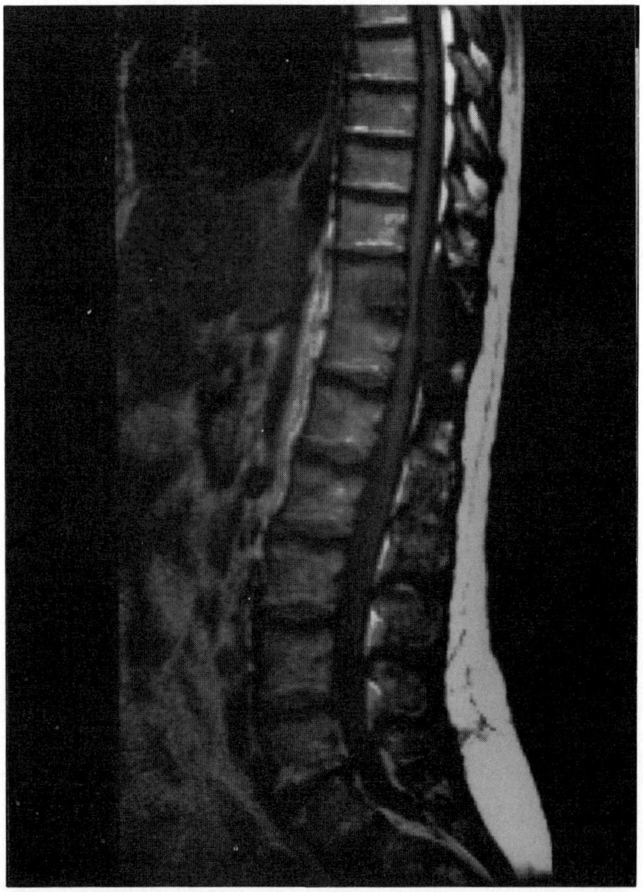

A

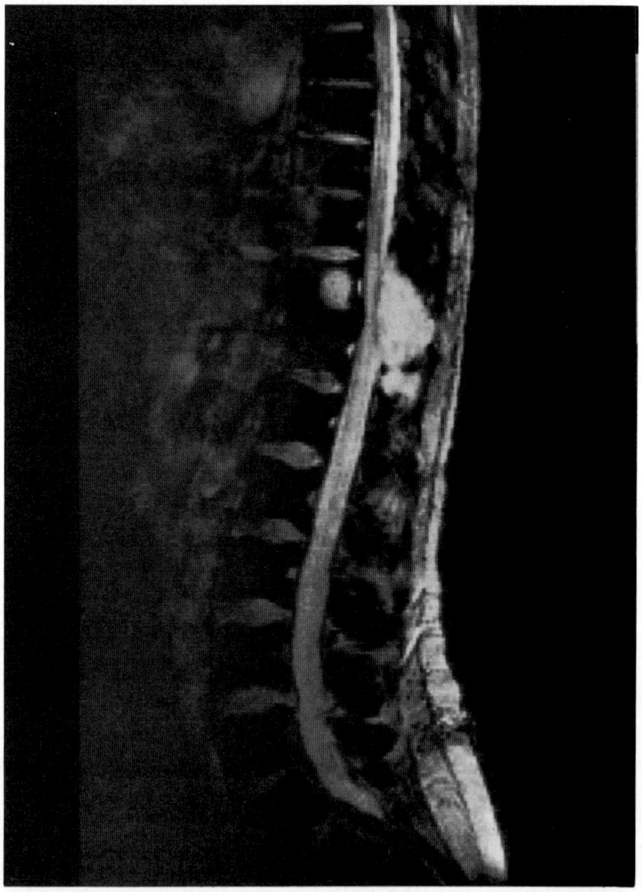

B

Figure 16-1

A patient presenting with paraparesis 2 years after surgery for breast carcinoma. **(A)** *T1-weighted image shows hypointense lesions in the vertebral body and posterior aspect of the spine at T10 to T11 with epidural cord compression. The fusion of the vertebral bodies of T10 and T11 is incidental.* **(B)** *The metastatic tissue appears bright on a T2-weighted gradient-echo sequence. Central cord hyperintensity is due to edema.*

focality also suggests metastatic disease, and the likelihood of detecting this feature increases with imaging of the entire spine.[10,16] Lymphomas occur more frequently as a single mass but have otherwise no specific signal characteristics.

Impingement on the spinal cord from primary tumors of the spine is rare. Benign tumors include osteochondroma, osteoid osteoma, vertebral hemangioma, osteoblastoma, aneurysmal bone cysts, giant-cell tumors, chordomas, and others. The two most common malignant neoplasms are osteosarcoma and chondrosarcoma. A tentative diagnosis may be reached by including age, location within the vertebra, MRI signal pattern, and findings on plain films in the consideration.[17]

Myelocompression from intradural neoplasms arises from meningioma and neurinoma in most instances. Although both tend to grow slowly, spinal cord symptoms may finally develop rather quickly following the breakdown of cord perfusion or a sudden increase in edema. The MRI characteristics of both tumors include low signal intensity on T1-weighted scans with marked contrast enhancement (Figs. 16-2, 16-3, and 16-4). Neurinomas extending through the intervertebral canal have a typical shape (Fig. 16-2). Widening of the neuroforamen and posterior scalloping of the vertebral body may be already seen on plain films. Centrally necrotic neurinomas enhance only in the periphery, which gives them a cystic appearance (Fig. 16-3). Meningiomas have a preponderance for women and tend to be located posterolaterally to the spinal cord. They can be easily overlooked on noncontrast scans because of a signal intensity that is similar to that of the cord on all sequences (Fig. 16-4). In contrast, very specific MRI signal characteristics are seen with lipomas or other fat-containing tumors (Fig. 16-5).

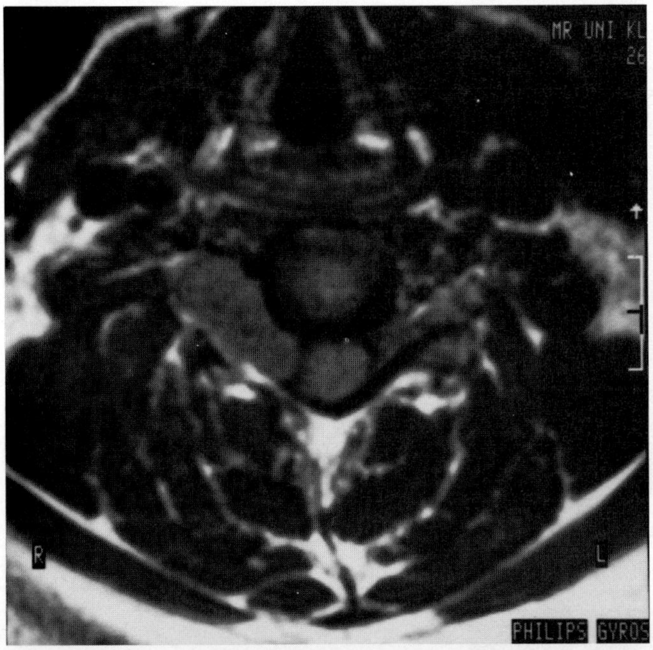

A

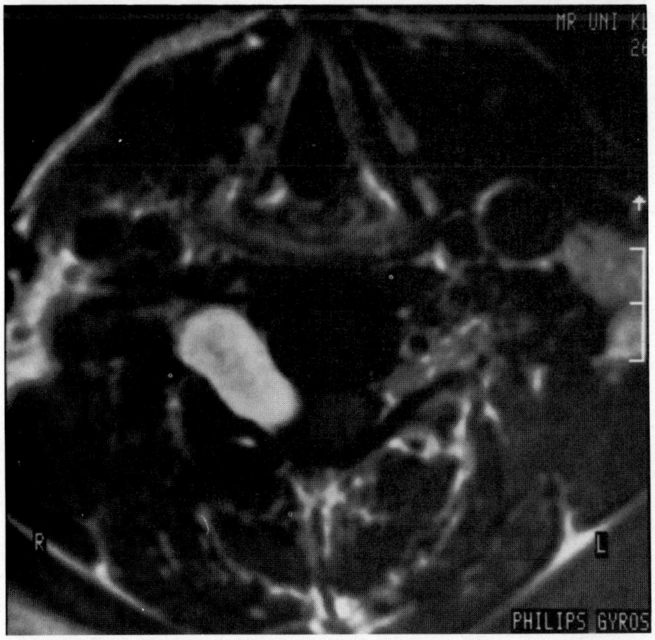

B

Figure 16-2
Neurinoma with dumbbell or hourglass shape in a markedly enlarged cervical neuroforamen. **(A)** *Precontrast scan and* **(B)** *postcontrast T1-weighted scan with marked enhancement.*

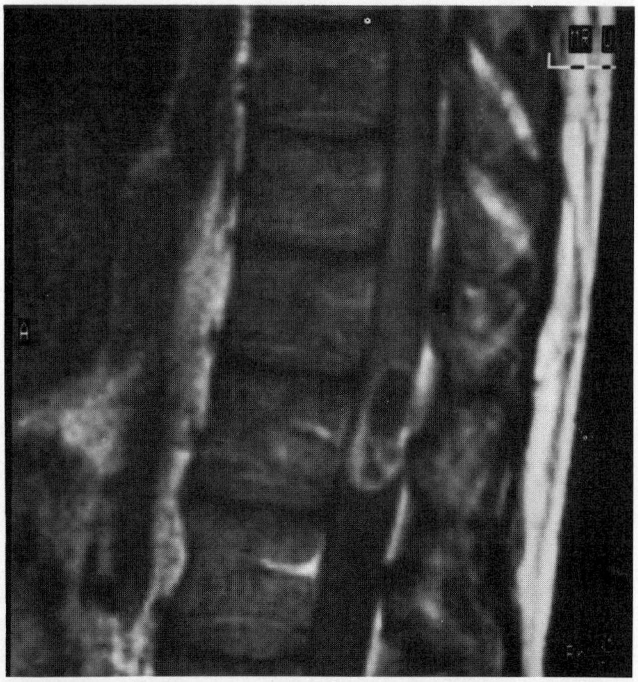

Figure 16-3
Neurinoma at the level of the conus medullaris with less typical appearance on contrast-enhanced study because of central necrosis.

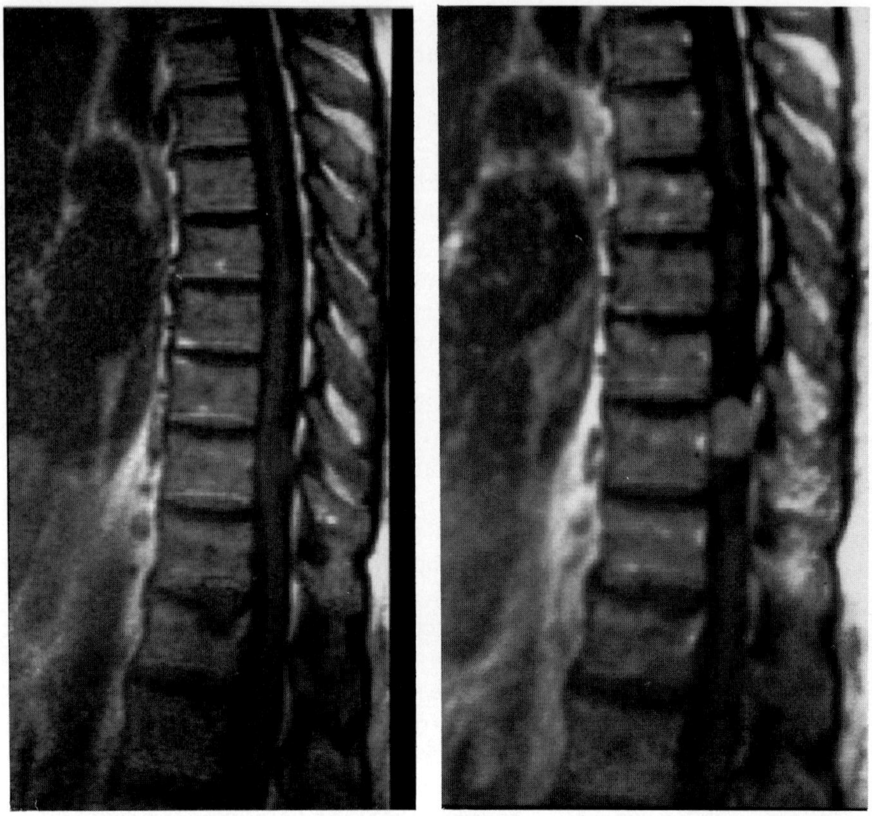

A B

Figure 16-4
Thoracic meningioma. **(A)** *Tumor located posterolateral to the cord can be easily overlooked on native scan but* **(B)** *shows marked contrast enhancement.*

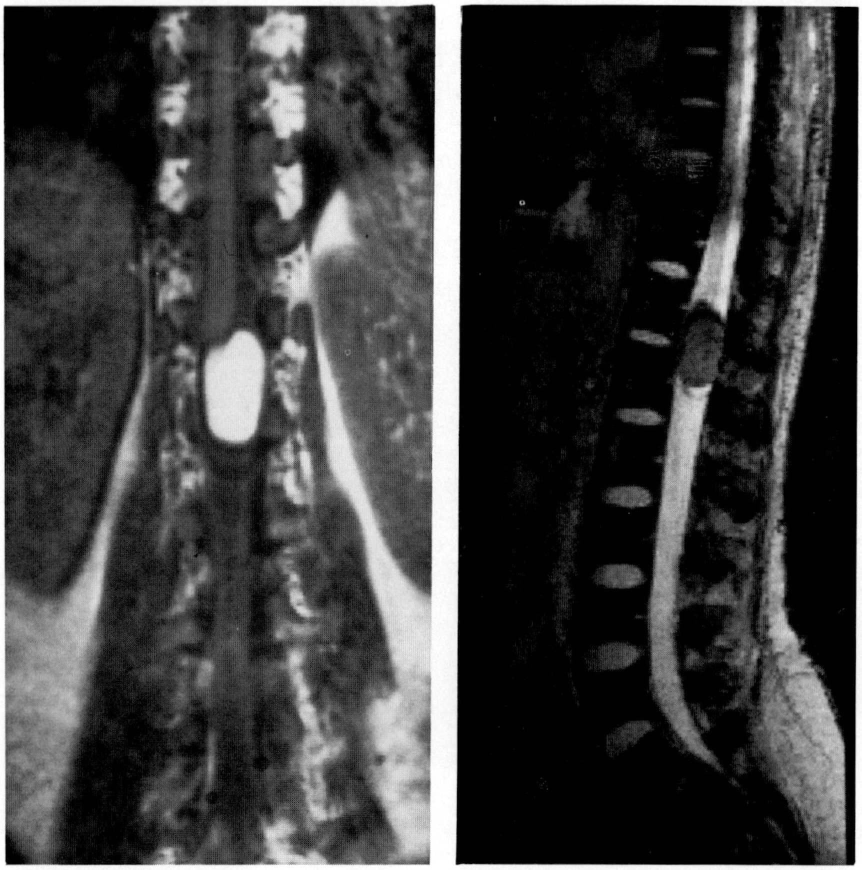

A B

Figure 16-5
Signal characteristics typical of a lipoma. **(A)** *T1-weighted coronal sequence shows displacement of the conus by a hyperintense, well-defined mass, which becomes* **(B)** *hypointense on the gradient-echo T2-weighted scan.*

Inflammation

Epidural abscesses compressing the spinal cord have a rather typical MRI appearance.[18] T1-weighted images may show an ill-defined spinal canal. After injection of contrast material, the area of inflammation densely enhances except for the necrotic, liquefied center of the abscess itself (Fig. 16-6A, B). Diffuse enhancement is noted before an abscess has formed. The entire inflammatory region and associated cord damage appear hyperintense on proton density and T2-weighted images (Fig. 16-6C). Abscesses tend to develop more often in the anterior part of the spinal canal and to involve multiple vertebral segments. Frequently, signal abnormalities and contrast enhancement extend into the adjacent vertebrae and disk spaces. The latter finding would be highly unusual for a neoplasm (Fig. 16-6A–C). It is sometimes difficult to decide, however, whether discitis and osteomyelitis are causes or consequences of the epidural inflammation.[15,19,20] Signal abnormalities within the spinal cord may stem from edema due to compression, from myelitis, or from ischemic damage because of vasculitis. Cord enhancement favors the latter two causes (Fig. 16-6C). *Staphylococcus aureus* is the most frequently identified microorganism among other bacteria, but granulomatous infections also need to be con-

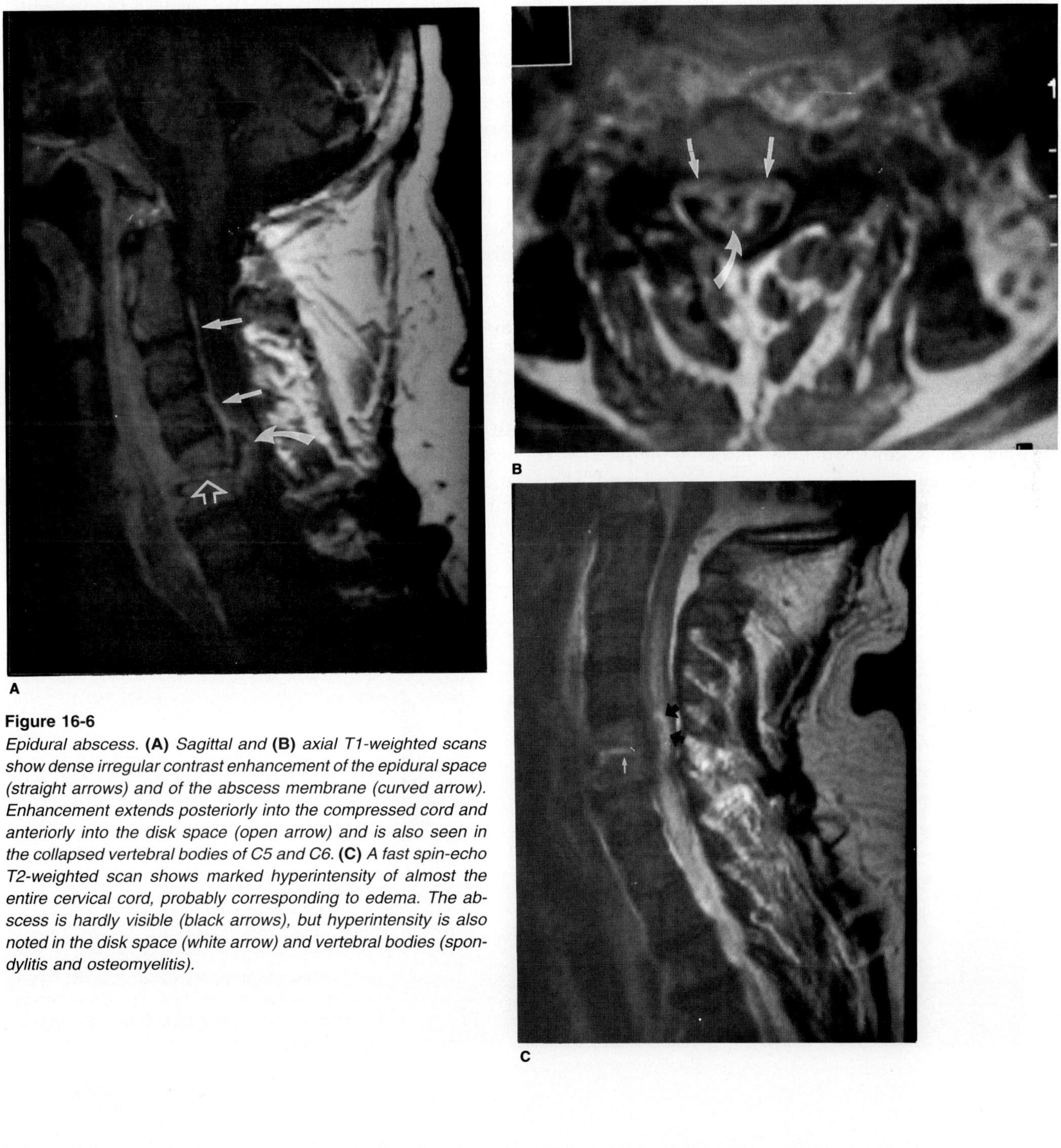

A

B

C

Figure 16-6

Epidural abscess. **(A)** *Sagittal and* **(B)** *axial T1-weighted scans show dense irregular contrast enhancement of the epidural space (straight arrows) and of the abscess membrane (curved arrow). Enhancement extends posteriorly into the compressed cord and anteriorly into the disk space (open arrow) and is also seen in the collapsed vertebral bodies of C5 and C6.* **(C)** *A fast spin-echo T2-weighted scan shows marked hyperintensity of almost the entire cervical cord, probably corresponding to edema. The abscess is hardly visible (black arrows), but hyperintensity is also noted in the disk space (white arrow) and vertebral bodies (spondylitis and osteomyelitis).*

sidered.[15,20] Often, focal back pain from spondylitis appears to precede spinal cord symptoms in association with or without an epidural abscess for several weeks. This mandates alertness for pyogenic spinal infection in patients at risk, such as elderly individuals with diabetes mellitus or previous nonspinal surgery, considering the ease of diagnosis by MRI and the availability of antibiotics to stop progression of infection before the development of serious neurologic deficits.[15,19] Sometimes the development of spinal cord symptoms in association with epidural infections can be related neither to cord compression nor to intramedullary signal changes.[21]

In patients with rheumatoid arthritis, retrodental pannus formation has to be thought of as another cause of "inflammatory" myelocompression (Fig. 16-7A,B).[22]

Degenerative Disease of the Spine

In rare cases, disk herniation may cause acute myelocompression. This process occurs preferentially in individuals with a narrow spinal canal. The MRI displays the compressive mass in continuity with the intervertebral disk space and as having similar signal intensity on all sequences or, when fragmented from the disk, in a position close above or below. Location of the mass in relation to the posterior longitudinal ligament and associated signal changes in the cord are best appreciated on T2-weighted images.

A progressive evolution of spinal cord symptoms and radiculopathy in association with pronounced degenerative changes of the cervical spine has been termed cervical spondylotic myelopathy. It appears to result from a combination of cord compression, motion-induced injury, and vascular compromise of the cervical cord. The MRI clearly shows the extent of spinal canal narrowing caused by bulging disks, osteophyte formation, and ligamentous thickening and the remaining diameter of the spinal cord (Fig. 16-8A–C). Focal hyperintensity within the spinal cord on T2-weighted scans at or slightly below the site of maximal impingement is seen in about half of the patients and reflects a wide range of histopathologic conditions, such as edema, ischemia, demyelination, gliosis, and necrosis. In a study of 668 patients, the frequency of this MRI finding was directly proportional to the degree of myelomalacia and compression of the spinal cord,[23] but focal intramedullary hyperintensity can also occur with mild compression only. Concomitant disruption of the blood-brain barrier is indicated by enhancement following contrast material injection. The prognostic significance of MRI changes of the spinal cord is not yet fully resolved. The results of some studies suggest a far less favorable outcome in those patients whose presurgical T2-weighted MRI displayed high signal intensity of the spinal cord at the level of compression. In those patients who improved nevertheless, focal hyperintensity tended to disappear.[23,24] Other investigators failed to find such correlation.[25] In part, this may reflect the variety of pathophysiologic processes causing high T2 signal intensity.[26] The range of recovery was also limited in those patients with marked cord atrophy preoperatively.[26] In patients with unsatisfactory improvement following surgery, MRI follow-up may be important to rule out remaining cord compression.

Trauma

In the acute setting of spinal trauma, plain radiography and CT are most often used to determine the occurrence of vertebral fractures and displacement of bony fragments into the spinal canal. These procedures can be

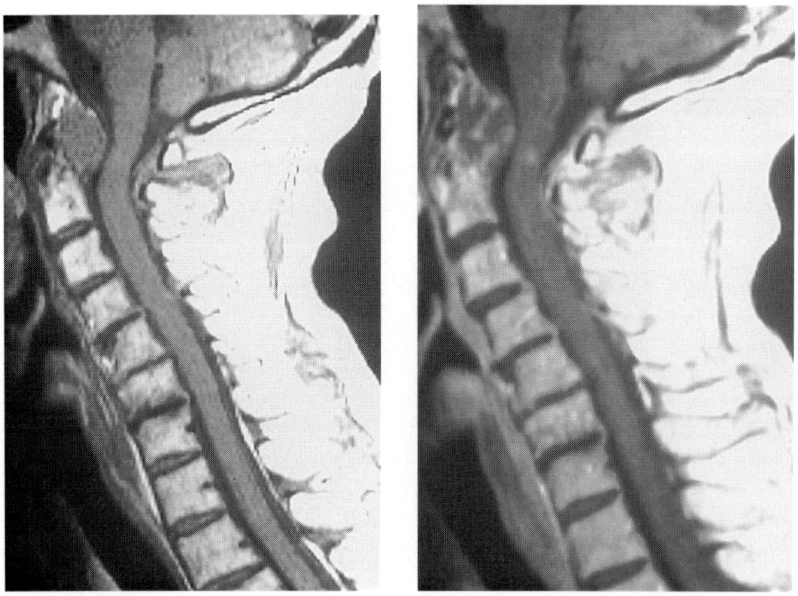
A B

Figure 16-7
A patient with rheumatoid arthritis and long tract signs. **(A)** *T1-weighted sagittal scan shows retrodental mass and mild compression with kinking of the upper cervical cord.* **(B)** *Following injection of Gd-DTPA, the pannus enhances and an area of focal enhancement is seen within the cord.*

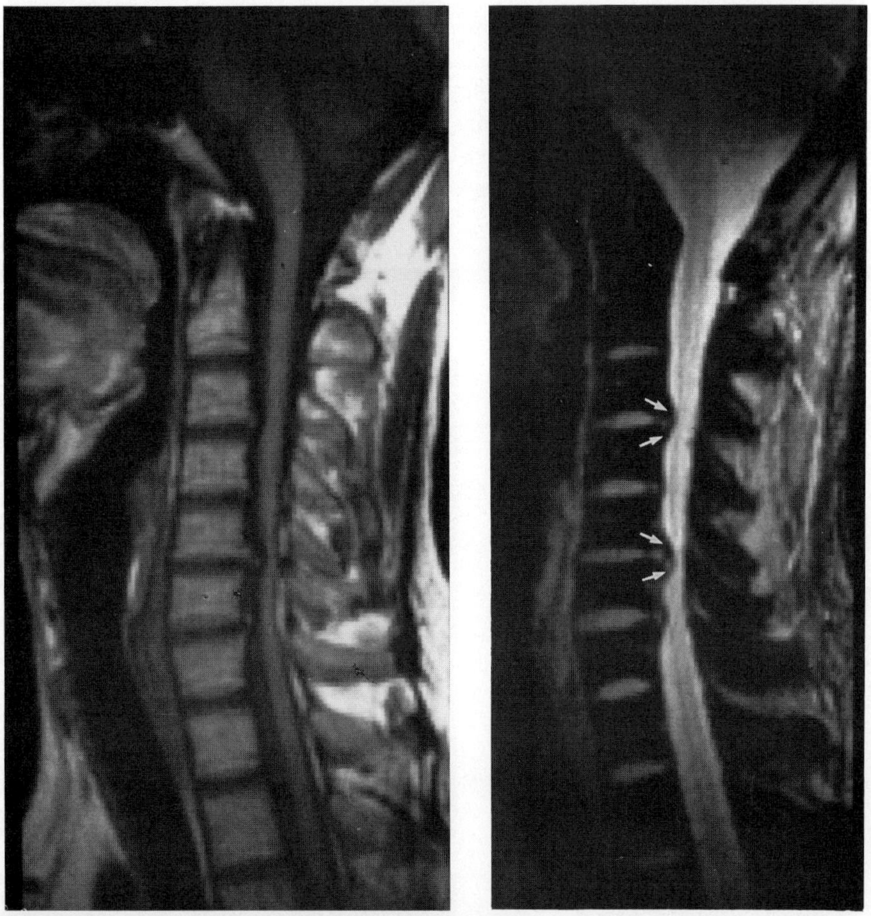

A B

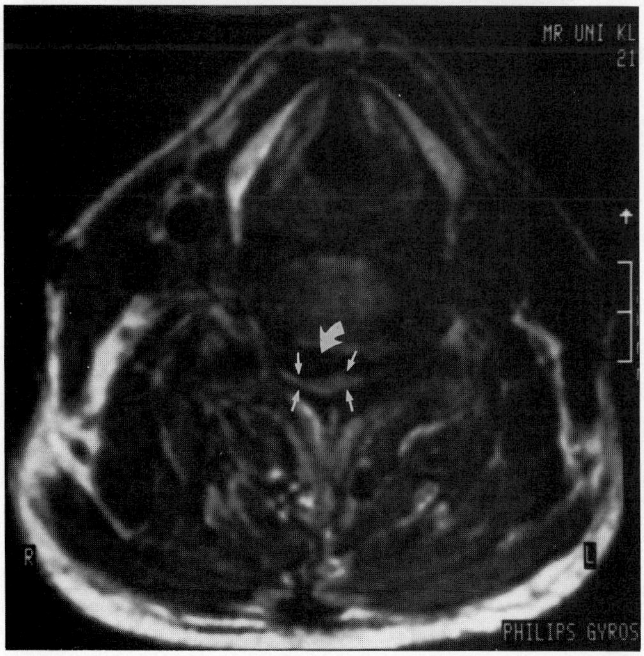

C

Figure 16-8

Cervical spondylotic myelopathy. **(A)** *T1-weighted and* **(B)** *gradient-echo T2-weighted scans show multisegmental narrowing of the spinal canal from bulging and herniated disks and osteophytes (arrows), with cord compression and atrophy. Findings are more accentuated on the gradient-echo sequence.* **(C)** *Axial scan at C5 to C6 highlights the extent of cord compromise (small arrows outline the cord) from herniation (curved arrow).*

easily applied even to critically ill patients. For those patients whose spinal cord symptoms still remain unexplained, MRI should subsequently be performed to rule out cord compression from soft tissues, such as a herniated disk, or at other levels than clinically or radiologically suspected. For the detection of small bony fragments, CT is superior, but only MRI can visualize changes in the traumatized cord itself.[27] The MRI findings may consist of the entire spectrum of pathologically described abnormalities, from macroscopically normal through cord swelling with edema, punctate or coalescent hemorrhages (Fig. 16-9A–D), and in the most se-

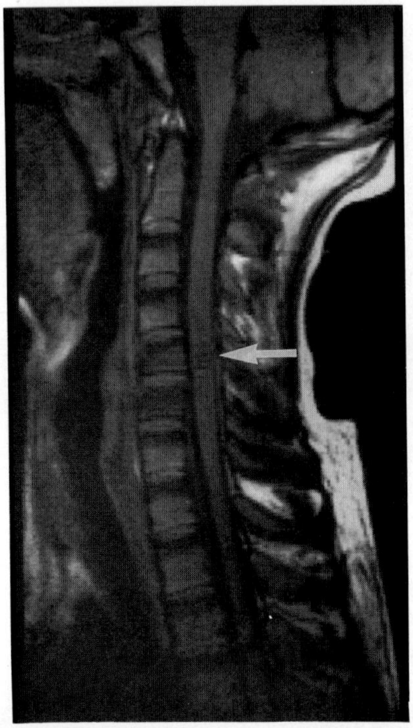

A

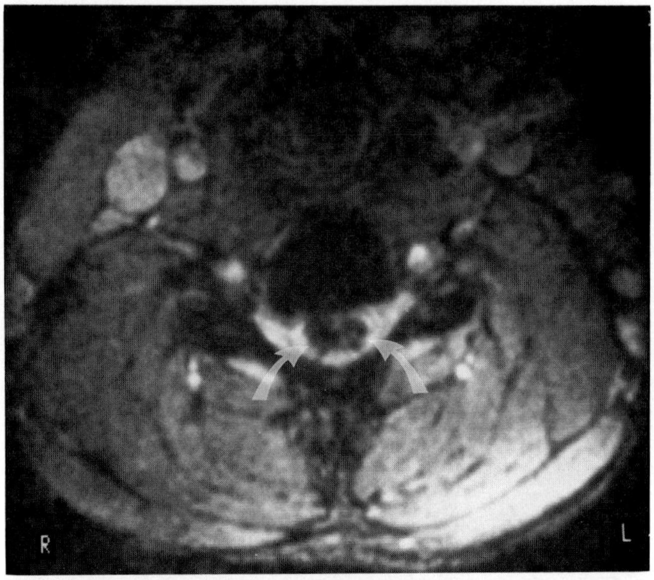

C

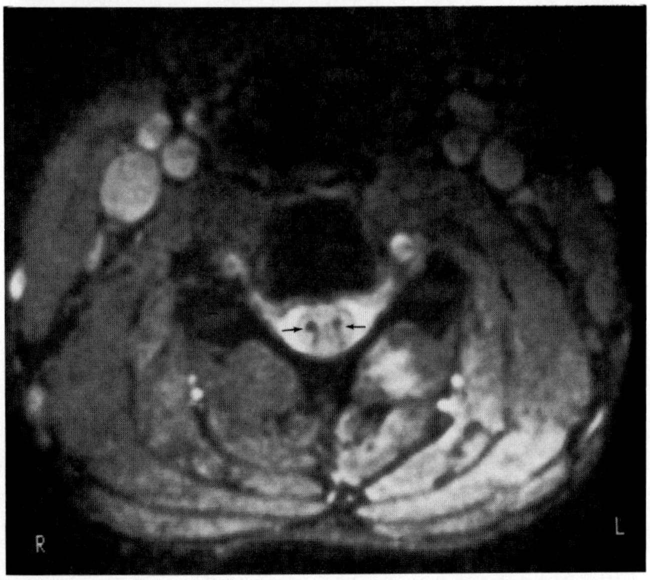

D

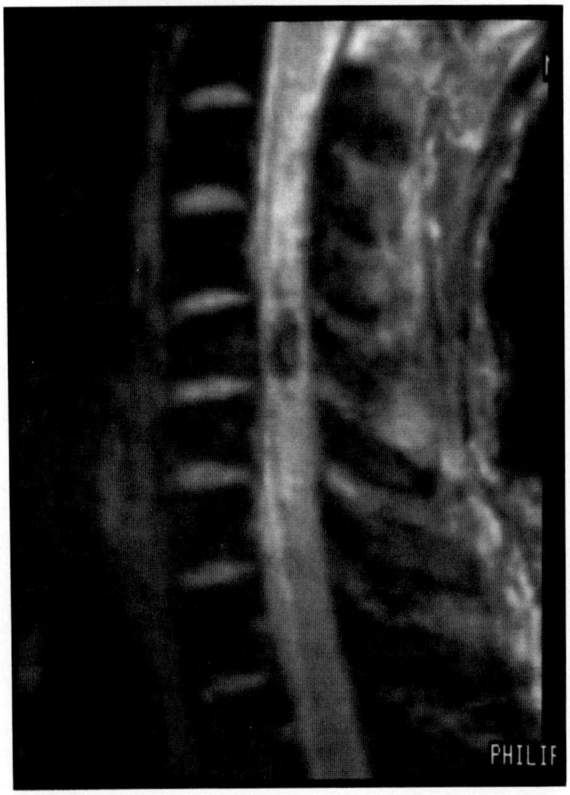

B

Figure 16-9

Acute study of a patient with tetraplegia a few hours after jumping into shallow water. Plain films were called unremarkable. **(A)** *T1-weighted images show an area of mildly reduced signal intensity in the spinal cord at the level of C5 (arrow). The vertebral bodies of C5 and C6 are minimally compressed and somewhat hypointense.* **(B)** *The intramedullary abnormality is markedly hypointense on a gradient-echo T2-weighted sequence, consistent with acute blood.* **(C)** *and* **(D)** *Axial scans confirm the central location of the hematoma (curved arrows) with extension along the gray matter (small arrows).*

vere cases, cord transsection. The prognostic significance of this information is high.[28–30] As expected, patients with cord transsection have no potential for recovery. Hemorrhage into the spinal cord, termed contusion by some, also carries a poor prognosis, but unexpected improvement has been reported.[31] Patients fare better who show cord hyperintensity on T2-weighted images only. The smaller this area, which presumably stems from edema and axonal disruption, the more likely is recovery.[28] Traumatic cord hemorrhages affect preferentially the more vascularized part of the spinal cord which is the central gray matter (Fig. 16-9C,D). However, this may not be the most frequent cause of a so-called central cord syndrome. In a series of 11 consecutive cases with paralysis affecting predominantly the upper extremities, there was no MRI evidence of hemorrhage in any of them, and the primary pathologic finding was diffuse axonal disruption within the lateral columns, probably including the pyramidal tracts.[32]

Neuroimaging is also important for patients in the aftermath of spinal trauma, since some of them may start to deteriorate even years after the injury. This syndrome is known as posttraumatic progressive myelopathy. Intramedullary cyst formation has been identified as the most frequent cause. In two large series of patients referred for MRI in the chronic stage of cord injury, posttraumatic syringomyelia was present in about 40 percent (Fig. 16-10). Another 25 to 30 percent had persistent cord compression (Fig. 16-11). Drainage of cysts exerting mass effect and decompression was able to prevent further deterioration of some of these patients.[33] Optimal vertebral realignment following the injury appears to be important for avoiding syrinx formation early on.[35] Sometimes, follow-up examinations are necessary to clearly separate progressive syringomyelia from CSF-filled spaces after myelomalacia. Development of intramedullary signal hyperintensity proximal to the fluid-filled cavity has been recently described as an early sign of syrinx progression.[36] Spinal cord atrophy is the most frequent long-term finding in patients with complete motor and sensory deficit following injury.[33]

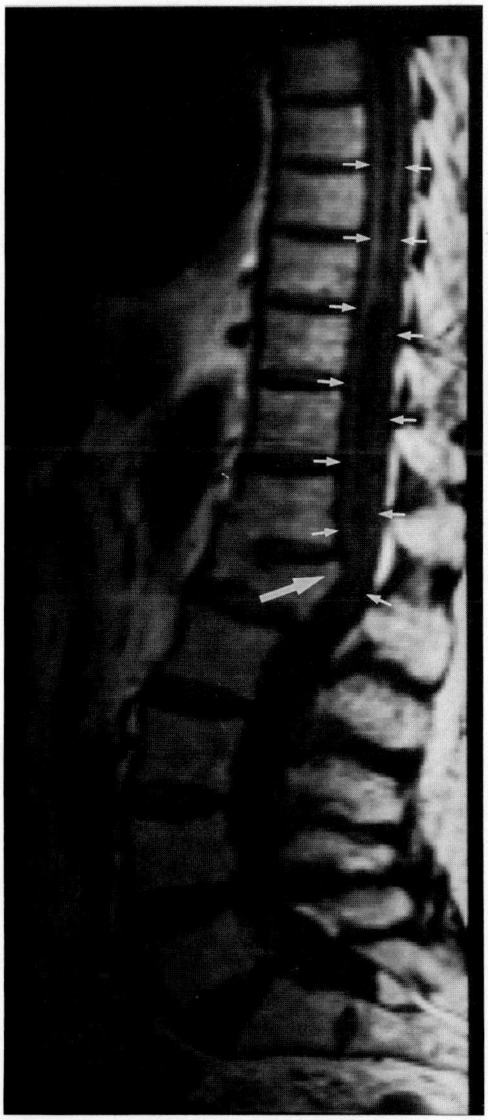

Figure 16-10

Posttraumatic syrinx after compression fracture of L1 with mild narrowing of the spinal canal (large arrow). The cavity extended over the entire cord, leaving only thin walls of cord tissue (marked with small arrows).

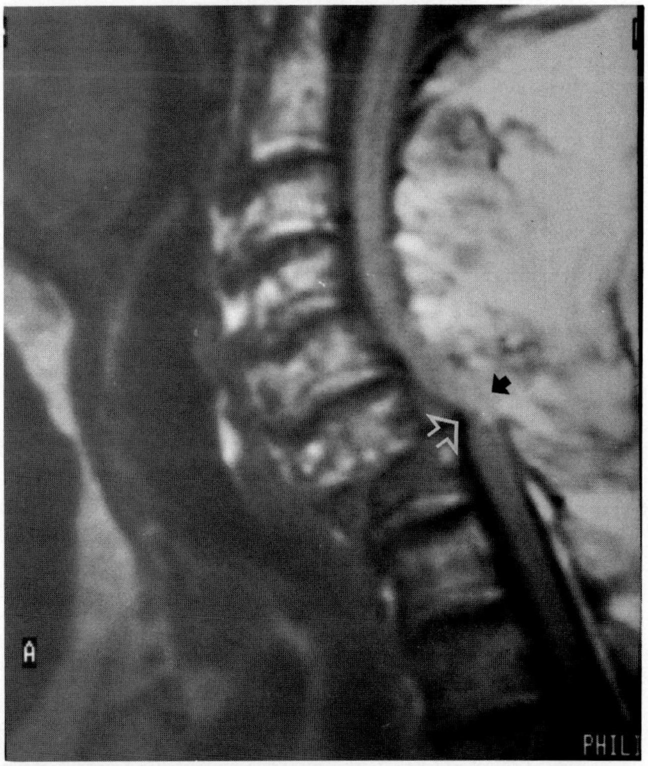

Figure 16-11

Increase of spasticity 15 years after cervical trauma. The MRI shows an old compression dislocation fracture with impingement of the cervical cord (arrows).

Spinal epidural hematoma is a rare consequence of trauma.[37] Nontraumatic causes include anticoagulant therapy, blood dyscrasias, and vascular anomalies. The MRI shows a biconvex mass dorsal to the thecal sac with signal characteristics of blood or its degradation products (Fig. 16-12A–C).[37,38] This allows one to estimate the age of the hematoma. In cord compression, immediate removal of the clot can be associated with complete neurologic recovery. Idiopathic dural herniation of the spinal cord is another infrequent cause of cord compression that needs to be considered.[39] Herniation usually occurs between the T2 and T8 levels. Patients present with long-standing, unexplained sensory symptoms and eventually develop a Brown-Sequard syndrome with or without motor changes.

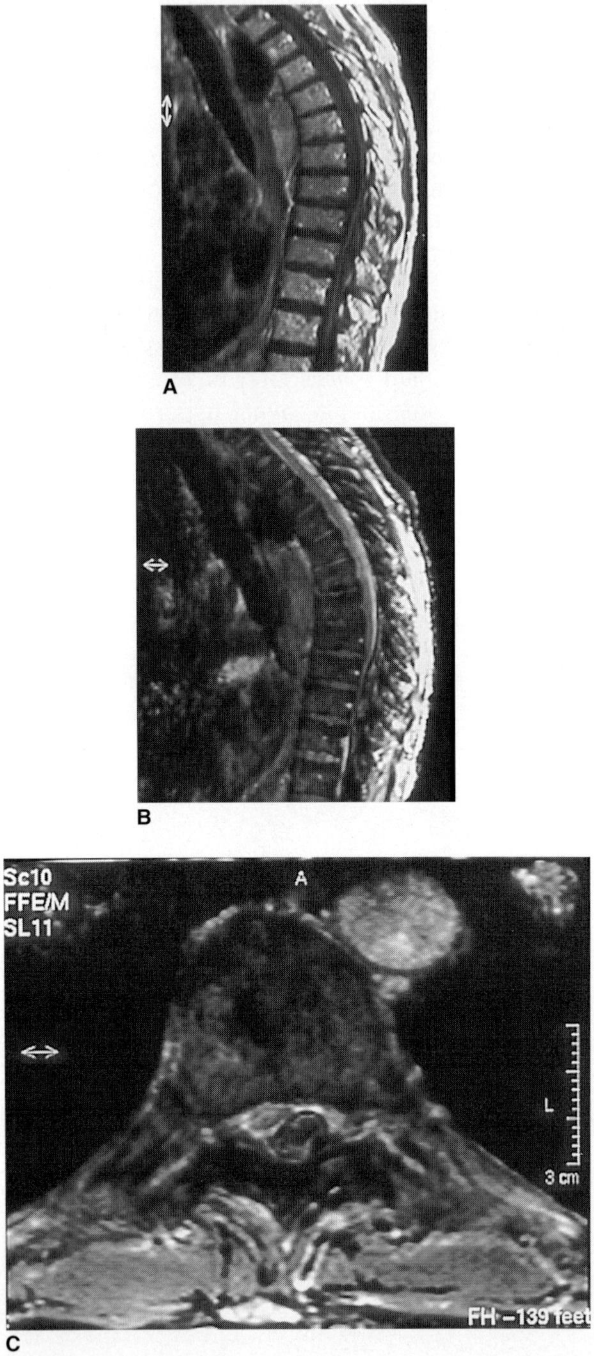

Figure 16-12
A patient with rapidly developing spastic paraparesis 1 week after a fall. **(A)** *Sagittal T1-weighted scan shows a biconvex epidural mass located dorsally from T6 to T10.* **(B)** *The lesion borders and its center appear black on gradient-echo T2-weighted images, which is consistent with acute bleeding.* **(C)** *Anterior dislocation and compression of the spinal cord is best seen on axial scans.*

NONCOMPRESSIVE SPINAL CORD DISORDERS

The MRI findings related to spinal cord disorders in the absence of compression can be grossly grouped into four morphologic categories: (1) the presence of intramedullary signal abnormalities with or without cord enlargement, (2) spinal cord cavitation, (3) cord atrophy, and (4) abnormalities of the spinal cord surface. These MRI patterns can serve to obtain a first diagnostic orientation.

Disorders with Abnormal Signal and Variable Enlargement of the Spinal Cord

The number of diseases associated with signal changes of the spinal cord is by far the largest. As in the brain, T2 hyperintensity of lesions prevails and is shared by many pathologic conditions. Location, size, and shape of signal abnormalities tend to be more specific. For a safe diagnosis, however, complementary investigations, follow-up studies, and clinical data, including type of onset, pattern, and course of symptoms, are frequently needed.

Inflammatory Diseases

Viral, bacterial, parasitic, and fungal infections of the spinal cord are known. In many cases, MRI shows appropriate lesions but clues as to the cause remain limited. Furthermore, variable timing of the imaging studies and variable aggressiveness of the inflammatory process are likely to explain many of the variations of MRI findings described. In general, nongranulomatous infections, such as from herpes zoster, echovirus, coxsackievirus, human T-lymphotropic virus type 1 (HTLV-1), and HTLV-3 appear to be relatively well separable from granulomatous diseases and tumor, since they tend to follow two patterns.[40] One pattern consists of diffuse swelling of the spinal cord that extends over multiple segments (Fig. 16-13). Contrast enhancement is mostly faint, diffuse, peripheral, or speckled, and the areas of cord enlargement appear diffusely hyperintense on T2-weighted scans (Fig. 16-14). Segments of normal-appearing cord may be interspersed, which would be atypical for a neoplasm. Acute transverse myelitis of noninfectious causes can share a similar appearance, however.[41,42] The other pattern of MRI findings in nongranulomatous myelitis consists of focal hyperintensity

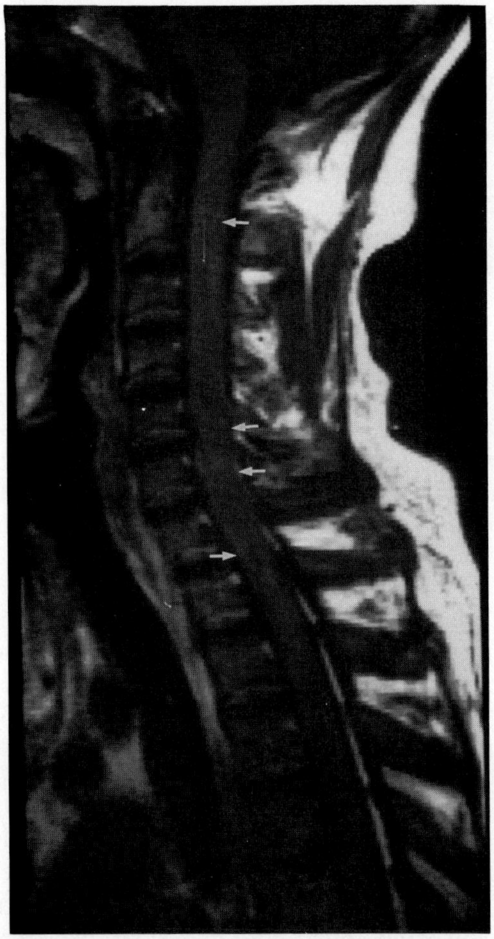

Figure 16-13
Myelitis of undetermined origin. The cord fills the cervical canal, and there is minimal speckled enhancement after application of contrast material (arrows).

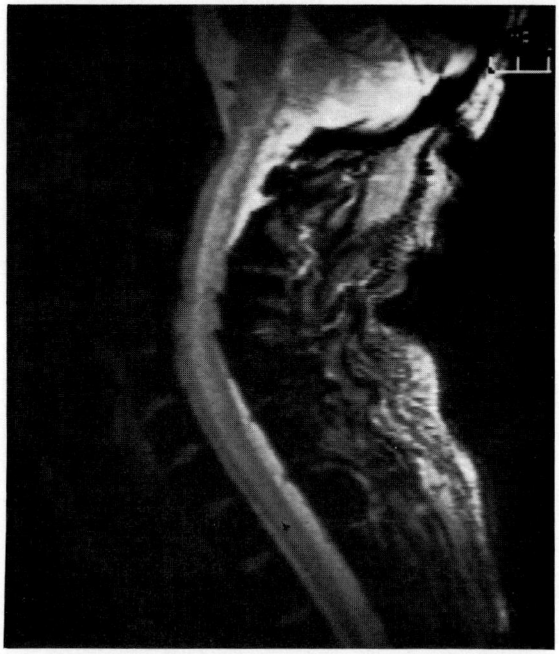

Figure 16-14
Diffuse hyperintensity and mild swelling of the spinal cord in a patient with viral myelitis.

on T2-weighted images and nodular enhancement without significant cord enlargement.[40] The absence of mass effect argues against a tumor in these cases, but focal demyelination can have an identical appearance. A normal MRI, especially early on, does not exclude myelitis. Furthermore, imaging findings need not correlate with the extent of the clinical deficit and most often cannot predict the patient's prognosis.

Marked swelling of the cord, focal hyperintensity on T2-weighted images, and nodular enhancement are seen with inflammation of granulomatous origin. Especially single foci, such as a tuberculoma, thus become indistinguishable from tumor.[40,43] Lesions of spinal cord sarcoidosis exhibit similar imaging findings but tend to occur at multiple sites.[44,45] Leptomeningeal spread can be the only abnormality in the initial phase of sarcoidosis.[45] The differential diagnosis of focal intramedullary T2 hyperintensity with cord swelling needs to include bacterial abscesses. A characteristic evolution of imaging findings with special emphasis on contrast-enhanced scans is diagnostically important.[46] A tumorlike appearance is also found in toxoplasmosis of the spinal cord and must be considered preferentially in immunocompromised patients.[47,48] AIDS-associated cytomegalovirus infection may have a similar appearance.[49]

Parasitic infections of the cord can be also well detected by MRI. Cysticercosis is characterized by fluid-filled mass lesions located within the cord, in the subarachnoid space, or at both locations, and sheetlike enhancement of the cord surface indicative of arachnoiditis has been noted in many cases. Associated intracranial disease is frequent.[50] The MRI findings in *Schistosoma* myelitis consist of mild cord enlargement with diffuse hyperintensity and heterogeneous enhancement after application of contrast material.[51]

Demyelinating Diseases

Multiple sclerosis (MS) is the most common demyelinating disease to affect the cord. At least 80 percent of MS patients have some form of spinal involvement at some point in their disease.[52] Characteristically, spinal cord plaques are located peripherally, rarely exceed two vertebral segments in length, and occupy less than half the cross-sectional area of the cord.[53] Acute plaques can produce mass effect, with swelling of the cord, and may enhance after the application of contrast material. In these instances, myelitis from another cause or sometimes even a tumor cannot be ruled out. The MS-related lesions are seen more frequently in the cervical than the thoracic cord and are most common in the mid-cervical region (Fig. 16-15A). Overall, it appears more difficult to define a typical MS lesion pattern for the spinal cord than for the brain because of limitations in

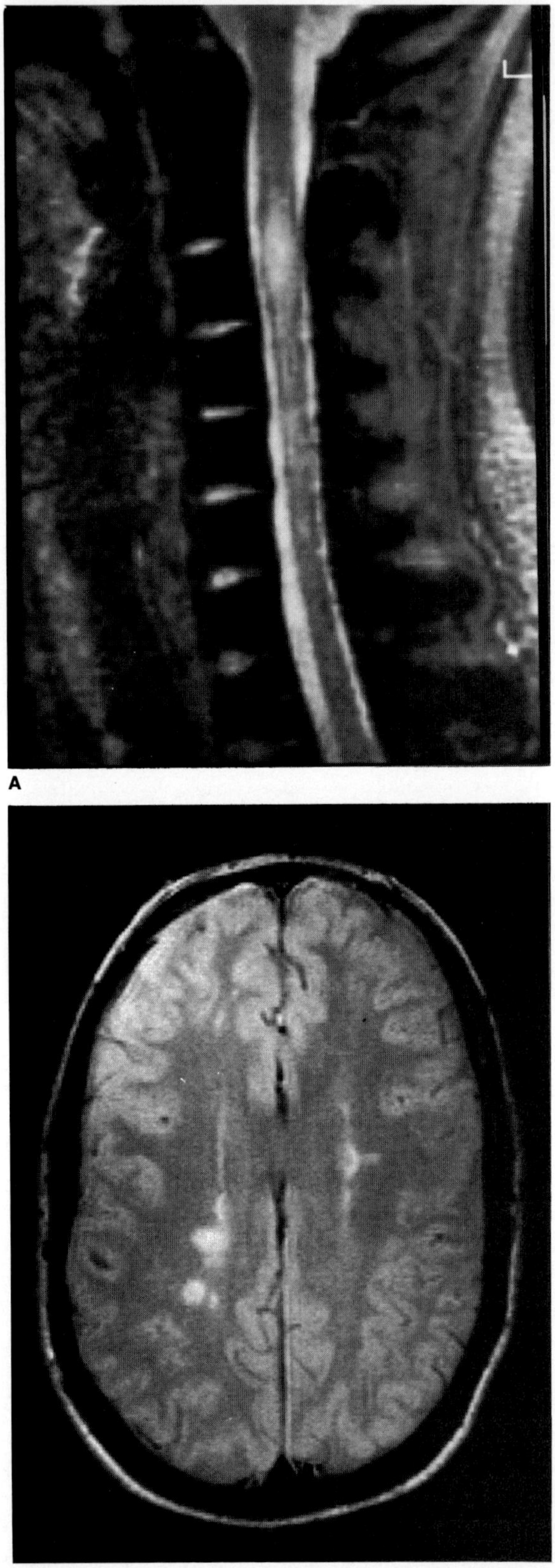

A

B

Figure 16-15

A 23-year-old female first presenting with spinal cord symptoms. **(A)** *T2-weighted MRI shows a large high-signal-intensity lesion with mild cord swelling at C3. The subtle signal differences below are more likely artifactual than true lesions on this gradient-echo sequence.* **(B)** *MRI of the head shows multiple high-signal-intensity lesions of the white matter, some in a periventricular location, which are suggestive of multiple sclerosis.*

relating plaques to the small anatomic structures involved.[4,54] Yet the detection of a lesion within the spinal cord gains specificity by the virtual absence of "incidental" lesions in normal individuals, in contrast to the brain.[55]

The possibility of missing demyelinating lesions on spinal MRI and the fact that their features are nonspecific argue for a complementary MRI study of the head in all patients with spinal cord symptoms as a possible sign of MS (Fig. 16-15B).[56–58] Concomitant presence of cerebral lesions in patients presenting with a spinal cord syndrome suggestive of MS also proves to be an excellent predictor of subsequent progression to clinically definite disease.[59] Conversely, spinal cord imaging may well support a clinical diagnosis of MS in the absence of significant brain lesions. Thorpe et al recently described a series of patients with definite or probable MS who had a normal or noncharacteristic brain study but evidence for demyelinating lesions on MRI of the spine.[60] These patients suffered predominantly from primary progressive MS or had a relapsing-remitting course with minimal disability. The authors suggest that the combination of brain and spinal cord examinations in all patients might increase the sensitivity of MRI for MS to nearly 100 percent using current technology. Intravenous injection of contrast material for delineating active cord lesions has remained less successful than in the brain[61] but may help to exclude other disorders.

Rarely, acute disseminated encephalomyelitis can also involve the spinal cord.[62] Lesions may resemble acute plaques of MS, but widespread enhancement should support a monophasic course of the disease. Extensive cord involvement can be also seen with neuromyelitis optica and is characterized by multiple scattered areas of enhancement within large swollen portions of the spinal cord (Fig. 16-16).[63,64] See Chap. 17 for a more complete discussion of MS.

Radiation Myelopathy

Radiation myelopathy with preferentially insiduous onset of symptoms is thought to result from either radiation-induced vascular changes or primary neuronal damage. It should be suspected when neurologic signs occur in a patient with irradiated cord, normal CSF, and no evidence of metastasis. The MRI findings depend on the time of scanning in relation to the onset of symptoms rather than on the interval to radiation therapy. In patients imaged less than 8 months after onset of symptoms, long segments of the cord demonstrate abnormal signal intensity with or without associated swelling and variable focal contrast enhancement. It is interesting to note that the location of blood-brain barrier breakdown appears to correlate best with neurologic symptoms.[65,66] When MRI is performed more than 3 years after the onset of symptoms, atrophy of the cervical cord has been noted without abnormal signal intensity.[65] In the acute phase, the differential diagnosis must include me-

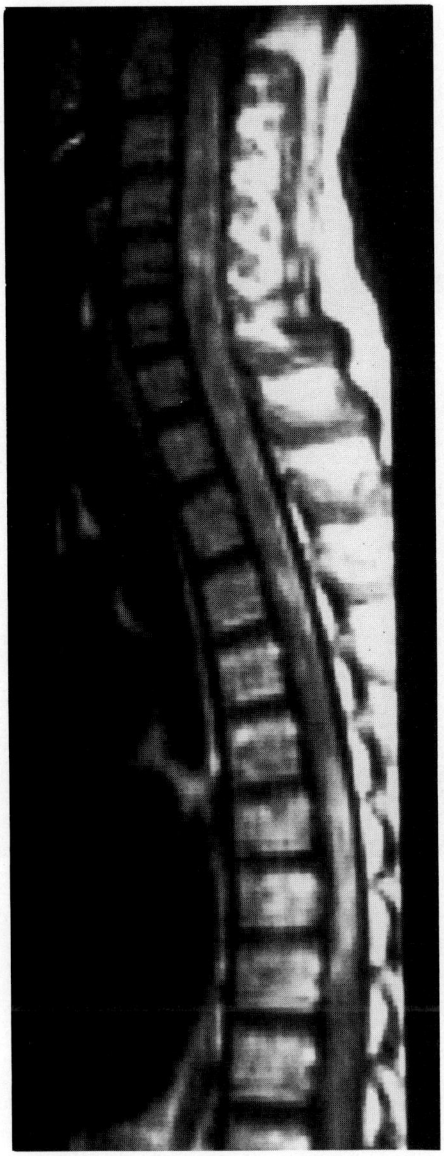

Figure 16-16
A patient with suspected neuromyelitis optica. Patchy contrast enhancement of the entire cervicothoracic spinal cord is most consistent with necrotic myelitis. (From Melhem and Wang.[43])

tastasis, tumor recurrence, and paraneoplastic necrotic myelitis.[67]

Vascular Diseases

Vascular lesions of the cord can be separated into infarcts and malformations. Because of the pattern of blood supply, infarcts usually involve the territory of the anterior spinal artery, a variable vertical extent of the ventral two-thirds of the spinal cord. The lower thoracic cord and conus medullaris are most frequently involved. Imaging findings in the acute stage include swelling of the cord at the injured levels with diffuse hyperintensity on T2-weighted sequences. Signal intensity on T1-weighted scans is normal or slightly reduced (Fig. 16-17A, B). In the subacute phase, contrast en-

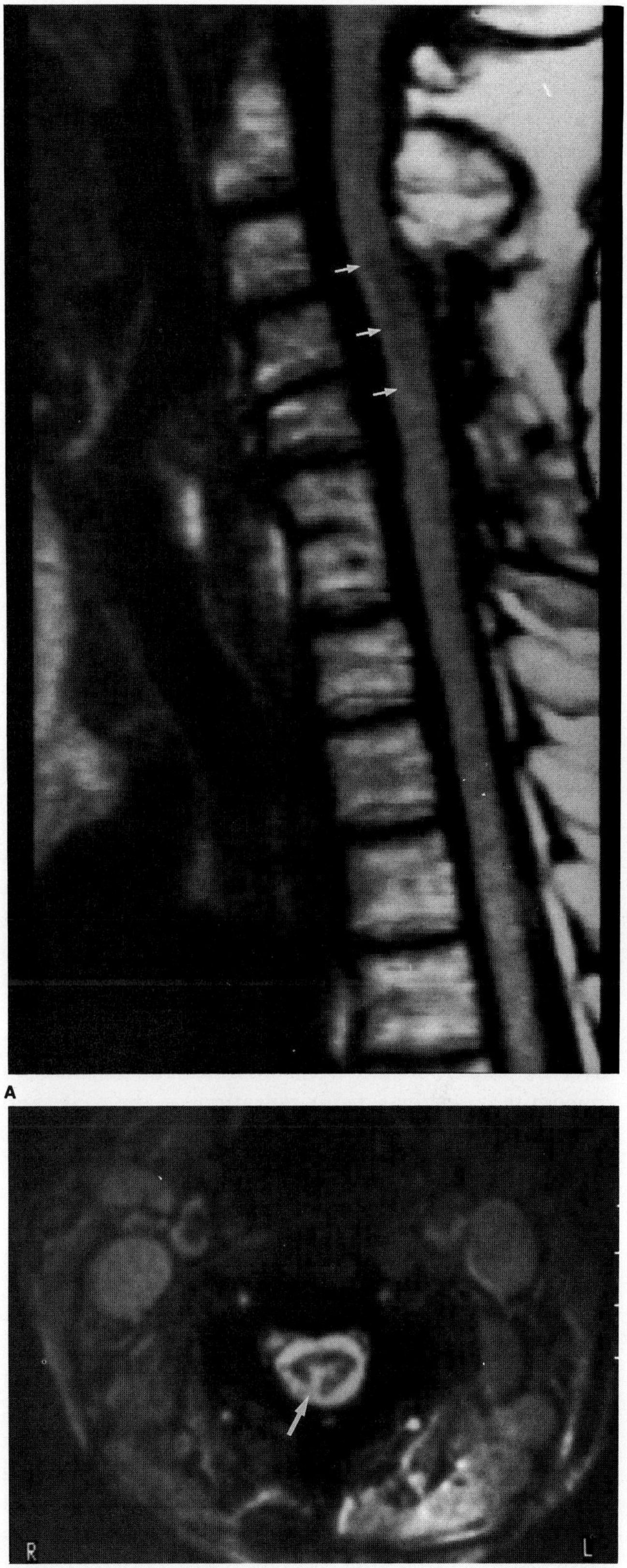

Figure 16-17
Spinal cord infarction at an unusual location after laminectomy. **(A)** *Acute sagittal T1-weighted scan shows mild hypointensity and swelling of the posterior portion of the mid-cervical medulla (arrows).* **(B)** *Axial scan after 1 year discloses remaining defect in the posterior column on the right (arrow), corresponding to a reduced sense of position and vibration.*

hancement can be demonstrated[68] and tends to reflect the angioarchitecture of the cord.[69] Concomitant infarcts to one or multiple vertebral bodies can be seen as areas of hyperintense signal on T2-weighted sequences and strongly support a diagnosis of cord ischemia.[70] In some cases, the cause of infarction, such as an aortic aneurysm, can be directly recognized on MRI as well.[70]

Venous infarction of the spinal cord is a possible consequence of impaired blood drainage in patients with dural arteriovenous fistulas. The MRI findings consist of changes in cord size and signal intensity, and contrast enhancement may persist over many months.[71] Middle-aged men are preferentially affected, and selective spinal angiography should be readily performed to avoid irreversible damage. Following verification of the fistula, it can be occluded by embolization or microsurgical procedures.[72] So-called subacute necrotizing myelopathy is also believed by some authors to result from impaired venous outflow. It is characterized clinically by a progressive course of para- or tetraparesis with sensory loss, at first dissociated and then complete, and loss of sphincteric control. Pathologic findings in the affected cord segments consist of severe necrosis of both gray and white matter and the presence of abnormal intraparenchymal vessels with thickened hyalinized walls. In histologically documented cases, MRI showed longstanding cord enlargement, diffuse signal abnormality, and rimlike enhancement (Fig. 16-18).[73] Thus, the enhancement pattern is somewhat different from that of intramedullary tumors, and the prolonged presence of cord changes excludes acute transverse myelitis.

Arteriovenous malformations (AVMs) can cause both ischemic and hemorrhagic lesions. Enlarged intradural vessels appear as black serpiginous structures on MRI but may be quite easily overlooked because of concomitant artifacts from pulsation of the CSF and blood vessels. They cause characteristic filling defects on the myelogram (Fig. 16-19A). Again, selective angiography is needed to precisely display the vascular supply and hemodynamics of a malformation and to plan treatment (Fig. 16-19B). The nidus of blood vessels from an intramedullary AVM is easily seen on MRI.[74,75] Arteriovenous malformations may also present with hemorrhage that follows the same pattern and time course of signal abnormalities as described for intracerebral hematomas (Fig. 16-20). Intramedullary cavernous hemangiomas typically consist of a dark rim of hypointensity that surrounds a small central focus of high signal intensity on both T1- and T2-weighted images.[76] The areas of hypointensity reflect hemosiderin deposition in most instances and thus become most apparent on a gradient-echo sequence. In case of less typical appearance, other features, such as a personal or family history of cavernous hemangiomas or the presence of similar lesions in the brain, may help in the differential diagnosis.[77] Results of spinal angiographic studies are always normal.[78]

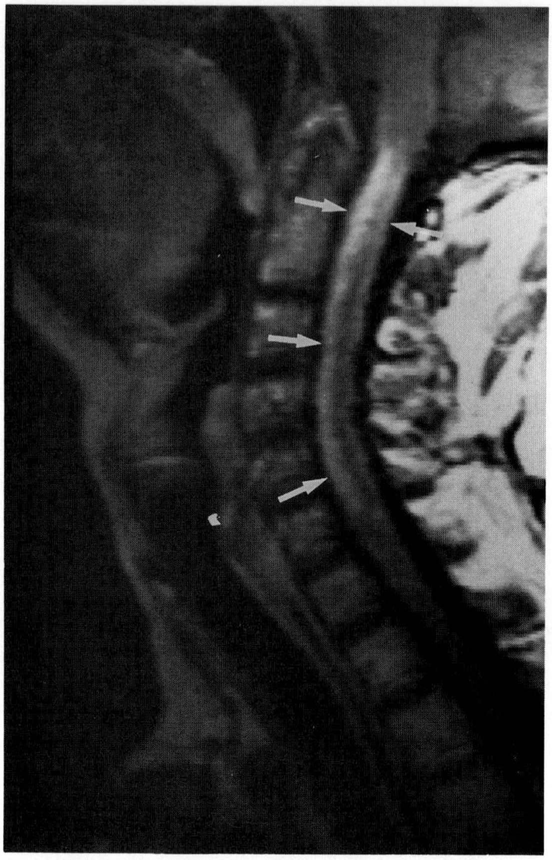

Figure 16-18
Rimlike enhancement (arrows) and cord swelling in a patient with pathologically proven subacute necrotizing myelopathy.

Neoplasms

Intramedullary tumors constitute about 5 percent of all spinal neoplasms in a general hospital setting. The vast majority are gliomas, with ependymomas and astrocytomas being most frequent. Ependymomas have a preponderance for the lower cord and filum terminale. Medulloblastoma, oligodendroglioma, ganglioneuroma, and neuroblastoma are rarely found. Mass effect with cord enlargement on T1-weighted images is seen in all of them. Signal abnormalities are variable, however. The solid portion of gliomas usually appears hyperintense on T2-weighted scans. Necrotic areas are further increased in signal intensity and are hypointense on T1-weighted scans. Bleeding into these pseudocysts may be identified from fluid levels and signal characteristics of blood products, such as methemoglobin or hemosiderin. Marked hypointensity at the tumor margins on both T1- and T2-weighted scans has been identified as a relatively firm pseudocapsule, which is suggestive of ependymoma (Fig. 16-21A,B).[79] Astrocytomas, in turn, more frequently undergo complete cystic degeneration.[80] Often, tumor extension cannot be estimated on MRI, since edema also appears bright on T2-weighted scans. In such instances, contrast mate-

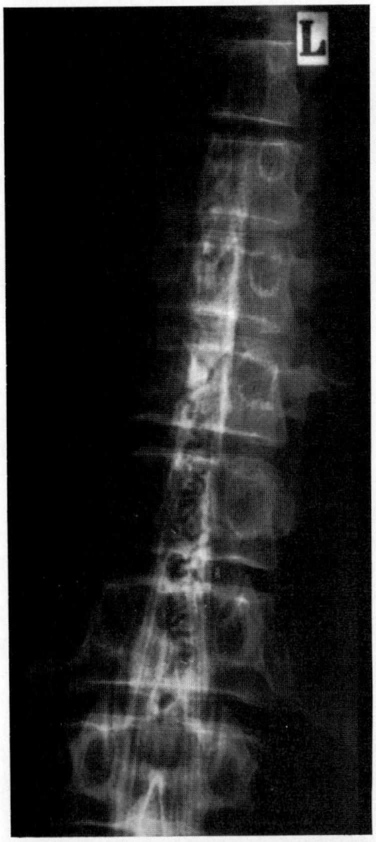

A

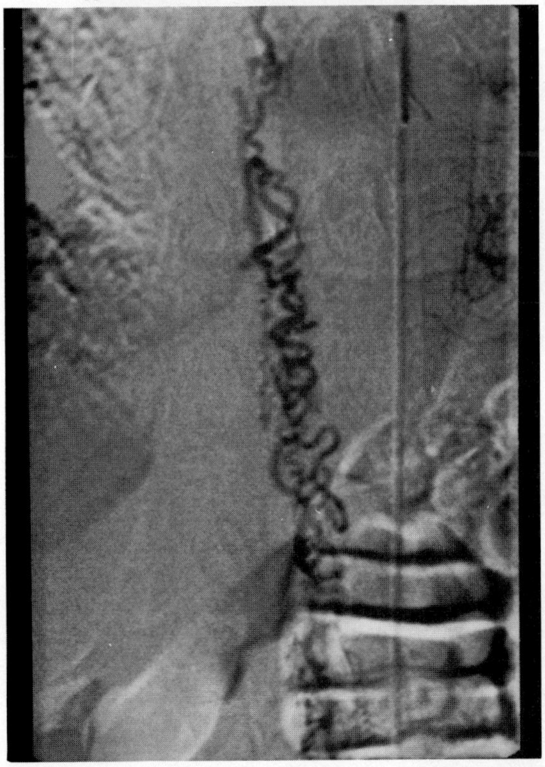

B

Figure 16-19
Intradural vascular malformation. **(A)** *Tortuous filling defects are seen on the myelogram.* **(B)** *Selective spinal angiography confirms an arteriovenous malformation. (Courtesy of Dr. Klein, Department of Radiology, Karl-Franzens University, Graz, Austria.)*

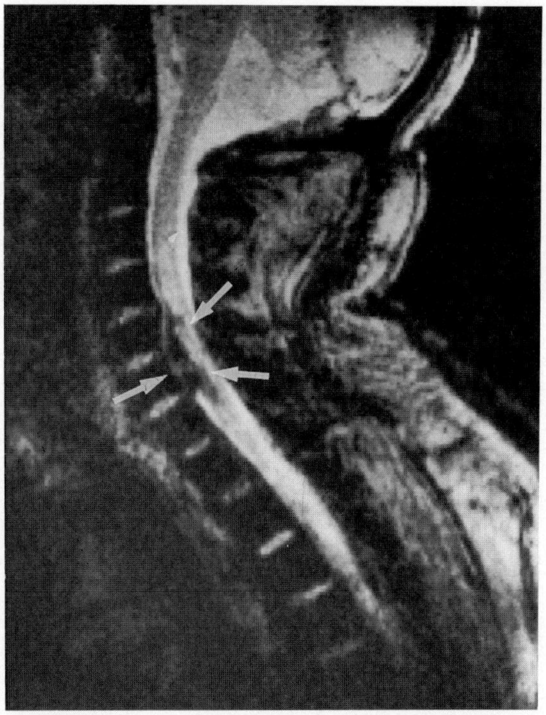

Figure 16-20
Acute bleeding from an arteriovenous malformation shown as focal hypointensity ventral to and extending into the cervical cord (arrows) on a gradient-echo T2-weighted sequence.

rial is helpful in localizing the tumor and should be given to every patient with a suspected neoplasm.[81] The areas of enhancement need not coincide with the actual boundaries of the infiltrative process. Unlike the brain, lack of contrast enhancement is unusual for gliomas of the spine. Even low-grade cord gliomas tend to show some enhancement (Fig. 16-22A,B). Contrast material also helps to evaluate the nature of associated cysts. Tumor cysts are generally surrounded by enhancement and located centrally. Cysts rostral and caudal of the tumor tend to be benign, which can be assumed from absence of contrast uptake in their walls.[82] Tumor spread over the CSF pathways can be also well recognized with injection of contrast material and occurs preferentially with medulloblastoma and ependymoma.[80]

Relatively typical MRI findings can be obtained in some nongliomatous tumors of the spinal cord. Hemangioblastomas are characterized by a cystic cavity with a markedly enhancing nodule in its wall. Despite a small size, they may produce extensive surrounding edema.[81] The signal characteristics of a lipoma have been described above (Fig. 16-5A,B).

Secondary seeding of metastasis into the spinal cord is a rare event. Lung and breast carcinoma are the two most commonly found primary tumors. The finding of a nodular enhancing mass helps to localize the lesion within the cord but is nonspecific (Fig. 16-23A,B).[83,84]

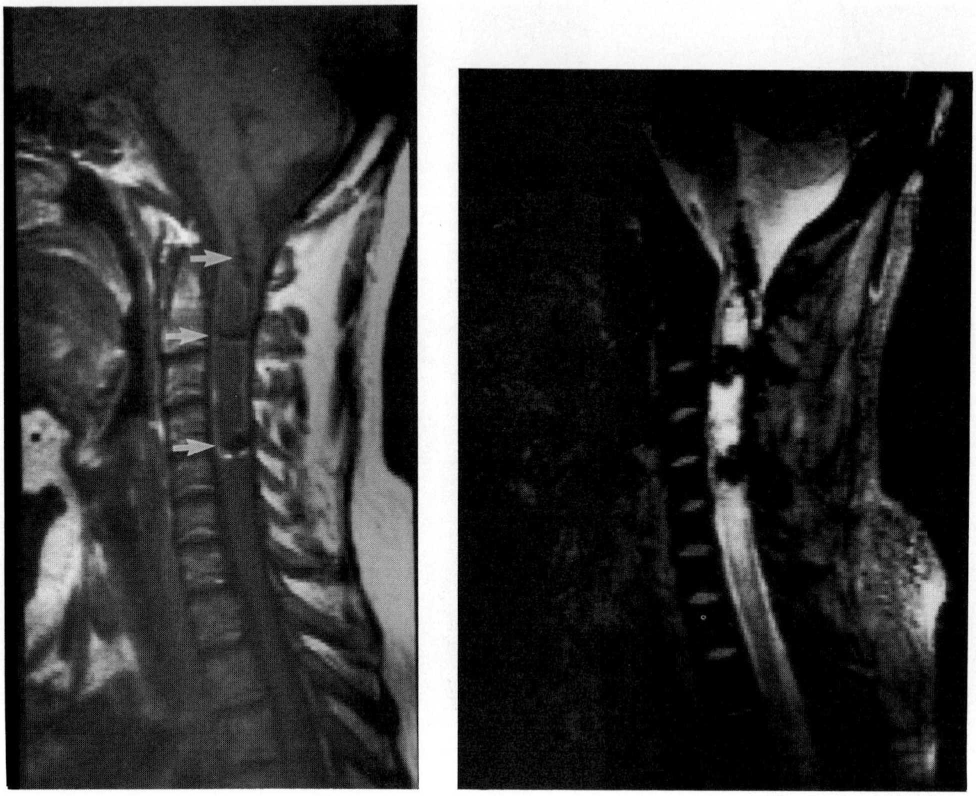

A B

Figure 16-21
Ependymoma. **(A)** *T1-weighted scan shows a longitudinal intramedullary lesion with minimal signal hypointensity. It is surrounded by marginal contrast enhancement (bright lines), and regions of more marked hypointensity are noted cranially, caudally, and in the upper third of the area with abnormal signal intensity (arrows).* **(B)** *These regions appear intensively hypointense and larger on the gradient T2-weighted sequence, suggesting hemosiderin. The remainder of the tumor and the adjacent edema are hyperintense.*

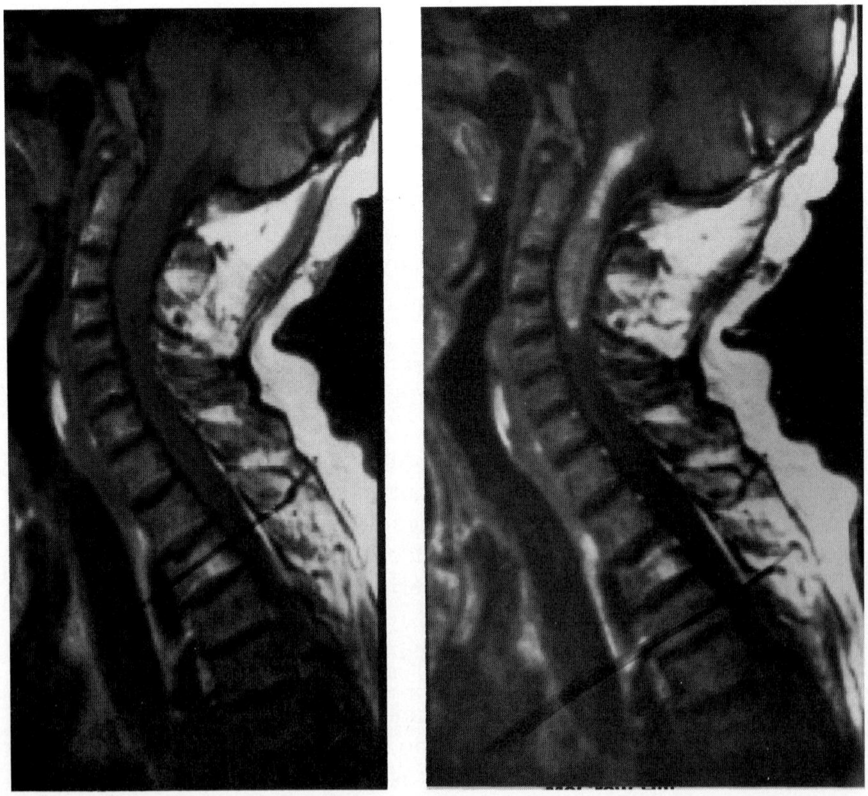

A B

Figure 16-22
Astrocytoma. **(A)** *Swelling of the cervical cord is seen; a focal lesion cannot be recognized.* **(B)** *Dense enhancement of a tumor that extends from the brainstem down to C4.*

and retrodental pannus in rheumatoid arthritis. *Spine* 22:1580–1583, 1997.
23. Takahashi M, Yamashita Y, Sakamoto Y, Kojima R: Chronic cervical cord compression: Clinical significance of increased signal intensity on MR images. *Radiology* 173:219–224, 1989.
24. Mehalic TF, Pezzuti RT, Applebaum BI: Magnetic resonance imaging and cervical spondylotic myelopathy. *Neurosurgery* 26:217–226, 1990.
25. Wada E, Ohmura M, Yonenobu K: Intramedullary changes of the spinal cord in cervical spondylotic myelopathy. *Spine* 20:2226–2232, 1995.
26. Kohno K, Kumon Y, Oka Y, et al: Evaluation of prognostic factors following expansive laminoplasty for cervical spinal stenotic myelopathy. *Surg Neurol* 48:237–245, 1997.
27. Quencer RM, Nunez D, Green BA: Controversies in imaging acute cervical spine trauma. *Am J Neuroradiol* 18:1866–1868, 1997.
28. Schaefer DM, Flanders AE, Osterholm JL, Northrup BE: Prognostic significance of magnetic resonance imaging in the acute phase of cervical spine injury. *J Neurosurg* 76:218–223, 1992.
29. Silberstein M, Tress BM, Hennessy O: Prediction of neurologic outcome in acute spinal cord injury: The role of CT and MR. *Am J Neuroradiol* 13:1597–1608, 1992.
30. Ramon S, Dominguez R, Ramirez L, et al: Clinical and magnetic resonance imaging correlation in acute spinal cord injury. *Spinal Cord* 35:664–673, 1997.
31. Wasenko JJ, Hochhauser L, Holsapple JW, et al: MR of post traumatic spinal cord lesions: Unexpected improvement of hemorrhagic lesions. *Clin Imaging* 21:246–251, 1997.
32. Quencer RM, Bunge RP, Egnor M, et al: Acute traumatic central cord syndrome. *Neuroradiology* 34:85–94, 1992.
33. Silberstein M, Tress BM, Hennessy O: Delayed neurologic deterioration in the patient with spinal trauma: Role of MR imaging. *Am J Neuroradiol* 13:1373–1381, 1992.
34. Curati WL, Kingsley DP, Kendall BE, Moseley IF: MRI in chronic spinal cord trauma. *Neuroradiology* 35:30–35, 1992.
35. Perrouin Verbe B, Lenne Aurier K, Robert R, et al: Post-traumatic syringomyelia and post-traumatic spinal canal stenosis: A direct relationship: Review of 75 patients with a spinal cord injury. *Spinal Cord* 36:137–143, 1998.
36. Jinkins JR, Reddy S, Leite CC, et al: MR of parenchymal spinal cord signal change as a sign of advancement in clinically progressive posttraumatic syringomyelia. *Am J Neuroradiol* 19:177–182, 1998.
37. Boukobza M, Guichard JP, Biossonet M, et al: Spinal epidural hematoma: Report of 11 cases and review of the literature. *Neuroradiology* 36:456–459, 1994.
38. Lovblad KO, Baumgartner RW, Zambaz BD, et al: Non-traumatic spinal epidural hematomas: MR features. *Acta Radiol* 38:8–13, 1997.
39. Hausman ON, Moseley IF: Idiopathic dural herniation of the thoracic spinal cord. *Neuroradiology* 503–510, 1996.
40. Gero B, Sze G, Sharif H: MR imaging of intradural inflammatory diseases of the spine. *Am J Neuroradiol* 12:1009–1019, 1991.
41. Tartaglino LM, Croul SE, Flanders AE, et al: Idiopathic acute transverse myelitis: MR imaging findings. *Radiology* 201:661–669, 1996.
42. Campi A, Filippi M, Comi G, Scotti G: Recurrent acute transverse myelopathy associated with anticardiolipin antibodies. *Am J Neuroradiol* 19:781–786, 1998.
43. Melhem ER, Wang H: Intramedullary spinal cord tuberculoma in a patient with AIDS. *Am J Neuroradiol* 13:986–988, 1992.
44. Nesbit GM, Miller GM, Baker HL Jr, et al: Spinal cord sarcoidosis: A new finding at MR imaging with Gd-DTPA enhancement. *Radiology* 173:839–843, 1989.
45. Junger SS, Stern BJ, Levine SR, et al: Intramedullary spinal sarcoidosis: Clinical and magnetic resonance imaging characteristics. *Neurology* 43:333–337, 1993.
46. Murphy KJ, Brunberg JA, Quint DJ, Kazanjian PH: Spinal cord infection: Myelitis and abscess formation. *Am J Neuroradiol* 19:341–348, 1998.
47. Poon TP, Tchertkoff V, Pares GF, et al: Spinal cord toxoplasma lesion in AIDS: MR findings. *J Comput Assist Tomogr* 16:817–819, 1992.
48. Quencer RM, Post MJ: Spinal cord lesions in patients with AIDS. *Neuroimaging Clin N Am* 7:359–373, 1997.
49. Moulignier A, Mikol J, Gonzalez Canali G, et al: AIDS-associated cytomegalovirus infection mimicking central nervous system tumors: A diagnostic challenge. *Clin Infect Dis* 22:626–631, 1996.
50. Leite CC, Jinkins JR, Escobar BE, et al: MR imaging of intramedullary and intradural-extramedullary spinal cysticercosis. *Am J Roentrenol* 169:1713–1717, 1997.
51. Dupuis MJ, Atroni S, Dooms GC, Gonsette RE: MR imaging of schistosomal myelitis. *Am J Neuroradiol* 11:782–783, 1990.
52. Kidd D, Thorpe JW, Thompson AJ, et al: Spinal cord MRI using multi-array coils and fast spin echo: II. Findings in multiple sclerosis. *Neurology* 43:2632–2637, 1993.
53. Tartaglino LM, Friedman DP, Flanders AE, et al: Multiple sclerosis in the spinal cord: MR appearance and correlation with clinical parameters. *Radiology* 195:725–732, 1995.
54. Fazekas F, Barkhof F, Filippi M: Unenhanced and enhanced magnetic resonance imaging in the diagnosis of multiple sclerosis. *J Neurol Neurosurg Psychiatry* 64(suppl):S2–S5, 1998.
55. Thorpe JW, Kidd D, Miller DH, et al: Spinal cord MRI using multi-array coils and fast spin-echo. I. Findings in normal controls. *Neurology* 43:2625–31, 1993.
56. Campi A, Filippi M, Comi G, et al: Acute transverse myelopathy: Spinal and cranial MR study with clinical follow-up. *Am J Neuroradiol* 16:115–123, 1995.
57. Papadopoulos A, Gouliamos A, Trakadas S, et al: MRI in the investigation of patients with myelopathy thought to be due to multiple sclerosis. *Neuroradiology* 37:384–387, 1995.
58. Fazekas F, Offenbacher H, Hartung HP: What is the role of ancillary investigations in establishing the diagnosis of multiple sclerosis? *Eur Neurol* 38:255–257, 1997.
59. O'Riordan JI, Thompson AJ, Kingsley DP, et al: The prognostic value of brain MRI in clinically isolated syndromes of the CNS: A 10-year follow-up. *Brain* 121:495–503, 1998.

60. Thorpe JW, Kidd D, Moseley IF, et al: Spinal MRI in patients with suspected multiple sclerosis and negative brain MRI. *Brain* 119:709–714, 1996.
61. Thorpe JW, Kidd D, Moseley IF, et al: Serial gadolinium-enhanced MRI of the brain and spinal cord in early relapsing-remitting multiple sclerosis. *Neurology* 46:372–378, 1996.
62. Caldemeyer KS, Smith RR, Harris TM, Edwards MK: MRI in acute disseminated encephalomyelitis. *Neuroradiology* 36:216–220, 1994.
63. Fazekas F, Schmidt R, Offenbacher H, Strasser-Fuchs S: MRI of neuromyelitis optica: Evidence for a distinct entity. *J Neurol Neurosurg Psychiatry* 57:1140–1142, 1994.
64. O'Riordan JI, Gallagher HL, Thompson AJ, et al: Clinical, CSF and MRI findings in Devic's neuromyelitis optica. *J Neurol Neurosurg Psychiatry* 60:382–387, 1996.
65. Wang PY, Shen WC, Jan JS: Magnetic resonance imaging in radiation myelopathy. *Am J Neuroradiol* 13:1049–1055, 1992.
66. Zweig G, Russell EJ: Radiation myelopathy of the cervical spinal cord: MR findings. *Am J Neuroradiol* 11:1188–1190, 1990.
67. Chouchair AK: Myelopathies in the cancer patient: Incidence, presentation, diagnosis and management. *Oncology* 5:25–37, 1991.
68. Mawad ME, Rivera V, Crawford S, et al: Spinal cord ischemia after resection of thoracoabdominal aortic aneurysms: MR findings in 24 patients. *Am J Neuroradiol* 11:987–991, 1990.
69. Friedman DP, Flanders AE: Enhancement of gray matter in anterior spinal infarction. *Am J Neuroradiol* 13:983–985, 1992.
70. Yuh WT, Marsh EE III, Wang AK, et al: MR imaging of spinal cord and vertebral body infarction. *Am J Neuroradiol* 13:145–154, 1992.
71. Larsson EM, Desai P, Hardin CW, et al: Venous infarction of the spinal cord resulting from dural arteriovenous fistula: MR imaging findings. *Am J Neuroradiol* 12:739–743, 1991.
72. Huffmann BC, Gilsbach JM, Thron A: Spinal dural arteriovenous fistulas: A plea for neurosurgical treatment. *Acta Neurochirurg* 135:44–51, 1995.
73. Mirich DR, Kucharczyk W, Keller MA, Deck J: Subacute necrotizing myelopathy: MR imaging in four pathologically proved cases. *Am J Neuroradiol* 12:1077–1083, 1991.
74. Dormont D, Gelbert F, Assouline E, et al: MR imaging of spinal cord arteriovenous malformations at 0.5 T: Study of 34 cases. *Am J Neuroradiol* 9:833–838, 1988.
75. Hojer C, Bewermeyer H, Assheuer J, et al: Diagnosis of spinal arteriovenous malformations by MRI at 1.0 T. *Clin Imaging* 20:79–84, 1996.
76. Fontaine S, Melanson D, Cosgrove R, Bertrand G: Cavernous hemangiomas of the spinal cord: MR imaging. *Radiology* 166:839–842, 1988.
77. Turjman F, Joly D, Monnet O, et al: MRI of intramedullary cavernous hemangiomas. *Neuroradiology* 37:297–302, 1995.
78. Canavero S, Pagni CA, Duca S, Bradac GB: Spinal intramedullary cavernous angiomas: A literature meta-analysis. *Surg Neurol* 41:381–388, 1994.
79. Nemoto Y, Inoue Y, Tashiro T, et al: Intramedullary spinal cord tumors: Significance of associated hemorrhage at MR imaging. *Radiology* 182:793–796, 1992.
80. Li MH, Holtas S: MR imaging of spinal intramedullary tumors. *Acta Radiol* 32:505–513, 1991.
81. Sze G, Stimac GK, Bartlett C, et al: Multicenter study of gadopentetate dimeglumine as an MR contrast agent: Evaluation in patients with spinal tumors. *Am J Neuroradiol* 11:967–974, 1990.
82. Chamberlain MC, Sandy AD, Press GA: Spinal cord tumours: Gadolinium-DTPA-enhanced MR imaging. *Neuroradiology* 33:469–474, 1991.
83. Fredericks RK, Elster A, Walker FO: Gadolinium-enhanced MRI: A superior technique for the diagnosis of intraspinal metastasis. *Neurology* 39:734–736, 1989.
84. Schiff D, O'Neill BP: Intramedullary spinal cord metastasis: Clinical features and treatment outcome. *Neurology* 47:906–912, 1996.
85. Small JA, Sheridan PH: Research priorities for syringomyelia: A National Institute of Neurological Disorders and Stroke workshop summary. *Neurology* 46:577–582, 1996.
86. Stovner LJ, Rinck P: Syringomyelia in Chiari malformation: Relation to extent of cerebellar tissue herniation. *Neurosurgery* 31:913–917, 1992.
87. Amer TA, el Shmam OM: Chiari malformation type I: A new MRI classification. *Magn Reson Imaging* 15:397–403, 1997.
88. Sherman JL, Barkovich AJ, Citrin CM: The MR appearance of syringomyelia: New observations. *Am J Neuroradiol* 7:985–995, 1986.
89. Mallucci CL, Stacey RJ, Miles JB, Williams B: Idiopathic syringomyelia and the importance of arachnoid webs, pouches and cysts. *Br J Neurosurg* 11:306–309, 1997.
90. Wessel K, Schroth G, Diener HC, et al: Significance of MRI-confirmed atrophy of the cranial spinal cord in Friedreich's ataxia. *Eur Arch Psychiatry Neurol Sci* 238:225–230, 1989.
91. Okumura R, Asato R, Shimada T, et al: Degeneration of the posterior columns of the spinal cord: Postmortem MRI and histopathology. *J Comput Assist Tomogr* 16:865–867, 1992.
92. Thorpe JW, Moseley IF, Hawkes CH, et al: Brain and spinal cord MRI in motor neuron disease. *J Neurol Neurosurg Psychiatry* 61:314–317, 1996.
93. Krabbe K, Nielsen JE, Fallentin E, et al: MRI of autosomal pure spastic paraplegia. *Neuroradiology* 39:724–727, 1997.
94. Waragai M, Takaya Y, Hayashi M: Serial MRI findings of chronic idiopathic ataxic neuropathy. *J Neurol Sci* 151:93–95, 1997.
95. Krol G, Sze G, Malkin M, Walker R: MR of cranial and spinal meningeal carcinomatosis: Comparison with CT and myelography. *Am J Radiol* 151:583–588, 1988.
96. Lim V, Sobel DF, Zyroff J: Spinal cord pial metastases: MR imaging with gadopentetate dimeglumine. *Am J Neuroradiol* 11:975–982, 1990.
97. Offenbacher H, Fazekas F, Reisecker F, et al: Superficial siderosis of the spinal cord: A rare cause of myelopathy diagnosed by MRI. *Neurology* 41:1987–1989, 1991.
98. Offenbacher H, Fazekas F, Schmidt R, et al: Superficial siderosis of the central nervous system: MRI findings and clinical significance. *Neuroradiology* 38:51–56, 1996.

CHAPTER 17

IMAGING MULTIPLE SCLEROSIS

Jack H. Simon
Lawrence Jacobs

Multiple sclerosis (MS) is an inflammatory demyelinating disease of the central nervous system (CNS) most frequently characterized by relapses and remissions of neurologic symptoms and signs. With repeated episodes over time, the remissions of neurologic deficits become less complete and the enduring deficits, with subsequent accumulation of physical disability, become more severe. After variable periods of time, the disease often enters a chronic-progressive stage, in which there is progressive worsening of neurologic signs without appreciable relapses and remissions.

Multiple sclerosis typically is a disease of young people, the usual age of onset being between 18 and 35 years. Life expectancy after disease onset is stated to be only modestly decreased, with some 75 percent of patients surviving 25 years.[1] However, disability during that period of time may become severe. The results of several series are variable, but 5 years after onset, about 20 percent of these patients are unable to walk, and within 10 years this number doubles.[1] Recent epidemiologic studies indicate that there are 250,000 to 300,000 MS patients in the United States and approximately 200 new cases are diagnosed each week.[2] The cost of medical care related to this disease, including rehabilitation and loss of productivity, is estimated to be in excess of 2.5 billion dollars annually.

Although there is no cure for MS, several recent treatments have been shown to modify the natural course of the relapsing-remitting disease. The β-interferons 1a[3] and 1b[4] and copolymer I[5] have received regulatory approval in the United States for treatment of relapsing MS. Definitive clinical trials have demonstrated that individual agents decrease the clinical relapse rate[3–5] and the progression of physical disability.[3,6] Based on magnetic resonance imaging (MRI), the β-interferons decrease both acute activity in the brain[3,6–10] and accumulation of lesions over time.[7,8,10,11] Other agents, at various stages of development and testing, also have been shown through MRI measurements of activity to have a promising impact on rate of lesion development.[12,13]

The diagnosis of MS ultimately depends on the clinical history and physical findings. However, the standard diagnostic criteria—detection of multiple lesions disseminated in the CNS (in space) and dissemination in time—may be difficult to achieve on a clinical basis. Correlation of lesions seen at autopsy with symptoms and signs that occurred during life is often impossible, since many lesions identified at autopsy are clinically silent. Moreover, there have been well-documented necropsy studies in which typical MS lesions were identified at autopsy in patients who had not experienced any neurologic deficit during their lifetimes and who had died from nonneurologic causes.[14,15]

Various laboratory tests have been developed that have helped to narrow the clinical differential diagnosis and increase diagnostic accuracy during life. Neuroimaging techniques have played a major role in that regard. In the mid-1970s, computerized tomography (CT) and myelography/CT became extremely helpful in excluding pathologic conditions that could mimic MS, such as neoplastic, vascular, or degenerative disease. Cerebral CT also sometimes demonstrated typical anatomic distributions, dissemination of disease in space, and mixed enhancement patterns, suggesting dissemination in time. As a result, CT improved one's ability to make an early diagnosis of MS.

The introduction of MRI into the clinical environment in the mid-1980s had a major impact on the diagnosis of MS patients. Magnetic resonance imaging detects the changes in water content that accompany CNS disease and is extremely sensitive in recognizing MS lesions at early stages, when they are often missed by other techniques. Magnetic resonance imaging has provided more specificity in diagnosis and more certain exclusion of other pathologic processes than any other of the previously used neuroimaging techniques singly or combined. Moreover, MRI has revealed that MS is a dynamic disease in which CNS lesions often evolve and resolve undetected by the clinical examination. Acute activity in relapsing MS can be detected about 4 to 10 times more frequently by MRI than by clinical symptoms and signs.[16–22]

This chapter outlines the major pathologic processes of the MS lesion that affect observations made by CT and MRI. It also considers the neuroimaging evaluation in terms of characteristic lesion distributions and differential diagnosis, and the role of MRI in evaluating new treatments, prognosis, and an individual's response to treatment. Finally, it discusses some important new technologies and their potential for improving diagnosis and advancing the understanding of the basic pathophysiology of MS.

NATURAL HISTORY OF MS BASED ON IMAGING

For practical purposes, MS lesion evolution in CNS tissue can be divided into three stages by MRI: (1) the acute inflammatory stage, characterized by a gadolinium-chelate- (or gadolinium) enhancing lesion that is also hyperintense on T2-weighted images (a T2 lesion); (2) a subacute stage, during which lesion enhancement eventually decreases and disappears and the T2 hyperintense area decreases but does not disappear; and (3) a chronic stage, during which relatively stable T2 lesions can be categorized by their variable degree of destructive changes.

Acute MS Lesions

Acute MS lesions in relapsing and secondary progressive MS are primarily inflammatory, with characteristic features including a mononuclear infiltrate, perivascular cuffing, and edema (Fig. 17-1, Plates 30 and 31).[23,24] The inflammatory infiltrate of the early MS lesion occurs along with a local disturbance in the blood-brain barrier, which is detected on MRI by gadolinium enhancement on T1-weighted images (Fig. 17-2)[25,26] or on CT imaging by using iodinated contrast agents.[27,28] It is fortunate that disruption of the blood-brain barrier can be readily imaged, since gadolinium enhancement provides a convenient marker for many of the early events in the inflammatory cascade[29–31] that ultimately leads to local demyelination and other tissue damage characteristic of MS. There is good evidence for a temporal correlation between the inflammatory lesion of MS and gadolinium enhancement. In one series,[26] 29 of 29 histologically proven active MS lesions could be shown as enhancing on prior imaging studies, while none of four inactive lesions enhanced. Macrophage infiltration was seen in 27 of 29 enhancing lesions. Gadolinium enhancement is a transient phenomenon and as such is a good marker for active (acute and early subacute) disease. Most lesions enhance for periods of 2 to 4 weeks, but enhancement can vary from less than 1 week to as long as 16 weeks.[19,32] Higher doses of CT[27,28] or MRI contrast material (triple dose) increase the detection of lesions.[33–35] While these enhancement patterns are typical of relapsing and secondary progressive MS, in primary progressive MS inflammation in individual lesions may be less marked, and correspondingly enhancement is also less commonly observed.[32,34,36]

In addition to onset of gadolinium enhancement in acute MS lesions, there is concurrent development of regional T2 hyperintensity overlapping the gadolinium-enhancing lesion and often extending beyond the borders of the gadolinium-enhancing lesion (Figs. 17-2 and

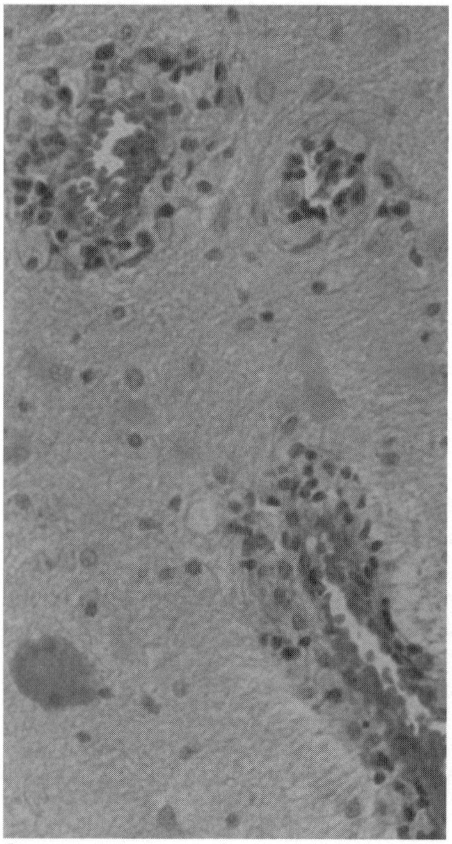

A

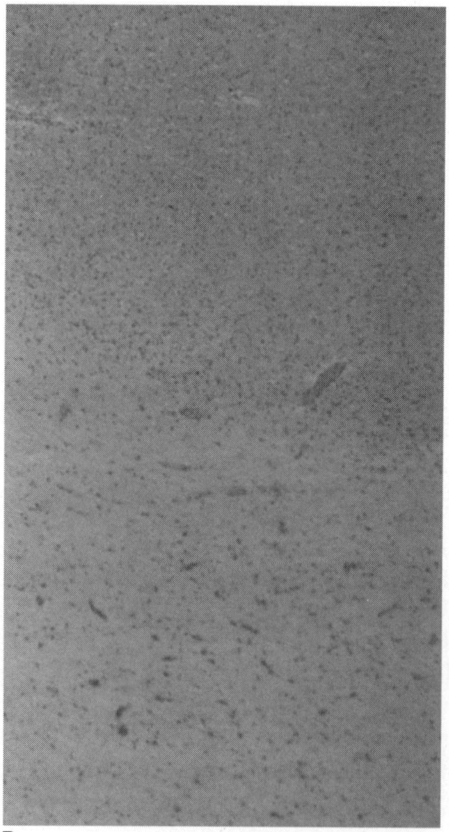

B

Figure 17-1 (Plates 30 and 31) *Photomicrographs of MS lesions.* **(A)** *Acute lesion showing round-cell infiltration surrounding venules. Magnification: 170×.* **(B)** *Chronic lesion at bottom appears pale compared with normal parenchyma at top because of demyelination and gliosis. Magnification: 40×. (Courtesy of Dr. P. Ostrow, Department of Pathology, Buffalo General Hospital, SUNY, Buffalo, NY.)*

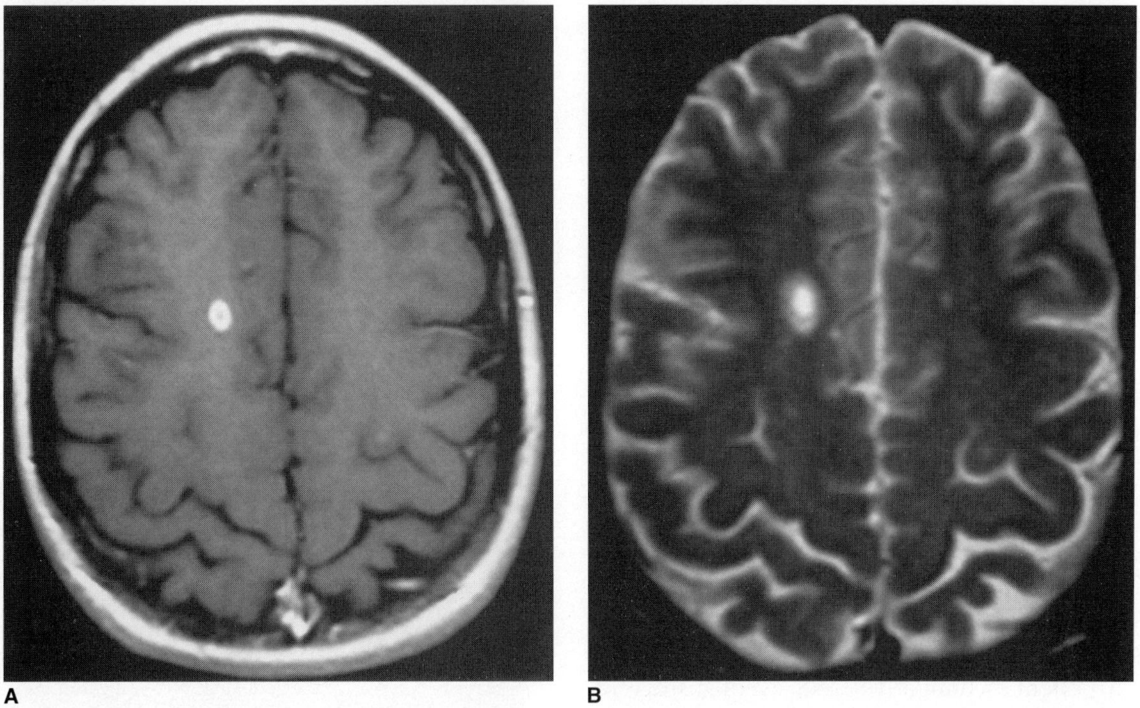

Figure 17-2
Acute enhancing MS lesion. **(A)** *The acute ring-enhancing MS lesion also shows a ring on* **(B)** *the T2-weighted image. The outer ring on the T2-weighted image is probably from edema, since it extends beyond the margin of the enhancing ring.*

17-3). In acute MS lesions, this so-called T2 lesion is believed to result from increased lesion fluid content with long T2 (more free water either in the intercellular spaces or between myelin lamellae) and edema surrounding the inflammatory lesion. These T2 lesions are relatively nonspecific. They represent lesions of varying severity and have signal intensity characteristics similar to those of other inflammatory, infectious, traumatic,

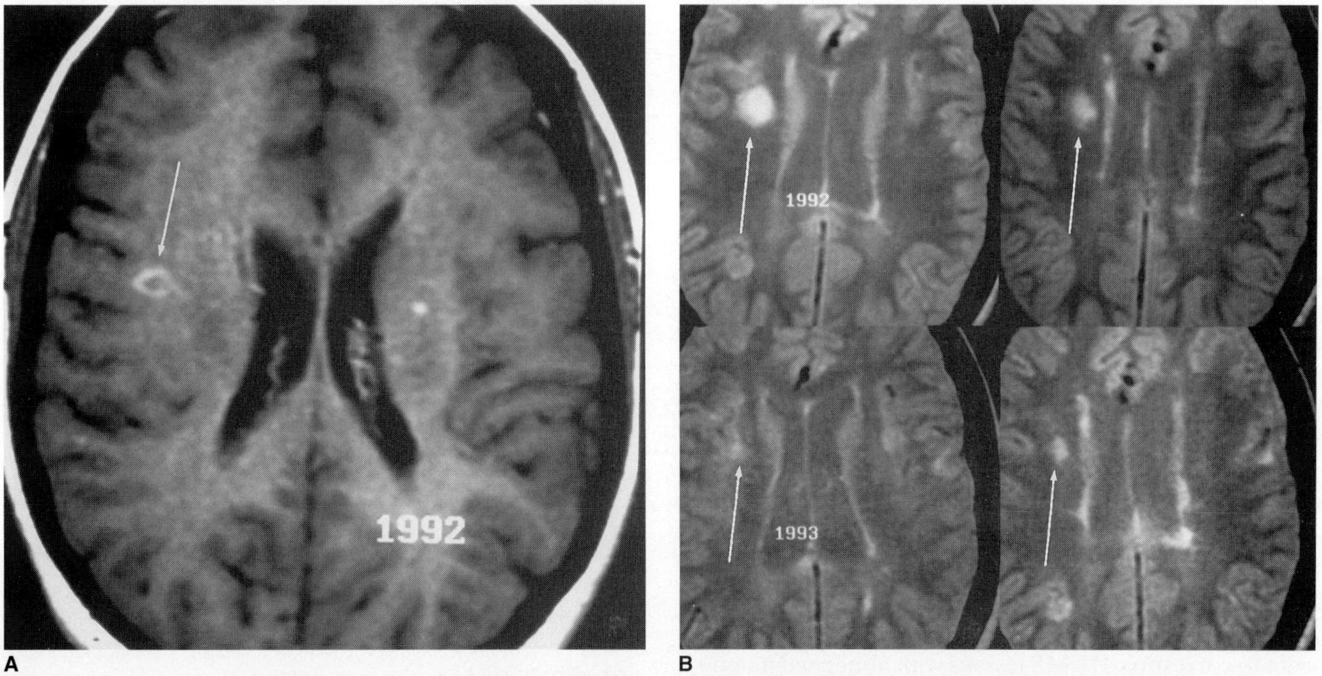

Figure 17-3
Natural history of individual MS lesion. **(A)** *A large right-sided acute enhancing lesion is seen on the T1-weighted series (arrow).* **(B)** *Consecutive images (top images) show the corresponding acute T2-hyperintense lesion (arrow). One year later (bottom images), the T2-hyperintense lesion has shrunk to less than one-fourth its initial volume (arrow).*

and neoplastic lesions in the CNS. Acute MS lesions are hypointense or isointense to normal white matter on T1-weighted images.

Early Subacute Stage

As the gadolinium enhancement in individual lesions decreases over a period of weeks,[37,38] the T2 hyperintense area also contracts.[39–41] In almost all cases with high-field imaging, these lesions regress to leave a smaller residual, or footprint, lesion about one-third to one-half its original size in most cases.[41] This T2 residual (Fig. 17-3) typically remains stable over a period of years (Fig. 17-4). The period of regression of the acute inflammatory lesion seen by MRI corresponds temporally to return to a normal or near-normal blood-brain barrier (return of endothelial tight-junction integrity), regression of edema and exudate, and conversion from the early inflammatory to the late inflammatory cellular milieu (macrophages). The residual T2 hyperintense lesions are the most popular of several potential measurements of a patient's cumulative CNS event history in phase III (definitive) clinical trials and natural history studies.[7,10,11,42]

Most hypointense T1 lesions evolve to isointensity with normal white matter over a period of weeks to months, while a subset of these lesions, for reasons that are not yet understood, evolve to permanent hypointensity on T1-weighted imaging sequences (Fig.17-5). A presumably unrelated observation is the appearance of a T1 hyperintense periphery in some MS lesions that may last for months (Fig. 17-6).

Chronic MS Lesions

Chronic MS lesions appear as focal or confluent regions of elevated signal intensity on T2-weighted MRIs (Fig. 17-4). These lesions do not appear to enhance unless there is superimposed new acute or recurrent activity, a phenomenon that is observed in a small fraction of lesions when followed by high-frequency (e.g., monthly) serial MRI.[19,43] The relative uniformity in appearance and signal characteristics of chronic MS lesions occurs in spite of variable underlying histopathologic conditions ranging from nearly normal to zones of myelin loss and reactive astrogliosis to the most severe lesions, characterized by axonal loss and severe astrogliosis.[44]

In contrast to the appearance by T2-weighted imaging, on T1-weighted imaging, chronic lesions separate into two groups and are either isointense to normal white matter or, in a smaller percentage of cases, hypointense (lower signal) to normal white matter (Fig. 17-5). The hypointense lesions, also now known as T1 holes,[45,46] seem to correspond to MS lesions with abnormal magnetization transfer ratios.[47] Preliminary studies suggest that these T1 holes do in fact correspond to regions of severe tissue destruction.[48]

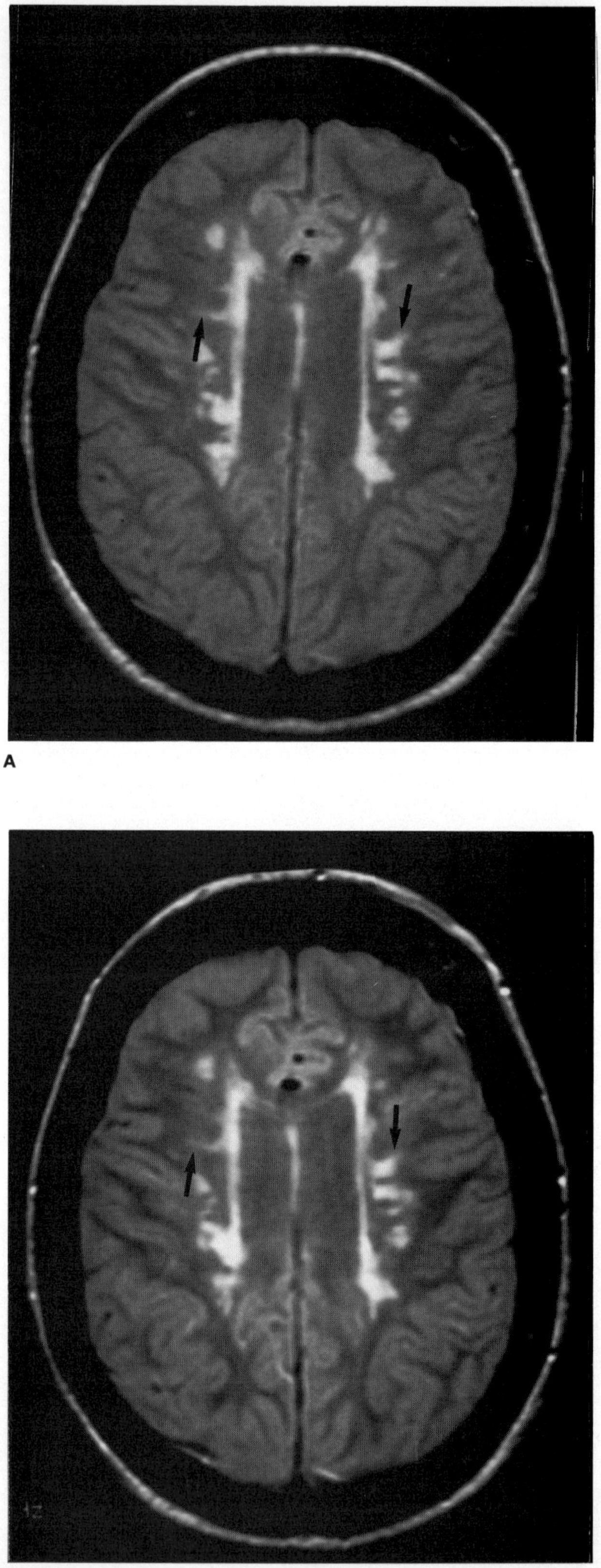

A

B

Figure 17-4
Stable T2-hyperintense lesions. **(A)** *Intermediate T2-weighted image (TR 2000/TE 30) from a 30-year-old MS patient shows multiple white matter ovoid lesions extending at right angles from the ventricular surface (arrows).* **(B)** *A study 1 year later shows that the majority of these periventricular lesions are stable.*

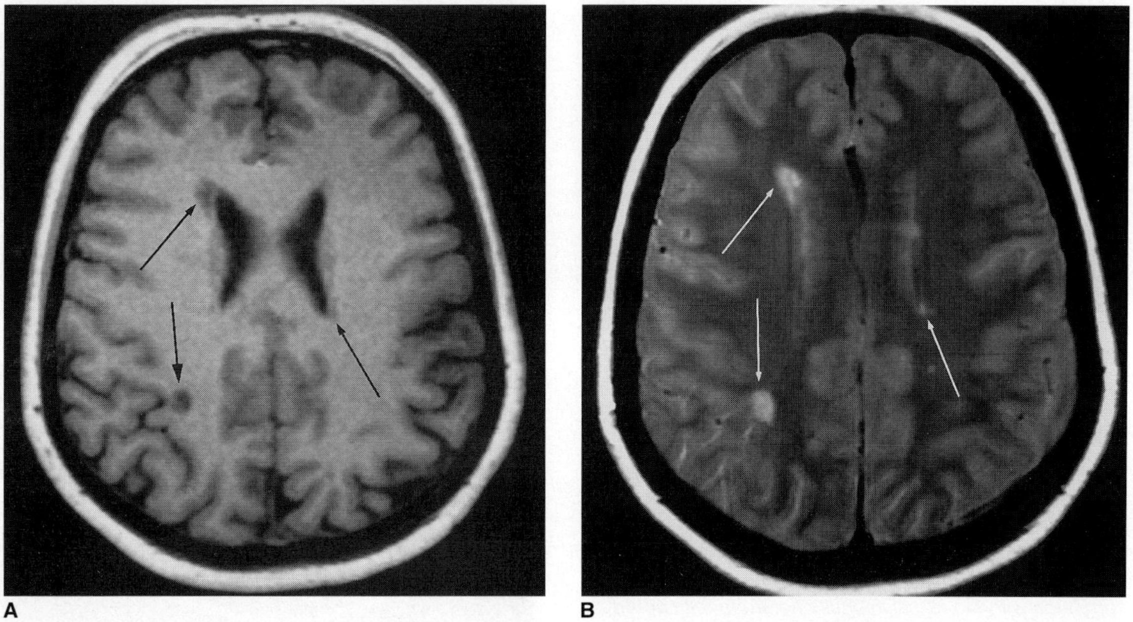

Figure 17-5
T1-hypointense lesions (T1 holes). **(A)** *Several focal hypointense lesions are seen on the T1-weighted series (arrows). These correspond to several of* **(B)** *the T2-hyperintense lesions. Many T2-hyperintense lesions have no appreciable T1-hypointense component (not shown). The areas of hypointensity on T1-weighted series are likely to be from a subset of lesions with severe disruption.*

While the major areas of involvement suggested by T2 hyperintensity are stable from month to month and in many cases over a period of years (Fig. 17-4), the natural history of the disease appears to be one of gradual accumulation of T2-hyperintense lesions by the addition of new T2 lesions and expansion of preexisting lesions. This expansion process over long intervals (years) outweighs the contraction of lesion area and the lesion volume oscillation that occur over months after individual acute events.[49] Based on population data from treatment trials in patients with relapsing MS, the expected increment in T2-lesion area or volume is on the order of 5 to 12 percent per year,[7,11] or a median of 0.45 to 0.7 mL/year.[7] Variation in lesion increment in individuals can be far greater, particularly in patients with only a few lesions, in whom increases on the order of 100 percent are not uncommon, and similarly large volume decreases may occur as acute lesions involute.

APPEARANCE OF MS BY CT AND MRI

Computerized Tomography

The most common abnormalities seen by brain CT consist of one or more of the following: (1) low-density white matter lesions, (2) ventriculomegaly and/or (3) cerebral cortical atrophy, (4) lesion enhancement, and, more rarely, (5) mass lesions.

Focal, hypodense lesions on brain CT have been reported in about 25 to 50 percent of MS patients (Fig. 17-7).[50,51] These lesions are typically located in the periventricular regions. Administration of intravenous contrast material may result in enhancement of acute white matter lesions, reflecting disruption of the blood-brain barrier, and thus provide physiologic as well as anatomic information about the lesion.[27,28,40,50] Enhanced CT studies, particularly those utilizing higher doses of CT contrast material,[27,28,40] were the first to convincingly demonstrate lesions fluctuating in size, location, and extent over time. However, CT is no longer utilized as a diagnostic test for MS because of its limited capacity for lesion detection and characterization compared to MRI (Fig. 17-8).

Magnetic Resonance Imaging

Magnetic resonance imaging has completely replaced CT in the assessment of MS patients because of its sensitivity to small changes in water concentration and water relaxation processes (the T1 and T2 relaxation rates), which are disturbed in acute and chronic MS lesions. Magnetic resonance imaging is not affected by dense bone-induced artifacts characteristic of CT, which, combined with its increased contrast resolution and multiplanar capabilities, makes it much more valuable than CT for assessing the brainstem.

Lesions in the brain are seen in about 85 to 95 percent of MS cases by MRI in most series, depending primarily on the imaging and diagnostic criteria used in each re-

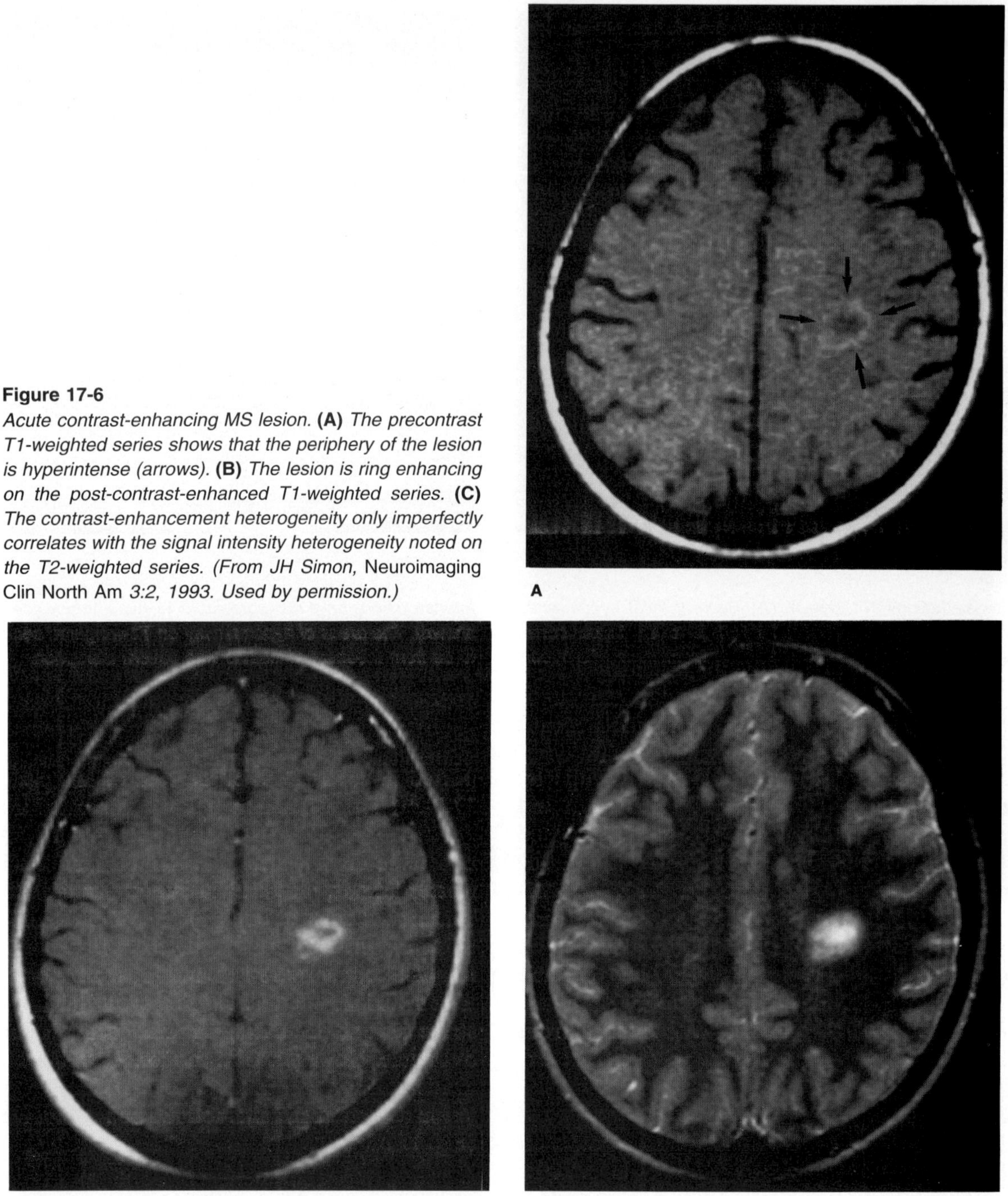

A

B

C

Figure 17-6
Acute contrast-enhancing MS lesion. **(A)** *The precontrast T1-weighted series shows that the periphery of the lesion is hyperintense (arrows).* **(B)** *The lesion is ring enhancing on the post-contrast-enhanced T1-weighted series.* **(C)** *The contrast-enhancement heterogeneity only imperfectly correlates with the signal intensity heterogeneity noted on the T2-weighted series. (From JH Simon,* Neuroimaging Clin North Am *3:2, 1993. Used by permission.)*

port. Standardized MRI diagnostic criteria have been proposed to improve the diagnosis of MS.[52–56] These criteria attempt to balance specificity and sensitivity[56] and have been tested primarily in research settings. Using strict Poser criteria[57] and only clinical features to classify cases, one or more focal brain lesions were seen in 113/114 (99 percent) of the cases in one series[58] and 197/200 (98.5 percent) in a second series,[59] suggesting that only about 1 percent of patients with well-established MS are likely to have completely normal brain MRI studies.[59]

General Lesion Features in the Brain

Typically, lesions start out as discrete, with well-defined margins. A frequently observed MS lesion pattern is the ovoid lesion that extends at right angles from the ventricular surface and occurs in as many as 86 percent

an individual patient's response to therapy. The success of these approaches may be partly due to the fact that, despite fluctuation of lesion numbers from week to week and month to month within individuals,[91] overall there is some stability in the enhancing lesion pattern, with some patients showing sustained periods of little or no activity (zero enhancing lesions) and others seeming to remain active with one or more lesions.[97] Recent large MRI studies confirm stability of activity patterns over periods from 6 months[98] to 1 to 2 years.[99]

In an individual patient evaluated by a clinical MRI study, a conservative appraisal could be that the observation of one or more enhancing lesions indicates that the patient shows evidence of active, inflammatory disease. However, because of the intraindividual variation in enhancing lesions over time, one observation does not exclude a significant decrease in activity, for example, through successful therapeutic intervention, nor does it exclude an increase. For patients with primary progressive MS, enhancing lesions in the brain are expected to be rare.[36]

There is no correlation between lesion load on T2-weighted images and the degree of clinical disability in individual MS patients. As a result, it is not uncommon to observe an MS patient in the clinic with a large T2 lesion volume who is only minimally disabled and another patient with minimal T2 lesions of the brain or spinal cord who is severely disabled. This MRI-disability discrepancy has also been seen in large study populations, where the correlation between T2 lesion load and expanded disability status scale (EDSS) was typically in the range of $r = 0.2$ to 0.3 in relapsing MS.[7,11,100,101] The MRI-disability discrepancy is most likely multifactorial: (1) T2 lesions are the consequence of a wide range of pathologic conditions (e.g., from edema to axonal loss); (2) there are imperfections in disability rating scales used in MS;[102] and (3) disability changes may be absent or limited during the short observation periods (1 to 3 years) typical of most large MS series. One of the frequently cited problems with the EDSS is its emphasis on ambulation and not upper-extremity function. Nevertheless, recent studies show that T2 lesion involvement in the spinal cord, where ambulation problems are expected, also correlates poorly with EDSS.[86] Despite the current controversy surrounding the discrepancy between T2 lesion load and disability and the failure of T2 lesions to meet the conservative definition of a surrogate marker of the disease,[102] it seems reasonable to suggest that an increase in the volume or number of T2 lesions over time reflects an increasing accumulation of MS lesions in the CNS and that stabilization of accumulation is a straightforward, important goal of a therapeutic intervention.

Another way of measuring the impact of MS on the brain is to determine its effect on cognitive function. Cognitive impairment is estimated to occur in about 43 percent of MS patients.[103] Several studies suggest that there is a modest correlation between abnormalities in neuropsychological test scores and MRI-based T2 lesion load scores and other MRI measures, such as cerebral atrophy.[103–108] Studies by Rao et al[104] suggest that there may be a critical threshold in the amount of pathology required to produce cognitive dysfunction. In one study,[104] 83 percent of MS patients with greater than 30 cm^2 lesion area were cognitively impaired, while only 22 percent with less than 30 cm^2 load were impaired. Change in lesion load may also correlate with change in information-processing speed, attention, and cognitive status.[108] The location of lesions may also predict, to some extent, the type of neuropsychological dysfunction seen in individuals.

Finally, several pilot and retrospective studies suggest that the gap between disability and quantitative MRI assessments can be narrowed if more tissue-specific MRI measures are utilized. Possible measures include the T1-hypointense lesion volume,[45,46,109] and change in T1-hypointense lesion volume,[45,46] change in new or enhancing lesions,[110] measures based on magnetization transfer indexes,[111,112] or *N*-acetylaspartate content.[113,114] In addition, MRI-based atrophy measurements may contribute to the understanding of disability in MS. For example, in one study,[115] a relatively high negative correlation ($r = -0.7$) was found for cross-sectional area of the spinal cord at the second cervical level and disability.

APPEARANCE OF EARLY MS

Very little is known about the earliest appearance of MS in the CNS. The best approximation to early disease comes from MRI studies in patients presenting with their first neurologic symptom resembling demyelination. From this group of patients, those with typical periventricular T2-hyperintense lesions are more likely to develop a second clinical event in 2 to 5 years, thereby meeting the criteria for a diagnosis of clinically definite MS.[116–120] Typical monosymptomatic presentations include spinal cord (partial transverse myelitis) and brainstem syndromes and optic neuritis. The number of such patients with T2 lesions at presentation depends on imaging criteria and scan quality but varies from about 25 to 60 percent.[116–117] Based on the largest published prospective trial, in patients presenting with monosymptomatic optic neuritis, about 25 percent have three or more white matter lesions by MRI.[119] In our experience, the lesions in the brain at first presentation are not distinguishable from those seen in relapsing or progressive MS, although the volume of lesion on average is about one-tenth to one-fifteenth that seen for modestly disabling relapsing MS.

Early-onset MS in the pediatric population has also been described[121] and is not known to show distinguishing MRI features. Since postinfectious and postvaccination acute disseminated encephalomyelitis occurs in children and may mimic MS, follow-up studies may be required to establish the correct diagnosis.

MR AS A PROGNOSTIC TEST IN MS

Although it is well accepted that monosymptomatic syndromes are often the first symptoms of MS, the strength of this relationship has been controversial. For example, for optic neuritis as a presenting symptom, 31 studies with follow-up for variable periods of time showed a conversion rate to clinically definite MS ranging from as low as 13 to as high as 88 percent.[122] More recent studies suggest that for all three monosymptomatic presentations the majority of patients (about two-thirds) are unlikely to develop clinical MS within a follow-up period of about 5 years. It has also become clear that simple MRI criteria (disseminated silent lesions) can be used to identify patients at higher risk of developing MS.[116–120]

The MRI factors that seem to increase the risk of MS in this first-onset group include (1) greater number or volume of T2 lesions,[52–56,116,117,119,120] (2) enhancing lesions,[55,56] (3) more typical MS patterns, including cerebellar or brainstem lesions,[52,53] (4) lesions greater than 6 mm in diameter,[52,53] and (5) juxtacortical lesions.[56]

In general, patients with no lesions in the brain (excluding the index lesion of optic nerve or brainstem in those presentations) at first presentation are at low but not zero risk of a subsequent attack and a diagnosis of clinically definite MS. Multiple relatively small studies with variable follow-up between 11 and 64 months suggested a risk on the order of 4 percent in this group. However, in the 5-year follow-up data from the Optic Neuritis Treatment Trial, the risk of clinically definite MS was greater, at 16 percent, in 202 patients without brain MRI lesions, the same risk as reported recently by Jacobs et al.[120]

For patients with an abnormal MRI study, the risk of MS has been reported to vary from 23 to 93 percent and averaged 44 percent in one summary report.[22] In the 5-year follow-up report from the optic neuritis treatment trial, the risk was 51 percent in the 89 patients with three or more MRI lesions.[119]

EFFECT OF THERAPY ON MS LESIONS BASED ON MR IMAGING

Corticosteroids

Corticosteroids remain the principal therapy for acute, symptomatic MS exacerbations[123] because they may decrease the severity and duration of symptoms, often dramatically over a period of hours. Although corticosteroid therapy may have a clinical impact over a 2-year period,[118] a long-term effect on development of clinically definite MS has not to date been detectable.[119]

High-dose parenteral corticosteroids may have a direct effect on the blood-brain barrier, resulting in closure within minutes to hours in acute MS lesions, based on imaging studies (Fig. 17-19).[16,124–126] This effect on the blood-brain barrier is transient, since many lesions reenhance after several days.[126] Over a period of weeks, lesion enhancement returns to expected levels.[126] Corticosteroids do not appear to affect T2-hyperintense lesions as markedly, and in some cases the T2-hyperintense lesion area may actually enlarge during the period of high-dose corticosteroid therapy.[125] As a practical issue, MRI studies conducted within days of high-dose intravascular corticosteroids are likely to show (falsely) fewer enhancing lesions and frequently no enhancing lesions, and this effect may last over a period of several weeks.

Beta-Interferons

Beta-interferon 1a (Avonex, Biogen, Inc.) and 1b (Betaseron, Berlex, Inc.) are currently approved for use in North America for relapsing MS and are widely used in Europe as well.[3,4] The β-interferons influence the blood-brain barrier, as indicated by their impact on enhancing lesions.[7–9] This effect is probably indirect through their influence on the immunologic and inflammatory cascade of events.

Serial monthly pilot MRI studies have shown a decrease in enhancing lesions within 1 week to 2 months of initiating treatment with β-interferon 1a[8] and 1b.[9,29] Long-term decreases in the number or volume of enhancing lesions have also been seen with continuous treatment over 6 months[8] and 1- and 2-year intervals.[3,7] Treatment also decreases the accumulation of T2-hyperintense lesion area[8,10,11] and volume,[7] the development of acute new T2 lesions,[10] and the 6-month[8] and 2-year accumulation of new T2-hyperintense lesions.[7]

Other Immunomodulatory Agents

A number of new treatments are being tested in phase I and II trials using MRI outcome criteria, principally those based on new lesions by enhancing lesion counts. To date, however, there has been a great deal of variability in trial design, entry characteristics, and utilization of appropriate control methodologies, which makes interpretation difficult. Greater standardization of trial design and analysis methods will improve the quality of studies over the next few years.[22] Nevertheless, pilot (phase I to II) trials suggest that the list of immunomodulatory agents that will affect development of acute MS lesions or long-term lesion accumulation is likely to increase rapidly over the next few years. Promising results have been reported using MRI criteria for such

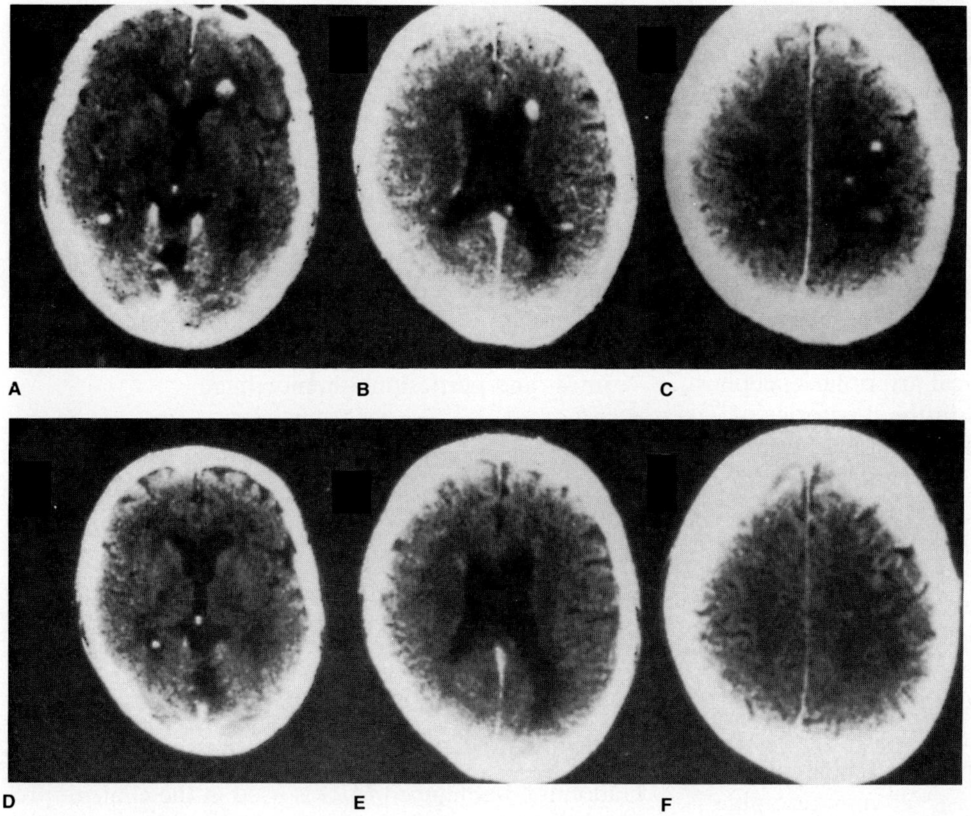

Figure 17-19
CT with intravenous contrast in patient with MS **(A–C)** *before and* **(D–F)** *after intravenous administration of high-dose methylprednisolone. Before administration or methylprednisolone, there were multiple contrast-enhancing white matter lesions, which disappeared almost completely when the study was repeated after treatment. (From R Troiano, M Hafstein, M Ruderman, et al,* Ann Neurol *15:257–263, 1984. Used by permission.)*

diverse agents as mitoxantrone,[12] linomide,[13] α-interferon,[127] campath-1H,[128] and cladribine.[129] Negative results or minimal effects based on MRI outcomes with other therapies have also been reported.[130,131] Screening of new therapies, fine-tuning of dose response, and evaluation of multiagent therapies are now feasible using MRI-based strategies. Phase I and II MRI-based trials can be completed relatively quickly (over periods of 6 months to 1 year) and in small cohorts (40 to 80 subjects) compared to definitive phase III clinical trials, which require a minimum of 2 to 3 years and typically several hundred subjects.[22] After preliminary evaluation using the phase I and II MRI-based trial design, MRI is likely to be used as a secondary outcome measure, based on a parallel groups study, and with annual measures of lesion burden as outcome.

The introduction and licensure of new MS therapies will no doubt be accompanied by an increasing interest in following the course of an individual's MS progression by brain MRI. Extrapolation of results from pilot and even definitive trial data can be hazardous, particularly in view of the known fluctuations in T2 lesion volume and enhancing lesion activity in individuals. Nevertheless, enhancing lesions imply continued activity and may someday be helpful ultimately in titrating dose or determining optimal combination therapy. Accumulation of new T2 lesions over time has similar implications.

DIFFERENTIAL DIAGNOSIS

Multiple sclerosis is a clinical diagnosis that cannot be made on imaging results alone. Lesions by imaging and a clinical picture remarkably similar to that of MS have been described in neurosarcoidosis,[132] Lyme disease, and the vasculitides.[133] Changes induced by aging,[134] diabetes, and hypertension may have features in common with MS, and, because of their frequency, some rare manifestations may overlap considerably with features expected for MS.

Overinterpretation of MRI studies should also be avoided, since there are patients with white matter lesions and monosymptomatic disease (e.g., optic neuritis) who may never develop other clinical symptoms or signs of MS.[135] The erroneous diagnosis of MS based solely on imaging findings has caused considerable suffering among patients who do not have the disease on clinical grounds but because of the MRI report suffer psychologically, have problems with family planning, and may encounter difficulties obtaining employment and insurance.

Differential diagnostic points for diseases with clinical or imaging features similar to MS have been recently reviewed in detail.[136] General considerations include the following:

1. *Apparently normal aging.* Kirkpatrick and Hayman[137] found white matter lesions in 80 percent of a

series of 15 brains from clinically healthy subjects aged 52 to 72, including atrophic periventricular demyelination in 8 and white matter infarcts in 2. Incidental white matter T2 hyperintensities occur frequently in the elderly population. Fazekas et al[52] proposed criteria for diagnosing an MS-like pattern; the criteria, which can be helpful in assessing the elderly brain, require two of the three following features: lesion size greater than or equal to 6 mm, lesions abutting ventricle bodies (surface), and lesions located infratentorially.

2. *Binswanger disease* (subcortical arteriolar encephalopathy). Watershed infarcts in the territories of deep perforating arterial branches affect both the periventricular white matter and centrum ovale. Apart from age and clinical presentation, this pattern may be distinguished from MS in some cases by associated lesions (lacunae) in the basal ganglia and absence of brainstem lesions. Small artery and arteriolar disease (e.g., hypertensive vascular disease) does not typically penetrate into the deep substance of the corpus callosum or affect subcortical U fibers, as does MS.[62]
3. *Vasculitides.* Conditions such as systemic lupus erythematosus and Behçet disease[133,138] may resemble MS clinically and by their white matter lesional pattern in the brain and spinal cord. The brain lesions of vasculitides tend to be mild in the periventricular compared with the more peripheral white matter, are more likely to involve cortical tissue or to show infarction in major vascular or discrete cortical territories, and may be associated with focal cortical atrophy.
4. *Migraine.* Lesions associated with migraine are said to involve the peripheral rather than the periventricular white matter. Patients with complicated migraine may have lesions involving the cerebellar or cerebral cortex.[139]
5. *Lyme disease (neuroborelliosis).* Lyme disease can mimic MS by clinical criteria, including optic neuritis and a relapsing course. Because Lyme disease is a treatable, often underdiagnosed entity, it is important to consider in endemic regions. Enhancement of the leptomeninges may be seen.[136]
6. *Acute disseminated encephalomyelitis (ADEM).* This monophasic acute inflammatory demyelinating disease of the CNS is usually distinguished from MS by its clinical course (single episode and acute onset including fever and headache) and history (preceding infection or vaccination and more frequent in childhood), but ADEM may sometimes relapse, similarly to MS. The location and characteristics of the lesions by MRI may be indistinguishable from MS.[140,141] Lesions in ADEM are more typically synchronously enhancing, which is rare for MS. Long-term serial follow-up, for example, at 6 months and 1 year, should in theory differentiate the monophasic pattern of ADEM from that of MS but will not be definitive in MS cases that become relatively inactive.
7. *Emboli.* With emboli, MRI patterns of abnormality may appear consistent with MS. However, unlike MS, emboli usually occur at the corticomedullary junction and sometimes produce vascular branch occlusive patterns that help in the differential diagnosis. Emboli may also be accompanied by small intra- and perilesional hemorrhage.
8. *Whipple disease.* In its early stages, Whipple disease can appear MS-like.[136] It can be treated with antibiotics.
9. *Malignancy, including metastases, and lymphomatosis.* Rarely, malignancy may produce lesional patterns similar to those of MS.[142]

CLINICAL IMAGING PROCEDURES

Gadolinium-Enhanced MRI

Gadolinium-enhanced MRI is used in the clinic to provide evidence of dissemination in time, to aid in the differential diagnosis, and to measure active disease in individuals.

Standard doses of any of the approved gadolinium-chelate MRI contrast agents (0.1 mmol/kg) are acceptable and appropriate for clinical imaging. Although cost-prohibitive in most cases, the use of triple rather than single doses results in convincing improvements in lesion detection and conspicuity. The increase in the numbers of lesions detected is on the order of 50 to 100 percent over conventional dosing routines.[33–35,143] T1-weighted magnetization transfer prepared imaging sequences also improve acute MS lesion contrast-to-noise ratios by as much as 50 percent.[143,144] When using this approach, precontrast magnetization transfer imaging series must be acquired and carefully evaluated, since chronic (nonenhancing) lesions may also appear hyperintense on both the pre- and post-contrast-enhanced series.[144]

Detection of T2-Hyperintense Lesions

The classic sequence for detection of MS in the brain has been the spin-echo sequence, but the fast spin-echo (turbo spin-echo) sequences are well-accepted replacements in the clinic, since they reduce scan time and provide comparable results.[145] Although dual-echo fast spin-echo imaging is most efficient, contrast on the first echo is not comparable to that achieved using a long-repetition-time, short-echo conventional spin-echo sequence. However, by using a short TR (e.g., 2000 to

2500 ms), short TE fast spin-echo series, and a long TR, long TE fast spin-echo series, one can mimic the usual imaging quality of the conventional spin echo and still maintain a strong time advantage.

Magnetic resonance imaging instrument field strength does not appear to be an important factor for MS diagnosis in the clinic.[146] In our experience, low-field (0.3 to 0.5 T) instruments will provide reliable diagnostic information in cooperative patients.

Fluid-attenuated inversion recovery and its fast variants (fast FLAIR and turbo inversion recovery) provide excellent MS lesion contrast in the supratentorial brain and improve detection and conspicuity of periventricular, immediate subcortical, and cortical lesions due to a minimized CSF signal. Fast FLAIR sequences may result in reduced lesion conspicuity in the posterior fossa[65] and spinal cord.[147] Improved commercial versions of FLAIR with minimized flow artifacts may make this the sequence of choice for MS lesion detection in the future.

T2-weighted echo-planar imaging can provide single slice images in 50 to 100 ms and full brain studies in seconds. Although echo-planar MRI studies will be helpful in the clinical evaluation of uncooperative patients, they are currently limited by large magnetic susceptibility artifacts near the skull base and paranasal sinuses.

ADVANCED AND EXPERIMENTAL METHODOLOGIES

Quantitative Relaxation

Magnetic resonance imaging based on standard T1- or T2-weighted images provides a convenient way to present brain images that provide a great deal of anatomic information (lesion distribution), some physiologic information (enhancement), and, because of sensitivity to T1 and T2 processes, additional sensitivity to small disturbances in the water milieu, allowing tissue characterization of, for example, T2-hyperintense lesions and T1 holes. Images can also be synthesized based on a more quantitative representation of the either the T1- or the T2-relaxation time or proton density.[148] Unfortunately, simple (monoexponential) relaxation maps do not separate new and mature lesions because of large overlapping values of T1 and T2.[38] Another approach attempts to sort out the various water compartments in cells, tissues, and other spaces by generating (multiexponential-based) maps of the various water components. The data for these tissue maps are generated using imaging studies using multiple narrowly spaced echoes from the fast spin-echo approach.[149] This approach may someday contribute to a finer biophysical and chemical characterization of the demyelination process in vivo.

Magnetization Transfer Imaging

Magnetization transfer imaging (MTI) takes advantage of the fact that in a conventional MRI instrument the exchange of magnetization between mobile water protons (those typically observed with MRI in the brain) and water protons organized by adjacent macromolecules that are typically MRI invisible can be conveniently measured. Magnetization transfer imaging seems to provide unique information, somewhat independent of that provided by T2-weighted imaging, believed to be related to the integrity of tissue in the MS brain, possibly related to structure of the membrane (myelin).[47,111,150–153]

Using a simple magnetization transfer (MT) index measure, strong MT effects are seen for normal white matter (e.g., 30 to 60 percent, depending on technique), while progressively less MT effect is seen with increasing tissue damage, ultimately approaching that of CSF, which shows essentially no (e.g., 0 to 2 percent) MT effect. Multiple sclerosis lesions have variably decreased MT ratios. Experimental validation in optic nerve,[150] lysolecithin-induced demyelination,[151] and an animal model for MS- experimental allergic encephalomyelitis,[152] suggests that the MT method provides some separation of the influence of edema from that of demyelination. The MT ratio in MS correlates modestly with loss of signal on T1-weighted imaging in a subset of lesions (T1 holes),[47] decreased *N*-acetylaspartate,[153] and clinical disability.[111]

Magnetic Resonance Spectroscopy

Magnetic resonance imaging is designed to detect and quantitate the major chemical species in brain tissue—the mobile water fraction—which is very abundant (the water concentration in the brain is about 55 moles/L).[154] Although fat protons are also abundant, with fat about 80 percent by dry weight in brain), the major lipid resonances ($-CH_2$ from methylene and $-CH_3$ from methyl groups) in cellular membrane including myelin normally have very short T2 relaxation times (about 50 μs) and are essentially MRI invisible, since signal decay occurs before the period of signal detection.[154]

Using conventional MRI instruments and radiofrequency pulses organized to eliminate the magnetic resonance signal from that of the water resonance, several far less abundant chemical species can be detected and quantitated in the brain, including species present in millimolar quantities, such as *N*-acetyl groups. With additional radiofrequency amplifiers and detection devices (properly tuned antennas), conventional MRI systems can detect 31phosphorus resonances, 13 carbon resonances, and resonances of other nuclei.

The most abundant hydrogen proton resonance detected by proton MRS is *N*-acetyl aspartate (NAA), which is a putative neuronal marker. The level of NAA is reduced in acute and chronic MS lesions when measured in absolute terms or as a ratio relative to creatine, in both acute and chronic MS lesions.[114,153,155–157] Although initially believed to reflect irreversible loss of neurons (and axons), NAA decreases are now thought to be from either neuronal loss or dysfunction, since reversible changes have been reported. The ratio of NAA to creatine has also been described as abnormally low in normal-appearing white matter in MS, but a recent report suggests that this finding may be attributed to elevated levels of creatine,[157] which is higher in astrocytes, oligodendroglia, and microglia.

Other resonances relevant to MS that can be detected by magnetic resonance spectroscopy include that of choline, levels of which may be elevated in acute MS,[156] and lipids, thought to be early markers in the course of lesion development.[158]

Diffusion MRI

Diffusion MRI or spectroscopy may improve the characterization of normal and abnormal white matter by providing quantitative information about the composition, shape, and orientation of water compartments in the CNS. The diffusion coefficient is abnormal in acute and chronic MS lesions,[159,160] and, based on animal demyelination models, diffusion MRI may be sensitive to early events in MS lesions.[161]

REFERENCES

1. Ebers GC, Paty DW. Natural history studies and applications to clinical trials, in Paty DW, Ebers GC, (eds): *Multiple Sclerosis.* Philadelphia, FA Davis, 1998, pp 192–228.
2. Multiple sclerosis, in *NIH Guide Grants Contracts* 22(2): 8–11, 1993.
3. Jacobs LD, Cookfair DL, Rudick RA, et al: Intramuscular interferon beta-1a for disease progression in relapsing multiple sclerosis. *Ann Neurol* 39:285–294, 1996.
4. IFNB Multiple Sclerosis Study Group: Interferon beta-1b is effective in relapsing-remitting multiple sclerosis: I. Clinical results of a multicenter, randomized, double-blind, placebo-controlled trial. *Neurology* 43:655–661, 1993.
5. Johnson KP, Brooks BR, Cohen JA, et al: Copolymer 1 reduces the relapse rate and improves disability in relapsing multiple sclerosis: Results of a phase III multicenter, double-blind placebo-controlled trial. *Neurology* 45: 1268–1276, 1995.
6. Rudick RA, Goodkin DE, Jacobs LD, et al: Impact of interferon beta-1a on neurologic disability in relapsing multiple sclerosis. *Neurology* 49:358–363, 1997.
7. Simon JH, Jacobs LD, Campion M, et al: Magnetic resonance studies of intramuscular interferon β-1a for relapsing multiple sclerosis. *Ann Neurol* 43:79–87, 1998.
8. Pozzilli C, Bastianello S, Koudriavtseva T, et al: Magnetic resonance imaging changes with recombinant human interferon-β-1a: A short-term study in relapsing-remitting multiple sclerosis. *J Neurol Neurosurg Psychiatry* 61:251–258, 1996.
9. Stone LA, Frank JA, Albert PS, et al: Characterization of MRI response to treatment with interferon beta-1b: Contrast enhancing MRI lesion frequency as a primary outcome measure. *Neurology* 49:862–869, 1997.
10. Paty DW, Li DKB, UBC MS/MRI Study Group, IFNB Multiple Sclerosis Study Group: Interferon beta-1b is effective in relapsing-remitting multiple sclerosis: II. MRI analysis results of a multicenter, randomized, double-blind, placebo-controlled trial. *Neurology* 43:662–667, 1993.
11. IFNB Multiple Sclerosis Study Group, University of British Columbia MS/MRI Analysis Group: Interferon beta-1b in the treatment of multiple sclerosis: Final outcome of the randomized controlled trial. *Neurology* 45:1277–1285, 1995.
12. Edan G, French and British Multiple Sclerosis Mitixantrone Trial Group: Demonstration of the efficacy of mitoxantrone (MTX) using MRI in MS patients with very active disease. *J Neuroimmunology* S1:16, 1995.
13. Andersen O, Lycke J, Tollesson PO, et al: Linomide reduces the rate of active lesions in relapsing-remitting multiple sclerosis. *Neurology* 47:895–900, 1996.
14. Gilbert JJ, Salder M: Unsuspected multiple sclerosis. *Arch Neurol* 40:533–536, 1983.
15. Phadke JG, Best PV: Atypical and clinically silent multiple sclerosis: A report of 12 cases discovered unexpectedly at necropsy. *J Neurol Neurosurg Psychiatry* 46:414–420, 1983.
16. Simon JH: Contrast-enhanced MR imaging in the evaluation of treatment response and prediction of outcome in multiple sclerosis. *J Magn Reson Imaging* 7:29–37, 1997.
17. Isaac C, Li DKB, Genton M, et al: Multiple sclerosis: A serial study using MRI in relapsing patients. *Neurology* 38:1511–1515, 1988.
18. Willoughby EW, Grochowski E, Li DKB, et al: Serial magnetic resonance scanning in multiple sclerosis: A second prospective study in relapsing patients. *Ann Neurol* 25:43–49, 1989.
19. Harris JO, Frank JA, Patronas N, et al: Serial gadolinium-enhanced magnetic resonance imaging scans in patients with early, relapsing-remitting multiple sclerosis: Implications for clinical trials and natural history. *Ann Neurol* 29:548–555, 1991.
20. Thompson AJ, Miller D, Youl B, et al: Serial gadolinium-enhanced MRI in relapsing/remitting multiple sclerosis of varying disease duration. *Neurology* 42:60–63, 1992.
21. Barkof F, Scheltens P, Frequin STFM, et al: Relapsing-remitting multiple sclerosis: Sequential enhanced MR imaging vs clinical findings in determining disease activity. *AJR* 159:1041–1047, 1992.
22. Miller DH, Albert PS, Barkhof F, et al: Guidelines for the use of magnetic resonance techniques in monitoring the treatment of multiple sclerosis. *Ann Neurology* 39:6–16, 1996.
23. Allen I: Pathology of multiple sclerosis, in Matthews WB, (ed): *McAlpine's Multiple Sclerosis,* 2d ed. London, Churchill Livingstone, 1991, pp 341–379.

24. Prineas JW: The neuropathology of multiple sclerosis, in Vinken PJ, Bruyn GW, Klawans HL (eds), Koetsier JC (co-ed): *Handbook of Clinical Neurology.* Amsterdam, Elsevier, 1985, 47(3):213–257.
25. Katz D, Taubenberger JK, Cannella B, et al: Correlation between magnetic resonance imaging findings and lesion development in chronic, active multiple sclerosis. *Ann Neurol* 34:661–669, 1993.
26. Nesbit GM, Forbes GS, Scheithauer BW, et al: Multiple sclerosis: Histopathologic and MR and/or CT correlation in 37 cases at biopsy and three cases at autopsy. *Radiology* 180(2):467–474, 1991.
27. Sears ES, McCammon A, Bigelow R, Hayman LA: Maximizing the harvest of contrast enhancing lesions in multiple sclerosis. *Neurology* 32:815–820, 1982.
28. Spiegel SM, Viñuela F, Fox AJ, Pelz DM: CT of multiple sclerosis: Reassessment of delayed scanning with high doses of contrast material. *AJNR* 6:533–536, 1985.
29. Calabresi PA, Tranquill LR, Dambrosia JM, et al: Increase in soluble VCAM-1 correlate with a decrease in MRI lesions in multiple sclerosis treated with interferon β-1b. *Ann Neurol* 41:669–674, 1997.
30. Giovannoni G, Lai M, Thorpe J, et al: Longitudinal study of soluble adhesion molecules in multiple sclerosis: Correlation with gadolinium enhanced magnetic resonance imaging. *Neurology* 48:1557–1565, 1997.
31. Trojano M, Avoilio C, Simone IL, et al: Soluble intercellular adhesion molecule-1 in serum and cerebrospinal fluid of clinically active relapsing-remitting multiple sclerosis. *Neurology* 47:1535–1541, 1996.
32. Lai HM, Hodgson T, Gawne-Cain M, et al: A preliminary study into the sensitivity of disease activity detection by serial weekly magnetic resonance imaging in multiple sclerosis. *J Neurol Neurosurg Psychiatry* 60:339–341, 1996.
33. Filippi M, Yousry T, Campi A, et al: Comparison of triple-dose versus standard dose gadolinium-DTPA for detection of MRI enhancing lesions in patients with MS. *Neurology* 46:379–384, 1996.
34. Silver NC, Good CD, Barker GJ, et al: Sensitivity of contrast enhanced MRI in multiple sclerosis: Effects of gadolinium dose, magnetization transfer contrast and delayed imaging. *Brain* 120:1149–1161, 1997.
35. Wolansky LJ, Bardini JA, Cook SD, et al: Triple-dose versus single dose gadoteridol in multiple sclerosis patients. *J Neuroimag* 4(3):141–145, 1994.
36. Thompson AJ, Polman CH, Miller DH, et al: Primary progressive multiple sclerosis. *Brain* 120:1085–1096, 1997.
37. Kermode AG, Tofts PS, Thompson AJ, et al: Heterogeneity of blood-brain barrier changes in multiple sclerosis: An MRI study with gadolinium-DTPA enhancement. *Neurology* 40:229–235, 1990.
38. Miller DH, Rudge P, Johnson G, et al: Serial gadolinium enhanced magnetic resonance imaging in multiple sclerosis. *Brain* 111:927–939, 1988.
39. Guttmann CRG, Ahn SS, Hsu L, et al: The evolution of multiple sclerosis lesions on serial MR. *Am J Neuroradiol* 16:1481–1491, 1995.
40. Koopsmans RA, Li DKB, Oger JJF, et al: The lesion of multiple sclerosis: Imaging of acute and chronic stages. *Neurology* 39:959–963, 1989.
41. Wiebe S, Lee DH, Karlik SJ, et al: Serial cranial and spinal cord magnetic resonance imaging in multiple sclerosis. *Ann Neurol* 32:643–650, 1992.
42. Simon JH: Magnetic resonance imaging of multiple sclerosis lesions: Measuring outcome in treatment trials. *West J Med* 164:502–509, 1996.
43. Smith ME, Stone LA, Albert PS, et al: Clinical worsening in multiple sclerosis is associated with increased frequency and area of gadopentetate dimeglumine-enhancing magnetic resonance imaging lesions. *Ann Neurol* 33: 480–489, 1993.
44. Barnes D, Munro PMG, Youl BD, et al: The long-standing MS lesion: A quantitative MRI and electron microscopic study. *Brain* 114:1271–1280, 1991.
45. Truyen L, van Waesberghe JHTM, van Walderveen MAA, et al: Accumulation of hypointense lesions ("black holes") on T_1 spin echo MRI correlates with disease progression in multiple sclerosis. *Neurology* 47: 1469–1476, 1996.
46. van Walderveen MAA, Barkhof F, Hommes OR, et al: Correlating MRI and clinical disease activity in multiple sclerosis: Relevance of hypointense lesions in short-TR/ short-TE (T_1-weighted) spin-echo images. *Neurology* 45: 1684–1690, 1995.
47. Loevner LA, Grossman RI, McGowan JC, et al: Characterization of multiple sclerosis plaques with T1-weighted MR and quantitative magnetization transfer. *Am J Neuroradiol* 16:1473–1479, 1995.
48. van Walderveen MAA, Scheltens Ph, Barkhof F et al: Histopathologic correlate of hypointense lesions on T1-weighted SE MR images in multiple sclerosis. *J Neurol* 243(suppl 2):S18, 1996.
49. Stone LA, Albert PS, Smith ME, et al: Changes in the amount of diseased white matter over time in patients with relapsing-remitting multiple sclerosis. *Neurolgy* 45: 1808–1814, 1995.
50. Jacobs L, Kinkel WR, Polachini I, Kinkel RP: Correlations of nuclear magnetic resonance imaging, computerized tomography, and clinical profiles in multiple sclerosis. *Neurology* 36:27–34, 1986.
51. Sheldon JJ, Siddharthan R, Tobias J. et al: MR imaging of multiple sclerosis: Comparison with clinical and CT examinations in 74 patients. *Am J Roentgenol* 145:957–964, 1985.
52. Fazekas F, Offenbacher H, Fuchs S, et al: Criteria for an increased specificity of MRI interpretation in elderly subjects with suspected multiple sclerosis. *Neurology* 38: 1822–1825, 1988.
53. Offenbacher H, Fazekas F, Schmidt R, et al: Assessment of MRI criteria for a diagnosis of MS. *Neurology* 43:905–909, 1993.
54. Paty DW, Oger JJF, Kastrukoff LF, et al: MRI in the diagnosis OF MS: A prospective study with comparison of clinical evaluation, evoked potentials, oligoclonal banding, and CT. *Neurology* 38:180–185, 1988.
55. Tas MW, Barkhof F, van Walderveen MAA, et al: The effect of gadolinium on the sensitivity and specificity of MR in the initial diagnosis of multiple sclerosis. *Am J Neuroradiol* 16:259–264, 1995.
56. Barkhof F, Filippi M, Miller DH, et al: Comparison of MRI criteria at first presentation to predict conversion to clinically definite multiple sclerosis. *Brain* 120:2059–2069, 1997.

57. Poser CM, Paty DW, Scheinberg L, et al: New diagnostic criteria for multiple sclerosis guidelines for research protocols. *Ann Neurol* 13:227–231, 1983.
58. Ormerod IEC, Miller DH, McDonald WI, et al: The role of NMR imaging in the assessment of multiple sclerosis and isolated neurological lesions: a quantitative study. *Brain* 110:1579–1616, 1987.
59. Miller DH: Spectrum of abnormalities in multiple sclerosis, in Miller DH, Kesselring J, McDonald W Ian, et al (eds): *Magnetic Resonance in Multiple Sclerosis.* Cambridge, Cambridge University Press, 1997, chap 3, pp 31–62.
60. Horowitz AL, Kaplan RD, Grewe G, et al: The ovoid lesion: A new MR observation in patients with multiple sclerosis. *Am J Neuroradiol* 10:303–305, 1989.
61. Giang DW, Poduri KR, Eskin TA, et al: Multiple sclerosis masquerading as a mass lesion. *Neuroradiology* 34:150–154, 1992.
62. Moody DM, Bell MA, Challa VR: The corpus callosum, a unique white matter tract: Anatomic features that may explain sparing in Binswanger disease and resistance to flow of fluid masses. *Am J Neuroradiol* 9:1051–1059, 1988.
63. Bastienello S, Bozzao A, Paolillo A, et al: Fast spin-echo and fast fluid-attenuated inversion recovery versus conventional spin-echo sequences for MR quantification of multiple sclerosis lesions. *Am J Neuroradiol* 18:699–704, 1997.
64. Filippi M, Yousry TA, Baratti C, et al: Quantitative assessment of MRI lesion load in multiple sclerosis: A comparison of conventional spin-echo with fast-fluid-attenuated inversion recovery. *Brain* 119:1349–1355, 1996.
65. Gawne-Cain ML, O'Riordan JI, Thompson AJ, et al: Multiple sclerosis lesion detection in the brain: A comparison of fast fluid-attenuated inversion recovery and conventional T2-weighted dual spin echo. *Neurology* 49: 364–370, 1997.
66. Barnard RO, Triggs M: Corpus callosum in multiple sclerosis. *J Neurol Neurosurg Psych* 37:1259–1264, 1974.
67. Lumsden CE: The neuropathology of multiple sclerosis, in Vinken PJ, Bruyn GW (eds): *Handbook of Clinical Pathology,* vol 9. Amsterdam, Elsevier, 1970, pp 217–309.
68. Simon JH, Holtas SL, Schiffer RB, et al: Corpus callosum and subcallosal-periventricular lesions in multiple sclerosis: Detection with MR. *Radiology* 160:363–367, 1986.
69. Simon JH, Schiffer RB, Rudick RA, Herndon RM: Quantitative determination of MS-induced corpus callosum atrophy in vivo using MR imaging. *Am J Neuroradiol* 8:599–604, 1987.
70. Gean-Marton AD, Vezina LG, Marton KI, et al: Abnormal corpus callosum: A sensitive and specific indicator of multiple sclerosis. *Radiology* 80:215–221, 1991.
71. Wilms G, Marchal G, Kersschot E, et al: Axial versus sagittal T2-weighted brain MR images in the evaluation of multiple sclerosis. *J Comput Assist Tomogr* 15:359–364, 1991.
72. Lee OH, Simon JH, Szumowski J, et al: Optic neuritis and orbital lesions: Lipid-suppressed chemical shift MR imaging. *Radiology* 179:543–546, 1991.
73. Miller DH, Newton MR, van der Poel JC, et al: Magnetic resonance imaging of the optic nerve in optic neuritis. *Neurology* 38:175–179, 1988.
74. Simon J, Szumowski J, Totterman S, et al: Fat suppression MR imaging of the orbit. *Am J Neuroradiol* 9:961–968, 1988.
75. Gass A, Barker GJ, MacManus DG, et al: High resolution magnetic resonance imaging of the anterior visual pathway in patients with optic neuropathies using fast spin echo and phased array local coils. *J Neurol Neurosurg Psychiatry* 58:562–569, 1995.
76. Simon JH, Rubinstein D, Brown M, et al: Quantitative contrast-enhanced MR imaging of the optic nerve. *Acta Radiol* 35:526–531, 1994.
77. Youl BD, Turano G, Miller DH, et al: The pathophysiology of acute optic neuritis. *Brain* 114:2437–2450, 1991.
78. Tien RD, Hesselink JR, Szumowski J: MR fat suppression combined with GD-DTPA enhancement in optic neuritis and perineuritis. *J Comput Assist Tomogr* 15: 223–227, 1991.
79. Plant GT, Kermode AG, Turano G, et al: Symptomatic retrochiasmal lesions in multiple sclerosis. *Neurology* 42: 68–76, 1992.
80. Brainin M, Reisner T, Neuhold A, et al: Topographical characteristics of brainstem lesions in clinically definite and clinically probable cases of multiple sclerosis. *Neuroradiology* 29:530–536, 1987.
81. Yousry TA, Filippi M, Becker C, et al: Comparison of MR pulse sequences in the detection of multiple sclerosis lesions. *Am J Neuroradiol* 18:959–963, 1997.
82. Oppenheimer DR: The cervical cord in multiple sclerosis. *Neuropathol Appl Neurobiol* 4:151–162, 1978.
83. Honig LS, Sheremata WA: Magnetic resonance imaging of spinal cord lesions in multiple sclerosis. *J Neurol Neurosurg Psychiatry* 52:459–466, 1989.
84. Tartaglino LM, Friedman DP, Flanders AE, et al: Multiple sclerosis in the spinal cord: MR appearance and correlation with clinical parameters. *Radiology* 195:725–732, 1995.
85. Simnad VI, Pisani DE, Rose JW: Multiple sclerosis presenting as transverse myelopathy. *Neurology* 48:65–73, 1997.
86. Kidd D, Thorpe JW, Thompson AJ, et al: Spinal cord MRI using multi-array coils and fast spin echo: II. Findings in multiple sclerosis. *Neurology* 43:2632–2637, 1993.
87. Campi A, Filippi M, Comi G, et al: Acute transverse myelopathy: Spinal and cranial MR study with clinical followup. *Am J Neuroradiol* 16:115–123, 1995.
88. Thorpe JW, Kidd D, Moseley IF, et al: Serial gadolinium-enhanced MRI of the brain and spinal cord in early relapsing-remitting multiple sclerosis. *Neurology* 46:373–378, 1996.
89. Losseff NA, Webb SL, O'Riordan JI, et al: Spinal cord atrophy and disability in multiple sclerosis: A new reproducible and sensitive MRI method with potential to monitor disease progression. *Brain* 119:701–708, 1996.
90. Thorpe JW, Kidd D, Moseley IF, et al: Spinal MRI in patients with suspected multiple sclerosis and negative brain MRI. *Brain* 119:709–714, 1996.
91. McFarland HF, Frank JA, Albert PA, et al: Using gadolinium-enhanced magnetic resonance imaging lesions to monitor disease activity in multiple sclerosis. *Ann Neurol* 32:758–766, 1992.
92. Atlas SW, Grossman RI, Savino PJ, et al: Internuclear ophthalmoplegia: MR-anatomic correlation. *Am J Neuroradiol* 8:243–247, 1987.

93. Gass A, Kitchen N, MacManus DG, et al: Trigeminal neuralgia in patients with multiple sclerosis: Lesion localization with magnetic resonance imaging. *Neurology* 49: 1142–1144, 1997.
94. Kaba S, Pullicino P, Jacobs L: MRI demonstration of the lesion causing continuous facial myokymia in MS. *Neurology* 43(suppl 2):A246, 1993.
95. Weinshenker BG: The natural history of multiple sclerosis, in Antel JP (ed): Multiple sclerosis. *Neurology Clinics* 13:119–146, 1995.
96. Nauta JJP, Thompson AJ, Brakhof F, Miller DH: Magnetic resonance imaging in monitoring the treatment of multiple sclerosis patients: Statistical power of parallel-groups and crossover designs. *J Neurol Sciences* 122:6–14, 1994.
97. Miller DH, Barkhof F, Nauta JFF: Gadolinium enhancement increases the sensitivity of MRI in detecting disease activity in multiple sclerosis. *Brain* 116:1077–1094, 1993.
98. Koudriavtseva T, Thompson AJ, Fiorelli M, et al: Gadolinium enhanced MRI predicts clinical and MRI disease activity in relapsing-remitting multiple sclerosis. *J Neurol Neurosurg Psychiatry* 62:285–287, 1997.
99. Simon JH, Jacobs L, Campion M, Multiple Sclerosis Collaborative Research Group: A longitudinal study of brain atrophy in relapsing MS. *Neurology* 1999, in press.
100. Goodkin DE, Rudick RA, VanderBrug Medendorp S, et al: Low-dose oral methotrexate in chronic progressive multiple sclerosis: Analyses of serial MRIs. *Neurology* 47:1153–1157, 1996.
101. Filippi M, Paty DW, Kappos L, et al: Correlations between changes in disability and T_2-weighted brain MRI activity in multiple sclerosis: A follow-up study. *Neurology* 45;255–260, 1995.
102. Whitaker JN, McFarland HF, Rudge P, Reingold SC: Outcomes assessment in multiple sclerosis clinical trials: A critical analysis. *Multiple Sclerosis* 1:37–47, 1995.
103. Rao SM, Leo GJ, Bernardin L, et al: Cognitive dysfunction in multiple sclerosis: I. Frequency, patterns and prediction. *Neurology* 41:685–691, 1991.
104. Rao SM, Leo GJ, Haughton VM, et al: Correlation of magnetic resonance imaging with neuropsychological testing in multiple sclerosis. *Neurology* 39:161–166, 1989.
105. Swirsky-Sacchetti T, Mitchell DR, Seward J, et al: Neuropsychological and structural brain lesions in multiple sclerosis: A regional analysis. *Neurology* 42:1291–1295, 1992.
106. Huber SJ, Paulson GW, Shuttleworth EC, et al: Magnetic resonance imaging correlates of dementia in multiple sclerosis. *Arch Neurol* 44:732–736, 1987.
107. Comi G, Filippi M, Martinelli V, et al: Brain MRI correlates of cognitive impairment in primary and secondary progressive multiple sclerosis. *J Neurol Sci* 132:222–227, 1995.
108. Hohol MJ, Guttmann CRG, Orav J, et al: Serial neurophyschological assessment and magnetic resonance imaging analysis in multiple sclerosis. *Arch Neurol* 54:1018–1025, 1997.
109. Giugni E, Pozzilli C, Bastianello S, et al: MRI measures and their relations with clinical disability and relapsing-remitting and secondary progressive multiple sclerosis. *Multiple Sclerosis* 3:221–225, 1997.
110. Khoury SJ, Guttmann CRG, Orav EJ, et al: Longitudinal MRI in multiple sclerosis: Correlation between disability and lesion burden. *Neurology* 44:2120–2124, 1994.
111. Gass A, Barker GJ, Kidd D, et al: Correlation of magnetization transfer ratio with clinical disability in multiple sclerosis. *Ann Neurol* 36:62–67, 1994.
112. Hiehle JF, Grossman RI, Ramer KN, et al: Magnetization transfer effects in MR-detected multiple sclerosis: Comparison with gadolinium-enhanced spin-echo images and non-enhanced T1-weighted images. *Am J Neuroradiol* 16:69–77, 1995.
113. DeStefano N, Matthews PM, Antel JP, et al: Chemical pathology of acute demyelinating lesions and its correlation with disability. *Ann Neurol* 38:901–909, 1995.
114. Davie CA, Barker GJ, Webb S, et al: Persistent functional deficit in multiple sclerosis and autosomal dominant cerebellar ataxia is associated with axonal loss. *Brain* 118:1583–1592, 1995.
115. Losseff NA, Webb SL, O'Riodan JI, et al: Spinal cord atrophy and disability in multiple sclerosis: A new reproducible and sensitive MRI method with potential to monitor disease progression. *Brain* 119:701–708, 1996.
116. Morissey SP, Miller DH, Kendall BE, et al: The significance of brain magnetic resonance imaging abnormalities at presentation with clinically isolated syndromes suggestive of MS: A five-year follow-up study. *Brain* 116:135–146, 1993.
117. Filippi M, Horsfield MA, Morrissey SP, et al: Quantitative brain MRI lesion load predicts the course of clinically isolated syndromes suggestive of multiple sclerosis. *Neurology* 44:635–641, 1994.
118. Beck RW, Cleary PA, Trobe JD, et al: The effect of corticosteroids for acute optic neuritis on the subsequent development of multiple sclerosis. *N Engl J Med* 329: 1764–1769, 1993.
119. Optic Neuritis Study Group: The 5-year risk of MS after optic neuritis: Experience of the optic neuritis treatment trial. *Neurology* 49:1404–1413, 1997.
120. Jacobs LD, Kaba SE, Miller CM, et al: Correlation of clinical, magnetic resonance imaging, and cerebrospinal fluid findings in optic neuritis. *Ann Neurol* 41:392–398, 1997.
121. Ghezzi A, Deplano V, Faroni J, et al: Multiple sclerosis in childhood: Clinical features of 149 cases. *Multiple Sclerosis* 3:43–46, 1997.
122. Perkin G-D, Rose FC: *Optic Neuritis and Its Differential Diagnosis.* Oxford, Oxford University Press, 1979, pp 246–248.
123. Weiner HL, Hohol MJ, Khoury SJ, et al: Therapy for multiple sclerosis. *Neurol Clin* 13:173–196, 1995.
124. Barkhof F, Hommes OR, Scheltens P, et al: Quantitative MRI changes in gadolinium-DTPA enhancement after high-dose intravenous methylprednisolone in multiple sclerosis. *Neurology* 41:1219–1222, 1991.
125. Burnham JA, Wright RR, Dreisbach J, et al: The effect of high-dose steroids on MRI gadolinium enhancement in acute demyelinating lesions. *Neurology* 41:1349–1354, 1991.
126. Miller DH, Thompson AJ, Morrissey SP, et al: High-dose steroids in acute relapses of multiple sclerosis: MRI evidence for a possible mechanism of therapeutic effect. *J Neurol Neurosurg Psychiatry* 55:450–453, 1992.
127. Durelli L, Bongioanni MR, Cavallo R, et al: Interferon alpha treatment of relapsing-remitting multiple sclerosis: Long-term study of the correlations between clinical and magnetic resonance imaging results and ef-

fects on the immune function. *Multiple Sclerosis* 1:S32–S37, 1995.
128. Moreau T, Thorpe J, Miller D, et al: Preliminary evidence from magnetic resonance imaging for reduction in disease activity after lymphocyte depletion in multiple sclerosis. *Lancet* 344:298–301, 1994.
129. Sipe JC, Romine JS, Koziol JA, et al: Cladribine in treatment of chronic progressive multiple sclerosis. *Lancet* 344:9–13, 1994.
130. van Oosten BW, Lai M, Hodgkinson S, et al: Treatment of multiple sclerosis with the monoclonal anti-CD4 antibody cM-T412. *Neurology* 49:351–357, 1997.
131. Wiles CM, Omar L, Swan AV, et al: Total lymphoid irradiation in multiple sclerosis. *J Neurol Neurosurg Psychiatry* 57:154–163, 1994.
132. Smith AS, Meisler DM, Weinstein MA, et al: High-signal periventricular lesions in patients with sarcoidosis: Neurosarcoidosis or multiple sclerosis? *Am J Neuroradiol* 10:485–490, 1989.
133. Miller DH, Ormerod IEC, Gibson A, et al: MR brain scanning in patients with vasculitis: Differentiation from multiple sclerosis. *Neuroradiology* 29:226–231, 1987.
134. Fazekas F, Kleinert R, Offenbacher H, et al: Pathologic correlates of incidental MRI white matter signal hyperintensities. *Neurology* 43:1683–1689, 1993.
135. Jacobs L. Munschauer FE, Kaba SE: Clinical and magnetic resonance imaging in optic neuritis. *Neurology* 41:15–19, 1991.
136. Kesselring J, Miller DH: Differential diagnosis, in Miller DH, Kesselring J, McDonald WI, et al (eds): *Magnetic Resonance in Multiple Sclerosis.* Cambridge, Cambridge University Press, 1997, pp 63–107.
137. Kirkpatrick JB, Hayman LA: White-matter lesions in MR imaging of clinically healthy brains of elderly subjects: Possible pathologic basis. *Radiology* 162:509–511, 1987.
138. Wechsler B, Dell'Isola B, Vidaihet M, et al: MRI in 31 patients with Behçet's disease and neurological involvement: Prospective study with clinical correlation. *J Neurol Neurosurg Psychiatry* 56:793–798, 1993.
139. Soges LJ, Cacayorin ED, Petro GR, et al: Migraine: Evaluation by MR. *Am J Neuroradiol* 9:425–429, 1988.
140. Epperson LW, Whitaker JN, Kapila A: Cranial MRI in acute disseminated encephalomyelitis. *Neurology* 38:332–333, 1988.
141. Andreula CF, Luciani NMR, Milella D: Magnetic resonance imaging in diagnosis of acute disseminated encephalomyelitis (ADEM). *Int J Neuroradiol* 3:21–34, 1997.
142. Case 31-1995: Case Records of the Massachusetts General Hospital. *N Engl J Med* 33:992–999, 1995.
143. van Waesberghe JHTM, Castelijns JA, Roser W, et al: Single-dose gadolinium with magnetization transfer versus triple-dose gadolinium in the MR detection of multiple sclerosis lesions. *Am J Neuroradiol* 18:1279–1285, 1997.
144. Mehta RC, Pike GB, Enzmann DR: Improved detection of enhancing and nonenhancing lesions of multiple sclerosis with magnetization transfer. *Am J Neuroradiol* 16:1771–1778, 1995.
145. Thorpe JW, Halpin S, MacManus DG, et al: A comparison between fast spin echo and conventional spin echo in the detection of multiple sclerosis lesions. *Neuroradiology* 36:388–392, 1995.
146. Lee DH, Vellet AD, Eliasziw M, et al: MR imaging field strength: Prospective evaluation of the diagnostic accuracy of MR for diagnosis of multiple sclerosis at 0.5 and 1.5 T[1]. *Radiology* 194:257–262, 1995.
147. Keiper MD, Grossman RI, Brunson JC, et al: The low sensitivity of fluid-attenuated inversion-recovery MR in the detection of multiple sclerosis of the spinal cord. *Am J Neuroradiol* 18:1035–1039, 1997.
148. Hendrick RE, Raff U: Image contrast and noise, in Stark DD, Bradley WG (eds): *Magnetic Resonance Imaging,* 2d edition. St. Louis, Mosby YearBook, 1992, pp 109–144.
149. Whittall KP, MacKay AL, Graeb DA, et al: In vivo measurements of T_2 distributions and contents in normal human brain. *Magn Reson Med* 37:34–43, 1997.
150. Lexa FJ, Grossman RI, Rosenquist AC: MR of wallerian degeneration in the feline visual system: Characterization by magnetization transfer rate with histopathologic correlation. *Am J Neuroradiol* 15:201–212, 1994.
151. Dousset V, Brochet B, Vital A, et al: Lysolecithin-induced demyelination in primates: Preliminary in vivo study with MR and magnetization transfer. *Am J Neuroradiol* 16:225–231, 1995.
152. Dousset V, Grossman RI, Ramer KN, et al: Experimental allergic encephalomyelitis and multiple sclerosis: Lesion characterization with magnetization transfer imaging. *Radiology* 182:483–491, 1992.
153. Kimura H, Grossman RI, Lenkinski RE, Gonzalez-Scarano F: Proton MR spectroscopy and magnetization transfer ratio in multiple sclerosis: Correlative findings of active versus irreversible plaque disease. *Am J Neuroradiol* 17:1539–1547, 1996.
154. Szumowski J, Simon JH: Proton chemical shift imaging, in Stark DD, Bradley WG (eds): *Magnetic Resonance Imaging,* 2d ed., St. Louis, Mosby YearBook 1992, pp 479–521.
155. Matthews PM, Pioro E, Narayanan S, et al: Assessment of lesion pathology in multiple sclerosis using quantitative MRI morphometry and magnetic resonance spectroscopy. *Brain* 119:715–722, 1996.
156. Matthews PM, Francis G, Antel J, et al: Proton magnetic resonance spectroscopy for metabolic characterization of plaques in multiple sclerosis. *Neurology* 41:1251–1256, 1991.
157. Rooney WD, Goodkin DE, Schuff N, et al: ^{1}H MRSI of normal appearing white matter in multiple sclerosis. *Multiple Sclerosis* 3:231–237, 1997.
158. Narayana PA, Wolinsky JS, Jackson EF, McCarthy M: Proton MR spectroscopy of gadolinium-enhanced multiple sclerosis plaques. *J Magn Reson Imaging* 2:263–270, 1992.
159. Christiansen P, Gideon P, Thomsen C, et al: Increased water self-diffusion in chronic plaques and in apparently normal white matter in patients with multiple sclerosis. *Acta Neurol Scand* 87:195–199, 1993.
160. Horsfield MA, Lai M, Webb SL, et al: Apparent diffusion coefficients in benign and secondary progressive multiple sclerosis by nuclear magnetic resonance. *Magn Reson Med* 36:393–400, 1996.
161. Richards TL, Alvord EC, He Y, et al: Experimental allergic encephalomyelitis in non-human primates: Diffusion imaging of acute and chronic brain lesions. *Multiple Sclerosis* 1:109–117, 1995.

CHAPTER 18

IMAGING THE BRAIN LESIONS OF ALCOHOLICS*

Steven J. Warach
Michael E. Charness

Alcoholics are subject to a wide range of neurologic disorders caused by nutritional deficiency, toxic effects of alcohol and its metabolites, liver disease, trauma, electrolyte abnormalities, and gestational exposure to alcohol. Many of the neurologic complications of alcoholism are associated with specific pathologic lesions that can be identified by neuroimaging. This chapter considers the use of computed tomography (CT) and magnetic resonance imaging (MRI) in the clinical evaluation of the neurologic complications of alcoholism. A discussion of the use of neuroimaging to investigate the pathogenesis of brain lesions in alcoholics may be found elsewhere.[1]

WERNICKE ENCEPHALOPATHY

Wernicke encephalopathy is a common neurologic disorder caused by thiamine deficiency. In the western world, most cases occur in alcoholics.[2] Clinical recognition of Wernicke encephalopathy is straightforward when alcoholics present with the classical triad of ataxia, oculomotor disorders, and encephalopathy. However, many patients lack one or more elements of this triad, and in some the major clinical feature may be lethargy or coma.[3] These presentations of Wernicke encephalopathy are frequently misdiagnosed, particularly in malnourished patients who do not drink alcohol. Autopsy studies suggest that the diagnosis of Wernicke encephalopathy is overlooked in a majority of patients found to have the acute and chronic lesions of this disorder.[4,5] Hence, neuroimaging may be useful in suggesting or supporting the diagnosis of Wernicke encephalopathy.

The characteristic lesions of Wernicke encephalopathy occur symmetrically in structures surrounding the third ventricle, aqueduct, and fourth ventricle.[2] The mamillary bodies are involved in virtually all cases, and the dorsomedial thalamus, locus ceruleus, periaqueductal gray matter, ocular motor nuclei, and vestibular nuclei are commonly affected. Acute Wernicke lesions can be identified by endothelial prominence, microglial proliferation, and, occasionally, petechial hemorrhages. In chronic lesions, there are demyelination, gliosis, and loss of neuropil with relative preservation of neurons. Atrophy of the mamillary bodies develops in up to 80 percent of cases after acute Wernicke encephalopathy and occurs rarely in other disorders.[2]

Abnormalities on CT scans or MRIs have been reported in small numbers of patients with acute Wernicke encephalopathy. The CT scan may show symmetrical, low-density abnormalities in the diencephalon and periventricular regions (Fig. 18-1)[6–8] that enhance after the injection of contrast material (Fig. 18-2).[9] Gross hemorrhages are uncommon in acute Wernicke encephalopathy but have also been detected by CT (Fig. 18-3).[10] Symmetrical areas of increased or decreased signal in the diencephalon, midbrain, and periventricular regions are relatively uncommon in other disorders and, when present in alcoholics, should strongly suggest the diagnosis of acute Wernicke encephalopathy. However, the paucity of reports of such findings would suggest that CT is an insensitive method for their detection. Hence, a normal CT scan does not exclude the diagnosis of acute Wernicke encephalopathy.

In general, MRI appears to be more sensitive than CT in detecting acute diencephalic and periventricular lesions.[11,12] Patients with acute Wernicke encephalopathy have exhibited areas of increased T2 signal surrounding the aqueduct and third ventricle and within the medial thalamus and mamillary bodies (Fig. 18-4), consistent with the localization of the pathologic lesions.[12,13] Corresponding areas of decreased T1 signal have also been detected (Fig. 18-5).[12] The alterations in T1 and T2 signal have been shown to resolve over months, leaving an enlarged aqueduct and third ventricle (Fig. 18-6).[12] These MRI abnormalities have been reported in small numbers of patients with acute Wernicke encephalopathy. The sensitivity of MRI in detecting these lesions has not been determined; hence, a normal MRI does not rule out acute Wernicke encephalopathy. We did not observe any abnormalities in the brainstem, thalamus, or aqueduct on transaxial T2-weighted images of two patients presenting with the classical triad of Wernicke encephalopathy.[14]

*The authors' work is supported by grants from NIAAA (AA06662 to MEC), NINDS (IK08NS01634-01 to SJW), and the Medical Research Service, Department of Veterans Affairs (MEC).

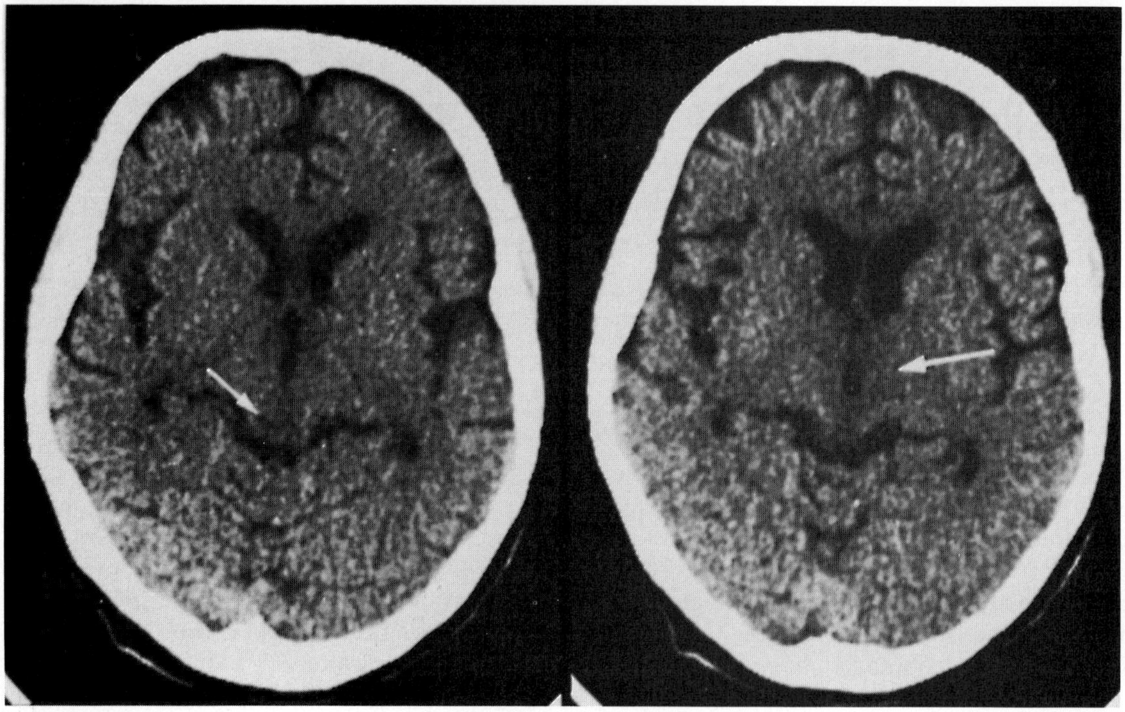

Figure 18-1
Acute Wernicke encephalopathy. CT scan showing symmetrical hypodensity in the periaqueductal gray matter and diencephalon. (From Hofmann et al.[8] Used by permission.)

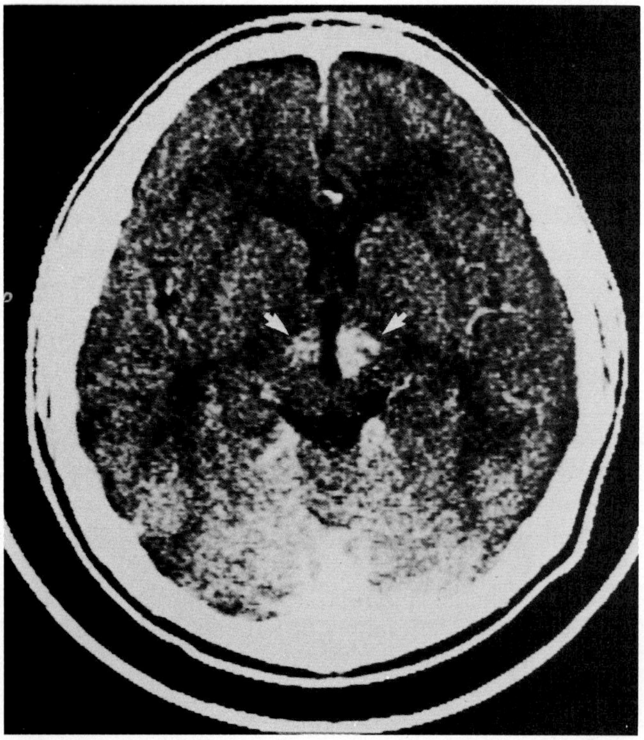

Figure 18-2
Acute Wernicke encephalopathy. CT scan showing symmetrical contrast-enhancing lesions in the thalamus bilaterally. (From Kitaguchi et al.[9] Used by permission.)

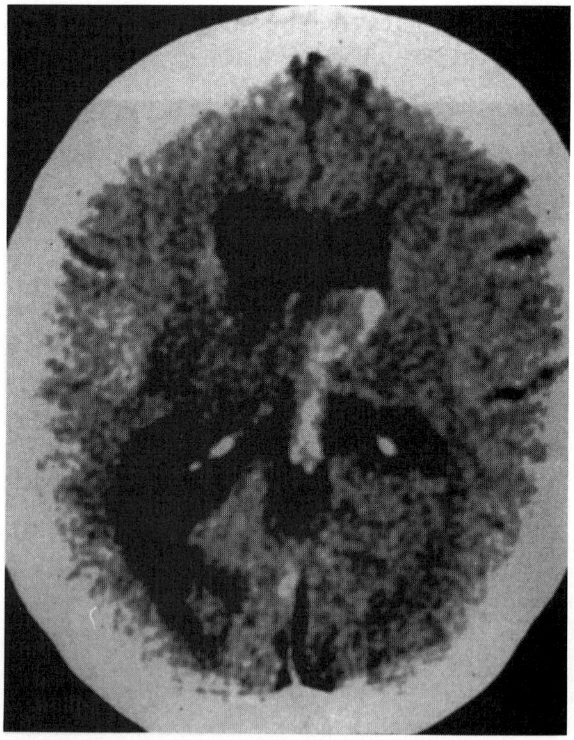

Figure 18-3
Acute Wernicke encephalopathy. CT scan showing patchy high-density abnormalities in the thalamus and fornices, consistent with hemorrhage. (From Roche et al.[10] Used by permission.)

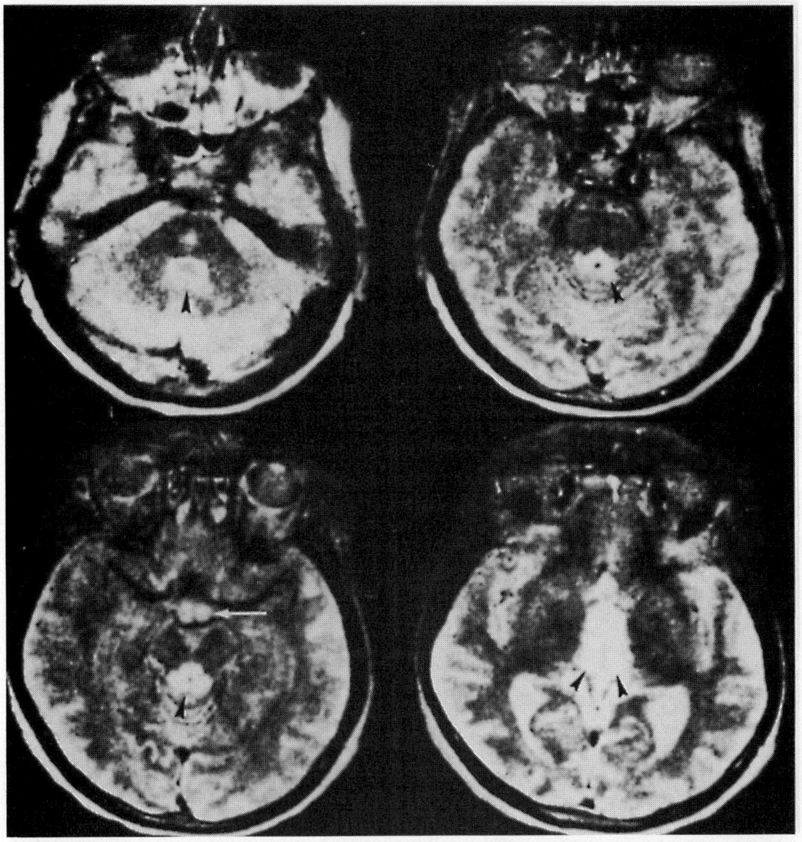

Figure 18-4
Acute Wernicke encephalopathy. MRI showing increased T2 signal surrounding the fourth ventricle (black arrow, top left) and aqueduct (black arrow, top right) and within the pertaqueductal gray (black arrow, lower left), mamillary bodies (white arrow, lower left), and thalamus (black arrows, lower right). (From Hofmann et al.[8] Used by permission.)

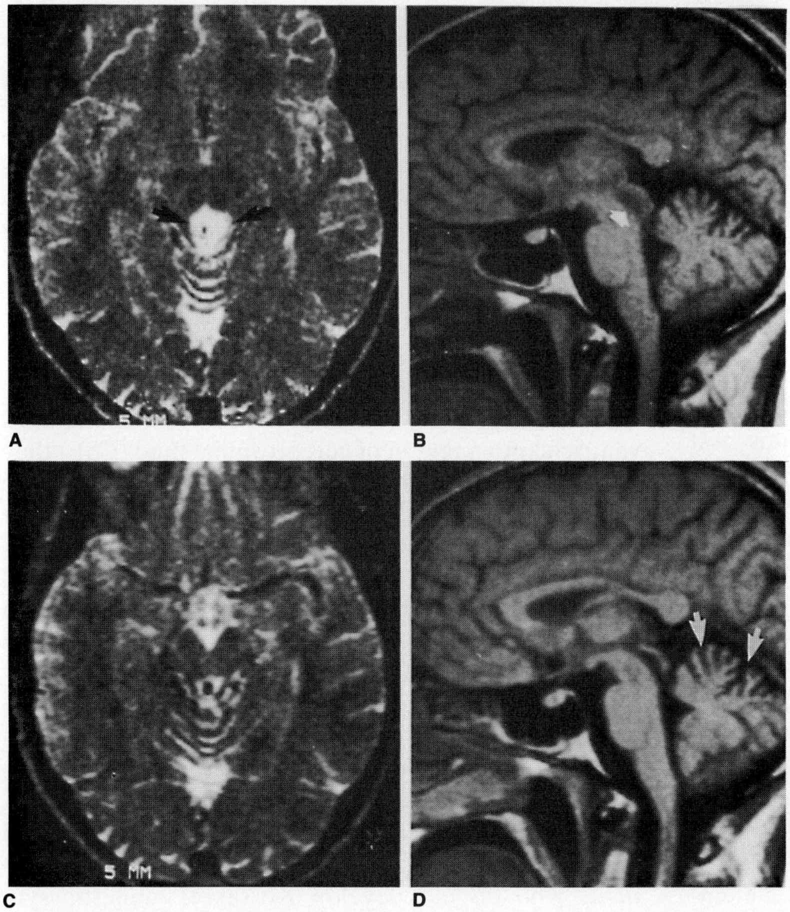

Figure 18-5
Resolution of MRI abnormalities of acute Wernicke encephalopathy. MRI shows areas of **(A)** *increased T2 signal (black arrows) and* **(B)** *decreased T1 signal (white arrow) in the periaqueductal gray matter. Nine months later, scans through the same region show* **(C and D)** *resolution of these abnormalities and* **(C)** *enlargement of the aqueduct. Note the presence of* **(D)** *anterior superior vermian atrophy (white arrow). (From Gallucci et al.[12] Used by permission.)*

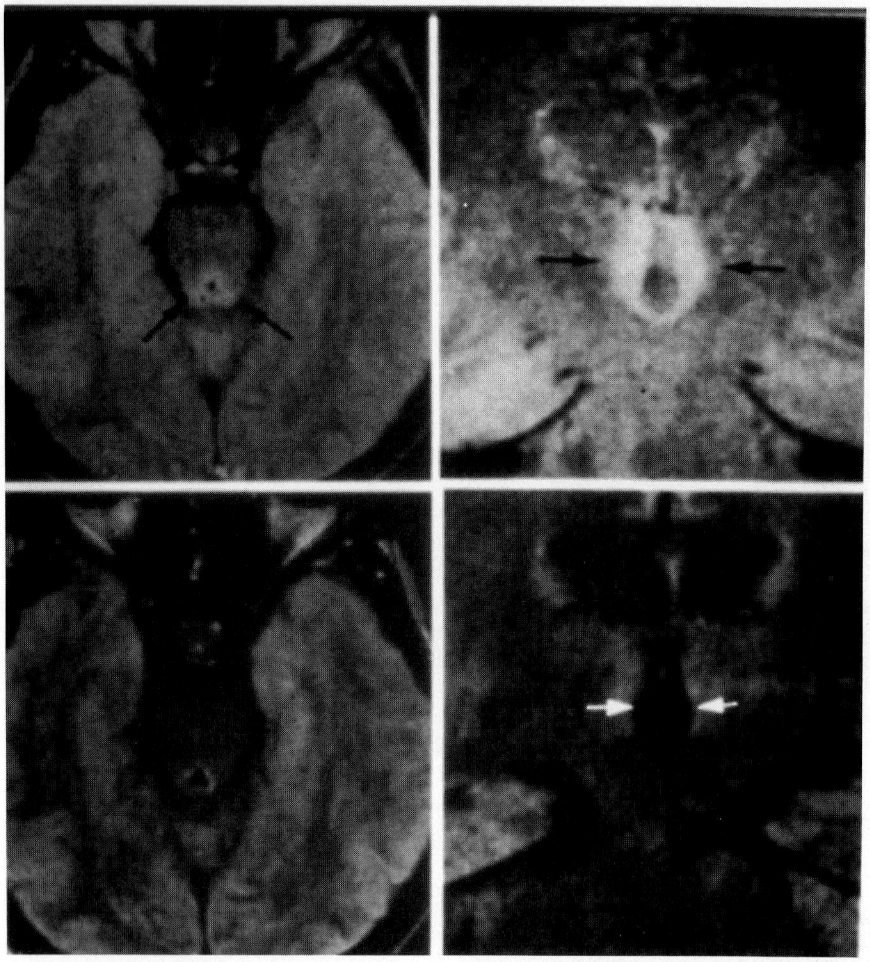

Figure 18-6
Resolution of areas of increased T2 signal in acute Wernicke encephalopathy. Increased T2 signal is seen surrounding the aqueduct (arrows, top left) and third ventricle (arrows, top right). A later study shows resolution of these abnormalities and enlargement of the aqueduct (lower left) and third ventricle (white arrows, lower right). (From Gallucci et al.[12] Used by permission.)

KORSAKOFF AMNESTIC SYNDROME

Approximately 80 percent of alcoholic patients recovering from classical Wernicke encephalopathy exhibit the selective memory disturbance of Korsakoff amnestic syndrome, which is characterized by marked deficits in anterograde and retrograde memory, apathy, an intact sensorium, and relative preservation of other intellectual abilities.[2] Korsakoff amnestic syndrome may also appear without an antecedent episode of Wernicke encephalopathy.[2,5] The memory disorder correlates best with the presence of histopathologic lesions[2] and areas of decreased density on CT scan[15] in the dorsomedial thalamus. However, Wernicke lesions have been confined to the mamillary bodies in one reported case of Korsakoff amnestic syndrome.[16]

Whereas Korsakoff amnestic syndrome is most readily recognized as a relatively selective disorder of anterograde and retrograde memory, some alcoholics with Wernicke lesions exhibit a more global abnormality of higher cognitive function. Torvik et al[4] identified Wernicke lesions at autopsy in 20 alcoholics who had been evaluated by psychiatrists during the course of their illness. Fifteen of the 20 patients were felt to have a global dementia, and only 5 had a circumscribed memory disorder; consequently, Korsakoff amnestic syndrome was diagnosed in only 3 of 20 patients, whereas Alzheimer disease was diagnosed in 8. The ability to image the chronic lesions of Wernicke encephalopathy would therefore be clinically useful in evaluating patients with selective memory loss or global dementia.

Mamillary body atrophy is a relatively specific pathologic abnormality that is found in a majority of patients with chronic lesions of Wernicke encephalopathy. Because the mamillary bodies protrude beneath the third ventricle into a region of cerebrospinal fluid (CSF) they are easily imaged by MRI, and their volume can be determined readily. A decrease in the volume of the mamillary bodies can be identified by MRI in approximately 80 percent of alcoholics with a history of classical Wernicke encephalopathy (Fig. 18-7)[14] and is not found in control subjects, Alzheimer patients, or alcoholics without a history of Wernicke encephalopathy.[14,17] Alcoholics with the Wernicke-Korsakoff syndrome have small mamillary bodies and normal hippocampal volumes, as determined by MRI, whereas the converse has been found in nonalcoholic amnestic patients.[18] A decrease in mamillary body volume may be found months after acute Wernicke encephalopathy in patients who do not develop Korsakoff amnestic syn-

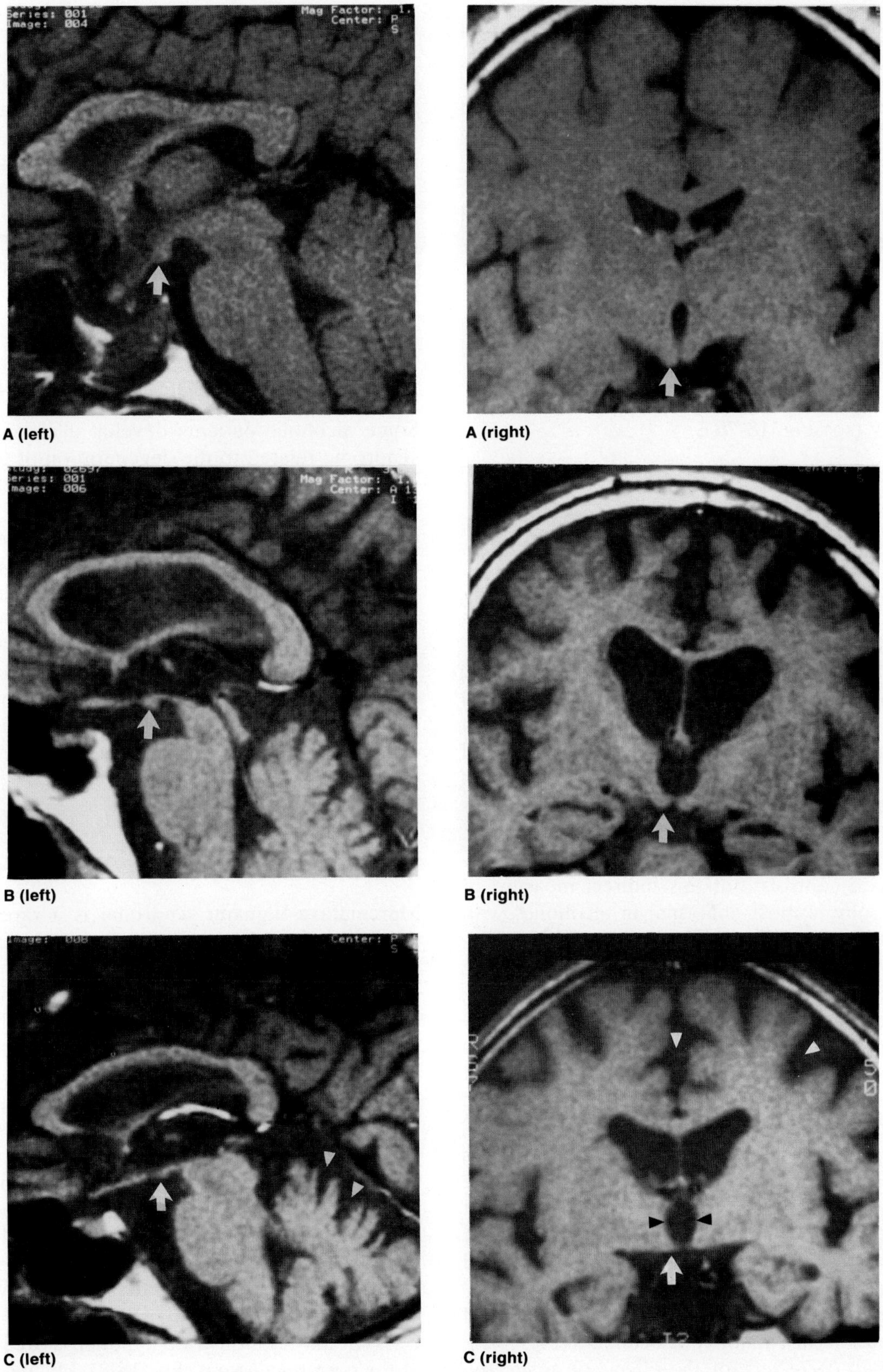

Figure 18-7

MRI of chronic Wernicke encephalopathy. **(A)** *Normal control subject.* **(B)** *Alzheimer disease.* **(C)** *Chronic Wernicke encephalopathy shown on T1-weighted sagittal (left) and coronal (right) images in the plane of the mamillary bodies (arrows). The Wernicke patient shows shrinkage of the mamillary bodies (arrows) and anterior superior cerebellar vermis (arrowheads) and enlargement of the third ventricle (black arrowheads), lateral ventricles, interhemispheric fissure (white arrowheads), and cerebral sulci (white arrowhead). Note that the Alzheimer patient exhibits greater cerebral atrophy and enlargement of the third and lateral ventricles than the Wernicke patient yet shows larger mamillary bodies. Images were acquired using TR 600, TE 25. (From Charness and DeLa Paz.[14] Used by permission.)*

drome; in contrast, one of our patients with marked memory loss had normal mamillary body volume.[14]

The finding of small mamillary bodies in a cognitively impaired patient should raise the question of alcoholism and malnutrition. The sequences required to properly demonstrate mamillary body atrophy are not those currently obtained on routine MRI studies of the brain. T1-weighted images including contiguous sagittal and coronal slices of 3 mm or less through the mamillary bodies should be requested in addition to routine views. Enlargement of the third ventricle and, by inference, shrinkage of the diencephalon has been reported in patients with chronic Wernicke encephalopathy (Figs. 18-6 and 18-7).[12,14] This finding is less specific than mamillary body atrophy in diagnosing chronic Wernicke encephalopathy (see Fig. 18-7B).

VENTRICULAR ENLARGEMENT AND COGNITIVE DYSFUNCTION IN ALCOHOLICS

Evidence that a direct neurotoxic effect of ethanol may contribute to chronic cognitive dysfunction in alcoholics has been adduced from imaging studies, neuropathologic observations, and animal experiments. Pathologic studies of the brains of alcoholics have provided mixed evidence of ethanol-induced cerebral atrophy.[2] Brain weight in alcoholics is reduced only slightly compared with that in nonalcoholics, and some workers find no differences at all.[2,14] Brain volume, estimated by the volume of the pericerebral space—the CSF-filled region between the brain and skull—is reduced in alcoholics compared with controls, but this indirect measure of cerebral atrophy is most abnormal in alcoholics with liver disease or Wernicke encephalopathy.[19] Quantitative morphometry suggests that alcoholics, including those with liver disease and Wernicke encephalopathy, lose a disproportionate amount of subcortical white matter compared with cortical gray matter.[20] This loss of cerebral white matter is also apparent when brains of nondemented alcoholics with liver disease are compared with those from patients with nonalcoholic liver disease; hence, liver disease cannot be the sole cause of this selective loss of brain tissue. The loss of cerebral white matter is evident across a wide range of ages, is not accentuated in the frontal lobes,[20] and is of sufficient magnitude (6 to 17 percent) to account for the associated ventricular enlargement.[21]

Both CT and MRI show enlargement of the cerebral ventricles and sulci in a majority of alcoholics (Fig. 18-7); however, when corrected for the effects of aging, the radiographic indexes do not correlate consistently with either the duration of drinking or the severity of cognitive impairment.[2,14] The ventricles and sulci become significantly smaller within about 1 month of abstinence,[22–24] whereas brain water, estimated by MRI[23] or chemical analysis,[25,26] does not change consistently. Based on these findings, it has been hypothesized that changes in brain parenchyma, but not brain water, may account for the reversible radiographic and cognitive abnormalities of alcoholics.[23,27] Reversible brain shrinkage, as determined by neuroimaging, has been documented after treatment of a number of other disorders, including anorexia nervosa and Cushing syndrome. The presence of ventricular enlargement on CT or MRI is too nonspecific a finding to suggest that a patient may be alcoholic.

ALCOHOLIC CEREBELLAR DEGENERATION

Some alcoholic patients develop a chronic cerebellar syndrome related to the degeneration of Purkinje cells in the cerebellar cortex.[28] Midline cerebellar structures—especially the anterior and superior vermis—are predominantly affected, a pattern that resembles the distribution of cerebellar pathology in Wernicke encephalopathy.[2] The diagnosis of alcoholic cerebellar ataxia is based on the clinical history and neurologic examination. The CT or MRI scans may, show cerebellar vermian atrophy (Figs. 18-5, 18-7, and 18-11), but one-half of alcoholic patients with this finding are not ataxic on examination.[29] Whether they represent subclinical cases in which symptoms will develop subsequently is unclear.

MARCHIAFAVA-BIGNAMI SYNDROME

Marchiafava-Bignami syndrome is a rare disorder of demyelination of necrosis of the corpus callosum and adjacent subcortical white matter that occurs predominantly in malnourished alcoholics.[2,14] In some cases there are associated lesions of Wernicke encephalopathy or selective neuronal loss and gliosis in the third cortical layer. A few cases have been described in nonalcoholics, demonstrating that ethanol alone is not responsible for the lesion. The course may be acute, subacute, or chronic and is marked by dementia, spasticity, dysarthria, and inability to walk. Patients may lapse into coma and die, survive for many years in a demented condition, or occasionally recover.[30] An interhemispheric disconnection syndrome has been reported in survivors.[30–32] The disorder was formerly diagnosed only at autopsy, but lesions can now be imaged using CT or MRI.[33] The CT scan may demonstrate hypodense areas in portions of the corpus callosum (Fig. 18-8). Magnetic resonance imaging typically shows areas of increased T2 signal (Figs. 18-9 and 18-10) or cystic areas of decreased T1 signal within the same regions (Fig. 18-10).[33] The abnormalities may be restricted to one region of the corpus callosum (Fig. 18-10) or may be present diffusely

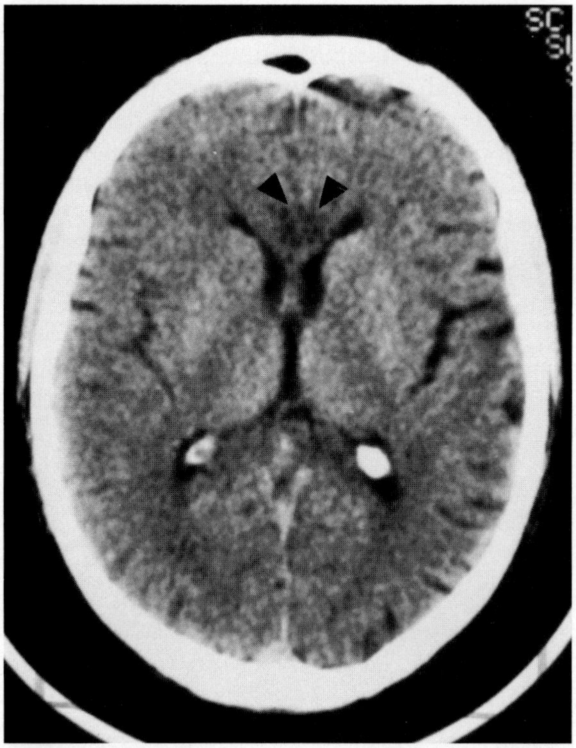

Figure 18-8
CT of Marchiafava-Bignami syndrome. There is a zone of hypodensity in the genu of the corpus callosum (arrowheads) between the anterior horns of the lateral ventricles. (Courtesy of Professor Jaques Thiébot, Centre Hospitalier Université de Rouen.)

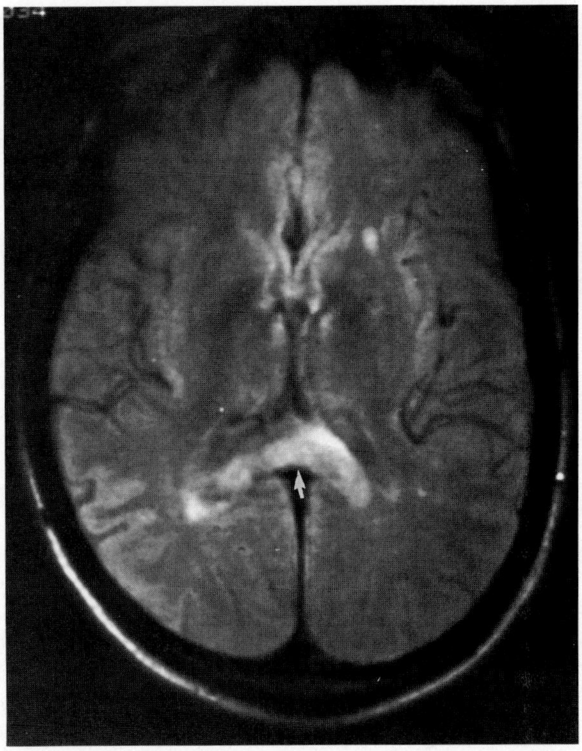

Figure 18-9
MRI of Marchiafava-Bignami syndrome. The splenium of the corpus callosum shows an area of increased T2 signal (arrow). (TR 2000, TE 40). (From Charness[48] Used by permission.)

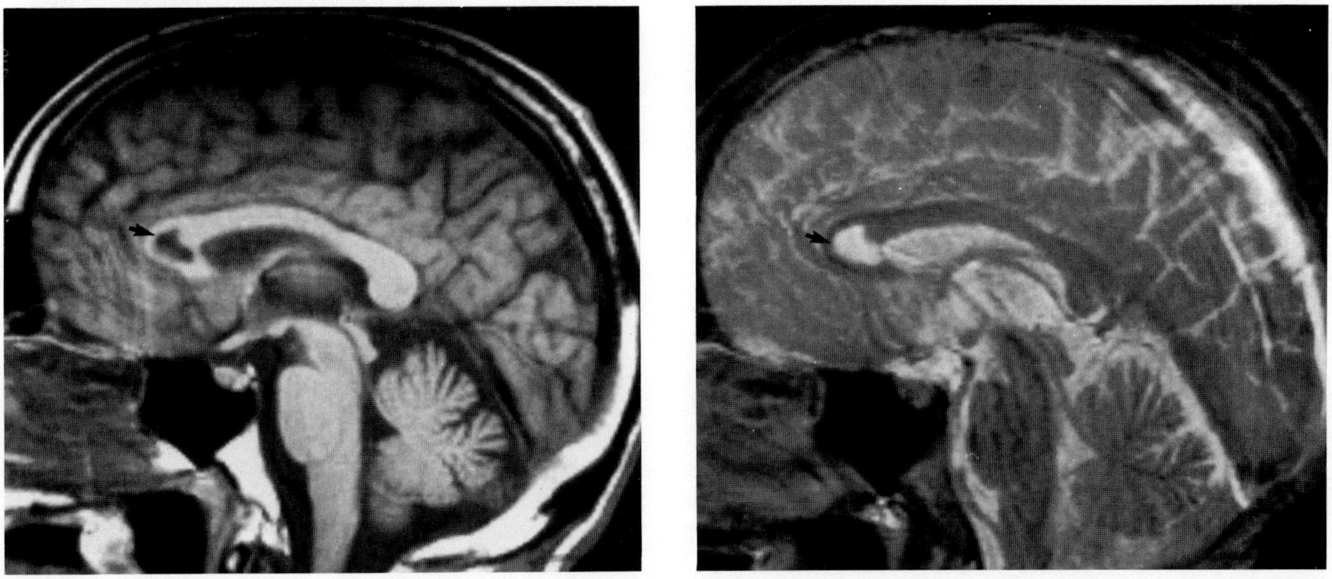

A **B**

Figure 18-10
MRI of Marchiafava-Bignami syndrome. **(A)** *T1-weighted image reveals a focal region of decreased signal within the anterior portion of the corpus callosum (arrow).* **(B)** *The corresponding T2-weighted image shows increased signal in the corresponding region. (Courtesy of Professor Jaques Thiébot, Centre Hospitalier Université de Rouen.)*

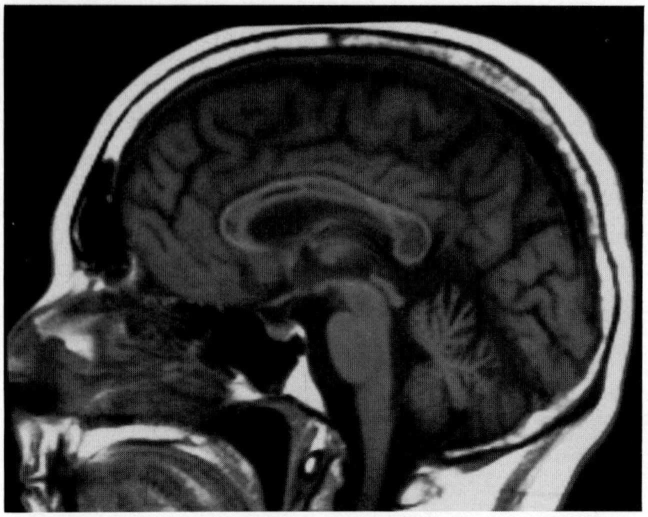

Figure 18-11
MRI of Marchiafava-Bignami syndrome. T1-weighted image shows a cystic region of decreased signal throughout the corpus callosum. There is also atrophy of the mamillary bodies and anterior superior cerebellar vermis. (Courtesy of Professor Jaques Thiébot, Centre Hospitalier Université de Rouen.)

throughout the corpus callosum (Fig. 18-11). The CT and MRI findings may persist after the resolution of clinical signs.[30]

CENTRAL PONTINE MYELINOLYSIS

Central pontine myelinolysis is a disorder of cerebral white matter that usually affects alcoholics but also occurs in nonalcoholics with liver disease, including Wilson disease, malnutrition, anorexia, burns, cancer, Addison disease, and severe electrolyte disorders, such as thiazide-induced hyponatremia.[2,34] Central pontine myelinolysis is frequently associated with a rapid correction of hyponatremia; however, the majority of cases occur in alcoholics, suggesting that alcoholism may contribute to the genesis of central pontine myelinolysis in as yet undefined ways.

The most common macroscopic lesion is a triangular region of pallor in the base of the pons. Approximately 10 percent of cases also show symmetrical extrapontine lesions, most frequently in the striatum, thalamus, cerebellum, and cerebral white matter.[35] Microscopic examination reveals demyelinated axons with preserved cell bodies except in the center of lesions, which may reveal cavitation. Symptoms and signs of central pontine myelinolysis may be absent[34] or obscured by associated conditions, such as ethanol withdrawal, Wernicke encephalopathy, or hepatic encephalopathy. Treatment of these disorders may lead to an initial improvement in mental status, followed within days by confusion, lethargy, and coma due to central pontine myelinolysis. Involvement of the corticospinal tracts causes paraparesis or quadriparesis, and demyelination of the corticobulbar tracts leads to dysarthria, dysphagia, and inability to protrude the tongue. The tendon reflexes may be increased, decreased, or normal, and Babinski signs may be present. Disorders of

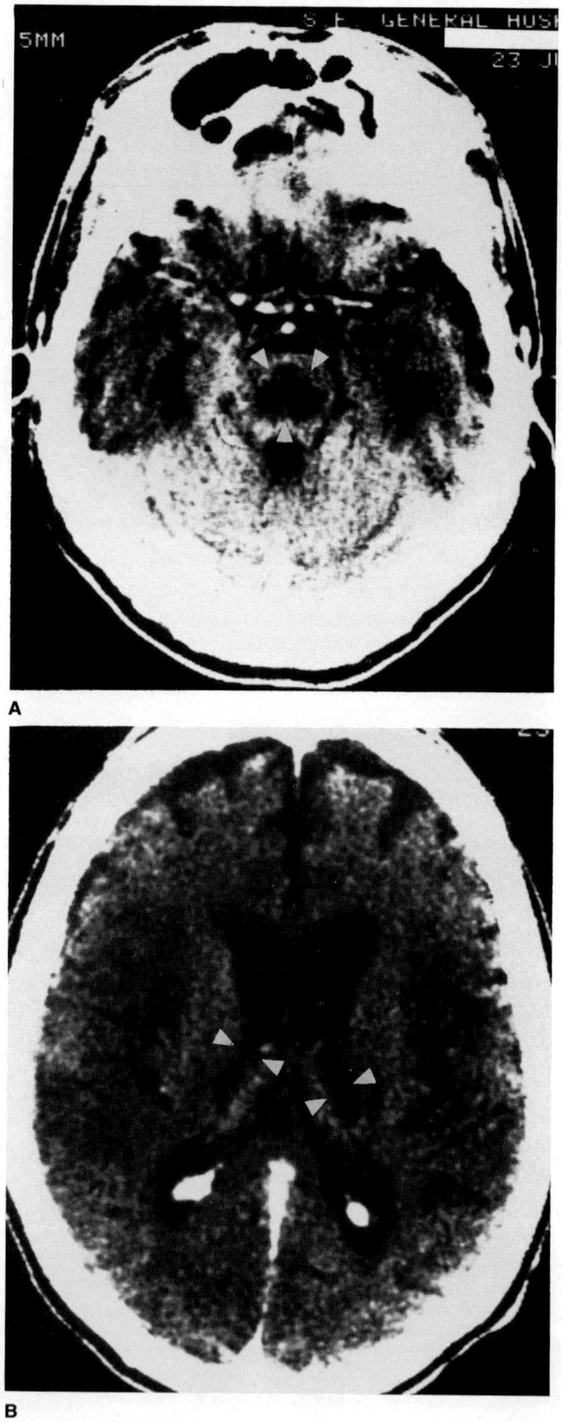

A

B

Figure 18-12
CT of pontine and extrapontine myelinolysis in an alcoholic man. There is **(A)** *a large lucent area in the central portion of the pons and* **(B)** *a symmetrical region of decreased signal intensity in the thalamus bilaterally (arrowheads). This patient's symptoms and signs appeared following rapid correction of hyponatremia.*

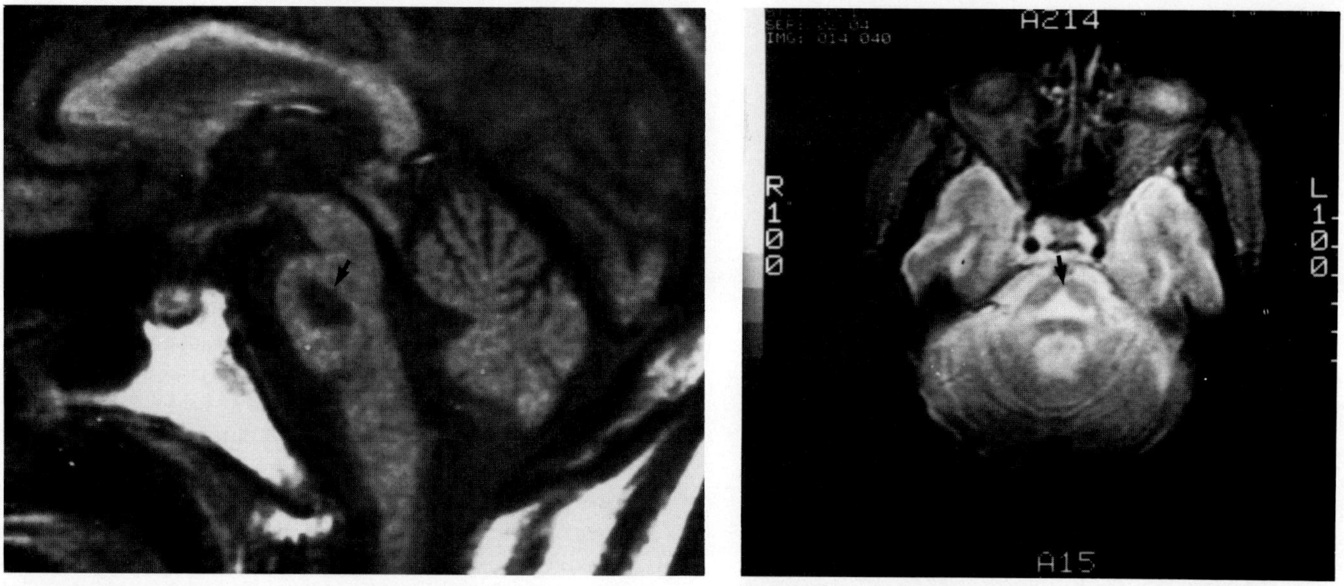

A B

Figure 18-13
MRI of central pontine myelinolysis in an alcoholic man. **(A)** *T1-weighted sagittal image (TR 600, TE 25) reveals a sharply delineated zone of decreased signal in the midpons.* **(B)** *An axial image through the same region shows a triangular area of increased T2 signal (TR 2000, TE 70). (From Charness.[45] Used by permission.)*

conjugate eye movement occur occasionally and may reflect extension of the lesion in the pons or associated Wernicke lesions. Disproportionate involvement of motor function may produce the "locked-in" syndrome, with only limited ability to move the limbs or face despite a normal level of consciousness.[36]

The lesions of central pontine myelinolysis can be visualized using CT scanning (Fig. 18-12) or MRI. While MRI is more sensitive than CT in imaging the pontine lesions, even MRI may be unremarkable early in the course of central pontine myelinolysis.[37] The most common MRI finding is an area of decreased T1 signal or increased T2 signal within the basis pontis (Figs. 18-13 and 18-14).[11,37] Symmetrical extrapontine abnormalities have also been detected by CT and MRI in patients suspected of having central pontine myelinolysis (Figs. 18-12 and 18-15).[37,38] Other disorders, such as multiple sclerosis, multi-infarct dementia, and encephalitis, may produce areas of increased T2 signal in the pons that resemble those of central pontine myelinolysis (Fig. 18-16) but also cause significant periventricular abnormalities and a distinctive clinical picture.[37] Serial CT or

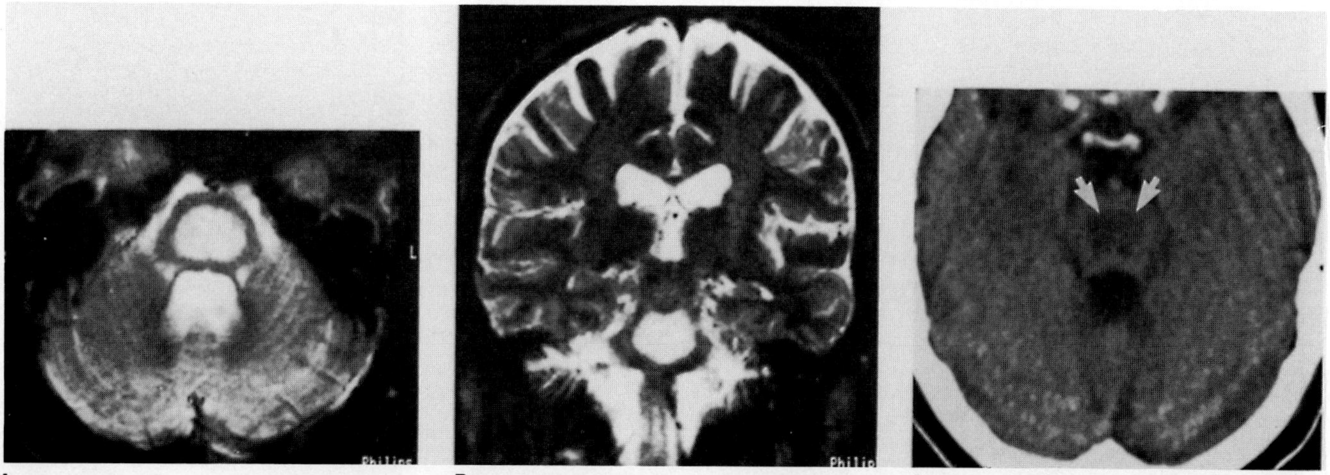

A B C

Figure 18-14
Corresponding CT and MRI images in a patient with central pontine myelinolysis. There is a large area of increased T2 signal intensity in the midpons seen in both **(A)** *axial and* **(B)** *coronal sections.* **(C)** *A corresponding axial CT image shows a similar region of decreased signal intensity (white arrows). (From Ostertun et al.[11] Used by permission.)*

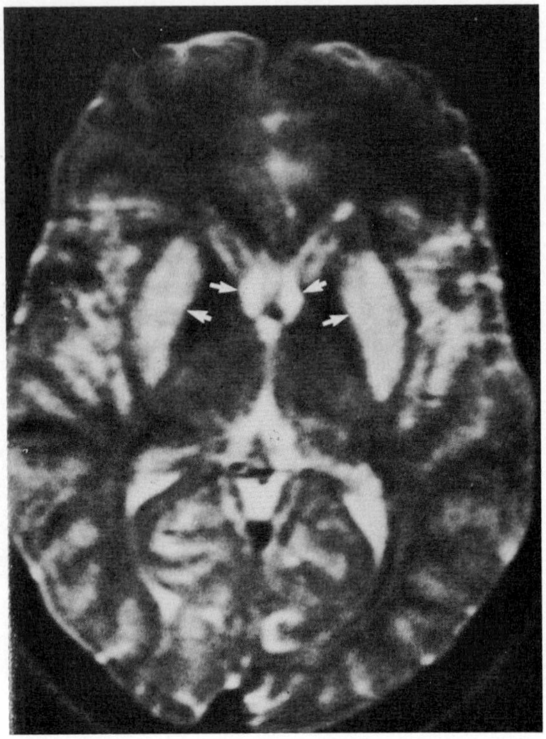

Figure 18-15
MRI showing symmetrical areas of increased T2 signal (arrows) in the striatum of a patient with pontine and extrapontine myelinolysis. (From Miller et al.[37] Used by permission.)

MRI studies indicate that the radiographic lesions of central pontine myelinolysis may resolve in parallel with a patient's recovery;[37] hence, the absence of lesions on MRI does not exclude a past episode of central pontine myelinolysis. Because small lesions of central pontine myelinolysis may be asymptomatic, typical MRI abnormalities can be an incidental finding in seriously ill patients.

ETHANOL NEUROTOXICITY IN THE DEVELOPING NERVOUS SYSTEM

Brain lesions in alcoholics may in some instances antedate birth. Alcoholism runs in families, and many alcoholics have been exposed to high concentrations of alcohol during critical stages of brain development. The fetal alcohol syndrome is characterized by pre- and postnatal growth retardation, microcephaly, neurologic abnormalities, facial dysmorphology, and other congenital anomalies.[39,40] More often, heavy intrauterine exposure to ethanol is associated with a constellation of less severe abnormalities, "fetal alcohol effects," including mental retardation, intrauterine growth retardation, and minor, ungrouped congenital anomalies involving the cutaneous, genitourinary, musculoskeletal, and cardiac systems.[40] Neuropathologic examination in fetal alcohol syndrome reveals microcephaly, cerebellar dysplasia, agenesis of the corpus callosum, and neuronal-glial heterotopias,[41,42] all lesions consistent with the decreased proliferation and disordered migration of neurons. Magnetic resonance imaging in a small number of children with fetal alcohol syndrome has identified agenesis or hypoplasia of the corpus callosum and selective reductions in the volume of the cerebrum, cerebellum, and basal ganglia (Fig. 18-17).[43,44] Agenesis of the corpus callosum occurs infrequently in the general population, and its presence on MRI in the retarded offspring of an alcoholic mother should suggest the possibility of a neurodevelopmental abnormality related to gestational alcohol exposure.

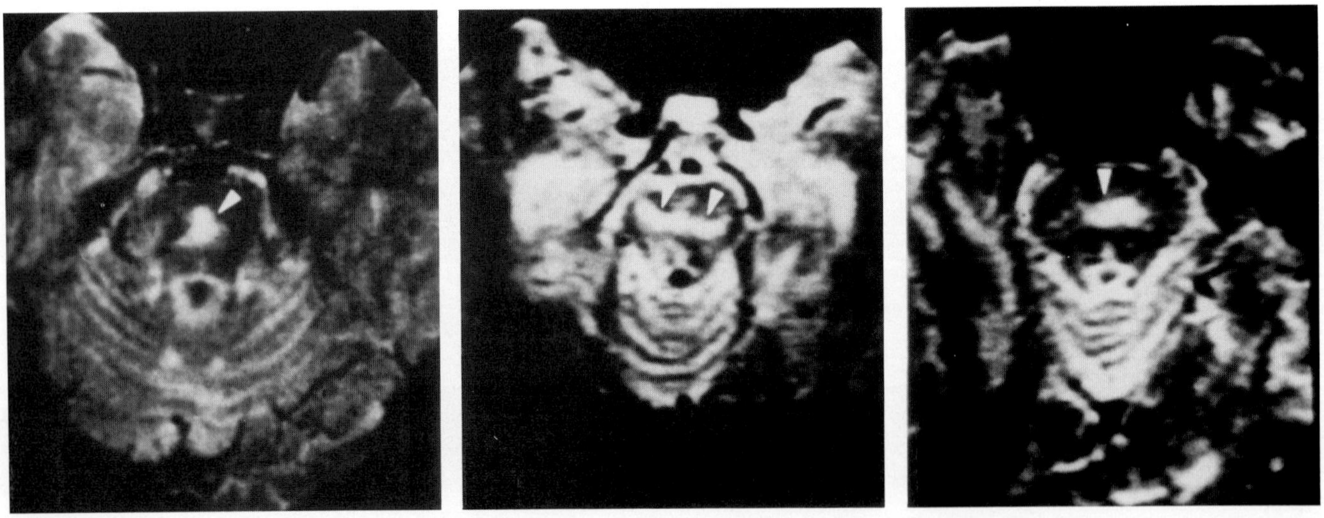

A B C

Figure 18-16
Midpontine areas of increased T2 signal in patients with **(A)** *dementia,* **(B)** *normal pressure hydrocephalus, and* **(C)** *brainstem infarction. None of these patients was believed to have central pontine myelinolysis. (From Miller et al.[37] Used by permission.)*

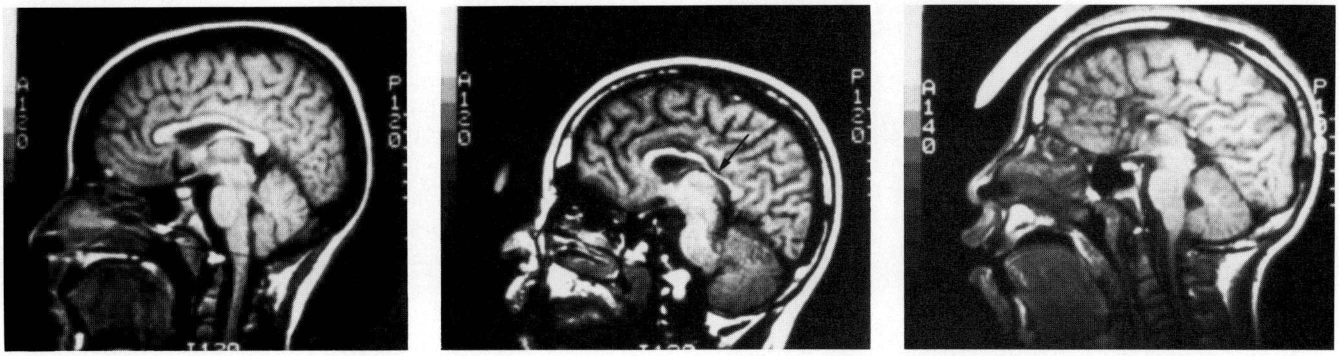
A B C

Figure 18-17
MRI showing agenesis of the corpus callosum after gestational exposure to alcohol. **(A)** *Normal 13-year-old female.* **(B)** *A 13-year-old male with fetal alcohol syndrome and focal thinning (arrow) of the corpus callosum.* **(C)** *A 14-year-old male with fetal alcohol syndrome and agenesis of the corpus callosum. (Courtesy of Dr. Edward P. Riley, San Diego State University.)*

THE ROLE OF NEUROIMAGING IN THE EVALUATION OF NEUROLOGIC DISORDERS IN ALCOHOLICS

Seizures

Generalized tonic clonic seizures occur in alcoholics, particularly during the first 48 h after the cessation of drinking. Seizures are brief, may recur within a period of 6 to 12 h, and are usually self-limited. If the patient has recovered completely within this period of time and has a clear history of recent alcohol withdrawal and a normal neurologic examination, then neuroimaging studies are unlikely to demonstrate a cerebral lesion.[45,46] In contrast, prolonged or widely separated seizures, focal seizures, prolonged postictal state, or a focally abnormal neurologic examination should prompt a search for correctable structural lesions, metabolic abnormalities, or infection. Computed tomography is an excellent means of excluding subdural hematoma (Fig. 18-18) or traumatic intracerebral hemorrhage.

Encephalopathy or Dementia

Alcoholics are at increased risk of developing large number of toxic, metabolic, and infectious disorders that produce encephalopathy. Because Wernicke encephalopathy is frequently overlooked and easily treated, thiamine should be administered parenterally to all encephalopathic patients, including those not felt to be alcoholic or malnourished. The presence of symmetrical diencephalic, midbrain, or periventricular abnormalities on T2-weighted MRIs may help suggest or confirm the diagnosis of acute Wernicke encephalopathy in atypical cases. In most demented patients, CT will be adequate to exclude mass lesions or multiple infarcts. In some cases, the contribution of alcoholism or nutritional deficiency to cognitive dysfunction will be unclear from the history and examination. For these patients, the finding of mamillary body atrophy on T1-weighted MRIs suggest that past thiamine deficiency has contributed to the clinical disorder. Rarely, such scans will also reveal evidence of Marchiafava-Bignami syndrome.

Gait Ataxia

Gait ataxia in a detoxified alcoholic may indicate Wernicke encephalopathy or alcoholic cerebellar degeneration. T2-weighted MRI may show evidence of ongoing thiamine deficiency, and T1-weighted images may demonstrate mamillary body atrophy. The midsagittal and parasagittal scans obtained to image the mamillary bodies will also provide a good view of the cerebellar vermis. While predisposed to toxic and nutritional cerebellar degeneration, alcoholics are not immune to other causes

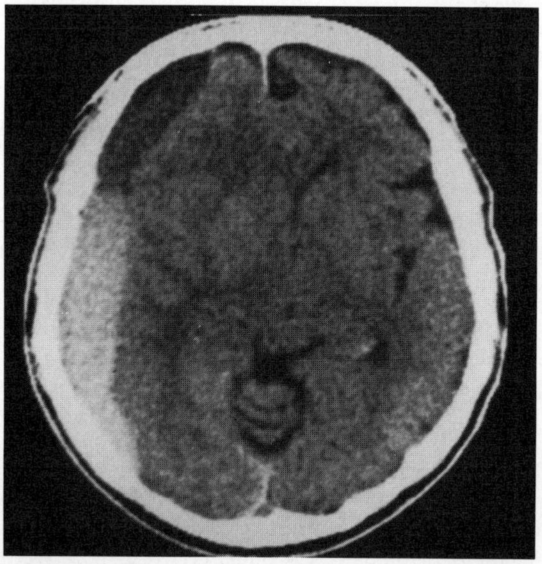

Figure 18-18
CT scan showing right subdural hematoma.

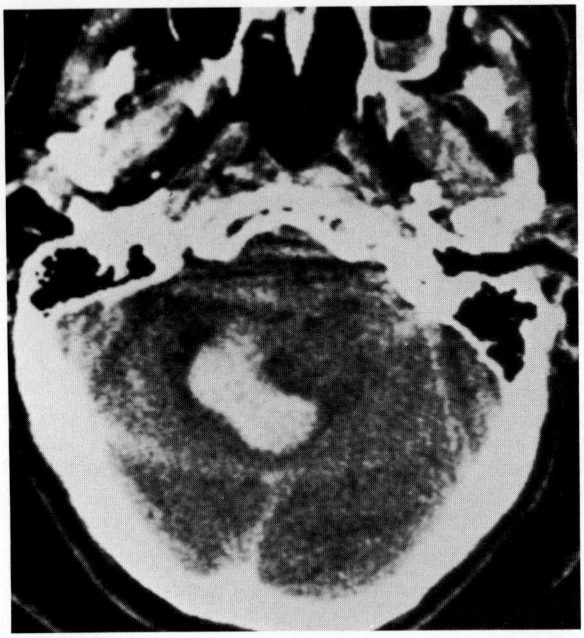

Figure 18-19
CT scan showing cerebellar hemorrhage in an ataxic alcoholic.

of cerebellar dysfunction. We have seen cerebellar hemorrhage overlooked in the emergency department in intoxicated alcoholics who present with gait ataxia and minimal headache (Fig. 18-19). Hence, one should carefully consider all causes of cerebellar dysfunction in alcoholics with gait ataxia and obtain imaging studies where appropriate.

Trauma

Alcoholics frequently present to emergency departments intoxicated and with evidence of external head trauma. It may be difficult in these cases to exclude on clinical grounds that their encephalopathy is caused by cerebral trauma. The encephalopathy associated with ethanol withdrawal can obscure the findings of subdural hematoma.[47] The decision to obtain a neuroimaging study will depend on particular details of the case; however, CT is now widely available and is a good screening test to exclude cerebral trauma. Bone windows should be carefully reviewed to identify basal skull fractures, which may predispose to meningitis.

REFERENCES

1. Zakhari S, Witt E (ed): *Imaging in Alcohol Research.* National Institute on Alcohol Abuse and Alcoholism Research monograph 21, DHHS publ (ADM)92-1890. Washington, Government Printing Office, 1992.
2. Victor M, Adams RA, Collins GH (ed): *The Wernicke-Korsakoff Syndrome and Related Disorders Due to Alcoholism and Malnutrition.* Philadelphia, FA Davis, 1989.
3. Charness ME, Simon RP, Greenberg DA: Ethanol and the nervous system. *N Engl J Med* 321:442, 1989.
4. Torvik A, Lindboe CF, Rodge S: Brain lesions in alcoholics: A neuropathological study with clinical correlation. *J Neurol Sci* 56:233, 1982.
5. Harper CG: The incidence of Wernicke's encephalopathy in Australia. A neuropathological study of 131 cases. *J Neurol Neurosurg Psychiatry* 46:593, 1983.
6. McDowell JR, LeBlanc HJ: Computed tomographic findings in Wernicke-Korsakoff syndrome. *Arch Neurol* 41: 453, 1984.
7. Mensing JWA, Hoogland PH, Sloof JL: Computed tomography in the diagnosis of Wernicke's encephalopathy: A radiological-neuropathological correlation. *Ann Neurol* 16:363, 1984.
8. Hofmann E, Friedburg H, Rasenack J, et al: Wernicke's encephalopathy on CT and MR (German). *ROFO* 148: 97, 1988.
9. Kitaguchi T, Kobayashi T, Tobimatsu S, et al: Computed tomography and magnetic resonance imaging in a young patient with Wernicke's encephalopathy. *J Neurol* 234: 449, 1987.
10. Roche SW, Lane RJ, Wade JP: Thalamic hemorrhages in Wernicke-Korsakoff syndrome demonstrated by computed tomography (letter). *Ann Neurol* 23:312, 1988.
11. Ostertun B, Dewes W, Hanisch E, Harder T: MR tomography and computer tomography of alcohol-induced brain tissue changes (German). *ROFO* 152:87, 1990.
12. Gallucci M, Bozzao A, Splendiani A, et al: Wernicke encephalopathy: MR findings in five patients (see comments). *Am J Roentgenol* 155:1309, 1990.
13. Yokote K, Miyagi K, Kuzuhara S, et al: Wernicke encephalopathy: Follow-up study by CT and MR. *J Comput Assist Tomogr* 15:835, 1991.
14. Charness ME, DeLaPaz RL: Mamillary body atrophy in Wernicke's encephalopathy: Antemortem identification using magnetic resonance imaging. *Ann Neurol* 22:595, 1987.
15. Shimamura AP, Jernigan TL, Squire LR: Korsakoff's syndrome: Radiological (CT) findings and neuropsychological correlates. *J Neurosci* 8:4400, 1988.
16. Pittella JE, de Castro LP: Wernicke's encephalopathy manifested as Korsakoff's syndrome in a patient with promyelocytic leukemia. *South Med J* 83:570, 1990.
17. Charness ME, DeLaPaz RL: Periodic alternating nystagmus in an alcoholic with small mammillary bodies. *Neurology* 38(suppl):421, 1988.
18. Squire LR, Amaral DG, Press GA: Magnetic resonance imaging of the hippocampal formation and mammillary nuclei distinguish medial temporal lobe and diencephalic amnesia. *J Neurosci* 10:3106, 1990.
19. Harper CG, Kril JJ: Brain atrophy in chronic alcoholic patients: A quantitative pathological study. *J Neurol Neurosurg Psychiatry* 48:211, 1985.
20. Harper CG, Kril JJ, Holloway RL: Brain shrinkage in chronic alcoholics: A pathological study. *Br Med J* 290:501, 1985.
21. de la Monte SM: Disproportionate atrophy of cerebral white matter in chronic alcoholics. *Arch Neurol* 45:990, 1988.
22. Carlen PL, Wortzman G, Holgate RC, et al: Reversible

cerebral atrophy in recently abstinent chronic alcoholics measured by computed tomography scans. *Science* 200: 1076, 1978.
23. Schroth G, Naegele T, Klose U, et al: Reversible brain shrinkage in abstinent alcoholics, measured by MRI. *Neuroradiology* 30:385, 1988.
24. Zipursky RB, Lim KO, Pfefferbaum A: MRI study of brain changes with short-term abstinence from alcohol. *Alcohol Clin Exp Res* 13:664, 1989.
25. Harper C, Krill JJ, Daly JM: Brain shrinkage in alcoholics is not caused by changes in hydration: A pathological study. *J Neurol Neurosurg Psychiatry* 51:124, 1988.
26. Harper CG, Kril JJ, Daly J: Does a "moderate" alcohol intake damage the brain? *J Neurol Neurosurg Psychiatry* 51:909, 1988.
27. Carlen PL, Wilkinson DA, Wortzman G, Holgate R: Partially reversible cerebral atrophy and functional improvement in recently abstinent alcoholics. *Can J Neurol Sci* 11:441, 1984.
28. Victor M, Adams RD, Mancall EL: A restricted form of cerebellar cortical degeneration occurring in alcoholic patients. *Arch Neurol* 76:579, 1956.
29. Hillborn M, Muuronen A, Holm L, Hindmarsh T: The clinical versus radiological diagnosis of alcoholic cerebellar degeneration. *J Neurol Sci* 73:45, 1986.
30. Delangre T, Hannequin D, Clavier E, et al: Maladie de Marchiafava-Bignami d'evolution favorable. *Rev Neurol (Paris)* 142:933, 1986.
31. Clavier E, Thiebot J, Delangre T, et al: Marchiafava-Bignami disease: A case studied by CT and MR imaging. *Neuroradiology* 28:376, 1986.
32. Rosa A, Demiati M, Cartz L, Mizon JP: Marchiafava-Bignami disease, syndrome of interhemispheric disconnection, and right-handed agraphia in a left-hander. *Arch Neurol* 48:986, 1991.
33. Kawamura M, Shiota J, Yagishita T, Mirayama K: Marchiafava-Bignami disease: Computed tomographic scan and magnetic resonance imaging. *Ann Neurol* 18:103, 1985.
34. Adams RD, Victor M, Mancall EL: Central pontine myelinolysis: A hitherto undescribed disease occurring in alcoholic and malnourished patients. *Arch Neurol* 81: 154, 1959.
35. Wright DG, Laureno R, Victor M: Pontine and extrapontine myelinolysis. *Brain* 102:361, 1979.
36. Messert B, Orrison WW, Hawkins MJ, Quaglieri CE: Central pontine myelinolysis: Considerations on etiology, diagnosis, and treatment. *Neurology* 29:147, 1979.
37. Miller GM, Baker HL, Okazaki H, Whisnant JP: Central pontine myelinolysis and its imitators: MR findings. *Radiology* 168:795, 1988.
38. Dickoff DJ, Raps M, Yahr MD: Striatal syndrome following hyponatremia and its rapid correction. *Arch Neurol* 45:112, 1988.
39. Streissguth AP, Landesman-Dwyer S, Martin JC, Smith DW: Teratogenic effects of alcohol in humans and laboratory animals. *Science* 209:353, 1980.
40. Rosett HL, Weiner L (ed): *Alcohol and the Fetus.* New York, Oxford, 1984.
41. Jones KL, Smith DW: Recognition of the fetal alcohol syndrome in early infancy. *Lancet* 2:999, 1973.
42. Clarren SK, Alvord EJ, Sumi SM, et al: Brain malformations related to prenatal exposure to ethanol. *J Pediatr* 92:64, 1978.
43. Mattson SN, Riley EP, Jernigan TL, Jones EK: Magnetic resonance imaging of children with fetal alcohol syndrome. *Alcohol Clin Exp Res* 16:369, 1992.
44. Gabrielli O, Salvolini U, Coppa GV, et al: Magnetic resonance imaging in the malformative syndromes with mental retardation. *Pediatr Radiol* 21:16, 1990.
45. Feussner JR, Linfors EW, Blessing CL, Starmer CF: Computed tomography brain scanning in alcohol withdrawal seizures: Value of the neurologic examination. *Ann Intern Med* 94:519, 1981.
46. Earnest MP, Feldman H, Marx JA, et al: Intracranial lesions shown by CT scans in 259 cases of first alcohol-related seizures. *Neurology* 38:1561, 1988.
47. Koranyi EK, Ravindran A, Seguin J: Alcohol withdrawal concealing symptoms of subdural hematoma: A caveat. *Psychiatr J Univ Ottawa* 15:15, 1990.
48. Charness ME: Brain lesions in alcoholics. *Alcohol Clin Exp Res* 17:2, 1993.

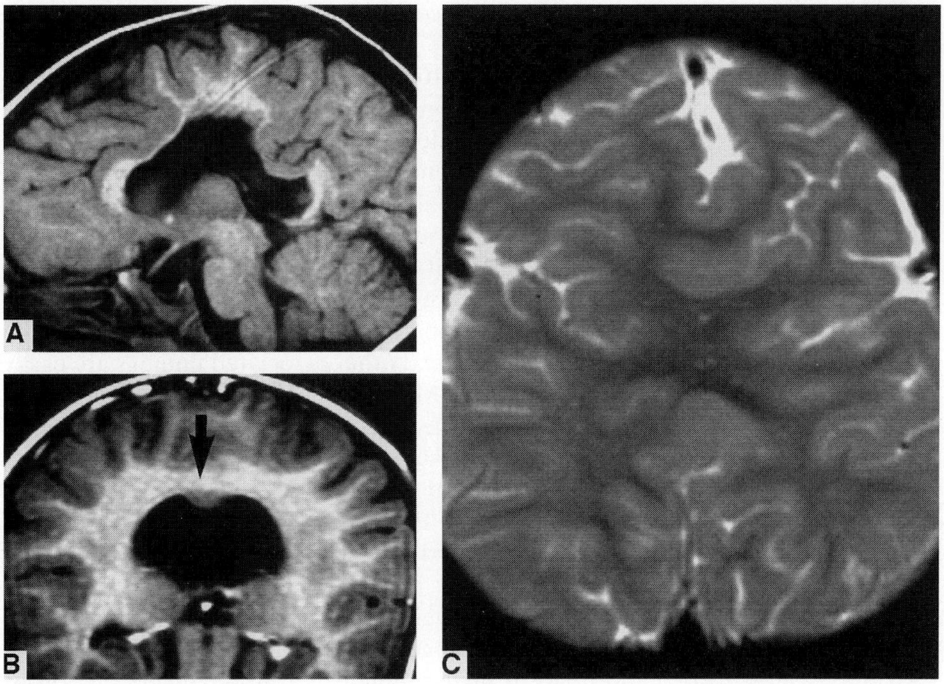

Figure 19-9
Dorsal lobar holoprosencephaly. Fusion of the gray and white matter is present only in the posterior frontal region (axial T2-weighted image, C). **(A)** *Sagittal T1-weighted image shows a dysplastic midcallosal body at the level of fusion.* **(B)** *On coronal T1-weighted image, the septum pellucidum is absent and there is a gray matter heterotopion in the subependymal region of the roof of the common ventricle (black arrow).*

is characterized by some fusion of the frontal white matter across the midline and a dysplastic anterior falx, although the posterior falx and interhemispheric fissure are well formed (Fig. 19-8). The frontal horns of the lateral ventricles show variable degrees of dysplasia. As in all forms of holoprosencephaly the septum pellucidum is absent. Dysplasia of the anterior corpus callosum is less severe than in the semilobar form.[45]

Finally, dorsal lobar holoprosencephaly, also termed middle interhemispheric fusion and syntelencephaly, is a recently described prosencephaly variant.[46] This form of prosencephaly is characterized by fusion of the cerebral hemispheres across the frontal convexities, with partially developed interhemispheric falx and fissure.[13] There is dysgenesis of the mid-callosal body at the level of hemispheric fusion, and, as in all cases of holoprosencephaly, there is absence of the septum pellucidum (Fig. 19-9).

Septo-optic Dysplasia

As initially described by DeMorsier, septo-optic dysplasia consists of optic nerve hypoplasia and absence or hypoplasia of the septum pellucidum (Fig. 19-10).[47] Ap-

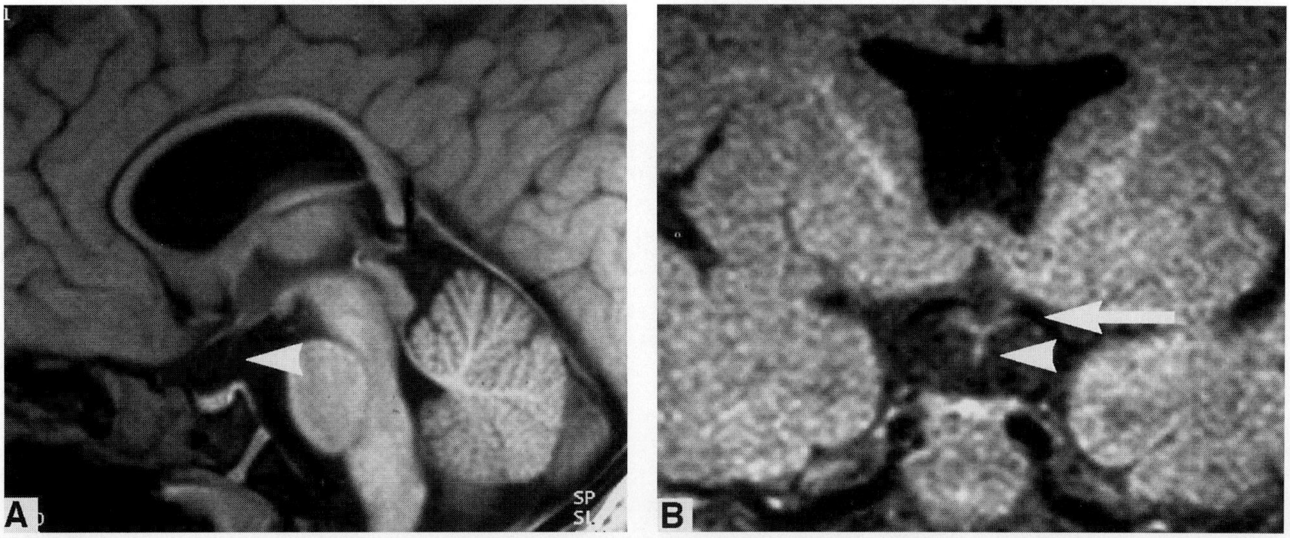

Figure 19-10
Septo-otpic dysplasia. **(A)** *T1-weighted sagittal and* **(B)** *coronal images demonstrate an absent septum pellucidum, a very thin infundibulum (white arrowheads), and a very small optic chasm (white arrows).*

proximately two-thirds of patients have hypothalamic-pituitary dysfunction manifested as growth retardation due to decreased secretion of growth hormone and thyroid-stimulating hormone.[48,49] However, the full triad of findings is not always seen: the septum pellucidum may be present in 40 percent of patients,[50] and up to 50 percent of patients do not have a hypoplastic optic nerve or chiasm.[51] Gray matter heterotopia and schizencephaly may be seen in up to 50 percent of patients with septo-optic dysplasia.[51]

Malformations of the Corpus Callosum

The sequence of development of the corpus callosum has received considerable attention in the neuroradiology literature lately. The manner in which this structure develops is important in differentiating anomalies of formation from destructive processes of the corpus callosum. The previously accepted theory stated that the corpus callosum developed from an anterior-to-posterior direction starting with the genu, followed by the body splenium and, finally, the rostrum.[52,53] However, recent phylogenetic, embryologic, and anatomic, studies suggest that the corpus callosum develops bidirectionally starting at the genu–anterior body junction;[54,55] furthermore, these studies showed that parts of the rostrum are actually among the first structures of the corpus callosum to develop.

The most common form of callosal hypogenesis is characterized by absent splenium. The rostral end of a hypogenetic corpus callosum may resemble a small genu; however, it is believed that this appearance is due to persistence of the fetal genu in its early, more posterior position.[54] Agenesis or hypogenesis of the corpus callosum and other associated findings are easily recognizable on MRIs (Fig. 19-11).[23,53,54,56] Sagittal and coronal images demonstrate absence or hypoplasia of the corpus callosum and typical steerhorn continuation of the lateral ventricles secondary to medially located bundles of Probst. In the absence of the corpus callosum, the third ventricle extends superiorly into the interhemispheric fissure, where an interhemispheric cyst may form. Sagittal images demonstrate a characteristic radial arrangement of midline sulci due to abnormally formed cingulate gyri. Anomalies of the corpus callosum are frequently accompanied by other brain

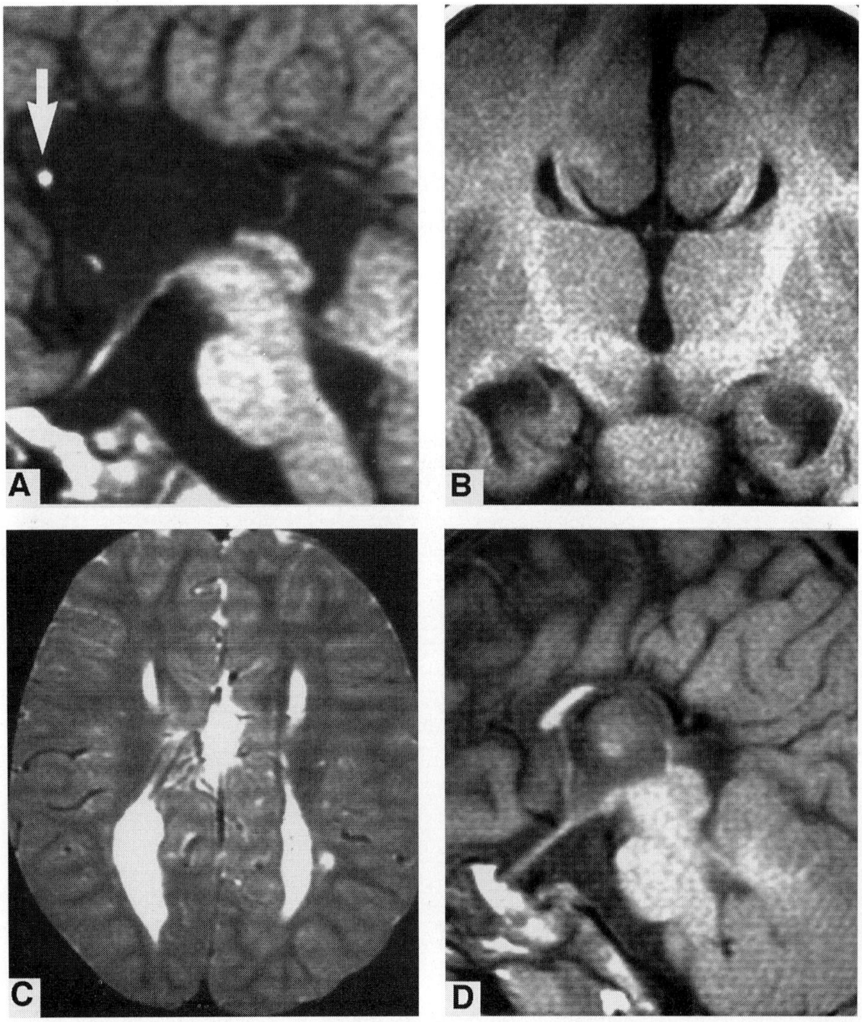

Figure 19-11
Agenesis and hypogenesis of the corpus callosum. T1-weighted **(A)** *sagittal and* **(B)** *coronal images and* **(C)** *an axial T2-weighted image show nearly complete agenesis of the corpus callosum (white arrows in* **A***).* **(D)** *A sagittal T1-weighted image in another patient shows severe hypoplasia of the corpus callosum. A coronal image shows a typical steerhorn configuration of the lateral ventricles caused by bundles of Probst along the superomedial margins of the ventricles, and extension of the third ventricle between the lateral ventricles. Axial images show colpocephaly and parallel course of the lateral ventricles.*

anomalies. Among the most commonly encountered anomalies are Chiari II malformation, Dandy-Walker malformation, neuronal migration abnormalities, and cephaloceles.[23,53,56]

Intracranial Lipoma

Intracranial lipoma arises from the developing subarachnoid space and may be associated with callosal agenesis or hypogenesis.[57] The most common location of an intracranial lipoma is the pericallosal region, followed by the suprasellar and quadrigeminal cisterns. Other sites include the sylvian fissure and cerebellopontine angle cistern (Fig. 19-12). Associated brain anomalies typically involve the corpus callosum, mamillary bodies, and superior vermis. Midline facial clefts and sincipital encephaloceles may also be seen with frontal interhemispheric lipomas.[58,59]

Intracranial lipomas are easily recognized by their short T1 and T2 relaxation. Sequences using fat-supression techniques demonstrate loss of signal intensity within these structures, which is diagnostic. Since lipomas originate in the primitive subarachnoid spaces, cranial nerves and subarachnoid vessels traverse intracranial lipomas. Flow voids representing subarachnoid vessels may be occasionally confused with areas of low signal intensity at the periphery of these tumors, which represent dystrophic calcifications in necrotic areas of the lipoma or adjacent brain tissue.

Dandy-Walker Complex

The Dandy-Walker complex, which represents a spectrum of abnormalities ranging from the Dandy-Walker malformation to the mega cistern magna, includes conditions with cerebellar hypoplasia and cystic malformations of the fourth ventricle.[60] The underlying abnormality in Dandy-Walker malformation and its variants is intrauterine obstruction at the level of the fourth ventricle leading to an enlarged, cystlike ventricle, which, due to its size, prevents fusion of the cerebellar hemispheres and formation of the vermis.

Imaging studies in patients with the Dandy-Walker malformation show a large posterior fossa with elevation of the torcular Herophili, a posterior fossa cyst, and hypoplasia of the vermis and cerebellar hemispheres (Fig. 19-13). A majority of patients have hydrocephalus. Other central nervous system (CNS) anomalies include callosal agenesis, occipital cephaloceles, and migrational disorders.[13]

The Dandy-Walker variant is a much less pronounced form of the malformation, consisting of a hypogenetic cerebellar vermis and cystic dilatation of the fourth ventricle. Hydrocephalus, torcular elevation, and vermian rotation are not typically seen in the Dandy-Walker variant. Patients with the Dandy-Walker variant have a lower incidence of supratentorial abnormalities and a better prognosis.[60]

The mega cisterna magna consists of the enlarged posterior fossa with a normal cerebellar vermis and

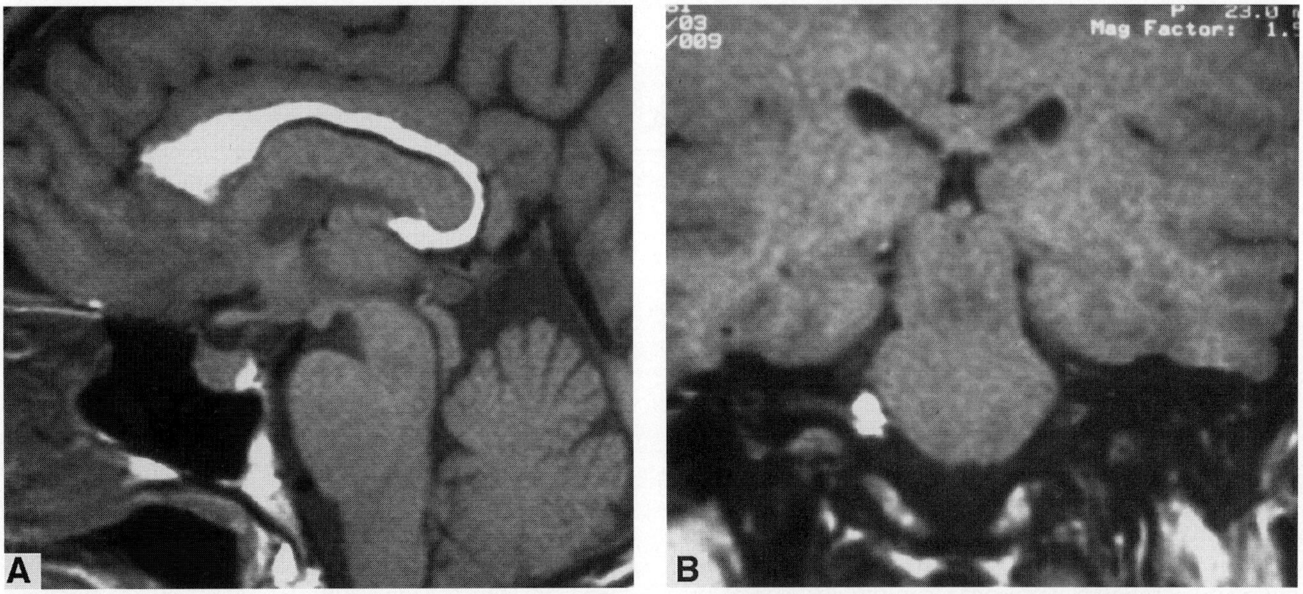

Figure 19-12
Intracranial lipomas. MRI is diagnostic of such an entity, demonstrating a structure of high T1 signal intensity. The most common locations include **(A)**, *the pericallosal region, the quadrigeminal and superior vermian cistern, the suprasellar cistern, and the sylvian fissure. Less commonly, lipomas may occur in such areas as* **(B)** *the cerebellopontine angle cistern. Because of interference with developing brain structures, the pericallosal lipomas is commonly associated with hypoplasia of the corpus callosum, as demonstrated in* **A. (B)** *A coronal T1-weighted image through the brainstem* **(B)** *demonstrates the concept of intracranial lipoma developing within the primitive subarachnoid space, with the cranial nerve VII–VIII complex traversing the small cerebellopontine angle lipoma.*

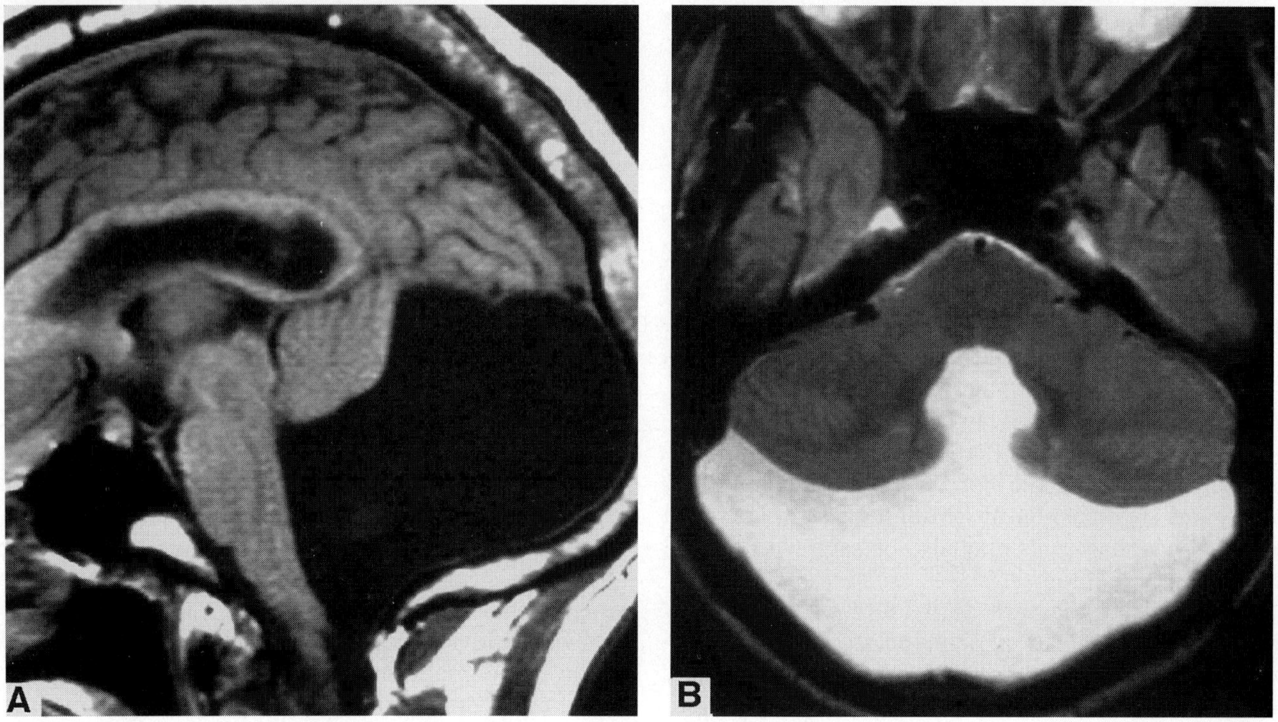

Figure 19-13
Dandy-Walker malformation. The typical features of the Dandy-Walker malformation are seen on **(A)** *sagittal T1-weighted and* **(B)** *axial T2-weighted images. A large CSF collection communicates with fourth ventricle, which is widely open posteriorly, and produces marked enlargement of the posterior fossa. The vermis is hypoplastic and malrotated superiorly.*

fourth ventricle. In contradistinction to an arachnoid cyst, a mega cisterna magna does not cause mass effect on the cerebellar vermis (Fig. 19-14).

Joubert Syndrome

Joubert syndrome is an uncommon congenital lesion presenting clinically with global developmental delay, respiratory abnormalities, and oculomotor disturbances.[61] Pathologically it consists of cerebellar vermian dysgenesis and disconnected cerebellar hemispheres. Characteristic features on MRI include brainstem hypoplasia, vermian dysgenesis, and a "bat-wing"–shaped fourth ventricle due to absence of the vermis and abnormal course of the middle cerebellar peduncles (Fig. 19-15).[62]

Rhombencephalosynapsis

Rhombencephalosynapsis is a rare abnormality of the posterior fossa consisting of the triad of fused dentate nuclei and cerebellar hemispheres in the absence of the cerebellar vermis. Associated anomalies include deficiency of the septum pellucidum, hydrocephalus, and thalamic fusion.[63] The condition is easily appreciated on MRI when the cerebellar folia appear fused across the midline without an intervening vermis (Fig. 19-16).

Abnormalities of Neuronal Migration

Following the period of structural development of the brain, neuroblasts of the germinal matrix undergo a period of proliferation, followed by neuronal migration from the germinal matrix to the overlying cortical mantle. Neuronal migration both precedes and occurs concurrently with the period of neuronal organization, when the normal cortical cytoarchitecture is formed. Cortical organization occurs in a well-organized manner, with the earliest migrating neuroblasts forming the deeper layers of the cortex and the later migrating neuroblasts organizing into the more superficial layers of the normal six-layered cortex.[64–68]

The stages of neuroblast proliferation, neuronal migration, and neuronal organization are commonly referred to as neuronal migration and occur all together between the second and fifth month of gestation. Numerous genetic, teratogenic, environmental, infectious, and ischemic insults may affect this period of brain development and lead to aberrancy of the normal cortical formation. Among the numerous abnormalities encountered are the lissencephalies (agyria and pachygyria), heterotopia (subependymal nodular heterotopia, focal heterotopia, and band heterotopia), cortical dysplasia (focal cleft of polymicrogyria and diffuse cortical dysplasia), schizencephaly, and unilateral megalencephaly. More recently, transmantle dysplasias have been de-

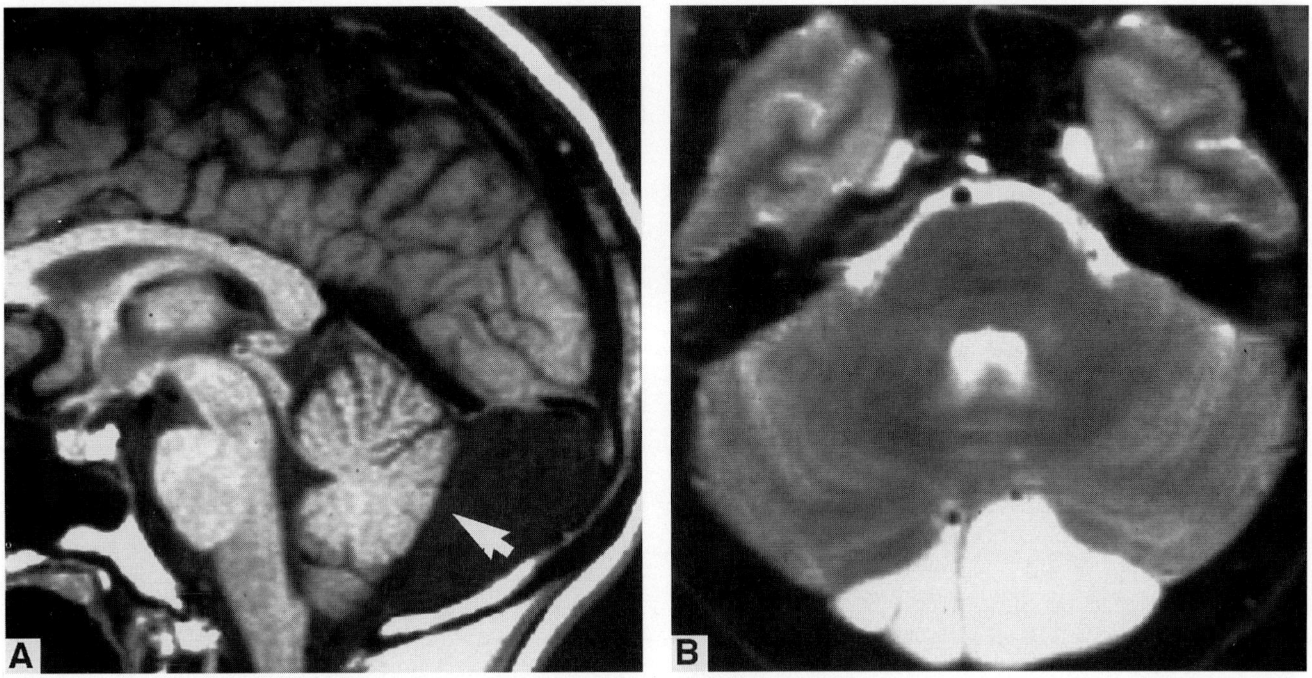

Figure 19-14
Posterior fossa arachnoid cyst. A fluid collection of CSF-like intensity is seen in the posterior fossa. In contradistinction to the Dandy-Walker malformation, the vermis is well formed, and the fourth ventricle does not communicate with this fluid collection. The mass effect on the vermis (white arrow) is typical of an arachnoid cyst but not seen with an enlarged cisterna magna. **(A)** *is T1 sagittal and* **(B)** *is T2 axial.*

scribed. These are very subtle heterotopias resulting from abnormalities of the radial glial elements that consist of thin neuronal migration anomalies extending through the white matter, from cortex to ventricular surface.[69] In addition, Kallmann syndrome (anosmia and hypogonadotrophic hypogonadism) is often included in disorders of neuronal migration due to disordered migration of cells from the olfactory placode to the future hypothalamic cell controlling reproductive neuroendocrinology.[70–73]

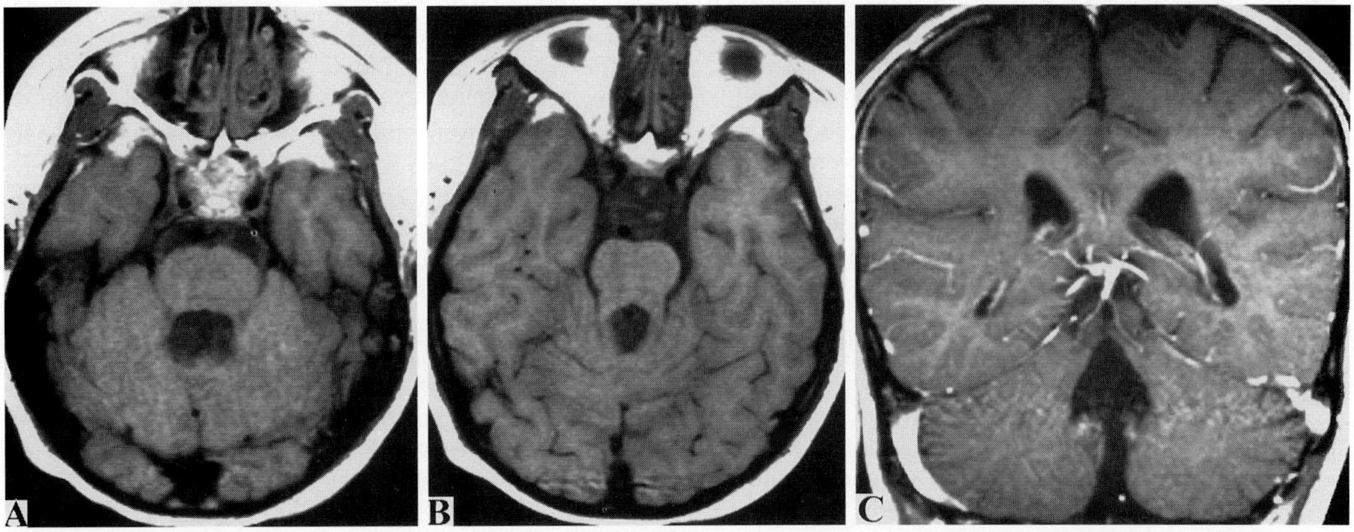

Figure 19-15
Joubert syndrome. **(A and B)** *T1-weighted axial and* **(C)** *coronal postgadolinium images demonstrate features of Joubert syndrome. The superior vermis is hypoplastic, and the cerebellar hemispheres are essentially disconnected. The fourth ventricle is enlarged at the level of the pons, with a characteristic "bat-wing"–shaped appearance. More cephalad, the horizontally arranged superior cerebellar peduncles are visible on the axial images.*

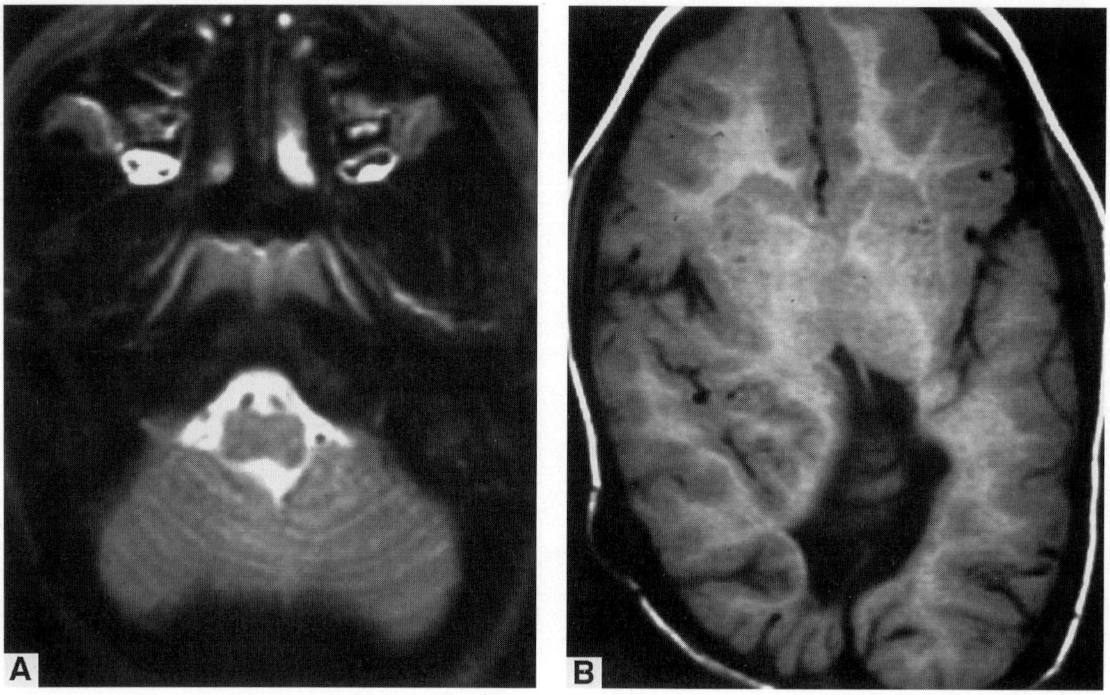

Figure 19-16
Rhombencephalosynapsis. **(A)** *An axial T2-weighted image demonstrates fusion of the cerebellar hemispheres, as seen by continuity of the folia across the midline.* **(B)** *More superiorly, an axial T1-weighted image shows the extremely hypoplastic vermis in a prominent superior cerebellar cistern. Note the associated hypoplasia of the corpus callosum and the prominent cortical dysplasia in the right posterior temporal and occipital lobe.*

These disorders are well described both on CT and MRI. These abnormalities are much more obvious on MRI due to the exquisite differentiation between gray and white matter structures. At our institution, we use a combination of three-dimensional MP-RAGE (TR 15 ms, TE 7 ms, flip angle 8°) and coronal two-dimensional inversion recovery images (TR 7000 ms, TE 60 ms, TI 225 ms, flip angle 180°) to bring out the subtle detail of these disturbances in neuronal migration. Routine transaxial spin-echo imaging is also performed, although it is important to recognize that subtle neuronal migration disturbances can be volume-averaged due to the thickness of slice and due to the axial plane of section. In particular, subtle nodules of subependymal heterotopia are easily obscured on axial imaging, as are transmantle dysplasias, due to scan thickness.

Lissencephaly

The most severe form of neuronal migration anomaly is lissencephaly, which results from an abnormality in neuronal migration between weeks 8 and 14 of gestation. This term is used interchangeably with agyria (“complete lissencephaly”) and pachygyria (“incomplete lissencephaly”) to refer to an abnormally smooth brain surface with complete lack of gyri or few, broad gyri, respectively. In recent years, the classification of lissencephalies has undergone considerable revision as genetic associations have been defined. For a review of such genetic associations, the reader is referred to recent articles.[9,74,75] Briefly, classical lissencephaly (previously type 1) includes patients with isolated lissencephaly, who have a chromosome 17 mutation, and patients with X-linked lissencephaly, which is related to subcortical band heterotopia.[76] Also included in this group are patients with the Miller-Dieker syndrome, which is due to a more extensive chromosome 17 mutation, and who have other craniofacial and brain anomalies in addition to lissencephaly.[76–78] As discussed above, agyria is best visualized on MRI on sequences that optimize gray-white matter differentiation, such as inversion recovery images. T2-weighted images are also useful in bringing out the subtle curvilinear hyperintensity of the cell-sparse layer within the abnormal four-layer cortex.[41,79] The cerebral cortex appears smooth and thickened, with shallow or absent sulci (Fig. 19-17). In the most severe forms, the cerebrum has been described as having a figure eight due to narrowing in its midportion by the vertically oriented sylvian fissures. Mild to moderate callosal hypogenesis is common in severe cases. In all cases of pachygyria and agyria, careful scrutiny of the less affected areas of the brain is suggested in order to identify subtle band heterotopia.

A second category of patients are those with cobblestone lissencephaly (previously type 2), which is a pri-

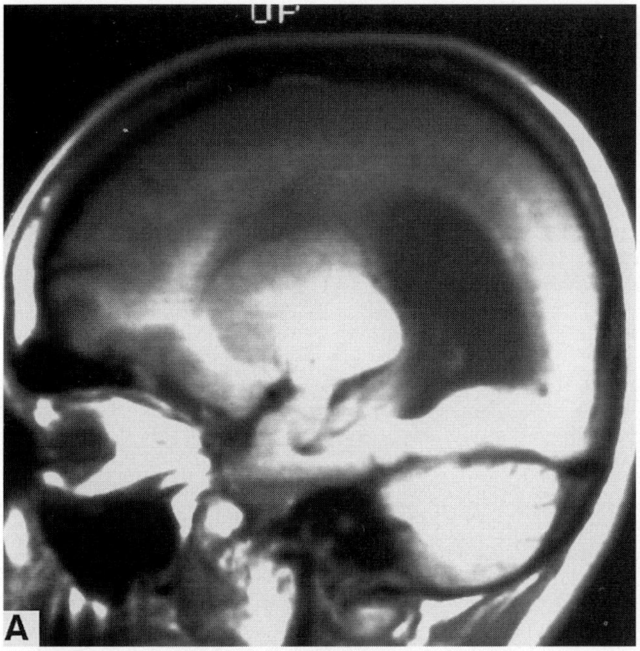

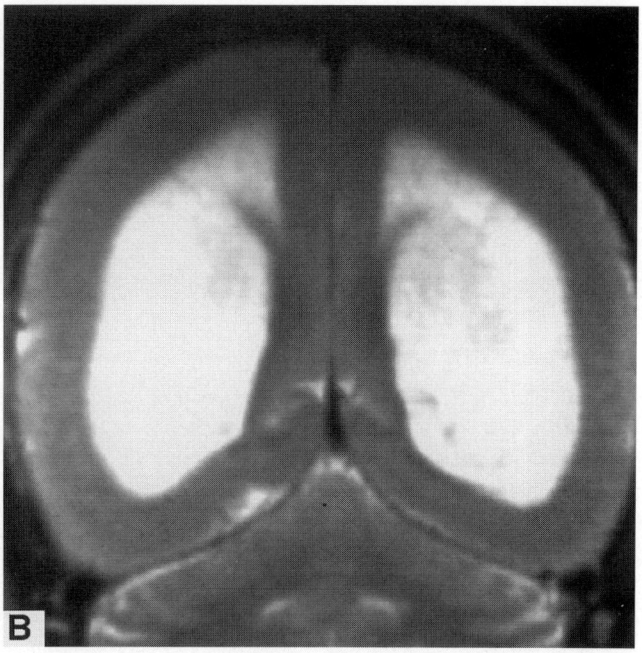

Figure 19-17
Lissencephaly. **(A)** *T1-weighted sagittal and* **(B)** *T2-weighted coronal images demonstrate abnormally smooth brain surface with thick cortex and thin underlying white matter. These features are typical of agyria.*

mary feature of disorders such as Fukuyama muscular dystrophy,[77] Walker-Warburg syndrome,[80] and muscle-eye-brain disease.[81] In cobblestone lissencephaly, the neuronal migration disorder is so extensive that neurons migrate through the developing cortex into the leptomeninges. This results in leptomeningeal glioneural heterotopia and studding of the cortical surface, hence the name *cobblestone lissencephaly*.[41,82] Because of the infiltration of the leptomeninges, communicating hydrocephalus is quite common, which distinguishes these patients from classic lissencephaly. Another distinguishing feature is the appearance of the cortex, which is not as thick in cobblestone lissencephaly as in classical lissencephaly. In addition, posterior fossa abnormalities are the rule, rather than the exception, in cobblestone lissencephaly.

Finally, lissencephaly may be seen in association with intrauterine cytomegalovirus infection, although this condition is more often associated with polymicrogyria than pachygyria.[83,84]

Children with lissencephaly present at birth with microcephaly, motor retardation, feeding problems, and hypotonia. Soon thereafter seizures and mental retardation become apparent. Life expectancy is less than 2 years.[79,85,86]

Gray Matter Heterotopia

Heterotopia refers to collections of ectopic neurons located in abnormal areas of the cerebral hemispheres secondary to arrest of migration between the germinal zone and the cortex. The precise cause of this anomaly is not known, but several causes have been proposed, including damage to the radial glial fibers, which serve as a scaffolding for neuronal migration,[87] premature differentiation of radial glial cells into astrocytes,[88] deficiency of chemotactic factors that guide and attract migrating neurons,[89] and genetic causes.[90–92]

Depending on its morphologic characteristics, two types of heterotopia are recognized: nodular heterotopia and band (or laminar) heterotopia. Nodular heterotopia, the more common of the two, presents with gray matter nodules, which may be located anywhere in the cerebral white matter and may be unilateral or bilateral. Clinical presentation of patients with subcortical heterotopia depends on the size of the gray matter nodules: patients with smaller nodules tend to present with seizures, while patients with large nodules present with earlier-onset seizures and developmental and intellectual delay.[93] The MRI demonstrates nodules of various sizes in the subcortical and periventricular white matter that follow gray matter signal intensity on all imaging sequences and do not enhance (Fig. 19-18). Mass effect may be seen with larger nodules. Subependymal heterotopia, another form of nodular heterotopia, presents with smaller gray matter nodules around the lateral ventricles as an isolated disorder or as part of a larger syndrome, such as a Chiari II malformation and cephaloceles. The lesions may be single, subtle, usually clustered around the trigones of the lateral ventricles, or numerous, giving an undulating appearance to the

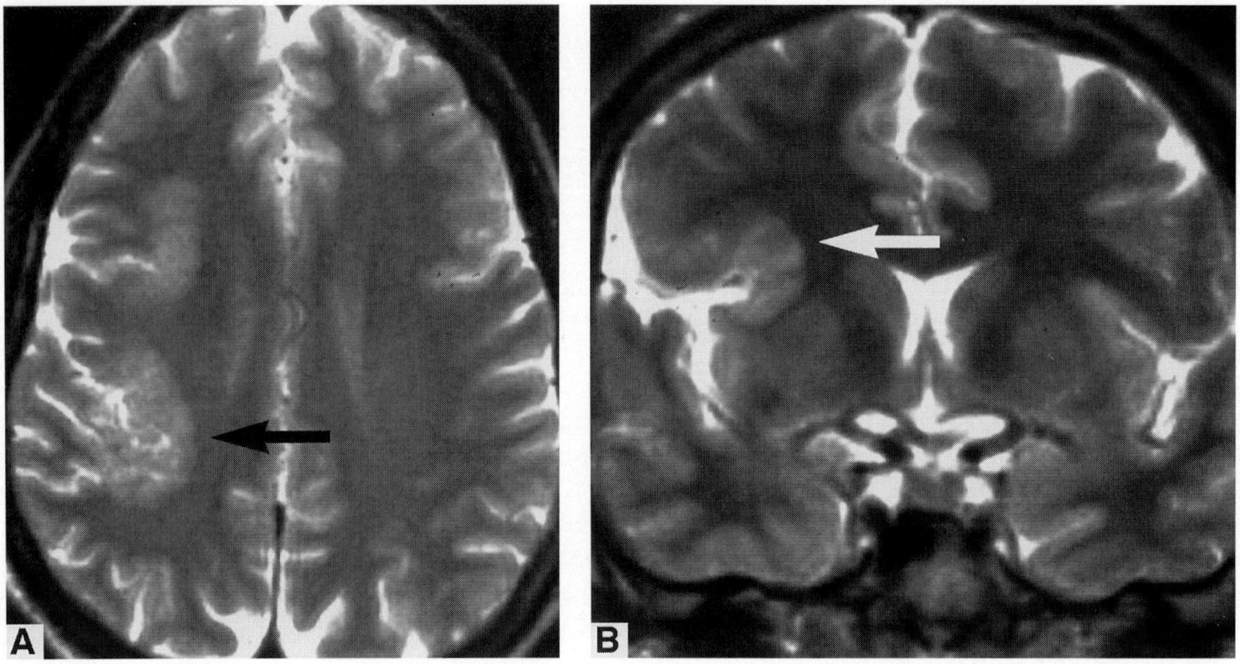

Figure 19-18

Nodular subcortical heterotopia. ***(A)*** *T2-weighted axial and* ***(B)*** *coronal images demonstrate two areas of cortical abnormality in the region of the anterior sylvian fissure and in the right posterior frontal area. The abnormally thick and nodular cortex is isointense to cortex elsewhere.*

ventricular wall (Fig. 19-19). It appears that the latter form of subependymal heterotopia is a different entity being transmitted as an X-linked disorder.[92,94] Unlike patients with the other disorders of neuronal migration, patients with periventricular nodular heterotopia often are of normal intelligence and function. If mental retardation or other symptoms are present, they are often related to associated disturbances of neuronal migration or associated brain anomalies.[93]

The rare band heterotopia is characterized by a band of gray matter within the centrum semiovale separated from the overlying cortex by a thin layer of white matter.[95] The cortex overlying the heterotopic gray matter may be normal or pachygyric (Fig. 19-20).[13] Patients usually present with seizures and motor and intellectual retardation, the severity of which correlate with the thickness of the subcortical band and the extent of cortical abnormalities.[96] The gene responsible for this malformation has been localized to the X chromosome,[75,91,97] and both familial[97,98] and sporadic[75] cases have been reported.

Unilateral Megalencephaly

Unilateral megalencephaly denotes a hamartomatous overgrowth of all or part of the cerebral hemisphere.[99] The CNS anomaly may occur in isolation or may be associated with hemihypertrophy of some or all of the body[100] and other conditions, such as tuberous sclerosis, Wilm's tumors, and cerebellar hemangioblastomas.[101–103] Patients usually have intractable seizures and are almost always hemiplegic and developmentally delayed.

Imaging studies show moderate to marked enlargement of the affected hemisphere (Fig. 19-21).[104,105] The cortex of the involved hemisphere is also abnormal, demonstrating migrational abnormalities and occasional calcifications.[105,106] Unilateral enlargement of the optic tract has also been reported.[107] Signal abnormalities of the white matter are present due to gliosis, abnormal myelination, and calcifications. The lateral ventricle is usually enlarged due to obstruction at the foramen of Monro.[42] Careful evaluation of the contralateral hemisphere is necessary, since heterotopia may be present (CL Truwit, personal observations).

Cortical Dysplasia

Cortical dysplasia includes a group of disorders characterized by abnormal organization of neurons resulting in multiple small gyri on the cerebral hemispheres. Several theories regarding potential pathogenic mechanisms leading to this disorder have been formulated, including interference with late stages of neuronal migration, a destructive cortical process, and disruption of neuronal migration.[41,42,108,109] Clinical presentation depends on the extent and location of the malformation, with extensive or bilateral lesions having more severe psychomotor retardation and earlier onset of seizures.[110]

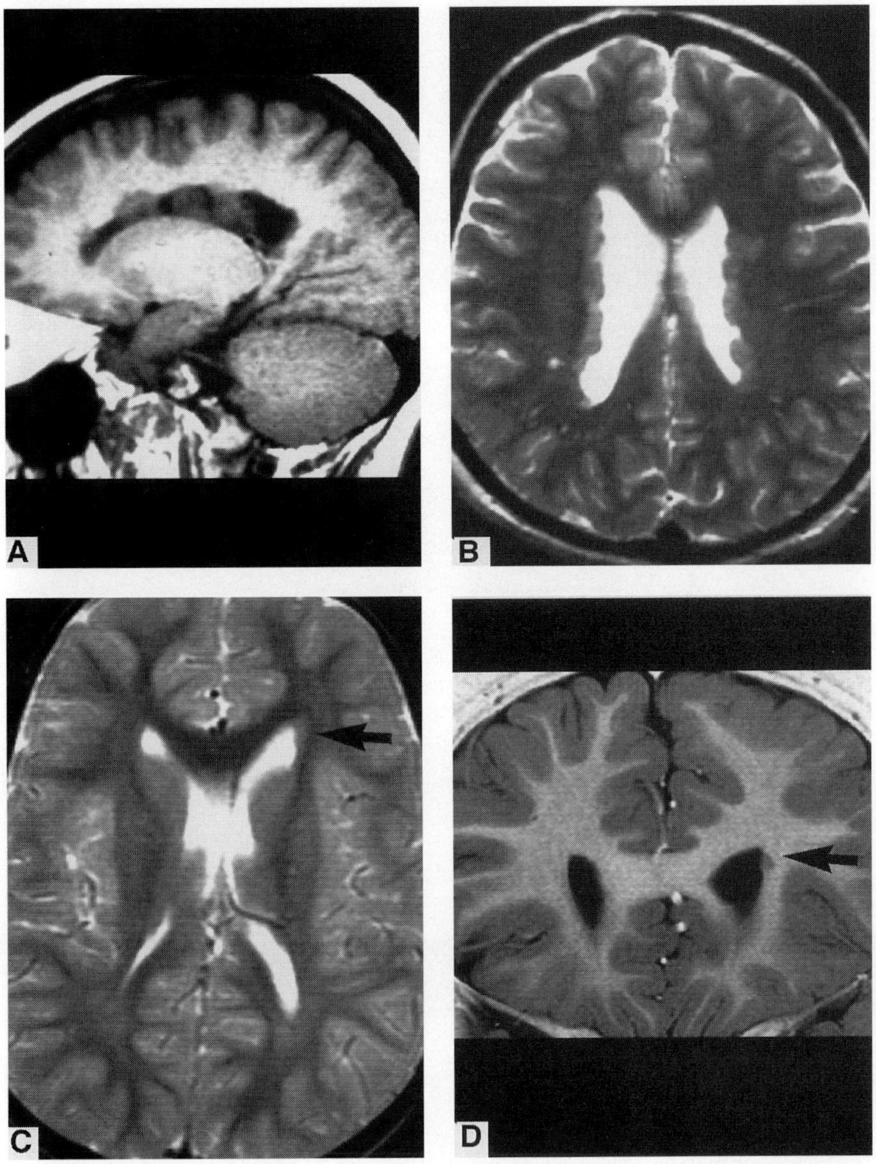

Figure 19-19
Periventricular nodular heterotopia. **(A)** *T1-weighted sagittal and* **(B)** *T2-weighted axial images in one patient demonstrate numerous small nodules, isointense to cortex, protruding from the walls of the lateral ventricles.* **(C)** *Axial T2-weighted image and* **(D)** *coronal inversion recovery image in another patient show subtle gray matter heterotopion adjacent to the frontal horn of the left lateral ventricle. Improved tissue contrast is obtained with the inversion-recovery sequence.*

At least three types of cortical dysplasia can be seen.[13] Focal polymicrogyric clefts, which most often occur in the posterior sylvian region, may be considered a form fruste of schizencephaly (Fig. 19-22). An almost pathognomonic finding is an anomalous venous drainage within the cleft (Fig. 19-22C). There is hypoplasia of the white matter of the involved hemisphere, and hypoplasia of the ipsilateral thalamus and cerebral peduncle due to a paucity of descending white matter tracts.

A second type of cortical dysplasia involves a cerebral hemisphere diffusely, and it may be bilateral (Fig. 19-23). Not uncommonly, this form of cortical dysplasia is a manifestation of in utero cytomegalovirus infection.[84]

Finally, the congenital bilateral perisylvian syndrome[111] is characterized by dysplastic and incomplete opercula, with widening, underdevelopment, and posterior extension of the sylvian fissure. Clinically, patients present with pseudobulbar palsy (oropharyngeal dysfunction and dysarthria), seizures, mental retardation, and delayed milestones.

Imaging studies demonstrate the dysplastic cortex as a thick, poorly sulcated band of cortex simulating pachygyria. Thin, 1.5-mm sections may be more helpful for detection of subtle irregularities at the gray-white matter junction. In a small number of patients, calcifications of the affected cortex may be seen. Abnormal T2 prolongation of the underlying white matter, thought to represent gliosis, may be seen.[13,112]

Schizencephaly

Schizencephaly describes gray matter-lined clefts that span the cerebral hemisphere, from the lateral ventricle

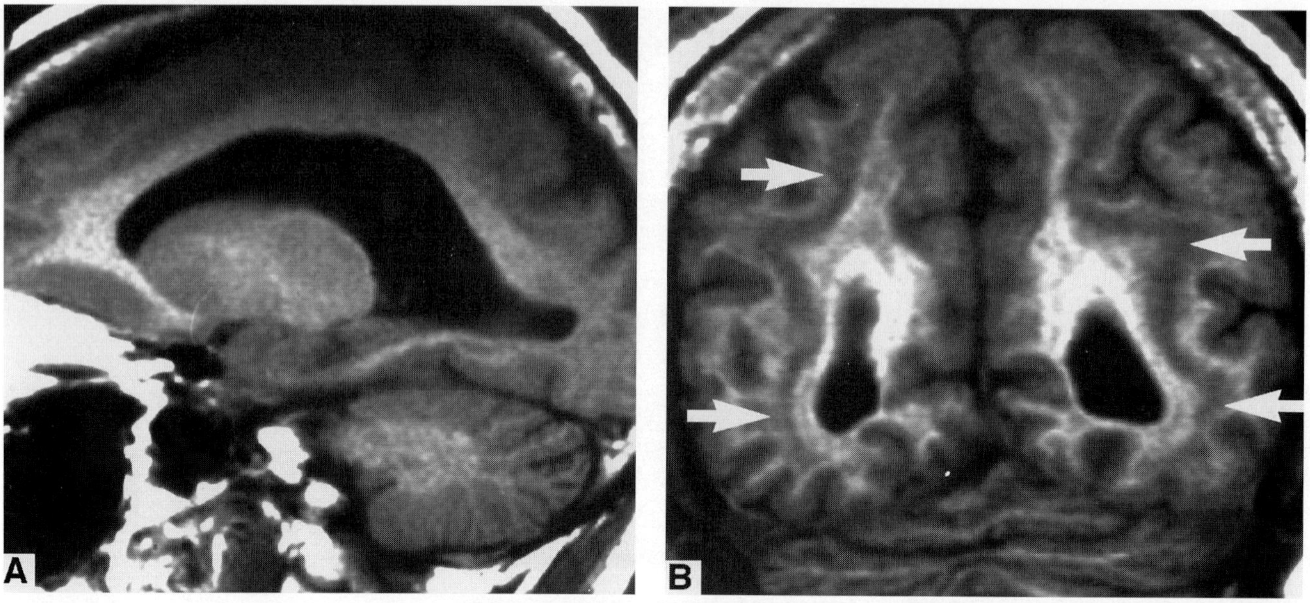

Figure 19-20

Band heterotopia. **(A)** *T1-weighted sagittal and* **(B)** *coronal images demonstrate a band of subcortical gray matter extending along the entire hemisphere and separated from the cortex by a thin layer of white matter. The frontal cortex is abnormally sulcated, but no definite pachygyria is seen. Sagittal images are useful for evaluating the extent of the band, while the coronal images produce a good estimation of the thickness of the band as well as the overlying cortex. (Courtesy of Dr. Douglas H. Yock, Jr.)*

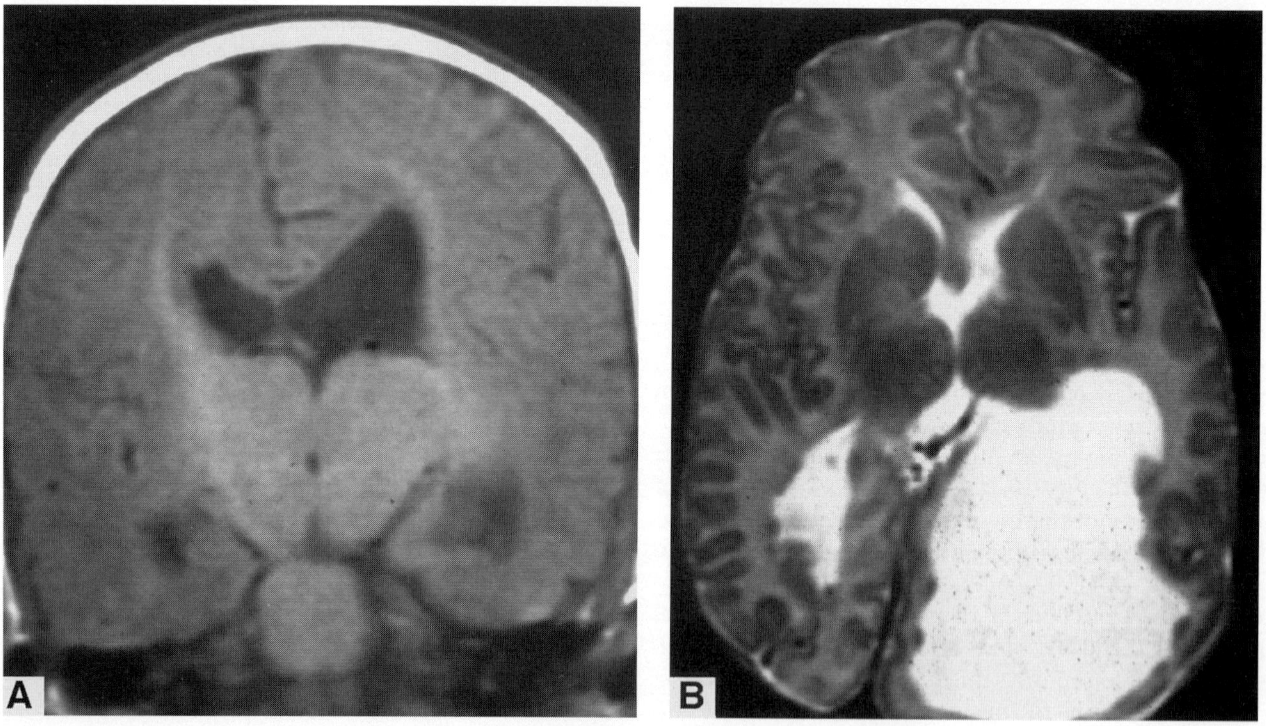

Figure 19-21

Unilateral megalencephaly. **(A)** *T1-weighted coronal and* **(B)** *T2-weighted axial images demonstrate enlargement of the left hemisphere compared with the opposite side. The atrium and occipital horns of the left lateral ventricle are especially enlarged. Nodules of heterotopic gray matter are present around the atria of both lateral ventricles.*

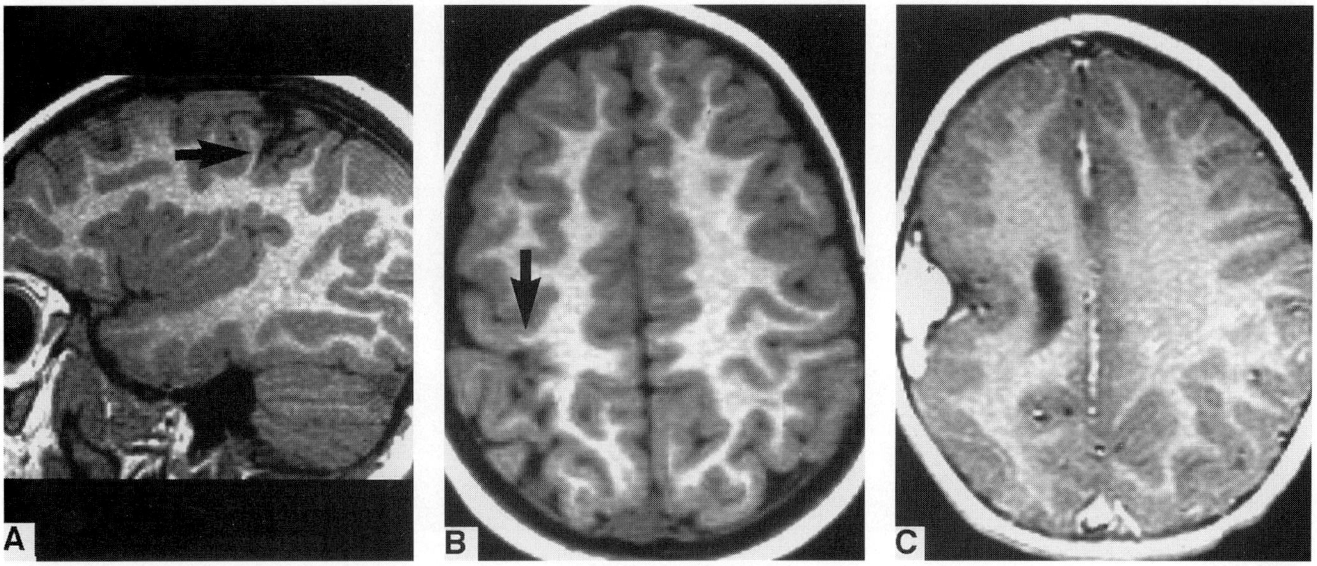

Figure 19-22
Focal polymicrogyria. **(A)** *T1-weighted sagittal and* **(B)** *axial images show an area of abnormally infolded cortex in the posterior right frontal area.* **(C)** *Another patient shown in T1 postgadolinium axial images demonstrates a similar, although more obvious, abnormality in the right frontal area. The strongly enhancing extra-axial structure adjacent to the dysplastic cortex represents an abnormal primitive draining vein. Such a vein is not uncommonly seen in the presence of focal polymicrogyria and should not be confused with a vascular malformation.*

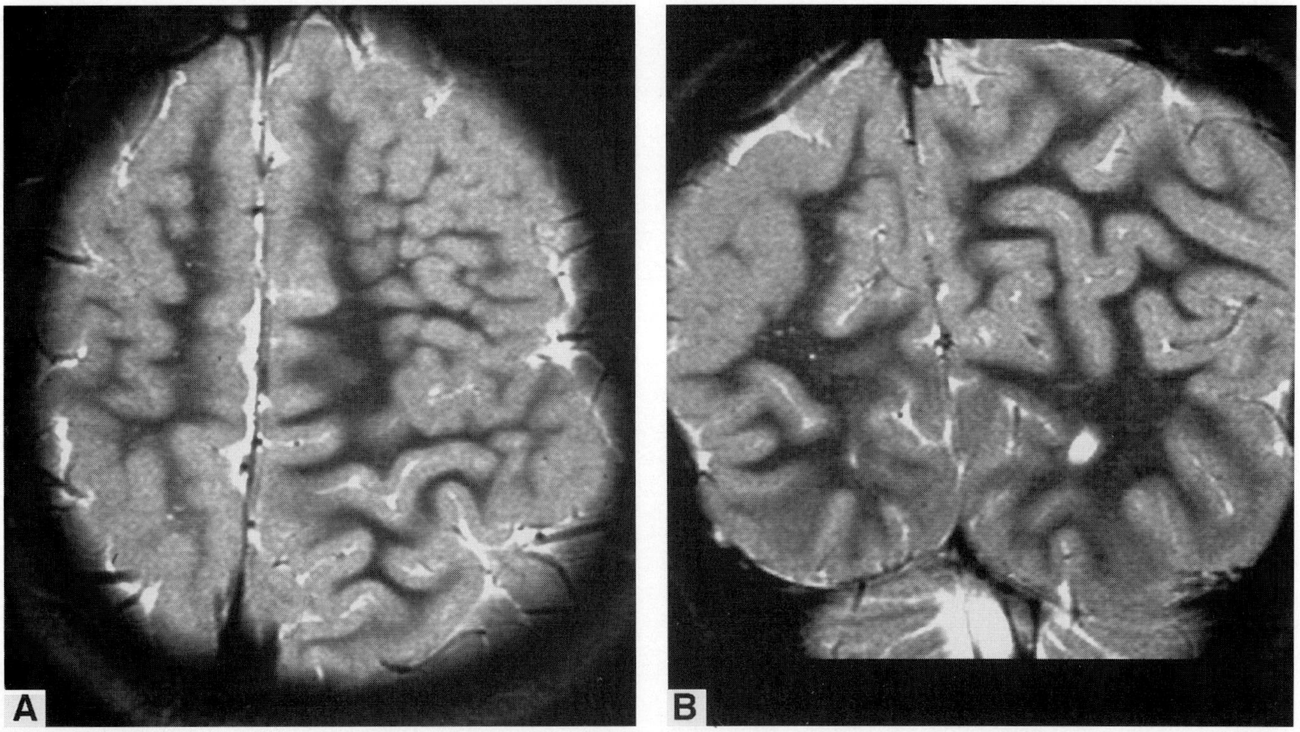

Figure 19-23
Bilateral polymicrogyria. **(A)** *Axial and* **(B)** *coronal turbo-inversion-recovery images demonstrate a thick and nodular cortex in both frontal regions. Decreased subcortical white matter and hypoplasia of the ipsilateral thalamus and cerebral peduncle (not shown) reflect the decreased white matter tracts that accompany the cortical dysplasia.*

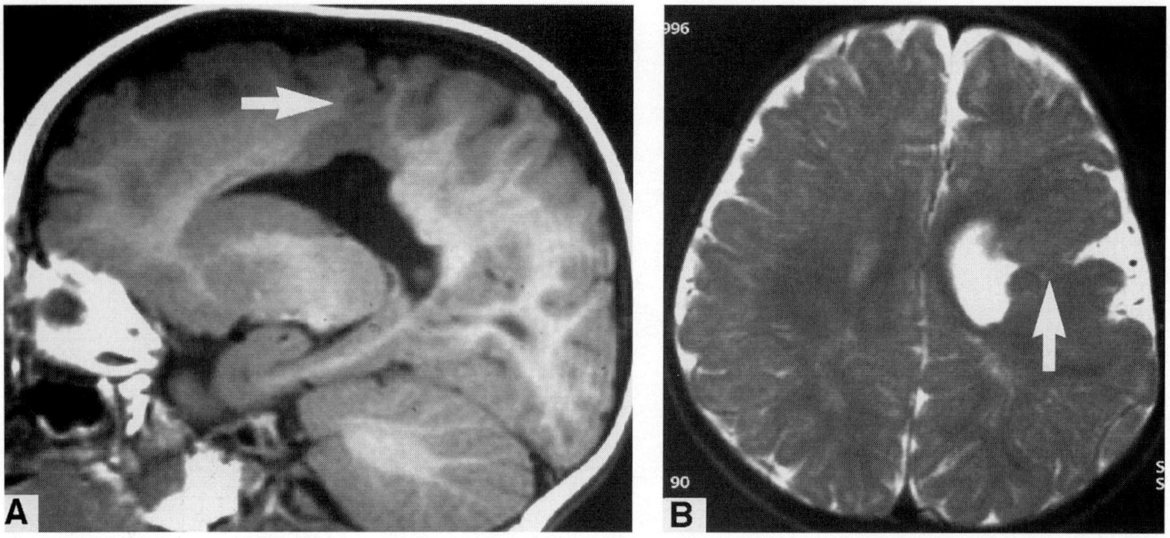

Figure 19-24
Closed-lip schizencephaly. **(A)** *T1-weighted sagittal and* **(B)** *T2-weighted axial images shown a transhemispheric layer of gray matter joining a cortical cleft to a ventricular dimple. No CSF is seen within the tract. These findings are characteristic of closed-lip schizencephaly.*

to the cerebral cortex. In most cases, the gray matter lining the cleft is polymicrogyric. The clefts may be unilateral or bilateral and are typically perisylvian, although they can appear anywhere in the brain. The adjacent cortex is dysplastic, usually demonstrating polymicrogyria, extending for a variable distance away from the cleft. Schizencephalic clefts may be "closed," with only a double layer of cortex seen extending from the brain surface to the ventricle.[113] A lateral ventricular "dimple" marks the pial-ependymal junction (Fig. 19-24).[113–115] Alternatively, an "open" cleft is filled by CSF from the lateral ventricle to the brain surface (Fig. 19-25).[114] Associated abnormalities include mild hypoplasia of the corpus callosum and absent or hypoplastic

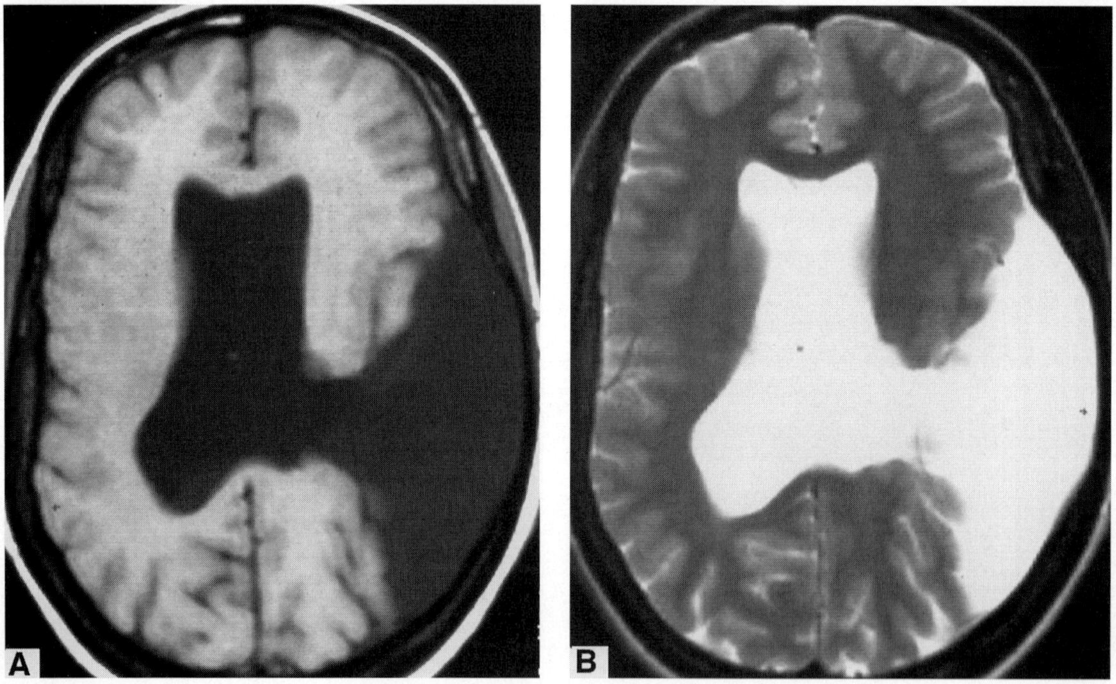

Figure 19-25
Open-lip schizencephaly. **(A)** *Axial T1-weighted and* **(B)** *T2-weighted images show a wide CSF-filled tract connecting the body of the left lateral ventricle to the subarachnoid space. The walls of the tract are lined by polymicrogyric gray matter. The subarachnoid space exerts mass effect both on the left hemisphere and on the overlying parietal bone, which is bowed. These findings, which have been long-standing, suggest the presence of an arachnoid cyst.*

septum pellucidum. A subset of these patients will have optic nerve hypoplasia, therefore meeting the criteria of septo-optic dysplasia (see the earlier discussion). The clinical presentation depends on the amount of involved brain.[115] Patients with a narrow, unilateral cleft usually have seizures and mild hemiparesis or visual difficulties, depending on the location of the cleft within the hemisphere. Patients with progressively larger clefts present with worse neurologic deficits, while patients with bilateral clefts tend to be severely retarded, with early epilepsy, severe motor deficits, and blindness.

Miscellaneous Developmental Anomalies

Aqueductal Stenosis

Aqueductal stenosis represents obstruction of the cerebral aqueduct and is usually due to a postnatal insult, such as bleeding, infection,[116] or compression by intrinsic brainstem tumors.[117,118] Less common causes include abnormal proliferation of periaqueductal tissues,[119] in utero infection or bleeding,[42,117] and chromosomal abnormalities.[120] Aqueductal stenosis may also be seen with Chiari II and Dandy-Walker malformations.[42]

Diagnosis is straightforward on MRI, since the proximal aqueduct tends to dilate and bulge posteriorly. In addition, there is enlargement of the lateral and third ventricles, with a normal-sized fourth ventricle (Fig. 19-26A). Occasionally, a thin web may be seen across the caudal end of the aqueduct restricting CSF flow into the fourth ventricle. Flow studies of CSF using a gated gradient-echo technique or phase-contrast slow-velocity MR angiogram demonstrate no flow through the aqueduct.[121,122] Discrimination between benign aqueductal stenosis and neoplastic aqueductal stenosis is critical. Cases of suspected aqueductal stenosis should be carefully studied with sagittal, contrast-enhanced T1-weighted images for the presence of third or fourth ventricular masses or neoplasms of the dorsal brainstem (Fig. 19-26B).

Chiari I Malformation

The Chiari I malformation is diagnosed by ectopia of the cerebellar tonsils greater than 5 mm below the foramen magnum.[123] This definition, however, is not strict, since the degree of inferior displacement of the cerebellar tonsils varies with age. Chiari I malformations may be

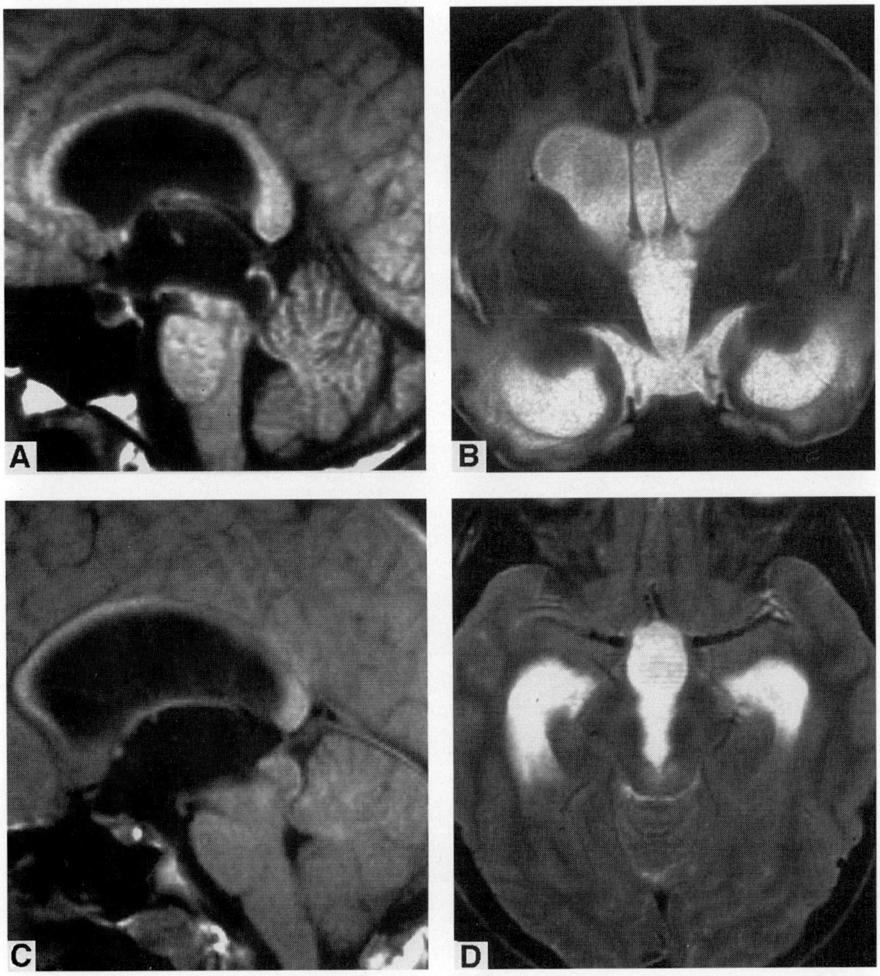

Figure 19-26
Aqueductal stenosis. **(A)** *T1-weighted sagittal and* **(B)** *T2-weighted coronal images demonstrate findings typical of benign aqueductal stenosis. The lateral and third ventricles are dilated, and the fourth ventricle is normal. The rostral end of the cerebral aqueduct is distended, and a thin membrane is seen across the caudal end of the aqueduct.* **(C)** *T1-weighted sagittal and* **(D)** *T2-weighted axial images in another patient show lateral and third ventricular hydrocephalus and a normal-appearing fourth ventricle. In contradistinction to the previous patient, the tectal plate is markedly enlarged and has abnormal T2 signal, suggesting a mass within the quadrigeminal plate.*

congenital or acquired. Congenital causes of Chiari I malformations include intrauterine hydrocephalus and craniocervical dysgenesis.[13] Acquired conditions include increased intracranial pressure due to mass lesions, and CSF diversion, such as ventriculoperitoneal shunting.[124] The flow of CSF through the foramen magnum is probably an important factor in the development of symptoms by patients with Chiari I malformations. Disturbances of CSF dynamics due to inadequate size of the foramen magnum may result in communicating hydrocephalus or cervical syringohydromyelia. Cervical syringes are not always seen on cranial MR scans, and therefore it is important to scan the cervical spine of patients with Chiari I malformations in order to exclude a lower cervical syrinx (Fig. 19-27).

PHAKOMATOSES

The phakomatoses are a heterogeneous group of congenital malformations affecting structures of ectodermal origin, including the CNS, skin, and retina. The most common disorders included in this group are neurofibromatosis types I and II, tuberous sclerosis, CNS angiomatosis, and encephalotrigeminal angiomatosis. Central nervous system involvement is seen with all these conditions.

Neurofibromatosis

There are at least two distinct types of neurofibromatosis, both of which are autosomal dominant. The gene responsible for neurofibromatosis type 1 (NF1, or von Recklinhausen disease) has been mapped to chromosome 17.[125,126] Type 1 disease represents approximately 90 percent of cases of neurofibromatosis, with an incidence of approximately 1 in 4000 births.[127] Diagnostic criteria for neurofibromatosis have been set by the National Institutes of Health consensus panels.[128]

Peripheral findings that are easily recognized clinically include café-au-lait spots, axillary and inguinal freckling, and hamartomas, or Lisch nodules, of the iris.[129] The incidence of CNS manifestations is between 15 and 50 percent and includes gliomas of the optic pathway, brainstem, and cerebrum, and areas of T2 signal hyperintensity in basal ganglia, brainstem, and cerebellar white matter.[130–133]

Optic pathway glioma is the most common primary brain tumor in NF1. These tumors are usually juvenile pilocytic astrocytomas and may involve the optic nerve, chiasm, or tract.[133] Other intracranial low-grade astrocytomas in patients with NF1 typically involve the tectum, brainstem, and cerebrum. Foci of T2 signal hyperintensity are often seen in characteristic locations in patients with NF1. These sites are the brainstem, cerebellar white matter, internal capsule, globus pallidus,

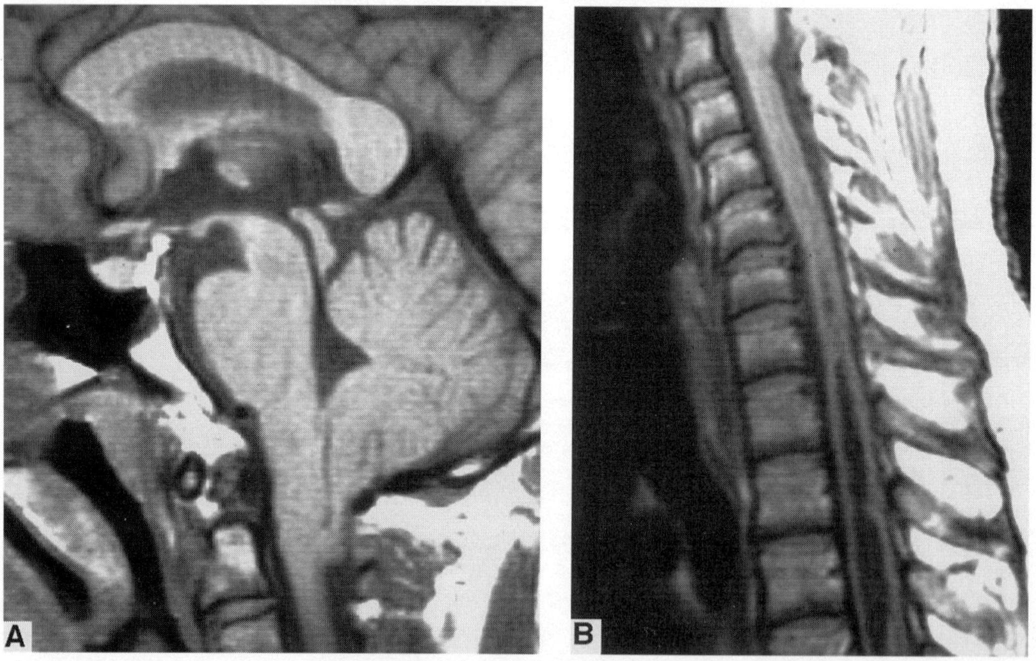

Figure 19-27

Chiari I malformation. Sagittal T1-weighted images through the **(A)** *brain and* **(B)** *the cervical thoracic spine show features of Chiari I hindbrain malformation. The peglike cerebellar tonsils are displaced inferiorly to the level of the C2–C3 intervertebral disk space. A large syrinx is evident within the mid and lower cervical spine and the upper thoracic spine. This case emphasizes the point that a screening examination of the entire cervical spine should be done in patients with Chiari I malformation, since the syrinx may not extend rostrally to be included on the sagittal views of the brain.*

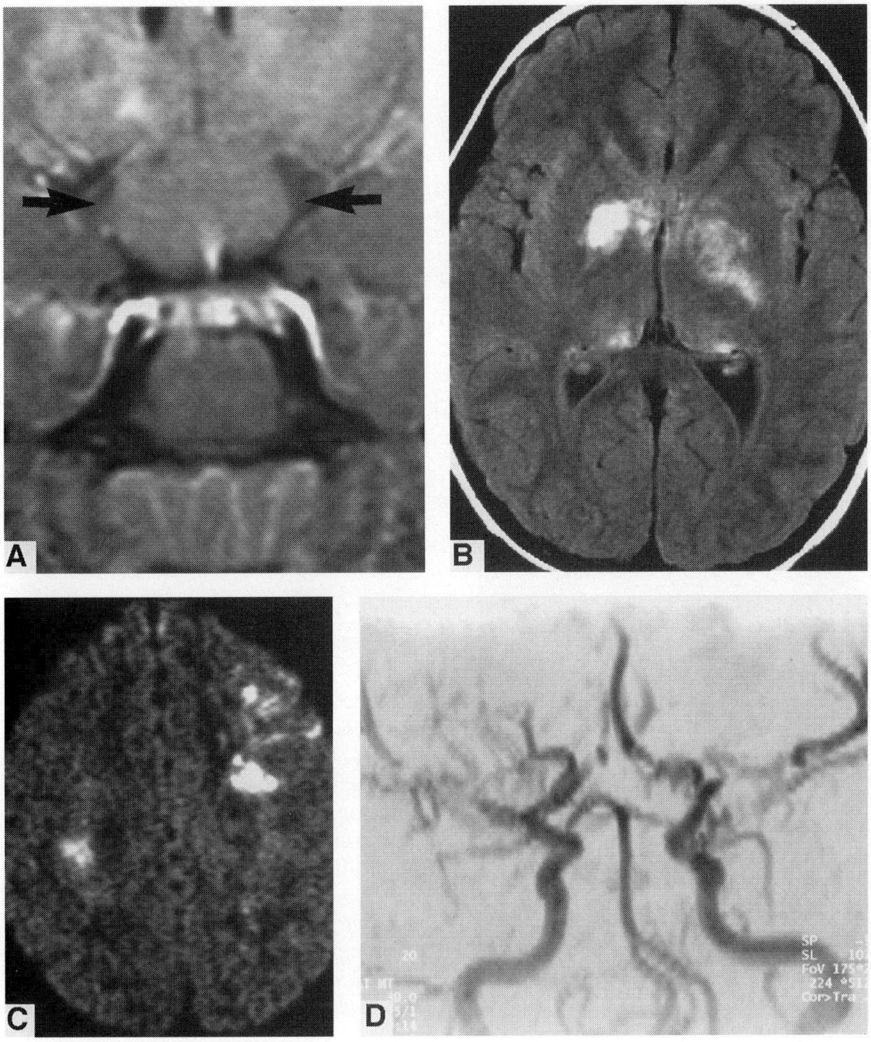

Figure 19-28
Neurofibromatosis type I. **(A)** *T1-weighted coronal postgadolinium image demonstrates markedly enlarged, nonenhancing optic chiasm in a patient with neurofibromatosis type I and optic glioma.* **(B)** *Axial turbo-FLAIR image shows characteristic foci of abnormal signal in the thalami as well as the globi pallidus bilaterally, representing hamartomatous lesions.* **(C)** *An axial diffusion-weighted image in another patient shows acute infarcts in the left frontal and right posterior frontal regions.* **(D)** *MRI angiogram of the same patient demonstrates significant stenosis of both middle cerebral arteries, with collateral vessels in the region of the right lenticulostriate arteries.*

posterior thalamus, and corpus callosum. They typically do not enhance and are thought to represent hamartomatous lesions (Fig. 19-28).[134,135] A characteristic lesion of NF1 involves the globus pallidus and demonstrates high T1 signal intensity, presumed to represent increased myelination.[136]

Other findings in NF1 include plexiform neurofibroma, a locally aggressive craniofacial tumor that arises from branches of the trigeminal nerve within the orbit.[137] Vascular dysplasia leading to occlusion of the internal carotid artery or its proximal branches and moyamoya syndrome may be idiopathic or may follow radiation therapy for optic glioma.[138] Finally, cranial bony abnormalities include absence of the greater wing of the sphenoid bone and skull defects along the lambdoid sutures.[139]

Neurofibromatosis type 2 (NF2) is much less common than NF1, with an overall incidence of approximately 1 in 50,000 births. It is transmitted as an autosomal dominant trait, with the gene locus mapped to chromosome 22.[140] In general, NF2 is considered a disorder of nerve coverings, with the major feature of the disease being bilateral acoustic schwannomas. Schwannomas of other cranial nerves, usually of the trigeminal and facial nerves, may be present. Multiple meningiomas are also characteristic findings.[134]

Tuberous Sclerosis

Tuberous sclerosis (also known as epiloia or Bourneville disease) is an autosomal dominant disease with deletions described on chromosomes 9 and 11, with an incidence of approximately 1 in 100,000 patients.[141–143] No racial or gender predilection has been detected. The classic triad of findings includes mental retardation (50 to 80 percent of patients), myoclonic seizures, and characteristic skin, although more comprehensive diagnostic criteria for this disease have been published.[144]

Unique intracranial lesions include subependymal nodules, peripheral hamartomas, and giant-cell tumors (Fig. 19-29). Peripheral hamartomas, also known as subcortical tubers, consist of disorganized neuronal and

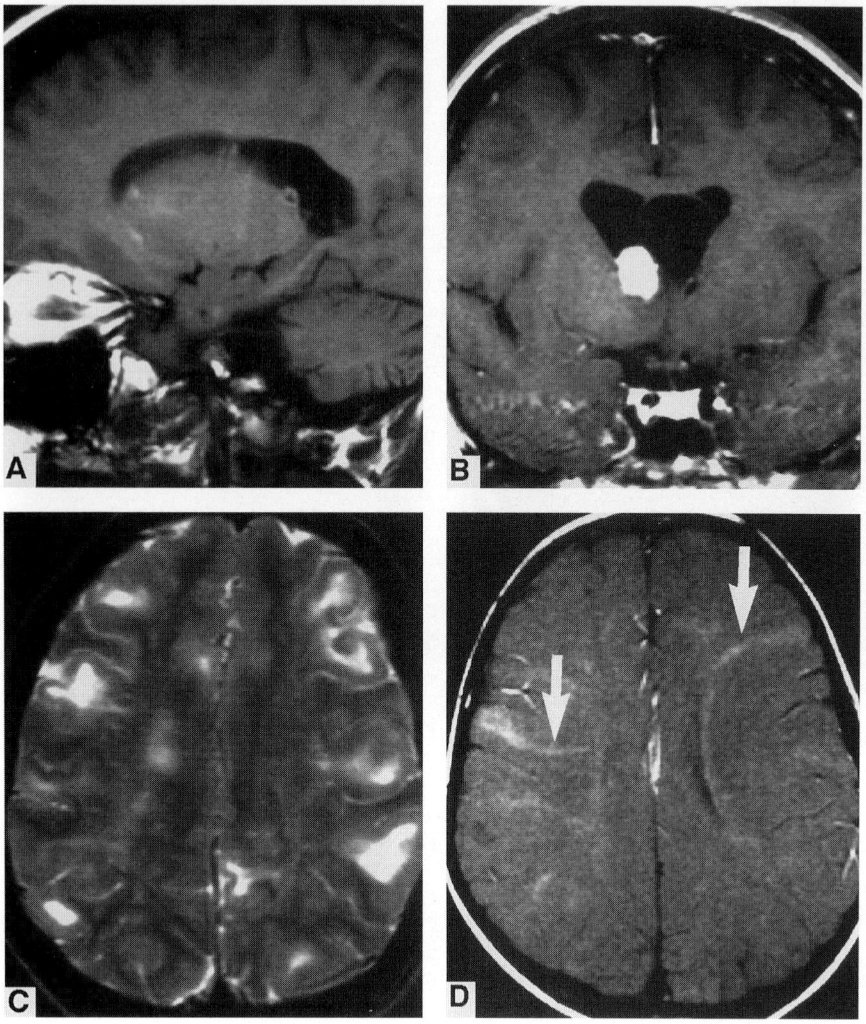

Figure 19-29
Tuberous sclerosis. **(A)** *T1-weighted sagittal and* **(C)** *T2-weighted axial images demonstrate subependymal nodules and subcortical tubers, respectively.* **(B)** *A T1-weighted coronal post-gadolinium image shows enhancing giant cell astrocytoma in the region of foramen of Monro, associated with hydrocephalus.* **(D)** *An axial turbo-FLAIR image shows curvilinear areas of increased signal intensity (white arrows) thought to represent radial glial fibers related to this migrational disorder. The patient also has cava septi pellucidi et vergae. (Courtesy of Douglas H. Yock, Jr.)*

glial elements and are the most characteristic lesions of tuberous sclerosis.[145] They are located throughout the white matter, although they have a predilection for the subcortical regions, where they appear as large, misshapen gyri that are hyperlucent on CT and bright on T2-weighted MRIs.[146–148] They demonstrate variable enhancement following infusion of paramagnetic contrast material, and they tend to calcify in older children and adults and therefore appear more conspicuous on CT.[144]

Occasionally, curvilinear bands of T2 signal hyperintensity may be seen extending from the ventricular surface to the cortical nodules; they are thought to represent residual tracks from abnormal migration of neuroblasts.[150] We found fluid-attenuated inversion-recovery (FLAIR) sequences to be useful in bringing out these white matter anomalies.

Subependymal nodules are histologically similar to subcortical tubers[145] but are smaller and occur along the walls of the lateral ventricles. They have a higher tendency to calcify, which allows distinction from heterotopic gray matter.[112] These lesions often enhance, and it is not uncommon to see several enhancing nodules around the foramen of Monro.[149] Stability in size and lack of symptoms differentiate these lesions from neoplasms.

Subependymal giant-cell astrocytoma is a benign, solitary neoplasm characteristically located at the foramen of Monro in patients with tuberous sclerosis.[151] The tumors usually demonstrate strong enhancement following contrast infusion, and, unlike the subependymal nodules, they tend to enlarge and become symptomatic. Due to the critical location of these tumors, patients present with hydrocephalus. Histologically, these tumors may be similar to the subependymal nodules and present a diagnostic problem; the radiologic assessment of an enlarging mass with associated hydrocephalus is crucial in differentiating a subependymal giant-cell astrocytoma from subependymal nodules.

Extracranial lesions of tuberous sclerosis involve multiple organ systems, including kidneys, lungs, heart, pancreas, liver, and bones.[144]

Sturge-Weber Syndrome

Sturge-Weber syndrome (SWS, also known as encephalotrigeminal angiomatosis) is a disease characterized by vascular malformations affecting the brain, eye, and soft tissues of the face. It is a sporadic disease with equal gender distribution. Clinically, patients present with midface angioma in the distribution of the trigeminal nerve, referred to as a port-wine stain. This is usually unilateral and consists of small, thin-walled vessels within the skin.[152] Infantile spasms develop in almost 90 percent of patients before 1 year of age. Other clinical manifestations include mental retardation, homonymous hemianopsia, and hemiparesis.[153]

Imaging of the brain reflects the pathologic process of SWS. It is believed that the pial and cutaneous angiomas result from persistence of primitive vascular channels in the subarachnoid space and impaired venous drainage.[137] The abnormal cortical vasculature leads to seizures, which in turn lead to cortical atrophy and calcifications. The CT scan demonstrates these gyriform calcifications in the subcortical white matter and cortex underlying the pial angioma, usually in the temporo-parieto-occipital lobes.[154] The pial angiomas are well seen on contrast-enhanced MRI, where they appear as enhancement over the surfaces of the gyri and in the subarachnoid spaces of the involved cortex[155,156] (Fig. 19-30). Other findings seen in SWS include accelerated myelination in areas underlying the leptomeningeal angioma,[157] enlargement of the ipsilateral choroid plexus,[158] and thickening and enhancement of the diploic space of the overlying calvaria as well as of the superficial soft tissues.[133]

Von Hippel-Lindau Disease

Von Hippel-Lindau disease (vHL, also known as CNS angiomatosis) is an autosomal dominant disease, with the gene mapped to chromosome 3.[159,160] The disease is characterized by multiple hemangioblastomas of the cerebellum, spinal cord, and retina and other visceral neoplasms. The presenting symptoms reflect the ocular, cerebellar, or spinal tumors, but most commonly patients present with visual complaints due to retinal angioblastomas (angiomas).

Cerebellar hemangioblastomas are seen in more than one half of patients with vHL and occur in the third and fourth decades.[161] More than two-thirds of tumors demonstrate the characteristic appearance, which is that of a posterior fossa cyst with a small peripheral nodule; its appearance, however, varies from cystic to entirely solid.[162] The tumor nodule is usually very vascular, demonstrating flow voids and intense enhancement on MRI. The cystic portion of the tumor usually follows CSF intensity, but may appear bright on T1- and T2-weighted images as a result of intracystic hemorrhage.

Spinal hemangioblastomas are uncommon and present as small, vascular, enhancing intramedullary lesions. This tumor is usually associated with a spinal cord syrinx.[163] Extra-CNS abnormalities are prominent in patients with vHL. The most common malignant neoplasms are renal cell carcinomas, which are multifocal

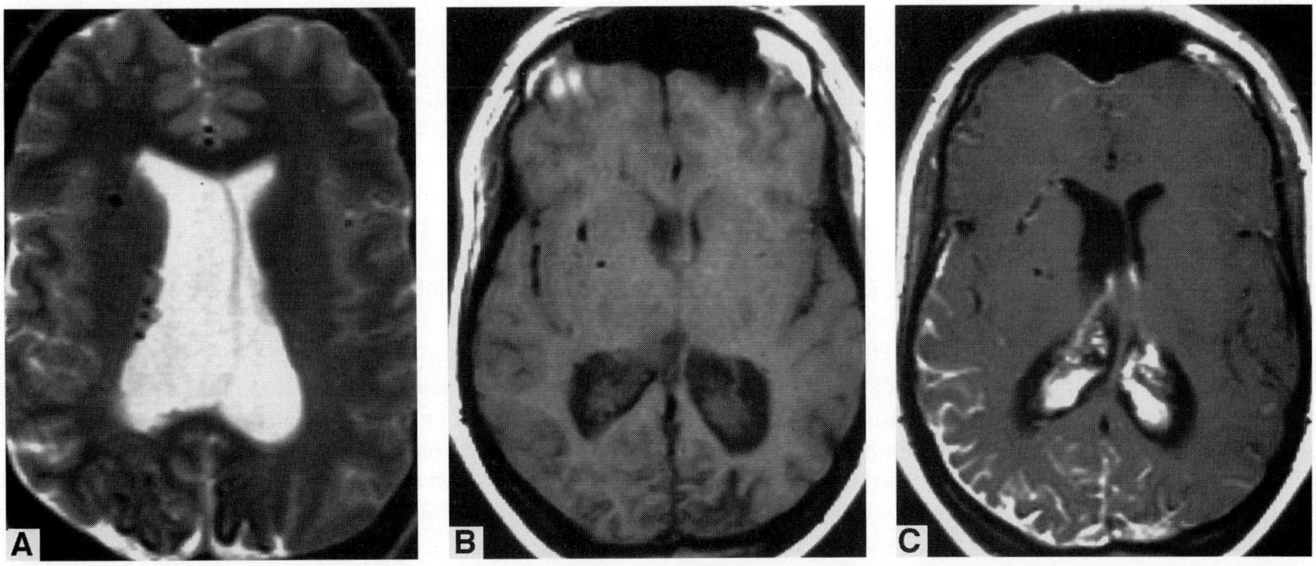

Figure 19-30
Sturge-Weber syndrome. **(A)** *Axial T2-weighted,* **(B)** *T1-weighted, and postgadolinium axial T1-weighted images demonstrate abnormal pial vessels as flow voids on precontrast images in the posterior temporal and occipital regions. Sulcal prominence reflects volume loss typically due to steal phenomenon and blood vessel pulsation. Following contrast administration, the exuberant pial vasculature is evident.*

and bilateral, and pheochromocytomas. Benign epithelial cysts develop in multiple organs.[159]

HYPOXIC-ISCHEMIC BRAIN INJURY

The pattern of injury seen in newborns with hypoxic-ischemic encephalopathy (HIE) depends on the gestational age of the patient and the severity of injury. Theories proposed to explain the difference in pattern of injury seen in preterm versus term infants are based on the distribution of metabolically active tissues in the brain and maturation of cerebral vasculature. It was shown that myelinated areas of the brain or those undergoing active myelination at the time of injury are metabolically most active and therefore most susceptible to hypoxic injury.[164–166] A second theory proposed to explain the preferential involvement of certain regions of the brain with HIE is related to the neurotoxic effect of excitatory amino acids, particularly glutamate. It was shown that cells mediating these neurotoxic effects via glutamate receptors are localized in maturing areas of the brain.[167]

Ischemic insults during the first and second trimesters of gestation interfere with the histogenesis and organogenesis of the developing brain. Such insults usually result in structural abnormalities of the brain, such as schizencephaly or polymicrogyria.[168]

The determining factor in the nature of the ischemic insult in the third-trimester preterm infant is the maturity of cerebral vasculature and location of border zones between arterial territories. Prior to 34 weeks of gestation, the superficial vessels over the brain surface are better developed than the deeper vessels. In these infants, the border zones between vascular territories are located deep in the periventricular white matter of the cerebral hemispheres.[12,169] This combination of factors leads to a more tenuous vascular supply in the periventricular white matter, which leads to the observed result of ischemic infarction in these infants: periventricular leukomalacia (PVL). A confounding factor in preterm infants is the presence of the germinal matrix, the area of formation of neuronal elements in the subependymal regions of the lateral ventricles that remains metabolically active until the third trimester. Hypoxia followed by reperfusion not uncommonly leads to hemorrhage from these highly vascularized structures. Depending on the extent of hemorrhage, germinal matrix bleeds have been graded I through IV for prediction of neurologic outcome.[170,171] Briefly, grade I hemorrhage is defined as bleeding into the germinal matrix. Grades II and III are defined as hemorrhages extending into the ventricular system without and with hydrocephalus, respectively. Grade IV hemorrhage is similar to grade III hemorrhage, but it includes an intraparenchymal hematoma as well. It is believed that the intraparenchymal hematoma in grade IV hemorrhage is due to bleeding within an area of venous infarction.[172,173] The proposed mechanism for this event is ventricular dilatation due to intraventricular clot, which causes increased intracranial pressure, leading to venous obstruction and infarction.

The sequela of HIE in premature infants (i.e., PVL and intracranial hemorrhage) are detected on ultrasound, CT, and MRI. Ultrasound is usually the first brain imaging modality used for premature, unstable patients. Acute germinal matrix hemorrhages appear as hyperechoic clot in the lateral wall of the lateral ventricle in the area of the caudothalamic groove. When echogenic clot is seen within the ventricle, a diagnosis of grade II or III germinal matrix hemorrhage can be made, depending on the absence or presence of ventricular dilatation. Acute intraparenchymal hemorrhage appears as hyperechoic clot within the brain parenchyma and is usually accompanied by mass effect with midline shift and effacement of the sulci and ventricles. Gradually the echogenicity of the clot decreases, and eventually encephalomalacia develops in this area.[174]

The most sensitive appearance of acute PVL on ultrasound is a diffuse increase in echogenicity in the periventricular regions that progresses to cavitation 2 to 6 weeks after the initial insult.[175–177] The CT scan may show nonspecific areas of low attenuation adjacent to the frontal horns and atria of the lateral ventricles.[112,178] Because of the high water content of nonmyelinated white matter, these areas may be difficult to appreciate on T2-weighted images. The decreased signal may be easier to detect on T1-weighted images, or, alternatively, very heavily T2-weighted images may be used.[112] In the chronic stages, MRI demonstrates the hallmarks of PVL, which are white matter atrophy in the peritrigonal regions, apposition of the posterior sylvian cortex to the trigone of the lateral ventricle, ventriculomegaly, thinning of the posterior body and splenium of the corpus callosum, and delayed myelination[179,180] (Fig. 19-31).

Maturation of the cerebral vasculature in term infants leads to a shift of the border zones to more peripheral regions of the cerebral convexities. In term infants, these border zones are located in parasagittal locations of the cortex and subcortical white matter, between the territories of the anterior and middle cerebral arteries and the middle and posterior cerebral arteries.[112] In addition, there is a second area of relative hypoperfusion: the sulcal depth in the parasagittal regions of the hemispheres.[169] Preferential damage to the depth of the sulci, while the crowns of the gyri remain relatively intact, leads to mushroom-shaped gyri, known as ulegyria.

Imaging studies reflect these developmental changes. Acute cortical and subcortical infarcts of the frontal and parieto-occipital lobes may appear as echogenic areas on ultrasound and hyperlucent regions on CT. As discussed above, these changes are best demonstrated as areas of decreased T1 signal intensity. The parasagittal ulegyria is readily detected on MRI, where the gyri

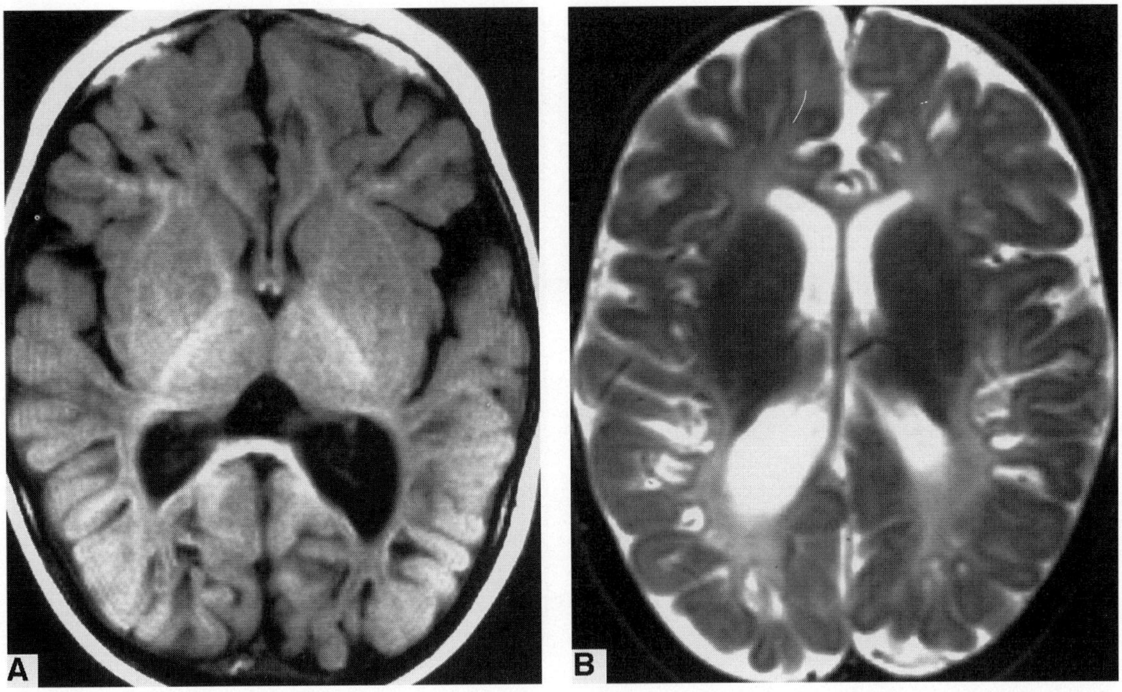

Figure 19-31
Periventricular leukomalacia. **(A)** *Axial T1-weighted and* **(B)** *T2-weighted images demonstrate extensive volume loss throughout the cerebral hemispheres. In addition, there is gliosis surrounding the atria and occipital horns of the lateral ventricles. The paucity of white matter reflected is posteriorly by the close proximity of the posterior sylvian fissure to the atrium of the lateral ventricle.*

have the characteristic mushroom shape described above (Fig. 19-32). T2-weighted images may show foci of subcortical hyperintensity at the base of the gyri where gliosis has occurred.[41,112] Subacute changes include hemorrhagic transformation of these infarcts and parenchymal enhancement following breakdown of the blood-brain barrier. Finally, the chronic stage of diffuse hypoxic injury is characterized by multicystic encephalomalacia, which develops in the mature brain capable of mounting a gliotic response[112] (Fig. 19-32).

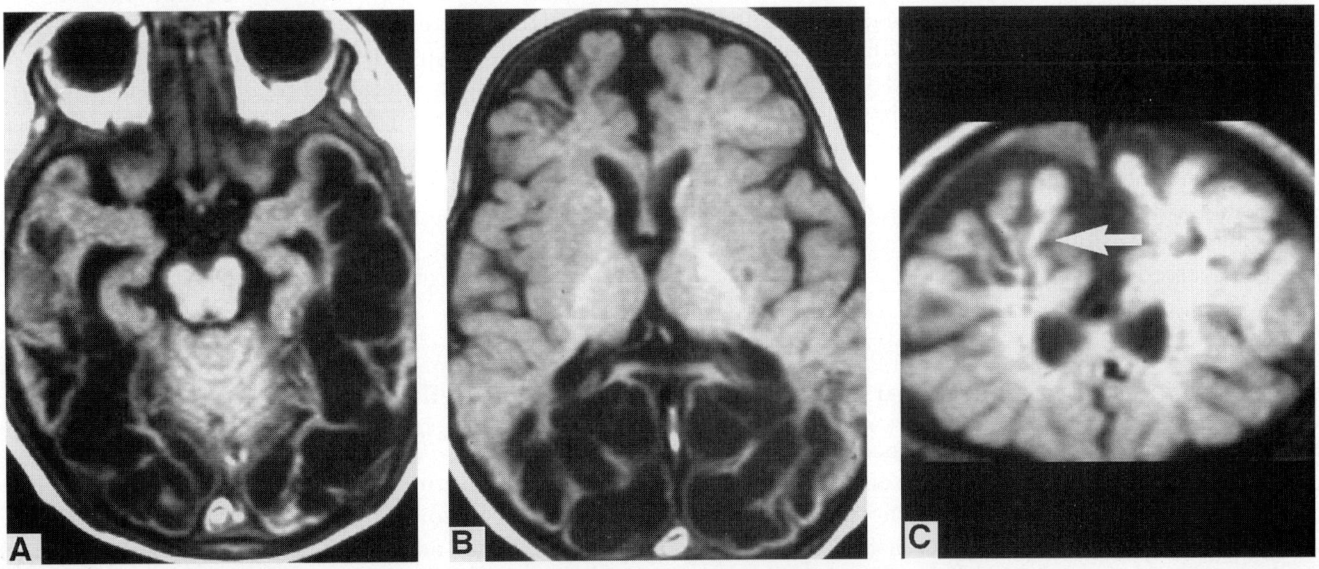

Figure 19-32
Multicystic leukomalacia and ulegyria. **(A and B)** *T1-weighted axial and* **(C)** *coronal images demonstrate extensive volume loss and CSF-filled cavities in both parieto-occipital areas and temporal regions, characteristic of multicystic encephalomalacia. Ulegyria, or the presence of mushroom-shaped gyri, is caused by volume loss at the depth of the sulci following subcortical ischemia and infarcts in term infants due to border zone ischemia at the depth of the sulcus.*

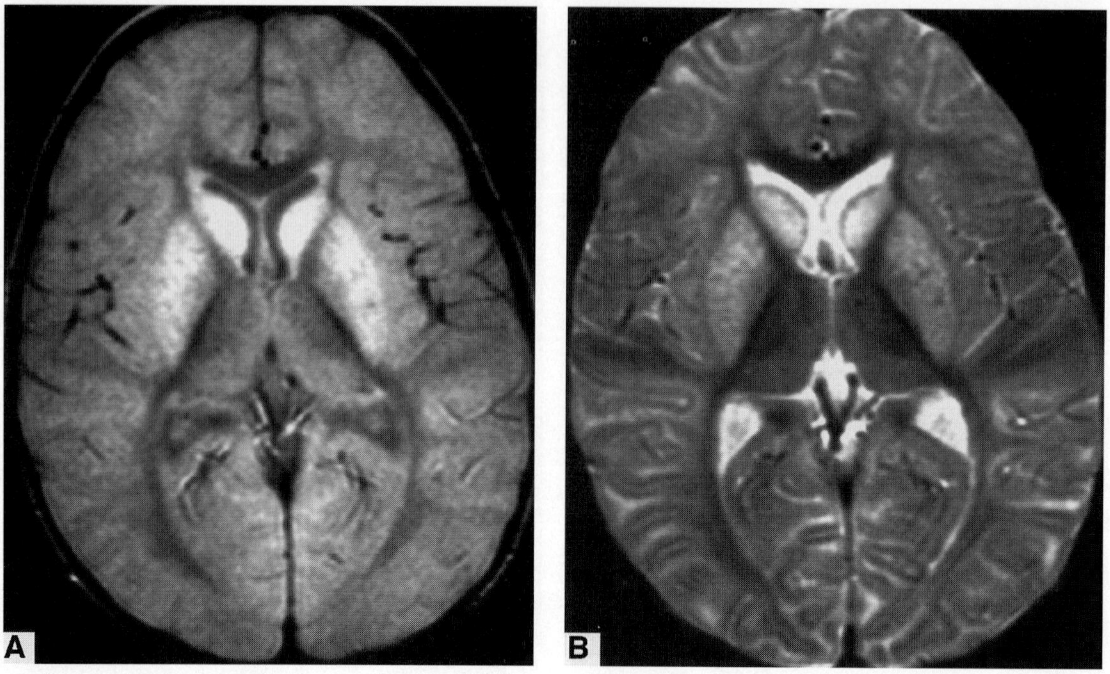

Figure 19-33
Profound asphyxia. **(A)** *Axial proton-density and* **(B)** *T2-weighted images show abnormally increased signal in the caudate and lenticular nuclei bilaterally due to severe anoxic injury in term infants.*

Pathologically, this process represents liquefactive necrosis of the cortex and underlying white matter with an astrocytic response that on imaging studies is characterized by variously sized, multiple, septated cystic cavities.[41,112]

Of special note is the pattern of injury that occurs in preterm and term infants who have suffered profound asphyxia. In this case, the injury is different from PVL and the border zone infarcts; it involves primarily the deep gray matter nuclei, namely, the thalami and basal ganglia, posterior mesencephalon, and descending corticospinal tracts (Fig. 19-33). The proposed explanation for this pattern of injury is dual and involves (1) increased metabolic activity of these structures and (2) increased local concentration of excitatory amino acids, both of which contribute to increased anoxic susceptibility, as discussed above.[112,181]

TOXIC AND METABOLIC BRAIN DISORDERS

Patients with toxic and metabolic brain disorders usually present with nonspecific symptoms (i.e., developmental delay, seizures, or focal neurologic symptoms). The final diagnosis is usually dependent on specific laboratory findings, since the imaging studies are usually nonspecific. The role of the radiologist is to offer a differential diagnosis that, when coupled with clinical findings, arrives at a more specific entity. For this purpose, among other things, careful evaluation of the pattern of myelination for the patient's age, as well as the appearance of the deep gray matter structures, is important. Myelination proceeds in an orderly fashion, which in a normal subject is very predictable. Extensive examples of normal myelination throughout development have been published.[112,182,183]

Disorders of the white matter fall into two categories. Demyelination is the loss of existing myelin and includes primary disorders, such as multiple sclerosis (MS) or other metabolic or neurodegenerative disorders, and secondary insults, such as ischemia, radiation therapy, or chemotherapy. Dysmyelination is the production of abnormal myelin. Dysmyelinating diseases are usually manifested by bilaterally symmetrical foci of abnormal signal, which initially affect the deep white matter preferentially. In contradistinction, demyelinating diseases demonstrate asymmetrical, sharply defined areas of abnormal signal with a more peripheral distribution.

Dysmyelinating Conditions

Adrenoleukodystrophy

Adrenoleukodystrophies are a group of disorders characterized by abnormal peroxisomal function involving the brain and adrenal gland caused by abnormal metabolism of long-chain fatty acids. X-linked adrenoleukodystrophy is seen exclusively in males and presents between the ages of 3 and 10 years. Presenting symptoms usually include behavorial problems, abnormal gait, and visual and auditory disturbances. The disease progresses rapidly to seizures, hypotonia, dementia, and blindness, and signs of adrenal failure are also noticeable.[184]

The MRI demonstrates confluent and symmetrical areas of long T1 and T2 relaxation times in the periventricular white matter around the atria of the lateral ventricles and the splenium of the corpus callosum[185,186] (Fig. 19-34). Occasionally, a thin band of enhancement is present at the anterior edge of the abnormal white matter, believed to represent the leading edge of the active demyelination. The CT scan demonstrates similar findings, with hypoattenuation of the posterior periventricular white matter and thin, peripheral enhancement. Other areas involved include the optic and auditory pathways. The cerebellar white matter, middle cerebellar peduncles, and descending pyramidal tracts can also be involved.[187] Proton spectroscopy of the abnormal white matter has shown promise in noninvasive diagnosis of this disorder.[188,189]

Metachromatic Leukodystrophy

Metachromatic leukodystrophy is a disorder of lysosomal function inherited in an autosomal recessive fashion and caused by deficiency of arylsulfatase A. The normal turnover of myelin is affected, leading to myelin breakdown and accumulation of cerebroside within lysosomes.[190] The most common form is the late infantile type, which presents at 1 or 2 years of age. Other variants include the congenital form, which presents at birth, as well as the juvenile and the adult forms. Initial symptoms include hypotonia, gait disorder, spasticity, and nystagmus, which progress to mental deterioration, blindness, decerebrate posturing, and death.[184]

Magnetic resonance imaging demonstrates symmetrical areas of T1 hypointensity and T2 signal hyperintensity in the deep white matter adjacent to the frontal horns and atria of the lateral ventricles. Enhancement of these lesions has not been reported. Involvement of the corpus callosum is also seen[191] (Fig. 19-35). As the disease progresses, the areas of abnormal signal coalesce and increase in size, and diffuse volume loss becomes apparent.

Krabbe Disease

Krabbe disease, or globoid cell leukodystrophy, is another autosomal recessive disorder of lysosomal function caused by deficiency of the galactocerebroside β-galactosidase. Patients usually present before 6 months of age with acute onset of intermittent fever, irritability, increased muscle tone, and hyperacusis.[190]

Imaging studies may be diagnostic. Early in the course of the disease, CT may demonstrate increased attenuation of the thalami, caudate nuclei, corona radiata, internal capsules, and brainstem,[192,193] which correlates with fine calcifications found in these structures at autopsy.[194] Magnetic resonance imaging demonstrates involvement of the cerebellar white matter, deep gray nuclei (dentate, basal ganglia, and thalamus), pyramidal tract, posterior aspect of the corpus callusum, and parieto-

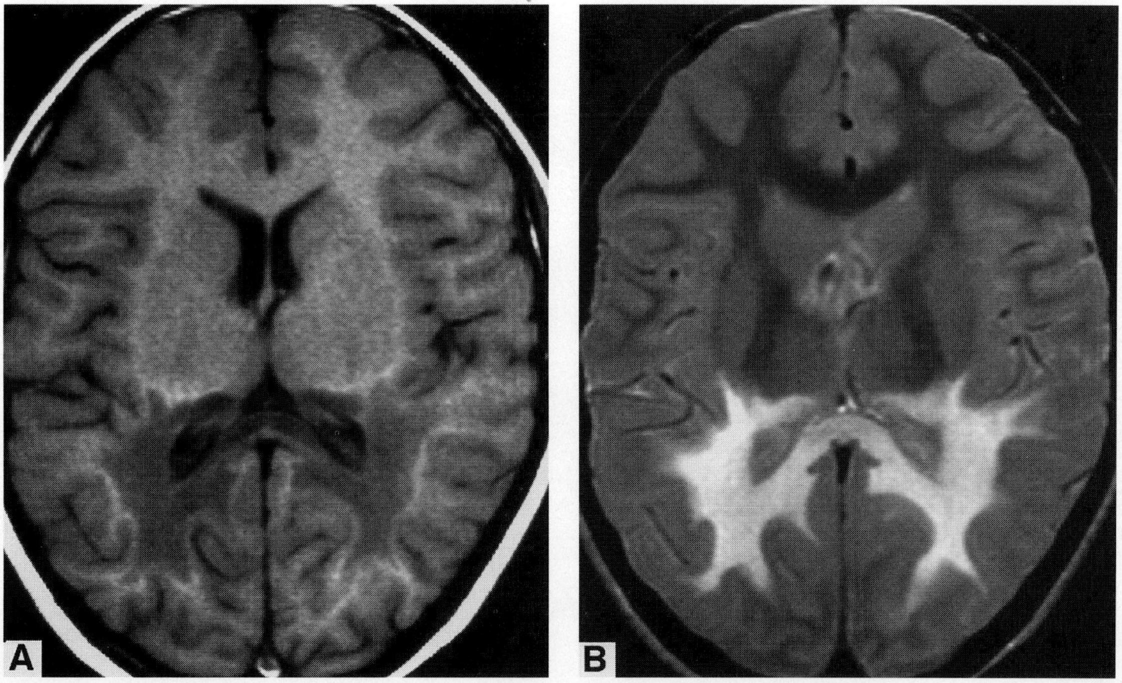

Figure 19-34
Adrenoleukodystrophy. Extensive white matter signal abnormality is seen on **(A)** *axial T1-weighted and* **(B)** *T2-weighted images in both posterior temporal and occipital regions and the corpus callosum. This extensive symmetrical pattern of involvement with posterior predilection is characteristic of adrenoleukodystrophy.*

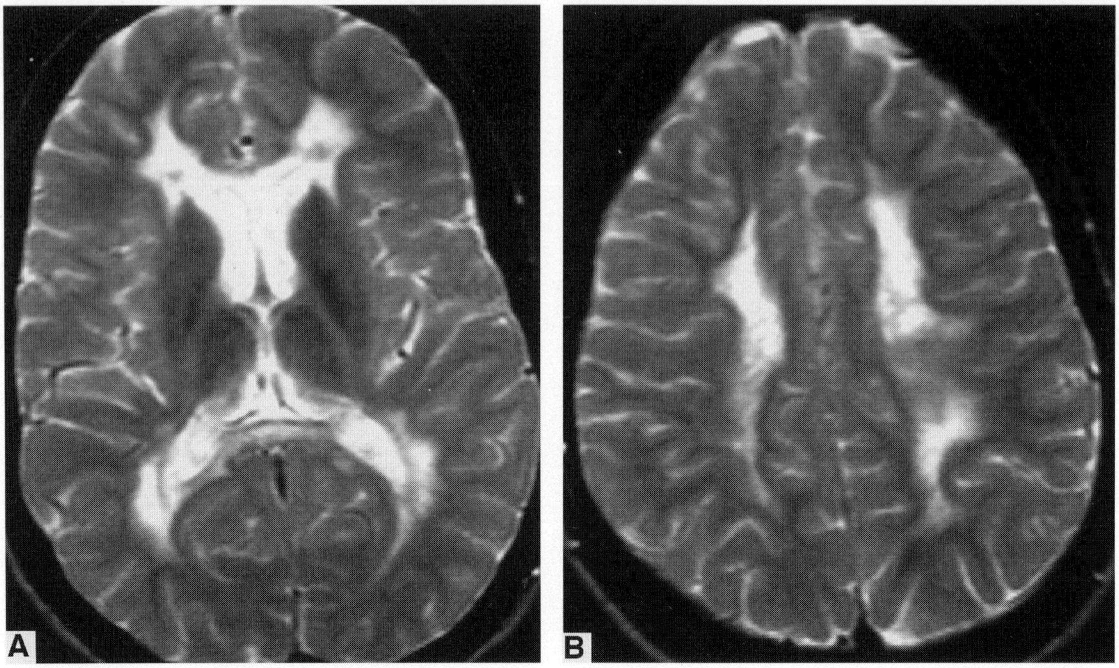

Figure 19-35
Metachromatic leukodystrophy. **(A and B)** *Axial T2-weighted images show coalescent, symmetrical areas of white matter signal abnormality around the frontal and occipital horns of the lateral ventricles.*

occipital white matter (Fig. 19-36) (DJ Loes, personal communication).[195]

Canavan Disease and Alexander Disease

Canavan disease and Alexander disease are two leukodystrophies that present with macrocephaly. Another common feature is preferential involvement of the peripheral white matter, in contradistinction to other leukodystrophies, which tend to spare the subcortical U fibers.

Canavan disease is an autosomal recessive disorder described initially in Jews of eastern Europe. In the most common infantile form, patients present at 2 to 4

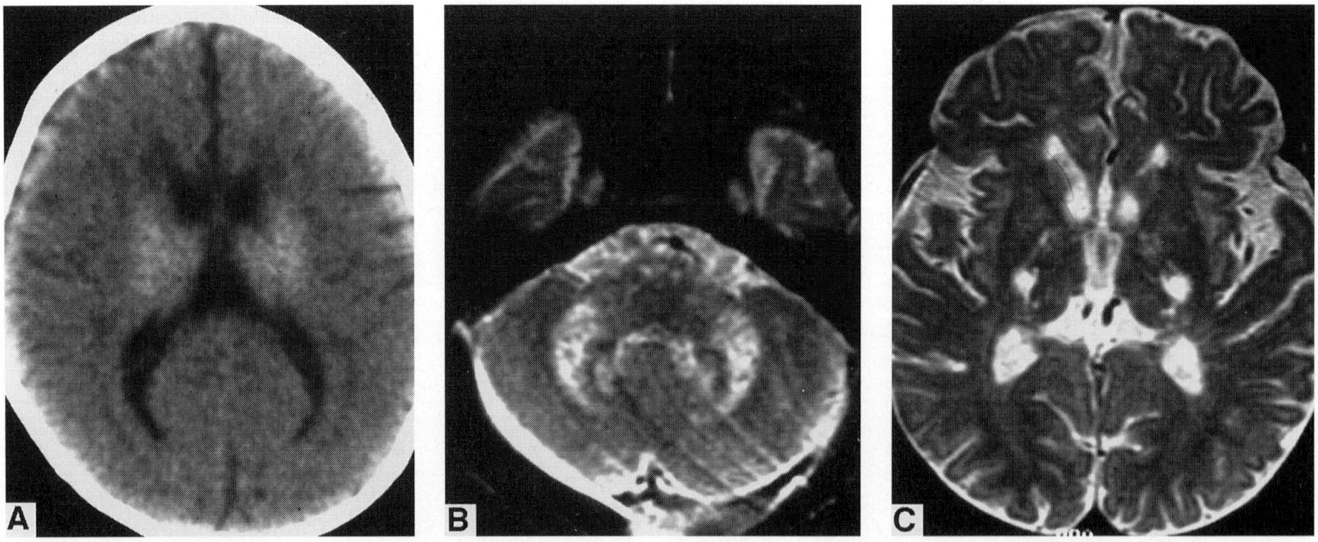

Figure 19-36
Krabbe disease. **(A)** *An unenhanced axial CT scan demonstrates the typical appearance of hyperdense thalami seen in Krabbe disease.* **(B and C)** *Axial T2-weighted images demonstrate involvement of the descending cortical spinal tracts, thalami, and dentate nuclei of the cerebellum. (Courtesy of Daniel J. Loes. Reprinted by permission of the* American Journal of Neuroradiology.*)*

months of age with hypotonia and macrocephaly. Symptoms progress with development of hypertonia, spasticity, seizures, vegetative state, and death by the age of 3 years.[12]

Imaging studies obtained at the onset of disease demonstrate T1 signal hypointensity and T2 signal hyperintensity of the subcortical U fibers throughout the cerebral hemispheres, although they are more prominent in the occipital lobes. The globi pallidi may also be involved.[112,190] A specific finding for this disease is a significant increase of the *N*-acetyl aspartate peak on proton spectroscopy and an absent choline peak.[196,197]

Alexander disease is a disease of unknown cause with onset before 2 years of age. Children present with seizures, psychomotor retardation, and macrocephaly, with death occuring in early childhood.[12,185] Findings on MRI demonstrate extensive areas of T2 signal hyperintensity involving the white matter, including the subcortical fibers, and the internal capsule. Frontal involvement is typical early in the disease, with extension of the demyelinating process posteriorly.[198] Magnetic resonance proton spectroscopy of abnormal white matter areas demonstrates decreased *N*-acetyl aspartate and lactate levels.[197]

Demyelinating Conditions

Multiple Sclerosis

Between 0.3 and 5.6 percent of all cases of MS present in childhood.[199] The usual age at presentation is in the early teenage years, although much younger patients have been reported.[200] The clinical presentation is similar to that of the adult form, with a clinical history of multiple neurologic deficits with a remitting and relapsing course. Common presenting symptoms include sensory or motor symptoms, optic neuritis, blurred vision, diplopia, or gait difficulty.[199] Laboratory findings that support the diagnosis of MS include oligoclonal bands in the CSF, CSF pleocytosis, and abnormal evoked potentials.[183] Imaging findings are similar in children and adults with MS. Magnetic resonance imaging is the most sensitive modality for demonstrating plaques in the brain or spinal cord. The demyelinating plaques appear as asymmetrical foci of T2 signal hyperintensity in the white matter of the brain, particularly in the periventricular areas, or the spinal cord. The typical appearance of perivenular plaques radiating from the ventricular surface ("Dawson's fingers") is seen in children as well as adults (Fig. 19-37). Active plaques demonstrate peripheral enhancement, which has been correlated with the presence of acute inflammation, and mass effect.[183,190] In our practice, sagittal proton-density and T2-weighted images are routinely obtained in suspected MS cases; these images demonstrate to great advantage lesions of the corpus callosum and the perivenular plaques.

Acute Disseminated Encephalomyelitis

Acute disseminated encephalomyelitis (ADEM) is an autoimmune demyelinating disease precipitated by a viral infection or postvaccination. The most common presentation includes seizures and focal neurologic deficits 7 to 14 days after the onset of viral illness or vaccination. Although most patients recover fully, 10 to 20 percent of patients die during the first week of disease or experience permanent neurologic damage.[201]

Magnetic resonance imaging demonstrates asymmetrical foci of demyelination, which appear as areas of T2 signal hyperintensity in the subcortical white matter of the cerebral hemispheres. The cerebellum, brainstem, and cervical cord can also be affected[202] (Fig. 19-38). The deep nuclei are usually involved in ADEM, which distinguishes this entity from MS.[203] Enhancement may be seen in the subacute phase of the disease, and it usually improves with improvement in the clinical course of the disease.[204]

Disorders of Lipid Metabolism

Disorders of lipid metabolism are characterized by abnormal sphingolipid metabolism and subsequent accumulation of membrane lipids within lysosomes. Both the white and gray matter structures are affected, although the white matter is involved to a greater degree.[185,190] Among diseases included in this category are Tay-Sachs disease, Sandhoff disease, Gaucher disease, and Fabry disease.

Imaging findings are often nonspecific. Generally, there are gray and white matter volume loss and areas of prolonged T2 relaxation of the white matter. More specific changes have been described in Tay-Sachs and Sandhoff diseases. Early changes consist of decreased attenuation of the caudate nuclei on CT and increased T2 signal intensity of the caudate heads and lentiform nuclei on MRI. In the late phase of the disease, there is shortening of the T1 and T2 relaxation values of the caudate nucleus and thalamus, along with extensive atrophy and cavitation of the cerebral and cerebellar white matter.[205–207]

Mucopolysaccharidoses

Mucopolysaccharidoses are a group of diseases characterized by an abnormality of the lysosomal enzymes responsible for degrading mucopolysaccharides. The clinical presentation varies among the individual types; however, CNS, visceral, and bony abnormalities are common.[184] As a result of abnormal accumulation of mucopolysaccharides, patients may have macrocephaly, with thickening of the meninges and inner table of the skull.

Imaging findings correlate with histopathologic abnormalities. The most prominent abnormality is dila-

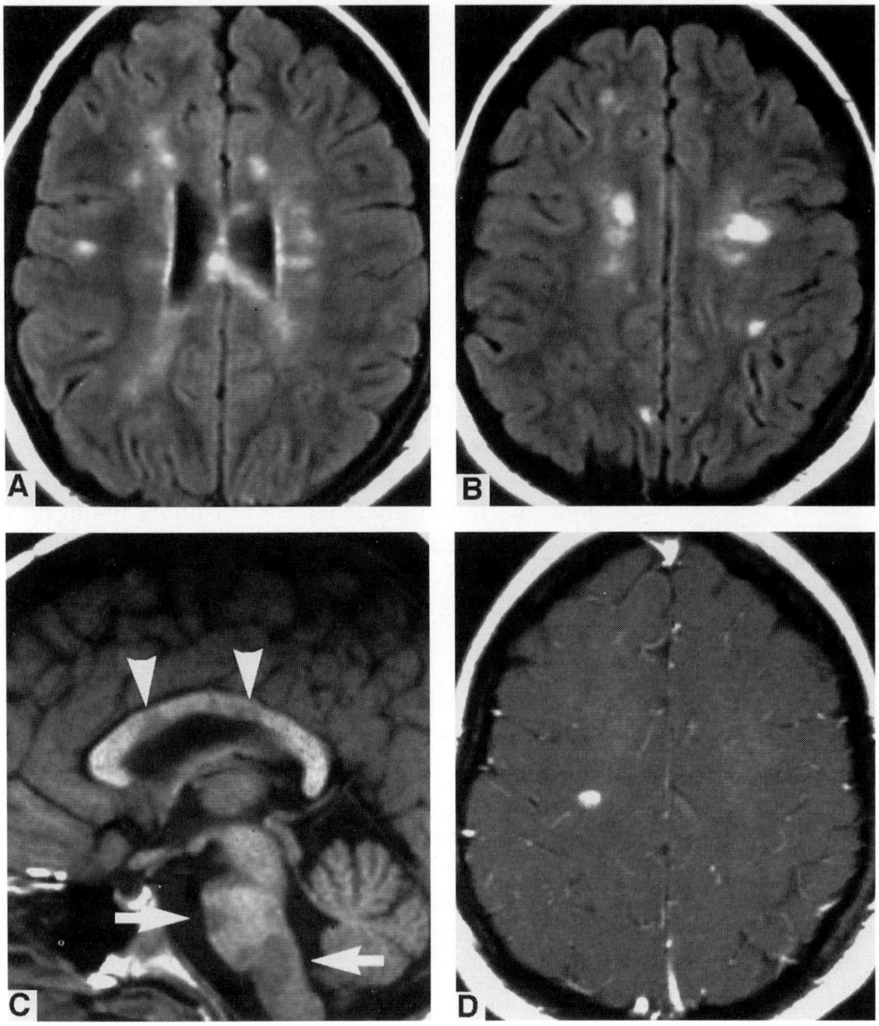

Figure 19-37
Juvenile MS. **(A and B)** *Axial turbo-FLAIR images demonstrate numerous foci of white matter abnormality in both cerebral hemispheres as well as the corpus callosum.* **(C)** *The involvement of the corpus callosum and the brainstem is also demonstrated on sagittal T1-weighted image.* **(D)** *An active enhancing plaque is seen following intravenous gadolinium administration. (Courtesy of Dr. Douglas H. Yock, Jr.)*

tation of the perivascular spaces due to accumulation of metabolites in foam cells within Virchow-Robin spaces (Fig. 19-39). The corpus callosum is also affected, and the basal ganglia may be involved in certain types of mucopolysaccharidoses.[208,209] Mucopolysaccharide deposition in the transverse ligament of the odontoid causes erosion of the dens and replacement of this structure by a "mucopolysaccharide cap." Involvement of the craniocervical junction results in atlantoaxial instability as well as compression of the cervicomedullary junction and communicating hydrocephalus.[210,211] Additional findings in patients with mucopolysaccharidoses include typical bone changes collectively known as dysostosis multiplex.[212] These changes include a dolichocephalic skull with widened diploic space, frontal bossing, and a J-shaped sella. Gibbous deformity of the spine consists of a hooklike configuration of the vertebral bodies at the thoracolumbar junction. Appendicular skeleton involvement includes the hips, phalanges, and long bones.

Mitochondrial Encephalomyelopathies

Mitochondrial encephalomyelopathies are a group of disorders characterized by deficiency or suspected abnormalities of mitochondrial enzymes leading to multisystem involvement, including the nervous system, muscular system, cardiovascular system, gastrointestinal system, and endocrine system.[112,213] Certain clinical features are common to this group of disorders, among which is muscle weakness, motor difficulty, cortical blindness, sensorineural hearing loss, and mental deficiency.[214] Laboratory findings generally show elevated level of serum lactate, which accumulates as a result of failure of aerobic metabolism. These findings are, however, not diagnostic, and patients with suspected mitochondrial disorders usually undergo skeletal muscle biopsy for diagnosis.[215]

Imaging studies demonstrate both white and gray matter abnormalities. The basal ganglia, cerebral cortex, and brainstem are usually more severely affected, prob-

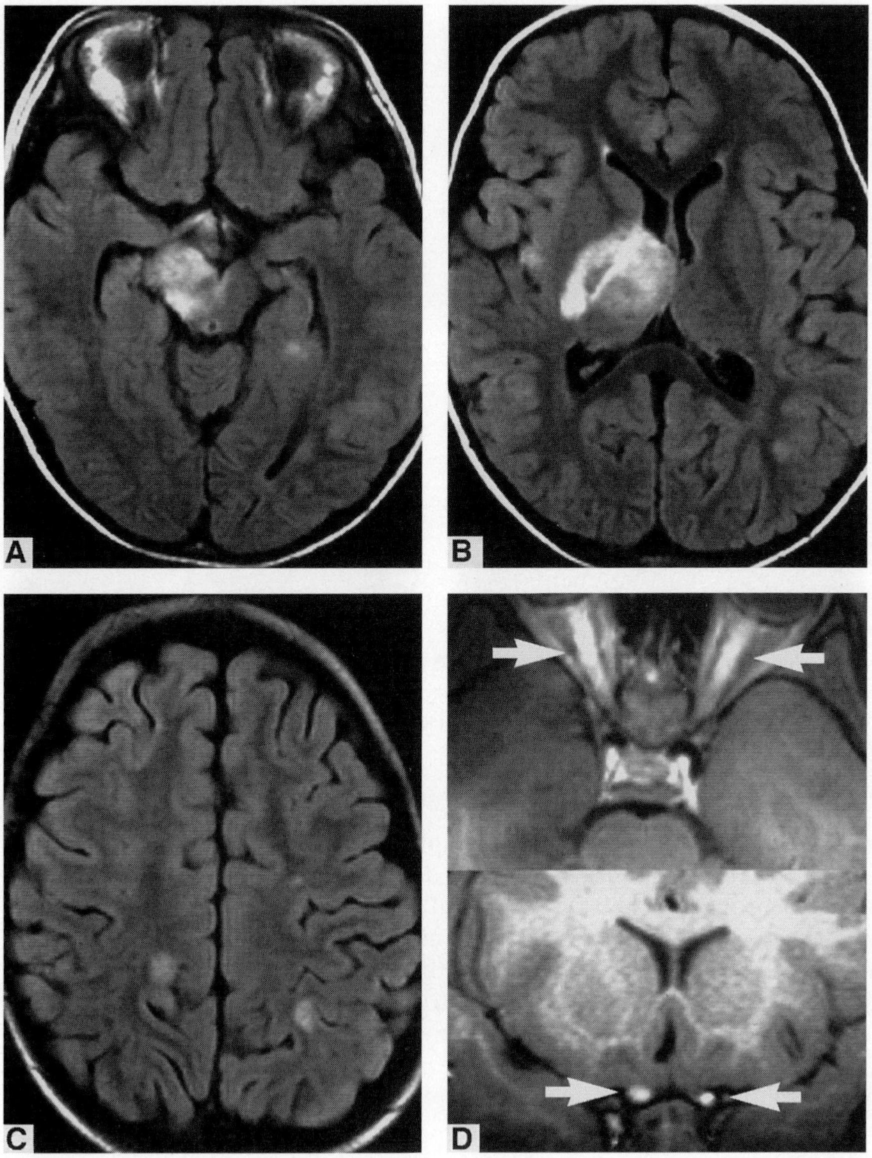

Figure 19-38
Acute demyelinating encephalomyelitis. **(A–C)** *Multifocal signal abnormality is seen on axial turbo-FLAIR images in the brainstem, basal ganglia, internal capsule, and deep and subcortical white matter. Diffuse enhancement of the intra-orbital segments of the optic nerves indicates bilateral optic neuritis on* **(D)** *axial and coronal T1-weighted post-gadolinium images.*

ably because of their higher metabolic activity. However, the combination of deep gray matter involvement and peripheral white matter involvement in young adults or children should suggest a diagnosis of mitochondrial encephalomyelopathy, especially when associated with an elevated lactate peak on proton magnetic resonance spectroscopy.[216,217]

The spectrum of imaging findings varies among the mitochondrial encephalomyelopathies. Subacute necrotizing encephalomyopathy (Leigh disease) occurs in infants and young children and demonstrates most severe involvement of the brainstem, substantia nigra, and basal ganglia.[218,219] The entities known as MELAS (myopathy, encephalopathy, lactic acidosis, and strokelike episodes) and MERRF (myoclonic epilepsy with ragged red fibers) present in older children and adults. A characteristic finding in MELAS is cortical infarcts with a predominantly posterior distribution, which leads to cortical blindness and hemiparesis [220] (Fig. 19-40). Patients with MERRF present with optic nerve atrophy and calcification of the globi pallidi and dentate nuclei on CT scans.[220]

Abnormalities of Amino Acid Metabolism

Disorders of amino acid metabolisms are rare and are usually due to the involvement of an abnormal enzyme in catabolism of proteins, with a resulting increased concentration of amino acids in serum and urine. These disorders can affect both the gray and white matter. Imaging findings usually demonstrate delayed myelination as well as reduction in the amount of myelin. Older patients may demonstrate cerebral and cerebellar atrophy. The imaging findings are nonspecific, and diagnosis

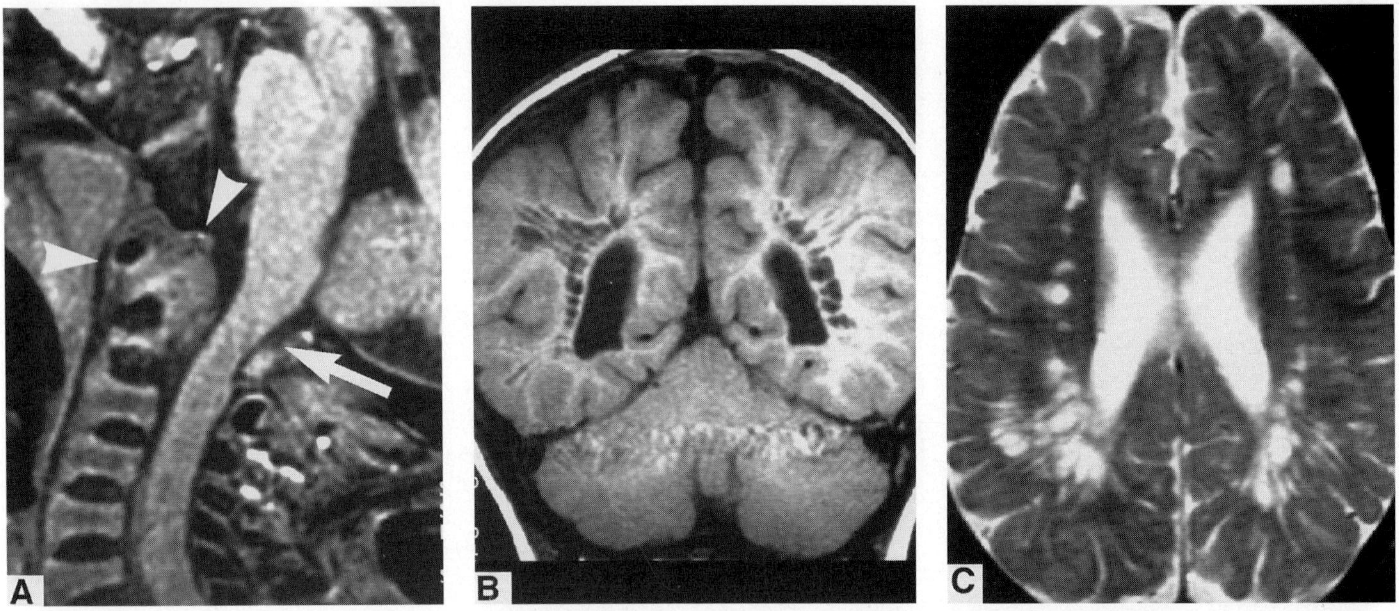

Figure 19-39
Hurler disease. **(A)** *A sagittal proton-density image through the craniocervical junction demonstrates a large mucopolysaccharide "cap" replacing most of the odontoid process (white arrowheads) and causing narrowing of the foramen magnum during extension.* **(B)** *T1-weighted coronal and* **(C)** *T2-weighted axial images demonstrate multiple CSF-containing spaces caused by accumulation of "foamy" cells within the perivascular spaces.*

is usually made based on demonstration of increased amino acids in blood and urine.[183]

Phenylketonuria is the most common of the disorders of amino acid metabolism. It is transmitted as an autosomal recessive trait and occurs in approximately 1 in 14,000 live births. Deficiency of phenylalanine hydroxylase leads to increased blood levels of phenylalanine, causing developmental delay, irritability, and seizures.[221] Imaging findings include delayed myelination followed by dysmyelination, which has a more posterior distribution involving the periatrial areas and optic radiations. Later in the course of disease, an abnormal signal in the white matter is noted in the frontal lobes as well.[222,223]

Maple syrup urine disease is caused by a defect in the breakdown of branched-chain amino acids, causing excretion of metabolites in the urine and giving it a characteristic maple syrup odor.[224] The most severe type of this disease has its onset in the first week of life, with difficulty in feeding, seizures, impaired consciousness, and rapid death if untreated.[224] Imaging studies demonstrate diffuse cerebral edema and diffuse white matter T2 hyperintensity. More focal findings of signal abnormality in the cerebellar white matter, brainstem, thalami, and basal ganglia reflect spongiform changes within these areas. As the disease progresses, diffuse atrophy of the entire brain is seen.[225]

Glutaric Aciduria Type I

This organic aciduria is related to deficiency of glutaryl coenzyme A dehydrogenase. Patients present with extrapyramidal symptoms, such as spasticity, choreoathetosis, ataxia, and distonia.[226] Metabolites tend to accumulate in the basal ganglia, preferentially in the caudate nucleus and putamen, with resulting T2 signal hyperintensity within these structures.[227,228] There are also frontotemporal atrophy and enlargement of the sylvian fissure, which may be due to formation of bilateral arachnoid cysts.[227,228] These fluid collections, however, may be partially reversible with appropriate therapy.

CONGENITAL INFECTIONS OF THE CNS

Congenital infections of the CNS are usually acquired by transplacental transmission or ascending cervical infection. A major determinant of the effect of the insult is the timing of infection. Early infections influence organogenesis and result in conditions such as hydranencephaly or schizencephaly. Infections occurring during the third trimester of gestation cause focal or widespread destructive changes. This section covers the pathologic conditions and imaging studies of congenital infections included under the acronym TORCH (toxoplasmosis, rubella, cytomegalovirus [CMV], and herpes).

Toxoplasmosis

Toxoplasmosis is caused by the protozoan *Toxoplasma gondii.* The incidence of infection is estimated to be 1 in 1000 to 1 in 3500 births.[232] Infections occurring very

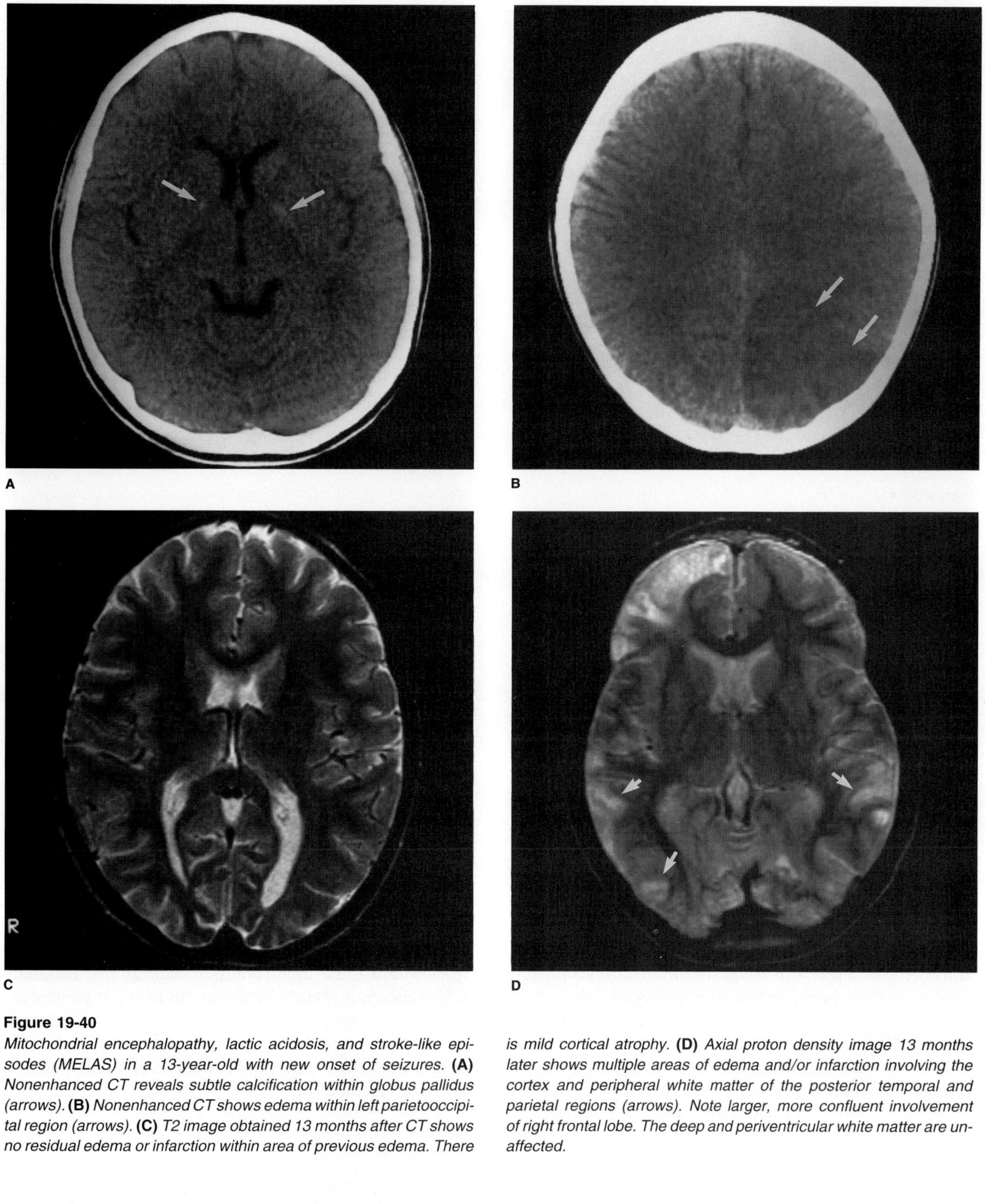

Figure 19-40
Mitochondrial encephalopathy, lactic acidosis, and stroke-like episodes (MELAS) in a 13-year-old with new onset of seizures. **(A)** *Nonenhanced CT reveals subtle calcification within globus pallidus (arrows).* **(B)** *Nonenhanced CT shows edema within left parietooccipital region (arrows).* **(C)** *T2 image obtained 13 months after CT shows no residual edema or infarction within area of previous edema. There is mild cortical atrophy.* **(D)** *Axial proton density image 13 months later shows multiple areas of edema and/or infarction involving the cortex and peripheral white matter of the posterior temporal and parietal regions (arrows). Note larger, more confluent involvement of right frontal lobe. The deep and periventricular white matter are unaffected.*

early during gestation result in spontaneous abortion, while late infections may have no detectable sequelae. The most severe clinical manifestations occur with infections acquired between the second and sixth months of gestation. CNS findings include bilateral chorioretinitis, hydrocephalus, seizures, mental retardation, and developmental delay.[233,234]

Imaging studies demonstrate periventricular as well as parenchymal calcifications and ventriculomegaly. The parenchymal calcifications tend to involve the basal gan-

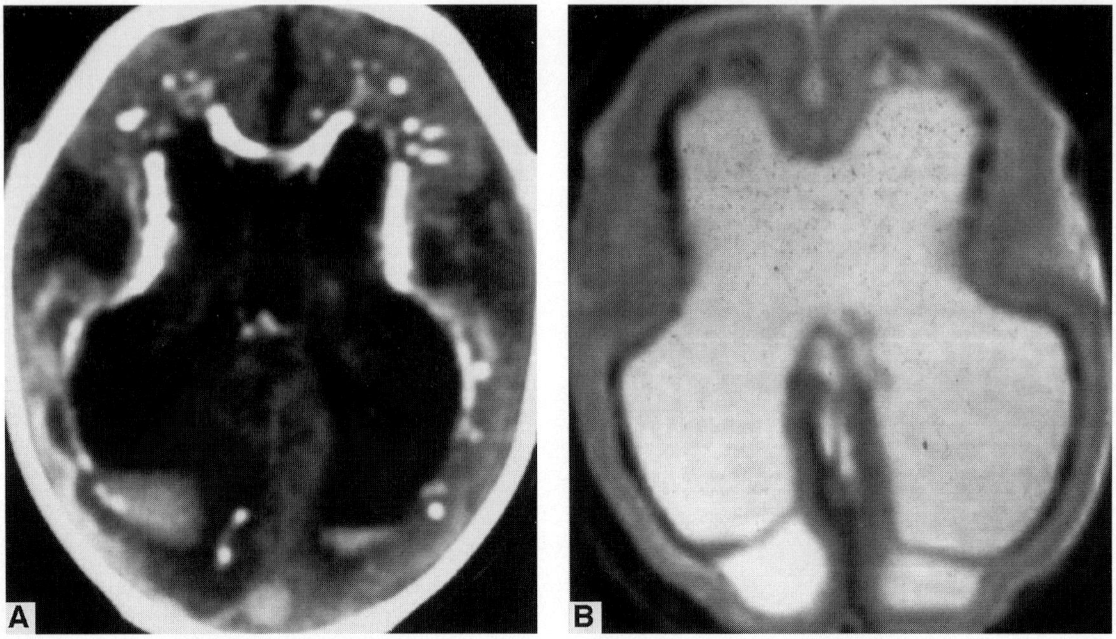

Figure 19-41
Cytomegalovirus infection. ***(A)*** *An unenhanced head CT scan demonstrates extensive periventricular calcifications typical of in utero CMV infection.* ***(B)*** *An axial T2-weighted image demonstrates the extensive periventricular calcifications as areas of marked T2-shortening. A small amount of blood from recent ventriculostomy is seen in the occipital horns of the lateral ventricles.*

glia, although they may be seen anywhere within the hemispheres. Regions of hypoattenuation in the cerebral white matter are seen on CT, and regions of T2 signal hyperintensity are seen on MRI, corresponding to areas of inflammation and gliosis[235] (Fig. 19-42). In contradistinction to CMV infection, migrational abnormalities are rarely seen in congenital toxoplasmosis infection.

Rubella

Congenital rubella in the western world is rare due to increased screening and immunizations. In utero infection occurs by transplacental spread of the virus, with the most severe involvement when the infection occurs during the second month of gestation.[236] Patients present with cataracts, micro-ophthalmia, glaucoma, chorioretinitis, choriomalformation, seizures, and deafness.[235,237]

The CT scan demonstrates calcification in the basal ganglia, cortex, and white matter, believed to be sequelae of a mineralizing vasculopathy similar to that seen with CMV.[235] Other findings include nonspecific white matter changes, probably reflecting neurovascular lesions, which persist into adulthood, and delayed myelination.[235,237] Migrational abnormalities may be seen in patients infected early in pregnancy.[112]

Cytomegalovirus

Human CMV is the most common viral infection in newborns. It is estimated that approximately 1 to 2 percent of all newborns are infected with CMV; however, less than 10 percent of these newborns will develop signs and symptoms of clinical infection. An additional 15 percent of infected infants will develop complications in the first few years of life.[229]

Clinically, CMV infections involve the reticuloendothial system, with resulting hepatosplenomegaly and petechial hemorrhages. Involvement of other organ systems produces congenital heart disease and inguinal hernias. Neurologic complications include intracranial calcifications, microcephaly, optic atrophy, chorioretinitis, and seizures.[230]

Imaging studies demonstrate periventricular calcifications in approximately 50 percent of patients (Fig. 19-41). Other findings depend on the timing of infection. Migrational abnormalities such as lissencephaly, schizencephaly, polymicrogyria, and severe ventriculomegaly are seen in patients affected in the first and second trimester, while parenchymal atrophy, hemorrhage, and calcifications may be seen in patients infected late during gestation.[83,84,231]

Herpes Simplex

Most congenital herpes simplex encephalitis is caused by type II herpes simplex virus. The infant acquires the infection either during birth, through mucosal contact with herpetic lesions, or as an ascending infection from the infected genital tract of the mother following rupture of the amniotic membranes. Incidence is estimated at 1 in 2000 to 1 in 5000 births, with CNS involvement in

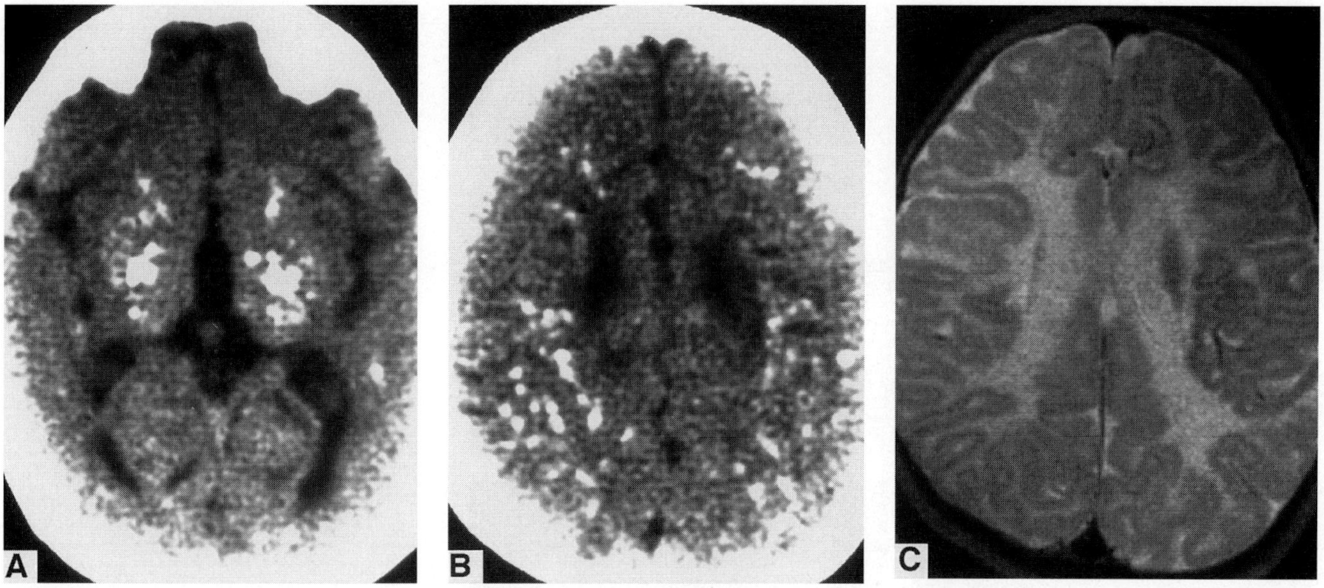

Figure 19-42
Toxoplasmosis. **(A and B)** *Noncontrast axial head CT scans demonstrate extensive parenchymal calcifications clustered in the thalami as well as in the subcortical and deeper white matter.* **(C)** *An axial T2-weighted image shows nonspecific white matter changes characterized by diffuse hyperintensity.*

approximately 30 percent of infected infants.[238] Infants develop lethargy, stupor, irritability, seizures, and coma 2 to 4 weeks after birth.

Acutely, the disease demonstrates abnormal white matter, which appears to be of low attenuation on CT and hyperintense on T2-weighted MRI.[239] A pattern described as specific to herpes encephalitis is increased attenuation of the cortical gray matter on CT and T1 signal hyperintensity on MRI, which are thought to represent cortical laminar necrosis and calcifications.[112,235] Dystrophic calcifications may occur in the basal ganglia, cortex, and periventricular white matter.[235] During the chronic stages, typical findings include diffuse volume loss and multicystic encephalomalacia.

HIV Encephalitis

Most of the HIV cases in the pediatric population are acquired by transplacental transmission of the virus from an infected mother.[240] Newborns are usually asymptomatic, but 80 to 90 percent of infected children develop neurologic symptoms before the age of 5 years.[241] Presenting symptoms include developmental delay, motor and intellectual regression, pyramidal tract signs, ataxia, and quadriparesis.[241]

The most common finding on imaging of HIV encephalitis is diffuse atrophy. Other frequent findings include basal ganglia and frontal subcortical calcifications.[242] Less common findings include intracranial hemorrhages, infarcts, and HIV-associated infections and neoplasms, such as progressive multifocal leukoencephalopathy and lymphoma, respectively.[112]

CEREBRAL TRAUMA

Neurologic trauma is a significant cause of morbidity and mortality in children. The incidence of head trauma is estimated at 220 per 100,000 children per year, with a mortality of 10 per 100,000 population.[243] The largest proportion of closed head injury is due to motor vehicle accidents. Other causes of head injury in pediatric patients include other accidental injuries as well as nonaccidental trauma (NAT).

Computed tomography is the first line of imaging in the evaluation of neurologic trauma in children as well as adults. Evaluation of bone windows and occasionally "subdural" windows is an important part of the evaluation of the head CT in trauma patients. Imaging findings include diffuse cerebral edema, extra-axial hematomas, and intra-axial contusions. These topics are not covered in this chapter (see Chap. 4). Instead, we will concentrate on types of injuries seen almost exclusively in the pediatric population, birth trauma, and NAT.

Birth Trauma

Birth trauma to the neonatal brain may occur during an uncomplicated vaginal delivery as well as during the use of instruments, such as during vacuum or forceps extraction. Subdural hematomas in the supratentorial compartment are usually due to tearing of the bridging veins. In the posterior fossa, subdural hematomas may be due to tearing of the tentorium cerebelli, dural venous sinuses, or bridging veins. Epidural hematomas are rare but may be seen with a highly traumatic deliv-

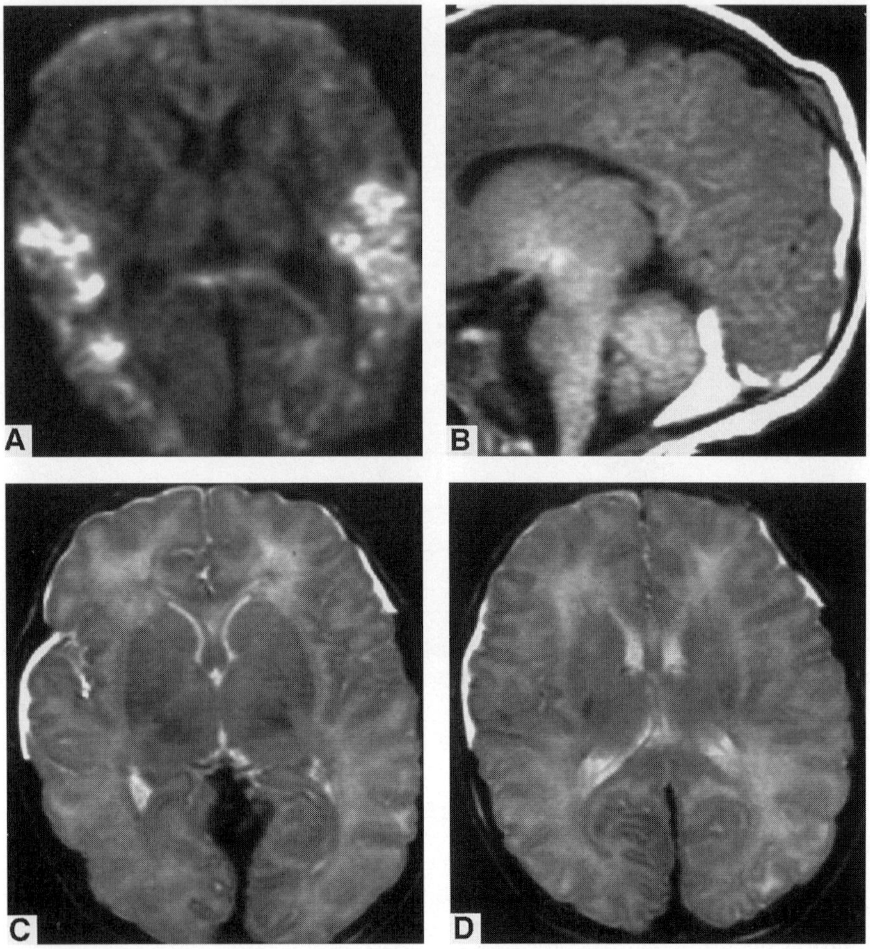

Figure 19-43
Birth trauma. **(A)** *An axial diffusion-weighted image demonstrates bilateral temporal and parieto-occipital infarcts in a newborn infant following prolonged labor.* (**B, C,** *and* **D**) *Subacute subdural hematomas demonstrating increased T1 and T2 signal intensity are present in the frontotemporal, occipital, and tentorial regions.*

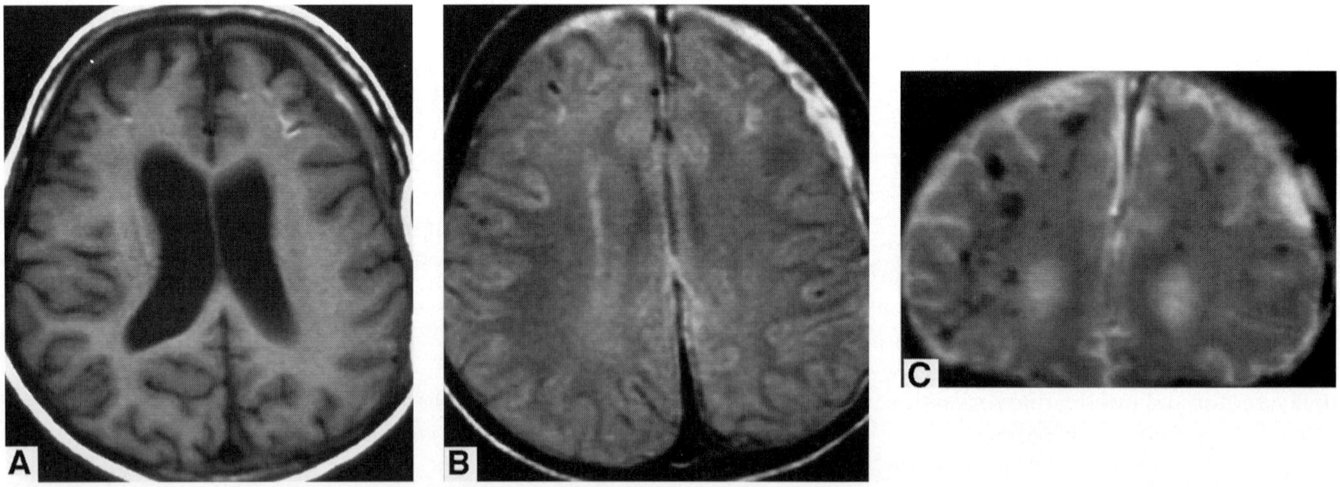

Figure 19-44
Nonaccidental trauma. **(A)** *Axial T1-weighted and* **(B)** *proton-density images demonstrate bifrontal subdural hematomas of different ages. The left frontal subdural hematoma, which has hyperintense components on T1-weighted images, is subacute and more recent than the contralateral hematoma. Curvilinear, gyriform T1 hyperintensity noted in the left frontal lobe is due either to cortical necrosis and subsequent calcification or to more acute hemorrhage.* **(C)** *A coronal gradient-echo image demonstrates innumerable foci or signal hypointensity due to "blooming" artifact from old blood products, reflecting extensive shear injury.*

ery. Ischemic brain injury may occur as a result of hypoxia due to a prolonged birth or other complicating factors, such as a hypercoagulable state (Fig. 19-43). Petechial hemorrhages may occur in infarcted areas or may result de novo from traumatic compression of the skull.[243]

Nonaccidental Trauma

Nonaccidental trauma is a common cause of craniocerebral injury, with approximately 13 percent of abused children showing evidence of head trauma.[244] This can result from blunt force, shaking injuries, or a combination of the two. Often, the radiologist has an important role in diagnosing unexplained trauma and establishing NAT as the cause of the clinically apparent injuries. Although nonspecific, the most common imaging findings of NAT are subdural hematomas over the cerebral convexities, followed by subarachnoid hemorrhage and cerebral hemorrhages.[245] Certain findings are highly specific for diagnosis of NAT, specifically bilateral subdural hematomas, hematomas of different ages, and posterior interhemispheric hematomas[246] (Fig. 19-44).

Cerebral infarction may be a consequence of NAT, resulting either from direct occlusion of the cervical vessels from strangulation or from intracranial vascular compromise secondary to diffuse cerebral edema and herniation. Imaging findings on CT and MRI are nonspecific, demonstrating loss of gray-white matter differentiation and gyral swelling with effacement of the sulci[243] (Fig. 19-44).

Computed tomography is highly sensitive for detection of acute subarachnoid hemorrhages and skull fractures and should be used in the acute setting. Magnetic resonance imaging is useful when injuries of varying ages are suspected as well as for the detection of subacute or chronic intraparenchymal hematomas or diffuse axonal injury. In addition, small hematomas near the vertex or along the tentorium, which may be missed by CT, are better demonstrated on MRI. Multiplanar spin-echo and gradient-echo MRI is useful for demonstration of old blood products and subacute hemorrhages, respectively, which may not be visible on CT.

ACKNOWLEDGMENTS

We want to thank Hiltje Loyd for manuscript preparation and Walt Gutzmer and Rhonda Dragan for photographic assistance.

REFERENCES

1. American Academy of Pediatrics Committee on Drugs: Guidelines for monitoring and management of pediatric patients during and after sedation for diagnostic and therapeutic procedures. *Pediatrics* 89:1110–1115, 1992.
2. Cohen MD: Pediatric sedation. *Radiology* 175:611–612, 1990.
3. American Academy of Pediatrics: Use of chloral hydrate for sedation in children. *Pediatrics* 92:471–473, 1993.
4. Nelson MD: Guidelines for the monitoring and care of children during and after sedation studies. *Am J Roentgenol* 160:581–582, 1993.
5. Shellock FG, Kanal E: *Magnetic Resonance: Bioeffects, Safety and Patient Management,* 2d ed. Philadelphia, Lippincott-Raven, 1996.
6. Warkany J, Passarge E, Smith LB: Congenital malformations in autosomal trisomy syndromes. *Am J Dis Child* 112:502–517, 1966.
7. Dominguez R, Aguire Vila-Coro A, Slopis JM, Bohan TP: Brain and ocular abnormalities in infants with in utero exposure to cocaine and other street drugs. *Am J Dis Child* 145: 688–695, 1991.
8. Gomez-Anson B, Ramsey RG: Pachygyria in a neonate with prenatal cocaine exposure: MR features. *J Comput Assist Tomogr* 18:637–639, 1994.
9. Dobyns WB, Truwit CL: Lissencephaly and other malformations of cortical development: 1995 update. *Neuropediatrics* 26:132–147, 1995.
10. Swayze VW, Johnson VP, Hanson JW, et al: Magnetic resonance imaging of brain anomalies in fetal alcohol syndrome. *Pediatrics* 99:232–240, 1997.
11. Van der Knaap MS, Valk J: Classification of congenital abnormalities of the CNS. *AJNR* 9:315–326, 1988.
12. Volpe JJ: *Neurology of the Newborn: Major Problems in Clinical Pediatrics,* 2d ed. Philadelphia, Saunders, 1987.
13. Truwit CL, Barkovich AJ: Disorders of brain development, in Atlas SW (ed): *Magnetic Resonance Imaging of the Brain and Spine.* Philadelphia, Lippincott-Raven, 1996.
14. Oi S, Saito M, Tamaki N, Matsumoto S: Ventricular volume reduction technique: A new surgical technique for the intracranial transposition of encephalocele. *Neurosurgery* 34:443–448, 1994.
15. Cohen MM, Lemire RJ: Syndromes with cephaloceles. *Teratology* 25:161–172, 1982.
16. Martinez-Lage JF, Martinez Robledo A, Poza M, Sola J: Familial occurrence of atretic cephaloceles. *Pediatr Neurosurg* 25:260–264, 1996.
17. Suwanwela C, Suwanwela N: A morphological classification of sincipital encephalomeningoceles. *J Neurosurg* 36:201–211, 1972.
18. Naidich TP, Zimmerman RA, Bauer BS, et al: Midface: Embryology and congenital lesions, in Som PM, Curtin HG (eds): *Head and Neck Imaging.* St. Louis, Mosby-Year Book, St. Louis, 1996, pp 3–60.
19. McLone DG, Knepper PA: The cause of Chiari II malformations. *Pediatr Neurosci* 15:1–12, 1996.
20. Naidich TP, Pudlowski RM, Naidich JB: Computed tomographic signs of the Chiari II malformation: II. Midbrain and cerebellum. *Radiology* 134:391–398, 1980.
21. Naidich TP, McLone DG, Fulling KH: The Chiari II malformation: IV. The hindbrain deformity. *Neuroradiology* 25:179–197, 1983.
22. Naidich TP, Pudlowski RM, Naidich JB: Computed tomographic signs of the Chiari II malformation: III. Ventricles and sulci. *Radiology* 134:657–663, 1980.

23. Barkovich AJ, Norman D: Anomalies of the corpus callosum: Correlation with other anomalies of the brain. *AJNR* 9:493–501, 1988.
24. Rajshekhar V, Chandy MJ: Computerized tomography-guided stereotactic surgery for brainstem masses: A risk-benefit analysis in 71 patients. *J Neurosurg* 82:976–981, 1995.
25. Yoshizato K, Kai Y, Kuratsu J, Ushio Y: Intramedullary epidermoid cyst in the brain stem: Case report. *Surg Neurol* 45:537–540, 1996.
26. Nassar SI, Haddad FS, Abdo A: Epidermoid tumor of the fourth ventricle. *Surg Neurol* 43:246–251, 1995.
27. Kallmes DF, Provenzale JM, Cloft HJ, McClendon RE: Typical and atypical MR imaging features of intracranial epidermoid tumors. *AJR* 169:883–887, 1997.
28. Tien RD, Felsberg GJ, Lirng JF: Variable bandwidth free-precession steady-state MR imaging: A technique for improving characterization of epidermoid tumor and arachnoid cysts. *AJR* 164:689–692, 1995.
29. Ikushima I, Korogi Y, Hirai T, et al: MR of epidermoids with a variety of pulse sequences. *AJNR* 18:1359–1363, 1997.
30. Modic MJ, Masaryk TJ, Ross JS. (eds): *Magnetic Resonance Imaging of the Spine.* St. Louis, Mosby, 1994.
31. Smith AS, Benson JE, Blaser SI, et al: Diagnosis of ruptured intracranial dermoid cyst: Value of MR over CT. *AJNR* 12:175–180, 1991.
32. DeMeyer W, Zeman W: Alobar holoprosencephaly (arhinencephaly) with median cleft lip and palate: Clinical, electroencephalographic and nosologic considerations. *Confin Neurol* 23:1–36, 1963.
33. DeMeyer W: Holoprosencephaly, in Myrianthopoulos N (ed): *Malformations.* New York, Elsevier, 1987, pp 225–244.
34. Hintz RL, Menking M, Sotos JF: Familial holoprosencephaly with endocrine dysgenesis. *J Pediatr* 72:81–87, 1968.
35. Khan M, Rozdilsky B, Gerrard JW: Familial holoprosencephaly. *Dev Med Child Neurol* 12:71–76, 1970.
36. Miyasaki K, Murao S, Nakamura K, Hashimoto Y: Congenital brain and facial anomalies in the D1 trisomy syndrome: Report of a case and review of literature. *Acta Pathol Jpn* 26:263–272, 1976.
37. Hunter AGW, Ray M, Longston C: Cebocephaly in an infant with trisomy 18. *J Med Genet* 14:291–292, 1977.
38. Gullotta F, Rehder H, Gropp A: Descriptive neuropathology of chromosomal abnormalities in man. *Hum Genet* 57:337–344, 1981.
39. Voiculescu I, Back E, Duncan AMV, et al: Trisomy 22 in a newborn with multiple malformations. *Hum Genet* 76:298–301, 1987.
40. Barr MJ, Hanson JW, Currey K, et al: Holoprosencephaly in infants of diabetic mothers. *J Pediatr* 192:565–568, 1983.
41. Friede RL: *Developmental Neuropathology,* 2d ed. Berlin, Springer-Verlag, 1989.
42. Kollias SS, Ball Jr WS: Congenital malformations of the brain, in Ball WS Jr (ed): *Pediatric Neuroradiology.* Philadelphia, Lippincott-Raven: Philadelphia. p. 91–174.
43. Leech RW, Shuman RM: Holoprosencephaly and related cerebral midline abnormalities: A review. *J Child Neurol* 1:3–18, 1986.
44. Barkovich AJ: Apparent atypical callosal dysgenesis: Analysis of MR findings in six cases and their relationship to holoprosencephaly. *AJNR* 14:431–440, 1990.
45. Fitz CZ: Holoprosencephaly and related entities. *Neuroradiology* 25:225–238, 1983.
46. Barkovich AJ, Quint DJ: Middle interhemispheric fusion: An unusual variant of holoprosencephaly. *AJNR* 14:431–440, 1993.
47. deMorsier G: Études sur les dysraphies crânio-encéphaliques: III. Agénésie du septum lucidum avec malformation du tractus optique: La dysplasie septo-optique. *Schweiz Arch Neurol Psychiatr* 77:267–292, 1956.
48. Izenberg N, Rosenblum M, Parks JS: The endocrine spectrum of septo-optic dysplasia. *Clin Pediatr* 23:632–636, 1984.
49. Morishima A, Aranoff GS: Syndrome of septo-optic dysplasia: The clinical spectrum. *Brain Dev* 8:233–239, 1986.
50. Stanhope R, Preece MA, Brook CGD: Hypoplastic optic nerves and pituitary dysfunction: A spectrum of anatomical and endocrine abnormalities. *Arch Dis Child* 59:111–114, 1984.
51. Barkovich AJ, Fram EK, Normal D: Septo-optic dysplasia: MR imaging. *Radiology* 171:189–192, 1989.
52. Rakic P, Yakovlev PI: Development of the corpus callosum and cavum septi in man. *J Comp Neurol* 132:45–72, 1968.
53. Kendall BE: Dysgenesis of the corpus callosum. *Neuroradiology* 25:239–257, 1983.
54. Kier EL, Truwit CL: The normal and abnormal genu of the corpus callosum: An evolutionary, embryologic, anatomic, and MR analysis. *AJNR* 17:1631–1641, 1996.
55. Kier EL, Truwit CL: The lamina rostralis: Modification of concepts concerning the anatomy, embryology, and MR appearance of the rostrum of the corpus callosum. *AJNR* 18:715–722, 1997.
56. Atlas SW, Zimmerman RA, Bilaniuk LT, et al: Corpus callosum and limbic system: Neuroanatomic MR evaluation of developmental anomalies. *Radiology* 160:355–362, 1986.
57. Truwit CL, Barkovich AJ: Pathogenesis of intracranial lipoma: An MR study in 42 patients. *AJNR* 11:665–674, 1990.
58. Naidich TP, McLone DG, Bauer BS, et al: Midline craniofacial dysraphism: Midline cleft upper lip, basal encephalocele, callosal agenesis, and optic nerve dysplasia. *Concepts Pediatr Neurosurg* 4:186–207, 1983.
59. Naidich TP, Osborn RE, Bauer B, Naidich MJ: Median cleft face syndrome: MR and CT data from 11 children. *J Comput Assist Tomogr* 12:57–64, 1988.
60. Barkovich AJ, Kjos BO, Norman D, Edwards MSB: Revised classification of posterior fossa cysts and cyst-like malformations based on results of multiplanar MR imaging. *AJNR* 10:977–988, 1989.
61. Joubert M, Eisenring JJ, Robb JP, Andermann F: Familial agenesis of the cerebellar vermis: A syndrome of episodic hyperapnea, abnormal eye movements, ataxia and retardation. *Neurology* 19:813–825, 1969.
62. Kendall B, Kingsley D, Lambert SR, et al: Joubert syndrome: A clinical-radiological study. *Neuroradiology* 31: 502–506, 1990.
63. Truwit CL, Barkovich AJ, Shanahan R, Maroldo TV: MR imaging of rhombencephalosynapsis: Report of

three cases and review of literature. *AJNR* 12:957–965, 1991.
64. McConnell S: Fates of visual cortical neurons in the ferret after isochronic and heterochronic transplantation. *J Neurosci* 8:945–974, 1988.
65. Marin-Padilla M: Early ontogenesis of the human cerebral cortex, in Peter A, Jones E (eds): *Cerebral Cortex: Development and Maturation of the Cerebral Cortex.* New York, Plenum Press, 1988, pp 1–34.
66. McConnell S: The generation of neuronal diversity in the central nervous system. *Annu Rev Neurosci* 14:269–300, 1991.
67. McConnell S, Kaznowski C: Cell cycle dependence of laminar determination in the developing cerebral cortex. *Science* 254:282–285, 1991.
68. Sarnat H: Role of the human fetal ependyma. *Pediatr Neurol* 8:163–178, 1992.
69. Barkovich AJ, Kuzniecky RI, Bollen AW, Grant PE: Focal transmantle dysplasia: A specific malformation of cortical development. *Neurology* 49:1148–1152, 1997.
70. Lightman S: Kallmann's syndrome. *J R Soc Med* 81:315–316, 1988.
71. Van Dop C, Burstein S, Conte FA, Grumbach MM: Isolated gonadotropin deficiency in boys: Clinical characteristics and growth. *J Pediatr* 111:684–692, 1987.
72. Schwanzel-Fukuda M, Bick D, Pfaff DW: Luteinizing hormone-releasing hormone (LHRH)-expressing cells do not migrate normally in an inherited hypogonadal (Kallmann) syndrome. *Brain Res* 6:311–326, 1989.
73. White BJ, Rogol AD, Brown KS, et al: The syndrome of anosomia and hypogonadotropic hypogonadism: A genetic study of 18 new families and a review. *Am J Med Genet* 15:417–435, 1983.
74. Dobyns WB, Elias ER, Newlin AC, et al: Causal heterogeneity in isolated lissencephaly. *Neurology* 42:1375–1388, 1992.
75. Dobyns WB, Andermann E, Andermann F, et al: X-linked malformations of cortical development. *Neurology* 47:331–339, 1996.
76. Dobyns WB, Reiner O, Carrozzo R, Ledbetter DH: Lissencephaly: A human brain malformation associated with deletion of the *LIS1* gene located at chromosome 17p13. *JAMA* 270:2838–2842, 1993.
77. Yoshioka M, Saiwai S, Kuroko S, Nigami H: MR imaging in Fukuyama-type congenital muscular dystrophy. *AJNR* 12:63–66, 1991.
78. Reiner O, Carrozzo R, Shen Y, et al: Isolation of a Miller-Dieker lissencephaly gene containing G protein B-subunit-like repeats. *Nature* 364:717–721, 1993.
79. Barkovich AJ, Koch T, Carrol C: The spectrum of lissencephaly: Report of ten cases analyzed by magnetic resonance imaging. *Ann Neurol* 30:139–146, 1991.
80. Takada K, Becker L, Takashima S: Walker-Warburg syndrome with skeletal muscle involvement: A report of three patients. *Pediatr Neurosci* 13:202–209, 1987.
81. Santavuori P, Somer H, Sainio K: Muscle-eye-brain disease. *Brain Dev* 11:147–153, 1989.
82. Brun A: Marginal glioneural heterotopias of the central nervous system. *Acta Pathol Microbiol Scand* 65:221–233, 1965.
83. Hayward JC, Titelbaum DS, Clancy RR, Zimmerman RA: Lissencephaly-pachygyria associated with congenital cytomegalovirus infection. *J Child Neurol* 6:109–114, 1991.
84. Barkovich AJ, Linden CL: Congenital cytomegalovirus infection of the brain: imaging analysis and embryologic considerations. *AJNR* 15:703–715, 1994.
85. Gastaut H, Pinsard N, Raybaud C, et al: Lissencephaly (agyria-pachygyria): Clinical findings and serial EEG studies. *Dev Med Child Neurol* 29:167–180, 1987.
86. de Rijk-van Andel J, Arts W, Barth P, Loonen M: Diagnostic features and clinical signs of 21 patients with lissencephaly type 1. *Dev Med Child Neurol* 32:707–717, 1990.
87. Barkovich AJ, Chuang SH, Norman D: MR of neuronal migration anomalies. *AJNR* 8:1009–1017, 1987.
88. Evrard P, de Saint-Georges P, Kadhim H, Gadisseux JF: Pathology of prenatal encephalopathies, in French J (ed): *Child Neurology and Developmental Disabilities.* Baltimore, Brookes, 1989, pp 153–176.
89. Rakic P: Contact regulation of neuronal migration, in Edelman G, Thiery J (eds): *The Cell in Contact: Adhesions and Junctions as Morphogenetic Determinants.* New York, Neuroscience Research Foundation, pp 67–91.
90. Ross ME, Allen KM, Srivastava AK, et al: Linkage and physical mapping of X-linked lissencephaly/SBH (XLIS): A gene causing neuronal migration defects in human brain. *Hum Mol Genet* 6:555–562, 1997.
91. des Portes V, Pinard JM, Smadja D, et al: Dominant X linked subcortical laminar heterotopia and lissencephaly syndrome (XSCLH/LIS): Evidence for the occurrence of mutations in males and mapping of a potential locus in Xq22. *J Med Genet* 34:177–183, 1997.
92. Fink JM, Dobyns WB, Guerrini R, Hirsch BA: Identification of a duplication of Xq28 associated with bilateral periventricular nodular heterotopia. *Am J Hum Genet* 61:379–387, 1997.
93. Barkovich AJ, Kjos BO: Gray matter heterotopias: MR characteristics and correlation with developmental and neurologic manifestations. *Radiology* 182:493–499, 1992.
94. Dobyns WB, Guerrini R, Czapansky-Beilman DK, et al: Bilateral periventricular nodular heterotopia with mental retardation and syndactyly in boys: A new X-linked mental retardation syndrome. *Neurology* 49:1042–1047, 1997.
95. Barkovich AJ, Jackson DE, Boyer RS: Band heterotopias: A newly recognized neuronal migration anomaly. *Radiology* 171:455–458, 1989.
96. Barkovich AJ, Guerrini R, Battaglia G, et al: Band heterotopia: Correlation of outcome with magnetic resonance imaging parameters. *Ann Neurol* 36:609–617, 1994.
97. Pinard J-M, Motte J, Chiron C, et al: Subcortical laminar heterotopia and lissencephaly in two families: A single X linked dominant gene. *J Neurol Neurosurg Psychiatry* 57:914–920, 1994.
98. Scheffer IE, Mitchell LA, Howell RA: Familial band heterotopias: An X-linked dominant disorder with variable severity (abstract). *Ann Neurol* 36:511, 1994.
99. Townsend JJ, Neilson SL, Malamud N: Unilateral megalencephaly: Hamartoma or neoplasm. *Neurology* 25:448–453, 1975.
100. Anlar B, Yalaz K, Erzen C: Klippel-Trenaunay-Weber syndrome: A case with cerebral and cerebellar hemihypertrophy. *Neuroradiology* 30:360, 1988.
101. Peserico A, Battistella P, Bertoli P, Drigo P: Unilateral

hypomelanosis of Ito with hemimegalencephaly. *Acta Paediatr Scand* 77:446–447, 1988.

102. Cumai R, Curatolo P, Mangano S, et al: Hemimegalencephaly and neurofibromatosis. *Neuropediatrics* 21: 179–182, 1990.
103. Hager B, Dyme I, Guertin S, et al: Linear nevus sebaceous syndrome: Megalencephaly and heterotopic gray matter. *Pediatr Neurol* 7:45–49, 1991.
104. Fitz CR, Harwood-Nash DC, Boldt DW: The radiographic features of unilateral megalencephaly. *Neuroradiology* 15:145–148, 1978.
105. Kalifa GL, Chiron C, Sellier N: Hemimegalencephaly: MR imaging in five children. *Radiology* 165:29–33, 1987.
106. Barkovich AJ, Chuang SH: Unilateral megalencephaly: Correlation of MR and pathologic characteristics. *AJNR* 11:523–531, 1990.
107. Davis RL, Nelson E: Unilateral ganglioglioma in a tuberosclerotic brain. *J Neuropathol Exp Neurol* 21:571–581, 1961.
108. McBride MC, Kemper TL: Pathogenesis of four-layered cortex in man. *Acta Neuropathol (Berl)* 57:93–98, 1982.
109. Barth PG: Disorders of neuronal migration. *Can J Neurol Sci* 14:1–16, 1987.
110. Barkovich AJ, Kjos BO: Nonlissencephalic cortical dysplasias: correlation of imaging findings with clinical deficits. *AJNR* 13:95–103, 1992.
111. Kuzniecky R, Andermann F, Guerrini R: Congenital bilateral perisylvian syndrome: Study of 31 patients, the CBPS Multicenter Collaborative Study. *Lancet* 341:698–612, 1993.
112. Barkovich AJ: *Pediatric Neuroimaging,* 2d ed. Philadelphia, Lippincott-Raven, 1996.
113. Yakolev PI, Wadsworth RC: Schizencephalies: A study of congenital clefts in the cerebral mantle: I. Clefts with fused lips. *J Neuropathol Exp Neurol* 5:116–130, 1946.
114. Yakolev PI, Wadsworth RC: Schizencephalies: A study of congenital clefts in the cerebral mantle: II. Clefts with hydrocephalus and lips separated. *J Neuropathol Exp Neurol* 5:169–206, 1946.
115. Barkovich AJ, Kjos BO: Schizencephaly: Correlation of clinical findings with MR characteristics. *AJNR* 13:85–94, 1992.
116. Ogata H, Oka K, Mitsudome A: Hydrocephalus due to acute aqueductal stenosis following mumps infection: Report of a case and review of literature. *Brain Dev* 14:417–419, 1992.
117. Jellinger G: Anatomopathology of non-tumoral aqueductal stenosis. *J Neurosurg Sci* 30:1–16, 1986.
118. Boydston WR, Sanford RA, Muhlbauer MS, et al: Gliomas of the tectum and periaqueductal region of the mesencephalon. *Pediatr Neurosurg* 17:234–238, 1991.
119. Fukumizu M, Becker LE, Takashima S: Periaqueductal microdysplasia in children with congenital aqueductal stenosis. *Clin Neuropathol* 13:46–52, 1994.
120. Willems PJ, Dijkstra I, Van der Auwera BJ, et al: Assignment of X-linked hydrocephalus to Xq28 by linkage analysis. *Genomics* 8:367–370, 1990.
121. Stehling MK, Firth JL, Worthington BS, et al: Observation of cerebrospinal fluid flow with echo-planar magnetic resonance imaging. *Br J Radiol* 64:89–97, 1991.
122. Kadowaki C, Hara M, Numoto M, et al: Cine magnetic resonance imaging of aqueductal stenosis. *Childs Nerv Syst* 11:107–111, 1995.
123. Barkovich AJ, Wippold FJ, Sherman JL, Citrin CM: Significance of cerebellar ectopia on MR. *AJNR* 7:795–799, 1986.
124. Payner TD, Pringer E, Berger TS, Crone KR: Acquired Chiari malformations: Incidence, diagnosis and management. *Neurosurgery* 34:429–434, 1994.
125. Barker D, Wright E, Nguyen K, Cannon P: Gene for von Recklinghausen neurofibromatosis is in the pericentromeric region of chromosome 17. *Science* 236:1100–1102, 1987.
126. Seizinger BR, Rouleau GA, Ozeluis LJ, Lane AH: Genetic linkage of von Recklinghausen neurofibromatosis to the nerve growth factor gene. *Cell* 49:589–594, 1987.
127. Gardeur D, Palmieri A, Mashaly R: Cranial computed tomography in the phakomatoses. *Neuroradiology* 25: 293–304, 1983.
128. National Institutes of Health Consensus Development Conference. Neurofibromatosis, Conference Statement. *Arch Neurol* 45:575–578, 1988.
129. Berg BO: Neurocutaneous disorders, in Berg BO (ed): *Neurologic Manifestations of Pediatrics,* Boston, Butterworth-Heinmann, 1992, pp 485–498.
130. Huson SM, Harper PS, Compston DAS: Von Recklinghausen's neurofibromatosis: A clinical and population study in southeast Wales. *Brain* 111:1355–1381, 1988.
131. DiMario FJ, Ramsby G, Greenstein R, et al: Neurofibromatosis type 1: Magnetic resonance imaging findings. *J Child Neurol* 8:32–39, 1993.
132. Sevick RJ, Barkovich AJ, Edwards MS, et al: Evaluation of white matter lesions in neurofibromatosis type 1: MR findings. *AJR* 159:171–175, 1992.
133. Smirniotopoulos JG, Murphy FM: Central nervous system manifestations of the phakomatoses and other inherited syndromes, in Atlas SW (ed): *Magnetic Resonance of the Brain and Spine.* Philadelphia, Lippincott-Raven, 1996, pp 773–802.
134. Aoki S, Barkovich AJ, Nishimura K, Kjos BO: Neurofibromatosis types 1 and 2: Cranial MR findings. *AJNR* 172:527–534, 1989.
135. Russell DS, Rubinstein LJ: Dysgenetic syndromes (phakomatoses) associated with tumors and hamartomas of the nervous system, in *Pathology of Tumors of the Nervous System.* Baltimore, Williams & Wilkins, 1989, pp 766–784.
136. Mirowitz SA, Sartor K, Gado M: High-intensity basal ganglia lesions on T1-weighted MR images in neurofibromatosis. *AJNR* 10:1159–1163, 1989.
137. Smirniotopoulos JG, Murphy FM: The phakomatoses. *AJNR* 13:725–736, 1992.
138. Sobata E, Ohkuma H, Suzuki S: Cerebrovascular disorders associated with von Recklinghausen's neurofibromatosis. *Neurosurgery* 22:544–549, 1988.
139. Binet EF, Kieffer SA, Martin SH, Peterson HO: Orbital dysplasia in neurofibromatosis. *Radiology* 93:829–833, 1969.
140. Seizinger BR, Martuza RL, Gusella JF: Loss of genes on chromosome 22 in tumorigenesis of human acoustic neuroma. *Nature* 322:664–667, 1986.
141. Sampson JR, Scahill SJ, Stephenson JBP, et al: Genetic aspects of tuberous sclerosis in the west of Scotland. *J Med Genet* 26:28–31, 1989.

142. Winship IM, Connor JM, Beighton PH: Genetic heterogeneity in tuberous sclerosis: Phenotipiccorrelations. *J Med Genet* 27:418–421, 1990.
143. Shepherd CW, Beard CM, Gomez MR, et al: Tuberous sclerosis complex in Olmsted county, Minnesota. *Arch Neurol* 48:400–401, 1991.
144. Gomez MR: *Tuberous Sclerosis.* New York, Raven Press, 1988.
145. Bender BL, Yunis EJ: The pathology of tuberous sclerosis. *Pathol Annu* 17:339–382, 1982.
146. Martin N, de Brouker T, Cambier J, et al: MR evaluation of tuberous sclerosis. *Neuroradiology* 29:437–443, 1987.
147. Altman NR, Purser RK, Donovan-Post MJ: Tuberous sclerosis: Characteristics at CT and MR imaging. *Radiology* 167:527–532, 1988.
148. Nixon JR, Houser OW, Gomez MR, Okazaki H: Cerebral tuberous sclerosis: MR imaging. *AJNR* 170:869–873, 1994.
149. Martin N, Debussche C, DeBroucker T, et al: Gadolinium-DTPA enhanced MR in tuberous sclerosis. *Neuroradiology* 31:492–497, 1990.
150. Iwasaki S, Nakagawa H, Kichikawa K, Fukusumi A: MR and CT of tuberous sclerosis: Linear abnormalities in the verebral white matter. *AJNR* 11:1029–1034, 1990.
151. Braffman BH, Bilaniuk LT, Naidich TP, et al: MR imaging of tuberous sclerosis: Pathogenesis of this phakomatosis, use of gadopentate dimeglumine, and literature review. *Radiology* 183:227–238, 1992.
152. Enjolras O, Riche MC, Merland JJ: Facial port-wine stains and Sturge-Weber syndrome. *Pediatrics* 76:48–51, 1985.
153. Pascual-Castroviejo I, Diaz-Gonzales C, Garcia-Melian R, et al: Sturge-Weber syndrome: Study of 40 patients. *Pediatr Neurol* 9:283–288, 1993.
154. Welch K, Naheedy MH, Abroms IF, Strand RD: Computed tomography of Sturge-Weber syndrome in infants. *J Comp Assist Tomogr* 4:33–36, 1980.
155. Schmauser I, Bittner R: MR-imaging findings in children with Sturge-Weber syndrome. *Neuropediatrics* 21:146–152, 1990.
156. Sugama S, Yoshimura H, Ashimine K, et al: Enhanced magnetic resonance imaging of leptomeningeal angiomatosis. *Pediatr Neurol* 17:262–265, 1997.
157. Adamsbaum C, Pinton F, Rolland Y, et al: Accelerated myelination in early Sturge-Weber syndrome: MRI-SPECT correlations. *Pediatr Neurol* 26:759–762, 1997.
158. Griffiths PD, Blaser S, Boodram MB, et al: Choroid plexus size in young children with Sturge-Weber syndrome. *AJNR* 17:175–180, 1996.
159. Horton WA, Wong V, Eldridge R: Von Hippel-Lindau disease: Clinical and pathological findings in nine families with 50 affected members. *Arch Intern Med* 136:769–777, 1976.
160. Latif F, Tory K, Gnarra J, et al: Identification of the von Hippel-Lindau disease tumor supressor gene. *Science* 260:1317–1320, 1993.
161. Jeffreys R: Clinical and surgical aspects of posterior fossa hemangioblastomata. *J Neurol Neurosurg Psychiatry* 38: 105–111, 1975.
162. Jeffreys R: Pathological and haematological aspects of posterior fossa hemangioblastomata. *J Neurol Neurosurg Psychiatry* 38:112–119, 1975.
163. Ho VB, Smirnitopoulos JG, Murphy FM, Rushing EJ: Radiologic-pathologic correlation: Hemangioblastoma. *AJNR* 13:1343–1352, 1992.
164. Chugani HT, Phelps ME, Mazziotta JC: Positron emission tomography study of human brain functional development. *Ann Neurol* 22:487–497, 1987.
165. Hasegawa M, Houdou S, Mito T, et al: Development of myelination in the human fetal and infant cerebrum: A myelin basic protein immunohistochemical study. *Brain Dev* 14:1–6, 1992.
166. Azzarelli B, Caldemeyer KS, Phillips JP, DeMyer WE: Hypoxic-ischemic encephalopathy in areas of primary myelination: A neuroimaging and PET study. *Pediatr Neurol* 14:108–116, 1996.
167. Greenmyre T, Penney JB, Young AB, et al: Evidence for transient perinatal glutamatergic innervation of globus pallidus. *J Neurosci* 7:1022–1030, 1987.
168. Choi BH, Ruess WR, Kim RC: Disturbances in neuronal migration and laminar cortical organization associated with multicystic encephalopathy in the Pena-Shokeir syndrome. *Acta Neuropathol (Berl)* 69:177–183, 1986.
169. Takashima S, Tanaka K: Development of the cerebrovascular architecture and its relationship to periventricular leukomalacia. *Arch Neurol* 35:11–16, 1978.
170. Papile LA, Burstein J, Burstein R, Koffler H: Incidence and evolution of subependymal intraventricular hemorrhage: A study of infants with births weights less than 1,500 grams. *J Pediatr* 92:529–534, 1978.
171. Van de Bor M, Ens-Dokkum M, Schreuder AM, et al: Outcome of periventricular-intraventricular hemorrhage at five years of age. *Dev Med Child Neurol* 35:33–41, 1993.
172. Volpe JJ: Intraventricular hemorrhage and brain injury in the premature infant: Neuropathology and pathogenesis. *Clin Perinatol* 16:361–386, 1989.
173. Volpe JJ, Edward B: Neuhauser lecture: Current concepts in brain injury in the premature infant. *AJR* 153: 243–251.
174. Babcock DS: Cranial sonography of the infant, in Ball WS Jr (ed): *Pediatric Neuroradiology,* Philadelphia, Lippincott-Raven, pp 1997, 37–67.
175. Schellinger D, Grant EG, Richardson JD: Cystic periventricular leukomalacia: Sonographic and CT findings. *AJNR* 5:439–445, 1984.
176. Dubowitz LMS, Bydder GM, Mushin J: Developmental sequence of periventricular leukomalacia: Correlation of ultrasound, clinical and nuclear magnetic resonance functions. *Arch Dis Child* 60:349–355, 1985.
177. Carson SC, Hertzberg BS, Bowie JD, Burger PC: Value of sonography in the diagnosis of intracranial hemorrhage and periventricular leukomalacia: A postmortem study of 35 cases. *AJNR* 11:677–684, 1990.
178. Ball WS Jr, Franz DN: Neonatal brain injury, in Ball WS Jr (ed): *Pediatric Neuroradiology.* Philadelphia, Lippincott-Raven, 1997, pp 239–272.
179. Baker LL, Stephenson DK, Enzmann DR: Endstage periventricular leukomalacia: MR imaging evaluation. *Radiology* 168:809–815, 1988.
180. Barkovich AJ, Truwit CL: MR of perinatal asphyxia: Correlation of gestational age with pattern of damage. *AJNR* 11:1087–1096, 1990.

181. Barkovich AJ: MR and CT evaluation of profound neonatal and infantile asphyxia. *AJNR* 13:959–972, 1992.
182. Barkovich AJ, Truwit CL: *Practical MRI Atlas of Neonatal Brain Development.* New York, Raven Press, 1990.
183. Ruggieri PM: Metabolic and neurodegenerative disorders and disorders with abnormal myelination, in Ball WS Jr (ed): *Pediatric Neuroimaging.* Philadelphia, Lippincott-Raven, 1997.
184. Diebler C, Dulac O: *Pediatric Neurology and Neuroradiology.* Berlin, Springer-Verlag, 1987.
185. Menkes JH: Metabolic diseases of the central nervous system, in Menkes JH (ed): *Textbook of Child Neurology.* Philadelphia, Lea & Febiger, 1985, pp 1–122.
186. Loes DJ, Hite S, Moser H, et al: Adrenoleukodystrophy: A scoring method for brain MR observations. *AJNR* 15:1761–1766, 1994.
187. Waragai M, Takaya Y, Hayashi M, et al: MRI of adrenoleukodystrophy involving primarily the cerebellum and brain stem. *Neuroradiology* 38:788–791, 1996.
188. Tzika AA, Ball WS Jr, Vigneron DB, et al: Childhood adrenoleukodystrophy: Assessment with proton MR spectroscopy. *Radiology* 189:467–480, 1993.
189. Rajanayagam V, Balthazor M, Shapiro EG, et al: Proton MR spectroscopy and neuropsychological testing in adrenoleukodystrophy. *AJNR* 18:1909–1914, 1997.
190. Valk J, van der Knapp MS: *Magnetic Resonance of Myelin, Myelination and Myelin Disorders.* Berlin, Springer-Verlag, 1989.
191. Demaerel P, Faubert C, Wilms G, et al: MR findings in leukodystrophy. *Neuroradiology* 33:368–371, 1991.
192. Kwan E, Drace J, Enzmann D: Specific CT findings in Krabbe disease. *AJNR* 143:665–670, 1984.
193. Baram TZ, Goldman AN, Percy AM: Krabbe disease: Specific MRI and CT findings. *Neurology* 36:111–115, 1986.
194. Feanny SJ, Chuang SH, Becker LE, Clarke JT: Intracerebral paraventricular hyperdensities: A new CT sign in Krabbe globoid cell leukodystrophy. *J Inherit Metab Dis* 10:24–27, 1987.
195. Barone R, Bruhl K, Stoeter P, et al: Clinical and neuroradiological findings in classic infantile and late-onset globoid cell leukodystrophy (krebbe's disease). *Am J Med Genet* 63:209–217, 1996.
196. Grodd W, Krageloh-Mann I, Petersen D, et al: In vivo assessment of *N*-acetylaspartate in brain in spongy degeneration (Canavan's disease) by proton spectroscopy (letter). *Lancet* 2:437–438, 1990.
197. Grodd W, Krageloh-Mann I, Klose U, Sauter R: Metabolic and destructive brain disorders in children: Findings with localized proton MR spectroscopy. *Radiology* 181: 173–181, 1991.
198. Schuster V, Horwitz AE, Kreth HW: Alexander's disease: Cranial MRI and ultrasound findings. *Pediatr Radiol* 21:133–134, 1991.
199. Duquette P, Murray TJ, Ebers GC, et al: Multiple sclerosis in childhood: Clinical profile in 125 patients. *J Pediatr* 111:359–363, 1987.
200. Shaw CM, Alvord ECJ: Multiple sclerosis beginning in infancy. *J Child Neurol* 2:252–256, 1987.
201. Sriram S, Steinman L: Postinfectious and postvaccinal encephalomyelitis. *Neurol Clin* 2:341–353, 1984.
202. Atlas SW, Grossman RI, Goldberg HI, et al: MR diagnosis of acute disseminated encephalomyelitis. *J Comput Assist Tomogr* 10:798–801, 1986.
203. Baum PA, Barkovich AJ, Koch TK, Berg BO: Deep gray matter involvement in children with acute disseminated encephalomyelitis. *AJNR* 15:1275–1283, 1994.
204. Caldmeyer KS, Harris TM, Smith RR, Edwards MK: Gadolinium enhancement in acute disseminated encephalomyelitis. *J Comput Assist Tomogr* 15:673–675, 1991.
205. Stalker HP, Han BK: Thalamic hyperdensity: A previously unreported sign of Sandhoff disease. *AJNR* 10 (suppl):82, 1989.
206. Yoshikawa H, Yamada K, Sakuragawa N: MRI in the early stages of Tay-Sachs disease. *Neuroradiology* 34: 394–395, 1992.
207. Mugikura S, Takahashi S, Higano S, et al: MR findings in Tay-Sachs disease. *J Comput Assist Tomogr* 20:551–555, 1996.
208. Rauch RA, Friloux LA, Lott IT: MR imaging of cavitary lesions in the brain with Hurler/Scheie. *AJNR* 10 (suppl):1–3, 1989.
209. Lee C, Dineen TE, Brack M, et al: Muccopolysaccharidoses: Characterization by cranial MR imaging. *AJNR* 14:1285–1292, 1993.
210. Parsons VJ, Hughes DG, Wraith JE: Magnetic resonance imaging of the brain, neck and cervical spine in mild Hunter's syndrome (mucopolysaccharidoses type II). *Clin Radiol* 51:719–723, 1996.
211. Hughes DG, Chadderton RD, Cowie RA, et al: MRI of the brain and craniocervical junction in Morquio's disease. *AJNR* 39:381–385, 1997.
212. Spranger JW, Langer LOJ, Wiedemann HR: *Bone Dysplasias.* Philadelphia, Saunders, 1974.
213. Lexa FJ, Trojanowski JQ, Braffman BH, Atlas SW: The aging brain and neurodegenerative diseases, in Atlas SW (ed): *Magnetic Resonance Imaging of the Brain and Spine.* Philadelphia, Lippincott-Raven, 1996, pp 803–870.
214. Tulinius MH, Holme E, Kristiansson B, et al: Mitochondrial encephalomyopathies in childhood: II. Clinical manifestations and syndromes. *J Pediatr* 119:251–259, 1991.
215. Egger J, Lake BD, Wilson J: Mitochondrial cytopathy: A multisystem disorder with ragged red fibers on muscle biopsy. *Arch Dis Child* 56:741–752, 1981.
216. Detre JA, Wang ZY, Bogdan AR, et al: Regional variation in brain lactate in Leigh syndrome by localized ^{1}H magnetic resonance spectroscopy. *Ann Neurol* 29:218–221, 1991.
217. Barkovich AJ, Good WV, Koch TK, Berg BO: Mitochondrial disorders: Analysis of their clinical and imaging characteristics. *AJNR* 14:1119–1137, 1993.
218. Montpetit VJA, Andermann F, Carpenter S, et al: Subacute necrotizing encephalomyelopathy. *Brain* 94:1–30, 1971.
219. Medina L, Chi TL, DeVivo DC, Hilal SK: MR findings in patients with subacute necrotizing encephalomyelopathy (Leigh syndrome): Correlation with biochemical defect. *AJNR* 11:379–384, 1990.
220. Allard JC, Tilak S, Carter AP: CT and MR of MELAS syndrome. *AJNR* 9:1234–1238, 1998.
221. Sweetman L, Haas RH: Abnormalities of amino acid metabolism, in Berg BO (ed): *Neurologic Aspects of Pediatrics.* Boston, Butterworth-Heinemann, 1992, pp 3–32.

222. Pearsen KD, Gean-Marton AD, Levy HL, Davis KR: Phenylketonuria: MRI of the brain with clinical correlation. *Radiology* 177:437–440, 1990.
223. Shaw DW, Maravilla KR, Weinberger E, et al: MR imaging of phenylketonuria. *AJNR* 12:403–406, 1991.
224. Naylor GW, Guthrie R: Newborn screening for maple syrup urine disease (branched chain ketoaciduria). *Pediatrics* 61:262–266, 1978.
225. Brismar J, Aqeel A, Brismar G, et al: Maple syrup urine disease: Findings on CT and MR scans of the brain in 10 infants. *AJNR* 11:1219–1228, 1990.
226. Bergman I, Finegold D, Garcia JC Jr, et al: Acute profound dystonia in infants with organic aciduria. *Pediatrics* 83:228–234, 1989.
227. Amir N, Elpeleg ON, Shalev RS, Christensen E: Glutaric aciduria type I: Enzymatic and neuroradiologic investigation of two kindreds. *J Pediatr* 114:983–989, 1989.
228. Iafolla AK, Kahler SG: Megalencephaly in the neonatal period as the initial manifestation of glutaric aciduria type I. *J Pediatr* 14:1004–1006, 1989.
229. Yow MD: Congenital and perinatal cytomegalovirus disease: A now problem. *J Infect Dis* 159:163–167, 1989.
230. Bale JF Jr, Murph JR: Infections of the central nervous system in the newborn. *Clin Perinatol* 24:787–806, 1997.
231. Boesch C, Issakainen R, Kewitz F, et al: Magnetic resonance imaging of the brain congenital cytomegalovirus infection. *Pediatr Radiol* 19:91–93, 1989.
232. Robertson JS: Toxoplasmosis. *Dev Ned Child Neurol* 4: 507–512, 1962.
233. Eichenwald HF: *Human Toxoplasmosis.* Baltimore, Williams & Wilkins, 1956.
234. Diebler C, Dusser A, Dulac O: Congenital toxoplasmosis: Clinical and neuroradiological evaluation of cerebral lesions. *Neuroradiology* 27:125–130, 1985.
235. Egelhoff JC: Infections of the central nervous system, in Ball WS Jr (ed): *Pediatric neuroradiology,* Philadelphia, Lippincott-Raven, 1997, pp 273–318.
236. Miller E, Craddock-Watson JE, Pollock TM: Consequences of confirmed maternal rubella infection at successive stages of pregnancy. *Lancet* 2:781–782, 1982.
237. Lane B, Sullivan EV, Lim KO, et al: White matter MR hyperintensities in adult patients with congenital rubella. *AJNR* 17:99–103, 1996.
238. Whitley RJ, Hutto C: Neonatal herpes simplex virus infection. *Pediatr Rev* 7:119–126, 1985.
239. Noorbehesht B, Enzmann DR, Sullinder W, et al: Neonatal herpes encephalitis: Correlation of clinical and CT findings. *Radiology* 162:813–819, 1987.
240. Belman AL: Acquired immunodeficiency syndrome and the child's central nervous system. *Pediatr Clin North Am* 39:691–714, 1992.
241. Epstein LG, Sharer LR, Goudsmit J: Neurological and neuropathological features of human immunodeficiency virus infection in children. *Ann Neurol* 23(suppl): 19–23.
242. Kauffman W, Sivit CJ, Fitz CR, et al: CT and MR evaluation of intracranial involvement in pediatric HIV infection: A clinical-imaging correlation. *AJNR* 13:949–957, 1992.
243. Beckett WW, Ball WS Jr: Craniocerebral trauma, in Ball WS Jr (ed): *Pediatric Neuroradiology.* Philadelphia, Lippincott-Raven, 1997, pp 443–487.
244. Merten DF, Osborne DRS, Radkowski MA, Leonidas JC: Craniocerebral trauma in the child abuse syndrome: Radiological observations. *Pediatr Radiol* 14:272–277, 1984.
245. Caffey J: The whiplash shaken infant syndrome: Manual shaking by the extremities with whiplash induced intracranial and intraocular bleedings, linked with residual permanent brain damage and mental retardation. *Pediatrics* 54:396–403, 1974.
246. Zimmerman RD, Russell EJ, Yurberg E, Leeds NE: Falx and interhemispheric fissure on axial CT: II. Recognition and differentiation of interhemispheric subarachnoid and subdural hemorrhage. *AJNR* 1:635–642, 1982.

PART FOUR

SPECIAL SECTION ON SPECIFIC IMAGING MODALITIES

DIFFUSION-PERFUSION MRI AND MAGNETIC RESONANCE SPECTROSCOPY IN CEREBROVASCULAR DISEASE

Wolf Schaebitz
Marc Fisher

Current imaging technology employing computed tomography (CT) and standard magnetic resonance imaging (MRI) techniques (T1- and T2-weighted images) has provided much important information for the diagnosis and management of cerebrovascular disorders. Deficiencies remain related to the inability of standard imaging to depict ischemic strokes at early time points, when patients initially present for medical evaluation.[1] Although CT scans are commonly performed shortly after patients arrive at the hospital because they will demonstrate hemorrhage, if present, it typically takes up to a day or longer for CT studies to accurately demonstrate the extent of an ischemic lesion. T1- and T2-weighted MRIs (T2 WIs) can reveal ischemic strokes earlier than CT but still typically require 8 to 12 h to accurately demonstrate the extent of an ischemic lesion. The availability of an imaging technique that could show ischemic lesions within minutes after onset would provide much useful information to the clinician and the radiologist. Recently a new MRI technique, diffusion-weighted imaging (DWI), became available. Both animal and human studies are available that demonstrate the feasibility and potential utility of DWI.

Diffusion-weighted imaging studies are derived by measuring the apparent diffusion coefficient (ADC) of water molecule protons on a voxel-by-voxel basis.[2] Signal intensity is directly related to these ADC measurements. Diffusion weighting of the MRI pulse sequence can be accomplished by adding short dephasing and rephasing magnetic field gradients onto standard pulse sequences (Fig. 20-1).[3] The extent of diffusion weighting of the sequences (b value) is related to the duration amplitude and temporal relationship of these gradients, and the b value directly influences ADC measurements. ADC values at standard b value vary in relationship to temperature and encumbrances to molecular motion of water protons. Thus, water protons in cerebrospinal fluid (CSF) move faster than they would in the extracellular space within brain parenchyma. CSF has a higher ADC and appears darker on DWI than brain parenchyma, while areas of lower ADC appear more intense, because signal intensity varies inversely with ADC (Fig. 20-2). Areas of ischemic brain injury have even lower ADC values than normal brain, related presumably to rapid accumulation of water intracellularly (cytotoxic edema) or reductions of cell membrane permeability to water movement.[4] These changes occur within minutes after ischemic brain injury and relate to severe reductions in blood flow and cellular metabolic compromise. Diffusion-weighted imaging can therefore provide confirmation of ischemic injury within minutes of onset.

Initial DWI studies in ischemic stroke models were performed by Moseley and colleagues beginning in the late 1980s. In a cat middle cerebral artery occlusion (MCAO) model, they observed hyperintense regions on DWI within 45 min after stroke onset, at which point T2 WI studies remained normal.[5] In a rat MCAO model, this group demonstrated DWI hyperintensity in ischemic regions within 14 min and reversal of these hyperintense regions when the animals were reperfused after 33 min of temporary ischemia.[4] Minematsu and colleagues quantitatively used DWI to evaluate ischemic lesion areas in the same MCAO model.[6] They demonstrated that lesion areas observed on DWI as early as 30 min after stroke onset were highly correlated with postmortem infarct areas in permanently occluded, nontreated animals (Fig. 20-3). Other groups have related the ADC changes observed with DWI to severe blood flow reductions and oubain-induced intracellular sodium and water accumulation.[7,8]

The ability of DWI to rapidly and quantitatively evaluate ischemic stroke suggested that it could be used to evaluate therapy in vivo. Kucharczyk et al. were the first investigators to perform such a study.[9] They qualitatively evaluated a purported sodium-calcium channel antagonist in a rat stroke model, giving varying drug doses 15 min after stroke onset. The DWI studies demonstrated smaller lesions in treated animals than in controls. Minematsu and colleagues used DWI to quantitatively evaluate the effects of reperfusion and cytoprotective therapy; both alone and in combination, employing the same rat stroke model as the other inves-

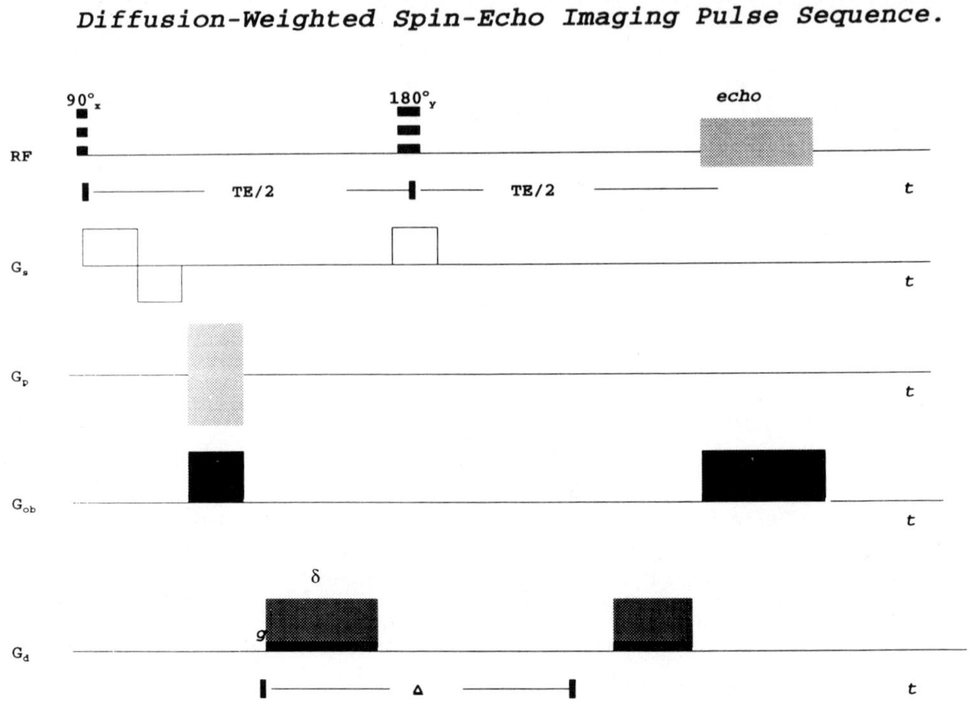

Figure 20-1
The pulse sequence for diffusion-weighted spin-echo imaging. (From Ann Neurol *32:115–122, 1992 Used by permission.)*

tigators. With mechanical reperfusion after 1 h of temporary occlusion, Minematsu et al. observed a significant (52 percent) reversal of hyperintense ischemic lesion areas when DWI studies obtained before and after reperfusion were compared (Fig. 20-4).[10] Reperfusion after 2 h had no significant effect on ischemic lesion size. When a noncompetitive NMDA antagonist was started 15 min after arterial occlusion, DWI studies beginning 30 min after ischemia documented a marked reduction in lesion size in vivo that was maintained over the 3-h imaging protocol (Fig. 20-5, Plate 32).[11] In a second study, using the same drug and delayed reperfusion after 3 h of temporary ischemia. DWI demonstrated not only the early reduction of ischemic lesion size by the cytoprotective agent but also the significant additive benefit of delayed reperfusion.[12]

In a recent study, ADC mapping was used to determine in vivo the neuroprotective effect of the glycine site antagonist ZD9379, which is potentially devoid of most side effects associated with competitive and noncompetitive NMDA antagonists.[13] Treatment started 30

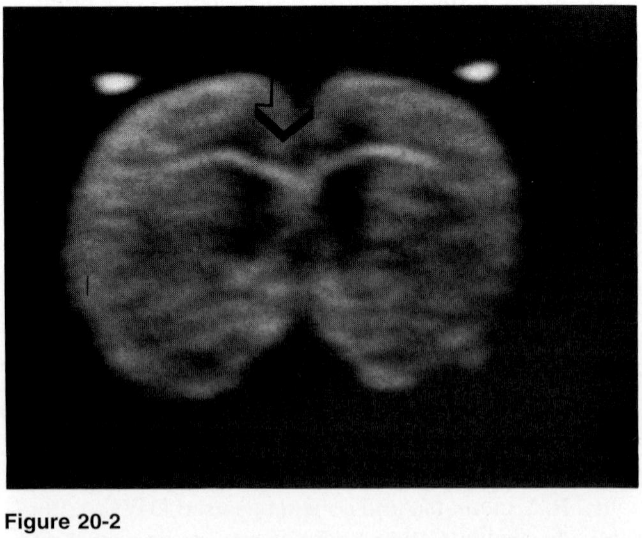

Figure 20-2
A DWI study depicting a coronal slice from a normal rat brain. The corpus callosum is lighter than the surrounding brain parenchyma because of anisoptropy (arrow).

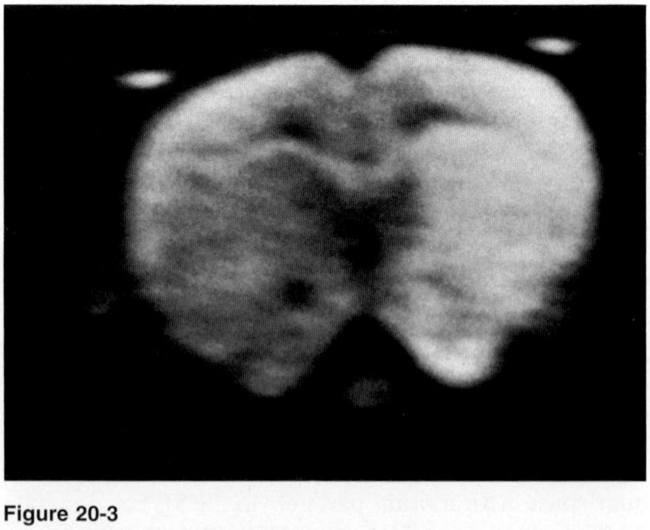

Figure 20-3
A coronal slice DWI obtained 30 min after MCAO. The area of hyperintensity represents the ischemic zone.

the ischemic lesion. Potential resolution of these abnormalities in the penumbra after acute human stroke has been demonstrated by spectroscopic imaging, suggesting that this technique may be able to identify patients for a therapeutic intervention on a biochemical basis.[42] Furthermore, choline elevation, primarily in the ischemic white matter, is thought to reflect the liberation of free trimethylamine resonances as myelin breakdown occurs.[42] In contrast, decreases in choline probably reflect a more chronic phase of infarction or ischemia not involving the white matter. ^{31}P MRS studies display high-energy phosphates, such as adenosine triphosphate (ATP), phosphocreatine, inorganic phosphates, and phosphomono- and diesters. With ischemia, high-energy phosphates rapidly decline and inorganic phosphates increase (Fig. 20-11), resulting in a decline of the phosphocreatine-to-inorganic phosphate ratio.[43] A reduction in pH also occurs with ischemia, leading to a small but detectable shift in the inorganic phosphate peak and the ability to determine pH changes. Therapeutic intervention with cytoprotective drugs has altered these changes in ^{1}H and ^{31}P MRS when they were given in an animal stroke model.[10] Sodium MRS studies are more difficult to perform but yield interesting information about global and focal ischemia in animal models.[44] A rapid rise in sodium signal was observed in both conditions, and it is likely that this increase in sodium is primarily intracellular. In focal ischemia, the increased sodium signal correlates well with areas of hyperintensity on DWI, implying that sodium and water enter ischemic cells together. Studies utilizing MRS take longer to perform than DWI and PI but offer the opportunity to determine what localized biochemical changes are occurring in focal brain ischemia and the effects of therapeutic measures.

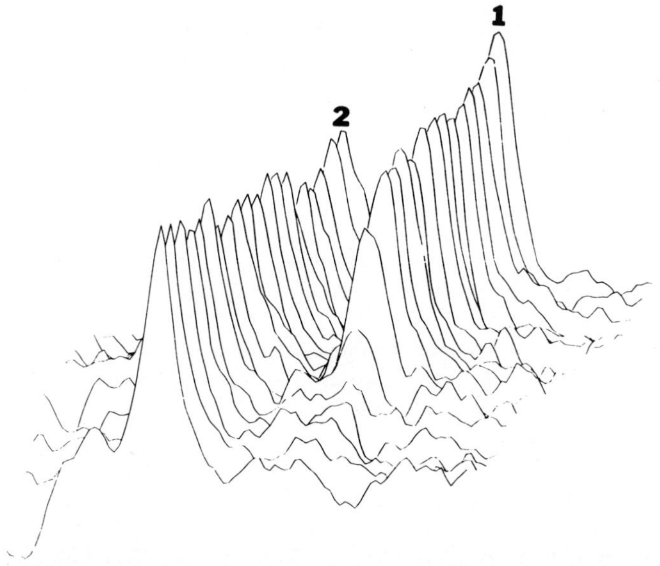

Figure 20-10
Sequential changes in ^{1}H-magnetic resonance spectra after cardiac arrest in a rat displaying an increase in lactate (1) and more gradual decline in N-acetyl aspartate (2) over 1 h. (From Ann Neurol *32:115–122, 1992. Used by permission.)*

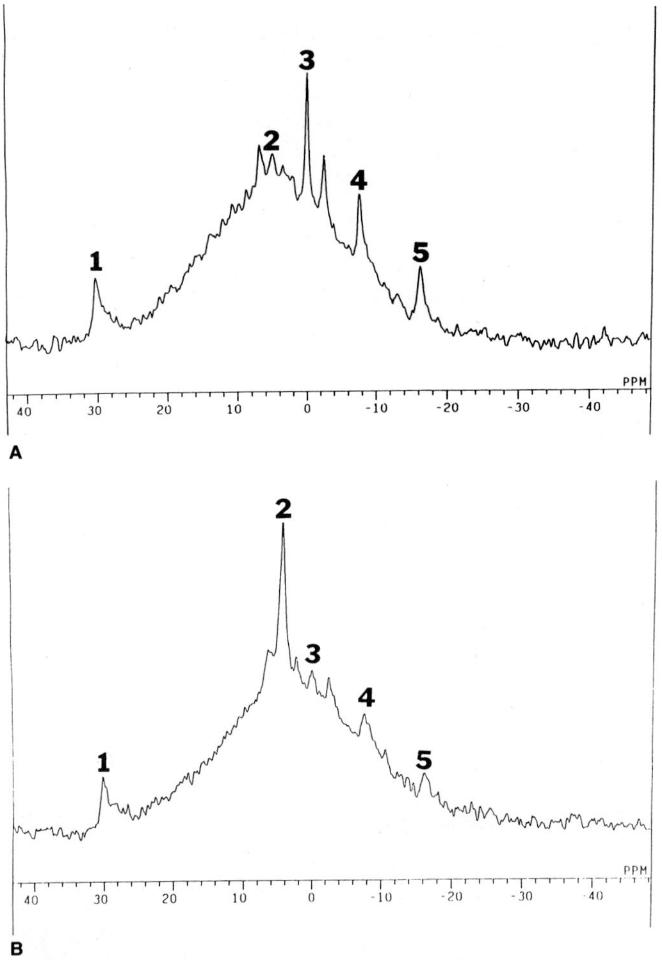

Figure 20-11
Phosphorus magnetic resonance spectra **(A)** *before and* **(B)** *30 min after bilateral common carotid artery occlusion in rats. The inorganic phosphate peak (2) rose, while phosphocreatine (3), x-adenosine triphosphate (4), and β-ATP levels (5) fell. (From* Ann Neurol *32:115–122, 1992. Used by permission.)*

REFERENCES

1. Bryan RL, Levy LM, Whitlow WD, et al: Diagnosis of acute cerebral infarction: Comparison of CT and MR imaging. *Am J Roentgenol* 157:585–597, 1991.
2. LeBihan D: Molecular diffusion nuclear magnetic resonance imaging. *Magn Reson Q* 7:1–30, 1991.
3. Fisher M, Sotak CH, Minematsu K, Li L: New magnetic resonance techniques for evaluating cerebrovascular disease. *Ann Neurol* 32:115–112, 1992.
4. Mintorovich J, Moseley ME, Chileuih L, et al: Comparison of diffusion and T2-weighted MRI for the early detection of cerebral ischemia and reperfusion in rats. *Magn Reson Med* 18:39–50, 1991.

5. Moseley ME, Kucharczyk J, Mintorovich J, et al: Diffusion-weighted MR imaging of acute stroke: Correlation of T2-weighted and magnetic susceptibility-enhanced MR imaging in cats. *Am J Neuroradiol* 11:423–429, 1990.
6. Minematsu K, Fisher M, Li L, et al: Diffusion-weighted magnetic resonance imaging: Rapid quantitative detection of focal brain ischemia. *Neurology* 42:235–240, 1993.
7. Busza AL, Allen KL, King MD, et al: Diffusion-weighted imaging studies of cerebral ischemia in gerbils: Potential relevance to energy failure. *Stroke* 23:1602–1613, 1992.
8. Benveniste H, Hedlund LW, Johnson GA: Mechanism of detection of acute cerebral ischemia by diffusion-weighted resonance spectroscopy. *Stroke* 23:746–754, 1992.
9. Kucharczyk J, Mintorovich J, Moseley ME, et al: Ischemic brain damage: Reduction by sodium-calcium ion channel modulator RS-87476. *Radiology* 179:221–227, 1991.
10. Minematsu J, Li L, Sotak CH, et al: Reversible focal ischemic injury demonstrated by diffusion-weighted magnetic resonance imaging. *Stroke* 23:1304–1311, 1992.
11. Minematsu K, Fisher M, Li L, et al: Effects of a novel NMDA antagonist on experimental stroke rapidly and quantitatively assessed by diffusion-weighted MRI. *Neurology* 43:397–403, 1993.
12. Minematsu K, Fisher M, Li L, Sotak CH: Diffusion and perfusion studies to evaluate a non-competitive NMDA antagonist and reperfusion in experimental stroke. *Stroke* 24:2074–2081, 1993.
13. Takano K, Tatlisumak T, Formato J, et al: Glycine site antagonist attenuates infarct size in experimental focal ischemia. *Stroke* 28:1255–1263, 1997.
14. Tatlisumak T, Takano K, Carano RAD, Fisher M: Effect of bFGF on experimental focal ischemia studied by DWI and PI. *Stroke* 27:2292–2298, 1996.
15. Warach S, Chien D, Li W, et al: Rapid diffusion imaging of acute cerebral infarction. *Neurology* 42:1717–1723, 1992.
16. Warach S, Gaa J, Siewart B, et al: Acute human stroke studied by whole echo-planar diffusion-weighted imaging. *Ann Neurol* 37:231–241, 1995.
17. Sorenson AG, Buonanno Gonzalez RG, et al: Hyperacute stroke: Evaluation with combined multisection diffusion-weighted and hemodynamically weighted echoplanar MR imaging. *Radiology* 199:391–401, 1996.
18. Marks MP, De Crespigny A, Lentz D, et al: Acute and chronic stroke: Navigated spin-echo diffusion-weighted MR imaging. *Radiology* 199:403–408, 1996.
19. Baird AE, Benfield BS, Schlaug G, et al: Enlargement of human cerebral ischemic lesion volumes measured by diffusion-weighted magnetic resonance imaging. *Ann Neurol* 41:581–589, 1997.
20. Lovblad KO, Baird AE, Schlaug G, et al: Ischemic lesion volumes in acute stroke by diffusion-weighted magnetic resonance imaging correlate with clinical outcome. *Ann Neurol* 42:164–170, 1997.
21. Lutsep HL, Albers GW, DeCrispigny A, et al: Clinical utility of diffusion-weighted resonance imaging in the assessment of ischemic stroke. *Ann Neurol* 41:574–580, 1997.
22. Warach S, Benfield A, Schlaug G, et al: Reduction of lesion volume in human stroke by citicoline detected by diffusion-weighted magnetic resonance imaging: A pilot study. *Ann Neurol* 40:527–528, 1996.
23. Dardzinski BJ, Fisher M, Sotak CH, et al: Apparent diffusion coefficient mapping of experimental focal cerebral ischemia using echo planar diffusion weighted imaging. *Magn Reson Med* 22:318–325, 1993.
24. Reith W, Hasegawa Y, Latour LL, et al: Multislice diffusion mapping for 3-D evolution of cerebral ischemia in rat stroke model. *Neurology* 45:172–177, 1995.
25. Takano K, Latour L, Formato JE, et al: Spreading depression contributes to the evolution of experimental focal brain ischemia evaluated by diffusion mapping. *Ann Neurol* 39:308–318, 1996.
26. Rosen BR, Belliveau JW, Chien D: Perfusion imaging by nuclear magnetic resonance. *Magn Reson Q* 5:263–281, 1989.
27. Stehling MK, Turner R, Mansfield P: Echo planar imaging: Magnetic resonance imaging in a fraction of a second. *Science* 254:43–50, 1991.
28. Belliveau JW, Rosen BR, Kantor HL, et al: Functional cerebral imaging by susceptibility contrast MR. *Magn Reson Med* 14:538–546, 1990.
29. Hamberg LM, MacFarlane R, Tasdemiroglu E, et al: Measurements of cerebrovascular changes in cats after transient ischemia using dynamic magnetic resonance imaging. *Stroke* 24:444–451, 1993.
30. Robert DA, Detre JY, Bolinger L, et al: Quantitative magnetic resonance imaging of brain perfusion at 1.5 T using steadystate inversion of arterial water. *Proc Natl Acad Sci U S A* 91:33–37, 1994.
31. Edelman RR, Siewert B, Darby DG, et al: Qualitative mapping of cerebral blood flow and functional localization with echo-planar MR imaging and signal targeting with alternating radio frequency. *Radiology* 192:513–520, 1994.
32. Moseley ME, Cohen Y, Mintorovitch J, et al: Early detection of regional cerebral ischemia in cats: Comparison of diffusion and T2-weighted MRI and spectroscopy. *Magn Reson Med* 14:330–346, 1990.
33. Warach S, Li W, Ronthal M, et al: Acute cerebral ischemia: Evaluation with dynamic contrast enhanced MR imaging and MR angiography. *Radiology* 182:41–47, 1992.
34. Siewert B, Schlaug G, Edelman RR, Warach S: Comparison of EPISTAR and T2-weighted gadolinium-enhanced perfusion imaging in patients with acute cerebral ischemia. *Neurology* 48:673–679, 1997.
35. Warach S, Li W, Ronthal M, Edelman RR: Acute cerebral ischemia: Evaluation with dynamic contrast-enhanced MR imaging and MR angiography. *Radiology* 182:41–47, 1992.
36. Welch KMA, Levine SR, Martin G, et al: Magnetic resonance spectroscopy in cerebral ischemia. *Neurol Clin* 10: 1–29, 1992.
37. Bruhn H, Frahm J, Gyngell ML, et al: Cerebral metabolism in men after acute stroke: New observation using localized NMR spectroscopy. *Magn Reson Med* 9:126–131, 1989.
38. Gideon P, Henriksen O, Sperling B, et al: Early time course of *N*-acetylaspartate, creatine and phosphocreatine, and compounds containing choline in the brain after stroke. *Stroke* 23:1566–1572, 1992.
39. Gideon P, Sperling B, Arlien-Soborg P, et al: Long-term follow-up of cerebral infarction patients with proton magnetic resonance spectroscopy. *Stroke* 25:967–973, 1994.
40. Graham GD, Blamire AM, Rothman DL, et al: Early

temporal variation of cerebral metabolites after human stroke: A proton magnetic resonance spectroscopic study. *Stroke* 24:1891–1896, 1993.

41. Petroff O, Graham GD, Blamire AM, et al: Spectroscopic imaging of stroke in humans: Histopathology correlates of spectral changes. *Neurology* 42:1349–1354, 1992.
42. Barker PB, Gillard JH, vanZijl PC, et al: Acute stroke: Evaluation with serial proton MR spectroscopic imaging. *Radiology* 92:723–731, 1994.
43. Bolas NM, Rajagopala B, Misumori F, Radda GK: Metabolic changes during experimental cerebral ischemia in hyperglycemic rats observed by ^{3}P and ^{1}H magnetic resonance spectroscopy. *Stroke* 19:608–614, 1988.
44. Lyon RC, Pekar J, Moonen CTW, McLaughlin AC: Double-quantum surface-coil NMR studies of sodium and potassium and the rat brain. *Magn Reson Med* 18:80–92, 1991.

CHAPTER 21

IMAGING OF STROKE WITH SPECT

Joseph C. Masdeu

Single photon emission computed tomography (SPECT), which was introduced into clinical medicine in the early 1980s, plays a role in the evaluation of patients with stroke. For the performance of SPECT, a flow tracer is tagged with a radionuclide and injected into the patient (Fig. 21-1). Through the use of a gamma camera and the techniques of computed tomography (CT), a three-dimensional image of the distribution of a radionuclide in the brain is obtained (Fig. 21-2).[1,2] Brain perfusion images obtained with SPECT can help differentiate an ischemic event from ictal or postictal phenomena such as Todd paresis. Initial data suggest that SPECT may be useful in predicting the likelihood of an early stroke after a transient ischemic attack (TIA) and in distinguishing between a lacunar stroke and a cortical stroke. After an acute stroke, early SPECT depicts the area of ischemia with greater accuracy than does either CT or magnetic resonance imaging (MRI). The extent and severity of ischemia can predict which patients are more prone to bleeding with intravenous thrombolytic therapy. Reperfusion of an arterial territory after thrombolysis can be documented less invasively with SPECT than it can with angiography. SPECT before and after the injection of acetazolamide has been used to assess the vascular reserve in patients with severe stenosis of the proximal vessels of the cerebrovascular tree or with vasospasm. Combined with transcranial Doppler studies, SPECT is useful in documenting ischemia after a subarachnoid hemorrhage (SAH). It also has been used to assess the effect on brain perfusion of arterial ligation intended to treat arteriovenous malformations (AVMs) or aneurysms.

In many of these clinical situations the information obtained with SPECT complements that obtained with CT, which is helpful in detecting intracranial hemorrhage, and MRI combined with magnetic resonance angiography (MRA), which provides information about structural damage to the brain as well as the situation of the vasculature. Newer techniques to study brain perfusion, such as MRI echo-planar imaging and contrast bolus on spiral CT, also can be used to detect ischemic areas very soon after the onset of a stroke.

NONISCHEMIC NEUROLOGIC DEFICITS

Occasionally, the clinical situation arises of differentiating ischemia from epilepsy as the cause of a neurologic finding, particularly in patients with a prolonged postictal deficit. Ischemia will cause an area of hypoperfusion on SPECT, whereas epileptic phenomena often are manifested by hyperperfusion (Fig. 21-3). Differentiating ischemia from epilepsy is critical as thrombolysis and other techniques for treating acute stroke become available. Increased perfusion of the hemisphere contralateral to the affected limbs also has been reported in some cases of infantile alternating hemiplegia[3] and cases of transient aphasia.[4] In migraine, decreased perfusion during the prodromal ischemic phase followed by hyperperfusion during the headache has been documented with Xe-133 SPECT.[5] SPECT also has been used to document decreased perfusion during the symptomatic phase of basilar migraine.[6]

Transient Ischemic Attack

SPECT may be useful in identifying patients who are at especially high risk for early stroke after a TIA. Bogousslavsky and coworkers[7] studied 12 patients with SPECT within a week after a TIA. Three of four patients who had a reduction in cerebral blood flow (CBF) >30 percent suffered an infarction in the first week after the TIA.[7] It is possible that patients with a negative SPECT had had a lacunar event, whereas those with a positive study are more likely to have experienced embolic ischemia with cortical involvement. However, Laloux and coworkers[8] did not find a correlation between stroke type and the likelihood of a post-TIA perfusion defect. Early recurrence is more common with embolic disease, often requiring anticoagulation, than it is with lacunar stroke.

The proportion of SPECT findings after a TIA is time-dependent. As many as 60 percent of TIA patients will have abnormalities if they are examined on the day of admission, 40 percent will have abnormalities by the second day,[9] and the number continues to fall during

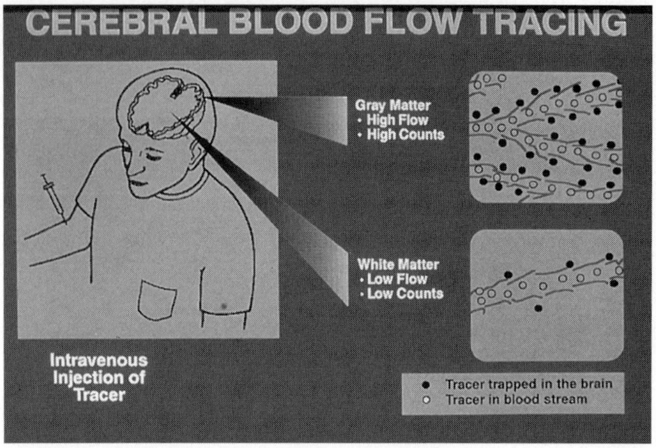

Figure 21-1 (Plate 35)
Injection of a SPECT perfusion agent. These agents, which are highly lipid-soluble, tend to penetrate the blood-brain barrier and remain trapped in the perivascular space for many hours, a long enough period to allow for imaging. Brain areas with high perfusion, such as the cerebral cortex, have higher counts than do those with lower perfusion, such as the white matter.

the first week after the event.[10] The sensitivity of SPECT imaging of TIAs can be improved with the addition of reactivity testing with acetazolamide, which also may provide information about the mechanism of ischemia.[11] For instance, failure of perfusion increase in a vascular territory suggests stenosis or occlusion of the artery supplying that territory (Fig. 21-4). Although not confirmed by a 1-year follow-up study,[12] the ability to identify patients with low flow states caused by asymptomatic carotid disease may permit the appropriate selection of cases for endarterectomy.

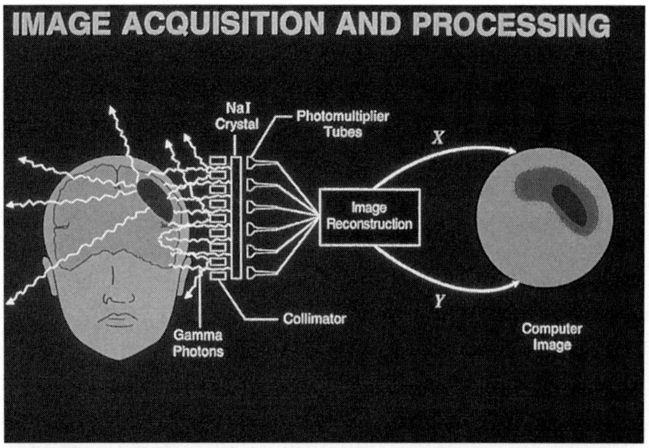

Figure 21-2 (Plate 36)
The distribution of a radionuclide in the brain is imaged by quantification of the photons that interact with sodium iodine (NaI) detectors. Careful collimation is essential for satisfactory image quality. Mathematical algorithms similar to the ones used with other CT techniques, including Fourier transform, are utilized to reconstruct the distribution of the isotope in the brain.

Decreases in cerebrovascular reserve, measured as a diminished dilatory response to CO_2 or acetazolamide, are an indicator of perfusion failure.[13] The long half-life of most SPECT agents imposes technical obstacles to this procedure for SPECT. These obstacles can be overcome partially by using multiple injections,[11] using reduced doses of radionuclides, and applying subtraction techniques.[14] When two isotopes are used, a technetium agent for a baseline blood flow measurement and an iodine agent for a postacetazolamide blood flow measurement, the separate distributions can be measured by using two windows on some modern three-head scanners. This greatly simplifies reactivity testing with SPECT and eliminates the need for multiple injections and subtraction techniques.[15]

These techniques are still predominantly investigational, but preliminary results suggest that reactivity testing may increase the sensitivity of detecting perfusion failure[16] and may have predictive value for early recurrent stroke or first stroke in asymptomatic patients.[17,18] The ability to determine accurately the stroke subtype and hemodynamic status with physiologic imaging is likely to become central to the management of patients with cerebrovascular disease.[19,20]

Acute Ischemic Neurologic Deficit

Precise information on which area of the brain is affected by ischemia cannot always be garnered from the clinical picture alone.[21,22] Information on the localization and extent of the lesion can be important for management. For instance, acute anticoagulation is not indicated for a lacunar stroke affecting deep structures but should be used with cardiogenic emboli, which generally cause cortical infarction. Consideration of stroke subtype is important in regard to treatment, recurrence, recovery, and mortality.[23–25] The need to differentiate stroke subtypes rapidly and accurately is becoming increasingly important as more specific stroke therapies are being evaluated. For instance, patients with deep ganglionic strokes on structural imaging and seizures have been shown on SPECT to have cortical involvement and therefore a higher likelihood of the etiology being embolic.[26] The demonstration of hemodynamically significant carotid stenosis in the setting of an acute infarct may prompt the use of revascularization as opposed to anticoagulation or thrombolytic therapy.

Early after a stroke, CT is helpful in defining hemorrhagic instances. However, in patients with ischemic stroke early CT is often negative. By 8 h after an infarction, about 20 percent of CT scans will be positive[27,28] and nearly 90 percent of SPECTs will be positive (Fig. 21-5).[10,27,29,30] Similar to positron emission tomography (PET), the defects seen on SPECT during the acute phase are usually equal to or larger than and better defined than the CT lesion.[26,31] Infarct location also de-

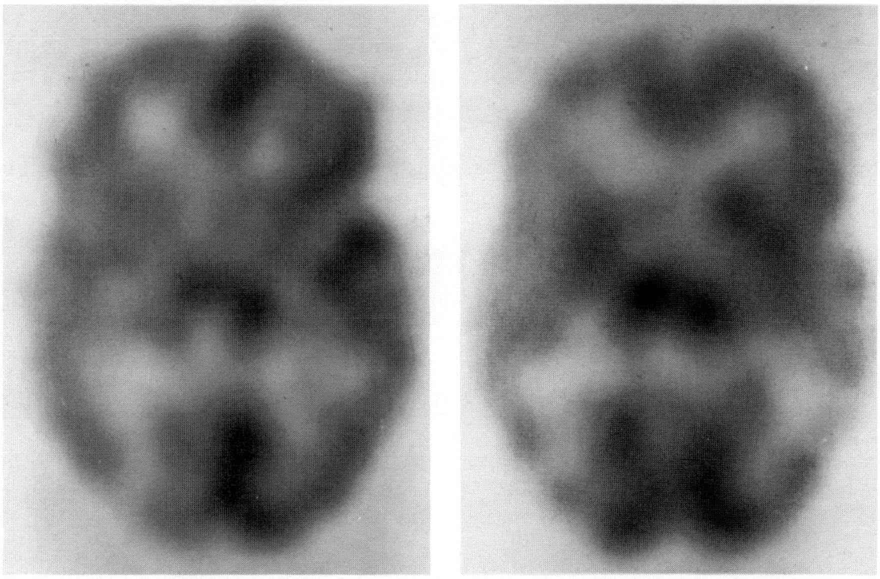

A B

Figure 21-3
Postictal hemiplegia. **(A)** *Axial SPECT showing increased perfusion of the left hemisphere obtained in a 58-year-old woman 26 h after she was found in the street with right-sided hemiplegia, global asphasia, and a gaze deviation to the left. Clinical findings persisted at the time of this SPECT. CT was negative. An electroencephalogram obtained 12 h before the SPECT had shown marked slowing over the left hemisphere but no epileptiform activity. Improvement ensued over a 1-week period, when the patient could give a history of having had a seizure disorder since her teens. Follow-up SPECT after the patient had improved showed symmetrical perfusion of the hemispheres* **(B)**.

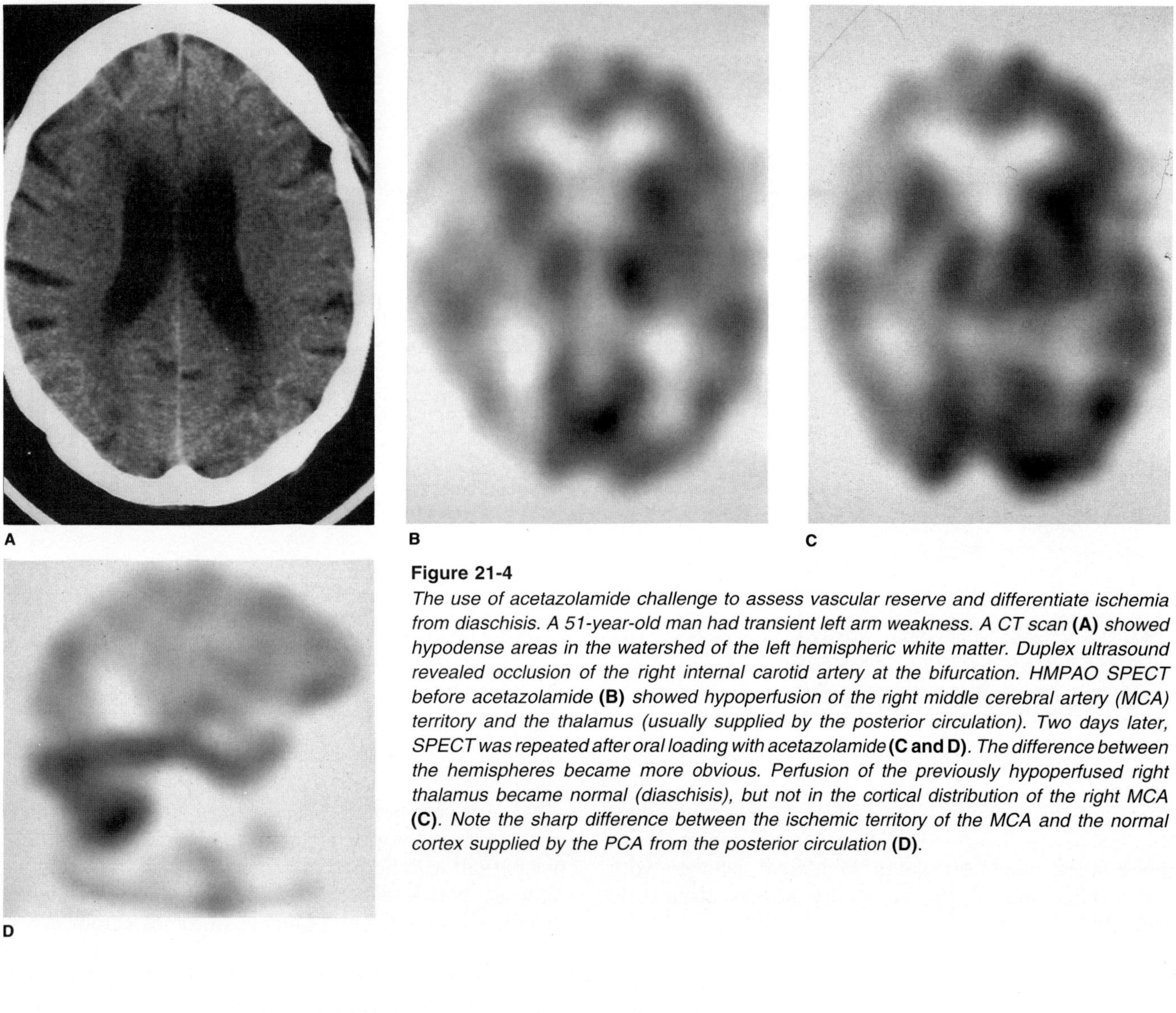

A B C D

Figure 21-4
The use of acetazolamide challenge to assess vascular reserve and differentiate ischemia from diaschisis. A 51-year-old man had transient left arm weakness. A CT scan **(A)** *showed hypodense areas in the watershed of the left hemispheric white matter. Duplex ultrasound revealed occlusion of the right internal carotid artery at the bifurcation. HMPAO SPECT before acetazolamide* **(B)** *showed hypoperfusion of the right middle cerebral artery (MCA) territory and the thalamus (usually supplied by the posterior circulation). Two days later, SPECT was repeated after oral loading with acetazolamide* **(C and D)**. *The difference between the hemispheres became more obvious. Perfusion of the previously hypoperfused right thalamus became normal (diaschisis), but not in the cortical distribution of the right MCA* **(C)**. *Note the sharp difference between the ischemic territory of the MCA and the normal cortex supplied by the PCA from the posterior circulation* **(D)**.

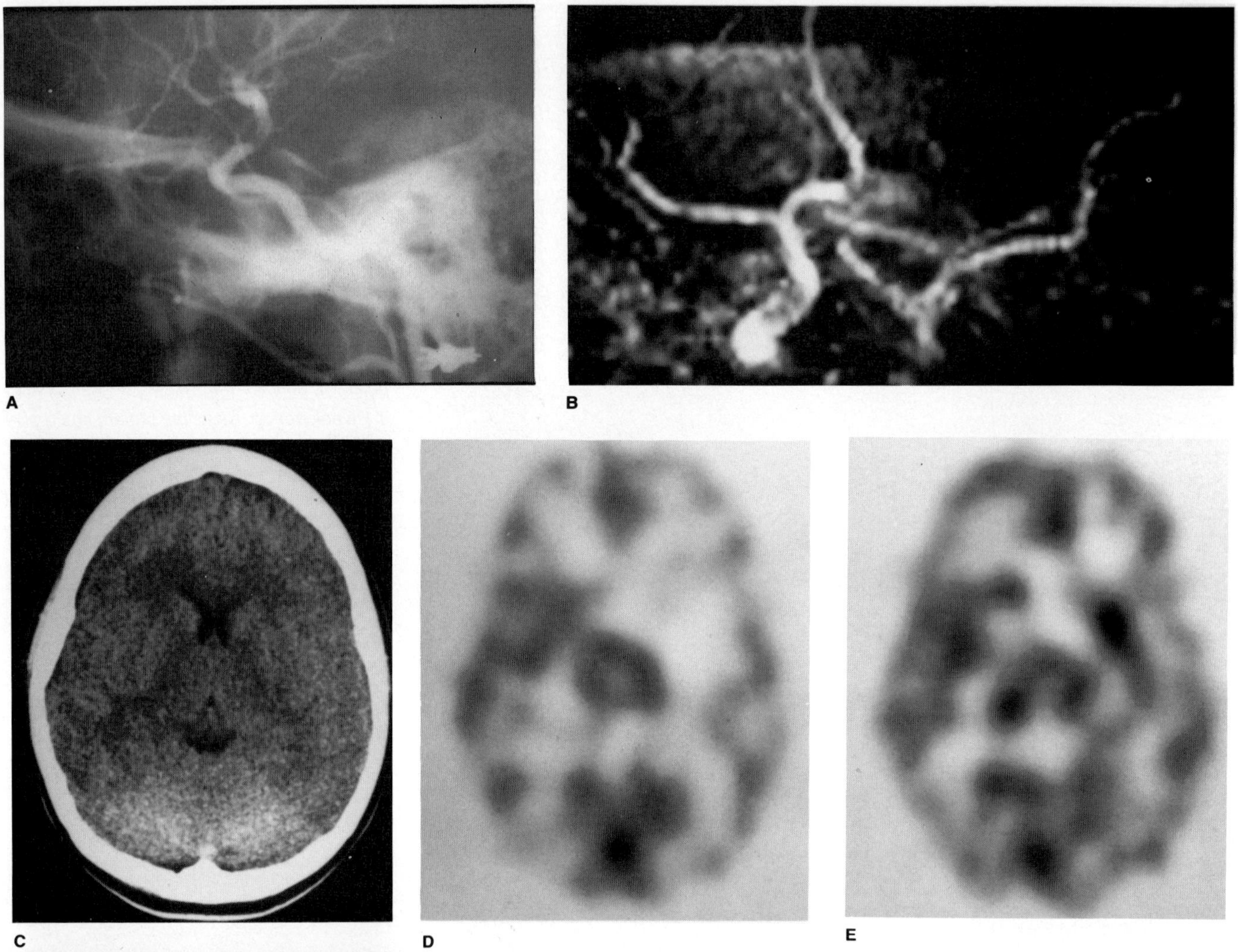

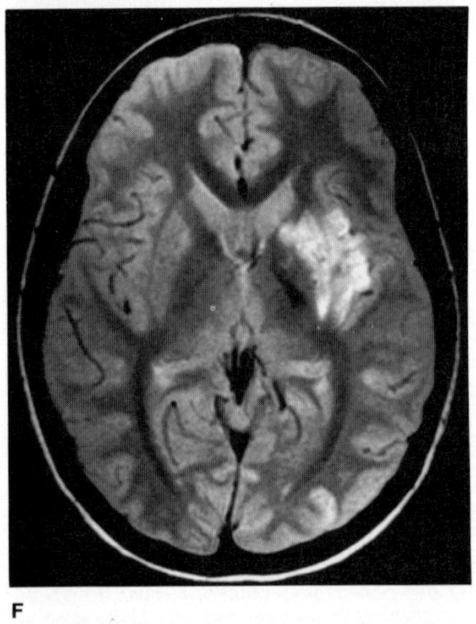

Figure 21-5

Acute stroke. A 23-year-old woman had a left putaminal infarct caused by dissection of the supraclinoid portion of the left internal carotid artery that was seen on lateral angiography **(A)** *and subsequently on MRA* **(B)**. *Early CT was negative* **(C)**. *Early SPECT at the same level as the CT showed hypoperfusion of the left basal ganglia and overlying frontal cortex* **(D)**. *Repeat SPECT 3 weeks after the event showed an area of hyperperfusion corresponding to the organizing cerebral infarction* **(E)**, *which was apparent on MRI* **(F)**.

termines the sensitivity of SPECT. In several studies, the sensitivity of early SPECT for cortical infarction has been in the neighborhood of 90 percent, whereas with subcortical infarcts the sensitivity hovers around 40 percent.[32,33]

MRA is very helpful in assessing acutely the situation of the major arteries supplying the brain, particularly in a patient with hemodynamic stroke caused by atheromatosis. It is less helpful when emboli have traveled distally to occlude the branches of major cerebral ves-

defect in transient ischemic attacks: A new clinically useful subgroup? *Stroke* 27:425–430, 1996.
9. Hartmann A: Prolonged disturbances of regional cerebral blood flow in transient ischemic attacks. *Stroke* 16:932–939, 1985.
10. De Roo M, Mortelmans L, Devos P, et al: Clinical experience with Tc-99m HM-PAO high resolution SPECT of the brain in patients with cerebrovascular accidents. *Eur J Nucl Med* 15:9–15, 1989.
11. Chollet F, Celsis P, Clanet M, et al: SPECT study of cerebral blood flow reactivity after acetazolamide in patients with transient ischemic attacks. *Stroke* 20:458–464, 1989.
12. Powers WJ, Tempel LW, Grubb RLJ: Influence of cerebral hemodynamics on stroke risk: One-year follow-up of 30 medically treated patients. *Ann Neurol* 25:325–330, 1989.
13. Bonte FJ, Devous MDS, Reisch JS, et al: The effect of acetazolamide on regional cerebral blood flow in patients with Alzheimer's disease or stroke as measured by single-photon emission computed tomography. *Invest Radiol* 24:99–103, 1989.
14. Momose T, Kosaka N, Nishikawa J, et al: A new method for brain functional study using Tc-99m HMPAO SPECT. *Radiat Med* 7:82–87, 1989.
15. Devous MD, Gassaway SK: Simultaneous SPECT imaging of Tc-99m- and I-123 labeled brain agents in patients using the PRISM scanner. *J Nucl Med* 31:877, 1990.
16. Burt RW, Witt RM, Cikrit DF, Reddy RV: Carotid artery disease: Evaluation with acetazolamide-enhanced Tc-99m HMPAO SPECT. *Radiology* 182:461–466, 1992.
17. Cikrit DF, Burt RW, Dalsing MC, et al: Acetazolamide enhanced single photon emission computed tomography (SPECT) evaluation of cerebral perfusion before and after carotid endarterectomy. *J Vasc Surg* 15:747–754, 1992.
18. Hasegawa Y, Yamaguchi T, Tsuchiya T, et al: Sequential change of hemodynamic reserve in patients with major cerebral artery occlusion or severe stenosis. *Neuroradiology* 34:15–21, 1992.
19. Weiller C, Ringelstein EB, Reiche W, Buell U: Clinical and hemodynamic aspects of low-flow infarcts. *Stroke* 22:1117–1123, 1991.
20. Prichard JW, Brass LM: New anatomical and functional imaging methods. *Ann Neurol* 32:395–400, 1992.
21. Foulkes MA, Wolf PA, Price TR, et al: The Stroke Data Bank: Design, methods, and baseline characteristics. *Stroke* 19:547–554, 1988.
22. Mohr JP, Barnett HJM: Classification of ischemic stroke, in Barnett HJM, Stein BM, Mohr JP, Yatsu FM (eds): *Stroke: Pathophysiology, Diagnosis, and Management,* Vol 2. New York, Churchill Livingstone, 1986, pp 281–291.
23. Bogousslavsky J, Regli F: Borderzone infarctions distal to internal carotid artery occlusion: Prognostic implications. *Ann Neurol* 20:346–350, 1986.
24. Sacco RL, Foulkes MA, Mohr JP, et al: Determinants of early recurrence of cerebral infarction: The Stroke Data Bank. *Stroke* 20:983–989, 1989.
25. Schroeder T: Hemodynamic significance of internal carotid artery disease. *Acta Neurol Scand* 77:353–372, 1988.
26. Giroud M, Dumas R: Role of associated cortical lesions in motor partial seizures and lenticulostriate infarcts. *Epilepsia* 36:465–470, 1995.
27. Bose A, Pacia SV, Fayad P, et al: Cerebral blood flow (CBF) imaging compared to CT during the initial 24 hours of cerebral infarction. *Neurology* 40(suppl 1):190, 1990.
28. Fieschi C, Argentino C, Lenzi GL, et al: Clinical and instrumental evaluation of patients with ischemic stroke within the first six hours. *J Neurol Sci* 91:311–321, 1989.
29. de Bruine JF, Limburg M, van Royen EA, et al: SPECT brain imaging with 201 diethyldithiocarbamate in acute ischaemic stroke. *Eur J Nucl Med* 17:248–251, 1990.
30. Podreka I, Suess E, Goldenberg G, et al: Initial experience with technetium-99m HM-PAO brain SPECT. *J Nucl Med* 28:1657–1666, 1987.
31. Lee RG, Hill TC, Holman BL, Clouse ME: N-isopropyl-(I-123)p-iodoamphetamine brain scans with single-photon emission tomography: Discordance with transmission computed tomography. *Radiology* 145:795–799, 1982.
32. Baird AE, Austin MC, McKay WJ, Donnan GA: Sensitivity and specificity of 99mTc-HMPAO SPECT cerebral perfusion measurements during the first 48 hours for the localization of cerebral infarction. *Stroke* 28:976–980, 1997.
33. Brass LM, Walovitch RC, Joseph JL, et al: The role of single photon emission computed tomography brain imaging with 99mTc-bicisate in the localization and definition of mechanism of ischemic stroke. *J Cereb Blood Flow Metab* 14:S91–S98, 1994.
34. Caplan L, Allam G, Teal P: The moving embolus. *J Neuroimaging* 3:195–197, 1993.
35. Alberts MJ, Faulstich ME, Gray L: Stroke with negative brain magnetic resonance imaging. *Stroke* 23:663–667, 1992.
36. Ramadan NM, Deveshwar R, Levine SR: Magnetic resonance and clinical cerebrovascular disease: An update. *Stroke* 20:1279–1283, 1989.
37. Moseley ME, Cohen Y, Mintorovitch J, et al: Early detection of regional cerebral ischemia in cats: Comparison of diffusion- and T2-weighted MRI and spectroscopy. *Magn Reson Med* 14:330–346, 1990.
38. Fisher M, Sotak CH, Minematsu K, Li L: New magnetic resonance techniques for evaluating cerebrovascular disease. *Ann Neurol* 32:115–122, 1992.
39. Brott TG, Gelfand MJ, Williams CC, et al: Frequency and patterns of abnormality detected by iodine-123 amine emission CT after cerebral infarction. *Radiology* 158:729–734, 1986.
40. Holman BL, Hellman RS, Goldsmith SJ, et al: Biodistribution, dosimetry, and clinical evaluation of technetium-99m ethyl cysteinate dimer in normal subjects and in patients with chronic cerebral infarction. *J Nucl Med* 30:1018–1024, 1989.
41. Seiderer M, Krappel W, Moser E, et al: Detection and quantification of chronic cerebrovascular disease: Comparison of MR imaging, SPECT, and CT. *Radiology* 170:545–548, 1989.
42. Alexandrov AV, Ehrlich LE, Bladin CF, Black SE: Clinical significance of increased uptake of HMPAO on brain SPECT scans in acute stroke. *J Neuroimaging* 6:150–155, 1996.
43. Tran-Dinh YR, Ille O, Guichard JP, et al: Cerebral post-ischemic hyperperfusion assessed by Xenon-133 SPECT. *J Nucl Med* 38:602–607, 1997.
44. Miller JH, Khonsary A, Raffel C: The scintigraphic appearance of childhood moyamoya disease on cerebral perfusion imaging. *Pediatr Radiol* 26:833–838, 1996.

45. Fukui M: Current state of study on moyamoya disease in Japan. *Surg Neurol* 7:138–143, 1997.
46. Companioni JM, Lassen NA, Tfelt-Hansen P, Friberg L: Delayed reflow of an ischemic infarct after spontaneous thrombolysis studied by CBF tomography using SPECT and Tc-99m HMPAO. *Am J Physiol Imaging* 6:167–171, 1991.
47. Alexandrov AV, Masdeu JC, Devous M Sr, et al: Brain single-photon emission CT with HMPAO and safety of thrombolytic therapy in acute ischemic stroke: Proceedings of the meeting of the SPECT Safe Thrombolysis Study Collaborators and the members of the Brain Imaging Council of the Society of Nuclear Medicine. *Stroke* 28:1830–1834, 1997.
48. Hanson SK, Grotta JC, Rhoades H, et al: Value of single-photon emission-computed tomography in acute stroke therapeutic trials. *Stroke* 24:1322–1329, 1993.
49. Alexandrov AV, Black SE, Ehrlich LE, et al: Simple visual analysis of brain perfusion on HMPAO SPECT predicts early outcome in acute stroke. *Stroke* 27:1537–1542, 1996.
50. Ayada Y, Tsuda Y, Takahashi T, et al: Volume of infarction and blood flow in cerebral embolism. *Angiology* 48:223–228, 1997.
51. Biller J, Godersky JC, Adams HP: Management of aneurysmal subarachnoid hemorrhage. *Stroke* 19:1300–1305, 1988.
52. Davis SM, Andrews JT, Lichtenstein M, et al: Correlations between cerebral arterial velocities, blood flow, and delayed ischemia after subarachnoid hemorrhage. *Stroke* 23:492–497, 1992.
53. Lewis DH, Eskridge JM, Newell DW, et al: Brain SPECT and the effect of cerebral angioplasty in delayed ischemia due to vasospasm. *J Nucl Med* 33:1789–1796, 1992.
54. Le Roux PD, Newell DW, Eskridge J, et al: Severe symptomatic vasospasm: The role of immediate postoperative angioplasty. *J Neurosurg* 80:224–229, 1994.
55. Caplan LR, Brass LM, DeWitt LD, et al: Transcranial Doppler ultrasound: Present status. *Neurology* 40:696–700, 1990.
56. Tranquart F, Ades PE, Groussin P, et al: Postoperative assessment of cerebral blood flow in subarachnoid haemorrhage by means of 99mTc-HMPAO tomography. *Eur J Nucl Med* 20:53–58, 1993.
57. Kimura T, Shinoda J, Funakoshi T: Prediction of cerebral infarction due to vasospasm following aneurysmal subarachnoid haemorrhage using acetazolamide-activated 123I-IMP SPECT. *Acta Neurochir (Wien)* 123:125–128, 1993.
58. Tran Dinh YR, Lot G, Benrabah R, et al: Abnormal cerebral vasodilation in aneurysmal subarachnoid hemorrhage: Use of serial 133Xe cerebral blood flow measurement plus acetazolamide to assess cerebral vasospasm. *J Neurosurg* 79:490–493, 1993.
59. Batjer HH, Devous MDS: The use of acetazolamide-enhanced regional cerebral blood flow measurement to predict risk to arteriovenous malformation patients. *Neurosurgery* 31:213–217, 1992.
60. Batjer HH, Devous MD, Seibert GB, et al: Intracranial arteriovenous malformation: Relationships between clinical factors and surgical complications. *Neurosurgery* 24:75–79, 1989.
61. Awad IA, Magdinec M, Schubert A: Intracranial hypertension after resection of cerebral arteriovenous malformations: Predisposing factors and management strategy. *Stroke* 25:611–620, 1994.
62. Chung TS, Lee JD, Suh JH, et al: Increased cerebral perfusion after detachable balloon embolization of carotid cavernous fistula on technetium-99m-HMPAO brain SPECT. *J Nucl Med* 34:1987–1989, 1993.

ULTRASOUND IN CEREBROVASCULAR DISEASE

Charles H. Tegeler
Disya Ratanakorn

OVERVIEW OF THE CLINICAL IMPERATIVE

The most important neurologic use of ultrasound (neurosonology) is in the clinical setting of stroke and cerebrovascular disease.[1] Stroke remains the third leading cause of death in the United States and is a key cause of disability in the elderly, with over 500,000 new or repeat strokes yearly and about 150,000 deaths.[2] The application of more specific preventive or therapeutic intervention demands better understanding of the ischemic mechanisms in the individual patient. Ultrasound is well suited to the noninvasive study of the cerebrovascular system to better identify potential ischemic mechanisms.

Of all the patients presenting with a stroke syndrome (acute focal neurologic deficit that persists for 24 h or more), 95 percent are due to vascular causes. Of all vascular causes, 80 to 85 percent are due to ischemic infarction and 15 to 20 percent are primary brain hemorrhages.[3,4] It is in the group with ischemic infarction that neurosonography plays a particularly important role. Many ischemic strokes are due to large-vessel cerebrovascular disease, mostly carotid atherosclerosis, and neurosonography provides a quick, safe, accurate, and cost-effective way of assessing the vascular system for potential ischemic causes.[5]

The NASCET Study,[6] VA Cooperative Study,[7] and European Study[8] all confirmed that patients with symptomatic, tight carotid stenosis of more than 70 percent linear stenosis have significantly better outcomes when treated with carotid endarterectomy and medical treatment than with medical treatment alone. The ACAS Study[9] demonstrated that carotid endarterectomy also benefits asymptomatic patients with 60 to 99 percent linear carotid stenosis. These studies provide a clinical mandate to identify tight carotid stenosis in patients with stroke or transient ischemic attack, as well as in patients without cerebrovascular symptoms, because of the direct implications for management. Yet this must be done in a safe, cost-effective manner so as not to place patients at undue risk or waste dwindling health care resources. Neurosonography can accurately identify patients with tight carotid stenosis in a safe, noninvasive, cost-effective manner, allowing more judicious use of the more costly, risky, or invasive angiographic procedures.[10–16]

In the intracranial circulation, identification of intracranial stenosis, intracranial collateral flow patterns in the presence of extracranial tight carotid stenosis or occlusion, and embolic signals is also important to guide the management of stroke patients. Embolic strokes due to cardiac or aortic causes account for 15 to 20 percent of all strokes, and diagnosis of a cardioembolic mechanism is a crucial clinical conclusion because it suggests a need for chronic anticoagulation, a potentially risky therapy.[17,18]

Intelligent use of ultrasound in cerebrovascular disease requires detailed knowledge of the basic principles and physics of ultrasound, the anatomy and pathophysiology of the cerebrovascular system, the ultrasound techniques used to assess structure and function and principles of interpretation, including the implications for management and quality-assurance requirements.[19–20] This chapter discusses the neurovascular ultrasound techniques, including their basic principles, clinical indications, and interpretation.

DOPPLER SONOGRAPHY

In ultrasound devices, a piezoelectric element in the transducer rapidly contracts and expands, converting electrical energy into acoustic energy, or sound waves. As the name *ultrasound* implies, the frequency (cycles per second, or hertz) of sound used in neurosonography is higher than the human audible range (20 to 20,000 Hz). Diagnostic ultrasound devices usually operate at frequencies of 2 to 10 million Hz (2 to 10 MHz).

The Doppler effect is the change or shift in the frequency or wavelength of a wave due to relative movement between the sound source or scatterer and the receiver (Fig. 22-1).[21] This phenomenon, first described by Christian Andreas Doppler in 1842 to explain the colored light of double stars, forms the basis for the hemodynamic assessment of vascular structures with ultrasound.

Applying Doppler's work to vascular ultrasound (see the Doppler equation below), the Doppler frequency shift, Fs, depends on the speed of blood flow, v, in meters per second; the angle between the sound beam and the direction of blood flow, or the angle of insonation, θ;

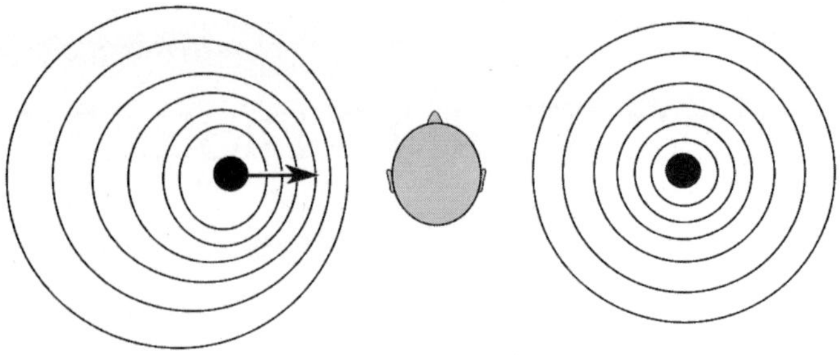

Figure 22-1
Doppler principle. A spectator (receiver) is hit by more waves per second (higher frequency) if the sound source is moving toward the spectator. (From Tegeler.[5] Used by permission.)

the transmitted frequency, f(t); and the speed of sound in the soft tissue, C, in meters per second. This change in Doppler frequency is the difference between the transmitted and received frequencies. The direction of flow relative to the transducer can be determined by whether the Doppler frequency shift is positive or negative.

$$\text{Fs (MHz)} = \frac{2 \times \text{v (m/s)} \times \text{f(t) (MHz)} \times \cos\theta}{\text{C (m/s)}}$$

$$\text{v (m/s)} = \frac{\text{Fs (MHz)} \times \text{C (m/s)}}{2 \times \text{f(t) (MHz)} \times \cos\theta}$$

$$\text{v (cm/s)} = \frac{\text{Fs (kHz)} \times 77}{\text{f(t) (MHz)} \times \cos\theta}$$

Because the equation uses the cosine of the angle of insonation, as the angle approaches 0° (sound beam parallel to the direction of flow), Fs will be maximal, whereas when the angle approaches 90° (right angle to the direction of flow), Fs decreases and approaches zero. The ideal Doppler angle of insonation is 0°, but in the body the angle of insonation may change dramatically depending on in situ anatomy. For vascular sonography, the magnitude of the Doppler shift is usually in thousands of hertz (kHz), and, since this shift is in the audible range, it can be heard. The direction of blood flow is determined by positive Doppler shift (flow toward the transducer) and negative Doppler shift (flow away from the transducer).

The use of blood flow velocity (v, in centimeters per second), rather than Doppler frequency shift (Fs in kilohertz), avoids potential confusion related to variance in f(t) or cosθ, by correcting for the transducer frequency and the angle of insonation. This provides a common language and a measure with which to compare results among various studies on the same patient and various equipment, laboratories, and scanning protocols. It is this blood flow velocity that is used to assess vascular hemodynamics and stenosis.

There are two broad categories of Doppler transducers: those that continuously transmit and receive (continuous-wave, or c-w, Doppler) and those that intermittently emit and receive a series of short pulses of sound (pulsed-wave, or p-w, Doppler). The use of c-w Doppler provides a sensitive evaluation of any moving target in the path of the sound beam and can accurately identify extremely high flow velocities. However, c-w Doppler is not able to localize the specific depth of the reflector (scatterer) at which the signal originated and often includes detection of the signals from undesired vascular structures, such as veins and small arteries. By transmitting discrete, brief pulses of sound and waiting for any scattered signals to return before emitting the next pulse, p-w Doppler transducers make use of the opportunity to vary the time of sampling in order to choose the specific depth of sampling (specific sample volume), as well as to localize the depth of signal origination. Since sound travels in soft tissue at a constant speed, the depth of a reflector can be determined by the use of the range equation:

$$\text{Depth (m)} = \frac{\text{propagation speed (m/s)} \times \text{round-trip travel time (s)}}{2}$$

While p-w Doppler allows discrete localization of the sample, the use of a series of sound pulses at a fixed rate (pulse repetition frequency, or PRF), rather than continuous sampling, means that it may not be able to accurately assess very high-frequency shifts generated by very high blood flow velocities. The PRF must be high enough to allow two samples from each cycle of the Fs, or erroneous readings might occur. This phenomenon, which in practical terms is similar to the appearance of the spokes of wagon wheels going in reverse in old western movies, is known as aliasing. Aliasing can occur when Fs exceeds one-half the PRF, a value also known as the Nyquist limit. On most devices, the PRF can be increased to eliminate aliasing, and, if not, for most current instruments aliasing usually does not occur until well above the velocity cut points for clinically important stenosis.

Even in normal vessels, because of laminar flow, the blood flowing in the vessels acts as many small reflectors or scatterers moving at a variety of speeds and directions, rather than as one single moving reflector. At any point in time, within the sample volumes used for Doppler sonography, there will be a "spectrum" of flow velocities (speed and direction). This spectrum can be visually displayed by use of the fast Fourier transform (Fig. 22-2).

The velocity spectrum can be analyzed for a number of specific parameters, including flow direction, peak systolic flow velocity (Vs), and end-diastolic flow velocity (Vd), as well as the characteristics of the velocity spectrum, such as the width or spread of the band or envelope of velocities, the shape of the margin of the envelope, or a variety of derived indexes, such as the acceleration time (systolic flow acceleration or systolic acceleration slope), the pulsatility, and the resistivity indexes. The most important parameters for clinical in-

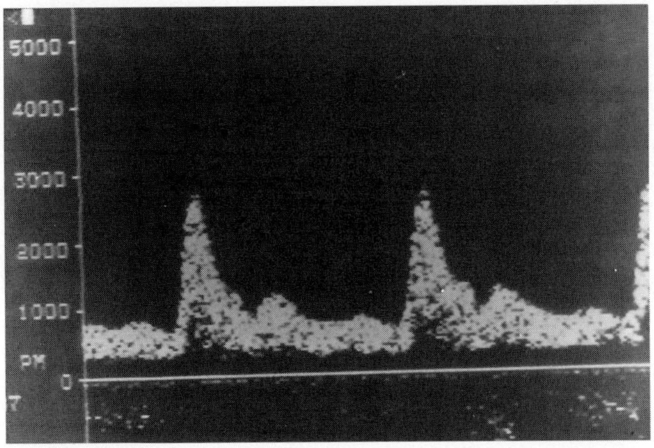

Figure 22-2
Spectral display of Doppler frequency shift (in hertz) information (Y axis) over time (X axis).

terpretation are Vs and Vd, but specific characteristics of the spectral waveform are also important in interpreting flow hemodynamics both proximally and distally to the point of interrogation. When using the same-sized sample volume, normal vessels have a compact, narrow, smooth velocity envelope, whereas vessels with disturbed flow demonstrate turbulence, with an increased variety of speeds and flow directions, resulting in broadening of the velocity spectrum, reversed flow depicted below the baseline, and an irregular margin of the acoustic envelope (Fig. 22-3). A jagged sawtooth margin correlates with a bubbling, gurgling audible signal.

Each vessel also has a characteristic spectral appearance, or fingerprint, based on the distal peripheral resistance. As a low-resistance system supplying the brain, which requires diastolic flow, the internal carotid artery has a quite different spectral appearance from the external carotid artery, which has high distal peripheral resistance (Figs. 22-4 and 22-5). With flow going to both the internal and external carotid arteries, the spectral pattern of the common carotid artery is a combination of the two. Specific spectral patterns can be used not only to help identify the insonated vessels but also to provide useful indirect information about pathologic conditions proximally and distally.

When stenosis occurs, characteristic hemodynamic changes detected by Doppler sonography can be used to estimate the severity of the stenosis. For very mild degrees of stenosis, which do not cause appreciable

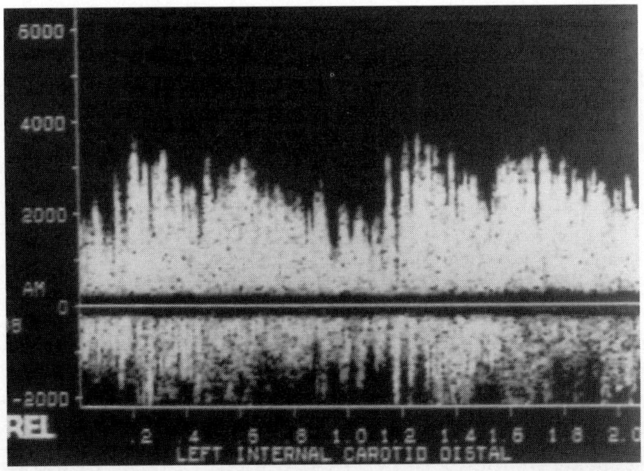

Figure 22-3
Doppler spectral display showing disturbed flow and turbulence in the left ICA beyond a tight stenosis.

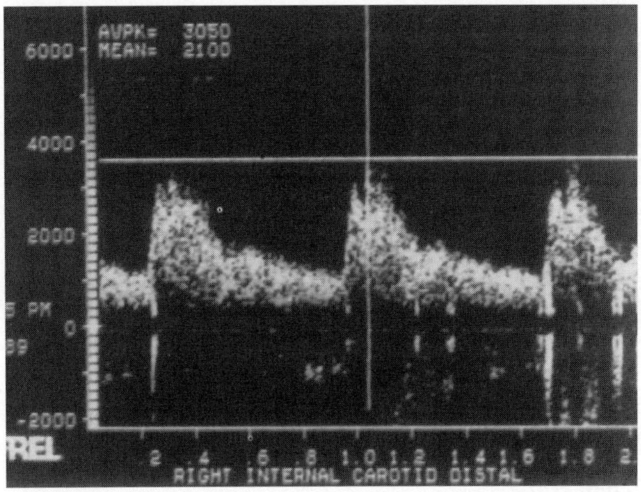

Figure 22-4
Spectral of the Doppler frequency shift from the right ICA. Note the gentler systolic upsloping, more rounded peak at systole, gradual fall-off, and persistent diastolic forward flow, due to a low-resistance distal vascular bed. Artifact is seen along the baseline.

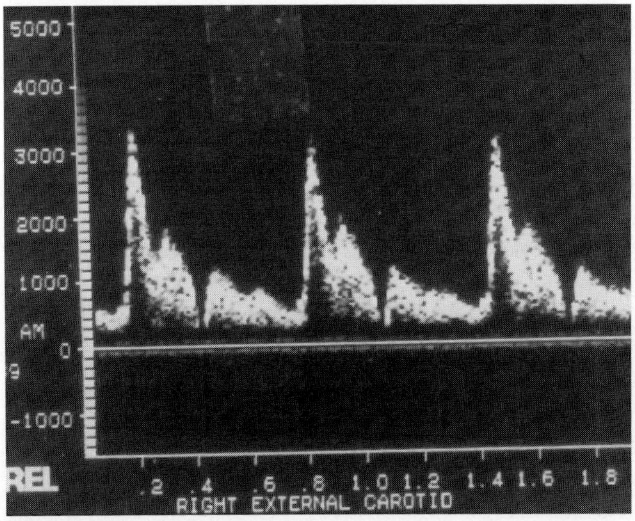

Figure 22-5
Spectral display of the Doppler frequency shift from the right external carotid artery. Note the sharp systolic upsloping, sharp peak, rapid fall-off, prominent dicrotic notch, and little diastolic forward flow, due to the higher resistance in the distal vascular bed it supplies.

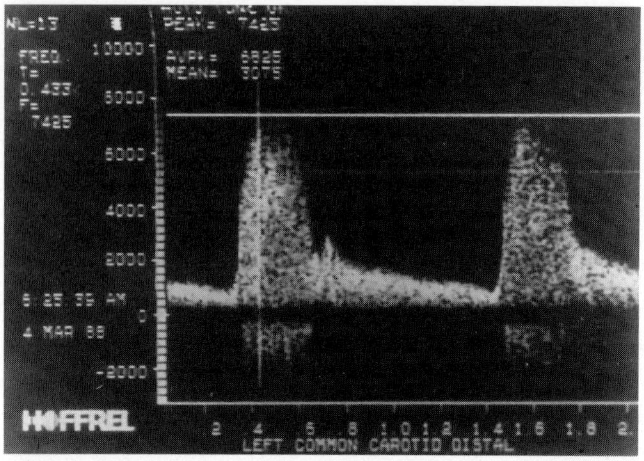

Figure 22-6
Doppler spectral display from a 50 to 75 percent carotid stenosis shows high peak systolic frequency shift, spectral broadening, and mild turbulence but normal diastolic frequency shift.

Table 22-1
Flow velocity criteria for grading carotid stenosis at Wake Forest University Baptist Medical Center

% stenosis, descriptor	*PSV, cm/s*	*EDV, cm/s*	*ICA : CCA ratio*
0–49, NSSF	<140	<40	<2
50–74, moderate	>140	<110	>2
75–94, severe	≥140	>110	>3
95–99, subtotal/string	Variable	Variable	Variable
Probable occlusion	No flow	No flow	Not applicable

Abbreviations: CCA, common carotid artery; EDV, end-diastolic velocity; ICA, internal carotid artery; NSSF, no significant stenotic flow; PSV, peak systolic velocity.

hemodynamic changes, there may be minimal or no apparent changes on Doppler velocities. As the stenosis worsens, the first hemodynamic effect is that of increased Vs across the narrowed region. Further narrowing causes additional increases in Vs, as well as development of a disturbed flow pattern or turbulence (Fig. 22-6). As stenosis becomes severe, even higher Vs can no longer maintain adequate flow volume; thus, Vd rises as well to try to meet the hemodynamic needs of the brain (Fig. 22-7). Further worsening of stenosis results in decreasing flow velocities and flow volume as the vessel approaches occlusion.

There are numerous published criteria to relate these changes in both the velocity and characteristics of flow, as identified by Doppler sonography, to severity of stenosis.[22–27] Most rely primarily on the peak systolic and diastolic velocities. Many also use the ratio of velocities in the internal carotid and the common carotid arteries as an important adjunct criterion (Table 22-1) for interpretation. Other parameters frequently used include side-to-side velocity differences, the spectral appearance of a high-resistance signal, and the visualization of extensive plaque by B-mode imaging as secondary criteria. Such criteria are used as guidelines for interpretation, not as inflexible, hard rules. Every patient is unique, and some flexibility and judgment regarding the overall clinical picture must go into the interpretation of the results. Whatever velocity criteria are used, there must be an ongoing program of quality assurance to ensure that, for specific sonographers, using specific equipment, interpreted by specific readers, the criteria are accurate.[28–31] This quality-assurance program should include formal correlation with results obtained using whatever modalities are available, including angiography, MRI angiography, and testing of pathologic specimens, as well as correlation with clinical outcome.

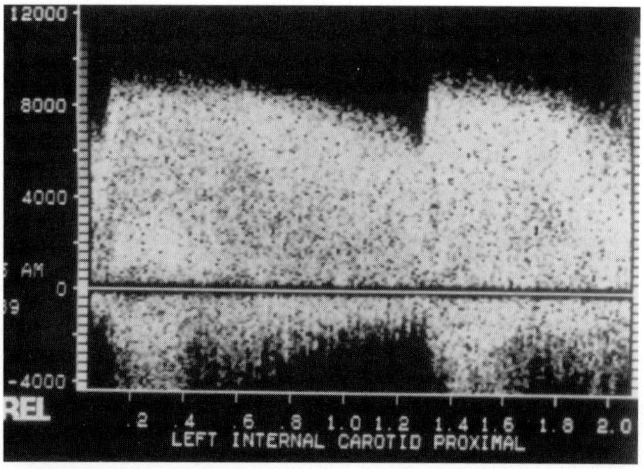

Figure 22-7
Doppler spectral display from a 75 to 95 percent carotid stenosis shows greatly increased systolic frequency shift, cutoff of peaks due to aliasing, spectral broadening, and turbulence, with very high diastolic frequency shift.

The most widely accepted method for measurement of angiographic stenosis is that used in both the ACAS and NASCET studies. This method compares the residual lumen at the narrowest point, with the vessel diameter measured distally, where the internal carotid artery has assumed a uniform diameter.[32] This measurement approach tends to underestimate stenosis relative to other measurement methods. There is a predictable relationship between diameter and area stenosis. For circular vessels with symmetrical stenosis, 50 percent diameter stenosis corresponds to 75 percent area stenosis, 70 percent diameter stenosis corresponds to 91 percent area stenosis, and 90 percent diameter stenosis corresponds to 99 percent area stenosis.[15] However, since severe carotid stenotic lesions are usually not circular or symmetrical, it is difficult to be certain of the most accurate diameter value. Most velocity criteria for ultrasound were developed using diameter stenosis, but ultrasound is actually assessing a hemodynamic parameter, regardless of the shape of the vessel or stenotic region. Thus, there is close correlation with methods that actually assess area stenosis. When used in a standard fashion, with an ongoing quality-assurance program and knowledge of the measurement and reporting methods, ultrasound is very accurate for identification of carotid stenosis and complements angiography.[5,12] Carotid ultrasonography should be considered the initial cerebrovascular test of choice for the study of patients with cerebral ischemia.[5,16,33,34]

B-MODE IMAGING

B-mode ("brightness-mode") imaging provides a two-dimensional gray scale image of the vascular structures and soft tissues based on the acoustic properties of the tissues. As a sound beam traverses the tissues, it is transmitted, bent, reflected, scattered, or absorbed as heat, based on the acoustic properties of the tissue, the interfaces between tissues, and the angle at which it strikes such interfaces.[19] The greater the magnitude of the difference in acoustic impedance between the adjacent tissues at an interface or boundary, the greater the reflection or scattering. Increased reflection or scattering results in the return of greater acoustic energy to the transducer. A digital memory encodes the signal intensity returning to the transducer at each point along the sound beam, displaying it as varying shades of gray. The more intense signals are displayed as brighter white, whereas absence of returning signal is displayed as black. A two-dimensional gray-scale image is created by mechanically or electronically sweeping a series of B-mode scan lines through a sector of the tissue in a single plane. These multiple scan lines are stored in the gray-scale memory and converted into a two-dimensional image (Fig. 22-8). Real-time B-mode imaging is achieved by updating the B-mode image 15 to 30 times each second, so fast that tissue appears to be moving in "real time." Such an image provides an anatomic assessment of the tissue based on the acoustic properties of the tissue being insonated.

Detail resolution is the ability of the ultrasound instrument to clearly distinguish two separate points. There are two aspects of detail resolution: axial and lateral resolution. Axial resolution, or the ability to identify separate points along the axis of the sound beam, is greatly dependent on transducer frequency. The higher the frequency, the better the axial resolution (the closer two points can be and still be clearly distinguished as separate points) and the better the details that can be displayed. Lateral resolution, or the ability to separate points in the direction perpendicular to the direction of the sound beam (across the scan lines), depends on the width and focusing of the sound beam. The narrower or better-focused the beam, the smaller the lateral resolution value and the better the ability to separate side-by-side points. Maximal resolution is certainly desirable to better visualize the vessel, atherosclerotic plaque, and the characteristics of carotid lesions. However, the higher the transducer frequency, the greater the attenuation (loss of acoustic energy as the sound moves through soft tissues), which causes decreased penetration to deeper structures. Lower-frequency transducers penetrate the tissue better, due to less attenuation, but have worse resolution. Thus, the best transducer for a specific task must be chosen based on both the required resolution capability and the depth of the structures to be studied. For carotid sonography, high-resolution B-mode imaging now implies transducer frequencies of 7.5 to 10 MHz.

B-mode imaging provides information regarding the soft tissue, the vessel wall, the vessel lumen, atherosclerotic plaque, and the pulsatile motion of the vessel wall or plaque. The residual lumen can be assessed by B-mode imaging in a longitudinal or an axial view of the vessel (Fig. 22-9), from which area stenosis can be

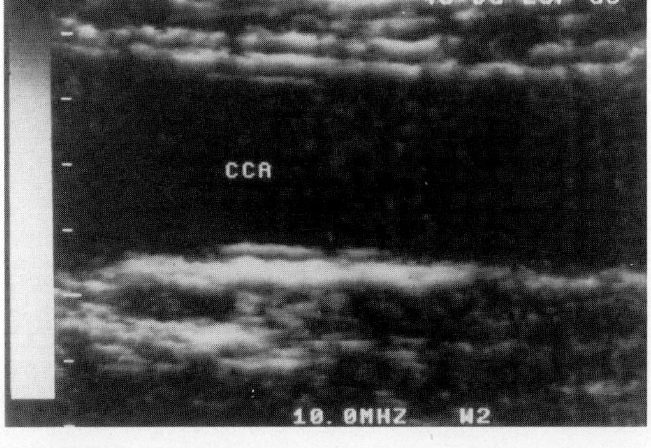

Figure 22-8
Gray-scale B-mode longitudinal image of the CCA.

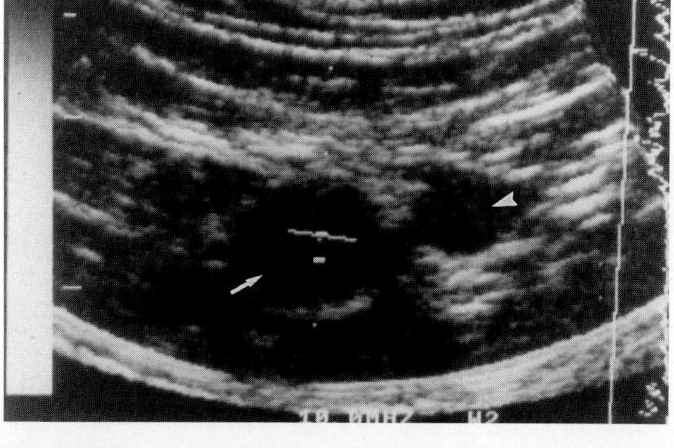

Figure 22-9
Gray-scale B-mode axial image of the internal (arrow) and external (arrowhead) carotid arteries.

evaluated. The earliest noninvasively measurable changes of the vessel wall caused by atherosclerosis may be thickening of the intima-media layers (IMT) of the arterial wall and increased stiffness of the vessel involved. Intima-media thickness can be accurately assessed to 0.1 to 0.3 mm.[35,36] The most reproducible parameter for IMT measurement is the mean difference of repeated measurements of the IMT of the common carotid artery segment using scanning from multiple planes. The median of the mean IMT values in defined segments of carotid arteries in a general population ranged between 0.5 and 1 mm at all ages, and less than 5 percent had mean IMT values exceeding 2 mm.[36] Normally, the vessel wall pulsates radially; however, longitudinal pulsation may occur in stiffened arteries with substantial hemodynamic impairment.

B-mode imaging has a unique ability to characterize specific plaque features in the carotid arteries. Plaque features routinely assessed include the distribution (e.g., concentric, eccentric, or length), surface features (e.g., smooth, irregular, or crater; Fig. 22-10), echodensity or calcification (Fig. 22-11), texture (e.g., homogenous, heterogenous, or intraplaque hemorrhage; Fig. 22-12), and the pulsation pattern (normal radial pattern, or longitudinal pattern). Longitudinal pulsation of the plaque suggests a possible increased risk of plaque rupture and thromboembolism. Surface features (craters or ulcers) have received the greatest attention. However, heterogeneity and echodensity now appear to be at least as important as surface features, especially early in the course of the disease process, for identifying high-risk plaques.

Plaques that are mostly homogenous and echogenic on B-mode imaging are primarily fibrous and represent more stable plaques, while plaques with prominent echolucent or anechoic regions (soft, dark, with lack of

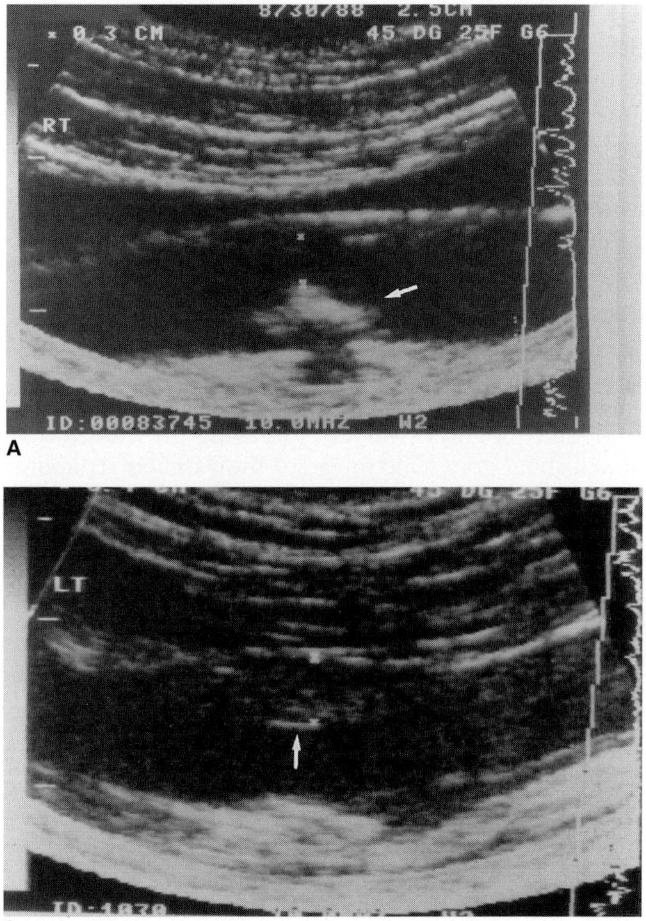

Figure 22-11
(A) *Calcified atherosclerotic carotid plaque with acoustic shadowing (arrow) seen on a longitudinal view by gray-scale B-mode imaging.* **(B)** *Hypoechoic, soft atherosclerotic plaque (arrow) seen on a longitudinal B-mode image of the ICA.*

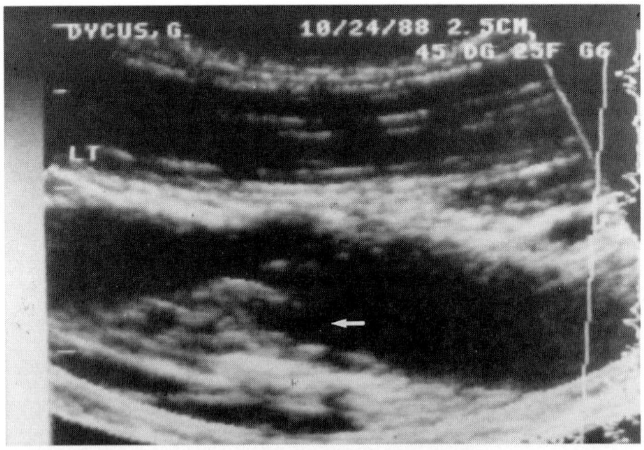

Figure 22-10
Gray-scale B-mode longitudinal image of an atherosclerotic plaque in the region of the carotid bifurcation. Note the crater on the proximal surface (arrow).

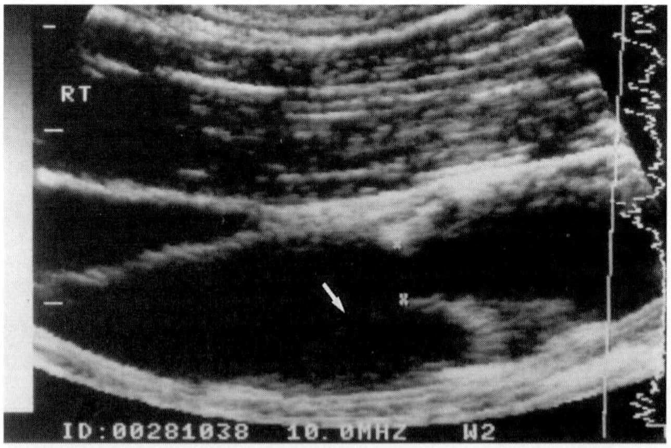

Figure 22-12
Hypoechoic region felt to represent intraplaque hemorrhage (arrow) in a carotid atherosclerotic plaque as seen on a longitudinal view by B-mode imaging.

echoes) are more likely to have high proportions of noncollagenized, noncalcified lipid material or intraplaque hemorrhage. Plaques that are heterogenous with marked surface abnormalities or possible intraplaque hemorrhage are often referred to as complex plaques. Heterogenous plaques and ulcerated plaques are considered to be unstable plaques with the possibility of causing cerebral or retinal ischemia.[37–40] Plaque features can be associated with identifiable risk factors. Echolucent carotid artery plaques are associated with elevated levels of triglyceride-rich lipoproteins in the fasting or postprandial state.[41] The sensitivity of B-mode imaging for detection of surface ulceration has been estimated at 77 percent in plaques of less than 50 percent linear stenosis and 41 percent for plaques of more than 50 percent linear stenosis, with no significant differences between B-mode carotid imaging and arteriography.[42] In the NASCET study, those patients with tight carotid stenosis randomized to the medical arm that had craters on angiography had worse outcomes than did those without craters. One author suggests that peak systolic velocity is significantly higher in patients with intraplaque hemorrhage, which may be one mechanism in causing cerebral ischemic symptoms.[43]

While most attention has focused on the hemodynamic aspects of carotid stenosis, plaque features should be considered in management decisions, especially in the setting of only moderate hemodynamic stenosis or recurrent symptoms. Ultrasonography currently provides the best opportunity to evaluate a variety of such plaque characteristics.[34] In addition, the use of new ultrasound techniques, such as densitometric analysis of carotid plaque composition[44] and 3-dimensional ultrasonography, to evaluate plaque volume[45] may add more information about plaque morphology and enable more precise study of the progression and regression of plaques following specific interventions.

DUPLEX ULTRASONOGRAPHY

Duplex ultrasonography is the combination of Doppler sonography and B-mode imaging within a single instrument and transducer, to allow visualization of high-resolution B-mode gray scale images of the vessels and simultaneous selective image-guided Doppler sampling (Fig. 22-13). This represents an advantage over using either modality separately, since the course of the vessel is also visualized and the angle of insonation can be determined, allowing more accurate calculation of blood flow velocity. Duplex sonography is now the standard method for carotid and vertebral sonography.

Carotid Artery Duplex Ultrasonography

The clinical indications for carotid duplex sonography may include known or suspected cerebral ischemia, evaluation of neck bruits (with or without symptoms), serial evaluation of known cerebrovascular disease, preoperative evaluation of patients with other types of vascular disease, postoperative follow-up after carotid endarterectomy, and assessment of pulsatile masses or other abnormal neck structures. Such methods are ideal to use as a safe and cost-effective screen for important carotid disease prior to the use of more expensive or potentially risky techniques such as angiography. When performed by trained sonographers using a standard protocol and with ongoing quality assurance, this method can approach 90 percent sensitivity and specificity for identification of important carotid stenosis[22–24,29]

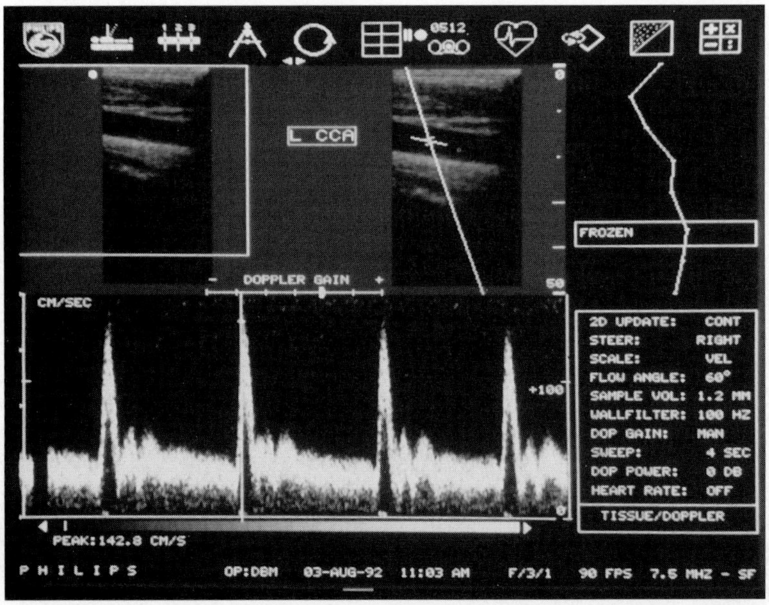

Figure 22-13

Carotid duplex sonography with B-mode image of the vessel to guide placement of the Doppler sample volume and to identify the angle of insonation relative to the direction of blood flow.

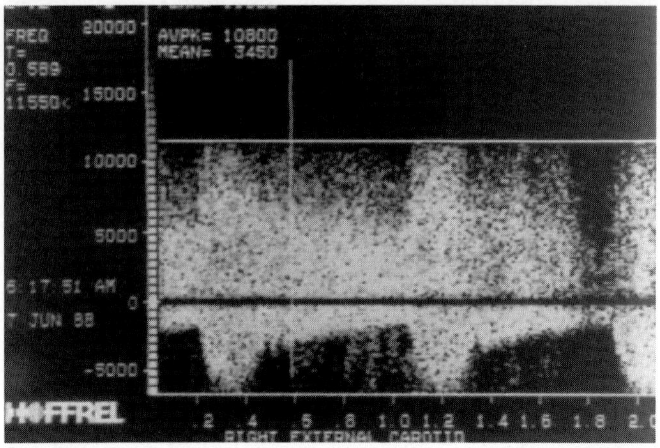

A

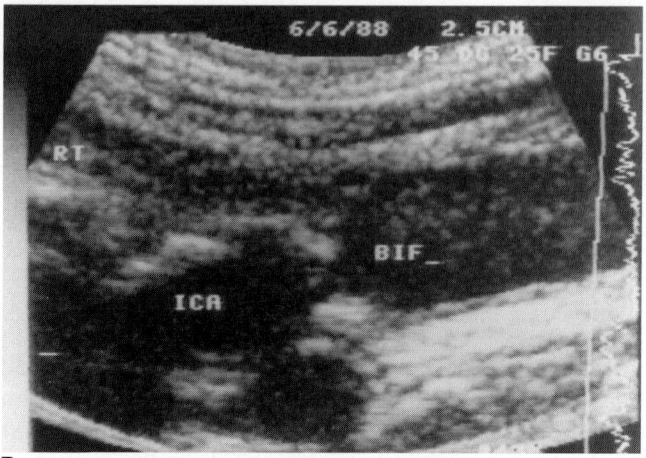

B

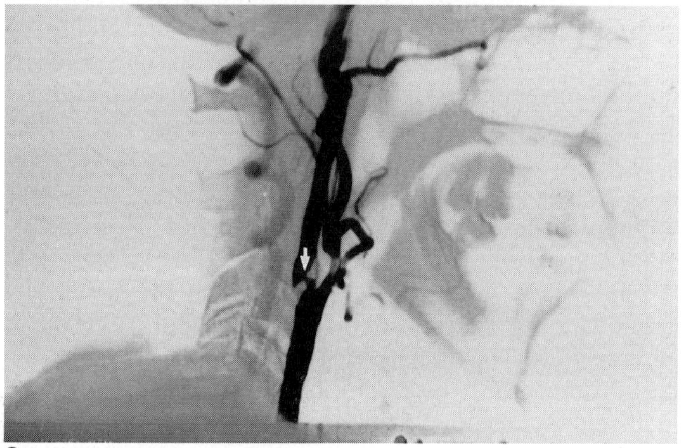

C

Figure 22-14

An elderly man presented with a right carotid transient ischemic attack. A carotid duplex examination identified a likely cause and helped to guide the additional workup and treatment. Abnormalities were seen on both Doppler and B-mode portions of the examination. **(A)** *Spectral Doppler display from the ICA shows very high frequency shift (velocity), both systolic and diastolic, with spectral broadening, suggesting a critical stenosis.* **(B)** *B-mode imaging reveals a complex plaque and apparent tight stenosis.* **(C)** *Cerebral angiography confirms a tight stenosis in the ICA (arrow).*

(Fig. 22-14A–C). The negative predictive value of the test is also high (95 percent).

The protocol for carotid duplex sonography varies among laboratories. However, certain components are crucial for an adequate examination, including examination of both carotids with Doppler velocity sampling of the proximal/mid and distal common carotid arteries (CCAs), the proximal and distal internal carotid artery (ICA), and the external carotid artery (ECA). If disease is detected, then additional Doppler sampling of the vessel proximal, at the point of, and distal to the stenosis should be included. B-mode real-time imaging of CCA, bifurcation (BIF), ICA, and ECA should include anterior, lateral, posterior, and transverse views or a circumferential scan at each level to include all of these views. Measurement of the plaque thickness and residual lumen in the CCA, BIF, ICA, and ECA are also performed. In our laboratory, we classify plaque severity (thickness) as minimal (1.1 to 2.0 mm), moderate (2.1 to 4.0 mm), or severe (greater than 4.0 mm). Carotid plaque and residual lumen are usually best measured in the posterolateral longitudinal view, since carotid plaque most often occurs on the posterior wall of the BIF and ICA, which are best visualized on a posterolateral view. This view also correlates best with the lateral view on carotid angiography. Color flow imaging and power Doppler are powerful additions to the interpretation of the studies (as discussed below). The potential limitations of carotid duplex sonography include a high carotid bifurcation, extremely deep vessels, or calcified plaques with acoustic shadowing, blocking the sound beam.

Vertebral Duplex Sonography

Cerebral ischemia in the posterior circulation is quite common. It is essential to evaluate the extracranial vertebral artery (VA) in routine carotid duplex sonography not only to detect locally abnormal flow in the VA, but also to detect hemodynamic changes due to proximal stenosis or occlusion, as can occur in the subclavian or innominate arteries. The VA can be insonated in the pretransverse and the intertransverse cervical segment C5–C6 in virtually all cases.[46] The VA origin can be imaged in 81 percent of cases on the right and in 65 percent of cases on the left.[46] The typical Doppler spectral pattern of the VA is a low pulsatile waveform, like that of the internal carotid artery (Fig. 22-15). The

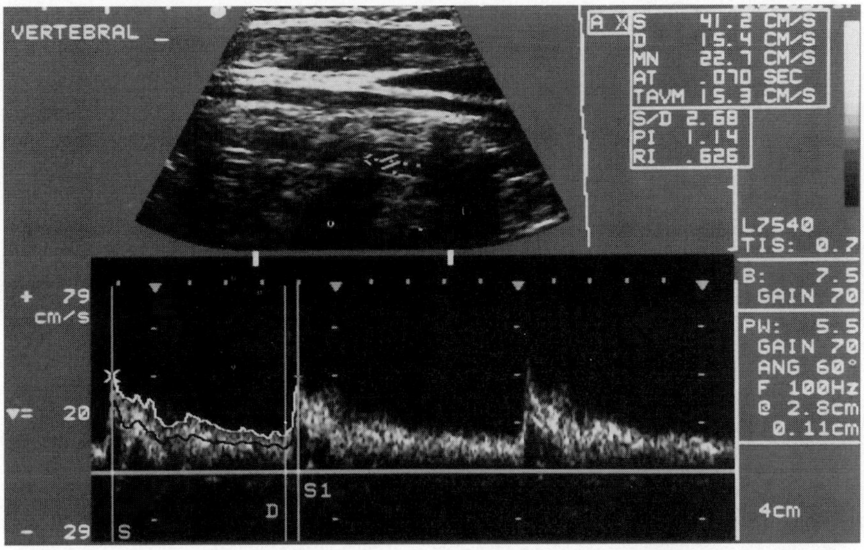

Figure 22-15
Duplex sonography of the normal VA.

average maximal systolic velocity is approximately 40 cm/s.[46] There are no accepted criteria for evaluation of extracranial VA stenosis. Vertebral duplex sonography is very useful in the evaluation of subclavian steal syndrome, which can be demonstrated by early systolic deceleration, alternating flow, or total reverse flow direction in the ipsilateral VA, depending on the stage of subclavian steal (Fig. 22-16). When combined with physiologic testing such as applying a blood pressure cuff or physical exercise of the arm, VA duplex sonography can help uncover or confirm steal phenomenon by revealing the change of the Doppler spectrum (Fig. 22-17). Monitoring of intracranial VA and basilar artery (BA) during this physiologic test can also help to identify patients with a true intracranial steal who may need vascular intervention.

COLOR FLOW IMAGING

Color flow imaging (CFI) provides color-coded flow velocity data based on both the speed and direction of flow and superimposes this information onto real-time gray-scale B-mode imaging.[47,48] Most CFI instruments obtain the flow velocity data by using Doppler methods and display a mean velocity value for particular points in the vessel. However, some instruments use time-domain processing based on the echoes contained in the B-mode image, with cross-correlation of echoes from adjacent scan lines, to detect and quantify flow velocity (color velocity imaging, or CVI). Such an approach allows color display of the instantaneous peak velocity and requires lower power levels than conventional Doppler color flow imaging approaches.[49]

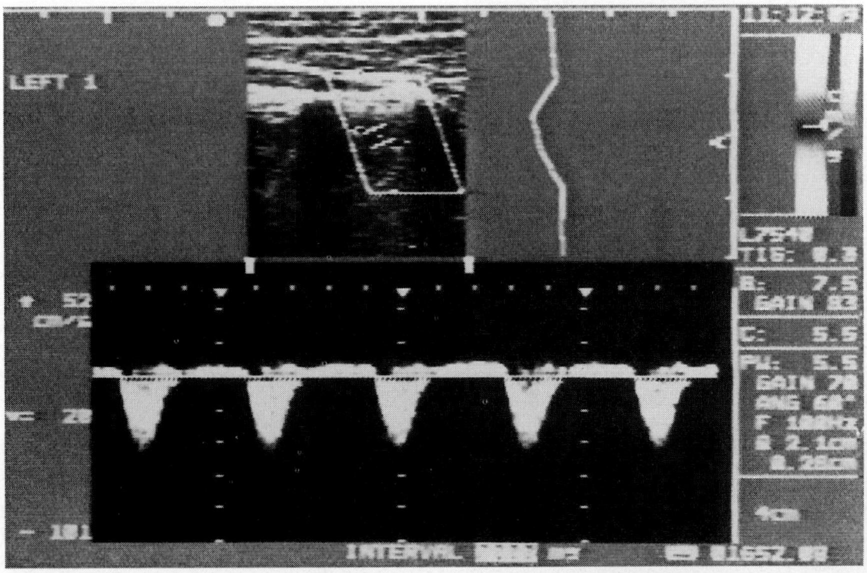

Figure 22-16
The VA duplex sonography shows alternating flow direction with reversal of flow in systole, suggesting an ipsilateral subclavian steal. (From CH Tegeler, D Ratanakorn, in M Fisher, J Bogousslavsky, eds: Textbook of Neurology: A Global Perspective, *Newton, MA, Butterworth-Heinemann, 1998. Used by permission.)*

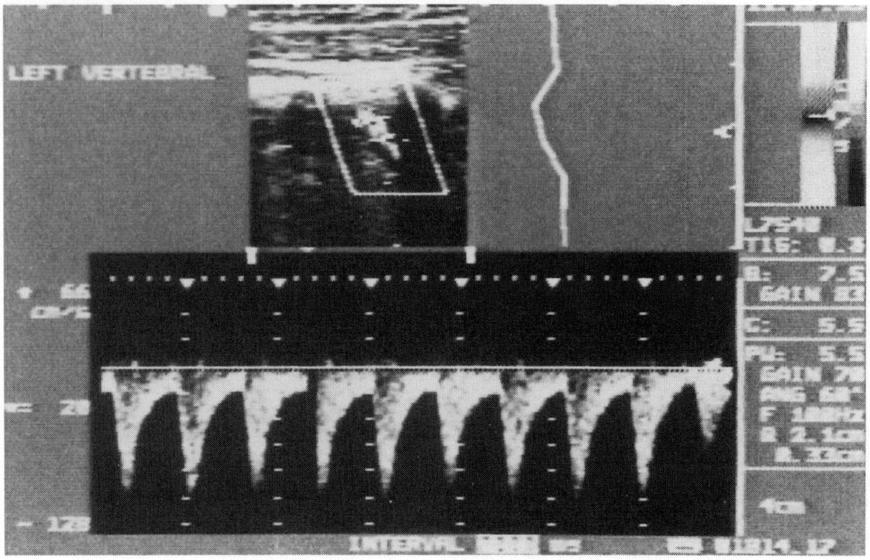

Figure 22-17
The same patient as shown in Fig. 22-16. After releasing a blood pressure cuff, the VA flow totally reverses and increases in velocity, suggesting more steal to the ipsilateral arm after physiologic testing.

Color flow imaging shows both anatomic and hemodynamic information simultaneously. However, the current color flow instruments cannot provide the same degree of quantitative hemodynamic data that duplex Doppler spectral analysis does. The use of CFI offers several potential advantages over gray-scale duplex sonography.[25,50,51] For example, CFI allows more rapid identification of the presence and direction of blood flow, and can serve as a road map to guide the placement of the sample volume for duplex Doppler velocity measurements, especially at the highest flow velocity jet in a stenotic area. Characterization of the surface of atherosclerotic plaques is improved with CFI. The presence or absence of color filling in an apparent "crater" suggests the presence of an open crater, as opposed to an intraplaque hemorrhage covered by a membrane (Fig. 22-18).[52] Similarly, a lack of flow, or "flow void," may identify a hypoechoic, soft plaque undetected by gray-scale B-mode imaging. Formerly a pitfall for gray-scale duplex sonography, critical stenosis that is near occlusion can be accurately identified by CFI (Fig. 22-19).[53] Such lesions, which create a "string sign" on angiography, were previously difficult to identify with certainty. Color flow imaging accurately differentiates between subtotal and total occlusion of the ICA with a sensitivity of 87 to 100 percent and a specificity of 84 percent, compared to conventional angiographic findings. Thus, angiography is necessary only when CFI findings are equivocal.[54–57] In addition, CFI can speed the examination and allows rapid understanding of many

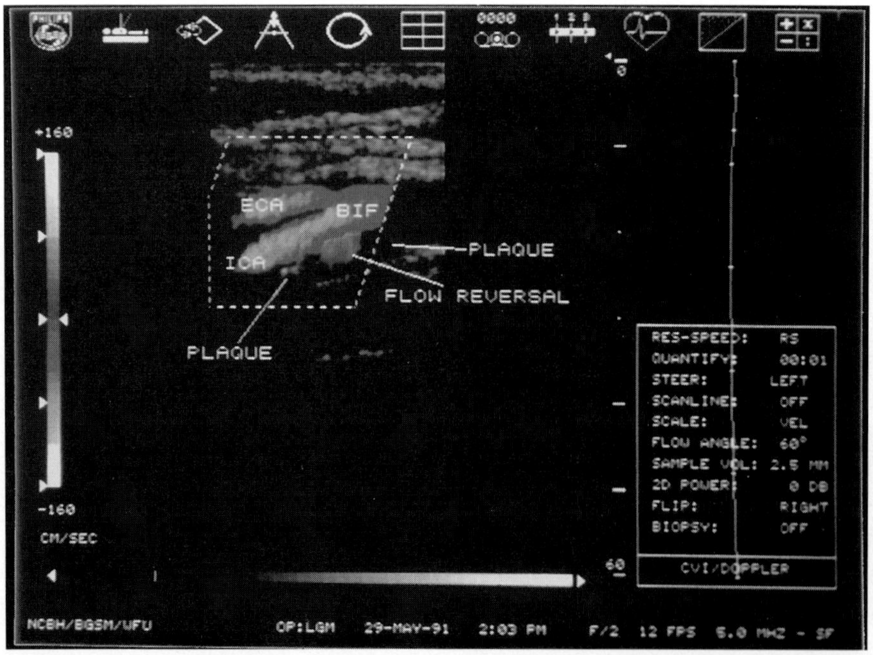

Figure 22-18 (Plate 39)
Color flow imaging with CVI demonstrating reversed flow in a crater on the surface of an atherosclerotic carotid plaque, confirming communication with the lumen, as opposed to an intraplaque hemorrhage with a membrane covering it.

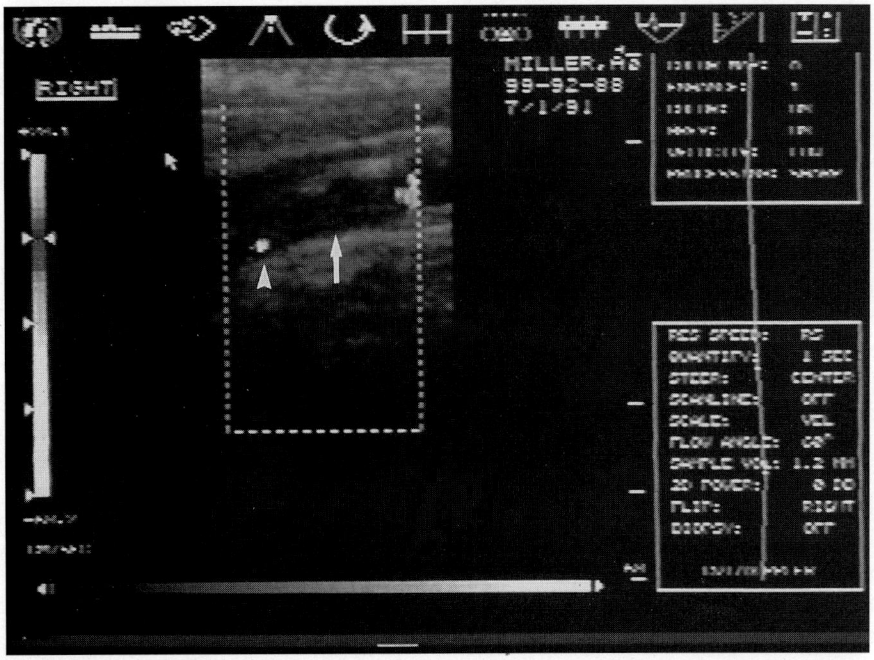

A

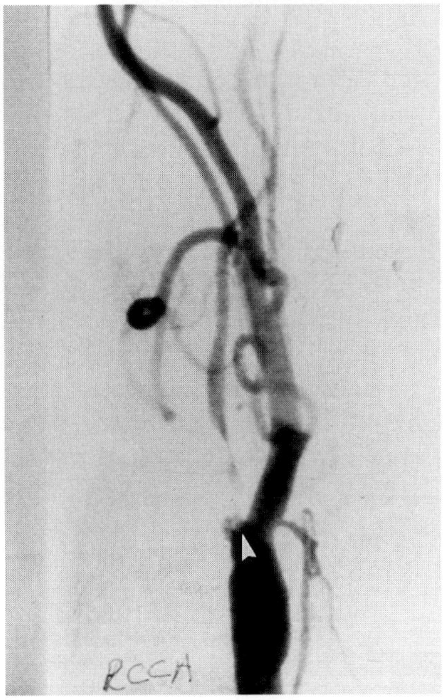

B

Figure 22-19 (Plate 40)
(A) *String or trickle of flow through a critical carotid stenosis (arrow), identified by color flow imaging distally (arrowhead).* **(B)** *Cerebral angiogram showing a string sign in the internal carotid artery (arrowhead).*

anomalous anatomic patterns, such as kinks or coils in the vessel (Fig. 22-20). Also, CFI is useful in identifying carotid dissection, carotid body tumors, and flow distal to a common carotid artery occlusion and in evaluating the vertebral arteries.[57–60] The addition of CFI probably adds about 5 percent to the overall diagnostic accuracy of the examination. Color flow duplex instruments with spectral Doppler duplex capability, rather than gray-scale duplex Doppler alone, are now used in most laboratories as the standard of practice.

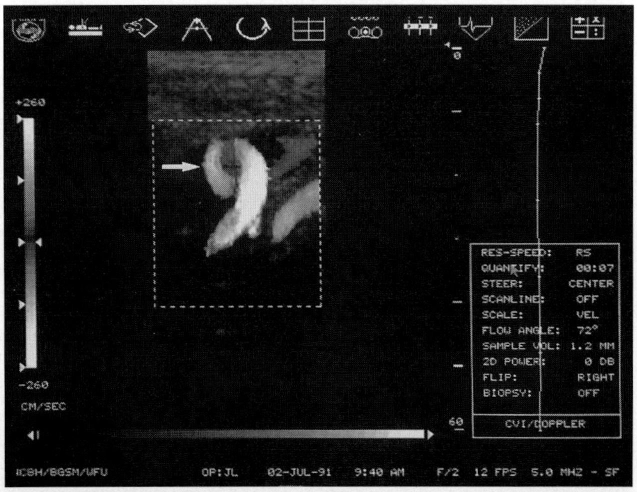

Figure 22-20 (Plate 41)
Complete coil in the ICA (arrow) as seen by color flow imaging. The diagnosis was not clear on gray-scale duplex imaging alone.

POWER DOPPLER IMAGING

Power Doppler imaging (PDI) is a Doppler technique that encodes an estimate of the integrated amplitude intensity of the Doppler spectrum in color rather than an estimate of the mean Doppler frequency shift, which is the parameter typically used in standard CFI.[61] The values encoded in the color display in PDI are a function of the amount of detectable blood flow at the point of insonation.[62] The advantages of PDI over CFI are its relative angle independence, no aliasing, and increased usable dynamic range of the ultrasound instrument, providing increased machine sensitivity to demonstrate flow by compensation for attenuation of the Doppler signal.[61,62] Thus, PDI is useful in detection of blood flow with nearly perpendicular angles of insonation and very low flow velocity. However, since PDI does not currently provide the direction or velocity of flow, it is still used in combination with CFI. Compared to CFI, PDI appears to more frequently and accurately identify stenosis, including measurement of the residual lumen in high-grade stenosis, as well as offering better differentiation of plaque surface morphology, largely free of artifacts such as shadowing, and better visualization of orbital vessels, intracranial aneurysms, and basal intracranial arteries.[63–68]

VOLUME FLOW RATE DETERMINATION

Most criteria for grading carotid stenosis are based on the flow velocity and percent stenosis. However, increased flow velocity in the extracranial carotid arteries may be due to other nonstenotic causes, such as a hypermetabolic state, collateral flow contralateral to high-grade carotid stenosis or occlusion, post–carotid endarterectomy hyperperfusion syndrome due to impaired intracerebral autoregulation, hyperemia due to treatment for subarachnoid hemorrhage, or intracranial arteriovenous malformation. Therefore, the identification of the volume flow rate (VFR) to the brain may be useful in these circumstances. There has previously been no method of noninvasively determining the ultimate cerebral hemodynamic parameter, VFR. Doppler methods have had difficulty in providing the instantaneous peak velocity across the entire vessel and in tracking changes in the flow lumen throughout the cardiac cycle. Color velocity imaging, a time-domain method of determining flow velocity, has already been described. Modifications of this technique now allow determination of the VFR (CVI quantification, or CVI-Q). An M-mode color display allows instantaneous assessment of the flow lumen and the velocity over time (Fig. 22-21). Assuming a circular vessel, these data can be integrated to derive the VFR. This method is valid and reliable in vitro, using a computer-controlled flow phantom.[69] With proper training and technique, CVI-Q has also been performed in volunteers. Using this technique, the VFR in the CCA in normal volunteers is 330 ± 60 mL/min for women and 375 ± 70 mL/min for men. In addition, VFR appears useful for grading carotid stenosis and evaluating cerebrovascular reserve in the internal carotid artery as well as for identifying feeders and for follow-up studies in intracranial arteriovenous malformation, quantification of hemodynamic changes in patients with subclavian steal phenomenon, and assessment of vasospasm in the patients with subarachnoid hemorrhage.[70,71] In addition, there is a correlation between the increase in the middle cerebral artery (MCA) mean flow velocity (Vm) and VFR of the CCA after CO_2 inhalation, allowing the evaluation of cerebral vasoreactivity in patients with inadequate acoustic temporal windows for transcranial Doppler sonography. The MCA Vm and the CCA VFR increase 6.1 and 5.3 percent per mmHg increase in end-expiratory CO_2, respectively, and MCA Vm increases 0.3 cm/s for each 1 mL/min increase in CCA VFR.[72] The CCA is quite accessible and reliable, but it is more difficult to obtain reliable

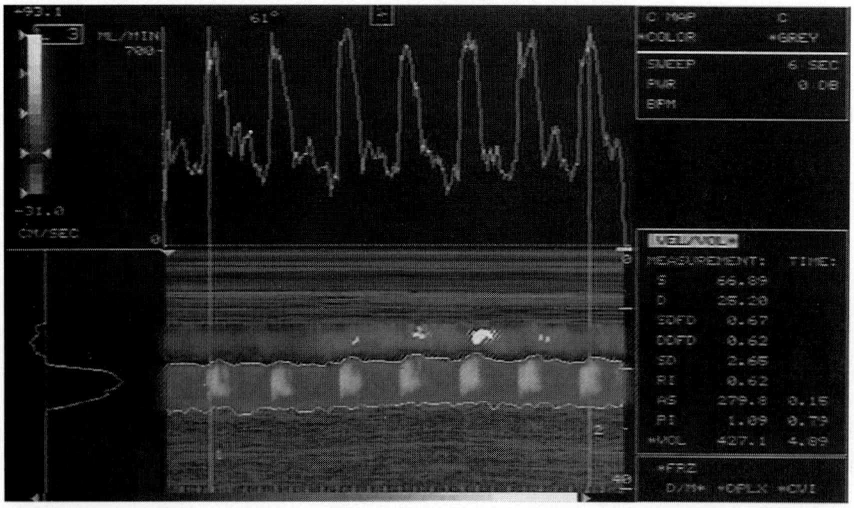

Figure 22-21 (Plate 42)
Display of the M-mode color format and volume flow rate calculation in the CCA obtained with color velocity imaging quantification.

data in the internal carotid arteries or vertebral arteries, owing to depth of the vessel, the angle of insonation, and the size of the vessels. The MCA VFR measured by this technique has been reported in normal subjects as a mean VFR of 139 ± 31 mL/min in the right and 173 ± 46 mL/min in the left.[73] This method has yet to be validated for the evaluation of intracranial hemodynamics.

TRANSCRANIAL DOPPLER SONOGRAPHY

The bony skull had long been considered an insurmountable obstacle to the use of ultrasound as a diagnostic tool to study the brain and its vasculature. This limitation of the acoustic properties of the skull is due to the marked attenuation of ultrasound energy by the skull. The classic paper by Dr. Rune Aaslid and colleagues, published in 1982,[74] reported the ability to use low-frequency (2 MHz) p-w Doppler sonography to noninvasively obtain flow velocity data from the basal cerebral arteries. Since then, this method has been widely used to study intracranial hemodynamic changes in a variety of clinical settings, especially in patients with stroke and cerebrovascular diseases. There are three standard acoustic windows for transcranial Doppler sonography (TCD): (1) the temporal acoustic window via the thin portion of temporal bone to study the middle, anterior, and posterior cerebral arteries, (2) the suboccipital acoustic window via the foramen magnum to study the vertebral and basilar arteries, and (3) the transorbital acoustic window via the optic foramen to study the ophthalmic artery and the ICA siphon. This method opens a new window to the understanding of cerebral hemodynamics.

In order to assess flow velocity and, in the absence of an image, to define the course of the vessels and allow correction for the angle of insonation, the conventional, or "blind," TCD method uses a 2-MHz p-w Doppler transducer and assumes a 0° angle of insonation for calculation of flow velocity. Identification of basal cerebral arteries is based on the direction of flow, the depth of the Doppler sample gate, the direction of the transducer, the flow velocity, and the characteristics of the Doppler spectral pattern. The criteria for normal TCD data are shown in Table 22-2.[75–77]

Clinical evaluation of the middle cerebral (MCA-M1 segment), anterior cerebral (ACA-A1 segment), and posterior cerebral arteries (PCA-P1 segment) is performed through the temporal acoustic window, which is located above the zygomatic arch, anterior to the ear. The MCA-M2, ACA-A2, and PCA-P2 segments are rarely identified because of the nearly 90° angle of insonation. The anterior and posterior communicating arteries are usually clearly identified only when they are functioning as collateral channels. Otherwise, the flow in these vessels is too low to detect. Insonation through the temporal window can also provide information on the contralateral MCA, ACA, and PCA in individuals with good acoustic temporal windows. Inadequate or absent temporal acoustic windows occur in approximately 15 percent of the population, especially in nonwhite women over 60 years of age,[78] which can limit the clinical use of this technique. The MCA signal, with flow toward the transducer, is first identified at a depth of between 45 and 60 mm. The vessel is then followed deeper, in increments of 5 mm or less, to define the maximal velocity for the MCA segment. The vessel is then followed deeper to the point of the bifurcation of MCA and ACA at a depth of about 65 mm, with flow away from the transducer in the ACA (Fig. 22-22). The

Table 22-2
Depth, velocity, and flow direction criteria and normal values for transcranial Doppler sonography of the basal cerebral arteries at Wake Forest University Baptist Medical Center

Artery	*Depth, mm*	*Mean velocity, cm/s*	*Flow direction from ipsilateral approach*
Middle cerebral	50–55	40–80	Toward
Anterior cerebral	65–70	35–60	Away
Posterior cerebral	60–65	30–55	Toward
Ophthalmic	40–55	15–30	Toward
ICA siphon	65–75	40–70	Variable
Vertebral	60–75	25–50	Away
Basilar	85–90	25–60	Away

Note: mean velocity is the time-averaged mean maximal velocity.
Abbreviation: ICA, internal carotid artery.

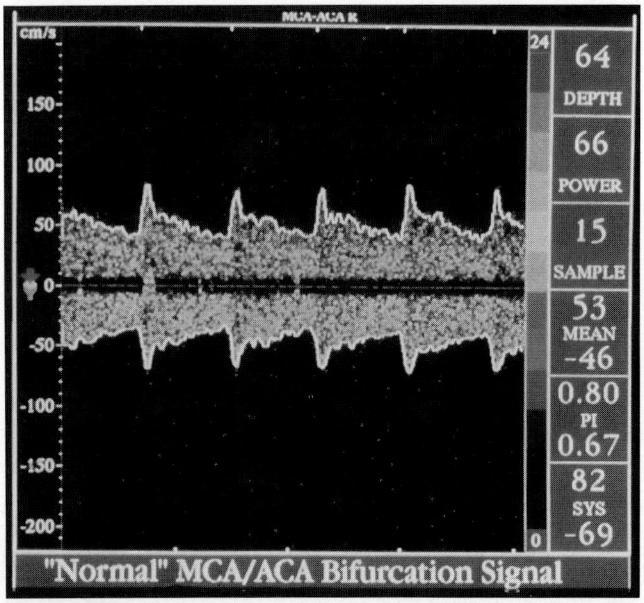

Figure 22-22
Transcranial Doppler spectrum obtained from the region of the bifurcation of the MCA and ACA at a depth of 64 mm.

ACA is followed deeper, and the maximal velocity is identified. The MCA/ACA bifurcation is again identified, and the transducer is pointed more inferoposteriorly to identify the PCA, usually with flow toward the transducer. The vessel is followed both deeper and more superficially until the maximal velocity is identified. Both the ACA and the PCA can often be followed deeply enough to identify the opposite ACA (flow toward the transducer) or PCA (flow away from the transducer), and the depth and position can be further adjusted to identify the opposite MCA (flow away from the transducer). The depth of the midline and contralateral MCA/ACA bifurcation are usually at 75 and 85 mm, respectively.

The vertebral and basilar arteries are studied by positioning the transducer over the suboccipital region in the midline or just lateral to the cervical paraspinal muscles, aiming the transducer superiorly, and searching for the VA signal (flow away from the transducer) at a depth of 45 to 75 mm. The head of the patient should be flexed to open the space between the atlas and the axis. When one VA is identified, the sample volume is moved to follow the vessel deeper in order to locate the basilar artery (flow away from the transducer at a depth of 75 to 120 mm). The right and left VA can be distinguished by angling the transducer to the right or left from the midline, or by approaching from the lateral position, as described above. The Doppler spectral velocity data are evaluated to identify the maximal velocity in each segment. Tortuosity of vessels is a frequent cause of technical difficulty in the suboccipital approach. The most common "normal" cause of apparent reversed flow in the region of the distal VA is mistaken insonation of the posterior inferior cerebellar artery, which actually flows toward the transducer at its takeoff at the depth of 75 mm. However, the signal usually cannot be followed proximally and distally.

Evaluation of the ophthalmic artery and ICA siphon requires reduction of Doppler power to 10 percent of maximal to avoid potential bioeffects on the lens and retina. The patient closes the eyelids, the ultrasound gel is applied to the closed lid, and the transducer is positioned over the superior lateral portion of the globe. Both the reduced power and the positioning help to avoid potential adverse effects, particularly on the lens. The transducer is pointed toward the optic foramen, and the normal ophthalmic artery is identified by flow toward the transducer at depths of 40 to 55 mm. The depth is increased to 55 to 70 mm to identify the Doppler signal from the distal ICA siphon, which may have flow toward or away from the transducer, depending on which portion is sampled. The transducer should not be directed too far medially, since this may result in the inadvertent sampling of the contralateral ACA instead of the ipsilateral carotid siphon.

Transcranial Doppler sonography is an operator-dependent procedure, especially using the conventional, or blind, TCD technique. It is crucial that the operators correctly identify the arteries being studied, accurately record flow velocities, and use the correct techniques, such as a small sample volume and optimal gain settings, which can help to avoid spectral mirror image artifact, a potential cause of erroneous interpretation of flow velocity data.[79] Interpretation of TCD results hinges primarily on flow velocity.[80–82] Most criteria have been based on time-averaged, mean-maximum velocity readings rather than the peak systolic velocity, as used in the extracranial circulation. Interpretation of TCD data requires consideration of variables that can affect the flow velocity values, such as age, arterial blood pressure, cardiac function, metabolic state, blood viscosity, P_{CO_2}, P_{O_2}, intracranial pressure, and drugs. Many pathologic conditions, such as intracranial atherosclerosis, intracranial dissection, vasospasm, or cerebral embolism, can cause vascular narrowing, resulting in increased flow velocities. However, physiologically increased flow velocities may be seen in young patients or may be associated with anemia, severely increased arterial blood pressure, hypermetabolic states such as hyperthyroidism, increased P_{CO_2}, or administrations of drugs such as acetazolamide.[83–86] Often, there are accompanying turbulence and disturbed flow, which help distinguish pathologic changes from normal or physiologically high-velocity variants. Decreased flow velocities may be due to an inadequate acoustic window or a poor angle of insonation but can also be seen with more proximal or extracranial stenosis or occlusion, poor cardiac function, poor distal cerebral blood flow, or a marked increase in intracranial pressure. Absence of a Doppler signal from a specific arterial segment in the presence of an adequate acoustic temporal window and technique, as evidenced by identification of other intracranial arterial segments, suggests occlusion of that arterial segment.

When interpreting flow velocity data, the velocities in all vessels insonated should be compared to identify both side-to-side differences and mean flow velocities in each vessel. Some have suggested that side-to-side differences in velocity for the MCA or ICA that exceed 14 percent be considered abnormal, with limits for side-to-side differences in velocity for the ACA and PCA being 24 and 34 percent, respectively.[87] Many would place the cutoff point for MCA side-to-side difference at a higher value (50 percent).

The spectral pattern might also suggest a diagnosis, as with the relatively high diastolic flow velocity due to the decreased distal resistance that accompanies arteriovenous malformations. A spectral pattern with very slow systolic flow acceleration (flattening of the systolic up slope) suggests significant proximal stenosis or occlusion.[88] A very high resistance pattern with no diastolic forward flow or even reversed diastolic flow, suggests increased intracranial pressure or even the lack of cerebral flow, as in cerebral circulatory arrest (brain death). However, the spectral pattern should be interpreted by comparing it with the other vessels studied, just as when interpreting flow velocity data. The direction of flow is also important, since reversal of flow may suggest collateralization.

The established clinical indications for TCD currently include the study of patients with known or suspected intracranial stenosis or occlusion, the assessment of collateral flow or hemodynamics in patients with intra- or extracranial stenosis or occlusion, the evaluation for vasospasm or vasoconstriction, especially following subarachnoid hemorrhage, the identification of arteriovenous malformations, and the evaluation of potential brain death.[89] Other applications of TCD include the measurement of cerebrovascular reserve, perioperative and periprocedural monitoring, evaluation of blood flow changes during tilt table testing, detection of the right-to-left intra- or extracardiac shunting, and study of cerebral blood flow in other conditions, such as migraine, epilepsy, meningitis, cerebral venous thrombosis, and sleep. In addition, TCD has been reported for use in assessment of cerebral blood flow changes induced by focal brain activation, defined as functional TCD, and evaluation of cerebral circulation in pilots and in astronauts.[90]

The TCD technique is safe, noninvasive, and reproducible, with no significant variations between the sides or between studies on different days, in normal subjects.[91] Thus, TCD can be performed repeatedly at frequent intervals to follow the evolution of processes causing abnormal cerebral hemodynamics. This aspect is particularly important in the setting of subarachnoid hemorrhage. Secondary development of vasospasm and its accompanying ischemic events are a major cause of mortality and morbidity after subarachnoid hemorrhage. By following flow velocities with TCD every few days, vasospasm can be detected early, prior to the onset of clinical ischemic symptoms, and patients at highest risk for complication can be identified so that preventive measures can be instituted without having to subject potentially unstable patients to multiple cerebral angiograms[92,93] (Table 22-3).

The TCD method has a unique ability to assess flow velocity changes in real time and to monitor such data for extended periods of time. Thus, there is an opportunity to perform a variety of maneuvers or apply physiologic stressors to assess cerebral hemodynamics. The simplest example is compression of the proximal CCA during TCD monitoring. The resulting distal hemodynamic changes can help to confirm the identity of the vessel being studied and/or assess the potential for collateral flow, which may help to determine whether it is likely that a shunt will be needed during carotid endarterectomy.[92] However, such compression maneuvers might precipitate embolization from friable carotid ulcerated plaques; therefore, compression is not usually performed in patients with recent neurologic symptoms.[93]

Table 22-3
Criteria for transcranial Doppler sonography in the diagnosis of MCA vasospasm in patients with subarachnoid hemorrhage at Wake Forest University Baptist Medical Center

Severity	*Mean velocity, cm/s*	*MCA/x-ICA*
Normal	<85	<3
Mild	<120	<3
Moderate	120–150	3–5
Severe	151–200	>6
Critical	>200	>6

Note: mean velocity is the time-averaged mean maximum velocity.
Abbreviations: MCA, middle cerebral artery; x-ICA, distal extracranial internal carotid artery by submandibular approach; MCA/x-ICA, ratio of these velocities.

Inhalation of a mixture of 5% CO_2 or intravenous injection of acetazolamide will dilate the intracerebral arterioles without changing the diameter of the large basal cerebral conduit arteries, such as the MCA. This should cause increased flow through the MCA (higher velocities), allowing evaluation of the cerebral vasoreactivity and cerebrovascular reserve.[94–97] The MCA flow velocity increases by as much as 52.5 percent during hypercapnia.[94] When 1000 mg of acetazolamide is given intravenously, MCA flow velocity reaches a plateau approximately 35 percent higher than baseline within 10 min and lasts more than 30 min before gradually decreasing.[95] Cerebral vasoreactivity testing can also be performed quite simply by having patients hold their breath or hyperventilate.[98,99]

The TCD method for evaluating cerebrovascular reactivity has been widely used in many clinical settings, especially in patients with severe stenosis or occlusion of the extracranial carotid arteries. In such patients, the brain vessels may already be maximally autoregulated (dilated) just to maintain adequate flow at rest. In this setting, an absent or impaired cerebral vasoreactivity suggests increased risk from any event that would compromise blood flow to that hemisphere. Such information may assist with management decisions regarding surgical intervention, such as extracranial to intracranial bypass surgery, carotid endarterectomy, or other revascularization techniques, as well as identify optimal target values for arterial blood pressure control to avoid hypoperfusion.

Other provocative tests can be done during TCD. Monitoring during changes in body position on a tilt table may help confirm poor cerebral perfusion as a cause of dizziness or syncope. In some patients, rotation of the head and neck may provoke symptoms of vertebrobasilar insufficiency, and TCD monitoring of the basilar artery flow velocity in these patients, correlated with clinical symptoms, offers a useful screening method for identifying patients with true position-related vertebrobasilar insufficiency. A reduction of basilar artery flow velocity during head turning of more than 20 percent from baseline is considered to be significantly abnormal. However, symptoms typically appear only in those whose basilar artery flow velocities drop more than 30 percent, followed by reactive hyperemia after the head returns to a neutral position.[100]

Embolus Detection

Transcranial Doppler ultrasonography can identify embolic signals in a variety of clinical settings. Cerebral embolization has been identified using TCD in patients with severe extracranial carotid stenosis, intracranial stenosis, and vertebrobasilar ischemia. It has also been used for detection of right-to-left shunting with air contrast injections, to identify cerebral emboli in patients with prosthetic heart valves, and during a variety of procedures, including carotid endarterectomy, cerebral angiography, carotid angioplasty, and cardiopulmonary bypass heart surgery. Identification of cerebral emboli has also been reported as a method of evaluating the effect of changes in anticoagulant treatment.[101–111] It is suggested that the presence of embolic signals at the time of ischemic stroke correlates with a greater risk of subsequent stroke, transient ischemic attack, or death.[112,113]

Such identification is possible because embolic material has a different acoustic impedance, or reflectivity, from that of the surrounding blood. As an embolic fragment passes through a Doppler beam, the higher acoustic impedance causes greater scattering of the Doppler energy than that caused by the surrounding red blood cells, with a more intense Doppler signal returning to the transducer. This "embolic signal" causes an audible pop or chirp, and appears as a transient high-intensity region within the Doppler spectral display (Fig. 22-23).

Very specific criteria have been developed to help define embolic signals. In vitro and in vivo data suggest a high sensitivity (greater than 90 percent) and excellent specificity (95 to 99 percent).[114–116] A new technique utilizing multigated Doppler ultrasound is now being used for TCD and embolus detection, and appears to have great promise as a way of differentiating true embolic signals from artifacts.[117] The use of various parameters, such as decibel threshold, velocity, duration, amplitude, and power increase of embolic signals, might enable discrimination among various embolic materials, which will be useful for selecting specific treatments for individual patients.[118] It appears to be possible to distinguish gaseous from solid embolic material in vitro and in vivo. The clear differentiation between sizes and types of solid embolic material remains problematic, particularly in clinical settings. The opportunity to perform embolus detection in patients with stroke may increase understanding of stroke mechanisms in general, while in specific patients it may help localize the embolic source, identify patients with higher risk even before a stroke, or provide a more objective way of evaluating the effect of preventive therapies. Embolus detection may become a standard part of the cerebrovascular examination.

TRANSCRANIAL COLOR FLOW IMAGING

Transcranial color flow imaging (TCCI) uses low-frequency transducers to obtain adequate penetration of the skull and enables simultaneous visualization of brain

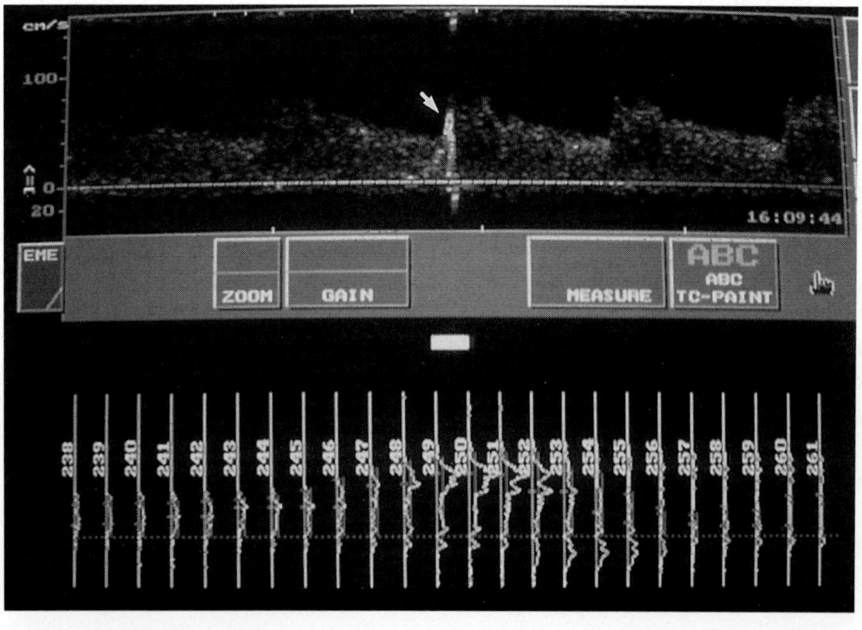

Figure 22-23 (Plate 43)
The MCA spectral waveform with an embolic signal (arrow).

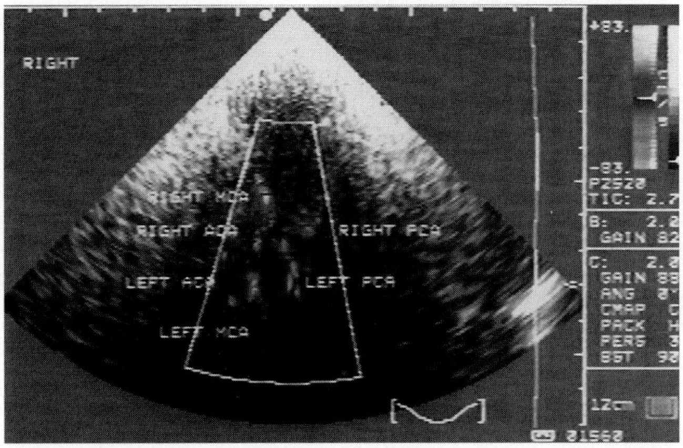

Figure 22-24 (Plate 44)
Transcranial color flow imaging of the basal cerebral arteries.

parenchyma (B-mode imaging) and blood flow in the basal cerebral arteries by color coding the flow velocity data (color duplex), as previously described for CFI in the extracranial vessels[119–121] (Fig. 22-24). The use of TCCI offers a number of potential advantages, compared with conventional TCD, including more rapid recognition of the acoustic window, more accurate identification of vessels, visually guided placement of the sample gate for spectral Doppler evaluation, visualization of multiple vessels simultaneously, and possibly improved understanding of collateral flow. Visualization of the course of the vessel also allows determination of the angle of insonation (rather than assuming a 0° angle); thus, angle-corrected flow velocities can be obtained.[122–124] Angle-corrected intracranial flow velocities are approximately 10 to 15 percent higher than uncorrected values in all the vessels insonated,[122] being 15 percent higher in the MCA, 18 percent in the ACA, 30 percent in the PCA, and 3 percent in the BA.[123] Overall, angle-corrected velocities are about 25 percent higher in about one-fourth of the vessels studied.[124] Nevertheless, current TCD velocity criteria are based on conventional TCD, using uncorrected velocity values. Thus, further studies are needed before angle-corrected values can be widely applied, in order to develop new criteria and to assess the clinical impact of using the higher, angle-corrected velocities.

In addition, TCCI may also allow noninvasive, bedside, ultrasonic "angiography" of the basal cerebral vessels that could be easily repeated after changes in the clinical picture or therapeutic interventions (e.g., thrombolytic therapy, balloon angioplasty, or embolization of arteriovenous malformation). In addition, TCCI may provide rapid and reliable data about various stroke subtypes and mechanisms immediately after onset.[125,126] The positive and negative predictive values of a pathologic flow pattern in patients with MCA infarctions or transient ischemic attacks are reported as 0.92 and 0.48, respectively, while those of a pathologic parenchymal echo pattern are 0.88 and 0.96, respectively.[125] While TCCI will not replace high-resolution imaging such as computed tomography or magnetic resonance imaging for the study of cerebral parenchymal lesions, it may be useful as a follow-up study. The potential for adding ultrasound contrast agents and three-dimensional ultrasonography could add greatly to the clinical utility of TCCI (as discussed below).

Power Doppler imaging has been successfully combined with TCCI. When compared to TCCI using the traditional flow velocity–encoded color, power Doppler TCCI has a more favorable signal-to-noise ratio and is relatively independent of angle and aliasing, allowing significant advantages in imaging small-caliber and low-flow arteries as well as those that run at unfavorable angles to the ultrasound beam.[127] Power Doppler TCCI offers better visualization of the M2 portion of MCA, the A2 portion of the ACA, and the P2 portion of the posterior cerebral artery (PCA)[8], as well as the anterior and posterior communicating arteries.

NEW DIRECTIONS IN NEUROSONOLOGY

Three-Dimensional Ultrasonography

Three-dimensional ultrasound images can now be reconstructed from a series of conventional two-dimensional ultrasound images obtained with either B-mode imaging alone, CFI, or power Doppler imaging. All three-dimensional techniques first require the acquisition of two-dimensional ultrasound data, which is stored in a computer and reconstructed into a three-dimensional format by off-line analysis from the stored data. It is imperative that the acquisition geometry be encoded to allow accurate three-dimensional reconstructions and to avoid distortions or artifacts. The three-dimensional ultrasound images are tomographically acquired at a high rate of 10 to 60 images per second, and the acquisitions can be triggered at appropriate phases of the electrocardiogram.[128] A new sensor-magnetic system, as opposed to earlier systems with mechanical arms, offers free-hand scanning, which promises to greatly increase the applicability and usefulness of three-dimensional sonography.[129]

Progression and regression of carotid plaques can be measured by conventional two-dimensional B-mode ultrasonography. However, three-dimensional ultrasound imaging may increase the reproducibility and precision of parameters such as plaque volume measurements, with reported intraexaminer variability between 2.8 and 4.1 percent, interexaminer variability between 4.2 and 7.6 percent, and follow-up measurement variability between 5.2 and 9.4 percent.[130] Atherosclerotic carotid plaques are also more precisely differentiated using three-dimensional power Doppler ultrasound, and plaque volume quantification is less affected by echo shadowing after three-dimensional reconstruction.[131] In addition, three-dimensional ultrasound facilitates imaging of intracranial vascular anatomy by clarifying spatial relationships and avoiding section artifact, as compared to two-dimensional ultrasound methods.[132]

Echo-Enhanced Ultrasound Imaging

Echo enhancement (ultrasound contrast) was first observed as an increase in ultrasound signal intensity after rapid intravenous injections of saline solution by Gramiak and Shah in 1968.[133] The mechanism of this echogenic effect is due to microscopic air bubbles that efficiently scatter ultrasound energy in all directions. Some of this energy is scattered back to the transducer, boosting the intensity of the signal from the blood.[134] For use in the arterial vessels, the echo-enhancing microbubbles should be sufficiently small (usually 2 to 10 μm in diameter) to cross the pulmonary capillary bed, should be stable enough to survive the cardiopulmonary circulation and to enhance the entire blood pool, and should resonate at diagnostic ultrasound frequencies.[135–137] Echo enhancement can increase the technical success rate of a suboptimal ultrasound examination by augmenting existing Doppler signals, reducing examination time, and allowing color imaging and pulsed Doppler detection of a greater number of vessels. The sonic energy scattered back to the transducer by the microbubbles also contains harmonics in which the stronger echoes occur at twice the transmitted frequency. It is now possible to have the ultrasound transducer transmit at one frequency (lower) and image at twice the transmitted frequency (higher). This method, known as harmonic imaging,[135] allows suppression of tissue signals (flash artifact). When combined with the use of ultrasound contrast agents, this technique improves the ability to image the contrast agent with minimal artifact and interference from tissue structures. This improves visualization of very small, low-flow vessels, including flow in moving tissue, without the flash artifact and rejection of solid tissue clutter (e.g., wall thump of the vessels) without the loss of flow data caused by filters.[135]

The evaluation of high-grade carotid stenosis with carotid CFI is often limited by acoustic shadowing from plaque calcification, extremely narrow residual lumen, and increased absorption of ultrasonic energy by heterogeneous atherosclerotic wall components. The use of intravenous transpulmonary echo-enhancement agents helps to overcome these problems and significantly improves visualization of the entire length of the stenotic residual flow lumen, with better demonstration of irregular or ulcerative plaques in patients with high-grade stenosis and more accurate interpretation of such lesions.[138]

Transtemporal insonation in TCD sonography can be thwarted by an insufficient signal-to-noise ratio, especially in elderly patients, who are much more likely to have inadequate or absent temporal acoustic windows. Transpulmonary stable air microbubble contrast agents, such as Levovist (galactose microparticle carrier, Schering, Germany), can safely and effectively improve the ability to obtain TCD data in such patients. The use of this agent enhances the Doppler signals by at least 3 dB above the native signal in up to 88.6 percent of patients, depending on the dose of the contrast agent.[139] With this approach for contrast-enhanced TCD, signal enhancement appears within 15 to 20 s and lasts for 2.5 to 4 min, depending on the dose of Levovist and the Doppler signal-to-noise ratio for the individual patient. Many other ultrasound contrast agents have been recently approved or are in clinical trials.

Contrast-enhanced TCCI allows detection of peripheral branches of the ACA, MCA, and PCA, as well as the posterior communicating and superior cerebellar arteries. The same technique can reveal the deep cerebral veins (i.e., inferior saggital sinus, internal cerebral veins, great cerebral vein of Galen, straight sinus, and the confluence sinuum) and the main infratentorial arterial branches (anterior inferior, posterior inferior, and superior cerebellar arteries) via the suboccipital window.[140] This technique has been used in the identification of transverse sinus venous thrombosis.[141] The addition of a transpulmonary ultrasound contrast agent may greatly broaden the diagnostic utility of TCCI in cerebrovascular diseases.

SUMMARY

Ultrasound methods provide a window for studying both the extracranial and the intracranial cerebrovascular systems in a safe, accurate, cost-effective manner. New developments promise improved ability to evaluate stroke mechanisms and allow more accurate noninvasive estimates of cerebral hemodynamics. Physicians caring for patients with cerebrovascular disease must have a working knowledge of these techniques, their strengths, weaknesses, indications, and interpretation. We currently use carotid ultrasound and TCD as the initial tests of choice to evaluate cerebrovascular disease, usually reserving magnetic resonance angiography, computed tomographic angiography, and especially conventional contrast angiography for those patients in whom noninvasive results are abnormal, conflicting, or technically inadequate. Finally, the use of *both* extracranial carotid or vertebral duplex sonography and TCD is preferred, since the combination offers a more complete assessment of the cerebral circulation than can be obtained with either test alone. This combination increases the likelihood that the noninvasive approach will provide clinically useful information.

REFERENCES

1. McKinney WM: The role of the neurologist in neurosonology. *J Child Neurol* 4(suppl):S3–S4, 1989.
2. American Heart Association: *1992 Heart and Stroke Facts*. Dallas, 1991, p 3.
3. Sherman DG, Dyken ML, Fisher M, et al: Antithrombotic therapy for cerebrovascular disorders. *Chest* 95 (suppl):140S–155S, 1989.
4. Cerebral Embolism Task Force: Cardiogenic brain embolism: The second report of the Cerebral Embolism Task Force. *Arch Neurol* 46:727–743, 1989.
5. Tegeler CH: Cardiac sources of embolism, in Feldmann E (ed): *Current Diagnosis in Neurology*. Philadelphia, Mosby-Yearbook, 1993, pp 41–47.
6. North American Symptomatic Carotid Endarterectomy Trial Collaborators: Beneficial effect of carotid endarterectomy in symptomatic patients with high grade carotid stenosis. *N Engl J Med* 325:445–453, 1991.
7. Mayberg MR, Wilson SE, Yatsu F, et al: Carotid endarterectomy and prevention of cerebral ischemia in symptomatic carotid stenosis. *JAMA* 266:3289–3294, 1991.
8. European Carotid Surgery Trialists' Collaborative Group: MCR European Carotid Surgery Trial: Interim results for symptomatic patients with severe (70-99%) or with mild (0-29%) carotid stenosis. *Lancet* 337:1235–1243, 1991.
9. Executive Committee for the Asymptomatic Carotid Atherosclerosis Study: Endarterectomy for asymptomatic carotid stenosis. *JAMA* 273:1421–1428, 1995.
10. Tegeler CH, Shi F, Morgan T: Carotid stenosis in lacunar stroke. *Stroke* 22:1124–1128, 1991.
11. Polak JF, Bajakian RL, O'Leary DH, et al: Detection of internal carotid artery stenosis: Comparison of MR angiography, color-Doppler sonography, and arteriography. *Radiology* 182:35–40, 1992.
12. Polak JF, Kalina P, Donaldson MC, et al: Carotid endarterectomy: Preoperative evaluation of candidates with combined Doppler sonography and MR angiography. *Radiology* 186:333–338,1993.
13. Health and Public Policy Committee, American College of Physicians: Diagnostic evaluation of the carotid arteries. *Ann Intern Med* 109:835–837, 1988.
14. Caplan LR: Stroke neuroimaging. *J Neuroimaging* 3:48–54, 1993.
15. Alexandrov AV, Bladin CF, Maggisano R, Norris JW: Measuring carotid stenosis: Time for a reappraisal. *Stroke* 24:1292–1296, 1993.
16. Moore WS, Mohr JP, Najafi H, et al: Carotid endarterectomy: Practice guidelines. *J Vasc Surg* 15:469–479, 1992.
17. Eckman MH, Levine HJ, Pauker SG: Decision analytic and cost-effectiveness issues concerning anticoagulant prophylaxis in heart disease. *Chest* 102(suppl):538S–49S, 1992.
18. Sherman DG, Dyken ML, Fisher M, et al: Antithrombotic therapy for cerebrovascular disorders. *Chest* 102 (suppl):529S–537S, 1992.
19. Kremkau FW: *Diagnostic Ultrasound: Principles and Instruments*, 4th ed. Philadelphia, Saunders, 1993.
20. Zweibel WJ: *Introduction to Vascular Ultrasonography*, 3d ed. Philadelphia, Saunders, 1992.
21. Tegeler CH, Ratanakorn D: *Physics and Principles of Transcranial Doppler Ultrasonography*. St Louis, Mosby-Yearbook, 1998.
22. Withers CE, Gosink BB, Keightley AM, et al: Duplex carotid sonography: Peak systolic velocity in quantifying internal carotid artery stenosis. *J Ultrasound Med* 9:345–349, 1990.
23. Beach KW, Lawrence R, Phillips DJ, et al: The systolic velocity criterion for diagnosing significant internal carotid artery stenosis. *J Vasc Technol* 13:65–68, 1989.
24. Robinson ML, Sacks D, Perlmutter GS, Marinelli DL: Diagnostic criteria for carotid duplex sonography. *Am J Roentgenol* 151:1045–1049, 1988.
25. Sumner DS: Use of color flow imaging technique in carotid artery disease. *Surg Clin North Am* 70:201–211, 1990.
26. Grant EG, Tessler FN, Perrella RR: Clinical Doppler imaging. *Am J Roentgenol* 152:707–717, 1989.
27. Zweibel WJ, Knighton R: Duplex examination of the carotid arteries. *Semin Ultrasound CT MR* 11:97–135, 1990.
28. Howard G, Chambless LE, Baker WH, et al: A multicenter validation study of Doppler ultrasound versus angiography. *J Stroke Cerebrovasc Dis* 1:166–173, 1991.
29. Smith LL, Anderson DC, Gramith F: A step-by-step guide for validation of carotid duplex studies. *J Vasc Technol* 17:17–22, 1993.
30. Gomez C, Kinkel P, Masdeu J, et al: American Academy of Neurology Guidelines for Credentialing in Neuroimaging: Report from the task force on updating guidelines for credentialing in neuroimaging. *Neurology* 49: 1734–1737, 1997.
31. Masdeu JC: The American Academy of Neurology Workshop on Neuroimaging Training: American Academy of Neurology Neuroimaging Training Guidelines. *Neurology* 49:1738–1740, 1997.
32. Fox AJ: How to measure carotid stenosis. *Radiology* 186:316–318, 1993.
33. Caplan LR: Diagnosis and treatment of ischemic stroke. *JAMA* 266:2413–2418, 1991.
34. Merritt CRB, Bluth EI: The future of carotid sonography. *Am J Roentgenol* 158:37–39, 1992.
35. Baldassarre D, Werba JP, Tremoli E, et al: Common carotid intima-media thickness measurement: A method to improve accuracy and precision. *Stroke* 25:1588–1592, 1994.
36. Howard G, Sharrett R, Heiss G, et al: Carotid artery intimal-medial thickness distribution in general populations as evaluated by B-mode ultrasound. *Stroke* 24: 1297–1304, 1993.
37. Gomez CR: Carotid plaque morphology and risk for stroke. *Stroke* 21:148–151,1990.
38. Sterpetti AV, Schultz RD, Feldhaus RJ, et al: Ultrasonographic features of carotid plaque and the risk of subsequent neurologic deficits. *Surgery* 104:652–660, 1988.
39. O'Farrell CM, Fitzgerald DE: Prognostic value of carotid ultrasound lesion morphology in retinal ischemia: Result of a long term follow up. *Br J Ophthalmol* 77:781–784, 1993.
40. Perez-Burkhardt JL, Gonzalez-Fajardo JA, Rodriguez E, Mateo AM: Amaurosis fugax as a symptom of carotid

artery stenosis: Its relationship with ulcerated plaque. *J Cardiovasc Surg* 35:15–18, 1994.
41. Gronholdt ML, Nordestgaard BG, Neilsen TG, Sillesen H: Echolucent carotid artery plaques are associated with elevated levels of fasting and postpandrial triglyceride rich lipoproteins. *Stroke* 27:2166–2172, 1996.
42. Comerota AJ, Katz ML, White JV, Grosh JD: The preoperative diagnosis of the ulcerated carotid atheroma. *J Vasc Surg* 11:505–510, 1990.
43. Beach KW, Hatsukami T, Detmer PR, et al: Carotid artery intraplaque hemorrhage and stenotic velocity. *Stroke* 24:314–319, 1993.
44. Beletsky VY, Kelly RE, Fowler M, Phifer T: Ultrasound densitometric analysis of carotid plaque composition: Pathoanatomic correlation. *Stroke* 27:2173–2177, 1996.
45. Delcker A, Diener HC, Wilhelm H: Influence of vascular risk factors for atherosclerotic carotid artery plaque progression. *Stroke* 26:2016–2022, 1995.
46. Bartels E, Fuchs H-H, Flugel KA: Duplex ultrasonography of vertebral arteries: Examination, technique, normal values, and clinical applications. *Angiology* 43:169–180, 1992.
47. Kremkau FW: *Doppler Ultrasound: Principles and Instruments*. Philadelphia, Saunders, 1995.
48. Kremkau FW: Principles and instrumentation, in Merritt CRB (ed): *Doppler Color Imaging*. New York, Churchill-Livingstone, 1992, pp 7–60.
49. Tegeler CH, Kremkau FW, Hitchings LP: Color velocity imaging: Introduction to a new ultrasound technology. *J Neuroimaging* 1:85–90, 1991.
50. Kiell CS, McPharlane M, Shepard AD, McManus MP: Efficacy of color flow Doppler in the diagnosis of carotid artery occlusion. *J Vasc Technol* 17:81–86, 1993.
51. Polak JF, Dobkin GR, O'Leary DH, et al: Internal carotid artery stenosis: Accuracy and reproducibility of color Doppler assisted duplex imaging. *Radiology* 173: 793–798, 1989.
52. Furst H, Hartl WH, Jansen I, et al: Color flow Doppler sonography in the identification of ulcerative plaques in patients with high-grade carotid artery stenosis. *Am J Neuroradiol* 13:1581–1587, 1992.
53. Steinke W, Kloetzsch C, Hennerici M: Carotid artery disease assessed by color Doppler flow imaging: Correlation with standard Doppler sonography and angiography. *Am J Neuroradiol* 11:259–266, 1990.
54. Sitzer M, Siebler M, Steinmetz H: Noninvasive evaluation of internal carotid stenosis with color Doppler assisted duplex imaging. *Clin Radiol* 51(suppl 1):24–27, 1996.
55. Lee DH, Gao FQ, Rankin R, et al: Duplex and color Doppler flow sonography of occlusion and near occlusion of the carotid artery. *Am J Neuroradiol* 17:1267–1274, 1996.
56. Mansour MA, Mattos MA, Hood DB, et al: Detection of total occlusion, string sign, and preocclusive stenosis of the internal carotid artery by color flow duplex scanning. *Am J Surg* 170:154–158, 1995.
57. Colquhoun I, Oates CP, Martin K, et al: The assessment of carotid and vertebral arteries: A comparison of CFI duplex ultrasound with intravenous digital subtraction angiography. *Br J Radiol* 65:1069–1074, 1992.
58. Bartels E, Flugel KA: Advantages of color Doppler imaging for the evaluation of vertebral arteries. *J Neuroimaging* 3:229–233, 1993.
59. Steinke W, Schwartz A, Hennerici M: Doppler color flow imaging of common carotid artery dissection. *Neuroradiology* 32:502–505, 1990.
60. Steinke W, Hennerici M, Aulich A: Doppler color flow imaging of carotid body tumors. *Stroke* 20:1574–1577, 1989.
61. Rubin JM, Bude RO, Carson PL, et al: Power Doppler US: A potentially useful alternative to mean frequency-based color Doppler US. *Radiology* 190:853–856, 1994.
62. Rubin JM, Adler RS, Fowlkes JB, et al: Fractional moving blood volume: Estimation with power Doppler US. *Radiology* 197:183–190, 1995.
63. Griewing B, Kessler CH, Doherty C: Power Doppler ultrasound examination of the intracerebral and extracerebral vasculature. *J Neuroimaging* 6:32–35, 1996.
64. Wardlaw JM, Cannon JC, Sellar RJ: Use of color power transcranial Doppler sonography to monitor aneurysmal coiling. *Am J Neuroradiol* 17:864–867, 1996.
65. Giovagnorio F, Quaranta L: Power Doppler sonography enhances visualization of orbital vessels. *J Ultrasound Med* 14:837–842, 1995.
66. Steinke W, Meairs S, Ries S, Hennerici M: Sonographic assessment of carotid artery stenosis: Comparison of power Doppler imaging and color Doppler flow imaging. *Stroke* 27:91–94, 1996.
67. Wardlaw JM, Cannon JC: Color transcranial "power" Doppler ultrasound of intracranial aneurysms. *J Neurosurg* 84:459–461, 1996.
68. Griewing B, Morgenstern C, Driesner F, et al: Cerebrovascular disease assessed by color flow and power Doppler ultrasonography: Comparison with digital subtraction angiography in internal carotid artery stenosis. *Stroke* 27:95–100, 1996.
69. Eicke BM, Tegeler CH, Howard G, Myers LG: In vitro reliability of flow volume measurements with color velocity imaging. *J Ultrasound Med* (abstract) 12:543, 1993.
70. Knappertz VA , Tegeler CH, Myers LG: Measurement using ultrasound time domains and color M mode analysis. *Ultraschall in der Medizin* 17:229–234, 1996.
71. Knappertz VA , Tegeler CH, Myers LG: Clinical cerebrovascular applications of arterial ultrasound volume flow rate estimates. *J Neuroimaging* 6:1–7, 1996.
72. Ratanakorn D, Greenberg JP, Meads DB, Tegeler CH: Middle cerebral artery flow velocity correlates with common carotid volume flow rate after CO_2 inhalation (abstract). *J Neuroimaging* 7:268, 1997.
73. Diedrich AL, McIntyre L, Tegeler CH: Middle cerebral artery volume flow rate with transcranial color velocity imaging quantification (abstract). *J Neuroimaging* 7:66, 1997.
74. Aaslid R, Markwalder TM, Nornes H: Noninvasive transcranial Doppler ultrasound recording of flow velocity in basal cerebral arteries. *J Neurosurg* 57:769–774, 1982.
75. Ringelstein EB, Kahlscheuer B, Niggemeyer E, Otis SM: Transcranial Doppler sonography: Anatomical landmarks and normal velocity values. *Ultrasound Med Biol* 16:745–761, 1990
76. Hennerici M, Rautenberg W, Sitzer G, Schwartz A:

Transcranial Doppler ultrasound for the assessment of the intracranial arterial flow velocity: I. Examination technique and normal values. *Surg Neurol* 27:439–448, 1987.

77. Rojanapongpun P, Drance S: Velocity of the ophthalmic arterial flow recorded by Doppler ultrasound in normal subjects. *Am J Ophthalmol* 115:174–180, 1993.
78. Ratanakorn D, Tegeler CH, Greenberg JP: Risks for inadequate temporal windows in transcranial Doppler sonography (abstract). *Neurology* 48:A156, 1997.
79. Ratanakorn D, Kremkau FW, Myres LG, et al: Effect of mirror-image artifact on transcranial Doppler interpretation (abstract). *J Neuroimaging* 7:251, 1997.
80. Petty GW, Weibers DO, Meissner I: Transcranial Doppler ultrasonography: Clinical applications in cerebrovascular disease. *Mayo Clin Proc* 65:1350–1364, 1990.
81. Gomez CR, Brass LM, Tegeler CH, et al: The transcranial Doppler standardization project: Phase I results. *J Neuroimaging* 3:190–192, 1993.
82. Babikian VL: Transcranial Doppler evaluation of patients with ischemic cerebrovascular disease, in Babikian VL, Wechsler LR (eds): *Transcranial Doppler Ultrasonography*. St Louis, Mosby-Yearbook, 1993, pp 87–104.
83. Dewitt LD, Rosengart A, Teal PA: Transcranial Doppler ultrasonography, in Babikian VL, Wechsler LR (eds): *Transcranial Doppler Ultrasonography*. St Louis, Mosby-Yearbook, 1993, pp 29–38.
84. Macko RF, Ameriso SF, Akmal M, et al: Arterial oxygen content and age are determinants of middle cerebral artery blood flow velocity. *Stroke* 24:1025–1028, 1993.
85. Gomez CR, McLaughlin JR, Njemanze PC, Nashed A: Effect of cardiac dysfunction upon diastolic cerebral blood flow. *Angiology* 43:625–630, 1992.
86. Adams RJ, Nichols FT, McKie V, et al: Transcranial Doppler: Influence of hematocrit in children with sickle cell anemia without stroke. *J Cardiovasc Technol* 8:97–101, 1989.
87. Sorteberg W, Langmoen IA, Lindegaard KF, Nornes H: Side-to-side differences and day-to-day variations of transcranial Doppler parameters in normal subjects. *J Ultrasound Med* 9:403–409, 1990.
88. Kelly RE, Namon RA, Jer-Juang S, et al: Transcranial Doppler ultrasonography of the middle cerebral artery in the hemodynamic assessment of internal carotid artery stenosis. *Arch Neurol* 47:960–964, 1990.
89. Therapeutics and Technology Assessment Subcommittee, American Academy of Neurology: Assessment: Transcranial Doppler. *Neurology* 40:680–681, 1990.
90. Pourcelot L, Lepoivre B, Ossard G, et al: Transcranial Doppler and +Gz acceleration modelling and applications (abstract) *J Neuroimag* 7:243, 1997.
91. Maeda H, Etani H, Handa N, et al: A validation study on the reproducibility of transcranial Doppler velocimetry. *Ultrasound Med Biol* 16:9–14, 1989.
92. Jorgensen LG, Schroeder TV: Transcranial Doppler for detection of cerebral ischemia during carotid endarterectomy. *Eur J Vasc Surg* 6:142–147, 1992.
93. Khaffaf N, Karnik R, Winkler W-B, et al: Embolic stroke by compression maneuver during transcranial Doppler sonography. *Stroke* 25:1056–1057, 1994.
94. Ringelstein EB, Sievers C, Ecker S, et al: Noninvasive assessment of CO_2-induced cerebral vasomotor response in normal individuals and patients with internal carotid artery occlusions. *Stroke* 19:963–969, 1988.
95. Piepgras A, Schmiedek P, Leinsinger G, et al: A simple test to assess cerebrovascular reserve capacity using transcranial Doppler sonography and acetazolamide. *Stroke* 21:1306–1311, 1990.
96. Maeda H, Matsumoto M, Handa N, et al: Reactivity of cerebral blood flow to carbon dioxide in various types of ischemic cerebrovascular disease: Evaluation by the transcranial Doppler method. *Stroke* 24:670–675, 1993.
97. Schneider PA, Rossman ME, Bernstein EF, et al: Noninvasive assessment of cerebral collateral blood supply through the ophthalmic artery. *Stroke* 22:31–36, 1991.
98. Hilgertner L, Majchrowski A: Breath holding and carotid compression test: A comparison of two methods for cerebrovascular reactivity assessment (abstract). *Cerebrovasc Dis* 6(suppl):18, 1996.
99. Markus HS, Harrison MJG: Estimation of cerebrovascular reactivity using transcranial Doppler, including the use of breath holding as the vasodilatatory stimulus. *Stroke* 23:668–673, 1992.
100. Petersen B, von Maravic M, Zeller JA, et al: Basilar artery blood flow during head rotation in vertebrobasilar ischemia. *Acta Neurol Scand* 94:294–301, 1996.
101. Siebler M, Sitzer M, Steinmetz H: Detection of intracranial emboli in patients with symptomatic extracranial carotid artery disease. *Stroke* 23:1652–1654, 1992.
102. Koennecke H-C, Mast H, Trocio SS, et al: Microemboli in patients with vertebrobasilar ischemia: Association with vertebrobasilar and cardiac lesions. *Stroke* 28:593–596, 1997.
103. Diehl RD, Sliwka U, Rautenberg W, Schwartz A: Evidence for embolization from a posterior cerebral artery thrombus by transcranial Doppler monitoring. *Stroke* 24:606–608, 1993.
104. Barbut D, Yao FS, Hager DN, et al: Comparison of transcranial Doppler ultrasonography to monitor emboli during cardiac bypass surgery. *Stroke* 27:87–90, 1996.
105. Gerraty RP, Bowser DN, Infeld B, et al. Microemboli during carotid angiography: Association with stroke risk factors or subsequent magnetic resonance imaging changes? *Stroke* 27:1543–1547, 1996.
106. Sturzenegger M, Beer J, Ries F: Monitoring combined antithrombotic treatments in patients with prosthetic heart valves using transcranial Doppler and coagulation markers. *Stroke* 26:63–69, 1995.
107. Gavrilescu T, Babikian VL, Cantelmo NL, et al: Cerebral microembolism during carotid endarterectomy. *Am J Surg* 170:159–164, 1995.
108. Markus HS, Clifton A, Buckenham T, Brown MM: Carotid angioplasty: Detection of embolic signal during and after the procedure. *Stroke* 25:2403–2406, 1994.
109. Leighton VJ, Tegeler CH, Hitchings LP, et al: Serial carotid artery embolus detection to evaluate effect of preventive therapy (abstract). *J Neuroimaging* 2:56, 1992.
110. Tegeler CH, Burke GL, Gillespie JA, Kitzman DW: Embolus detection helps localize embolic source (abstract). *Stroke* 24:508, 1993.
111. Chimowitz MI, Nemec JJ, Marwick TH, et al: Transcranial Doppler ultrasound identifies patients with right-to-

left cardiac or pulmonary shunts. *Neurology* 41:1902–1904, 1991.

112. Tegeler CH, Burke GL, Dalley GM, Stump DA: Carotid emboli predict poor outcome in stroke (abstract). *Stroke* 24:186, 1993.
113. Sliwka U, Lingnau A, Stohlmann W-D, Schmidt P, et al: Prevalence and time course of microembolic signals in patients with acute stroke: A prospective study. *Stroke* 28:358–363, 1997.
114. Markus HS, Brown MM: Differentiation between different pathological cerebral embolic materials using transcranial Doppler in an in vitro model. *Stroke* 24:1–5, 1993.
115. Tegeler CH, Stump DA, Bennett JB, Burke GL: In vitro Doppler emboli detection monitoring with simultaneous B-mode imaging (abstract). *Stroke* 23:474, 1992.
116. Markus H, Loh A, Brown MM: Computerized detection of cerebral emboli and discrimination from artifact using Doppler ultrasound. *Stroke* 24:1667–1672, 1993.
117. Molloy J, Markus HS: Multigated Doppler ultrasound in the detection of emboli in a flow model and embolic signals in patients. *Stroke* 27:1840–1843, 1996.
118. Markus HS, Molley J: Use of decible threshold in detecting Doppler embolic signals. *Stroke* 28:692–695, 1997.
119. Bogdahn U, Becker G, Winkler J, et al: Transcranial color-coded real time sonography in adults. *Stroke* 21: 1680–1688, 1990.
120. Kaps M, Seidel G, Bauer T, Behrmann B: Imaging of the intracranial vertebrobasilar system using color-coded ultrasound. *Stroke* 23:1577–1582, 1992.
121. Martin PJ, Evans DH, Finst P, Naylor AR: Transcranial color-coded sonography of the basal cerebral circulation: Reference data from 115 volunteers. *Stroke* 25:390–396, 1994.
122. Schoning M, Buchholz R, Walter J: Comparative study of transcranial color duplex sonography and transcranial Doppler sonography in adults. *J Neurosurg* 78:776–784, 1993.
123. Bartels E, Flugel KA: Quantitative measurements of blood flow velocity in basal cerebral arteries with transcranial duplex color flow imaging: A comparative study with conventional transcranial Doppler sonography. *J Neuroimaging* 4:77–81, 1994.
124. Eicke BM, Tegeler CH, Dalley GM, Myers LG: Angle correction in transcranial Doppler sonography. *J Neuroimaging* 4:29–33, 1994.
125. Seidel G, Kaps M, Gerriets T: Potential and limitations of transcranial color-coded sonography in stroke patients. *Stroke* 26:2061–2066, 1995.
126. Becker G, Lindner A, Hofmann E, Bogdahn U: Contribution of transcranial color-coded real time sonography to etiopathogenetic classification of middle cerebral artery stenosis. *J Clin Ultrasound* 22:471–477, 1994.
127. Kenton AR, Martin PJ, Evans DH: Power Doppler: An advance over color Doppler for transcranial imaging? *Ultrasound Med Biol* 22:313–317, 1996.
128. Rankin RN, Fenster A, Downey DB, et al: Three-dimensional sonographic reconstruction: Techniques and diagnostic applications. *Am J Roentgenol* 161:696–702, 1993.
129. Picot PA, Rickey DW, Mitchell R, et al: Three-dimensional color Doppler imaging. *Ultrasound Med Biol* 19: 95–104, 1994.
130. Delcker A, Diener HC: Quantification of atherosclerotic plaques in carotid arteries by three-dimensional ultrasound. *Br J Radiol* 67:672–678, 1994.
131. Griewing B, Schminke U, Morgenstern C, et al: Three-dimensional ultrasound angiography (power mode) for the quantification of carotid artery atherosclerosis. *J Neuroimaging* 7:40–45, 1997.
132. Lyden PD, Nelson TR: Visualization of the cerebral circulation using three-dimensional transcranial power Doppler ultrasound imaging. *J Neuroimaging* 7:35–39, 1997.
133. Gramiak R, Shah PM: Echocardiography of the aortic root. *Invest Radiol* 3:356–366, 1968.
134. Meltzer RS, Tickner G, Sahines TP, et al: The source of the ultrasound contrast effect. *J Clin Ultrasound* 8:121–127, 1980.
135. Burns P: Overview of echo-enhanced vascular ultrasound imaging for clinical diagnosis in neurosonology. *J Neuroimaging* 7(suppl 1):S2–S14, 1997.
136. Schliff R: Developments in echo-enhancing agents. *Clin Radiol* 51(suppl 1):5–7, 1996.
137. Cosgrove D: Why do we need contrast agents for ultrasound? *Clin Radiol* 51(suppl 1):1–4, 1996.
138. Sitzer M, Siebler M, Rose G, et al: Characteristics and clinical value of an intravenous echo-enhancement agent in evaluation of high-grade internal carotid stenosis. *J Neuroimaging* 7(suppl 1):S22–S25, 1997.
139. Ries F, Honisch C, Lambertz M, Schlief R: A transpulmonary contrast medium enhances the transcranial Doppler signal in humans. *Stroke* 24:1903–1909, 1993.
140. Bogdahn U, Becker G, Schlief R, et al: Contrast-enhanced transcranial color-coded real time sonography: Results of a phase-two study. *Stroke* 24:676–684, 1993.
141. Ries S, Steinke W, Neff KW, Hennerici M: Echocontrast-enhanced transcranial color-coded sonography for the diagnosis of transverse sinus venous thrombosis. *Stroke* 28:696–700, 1997.

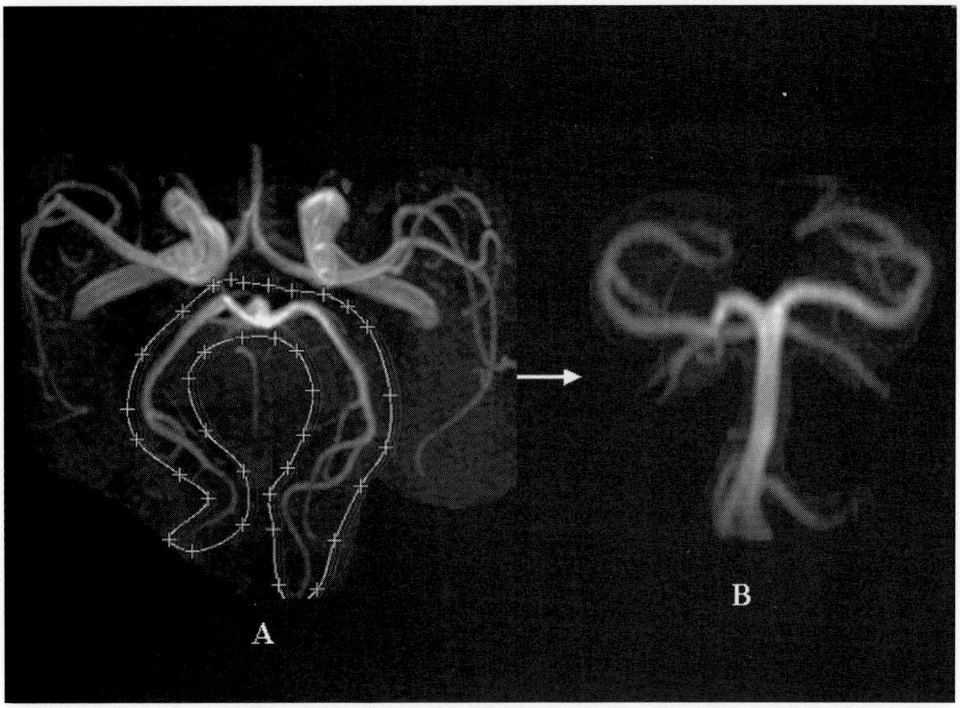

Figure 23-6
(A) *Targeted MIP submental vertex view from which the basilar artery is processed as another targeted MIP.* **(B)** *Coronal view of basilar artery after targeted MIP. (Technique: 3D TOF, single slab, ramped RF pulses.)*

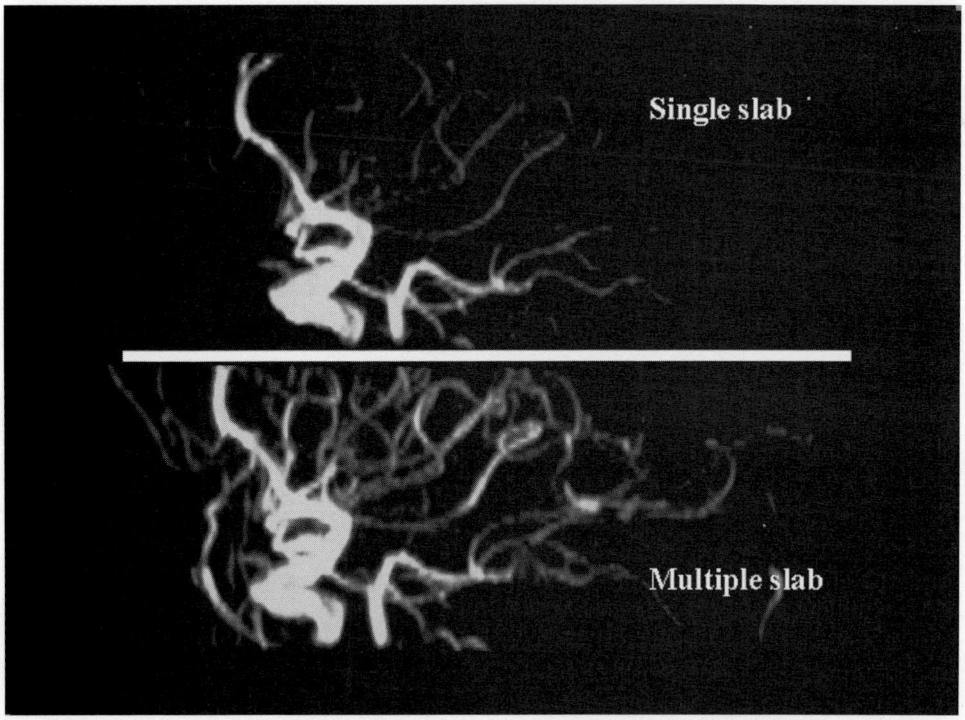

Figure 23-7
Intracranial arteriogram, 3D TOF MRA, lateral view. A single slab is at the top, and multiple slabs are at the bottom. Note the greater number and better visualization of small vessels in the multiple-slab technique due to less saturation.

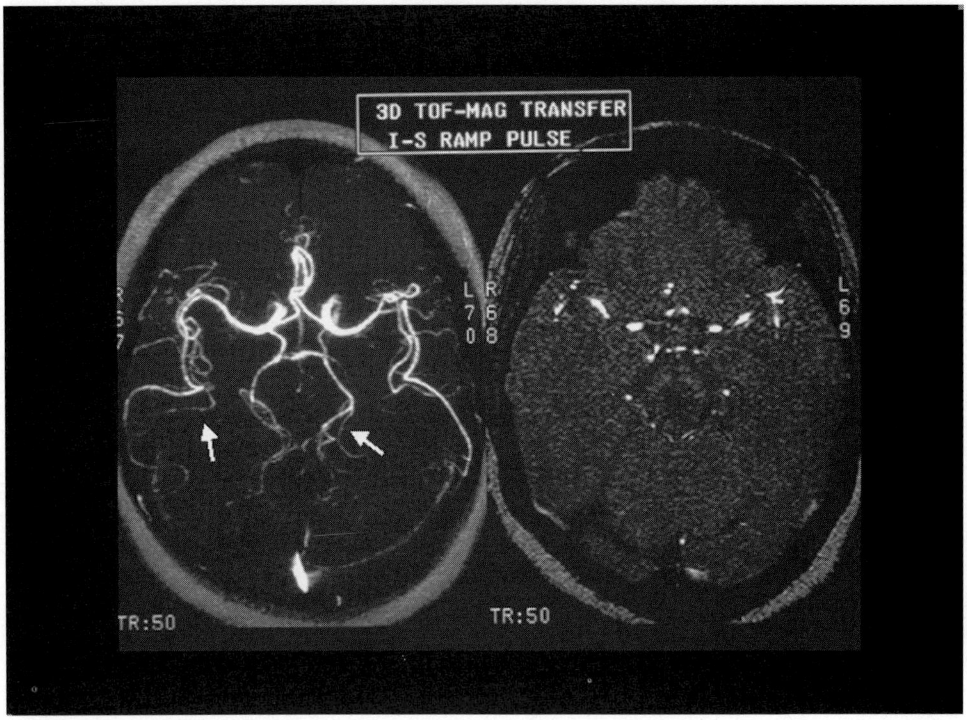

Figure 23-8
Intracranial arteriogram, 3D TOF with inferior to superior ramped RF pulses, Submental view (SMV). Note the excellent suppression of background in the source image with MTC, which permits visualization of distal small vessels (arrows).

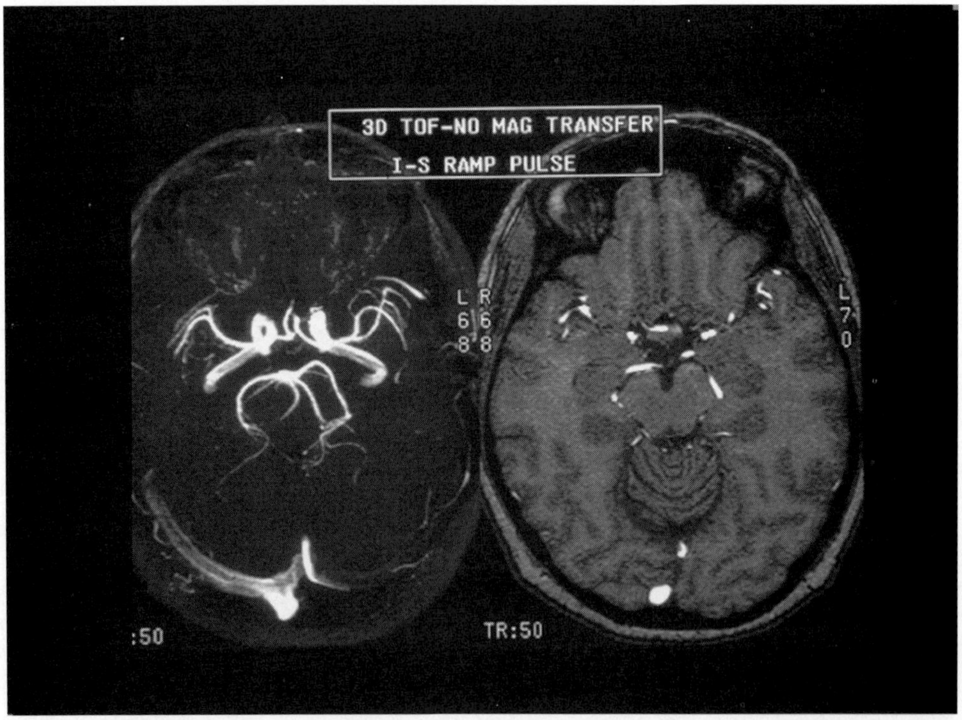

Figure 23-9
Intracranial arteriogram, 3D TOF without magnetization transfer pulse and with inferior-to-superior ramped RF pulses, SMV view. Note that the background is not as well suppressed and that distal vessel detail is not as well visualized as in Fig. 23-8.

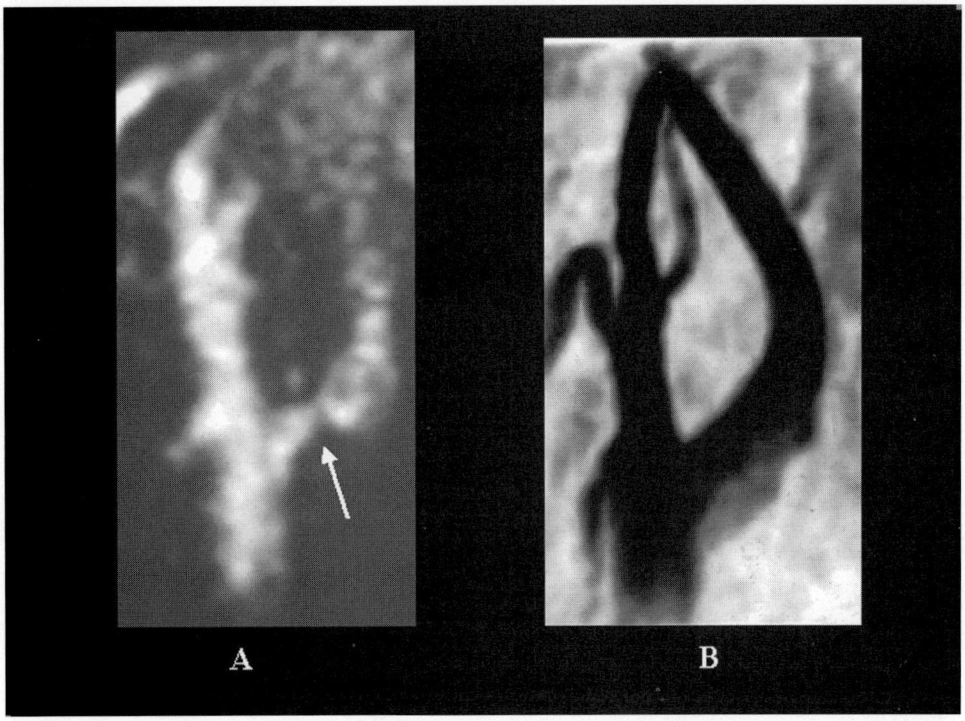

Figure 23-25
(A) *Artifactual left internal carotid stenosis caused by motion artifact and poor background suppression in 3D TOF single slab technique (arrow).* **(B)** *Normal left carotid bifurcation in the same patient obtained with sedation and better background suppression.*

Table 23-1
Time-of-flight angiography

	Advantages	*Disadvantages*
General	Reprojection and subvolumes possible Presaturation works well	Thrombus may simulate flow Tortuous vessels give less contrast
2D TOF	Sensitive to slow flow Reasonable scan times No saturation effects	Thick slices Large voxels; more intravoxel dephasing Motion artifacts Insensitive to in-plane flow Long TE
3D TOF	Short scan times High spatial resolution Very short TE Good signal to nerve ratio (SNR) Small voxels Less dephasing (due to small voxels, short TE) Sensitive to in-plane flow (small flip angle)	Insensitive to slow flow Field distortion artifacts (air, bone) Limited vessel track (<70 mm) Sensitive to motion Less static background suppression

the minds of clinicians, which translates into frequent requests to image this anatomic region. Hence, in patients who undergo routine MRI as part of a stroke workup, adding 5 to 10 min for a MRA of the carotid arteries is feasible, and the information obtained is useful. Ultrasound has been a reliable noninvasive screening test for imaging the carotid bifurcation, but this technique is not without limitations.[35] With ultrasound, there is difficulty in distinguishing high-grade stenosis from occlusion. Tandem lesions may be missed above the bifurcation, and the origin of the common carotid artery is not routinely accessible by this technique. Although these possibilities were not addressed in the early days of MRA, further developments in the technique now allow reliable imaging of the cerebrovascular system from the origin of the aortic arch to the intracranial branches.

Several MRA techniques have been proposed to assess the carotid bifurcation, including 2D TOF with superior saturation and single- and multiple-slab 3D TOF with standard and spatially varying or ramped RF excitation pulses.[5,8,36–38] The best results are obtained with the acquisition of thin, contiguous sections oriented as perpendicularly as possible to the vessel in order to maximize inflow-related enhancement. Once individual axial images are acquired and stacked, MIP processing of limited volumes of interest containing individual vessels is essential if one is to obtain accurate views of

Table 23-2
Phase-contrast angiography

	Advantages	*Disadvantages*
General	Variable velocity encoding allowing depiction of slow and fast flow Excellent background suppression Minimized saturation effects Differentiation between flowing and stationary blood (hemorrhage) Directional flow images	Long TE Presaturation less effective More turbulence effects
2D PCA	Short scan time (one or few slices) Useful as survey	No projection images Large voxels due to thick slice
2D cine-PCA	Variable velocity encoding Time resolution Hemodynamic flow information	Needs cardiac triggering Longer scan times
3D PCA	Small voxels Reprojection and subvolumes possible	Long scan time Motion sensitive Field distortion artifacts (air, bone)

the bifurcation that might otherwise be obscured by neighboring overlapping vessels.

Several blinded-reader studies have been published comparing MRA with conventional arteriography in the detection of luminal carotid stenosis[39–45] (Fig. 23-26). The results, based mostly on 2D TOF MRA, indicate high sensitivity (greater than 90 percent) and high negative predictive value (greater than 90 percent) for detecting narrowing greater than 70 percent [i.e., surgical stenosis, based on the North American Symptomatic Carotid Endarterectomy Trial (NASCET) criteria]. Also noted was an overestimation of stenosis by the technique, resulting in lower specificity and lower positive predictive value for detecting surgical narrowing of the carotid bifurcation[46] (Fig. 23-27).

Although MRA has shown higher sensitivity, higher negative predictive value, lower specificity, and lower positive predictive value in the 70 to 90 percent category of stenosis when compared to ultrasound, the differences were not statistically significant. Magnetic resonance angiography appears superior in detecting complete occlusion, reaching 100 percent sensitivity and specificity, compared to 83.3 percent sensitivity and 96.7 percent specificity for ultrasound[45] (Fig. 23-28).

When utilizing 2D TOF MRA, tight stenosis of the proximal internal carotid commonly shows as complete signal loss and reconstruction of the vessel above, denoting patency (Fig. 23-29). In fact, in 2D TOF MRA this pattern had been equated with tight stenosis leading to turbulent flow, intravoxel dephasing, and signal loss. One study, however, demonstrated a number of cases with less than 70 percent strenosis (i.e., nonsurgical until recently), which may still exhibit marked signal loss, as observed in the 70 to 99 percent stenosis group.[45]

Table 23-3
Gadolinium-enhanced MRA

	Advantages	*Disadvantages*
General	T1 weighting Reprojection and subvolumes possible Minimal saturation effects Good suppression of background (short TEs and large flip angle)	Thrombus may simulate flow High performance gradients needed for short TR/TE Moderate spatial resolution (192–256) Presaturation less effective
2D Gd MRA	Use restricted by very short TR/TEs and thin slices	
3D Gd MRA	Very short scan times (5–7 s) Temporal resolution Very short TE Good SNR Less dephasing (short TE) Sensitive to in-plane flow Coronal acquisition with good coverage without saturation	Poor temporal resolution for high-resolution intracranial studies

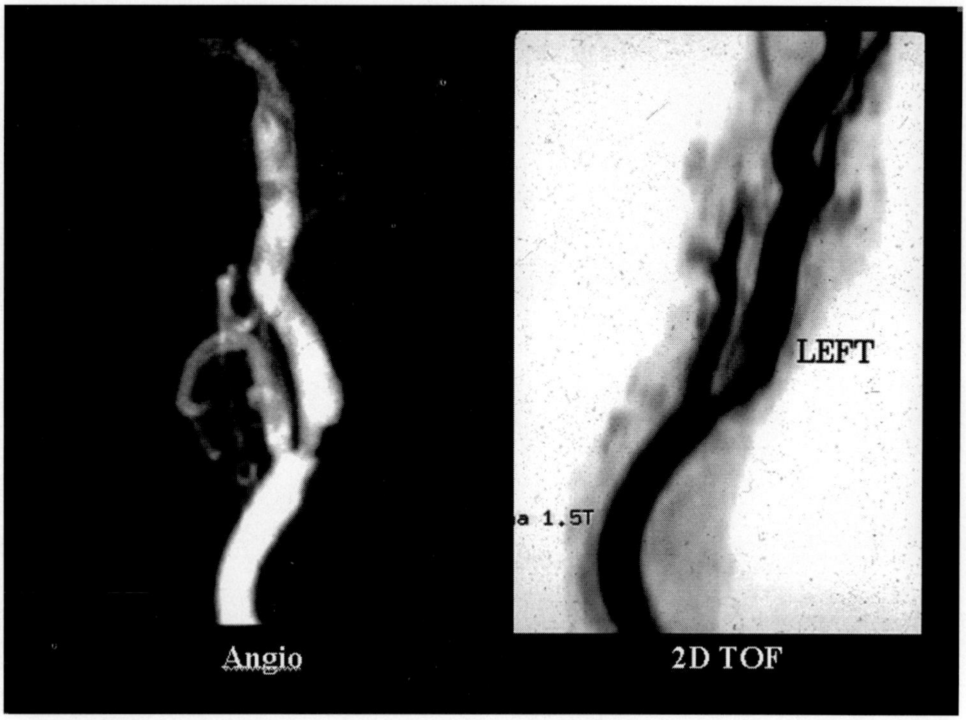

Figure 23-26
Moderate carotid stenosis accurately depicted by 2D TOF MRA, as compared to conventional angiogram.

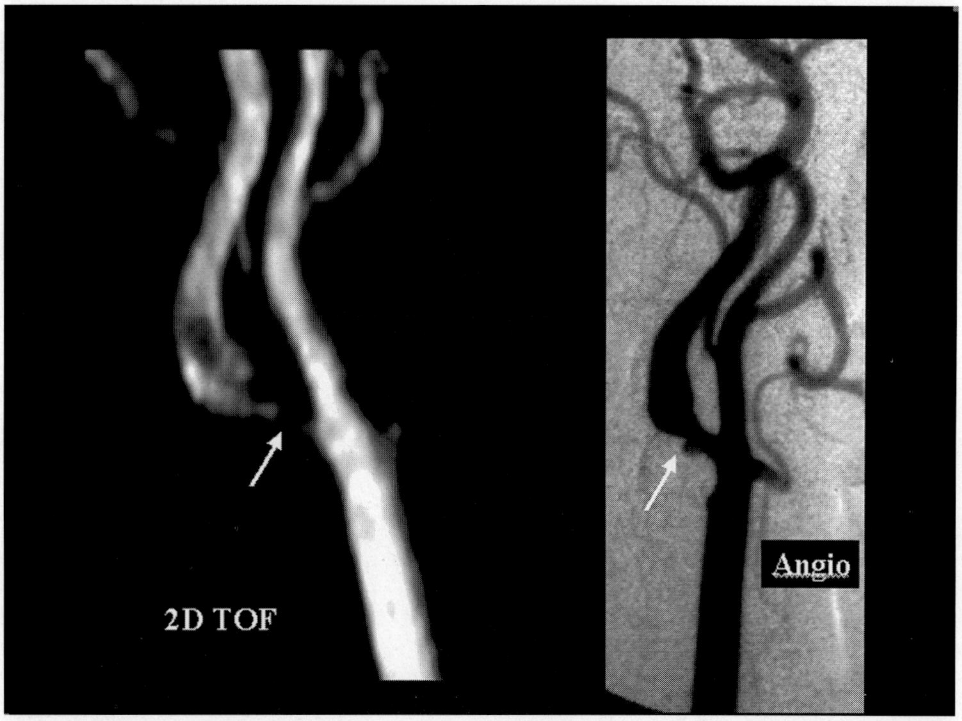

Figure 23-27
Overestimation of carotid stenosis by 2D TOF MRA. The area of stenosis is shown in 2D TOF MRA as flow gap, a sign that was thought to indicate greater than 70 percent stenosis. By conventional angiography, the stenosis is moderate, about 55 percent. There is also a small ulcer at the posterior wall of the internal carotid artery (arrow). Overestimation of carotid stenosis by 2D TOF MRA is frequent and in this case was exacerbated by a long TE of 9 ms.

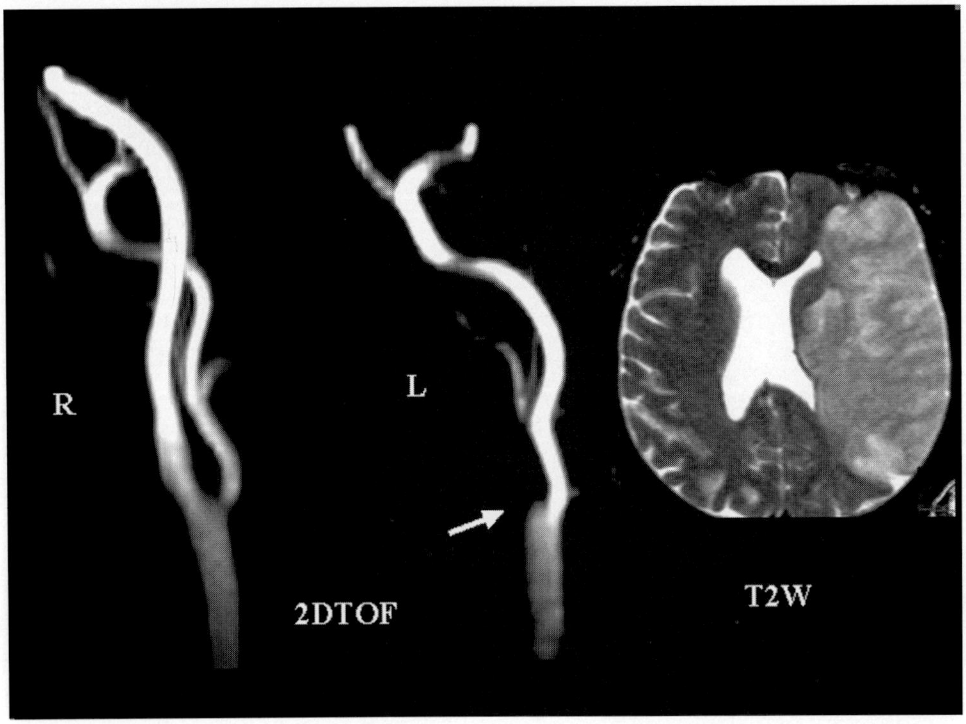

Figure 23-28
Carotid occlusion, 2D TOF MRA. The arrow points to the occluded internal carotid artery on the left associated with an infarction in the left MCA distribution, as shown by T2-weighted MRI of the brain. On the right, the carotid bifurcation is normal.

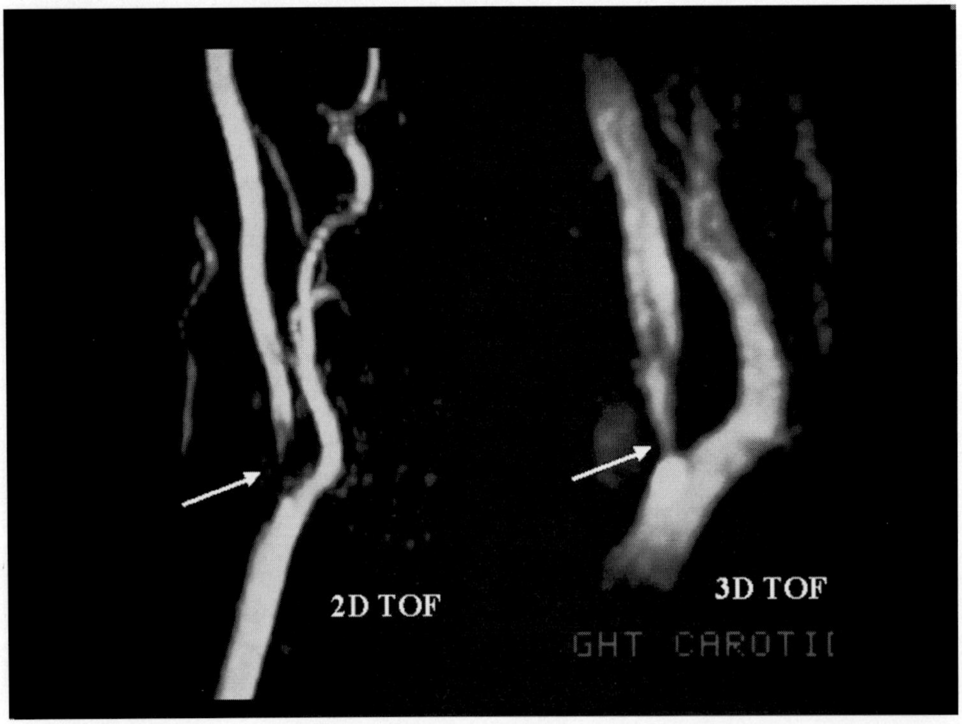

Figure 23-29
Severe carotid stenosis shown by 2D TOF MRA as flow gap with normal-appearing vessel above. 3D TOF MRA depicts stenosis more accurately than does 2D TOF due to its smaller voxel size and shorter TE, which reduce intravoxel dephasing. TR, TE, and voxel size are 32 ms, 7.7 ms, and 1.62 mm^3, respectively, for 2D TOF MRA and 35 ms, 6.9 ms, and 48 mm^3 for 3D TOF MRA.

Circumstances other than focal stenosis may also lead to varying degrees of signal loss at or near the common carotid bifurcation. The high flip angles of 2D TOF MRA quickly saturate in-plane flow of the horizontal, nonstenotic, proximal internal carotid artery, leading to marked signal loss and thus mimicking tight stenosis, as seen in Fig. 23-20. Also, a tortuous, convoluted segment of the vessel that reverses the direction of flow will be nulled by the superior saturation pulse of 2D TOF MRA and thus may show a segmental signal loss, mimicking stenosis, as seen in Fig. 23-21. At the level of the proximal posterolateral wall of the internal carotid or carotid bulb, local, complex, recirculating, relatively stagnant blood flow may lead to signal loss and artifactual stenosis, as seen in Fig. 23-23.[47] In most cases, the luminal narrowing is minimal and clinically insignificant.

Signal loss in regions of stenosis with complex flow is magnified by the relatively long TE (7 ms) and the large voxel (1.62 mm^3) of typical 2D TOF acquisitions. In 3D TOF MRA, these parameters can be scaled down to 2.3 ms and 0.1 mm^3, respectively, while maintaining a good signal-to-noise ratio. Saturation, which plagues single 3D acquisitions with long coverage, can be corrected by acquiring multiple thin slabs at the expense of prescribing excessively long acquisition times. A compromise is to start with a 2D TOF MRA that rapidly examines long segments and accurately depicts normal carotid arteries, followed by a single high-resolution 3D TOF slab at the bifurcation if significant stenosis is suspected. This combined approach improves both the specificity and the positive predictive value of MRA[48–50] (Figs. 23-30, 23-31, and 23-32).

Our current approach uses a combination of 2D TOF (2-mm thick slices) and ramped (to minimize saturation) single-slab 3D TOF technique through stenotic segments, which are then processed by subvolume MIP for a total acquisition time of approximately 10 min. The 3D slab is positioned perpendicular to the vessel in order to maximize flow-related enhancement. In some cases, we grade stenosis in individual sections as well as multiplanar reformatted images and compare measurements obtained from MIP images according to the NASCET method.[51] In the detection of 70 to 99 percent stenosis, the combination 2D and 3D TOF techniques yields a sensitivity of 94 percent, a specificity of 85 percent, and accuracy of 88 percent.[50] The combination of MRA and ultrasound raises the sensitivity to 100 percent, the specificity to 91 percent, and the accuracy to 94 percent, obviating the need for conventional contrast angiography in a majority of cases.[50,52] First-pass Gd MRA appears better than conventional 2D and 3D TOF in the depiction of stenosis of the extracranial circulation[25] (Figs. 23-33 through 23-41).

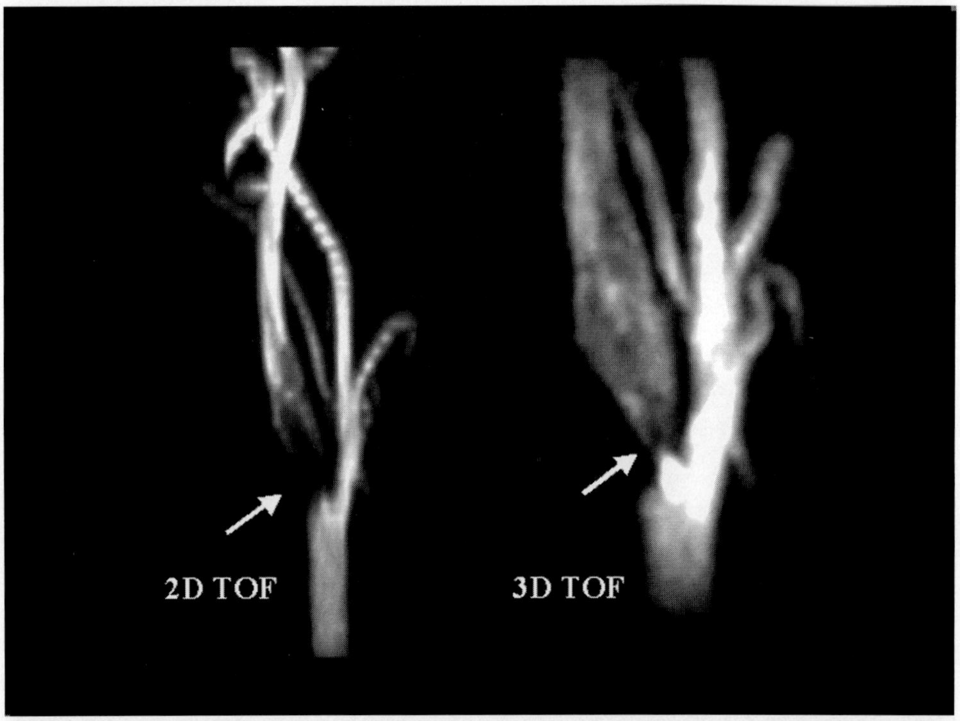

Figure 23-30
Severe internal carotid stenosis shown as flow gap in 2D TOF MRA and better depicted with 3D TOF MRA, ramped RF pulses. Shorter TE and smaller voxel size of 3D TOF acquisitions result in less intravoxel dephasing and, therefore, more accurate depiction of focal stenosis.

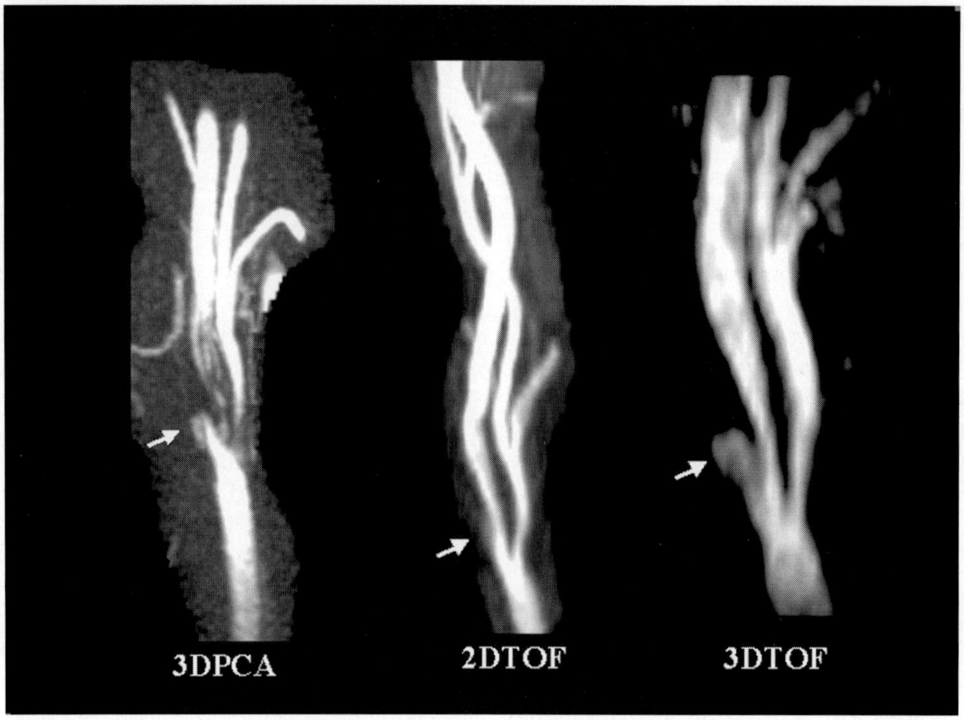

Figure 23-31
Carotid stenosis (70 percent) and ulcer (arrow). Ulcer and stenosis are better depicted by 3D TOF technique. There is not enough resolution to depict the ulcer in the 2D TOF acquisition. The ulcer is also well depicted by 3D PCA. In general, MRI has a low sensitivity for detecting ulcerated plaques at the carotid bifurcation.

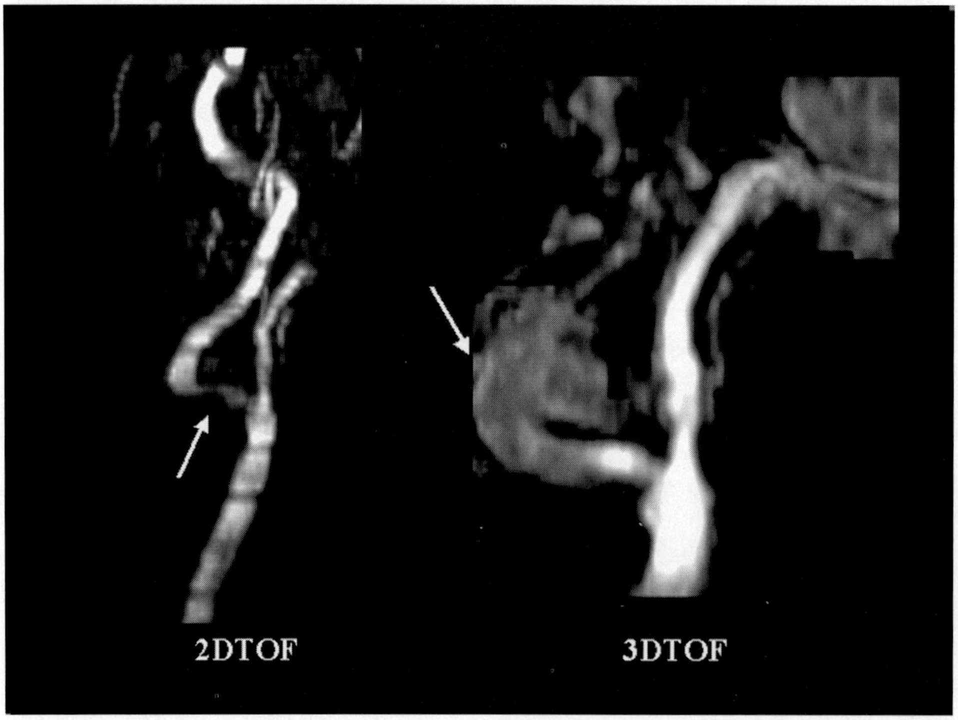

Figure 23-32
Carotid stenosis. In 2D TOF MRA, stenosis appears severe (arrow). In single-slab 3D TOF MRA with ramped RF pulses, stenosis appears mild, but the distal carotid artery cannot be clearly separated from the background, which is poorly suppressed (arrow).

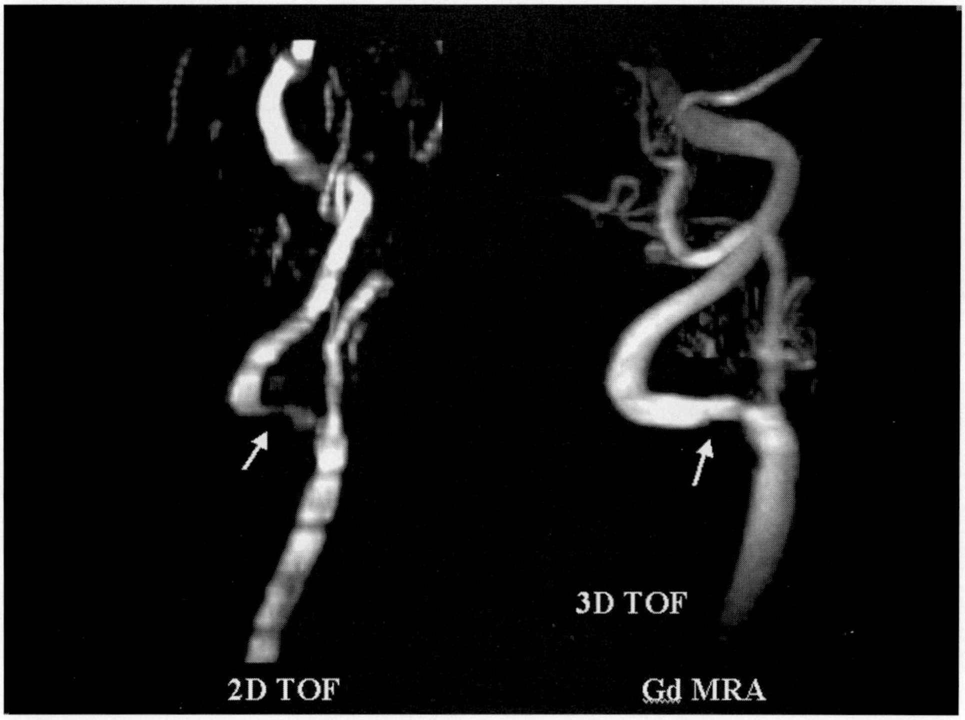

Figure 23-33
2D TOF compared to gadolinium-enhanced 3D MRA obtained with a local coil, of the same case as in Fig. 23-32. Stenosis is much better depicted by Gd MRA (arrow). It is only mild to moderate in degree. Note the poor quality of the 2D TOF due to movement artifact and overestimation of the stenosis typical of this type of acquisition (arrow). The short acquisition time of 3D TOF gadolinium-enhanced MRA (7 s) eliminates movement artifact.

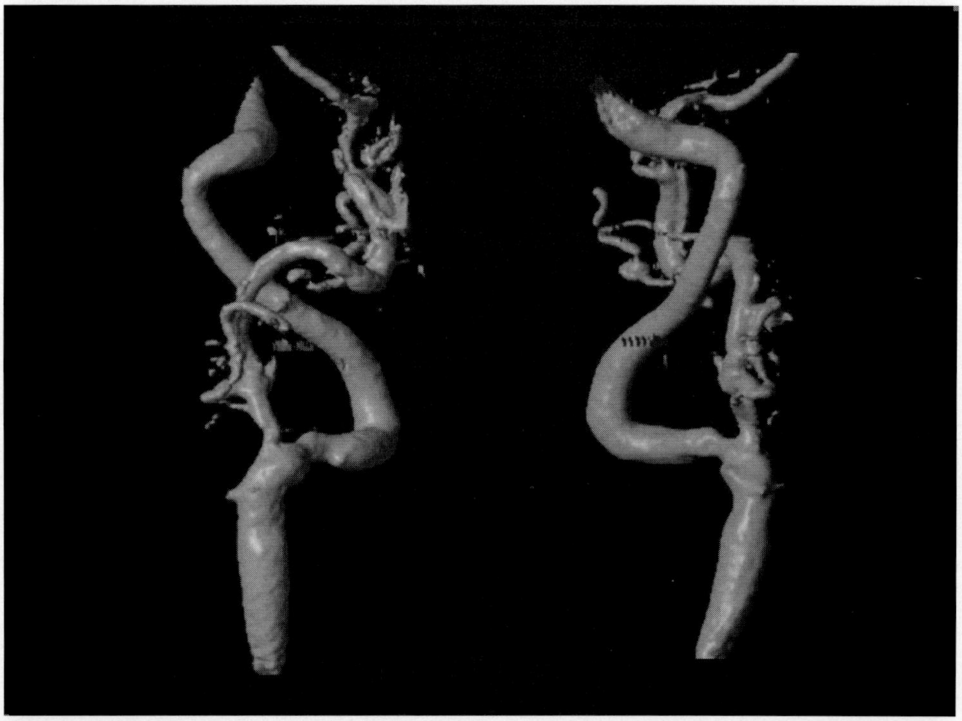

Figure 23-34 (Plate 46)
3D volume-rendered Gd MRA of the case depicted in Figs. 23-32 and 23-33. Note the excellent depiction of the carotid bifurcation.

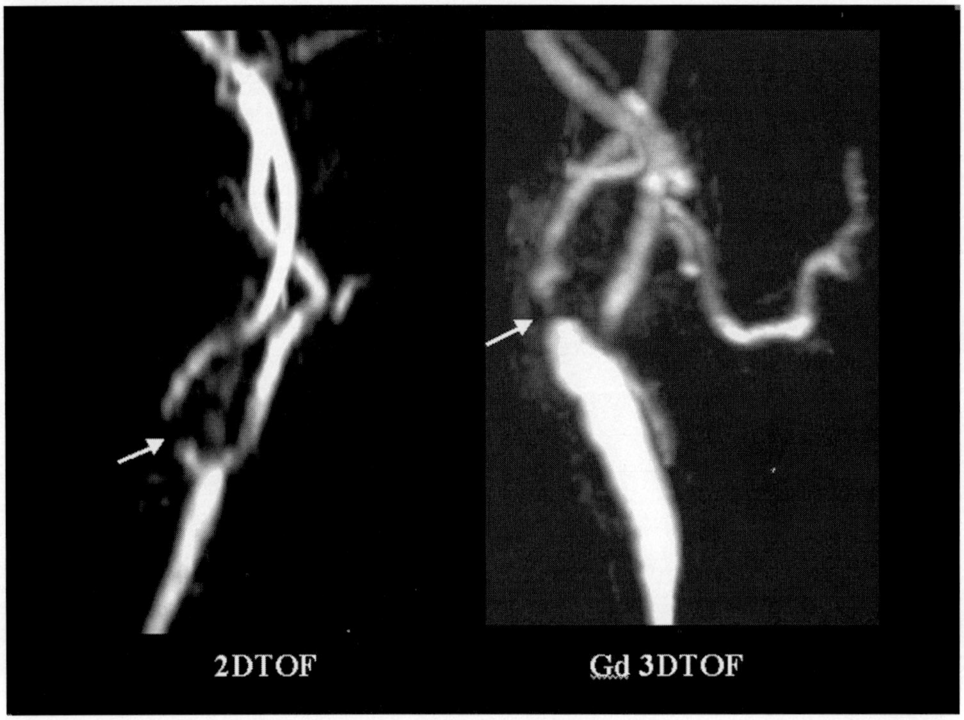

Figure 23-35
Severe carotid stenosis, 2D TOF compared to gadolinium-enhanced 3D TOF MRA. The 2D TOF image overestimates the stenosis, showing it as flow gap (arrow). Stenosis is better depicted by 3D Gd MRA and appears very severe (arrow). It was confirmed surgically.

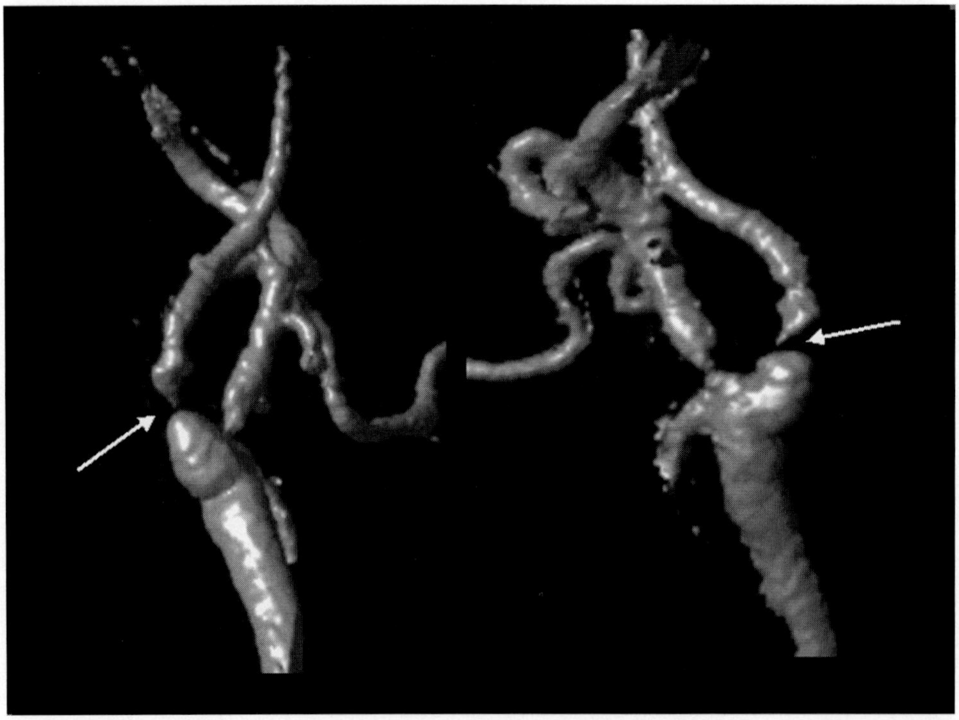

Figure 23-36 (Plate 47)
3D volume-rendered gadolinium-enhanced 3D TOF MRA of the case depicted in Fig. 23-35 showing marked stenosis of both the external and internal carotid arteries (arrows).

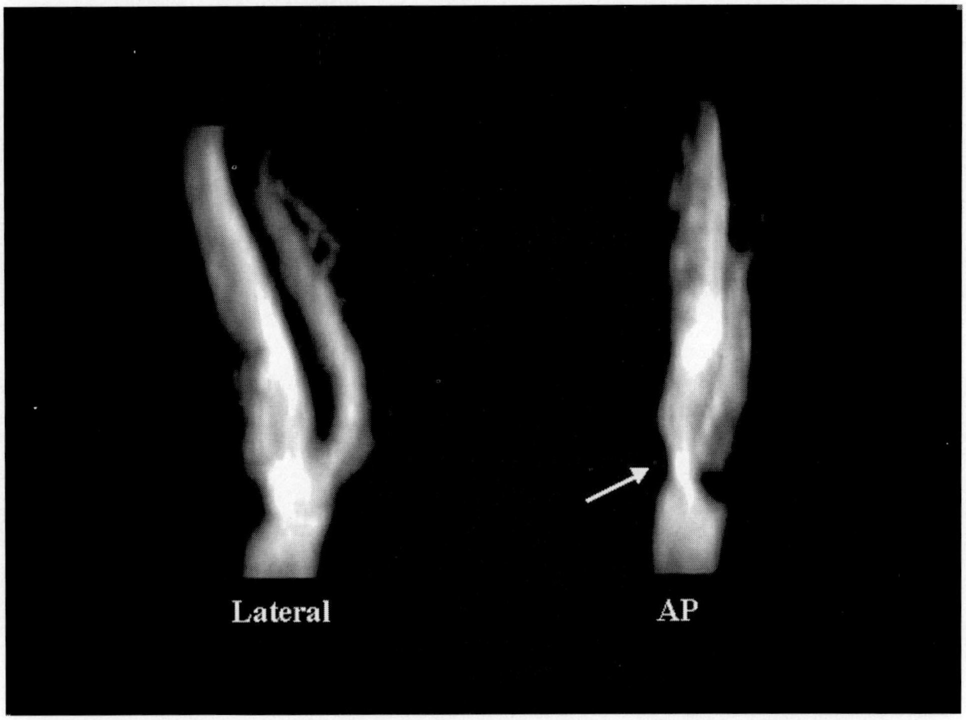

Figure 23-37

Moderate "pancake-like" carotid stenosis, 3D TOF MRA with ramped RF pulses. Stenosis is seen only in the AP view (arrow). In the lateral view, there appears to be no stenosis, since the plane of the angiographic projection is the same as that of the plaque.

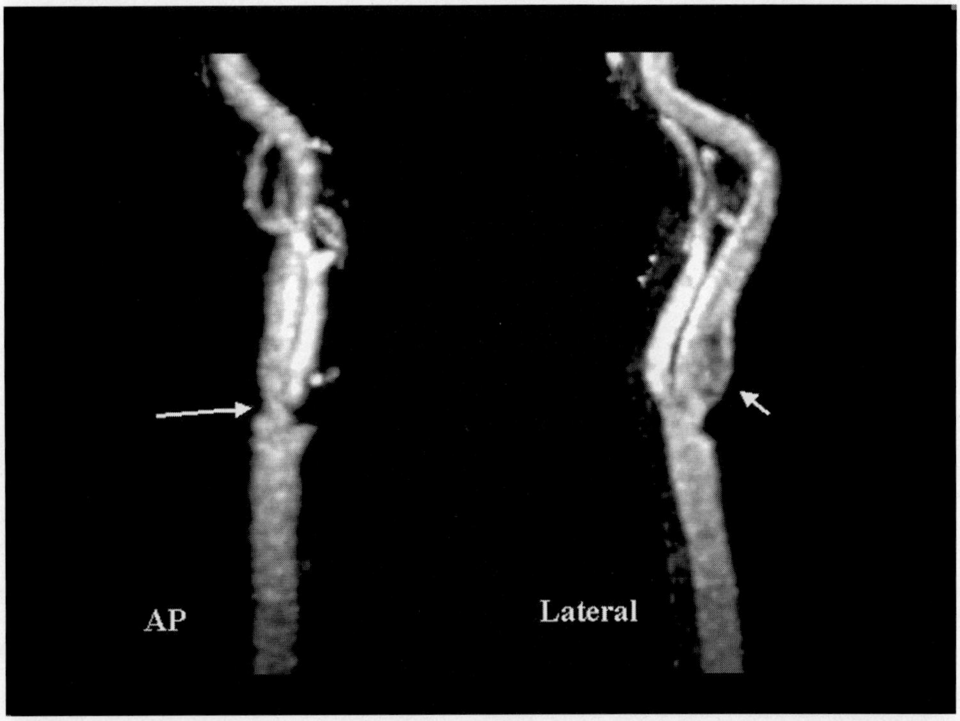

Figure 23-38

AP and lateral projections of Gd MRA in the case depicted in Fig. 23-37. Again, stenosis is seen in AP but not in lateral projection.

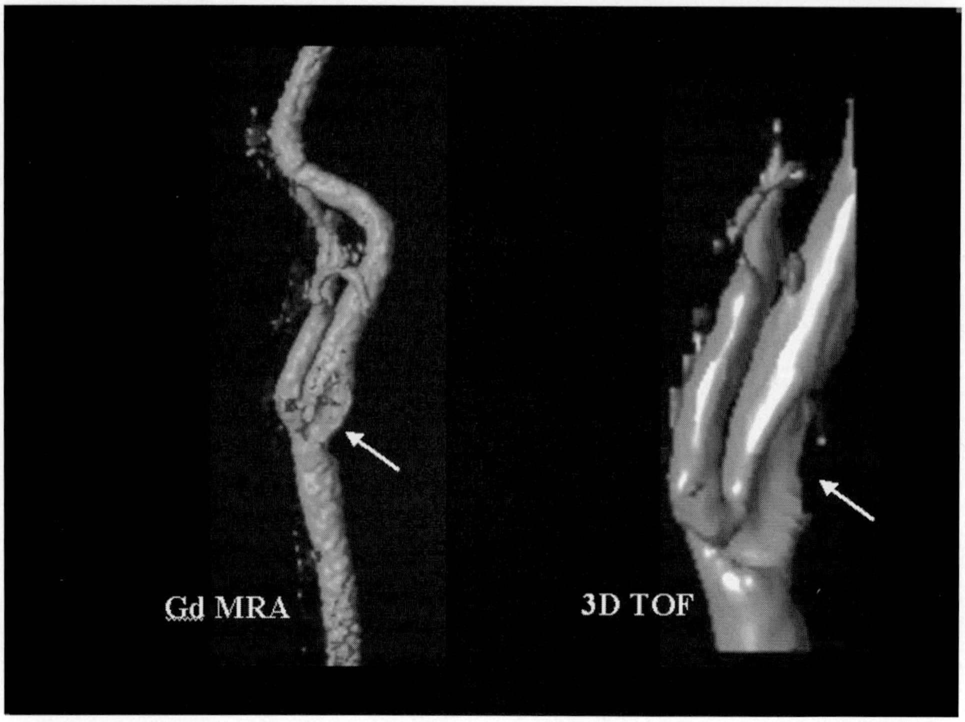

Figure 23-39 (Plate 48)
Carotid stenosis, moderate, same case as in Figs. 23-37 and 23-38. En face view of internal carotid plaque in volume-rendered gadolinium-enhanced 3D TOF MRA (arrow). Close-up view of a volume-rendered standard 3D TOF MRA showing detailed view of plaque at the internal carotid origin (arrow).

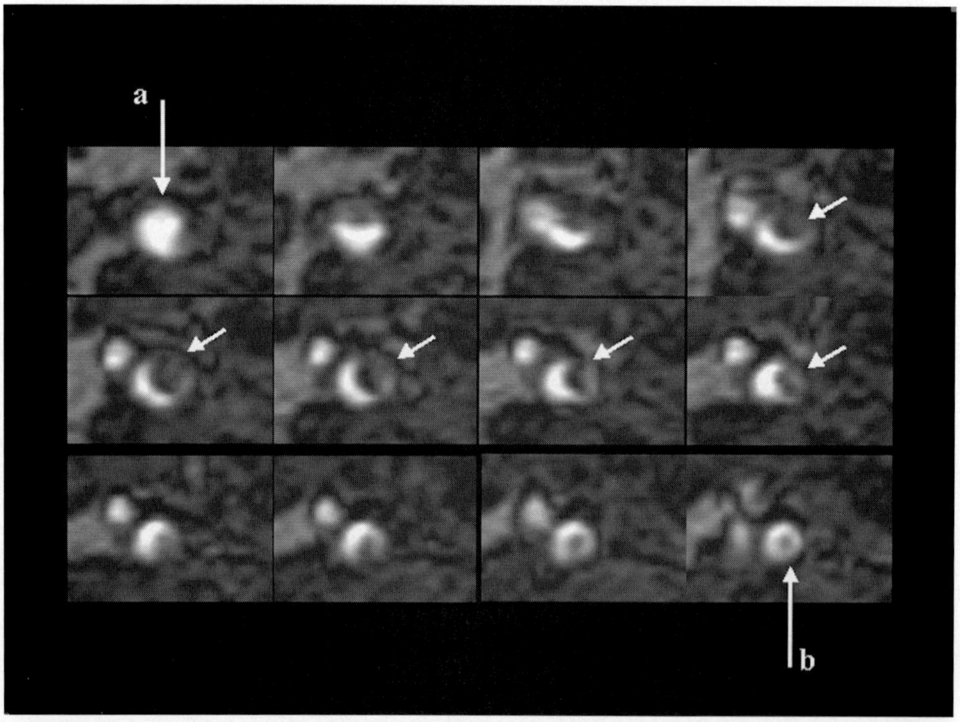

Figure 23-40
Carotid stenosis in the same patient as depicted in Fig. 23-39. The source image for 3D TOF MRA shows calcified plaque at the origin of the internal carotid artery (short arrows). Arrows a and b indicate the common and distal internal carotid arteries, respectively. Plaque flattens the arterial lumen, causing stenosis of approximately 50 percent.

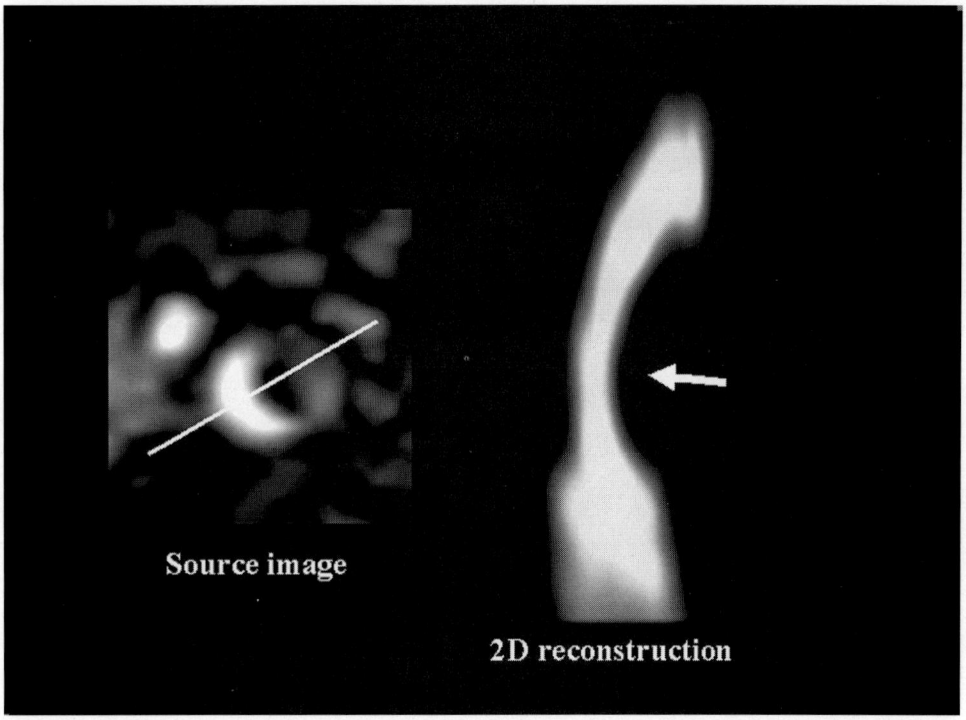

Figure 23-41
Carotid stenosis, 2D planar reconstruction, in the same case as depicted in Figs. 23-37 through 23-40. The line in the source image indicates the 2D reconstruction plane showing moderate carotid stenosis (arrow). Examination of source images as well as multiplanar reconstructions improve accuracy of MRA in grading stenosis.

Conventional TOF MRA combined with MRI is quite sensitive and specific in the detection of cervicocranial artery dissection, displaying it as a tapered stenosis string sign on MRA and at times the subintimal clot in MRI (Fig. 23-42). Its sensitivity and specificity is comparable to that of conventional angiography.[53]

The region of the aortic arch and origin of brachiocephalic vessels is difficult to image by MRA.[23] Ideally in this situation, a gated, efficient TOF technique is needed to eliminate motion artifact from pulsatility and to position saturation pulses and a surface coil with good sensitivity. Good-quality aortic arch studies acquired with a gated fast TOF technique depicting the origins of the carotid and subclavian arteries can be obtained, but no technique has systematically and reliably pictured the origin of the vertebral arteries (Fig. 23-43). In the appropriate clinical setting, it is important to investigate and detect lesions at this site because they are amenable to treatment by percutaneous angioplasty. It is hoped that the use of first-pass Gd MRA will improve the sensitivity and specificity for detecting occlusive disease of the extracranial circulation at the aortic arch level, but systematic and comparative studies are not yet available[20] (Figs. 23-44 and 23-45). Subclavian artery steal phenomenon is best demonstrated by a directional-weighted phase-contrast acquisition to depict reversed flow in the vertebral artery.[13]

Intracranial Circulation

Intracranial Aneurysms

The use of MRA in the detection of intracranial aneurysms was greeted with enthusiasm by neuroimagers. Several studies have been published on this subject.[54–58] An early study by blinded readers utilizing 3D TOF claimed a sensitivity of 67 percent for MRA alone and 86 percent for MRA plus individual sections plus spin-echo studies in aneurysms mostly greater than 5 mm in size.[54] A more recent study by blinded readers reported a much lower overall sensitivity of 55.6 percent despite using a high-resolution 3D TOF technique.[59] Prospectively in this study, the overall sensitivity for 3D PCA was even lower, at 44.4 percent. Size was considered critical: for aneurysms greater than 5 mm, the sensitivity was 87 percent for 3D TOF MRA and 75 percent for 3D PC MRA, whereas for aneurysms smaller than 5 mm, the sensitivity was 9 percent for 3D TOF MRA and 0 percent for 3D PC MRA (Figs. 23-46 and 23-47). Retrospectively, all but 2-mm aneurysms (25 of 27) were identified in this study. Adding MTC and ramped RF pulses to 3D TOF MRA raises the sensitivity for aneurysms smaller than 5 mm to about 71 percent.[60]

Intracranial aneurysms occur in 1 to 14 percent of the population,[61] presenting most commonly as subarachnoid hemorrhage, a condition associated with high mor-

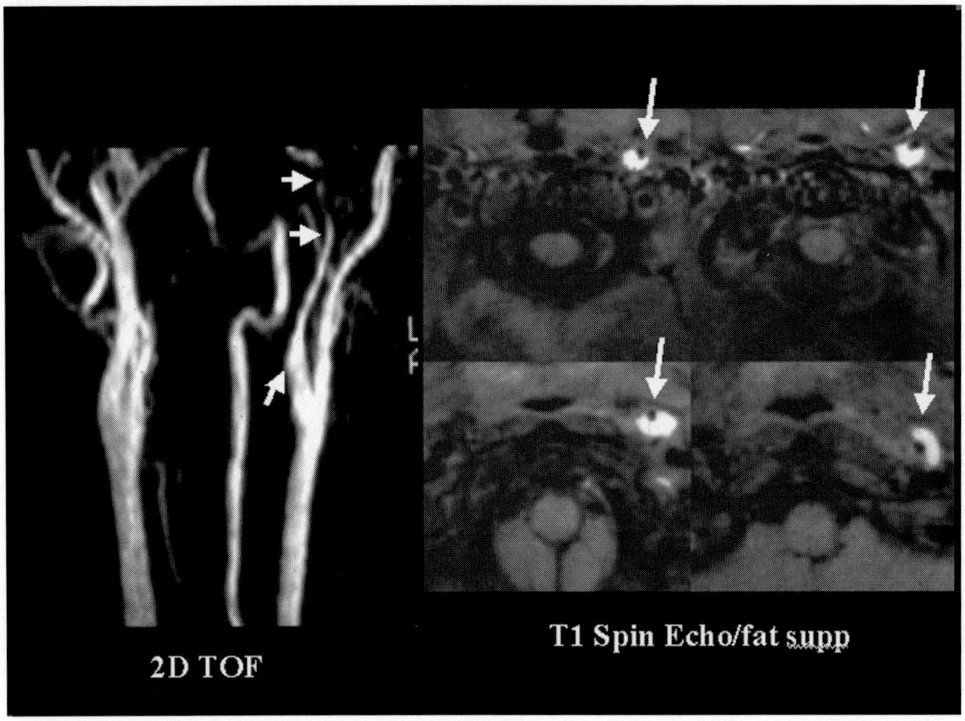

Figure 23-42
Carotid dissection shown on 2D TOF MRA as a long, tapered segment of stenosis (short arrows). In this T1-weighted spin-echo image with fat suppression, the arrows point to a narrow lumen (dark flow void) surrounded by subintimal clot, which appears bright (methemoglobin).

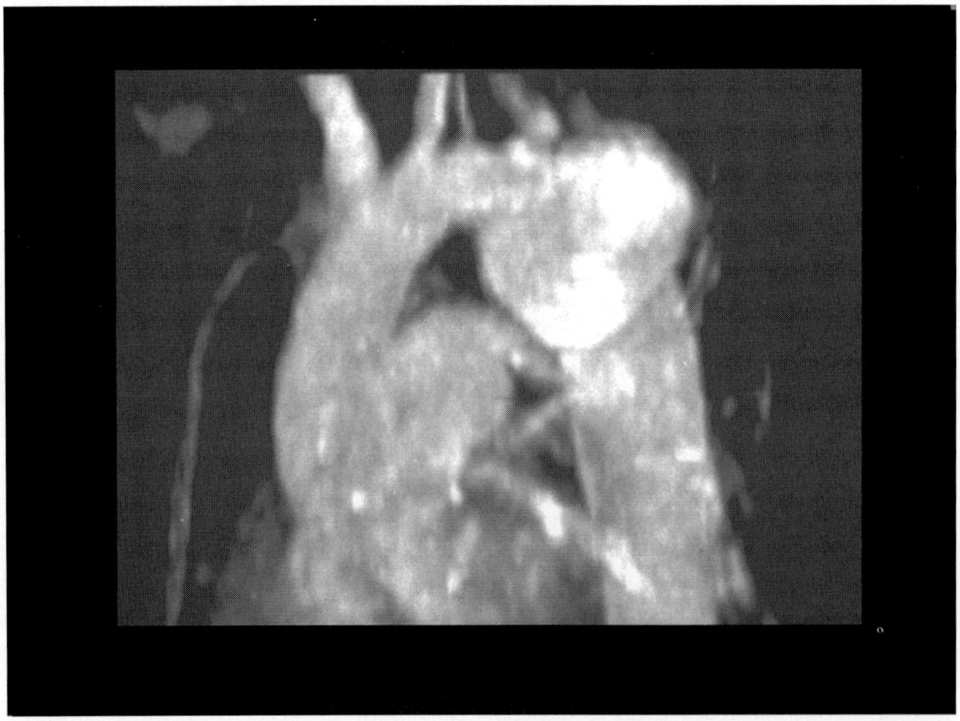

Figure 23-43
Aortic arch aneurysm shown by gated 2D TOF MRA, acquisition time 14 min.

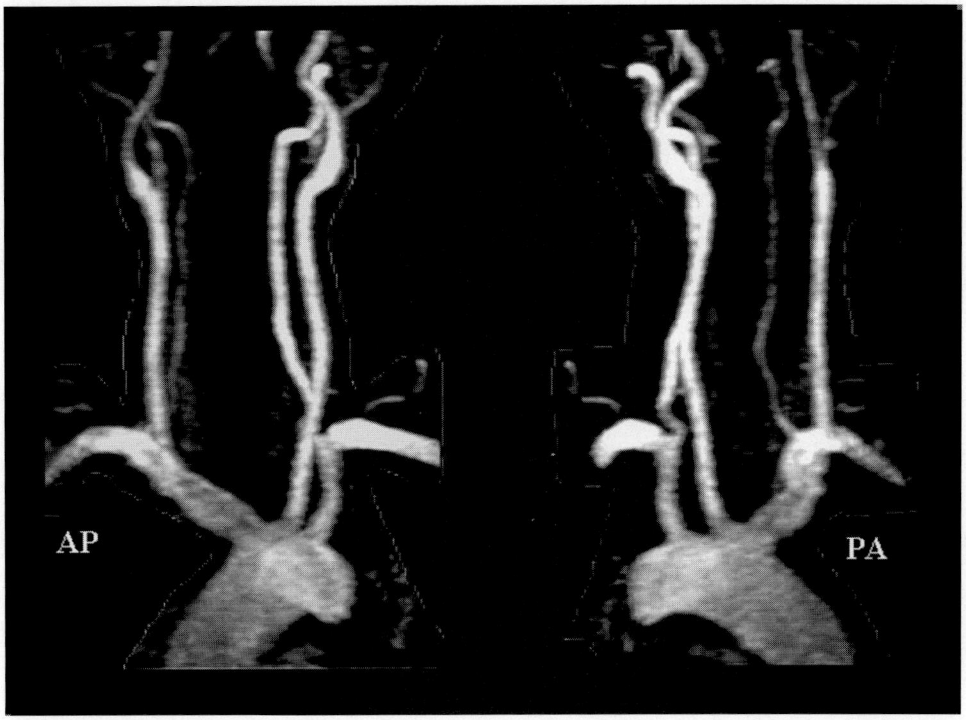

Figure 23-44
First pass gadolinium-enhanced 3D TOF MRA of the aortic arch and brachiocephalic vessels, normal study, acquisition time 7 s.

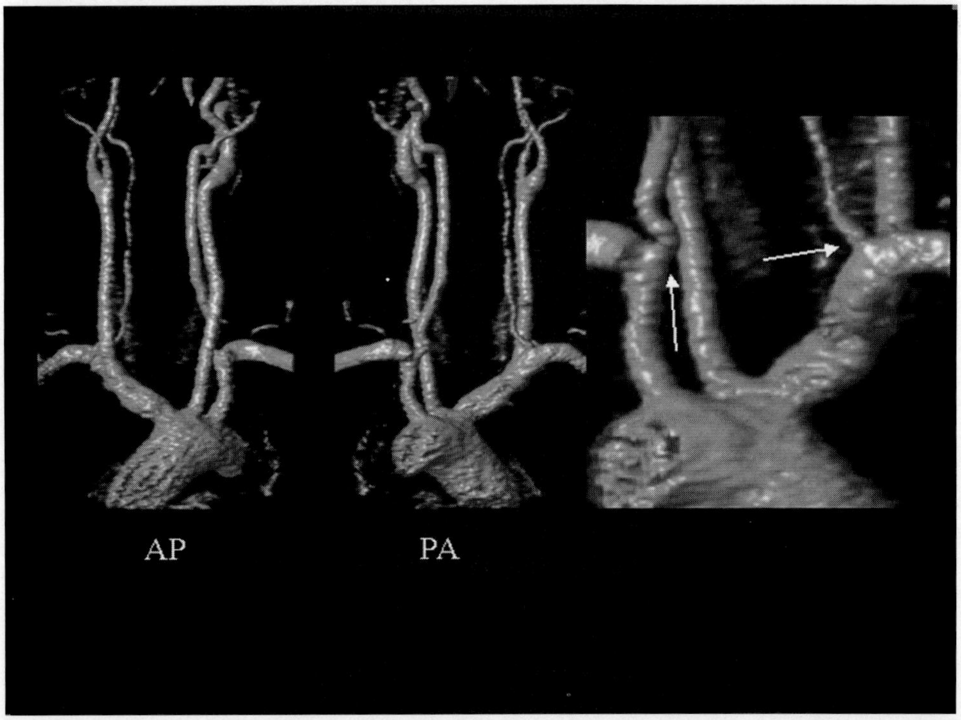

Figure 23-45 (Plate 49)
Volume-rendered display of normal first-pass gadolinium-enhanced 3D TOF MRA of the aortic arch in the same case as depicted in Fig. 23-44. Note the clear depiction of the vertebral artery origins (arrows).

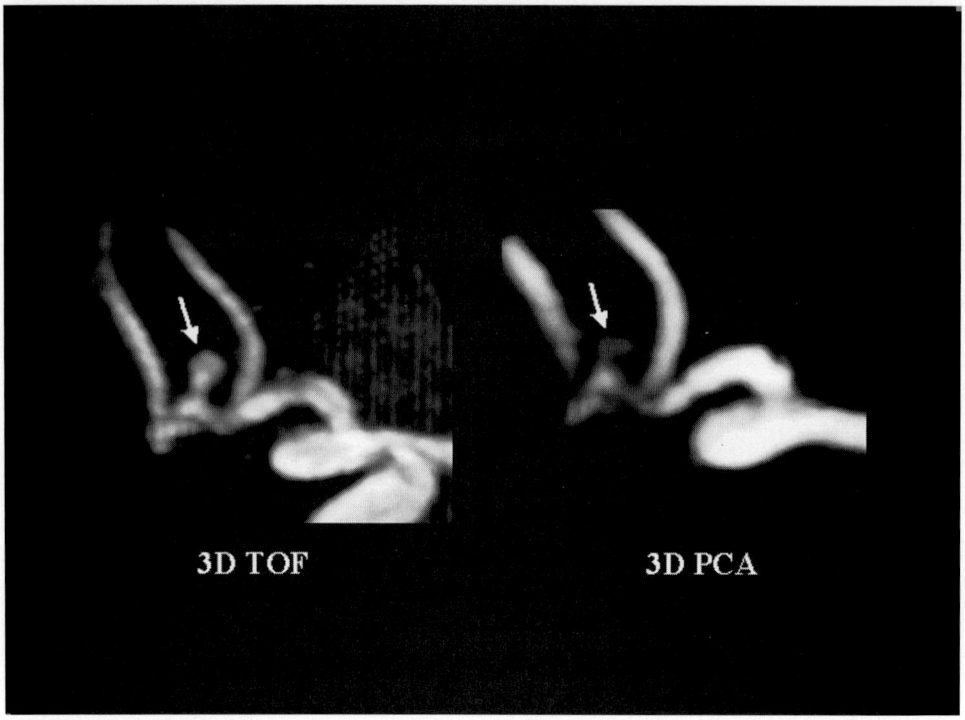

Figure 23-46
Anterior communicating artery aneurysm, 6 mm, well demonstrated by 3D TOF MRA. In 3D PCA, the aneurysm is poorly depicted. For small aneurysms (less than 5 mm), PCA has poor sensitivity.

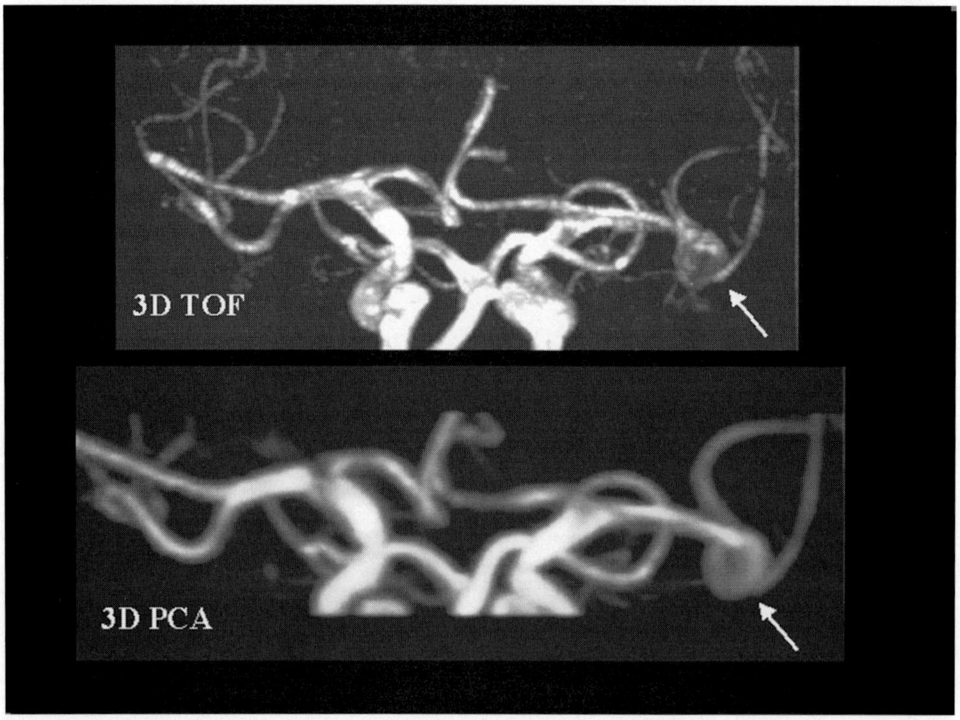

Figure 23-47
Large left MCA bifurcation aneurysm as shown by 3D TOF MRA. The same aneurysm is shown slightly better by 3D PCA with velocity encoding at 30 cm/s. Better visualization of large aneurysms by 3D PCA in some cases is attributed to less saturation effect in phase-contrast acquisitions.

bidity and mortality rates. What role does MRA play in patients with subarachnoid hemorrhage? Initially none, given that (1) patients with subarachnoid hemorrhage are best treated by careful monitoring in a neurosurgical intensive care unit, (2) all will require a formal angiogram before contemplating surgery, and (3) the sensitivity of MRA for detecting intracranial aneurysms is lower than that of the gold standard, catheter angiography.

Patients who stabilize and who have had negative catheter angiogram results may then undergo MRI and MRA as part of their workup. This may change, however, with the introduction of fluid-attenuated inversion recovery (FLAIR), a T2-weighted acquisition method that appears more sensitive than CT in the detection of acute subarachnoid hemorrhage[62] (Fig. 23-48). Occasionally an aneurysm may be hidden by the parent artery, making its visualization difficult with conventional angiography, and MRA may be helpful in such cases (Figs. 23-49 through 23-53). A concern, however, remains for the small aneurysm that occasionally may not be visualized by MRA, and therefore all patients presenting with subarachnoid hemorrhage must have a conventional angiogram (Figs. 23-54, 23-55, and 23-56).

A focal parenchymal collection of subacute blood may appear bright (methemoglobin) and simulate an aneurysm in 3D TOF MRA. A PCA acquisition will help in the differentiation of stationary versus flowing blood (Figs. 23-57 and 23-58). Vessel loops can also be confused with aneurysms despite the use of multiple views and 3D rendering techniques. An MRA-based 3D volume rendering of intracranial aneurysms is useful in the presurgical planning of aneurysm surgery, since it is able to display aneurysm orientation and relationship to parent vessels better than conventional 2D biplanar conventional angiography[63] (Figs. 23-59 through 23-65).

What about patients suspected of having had subarachnoid hemorrhage (high or low suspicion) in whom the diagnosis of this event cannot be established with certainty? Choosing to do MRA instead of a catheter angiogram in this situation must take into account the high fatality rate of untreated ruptured intracranial aneurysm and that missing it is a life-threatening situation. In view of the aforementioned sensitivity of MRA for detecting intracranial aneurysms, one can safely state that the technique cannot exclude aneurysms in this clinical category. Conversely, MRA is a useful technique for detecting unruptured intracranial aneurysm in clinical conditions where its incidence is increased, such as in polycystic kidney disease. Before the advent of MRA, the incidence of intracranial aneurysm in polycystic kidney disease from postmortem findings was estimated to vary from 7 to 40 percent. An MRA study of 93 patients with polycystic kidney disease puts the overall incidence at 11.7 percent and the incidence for patients with a family history of aneurysms at 25.8 percent.

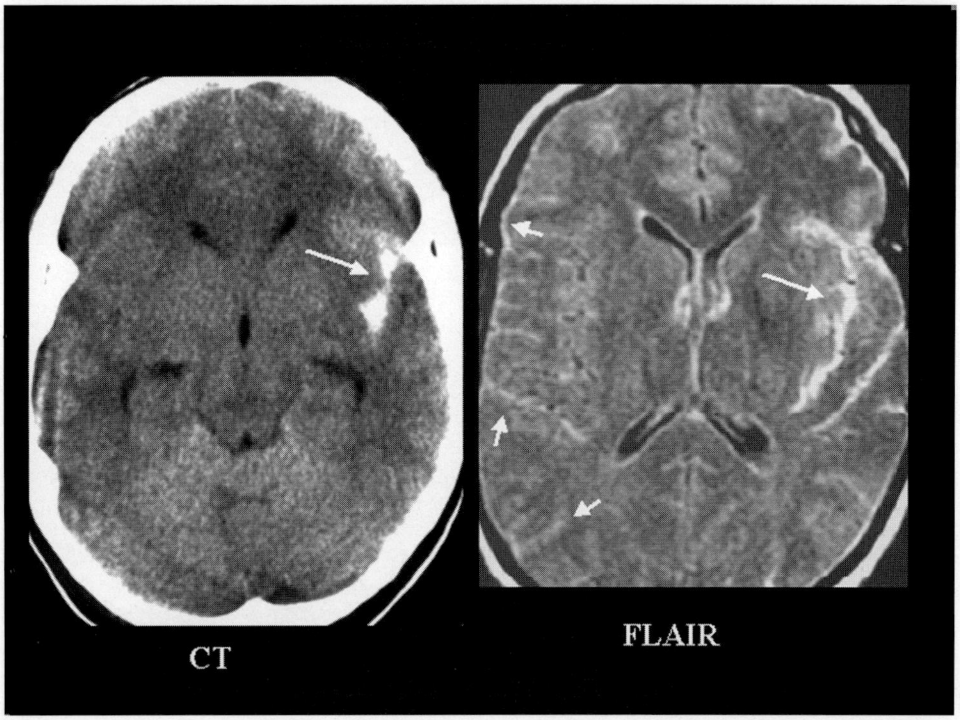

Figure 23-48

Acute subarachnoid hemorrhage presenting on CT as a clot in the left sylvian fissure. Blood in the left sylvian fissure is just as well demonstrated by fluid-attenuated inversion recovery (FLAIR). FLAIR is more sensitive than CT in detection of acute subarachnoid hemorrhage. The short arrows in the FLAIR image point to blood in the subarachnoid space that was not visualized by CT.

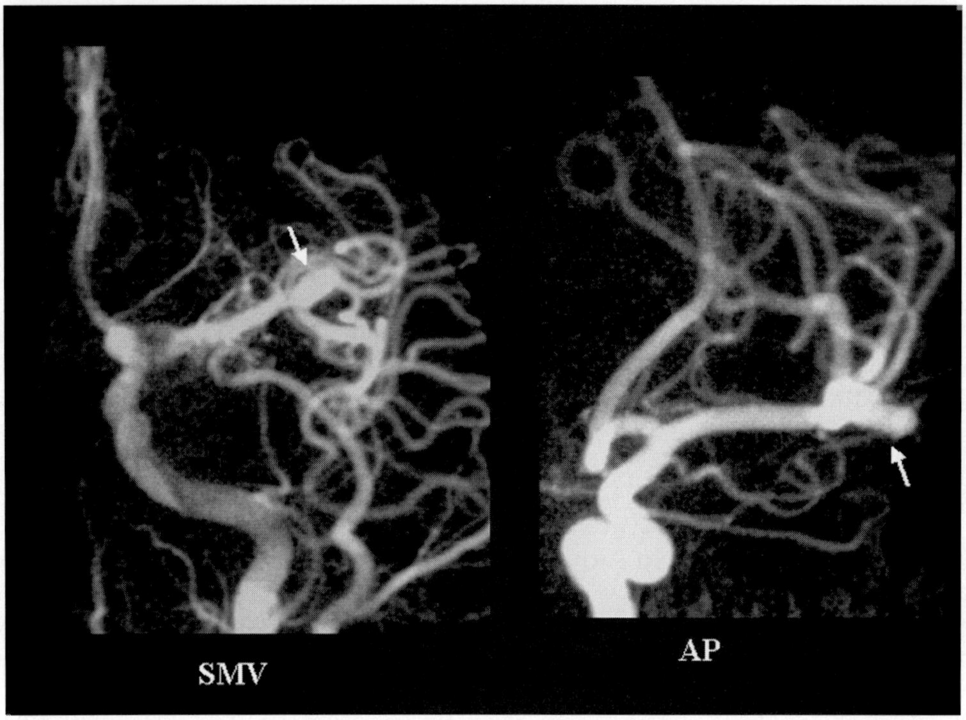

Figure 23-49
Conventional angiogram of the same patient as depicted in Fig. 23-48. Submental vertex and AP views demonstrate a sizable left MCA bifurcation aneurysm (arrows) in this left-selective common carotid injection.

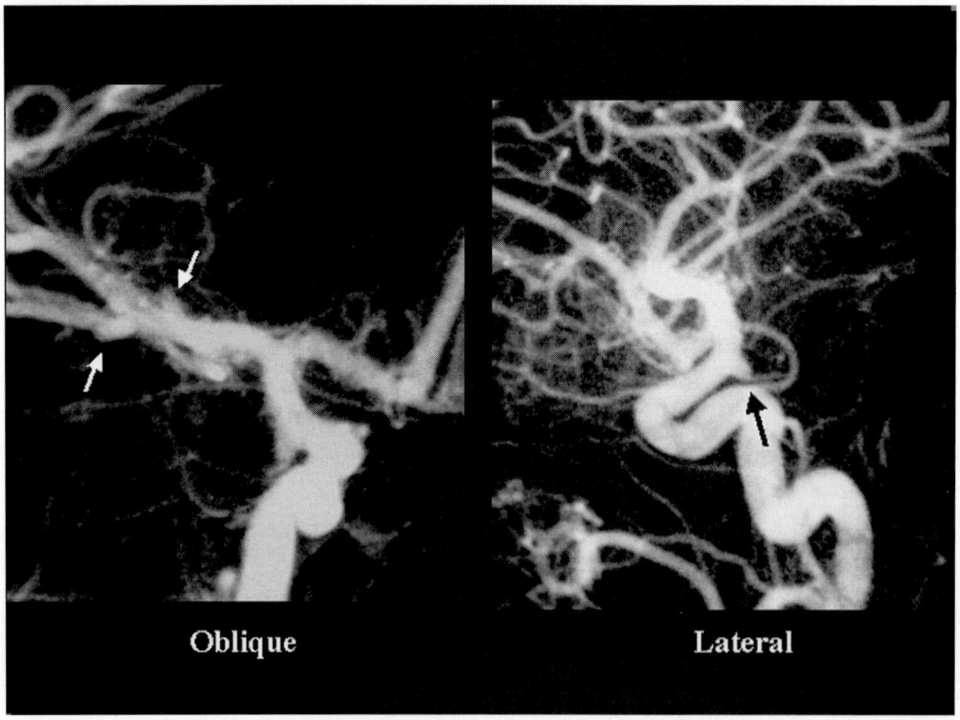

Figure 23-50
Right carotid injection, oblique and lateral views, in the same patient as depicted in Figs. 23-48 and 23-49. The short arrows in the oblique views point to two small aneurysms in the region of the MCA bifurcation. The black arrow in the lateral views shows infundibular dilatation of the posterior cerebral artery. No other aneurysms were clearly identified in the conventional angiogram.

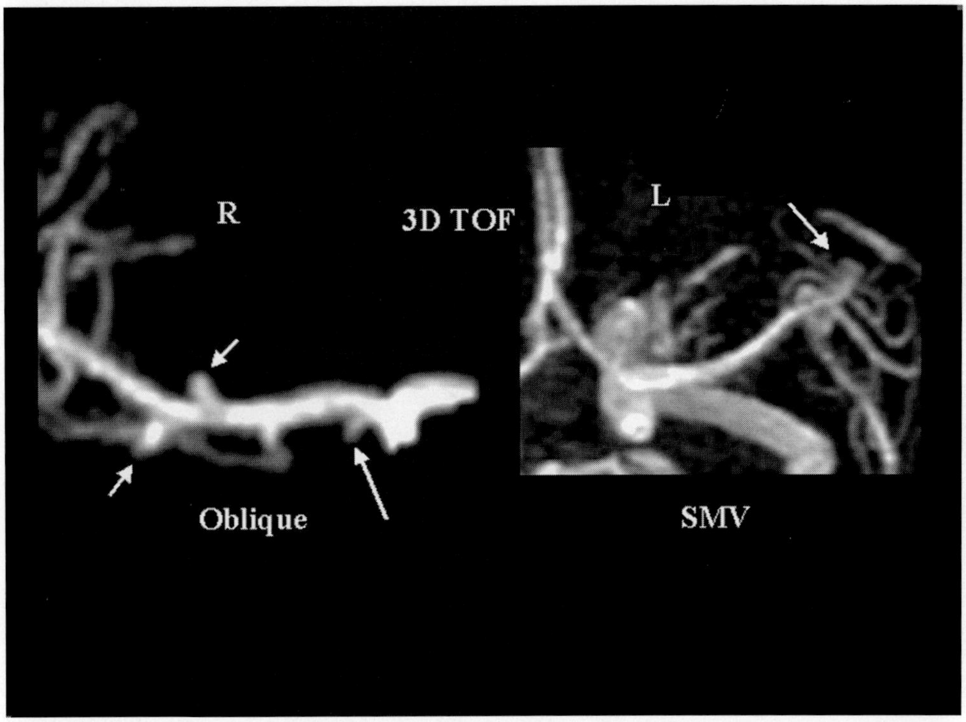

Figure 23-51

3D TOF MRA of the right internal carotid artery and the MCA in the same patient as depicted in Figs. 23-48 through 23-50. In oblique view, short arrows point to small aneurysms in the region of the MCA bifurcation as detected by conventional angiogram. Long arrow in oblique view points to aneurysm behind right internal carotid which was not clearly detected by conventional angiogram. Left SMV view shows large aneurysm of the left MCA bifurcation which bled (arrow).

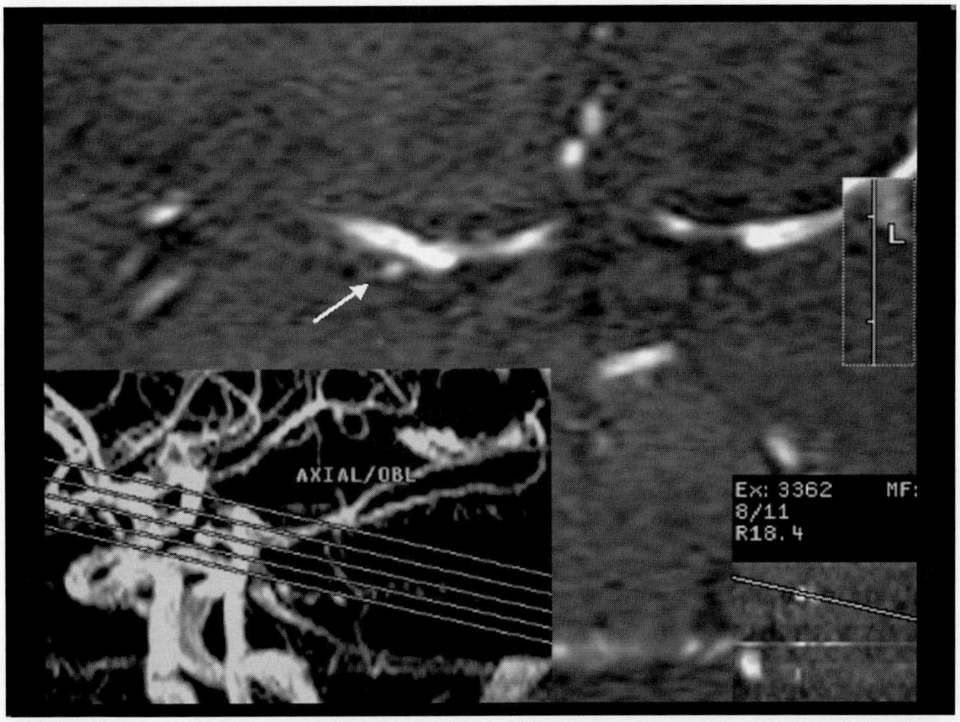

Figure 23-52

Source views, axial plane for 3D TOF MRA in the same patient as depicted in Figs. 23-48 through 23-51. The arrow points to an aneurysm in the region of the right upper internal carotid artery, as shown by the long arrow in the right oblique view of Fig. 23-51. The inset image in the lower left corner illustrates the plane of reconstruction for source views.

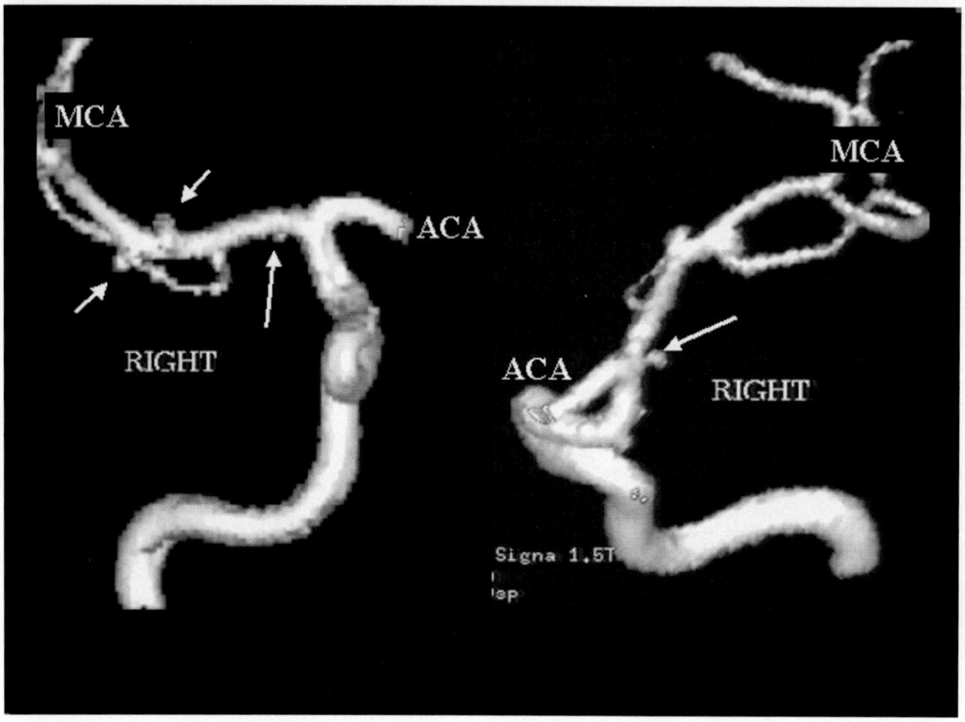

Figure 23-53
The same patient as depicted in Figs. 23-48 through 23-52. Surface-rendered reconstructions of the right carotid artery and intracranial branches. Short arrows point to small aneurysms in the region of the right MCA bifurcation. Long arrows point to a small aneurysm behind the right internal carotid that was not visualized by conventional angiogram. All aneurysms were found to be present at the time of surgery. 3D volume surface-rendered reconstructions are useful in displaying small aneurysms that may be hidden by the parent artery in the limited number of views of conventional angiography.

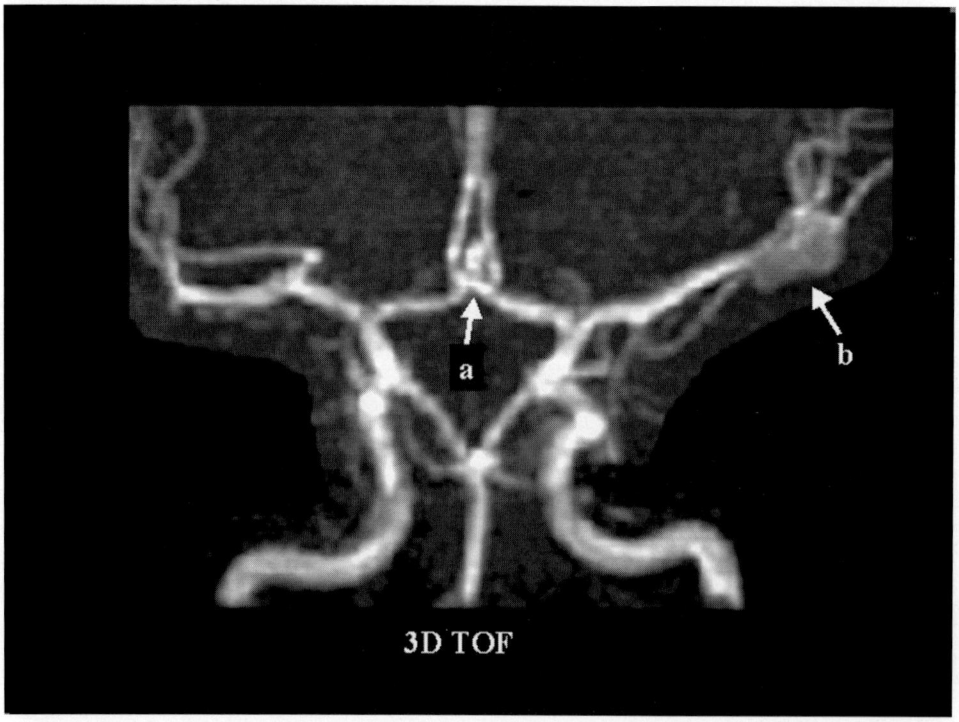

Figure 23-54
Multiple aneurysms. 3D TOF single-slab MRA shows a small anterior communicating aneurysm (arrow a*) and a large MCA aneurysm on the left (arrow* b*). No other aneurysms are seen in this view.*

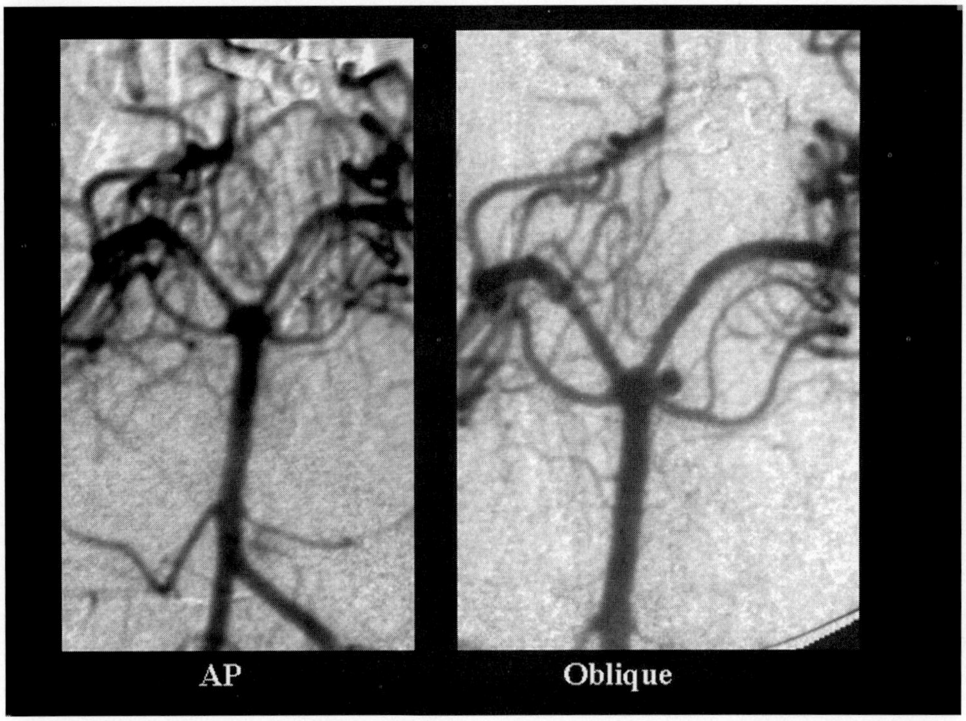

Figure 23-55
Conventional angiogram, AP and slightly oblique views of basilar artery, showing small aneurysm at the space between the posterior cerebral and the superior cerebellar artery on the left (black arrow) in the same patient as depicted in Fig. 23-54.

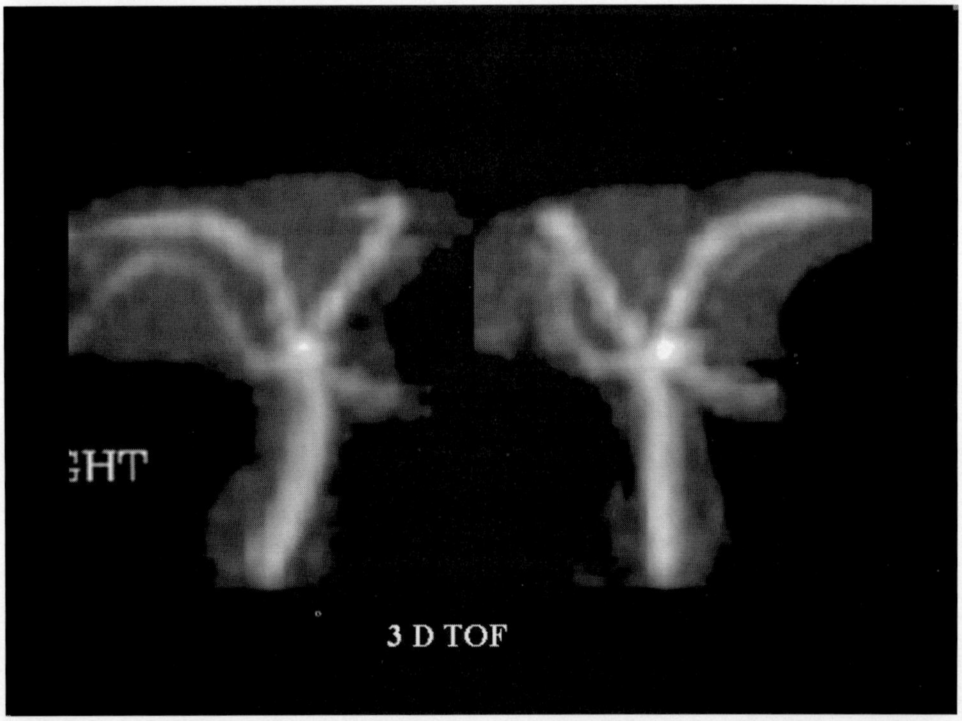

Figure 23-56
3D TOF MIP reconstruction of the basilar artery fails to show definite aneurysmal formation, as demonstrated by conventional angiography in Fig. 23-55. The catheter angiogram is still the gold standard for imaging intracranial aneurysms.

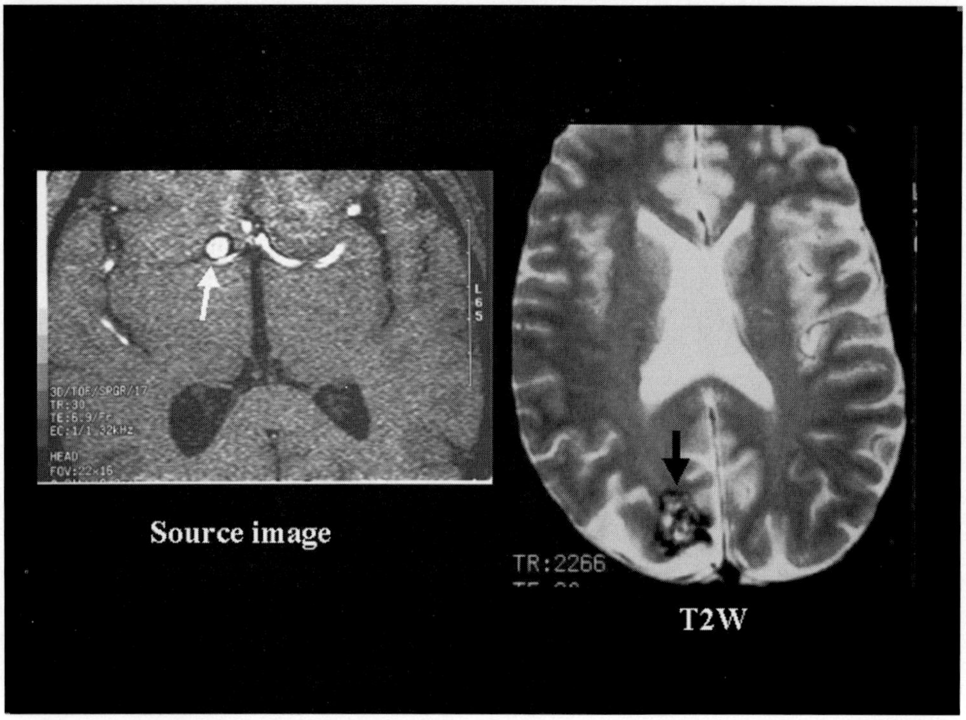

Figure 23-57

Subacute hemorrhage mimicking an aneurysm. The subacute hemorrhage shows as a roundish area of brightness (methemoglobin) near the MCA trunk in the source image (white arrow). The hemorrhage was from cavernous angioma, seen also in right parieto-occipital junction, as shown by T2-weighted imaging (black arrow).

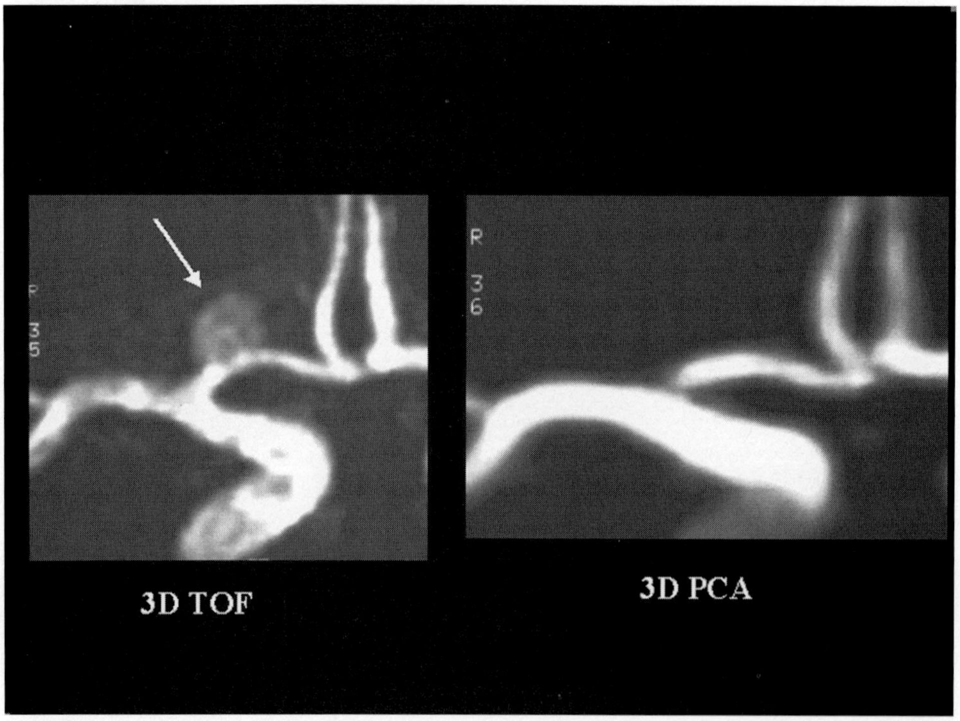

Figure 23-58

Subacute hemorrhage mimicking an aneurysm on 3D TOF MRA (white arrow) in the same case as depicted in Fig. 23-57. 3D PCA shows no evidence of aneurysmal formation owing to subtraction of background, including stationary blood.

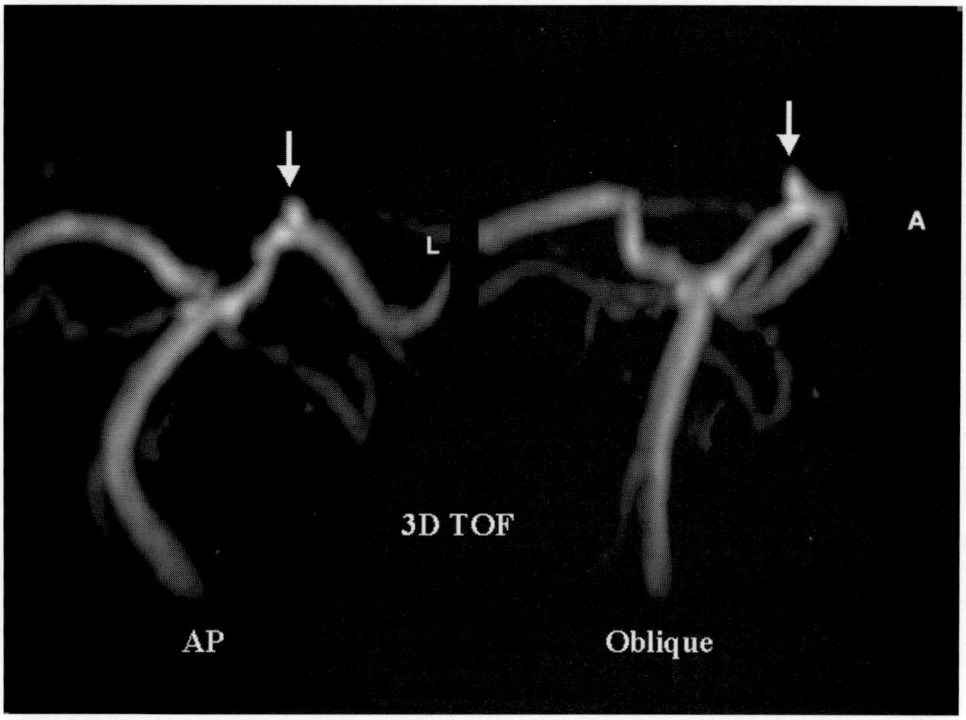

Figure 23-59
AP and oblique views of a single-slab 3D TOF MRA showing an aneurysm in the P2 segment of the posterior cerebral artery on the left (arrows). It is important to differentiate an aneurysm of this size from a tightly wound vessel loop.

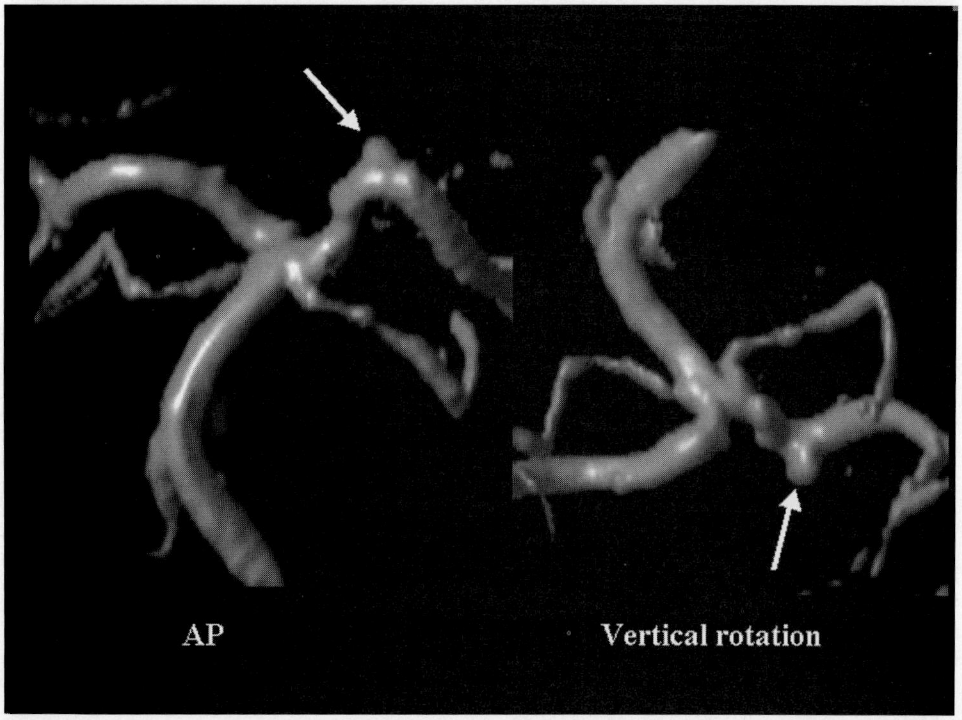

Figure 23-60 (Plate 50)
The volume-rendered reconstruction from 3D TOF MRA, AP view, shows an aneurysm (arrow) in the P2 segment of the left posterior cerebral artery in the same patient as depicted in Fig. 23-59. The vessel has been flipped in the vertical plane, and it continues to show aneurysmal dilatation at the P2 segment on the left (arrow). This aneurysm was confirmed at the time of surgery.

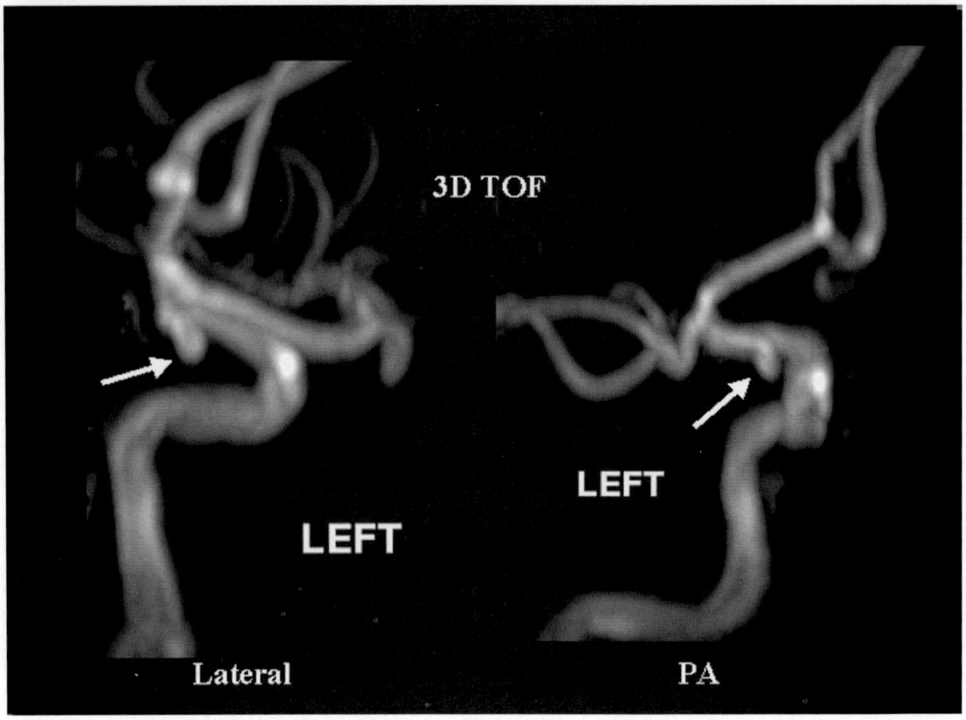

Figure 23-61
Vessel loop mimicking an aneurysm in the same patient as depicted in Figs. 23-59 and 23-60. 3D TOF MRA of the left carotid artery and the intracranial branches. In the lateral view, there is a possible aneurysm formation in the region of the posterior communicating artery (arrow). The PA view continues to show a possible aneurysmal formation in the region of the posterior communicating artery (arrow).

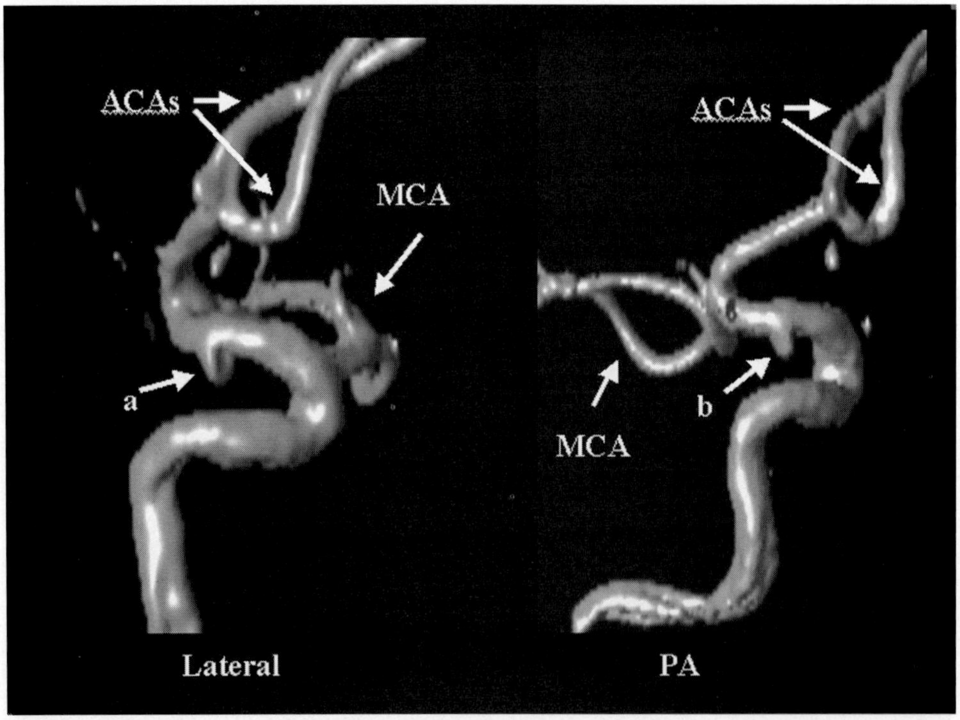

Figure 23-62 (Plate 51)
Vessel loop mimicking an aneurysm in the same patient as depicted in Figs. 23-59 through 23-61. In this volume-rendered reconstruction from 3D TOF MRA of the left carotid and intracranial branches, arrow a *in the left view and arrow* b *in the PA view continue to show a possible aneurysm in the region of the posterior communicating take-off. This was proven to be a tightly wound posterior communicating artery at time of surgery.*

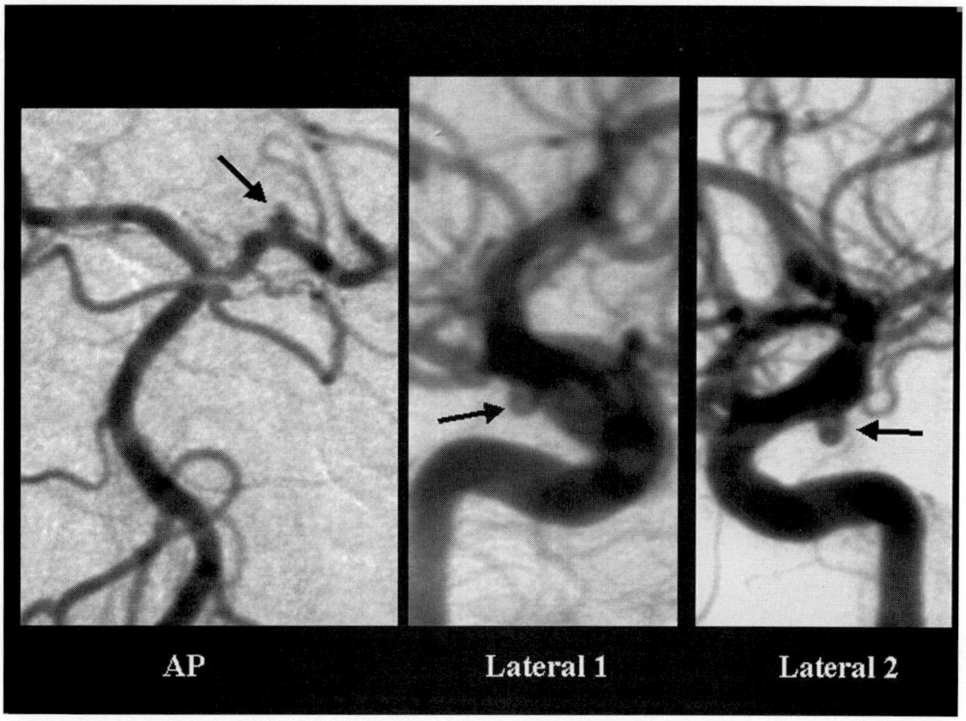

Figure 23-63

Vessel loop mimicking an aneurysm in the same patient as depicted in Figs. 23-59 through 23-62. In this catheter angiogram, the AP view shows an aneurysm in the P2 segment on the left (black arrow). Lateral view 1 of the left internal carotid artery shows a vessel loop, which could not be completely differentiated from an aneurysm at the time of conventional angiography. Lateral view 2 of the internal carotid artery also shows an aneurysm-like structure in the region of the posterior communicating artery. At the time of angiography, this could not clearly be differentiated from a true aneurysm. It was proven at the time of surgery to be a tightly wound loop of the posterior communicating artery. Fortunately, the surgical approach was the same for definite left posterior cerebral aneurysm and possible left posterior communicating artery aneurysm.

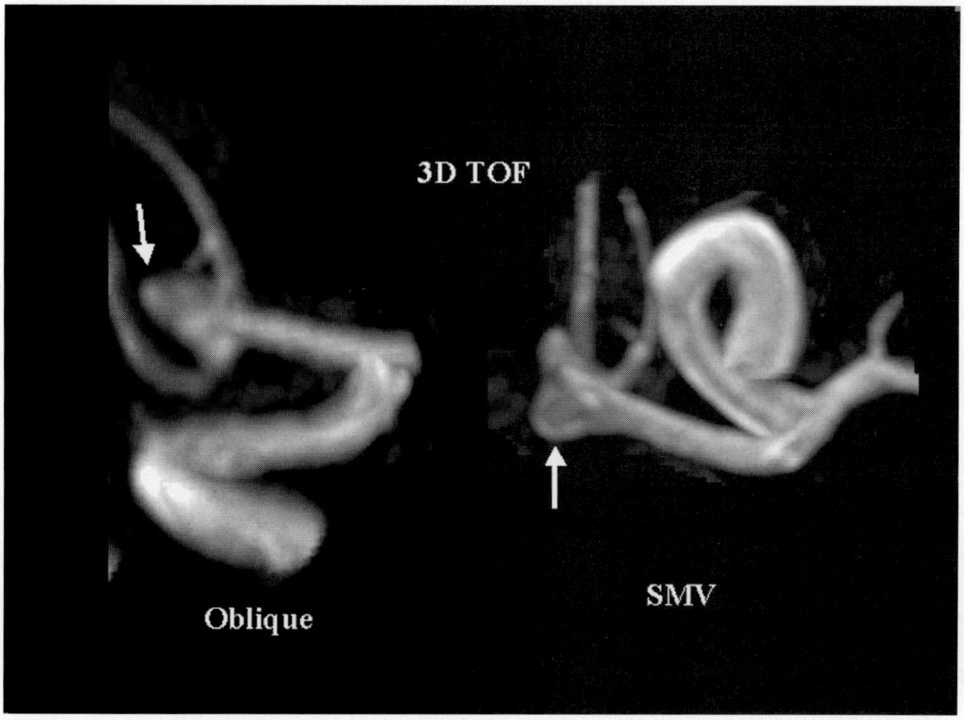

Figure 23-64

ACA aneurysm. Targeted MIP of the left carotid and anterior cerebral arteries shows an aneurysm in the region of the anterior communicating in oblique and submental vertex views.

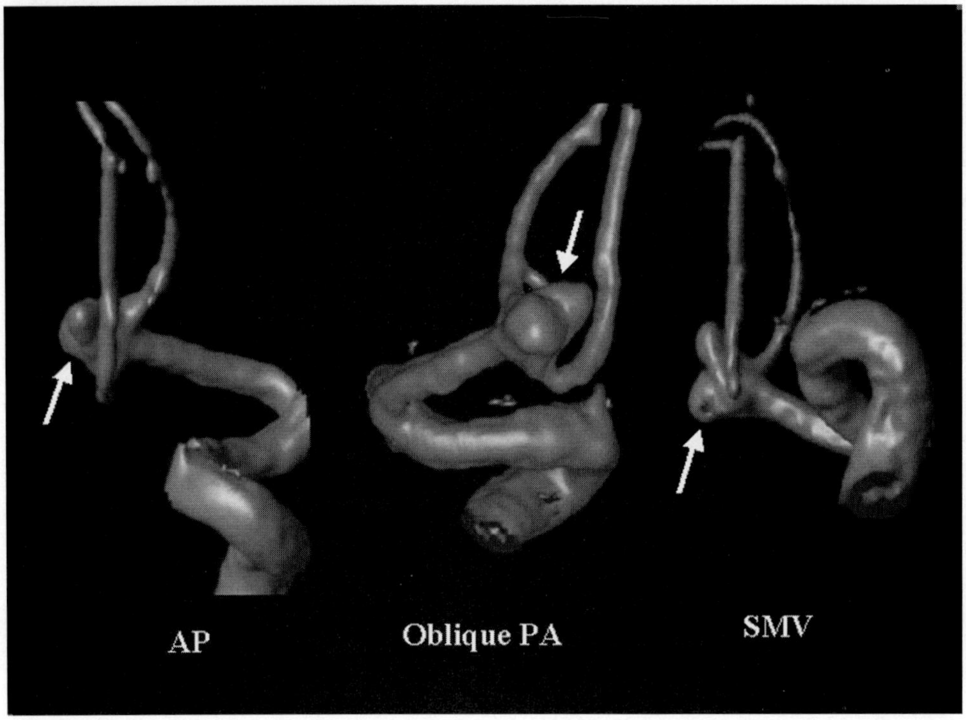

Figure 23-65 (Plate 52)
ACA aneurysm. 3D volume-rendered reconstruction from the targeted MIP of Fig. 23-64 in AP, oblique PA, and SMV views. Note that the aneurysm is clearly defined as bilobed, and its precise relationship to both A2 segments of the anterior cerebral arteries is well defined in this reconstruction.

Improvements in MRA spatial resolution and shorter echo times with new high-performance gradients have raised the technique's sensitivity, but it does not yet equal that of conventional catheter angiography and therefore it cannot replace it completely in the presurgical planning of intracranial aneurysm.

Vascular Malformations

Intracranial vascular malformations include four basic types: arteriovenous malformations (AVMs), cavernous angiomas, venous angiomas, and capillary telangiectasias. Of these, only AVMs are detected by MRA consistently and will be the subject of this discussion. The other three malformations are more likely to show in regular MRIs than in MRAs.

Brain parenchyma AVMs consist of a network of abnormal vasculature made up of arterial feeders, collaterals, an AVM nidus, and enlarged draining venous channels without an intervening capillary bed. Eighty-five percent are supratentorial and 15 percent are infratentorial. Among the vascular malformations, AVMs are the most likely to become symptomatic, with 50 percent of patients presenting with acute hemorrhage and 25 percent presenting with seizures.[65] There is a 2 to 4 percent cumulative yearly risk for hemorrhage, with significant mortality and morbidity for each hemorrhagic event.[66] These lesions are treated aggressively by surgical excision, endovascular therapy, and radiotherapy alone or in a combined approach. An important step in the therapeutic planning for AVMs is the angiographic study of the lesion to define the vascular nidus, feeding arteries, draining veins, and associated aneurysms. All these abnormalities can be precisely defined only by catheter angiography. Both MRA and MRI will show a tangle of vessels, or nidus, but in difficult cases they cannot define all relevant features with sufficient clarity to obviate the need for a catheter angiography study (Fig. 23-66). It is possible to separate arterial feeders and draining veins in a general sense by utilizing 2D slab PCA with various velocity-encoding settings (Figs. 23-67 and 23-68). Whether or not this technique will consistently find all arterial feeders and draining veins remains to be determined. Conversely, if one adheres to the theory that AVMs with a nidus smaller than 3 cm are best treated with radiotherapy,[67,68] then demonstrating the nidus with a MRI/MRA combined study may be the only diagnostic test required.

The sensitivity of PCA to slow flow can be exploited in the depiction of spinal cord AVMs (Fig. 23-69). Spinal arteriovenous (AV) fistulas can also be demonstrated by MRI and MRA (Fig. 23-70). Phase-contrast cine-MRA has been used to quantify increased flow rates in parent arteries of AVM feeders.[69]

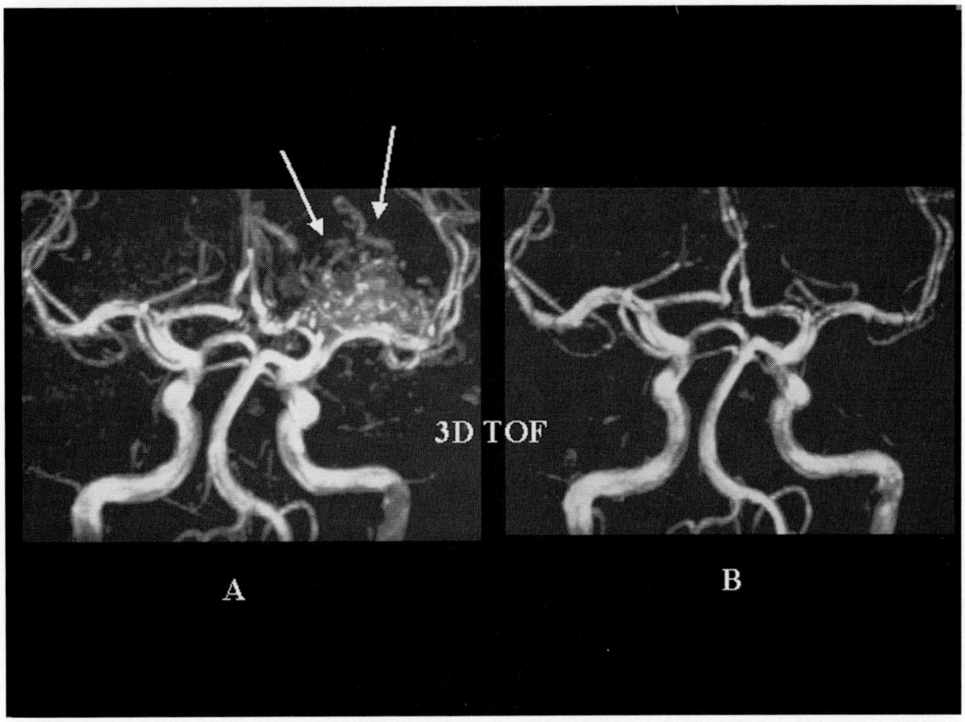

Figure 23-66

(A) *Large deep left hemispheric AVM, shown by 3D TOF MRA as tangled vessels (arrows). Feeders and draining vessels are not individually shown.* **(B)** *The same patient 2 years later after gamma-knife treatment. 3D TOF MRA shows that the AVM has obliterated.*

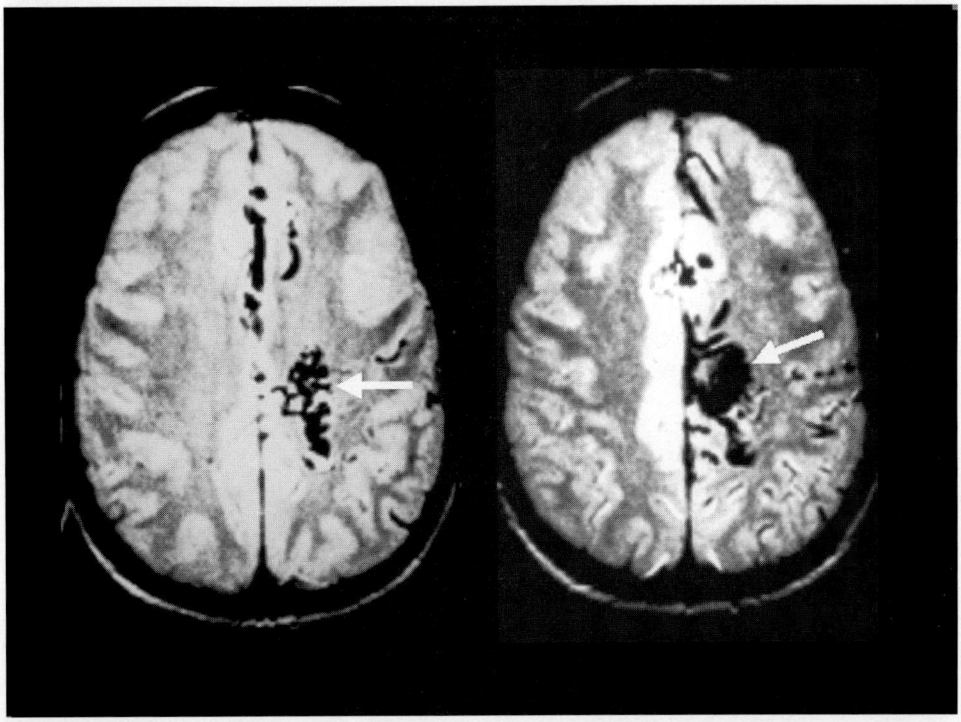

Figure 23-67

Proton-density MRI slices showing a mesioparietal AVM as a latticework of flow void spaces (arrows).

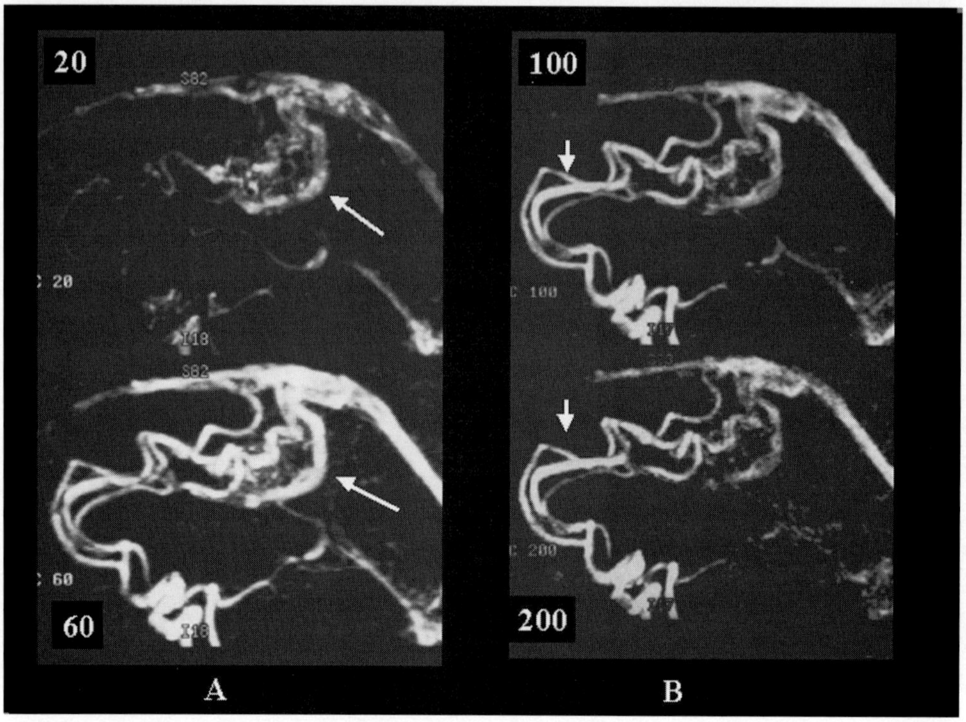

Figure 23-68

(A) *AVM in the mesioparietal lobe in the same patient as depicted in Fig. 23-66. Sagittal thick-slab 2D PCA had* V_{enc} *set at 20 and 60 cm/s, to emphasize draining veins (long arrows).* **(B)** *Increasing the* V_{enc} *to 1200 and 200 cm/s emphasizes arterial feeders (short arrows).*

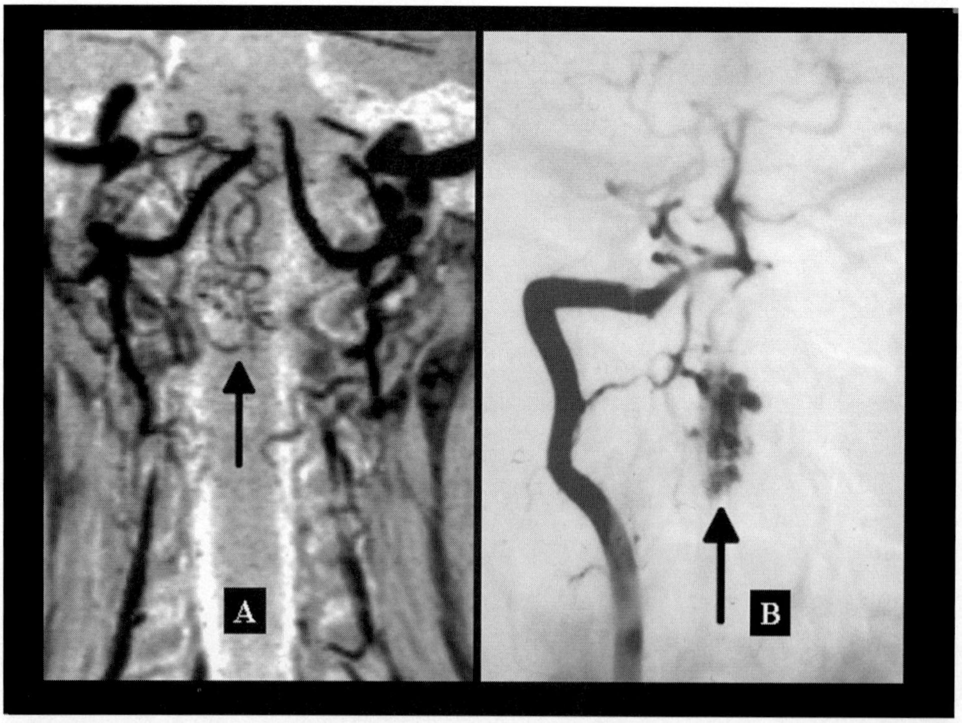

Figure 23-69

(A) *Glomus AVM of the cervical spinal cord. In this postcontrast 3D PCA, a glomus AVM is shown as a tangle of vessels fed from the right vertebral artery branch (arrow).* **(B)** *Right vertebral contrast angiogram showing nidus of glomus AVM and feeders from right vertebral artery (arrow).*

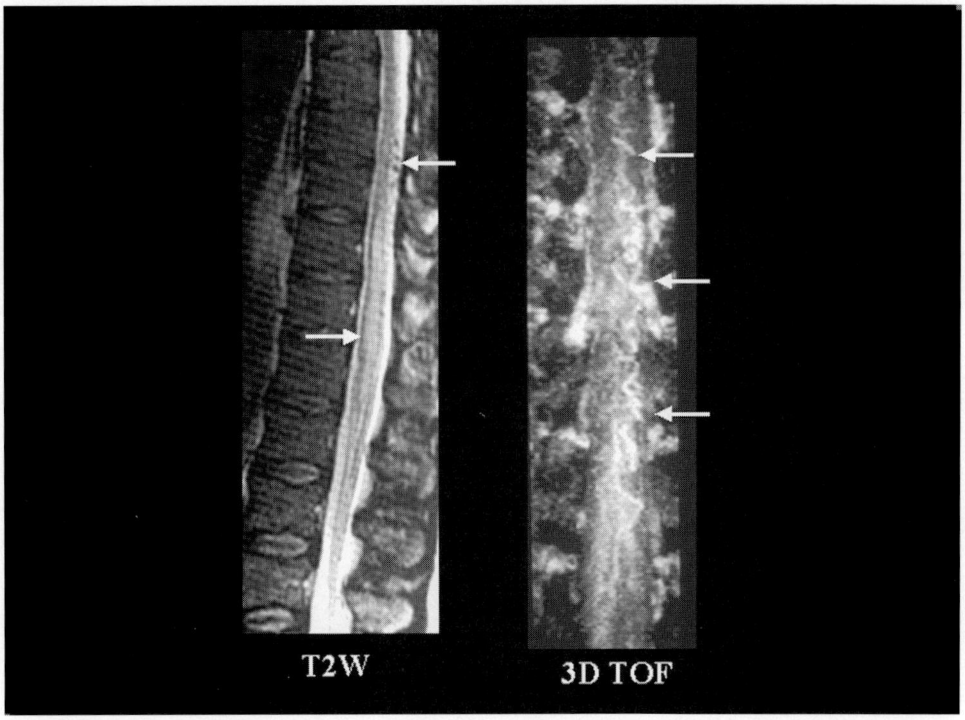

Figure 23-70
AV fistula. T2-weighted sagittal MRI shows hyperintensity involving the lower thoracic cord from congestive myelopathy caused by an AV fistula of the lower thoracic cord (arrows). Postcontrast 3D TOF MRA shows dilated venous channels from the AV fistula overlying the surface of the cord (arrows).

Occlusive Disease

Several studies have reported on the ability of MRA to demonstrate intracranial occlusive disease.[70–73] Since the 3D TOF technique is shorter in acquisition time and offers greater resolution compared to PCA, it has been the dominant method employed in patients with intracranial arterial occlusive disease.

Three-dimensional TOF MRA depicts stenosis of the proximal intracranial vasculature with a tendency for overestimation, as segmental narrowing, nonvisible vessels, and decreased distal vessel signal intensity[71,74,75] (Figs. 23-71 through 23-74). Findings of embolism or atherothrombotic occlusion in MRA include cut-off vessels, nonsegmental visualization with distal visualization, and decreased signal intensity distal to the embolus[71] (Figs. 23-75, 23-76, and 23-77).

Directional-weighted phase-contrast images can show directional flow about the circle of Willis and may be used when determining patterns of collateral circulation in cases of intracranial occlusion (Figs. 23-78, 23-79, and 23-80).

From these studies it is clear that MRA can consistently demonstrate intracranial arterial occlusive disease and that in the appropriate clinical setting it is reasonable to assume that there is a relationship between imaging and clinical findings. However, because artifacts in MRA can mimic pathologic conditions that simulate intracranial arterial occlusive disease, caution should be exercised in the interpretation of these images. For instance, in a significant number of cases, there is signal loss noted at the petrous and siphon carotid regions from magnetic susceptibility and turbulence that mimics stenosis at these sites respectively (Figs. 23-81, 23-82, and 23-83).

Since the technique employed has a direct relationship to the frequency of visualization of intracranial vessels, the study's spatial resolution and other parameters will have to be scrutinized before ascribing clinical importance to an imaging finding. With voxels between 0.7 and 1.5 mm^3, one can consistently identify first- and second-order intracranial branches, provided multiple slabs are acquired to minimize saturation.[76,77] Current techniques allow for voxels as small as 0.1 mm^3, but the effect of this ultrahigh resolution on the frequency of vessel visualization has not been studied systematically. Also, the presence of motion artifact that mimics intracranial arterial occlusive disease should always be a consideration when interpreting MRIs. Despite the aforementioned limitations of the technique, a technically sound, good-quality normal intracranial MRA is of great value in the setting of ischemic cerebrovascular disease and obviates the need for invasive angiography in many instances.

The sensitivity and specificity of 3D TOF MRA for

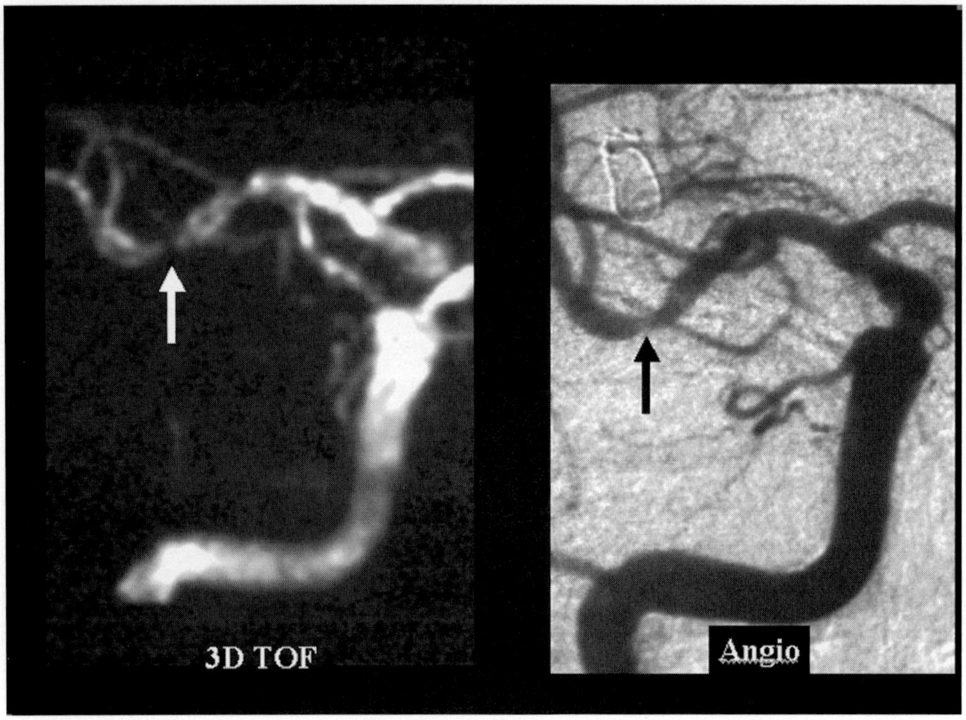

Figure 23-71
Right MCA stenosis shown by marked focal signal loss in 3D TOF MRA (white arrow). Stenosis appears severe in this technique. A conventional angiogram shows stenosis as moderate (black arrow).

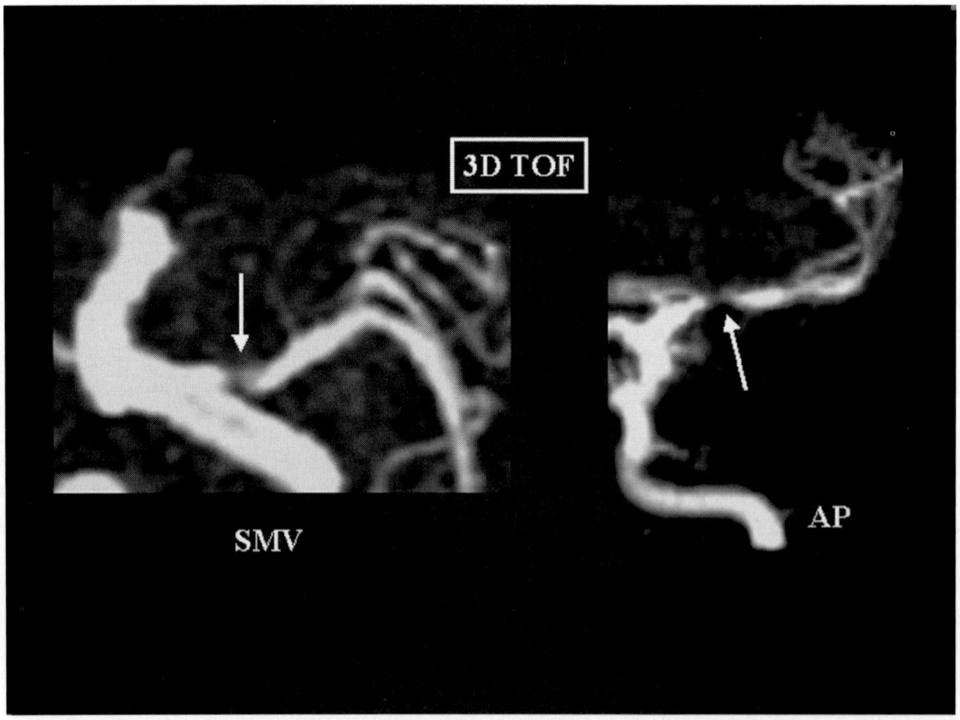

Figure 23-72
Left MCA stenosis shown in 3D TOF MRA as focal signal loss in SMV and AP views (arrows).

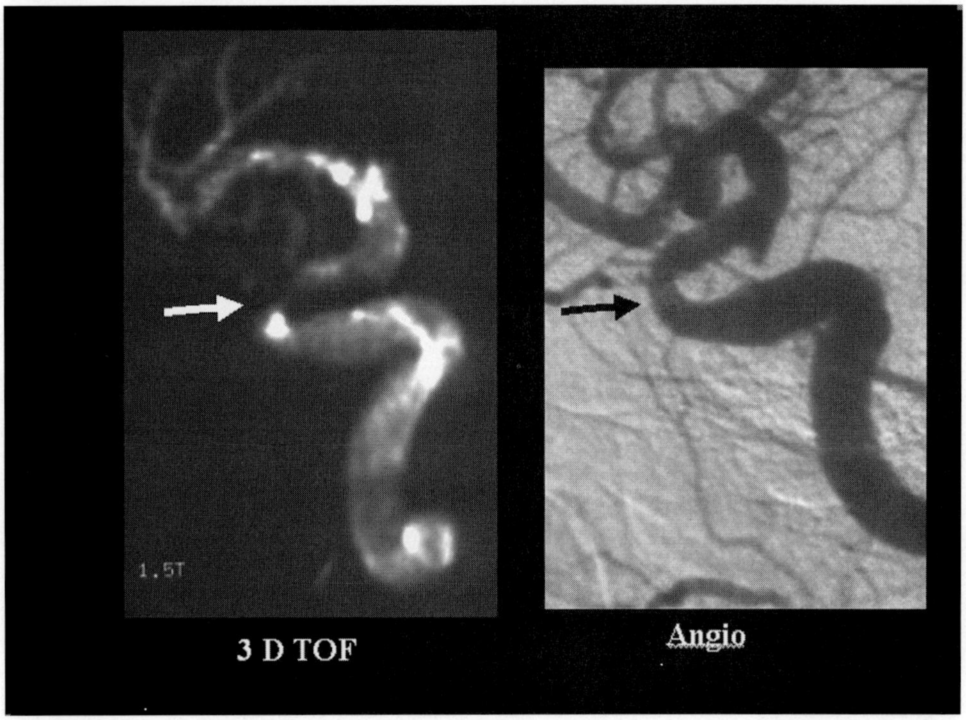

Figure 23-81
Siphon stenosis overestimated by 3D TOF MRA (white arrow) as compared to conventional angiography, where stenosis is mild (black arrow).

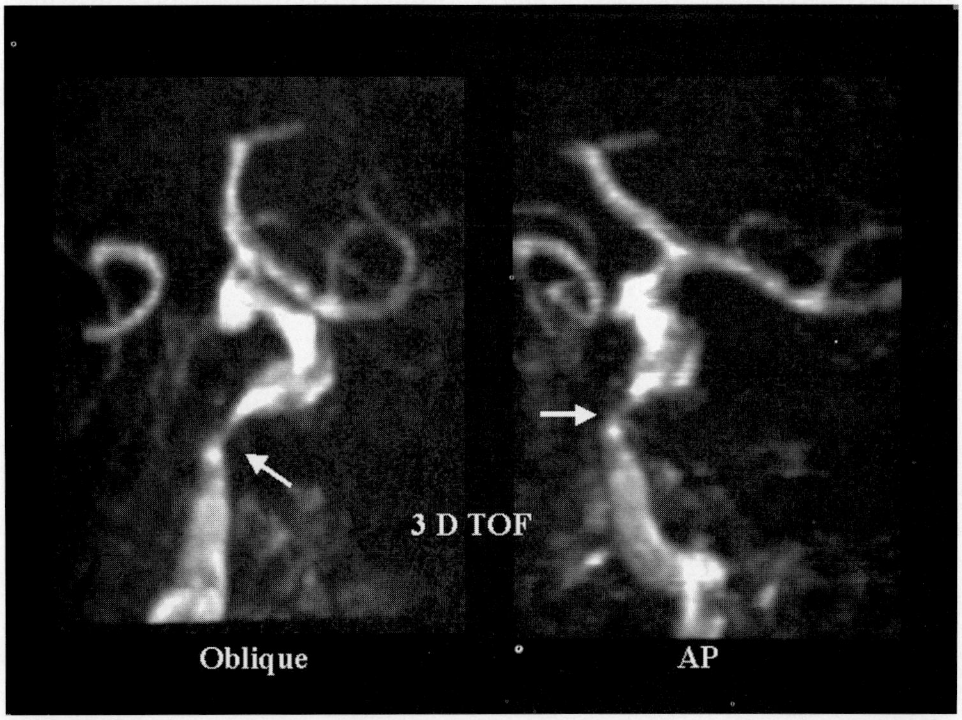

Figure 23-82
Siphon stenosis in the proximal segment shown as severe by single-slab 3D TOF MRA in oblique and AP views (arrows).

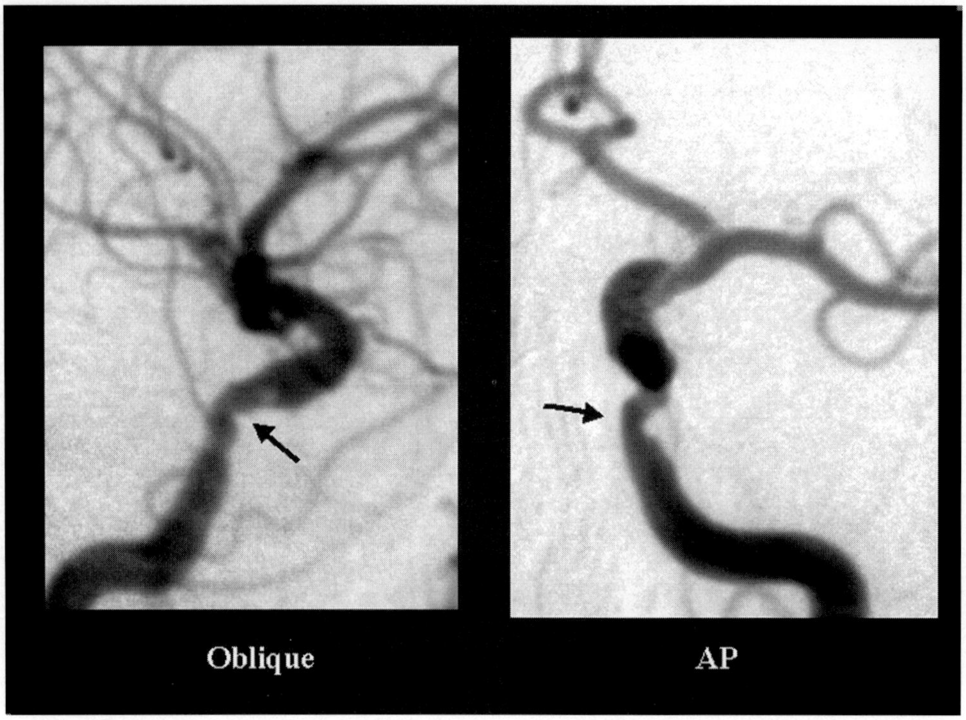

Figure 23-83

Siphon stenosis in the same patient as depicted in Fig. 23-82, shown as mild by conventional angiogram in oblique and PA views (black arrows). MRA has a tendency to overestimate stenosis in the region of the cavernous sinus and petrous carotid arteries due to turbulent flow and magnetic susceptibility, respectively, in these regions.

detecting arterial intracranial occlusive disease vary according to the vessel territory as well as the technique employed. Initial studies listed an overall sensitivity and specificity of 85 and 88 percent, respectively, for the middle cerebral artery (MCA) and 95 and 97 percent, respectively, for the intracranial internal carotid.[78] The same range has been reported in a more recent study despite the use of a higher-resolution technique with ramped RF pulses.[79] Sensitivity and specificity can be increased further if one carefully inspects the source images.[80] A sensitivity of 97 percent and specificity of 98 percent have been reported for stenocclusive disease of the distal vertebral and basilar artery trunks[81] (Figs. 23-84 and 23-85).

Intracranial venous occlusive disease is optimally evaluated by MRI and MRA.[82] Thrombus can be easily detected in MRI and absent flow documented by MRA (Figs. 23-86 through 23-92). When utilizing TOF MRA, however, a subacute thrombus that is bright (methemoglobin) can mimic flow. In this situation, a quick 2D slab PCA will demonstrate absent flow.

Table 23-4 summarizes the clinical applications of MRA, and Table 23-5 lists MRA protocols we currently utilize.

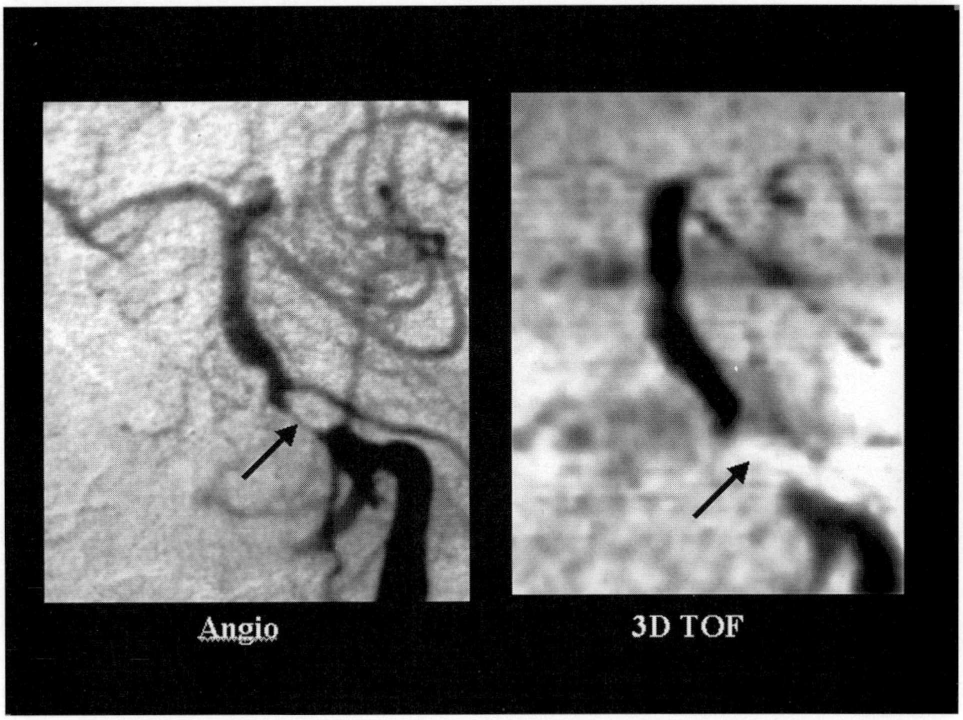

Figure 23-84
Severe inferior basilar artery stenosis shown as a string sign on a conventional angiogram (arrow). 3D TOF MRA depicts focal stenosis as signal void, indicative of very slow flow and severe stenosis (arrow).

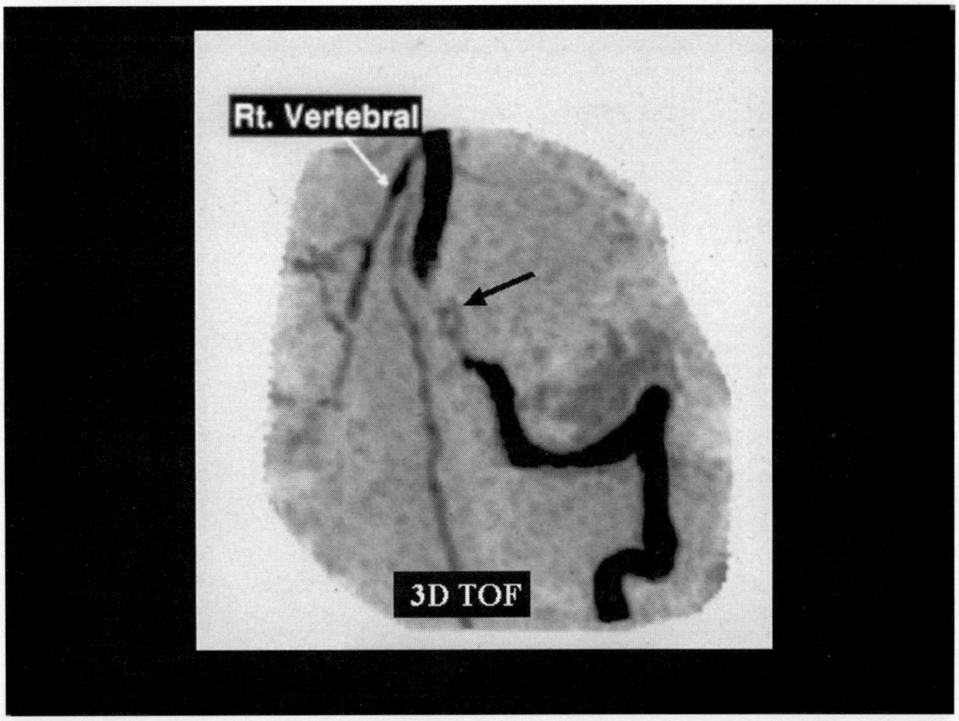

Figure 23-85
Severe distal vertebral artery stenosis on the left shown as segmental signal loss in 3D TOF MRA (black arrow). Note the rudimentary right vertebral artery (white arrow). MRA has excellent sensitivity for detecting stenosis of main trunks of the vertebrobasilar system.

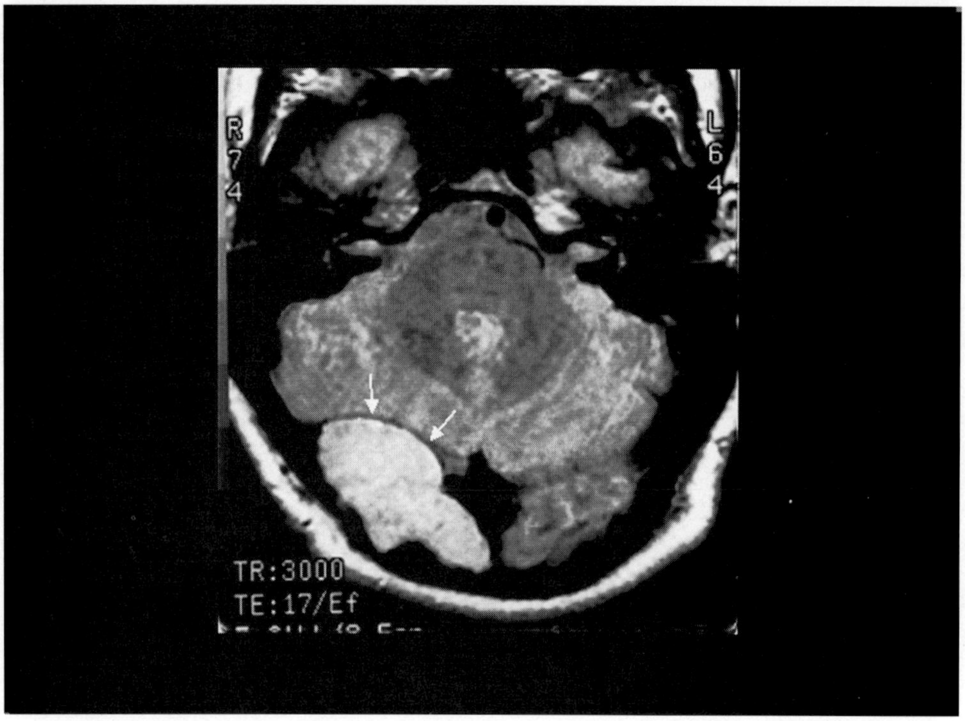

Figure 23-86
Epidermoid of the posterior fossa in a proton-density MRI (arrows) located next to the right lateral sinus.

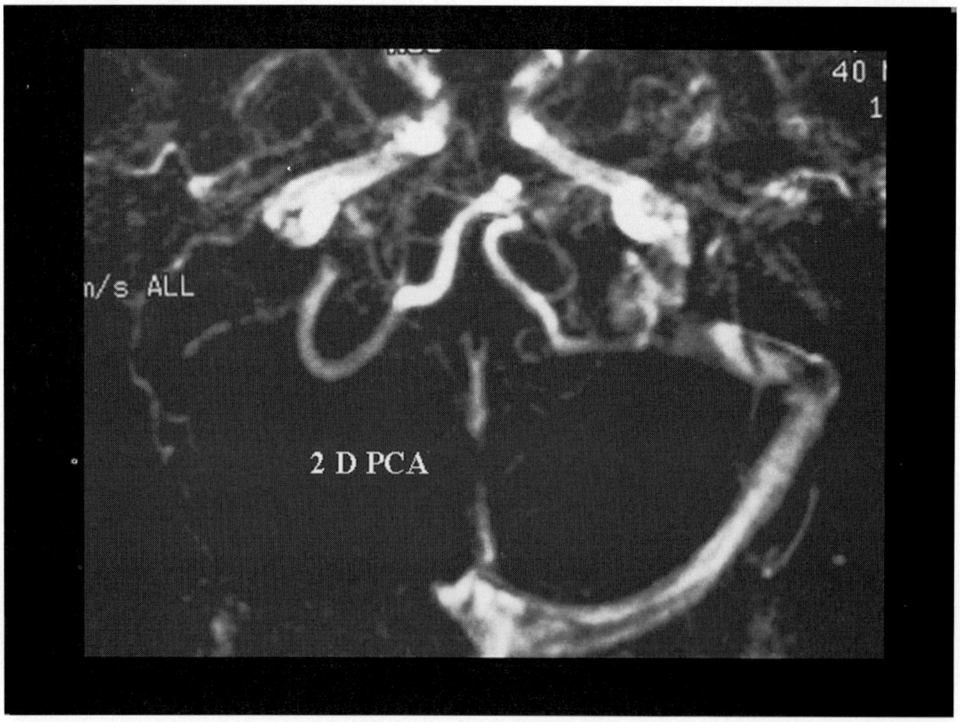

Figure 23-87
Epidermoid in the same patient as depicted in Fig. 23-86. The occluded right lateral sinus is shown by transverse thick-slab 2D PC MRA. The left lateral sinus is patent. V_{enc} was set at 20 cm/s to image slow flow.

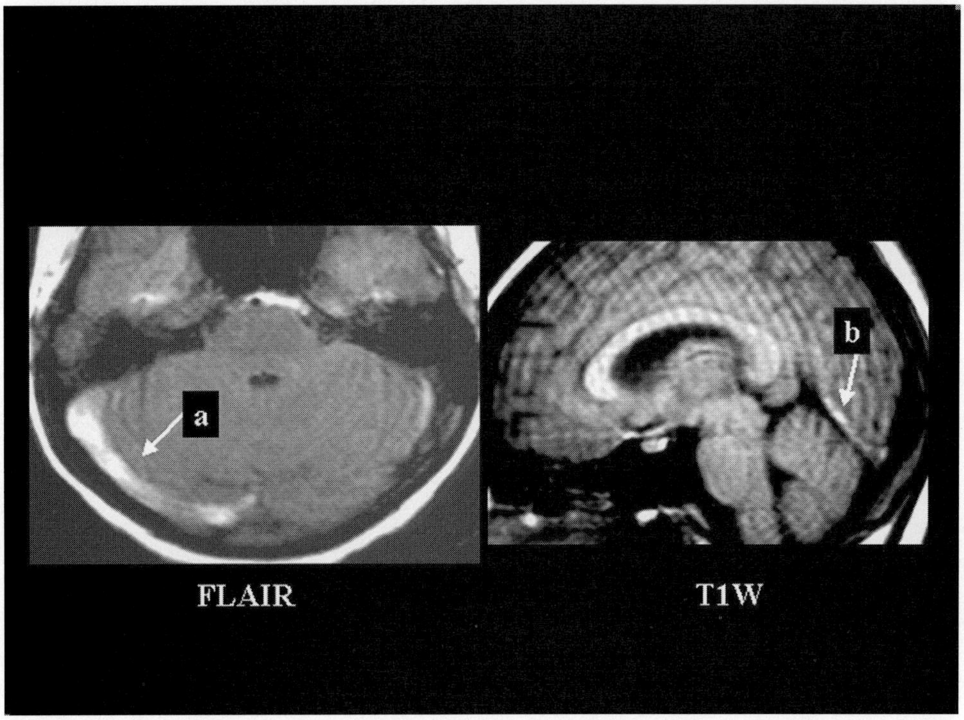

Figure 23-88

Right lateral sinus and straight sinus occlusion shown by hyperintense clot in FLAIR (arrow a*) and hyperintense clot in T1-weighted images (arrow* b*), respectively. Conventional MRI is excellent in depicted occlusion of major intracranial sinuses.*

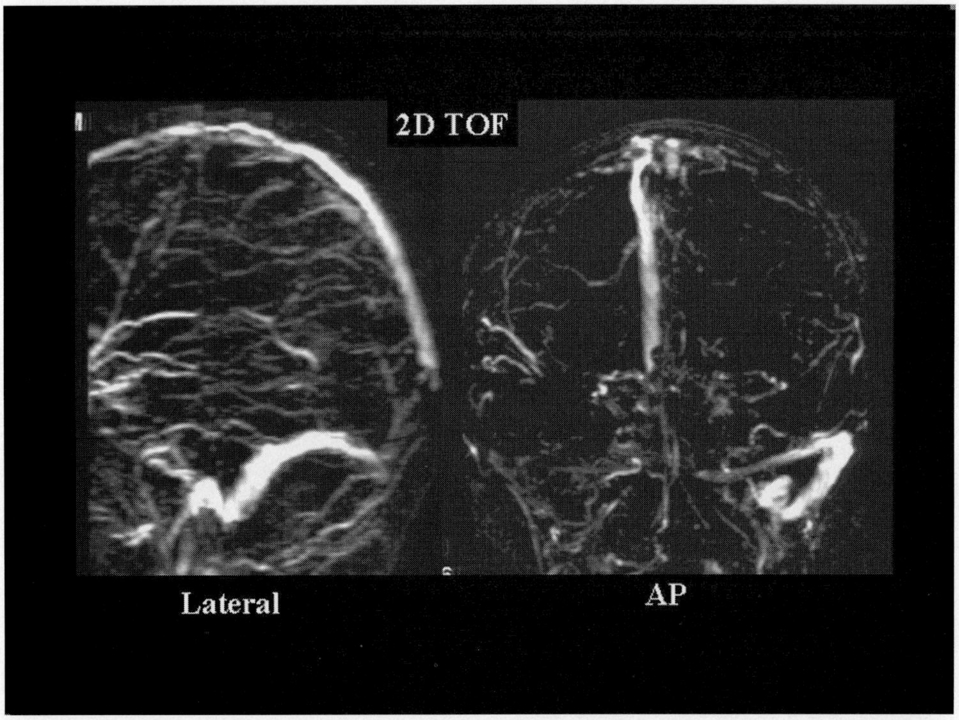

Figure 23-89

Straight sinus and right lateral sinus occlusion shown by 2D TOF MRA in the same patient as depicted in Fig. 23-88. Images are acquired in the coronal plane with inferior saturated pulse to knock our arterial flow. Note the absent straight sinus and vein of Galen in the lateral view and the absent right lateral sinus in the AP view.

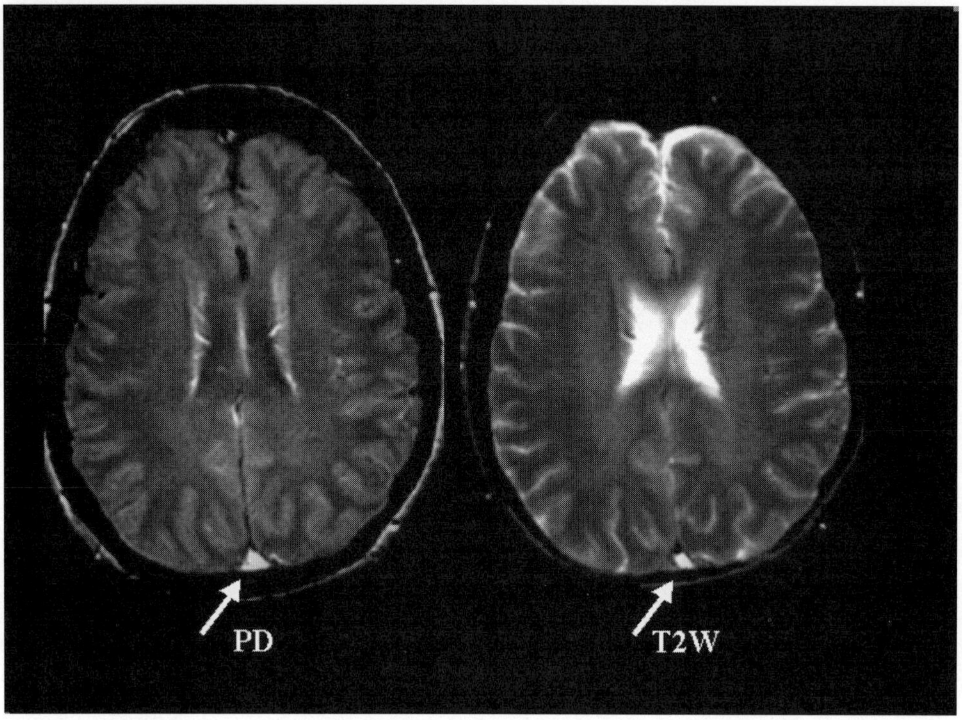

Figure 23-90

Superior sagittal sinus occlusion shown as a hyperintense clot in proton-density and T2-weighted images (arrows).

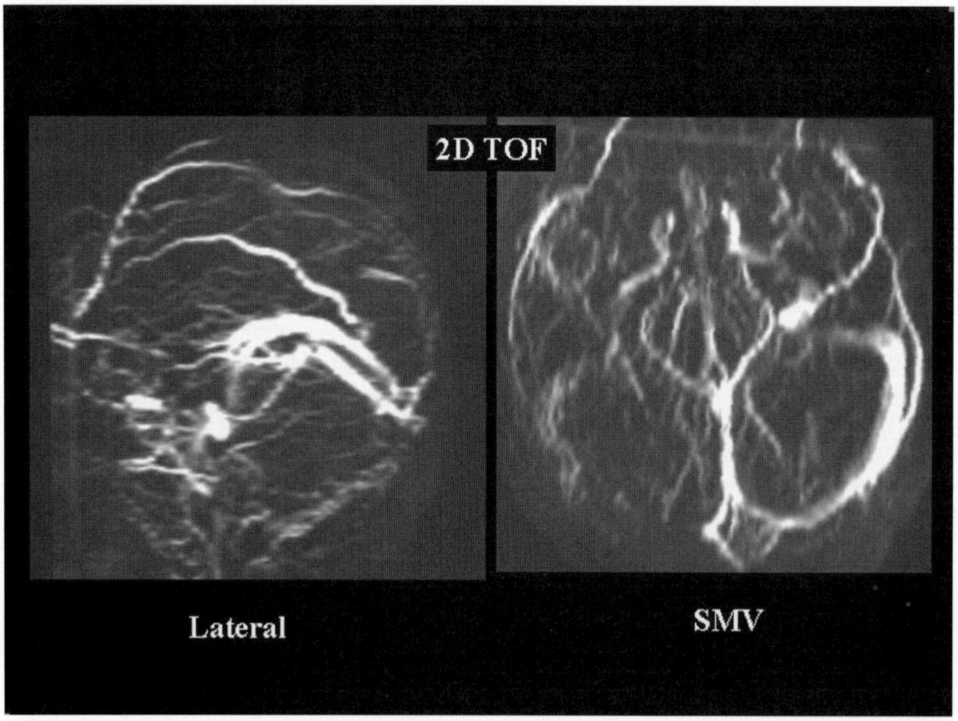

Figure 23-91

Sagittal sinus and right lateral sinus occlusion shown in 2D TOF in the same case as depicted in Fig. 23-90. Note the absent flow in the superior sagittal sinus in the lateral view and the absence of flow in the right lateral sinus in the SMV view. Images are acquired in the coronal plane with inferior saturated pulse to eliminate arterial flow.

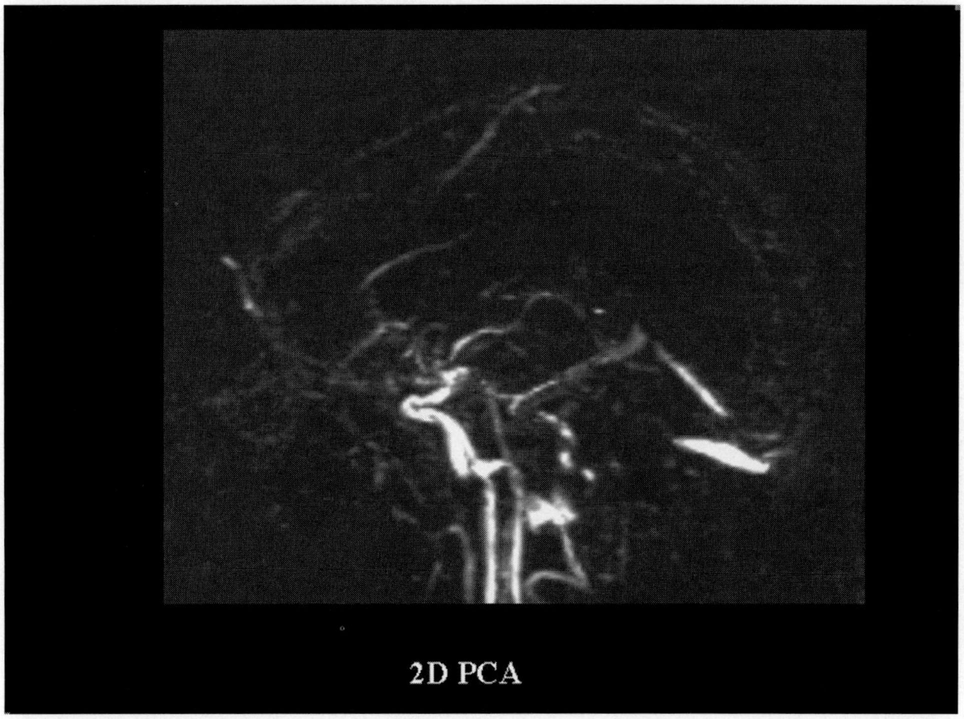

Figure 23-92
Superior sagittal sinus occlusion in the same patient as depicted in Fig. 23-91, 2D thick slab PCA. Note the complete absence of flow in the region of the superior sagittal sinus. Acquisition time is less than 1 min for this technique, which has excellent sensitivity for detecting intracranial venous sinus occlusion.

Table 23-4
Clinical applications of MRA

	Time of Flight MRA	*Phase Contrast MRA*	*Gadolinium-Enhanced MRA*
2D	Carotid bifurcation Venous sinuses Aortic arch (gated)	Sagittal sinus AVMs Vertebrobasilar system Directional flow Cineflow analysis	
3D	Aneurysm Circle of Willis Intracranial stenosis, occlusion Basilar stenosis Aortic arch	Intracranial occlusion Basilar stenosis Directional flow	Aortic Arch Carotid origin/bifurcation Vertebral origins

Table 23-5
MRA protocols

Series name	*ECA Coronal 2D PCA*	*ECA Axial 2D TOF*	*ECA Axial 3D TOF Tone*	*ECA Dynamic carotid*	*ICA Axial 3D TOF Tone*	*ICA Axial 3D PCA*
Geometry*						
FOV, mm	200	210	210	200	200	200
RFOV	80	75	65	50	75	80
Matrix	256	256	256	256	256	256
Scan, %	80	50	50	100	75	80
REST	None	1-SUPR	1-SUPR	None	None	None
Stacks	1 slice	1	1 Chunk	1	1	1
Number of slices	1	60	64	28	100	75
Slice thickness	35	3	0.8	0.7	0.7	1.0
Contrast†						
Scan mode	2D	M2D	3D	3D	3D	3D
Pulse sequence	FFE	FFE	FFE	FFE	FFE	FFE
TR	22.2	13.4	10.7	7	30	11.6
TE	7.6	3.5	2.8	1.9	2.9	5.5
Flip angle	20	70	20	60	25	15
Motion‡						
Flow compensation	No	Yes	Yes	No	Yes	Yes
NSA	4	2	2	2	1	1

*Scan geometry.
†Contrast parameters.
‡Motion suppression.
Note: Philips ACS-NT 1.5T–22mT/m gradients.
Definitions: ECA, extracranial angiogram; FFE, fast-field echo (gradient echo); FOV, field of view; ICA, intracranial angiogram; MTC, magnetization transfer contrast; NSA, number of signal averages; REST, saturation pulses in the field of view; RFOV, rectangular field of view; SUPR, superior; TE, echo time; TONE, tilted optimized nonsaturating excitation or ramped RF; TR, repetition time.

CONCLUSION

Magnetic resonance angiography has greatly benefited from advancements in hardware and software, and today the technique is more than just a screening tool in the study of patients affected by cerebrovascular disease. In extracranial occlusive disease, MRA is rapidly becoming the only test needed for diagnosis and treatment decisions in the large majority of patients.

Intracranial aneurysms are well displayed by MRA, but limitations remain in this clinical setting, such as difficulty imaging aneurysms smaller than 5 mm and false-positive results in cases of tightly wound vessel loops. For these reasons, conventional angiography remains the gold standard in cases of acute subarachnoid hemorrhage until further progress in spatial resolution is achieved with MRA and a consistent higher sensitivity is documented for the technique. Conversely, MRA is an excellent technique for detecting asymptomatic aneurysms because of its high sensitivity for aneurysms measuring more than 5 mm and the fact that smaller aneurysms in this category may be observed rather than treated surgically. In addition, MRA can be used as a guide for optimizing views during conventional angiography and for assisting in the visualization of aneurysm necks and their relationship to parent and neighboring vessels.

The variable sensitivity and specificity of MRA in the detection of arterial intracranial occlusive disease somewhat limits its usefulness as the only test needed for a treatment decision in this clinical setting. This is especially true in the petrous and carotid siphon regions, since overestimation of stenosis may result due to magnetic susceptibility and turbulent flow, respectively, in those locations. Intracranial occlusive disease of the major venous sinuses is optimally displayed by MRA in conjunction with conventional MRI, and there is no need to perform invasive angiography in this clinical setting. Finally, MRA is best utilized when performed by personnel familiar not only with disease states but also with the great number of disease-mimicking artifacts inherent in the technique.

REFERENCES

1. Weeden VJ, Rosen BR, Chesler O, et al: MR velocity imaging by phase display. *J Comput Assist Tomogr* 9:530–536, 1985.

with decreasing VOI size. In some settings smaller VOIs may be justified, but at a cost of longer measurement times.

2. The VOI should be positioned in a region well suited for the desired diagnosis. A list of recommended positions is given in Table 24-1.
3. A standardized routine with respect to measurement parameters and patient positioning should be followed rigorously.
4. The protocol should be standardized, including decisions on whether to perform MRS before or after major MRI sequences and before or after gadolinium (Gd) injection. The possibility of performing ^{1}H MRS after Gd injection has been a matter of discussion because it has been thought that Gd affects the spectral resolution. In the experience of Cousins and associates (personal communication), post-Gd MRS (both short and long TE) does not cause problems.

The New Neurochemistry

Figure 24-1 depicts some of the neurochemical pathways that have become more relevant since the advent of neuro-MRS. The major peaks of the ^{1}H MR spectrum, corresponding to *N*-acetylaspartate (NAA), total creatine [Cr; includes phosphocreatine (PCr)], total choline (Cho; includes phosphorylcholine and glycerophosphorylcholine), *myo*-inositol (mI), and glutamate plus glutamine (GIx), were encountered only infrequently in neurochemical discussions of physiology and disease before the advent of MRS. They now join glucose uptake and oxygen consumption as the most easily measured neurochemical events and must become increasingly important in neurologic discussions.

INTERPRETATION

The MR Spectrum

A Brain Spectrum Presents a Sum of "Metabolite Spectra"

The ^{1}H MR spectrum of the normal human brain is most readily understood by referring to Fig. 24-2. Each metabolite has a "signature"[4,5] that, when added to the other major metabolites, results in a complex spectrum of overlapping peaks. Although such spectra are familiar, it is crucial to adopt a rigorous approach to acquiring and interpreting spectra so that they can form the basis of a clinical report.

Peak Ratios

One useful approach to differential diagnosis consists of noting each cerebral metabolite within the ^{1}H brain spectrum and determining whether it is elevated, reduced, or unchanged in relation to the reference, usually Cr. In determining whether the ratios are normal, they

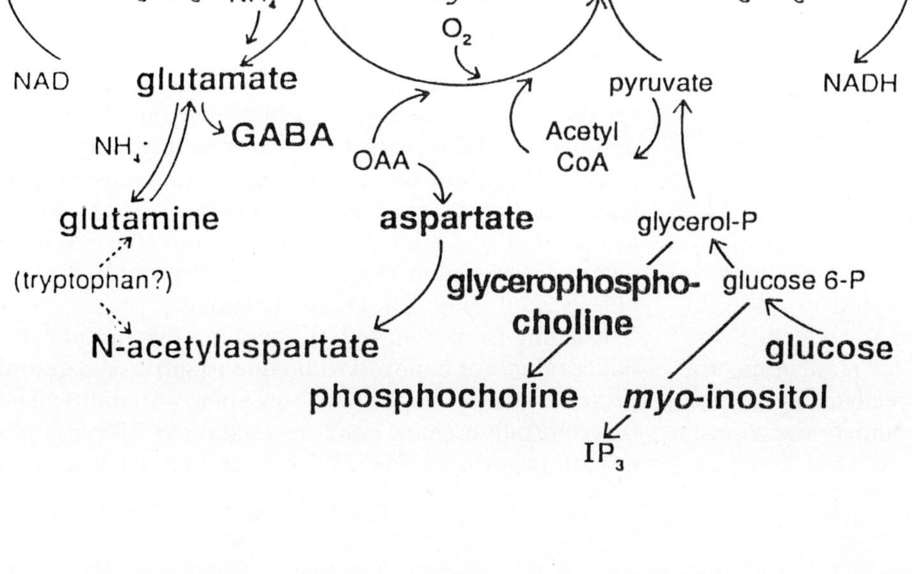

Figure 24-1
Neurochemical pathways relevant to the advent of neuro-MRS.

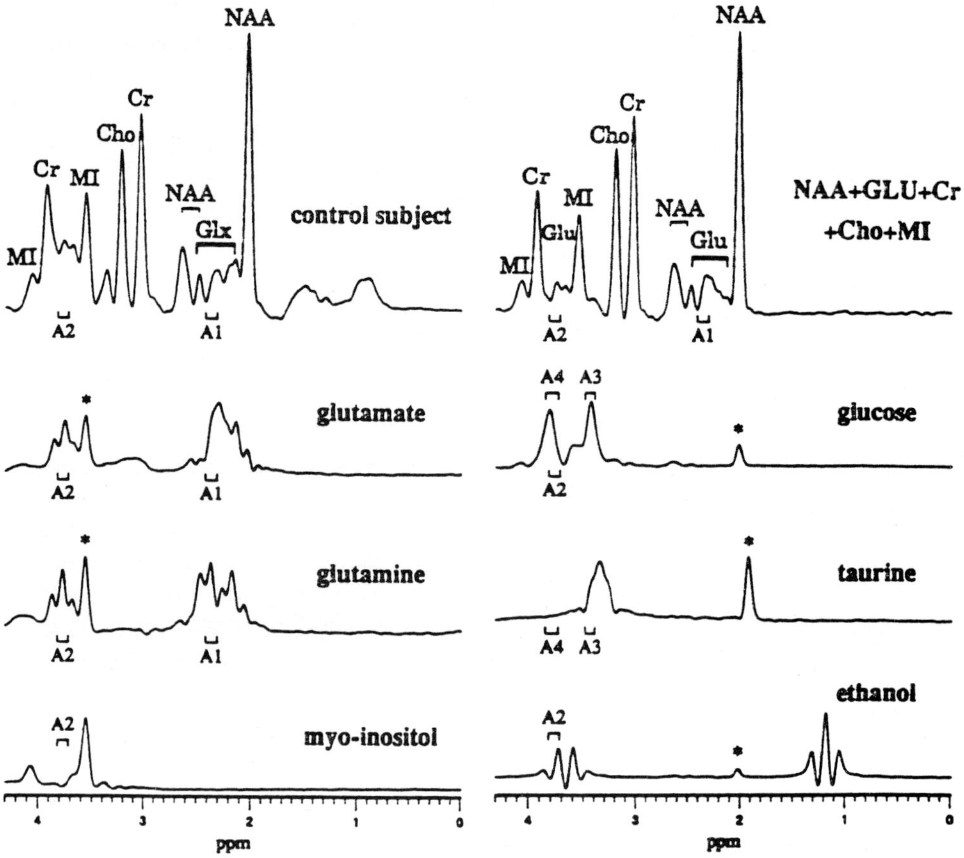

Figure 24-2

Localized in vivo and in vitro ^{1}H MR spectra obtained with a stimulated echo sequence at 1.5 T illustrate the identification of cerebral metabolites. At the top left is a normal brain spectrum (the sum of results from 10 age-matched control subjects). At the top right is a reference spectrum from an aqueous solution composed of 36.7 mM/L NAA, 25 mM/L Cr, 6.3 mM/L choline chloride, 30 mM/L Glu, and 22.5 mM/L mI (adjusted to pH 7.15 in a phosphate buffer). The remaining spectra were recorded from solutions of individual biochemicals. To simulate in vivo conditions, all spectra were subjected to a line-shape transformation yielding gaussian peaks of approximately 4-Hz line width. The integration ranges used to detect changes in the cerebral levels of Glx (Glu or Gln) (A1 + A2) and glucose (A3 + A4) are indicated. The peaks labeled originated from glycine, NAA, or acetate, which were added to the various solutions as chemical shift references (the methyl peak of NAA was set to 2.02 ppm). All spectra were scaled individually and cannot be used for direct quantitation.*

should be compared to age and regionally matched normal ratios (see the section on metabolites, below). Table 24-2 contains an abbreviated list of differential diagnostic uses of MRS based on these metabolites considered individually.

Pattern Recognition in Neurospectroscopy

An alternative approach is that of pattern recognition, taking account of the fact that several metabolite concentrations may be abnormally elevated or reduced within a single pathology. To be most productive, the radiologist should adopt a "routine" for reading spectra rapidly, identifying patterns, and recognizing at the same time any artifacts that may invalidate the clinical interpretation.

Reading MRS

Metabolites Detected by MRS

Figure 24-3, which shows raw PROBE spectra (as seen on the MR display screen) obtained from the region denoted by the box on the corresponding single axial images, illustrates the normal cerebral metabolite pattern found in the gray matter occipital cortex (GM) of an infant (Fig. 24-3A, 1 day old), a child (Fig. 24-3B, 8 years old), an adult (Fig. 24-3C, 31 years old), and an elderly adult (Fig. 24-3D, 83 years old).

Reading from right to left, there are two broad resonances that are believed to be due to intrinsic cerebral proteins and/or lipids that show some variability. The first and tallest sharp peak, resonating at 2.0 parts per million (ppm) (see Fig. 24-2 for the frequency scale in

Table 24-2
Differential diagnostic uses of MRS

Metabolite (normal cerebral concentration)	Increased	Decreased
Lactate (Lac) (~1 m*M*; not "visible")	(often) Hypoxia, anoxia, near drowning, stroke, hypoventilation (inborn errors of TCA, etc.), Canavan, Alexander, hydrocephalus	(Unknown)
N-acetylaspartate (NAA) (5, 10, or 15 m*M*)	(rarely) Canavan	(Often) Developmental delay, infancy, hypoxia, anoxia, ischemia, ICH, herpes II encephalitis, near drowning, hydrocephalus Alexander, epilepsy, neoplasm, MS, stroke, normal-pressure hydrocephalus, (diabetes mellitus) closed head trauma)
Glutamate (Glu) and/or glutamine (Gln)		(unknown)
(GIu = (?) 10 m*M*; GIn = (?) 5 m*M*)	Chronic hepatic encephalopathy (HE), acute HE, hypoxia, near drowning, OTC deficiency	Possibly Alzheimer disease
Myo-inositol (mI) (5 m*M*)	Neonate, Alzheimer disease, diabetes mellitus, recovered hypoxia, hyperosmolar states	Chronic HE, hypoxic encephalopathy, stroke, tumor
Total creatine (Cr) (8 m*M*)	Trauma, hyperosmolar, increasing with age	Hypoxia, stroke, tumor, infant
Glucose (GIc) (~m*M*)	Diabetes mellitus (?) parenteral feeding (G), (?) hypoxic encephalopathy	Not detectable
Choline (Cho) (1.5 m*M*)	Trauma, Diabetes, "white" versus "gray" neonates, after liver transplant, tumor, chronic hypoxia, hyperosmolar, elderly normal, (?) Alzheimer disease	Asymptomatic liver disease, HE, stroke nonspecific dementias
Acetoacetate, acetone, ethanol, aromatic amino acids, xenobiotics (propanediol, mannitol)	Detectable in specific settings	

ppm), is assigned to the neuronal marker NAA. The next cluster of small peaks consists of the coupled resonances of β- and γ-GIx (α-, β-, and γ- refer to different regions within the glutamine and glutamate molecules). However, the tallest peak of this cluster, at approximately 2.6 ppm, is actually a second resonance of NAA. The second tallest resonance (at ~3 ppm) is Cr, and adjacent to this is another prominent but smaller peak assigned to Cho. The Cho/Cr ratio of about 0.5 in spectra B through D in Fig. 24-3 is characteristic of gray matter.[45] The small peak to the left of Cho, which is seen clearly only in spectra B and D, is *scyllo*-inositol (sI). However, in spectrum C, sI is hard to identify because of the presence of glucose, which has a very similar frequency and appears as a shoulder to the left of sI in this spectrum. The common appearance of glucose in ^{1}H spectra often makes the detection of sI difficult.

The prominent peak at 3.6 ppm is assigned to mI. To the left of mI, two small peaks of the α-GIx triplet are clearly seen. The third peak of the triplet appears as a poorly resolved shoulder to the right of the last prominent spectral peak, which is a second resonance of Cr. To the left of the second Cr peak is a second peak of mI (at 4.1 ppm). This mI peak is not always readily identifiable. Variations in the degree of water suppression affect the peak intensities of metabolites closest to the water frequency at 4.7 ppm: the second Cr peak and its immediate neighbors (compare spectra B, C, and D). Normally, this effect of water suppression has no influence on the diagnostic value of spectra.

A dramatically different spectrum was obtained from

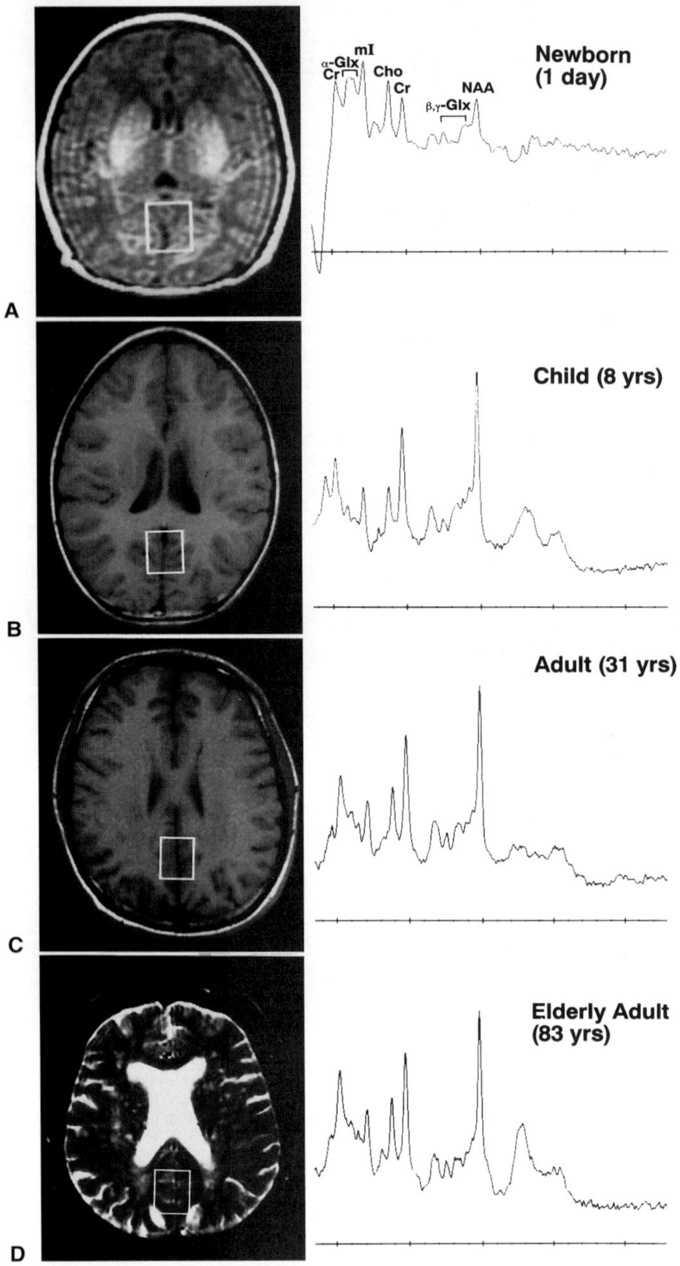

Figure 24-3
(A–D) *PROBE spectra as they appear on the screen. They illustrate normal age-related changes.*

a normal newborn infant (Fig. 24-3A) 36 h postnatal. At first glance, the most striking difference between Fig. 24-3A and Fig. 24-3B–D is the elevated baseline, which is attributable to the effect of water suppression and therefore is not significant. The important difference is that the heights of the NAA, Cho, Cr, and mI peaks are reversed. From left to right, there is a suggestion of a lactate (Lac) doublet, a small NAA resonance, an unremarkable β,γ-Glx region, and a Cr peak of equal intensity to NAA. Cho, in contrast to adult spectra, exceeds Cr, while mI is the most prominent peak. These are normal NAA/Cr, Cho/Cr, and mI/Cr ratios compared with age-related healthy infants.[46]

Identifying Lactate

Significant contributions from Lac are easily identified from a stimulated echo acquisition mode (STEAM) (TE = 30 ms) or a point resolved spectroscopy (PRESS)

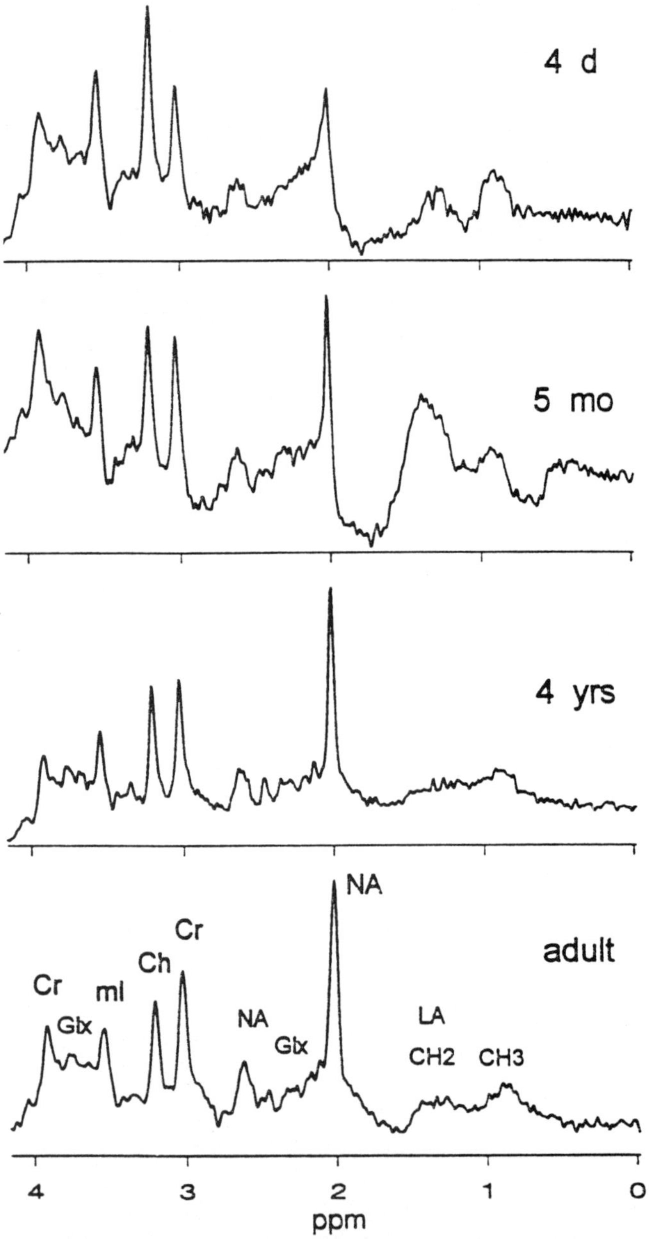

Figure 24-4
Typical cerebral ^1H MR spectra from subjects of different ages. Relative amplitudes of the main peaks in short echo time stimulated echo acquisition mode (STEAM) spectra vary drastically with age. Spectra were obtained from a periventricular area in the parietal cortex. Acquisition parameters: 30 ms echo time (TE), 1.5 s repetition time TR, 144–256 averages, voxel sizes 8–10 cm^3 for children and 2–16 cm^3 for adults. (Modified from Ref. 46.)

spectrum. Qualifications are (1) a doublet peak at 1.33 ppm and (2) the two narrow peaks of the doublet that are separated by 7 Hz (or, at 1.5 tesla, separated by 0.11 ppm). A broad peak at 1.33 ppm should not automatically be attributed to Lac; it is more likely to be lipid. Overlapping lipid is usually not a problem, since Lac will appear as two narrow peaks. However, poor resolution may make it difficult to distinguish Lac from lipid, in which case a longer TE (135 or 270 ms) or editing schemes can be helpful. One useful scheme is shown in Fig. 24-23A.

MRS IN NEONATOLOGY AND PEDIATRICS

Developmental Disorders

Normal Development

The evolution of MRS changes in the newborn brain, from in utero (in a single near-term fetus)[47] to postpartum 50-plus weeks of gestational age, has been well described (Fig. 24-4).[46] The findings add significantly to the information routinely obtained with MRI. Van der Knaap and coworkers correlated the evolution of MRS changes with the development of myelination,[43] but without short echo time spectra with which to define changes in mI. Normative curves for normal development that have been established for two cerebral locations (Fig. 24-5) confirm earlier published long echo time and ^{31}P findings and unpublished data.[46–48] *Myo*-inositol dominates the spectrum at birth (12 m*M*/kg), while Cho is responsible for the strongest peak in older infants (2.5 m*M*/kg). Cr (including PCr) and NAA are at significantly lower concentrations in the neonate than in the adult (Cr~6 and NA~5 m*M*/kg). NAA and Cr increase, while Cho and particularly mI decrease during the first few weeks of life (Table 24-3).[46] Increased NAA and Cr are determined by gestational age, whereas the falling concentration of mI correlates best with postnatal age (Fig. 24-6). Absolute metabolite concentrations depend on metabolite T1 and T2 relaxation. Whereas T1 values alter significantly with age for the metabolites NAA, Cr, and mI, the value for Cho is not altered. T2 of NAA does appear to show important changes between newborns and adults, whereas that of Cr, Cho, and mI seems to be unimportant.

Absolute quantitative ^{1}H MRS is expected to be of particular value in the diagnosis and monitoring of pathology in infants (Fig. 24-6),[46] since metabolite ratios are often misleading. This may be particularly useful in the period before myelination is apparent in the developing brain.

MRS of Inborn Errors

Inborn errors of metabolism, although relatively rare individually, together make up a large proportion of pediatric clinical practice. Extensive reviews of MRI discuss pattern recognition in differential diagnosis. Something similar can be done for MRS. Figures 24-7 and 24-8 draw together examples of common inborn

Table 24-3
Absolute concentrations of different age groups in m*M*/kg brain tissue (mean ± 1 SEM) and significance tests for the differences found

Group	n (ROIs)*	GA, weeks	pn age, weeks	NAA	Cr	Cho	mI
<42 GA	11	38.7 ± 0.7	3.9 ± 1.6	4.82 ± 0.54	6.33 ± 0.32	2.41 ± 0.11	10.1 ± 1.1
42–60 GA	8	50.2 ± 1.8	9.3 ± 1.9	7.03 ± 0.41	7.28 ± 0.28	2.23 ± 0.06	8.52 ± 0.92
≤2 pm	6	40.0 ± 1.0	0.8 ± 0.2	5.52 ± 0.64	6.74 ± 0.43	2.53 ± 0.12	12.4 ± 1.4
2–10 pn	7	41.9 ± 1.5	3.8 ± 0.9	5.89 ± 0.21	6.56 ± 0.44	2.16 ± 0.09	7.69 ± 0.62
Adult	10		1440 ± 68	8.89 ± 0.17	7.49 ± 0.12	1.32 ± 0.07	6.56 ± 0.43
p < 42 GA versus adult				<0.0001	<0.0001	<0.0001	0.001
p < 42 GA versus 42–60 GA				0.0007	0.02	0.07	0.10
*p*42–60 GA versus adult				<0.0001	0.16	<0.0001	0.0003
p < 2 pn versus adult				<0.0001	0.005	<0.0001	<0.0001
p < 2 pn versus 2–10 pn				0.7	0.8	0.02	0.004
*p*2–10 pn versus adult				<0.0001	0.001	<0.0001	0.007

Source: Modified from Ref. 46.
Note: Minima and maxima are highlighted in bold.
* ROI = region of interest; GA = gestational age, pn = postnatal (age); NAA = *N*-acetylaspartate; Cr = creatine; Cho = choline; m*I* = *myo*-inositol.

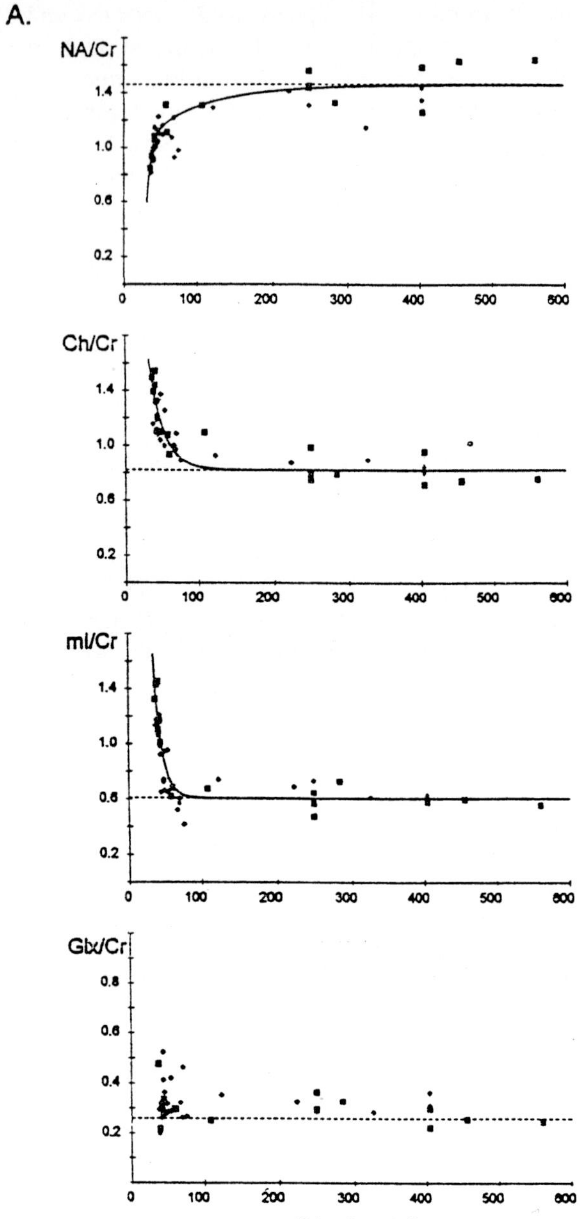

Figure 24-5
Time courses of metabolite peak amplitude ratios versus gestational age of the subject. **A** *and* **B** *contain the normative curves for the parietal (mostly white matter) and occipital (predominantly gray matter) locations, respectively. The curves are well defined for the first year of life, when the most dramatic changes take place. The normative curves are specific for the acquisition parameters used. (Modified from Ref. 46.)*

errors. Despite profound methodologic differences, in each case the MR spectrum is diagnostic. MRS may fill in part of the gap in the diagnostic workup of inborn errors of metabolism. MRS data in lysosomal and peroxisomal disorders are limited, and generally nonspecific abnormalities related to the loss of myelin or neuronal damage have been described. Nevertheless, even these preliminary data may carry important information and reveal distinct patterns of metabolic disturbances involving the neuronal marker NAA (Fig. 24-7), Lac, and separate abnormalities of Cho, Cr, mI, and sI that may point to a significant new role for MRS in the critical area of the diagnosis of inborn errors. Especially in atypical and nondiagnostic MRI findings, the demonstration of an elevation of cerebral Lac or other substances may constitute a lead in the diagnostic workup.

Three types of spectroscopic abnormalities are seen in inborn metabolic errors: (1) nonspecific spectroscopic

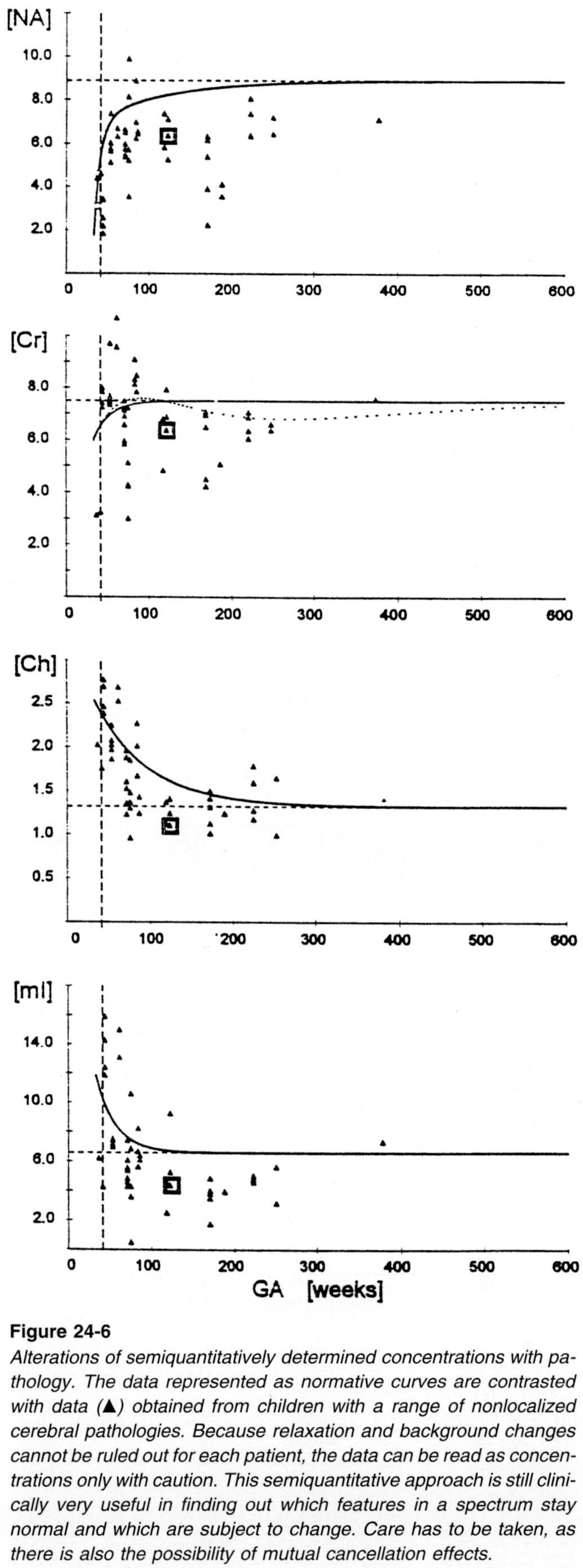

Figure 24-6

Alterations of semiquantitatively determined concentrations with pathology. The data represented as normative curves are contrasted with data (▲) obtained from children with a range of nonlocalized cerebral pathologies. Because relaxation and background changes cannot be ruled out for each patient, the data can be read as concentrations only with caution. This semiquantitative approach is still clinically very useful in finding out which features in a spectrum stay normal and which are subject to change. Care has to be taken, as there is also the possibility of mutual cancellation effects.

abnormalities related to MRI-visible brain damage, including demyelination or atrophy, (2) generic (nonspecific) spectroscopic changes that largely are not associated with particular changes in MRI, for instance, loss of the neuronal marker NAA, loss of high-energy metabolites, accumulation of Lac, and changes in glutamine/glutamate, and (3) specific spectroscopic abnormalities that are directly related to the chemistry of the inborn error under investigation, such as phenylalanine in phenylketonuria and glycine in hyperglycemia. All these changes may be associated with MRI abnormalities.

Nonspecific cerebral damage in inborn errors of metabolism may consist of disturbance of brain maturation, demyelination, or neuronal degeneration. The neuronal damage and loss accompanying demyelination are reflected in a decrease in NAA in the ^{1}H spectra. In active demyelination, an elevation of Cho and Lac has been reported repeatedly, in addition to elevation of fatty acids, presumably representing the breakdown products of myelin.

In neuronal degenerative disorders, neuronal damage is reflected in a decrease in NAA, which is present in the cytosol of neurons and probably is lost early in neuronal dysfunction. In infarction, a decrease in NAA occurs within minutes or hours, whereas the removal of dead neurons starts only after days.

MRS is a sensitive and valuable extension to the diagnostic information offered by MRI. As a quantitative method it is more sensitive than MRI to subtle changes in disease. Because metabolic abnormalities precede many of the MRI changes, these MRS findings may be of value as early diagnostic indicators in siblings screened for a disease or in monitoring treatment.

Spectroscopic changes that are characteristic of a particular inborn error or a subclass of inborn errors are now recognized. Examples (Figs. 24-7 and 24-8) include elevated glutamine in hyperammonemia, elevation of sI in some peroxisomal disorders,[49] and highly elevated NAA in Canavan disease.[50] Others, assigned with less certainty at present, include a peak at 0.9 to 1 ppm assigned to branched-chain amino acids and oxo acids in maple syrup urine disease,[51,52] a peak at 3.55 ppm assigned to glycine in nonketotic hyperglycinemia,[53] and a peak of unknown origin at 1.1 ppm that possibly has been confounded with that of propanediol (see the section on the detection of xenobiotics below), in propionic acidemia.[52] Lac is typically elevated in many mitochondrial disorders[50] but is elevated in several other conditions, such as hypoxia-ischemia and inflammation.

Both MRI and MRS may be of help in screening of children with a suspected inborn error of metabolism to provide clues for the diagnosis and give direction to the biochemical investigations. As carriers often have minor metabolic abnormalities that do not lead to structural damage, MRS may be of greater use than MRI. The potential for MRS in monitoring possible treat-

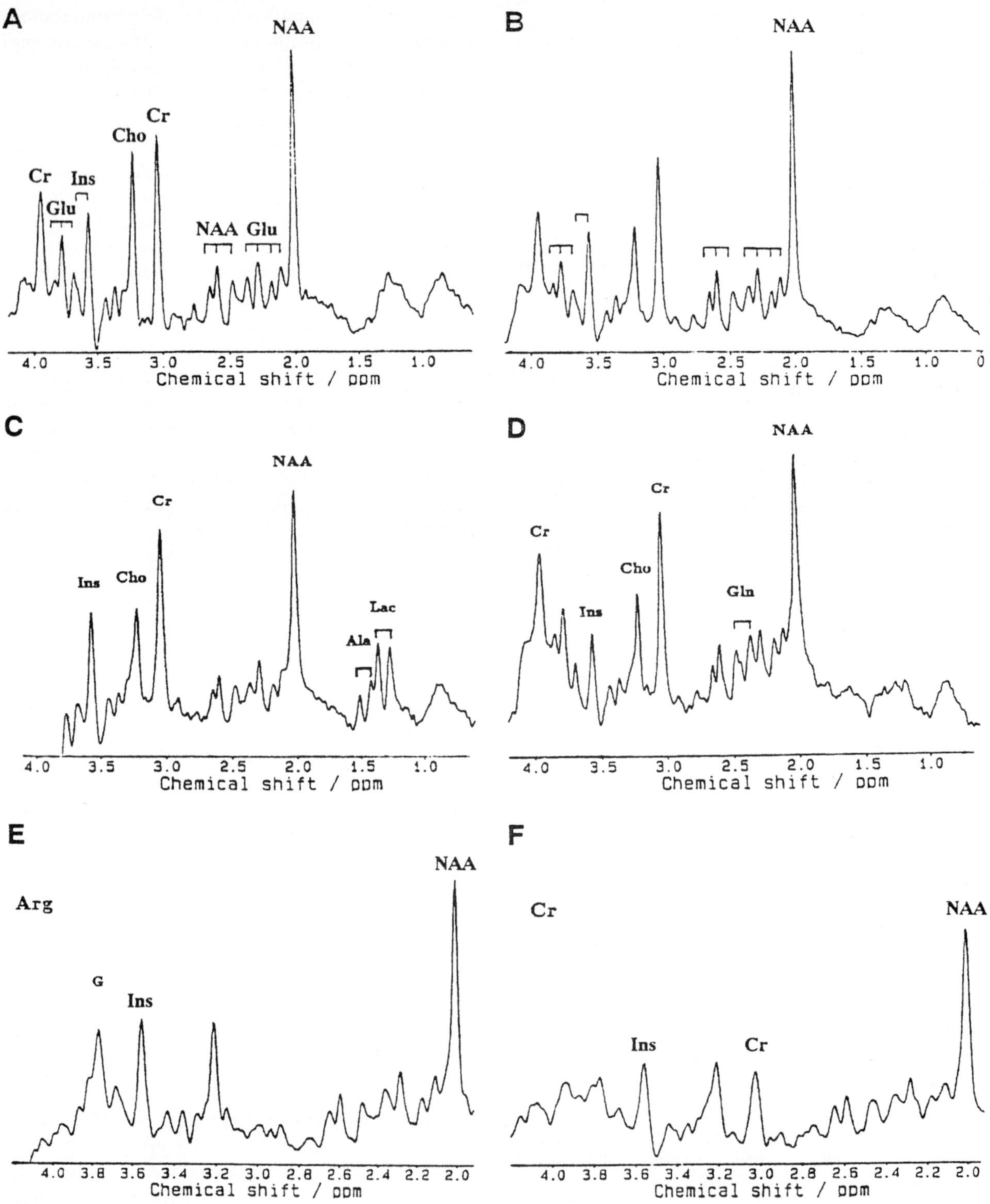

Figure 24-7

Inborn errors. Examples at 2 T, 20 ms TE (short echo). All spectra are courtesy of Dr. Jens Frahm. **(A)** *Normal gray matter at 4 months.* **(B)** *Normal gray matter at 2 years.* **(C)** *Leigh disease: white matter at 11 months.* **(D)** *Zellweger syndrome variant: gray matter at 15 months.* **(E)** *Guanidinoacetate methyltransferase deficiency (Frahm-Hanefeld syndrome) with total Cr deficiency. (*__F__*, inset) Partially restored after treatment.*

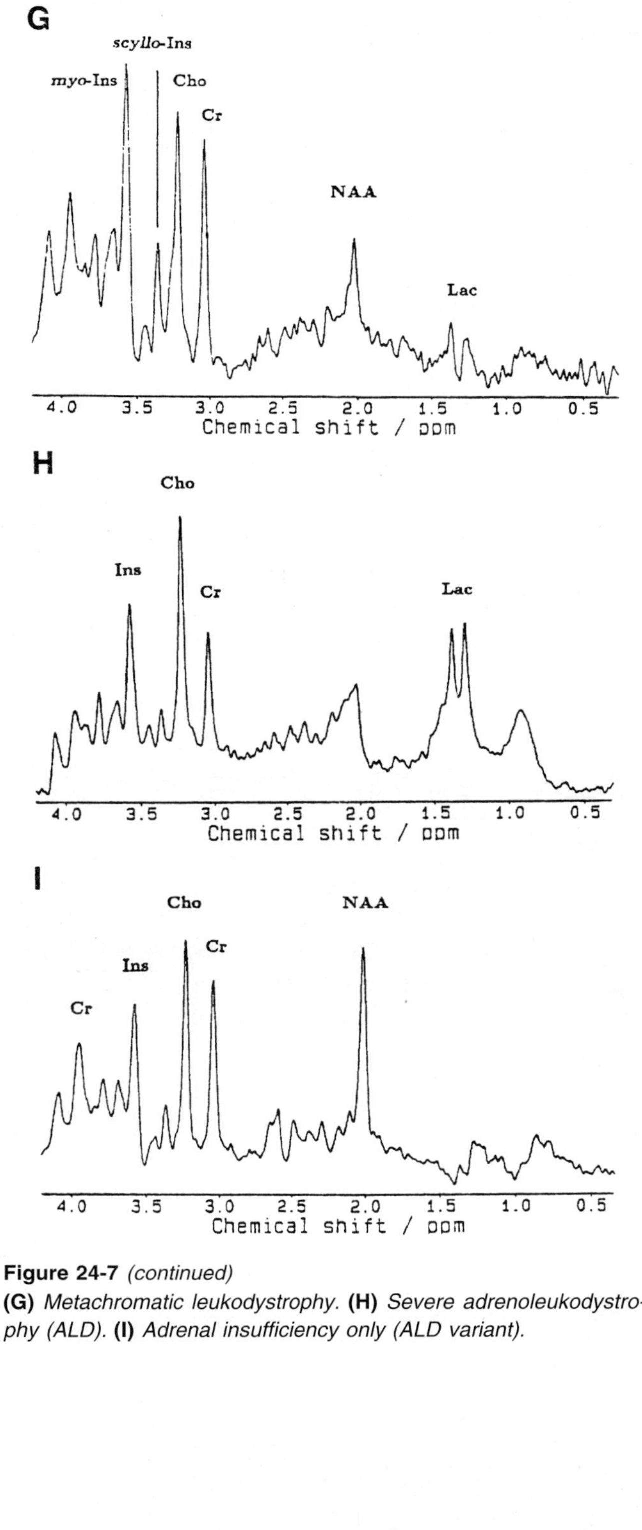

Figure 24-7 *(continued)*
(G) *Metachromatic leukodystrophy.* **(H)** *Severe adrenoleukodystrophy (ALD).* **(I)** *Adrenal insufficiency only (ALD variant).*

ments of inborn errors has been illustrated in adrenoleukodystrophy (ALD) patients receiving bone marrow transplantation.[54]

Leukodystrophies

The term *leukodystrophy* covers both adult and infantile white matter diseases; both are dealt with in this section. Undifferentiated white matter disease appears to be rare. The MRS patterns have not been described in any large series of patients. In children, ALD, metachromatic leukodystrophy, Canavan disease, Alexander disease, and "vanishing white matter" disease (Fig. 24-9)[55–57] have been characterized to some extent by ^{1}H MRS. All result in impressive changes in the ^{1}H spectrum, including a minor change in sI in a preclinical case of ALD through NAA depletion, increased Cho/Cr, increased mI/Cr, the presence of Lac in affected ALD patients, and universal depletion of all regular metabolites in vanishing white matter disease.

In ALD, the major MRS disturbances can be observed earlier than can the MRI changes. The MRS changes are first detected in the regions of the brain that are later most affected in MRI, but they finally appear in all regions of the brain. The early detection of the onset of the disease makes MRS a useful tool for deciding when to start treatments such as bone marrow transplantation. Rajanayagam and coworkers,[54] recently used MRS to monitor ALD patients after bone marrow transplantation. They observed a partial normalization of the MR spectrum in the patients who improved clinically.

Abnormal Development

In inborn errors there are two broad categories of central nervous system (CNS) involvement[43]: primarily structural and primarily functional abnormalities. Inborn errors of metabolism are presumably present from the beginning of embryonic genesis, and so a number of them lead to disturbances of normal brain development. Zellweger syndrome, Pelizaeus-Merzbacher disease, glutaric aciduria type I, aminoacidopathies, phenylketonuria, metachromatic leukodystrophy, globoid cell leukodystrophy (Krabbe disease), and gangliosidoses are some of the inborn errors of metabolism in which (it is presumed) the anatomic abnormality by which they are recognized in MRI results primarily from metabolic interference with normal brain development. In a recent example,[58] an infant with an abnormal thirst control mechanism presented with hypernatremia, a markedly "hyperosmolar" brain chemistry on MRS examination (see "The Hyperosmolar State," page 761), and was discovered at the same time to have a minor and incomplete holoprosencephaly on MRI. Presumably, the anatomic defect underlay the complex biochemical disorder uncovered by MRS.

However, many of the primary defects are in pathways involving macromolecules or membrane lipids that are invisible to MRI. Unless the inborn error of metabolism results in the accumulation of a low-molecular-weight species that is detectable in conventional or edited versions of MRS, the underlying biochemical disorder will not be apparent.

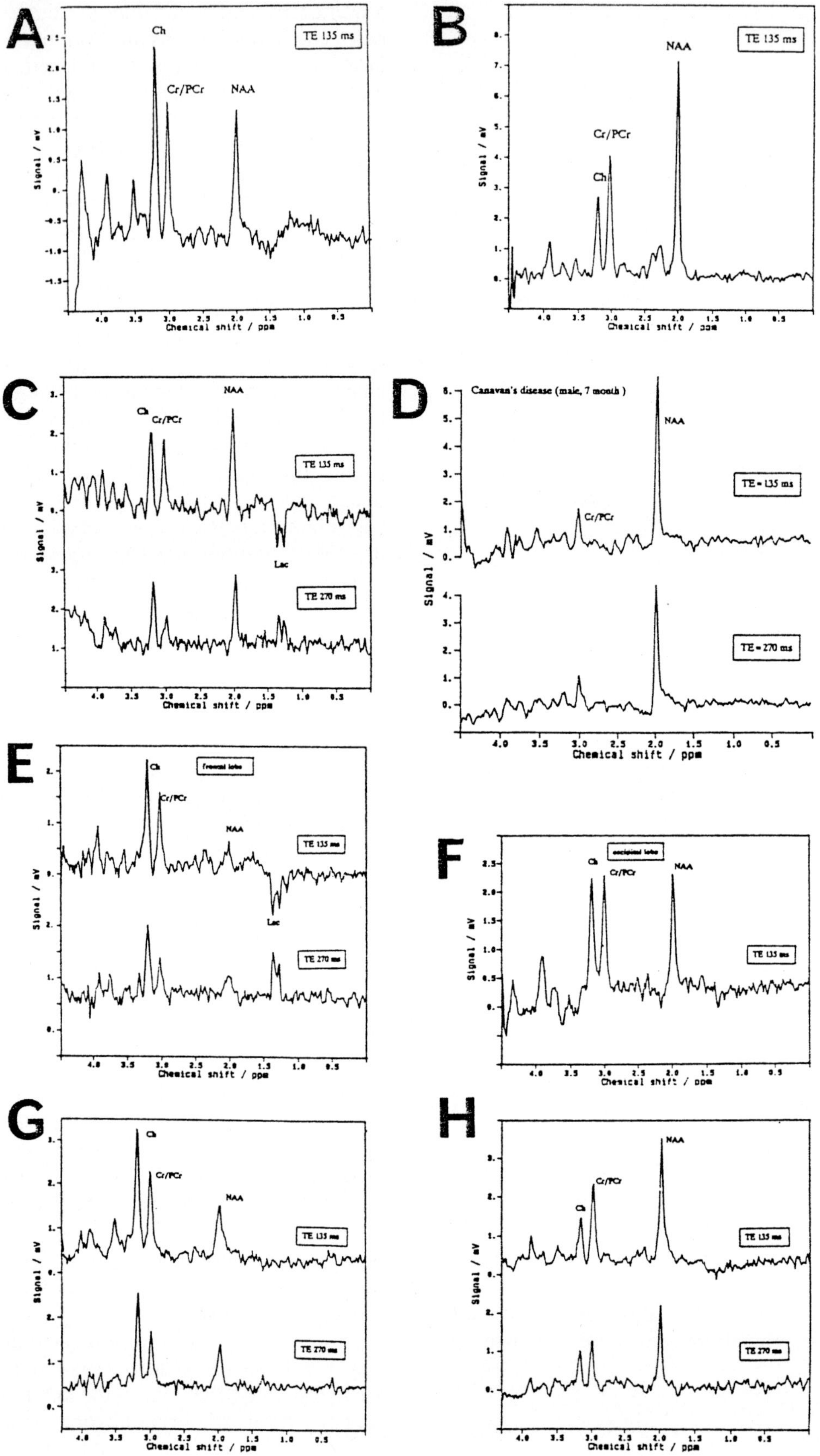
A
Ch
Cr/PCr
NAA
TE 135 ms
Signal / mV
Chemical shift / ppm
B
NAA
Cr/PCr
Ch
TE 135 ms
Signal / mV
Chemical shift / ppm
C
Ch
Cr/PCr
NAA
TE 135 ms
Lac
TE 270 ms
Signal / mV
Chemical shift / ppm
D
Canavan's disease (male, 7 month)
NAA
TE = 135 ms
Cr/PCr
TE = 270 ms
Signal / mV
Chemical shift / ppm
E
Ch
Cr/PCr
NAA
TE 135 ms
Lac
TE 270 ms
Signal / mV
Chemical shift / ppm
F
occipital lobe
Ch
Cr/PCr
NAA
TE 135 ms
Signal / mV
Chemical shift / ppm
G
Ch
Cr/PCr
NAA
TE 135 ms
TE 270 ms
Signal / mV
Chemical shift / ppm
H
NAA
Cr/PCr
Ch
TE 135 ms
TE 270 ms
Signal / mV
Chemical shift / ppm

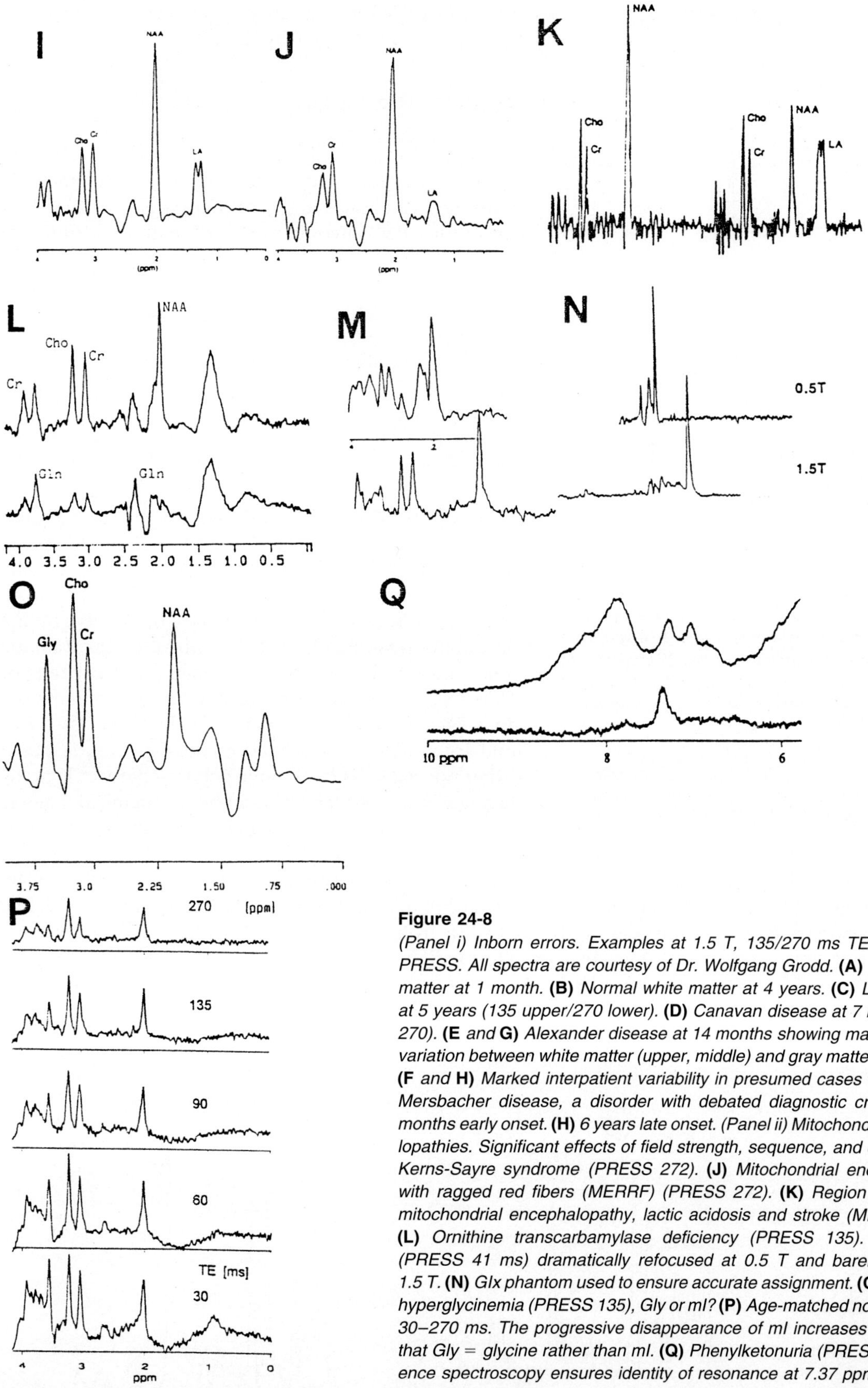

Figure 24-8

(Panel i) Inborn errors. Examples at 1.5 T, 135/270 ms TE (long echo), PRESS. All spectra are courtesy of Dr. Wolfgang Grodd. **(A)** *Normal white matter at 1 month.* **(B)** *Normal white matter at 4 years.* **(C)** *Leigh disease at 5 years (135 upper/270 lower).* **(D)** *Canavan disease at 7 months (135/270).* **(E** *and* **G)** *Alexander disease at 14 months showing marked regional variation between white matter (upper, middle) and gray matter (lower 135).* **(F** *and* **H)** *Marked interpatient variability in presumed cases of Pelizaeus-Mersbacher disease, a disorder with debated diagnostic criteria.* **(F)** *17 months early onset.* **(H)** *6 years late onset. (Panel ii) Mitochondrial encephalopathies. Significant effects of field strength, sequence, and echo time.* **(I)** *Kerns-Sayre syndrome (PRESS 272).* **(J)** *Mitochondrial encephalopathy with ragged red fibers (MERRF) (PRESS 272).* **(K)** *Region variations in mitochondrial encephalopathy, lactic acidosis and stroke (MELAS) (CSI).* **(L)** *Ornithine transcarbamylase deficiency (PRESS 135).* **(M)** *Normal (PRESS 41 ms) dramatically refocused at 0.5 T and barely present at 1.5 T.* **(N)** *Glx phantom used to ensure accurate assignment.* **(O)** *Nonketotic hyperglycinemia (PRESS 135), Gly or mI?* **(P)** *Age-matched normal STEAM 30–270 ms. The progressive disappearance of mI increases the certainty that Gly = glycine rather than mI.* **(Q)** *Phenylketonuria (PRESS 20). Difference spectroscopy ensures identity of resonance at 7.37 ppm.*

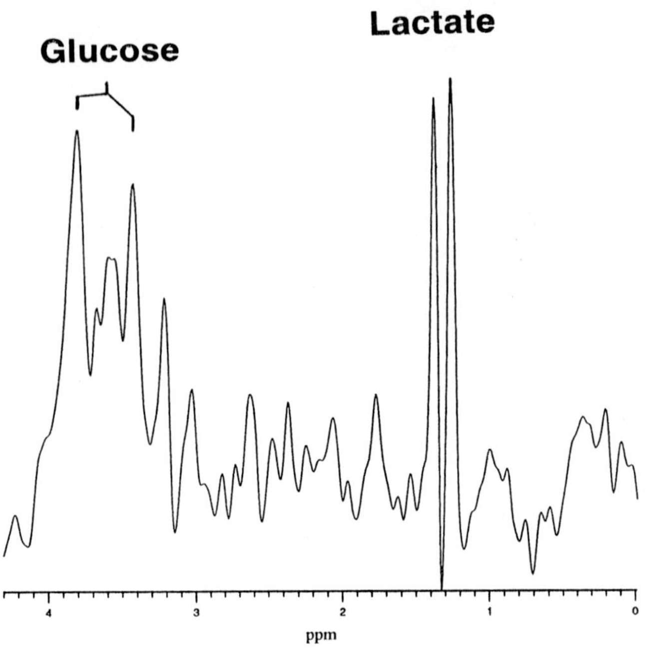

Figure 24-9
MR spectrum from an occipitoparietal location in a patient (M 21 months) who fits the pattern of Schiffman disease[55–57]: universally very low concentration of the usual metabolites and presence of Lac and glucose. The "white matter" spectrum is simiilar to a spectrum of CSF. The possibility that the VOI contains mostly CSF is supported by the assay of water compartments, which measured at 75 percent fraction of CSF in the VOI. The patient had a female sibling who died of a similar condition.

Preshunt Surgery Evaluation in Hydrocephalus

Hydrocephalus is a significant neurosurgical emergency in infants that often is treated by ventricular shunt surgery. Since ventricular shunt surgery is not benign, differentiation between atrophy, metabolic disease, and true hydrocephalus, all of which present as ventricular dilatation, is vital. MRS aids this differentiation. MRS is normal in hydrocephalus.[59] Metabolic diseases result in abnormal MRS, particularly reduced NAA/Cr and the appearance of Lac (Fig. 24-10).

Neonatal Brain Injury

Shaken Baby Syndrome

Shaken baby syndrome results in major, often fatal head injury and can cause a severe neurologic deficit. MRS can predict the outcome in shaken baby syndrome, as is illustrated in Fig. 24-11. A further role of MRS in shaken baby syndrome involves sequential examinations that assist in understanding the mechanisms of the brain damage that cannot be explained easily by the physical insult alone. A cascade of biochemical changes that occur after the insult may be treatable or can be interrupted.[60]

Neonatal Hypoxia

An example of an essentially normal brain spectrum after what was presumed to be severe perinatal hypoxic encephalopathy is shown in Fig. 24-12. This example, which is indicative of an important role for ^{1}H MRS in predicting a good outcome in the face of unduly gloomy clinical impressions, serves as a contrast to the dramatic abnormalities that are detected regularly by means of ^{1}H MRS in newborns with true hypoxic encephalopathy (Fig. 24-13); NAA is depleted, while Cho, Lac, and lipid accumulate in both cerebral hemispheres despite a rather normal MRI. Anatomic heterogeneity of hypoxic damage and the progression of the biochemical damage over time are illustrated in Fig. 24-14. Progressive loss of NAA, Cr, and mI with time reflects the evolution of hypoxic damage between days 5, 12, and 42 after birth. The occipital (gray) region is the most severely affected, and the frontal the least, while the parietal cortex is intermediate. This patient clearly demonstrates the general point that lipid is one of the metabolic markers of cerebral hypoxia in neonates.

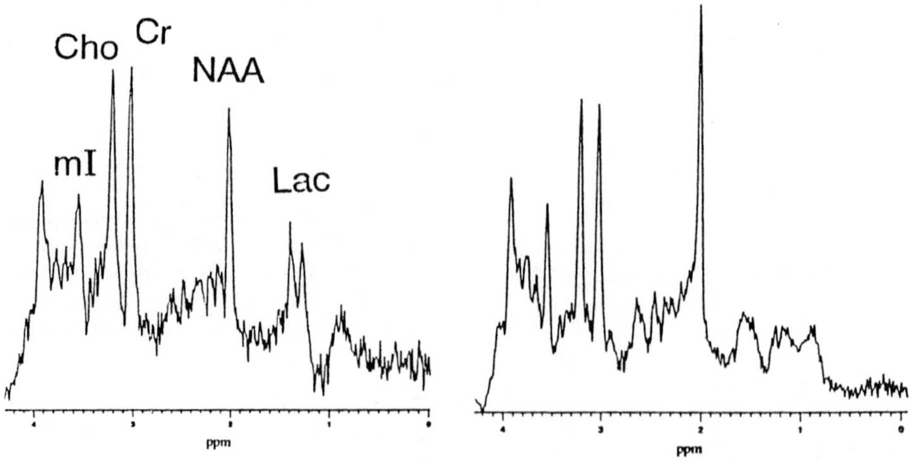

Figure 24-10
MRS before shunt in two infants who both had shunt surgery performed illustrates how MRS can differentiate metabolic disease from true hydrocephalus. One infant (left, abnormal spectrum) had a bad outcome from the surgery, and one (right, normal spectrum) had successful surgery.

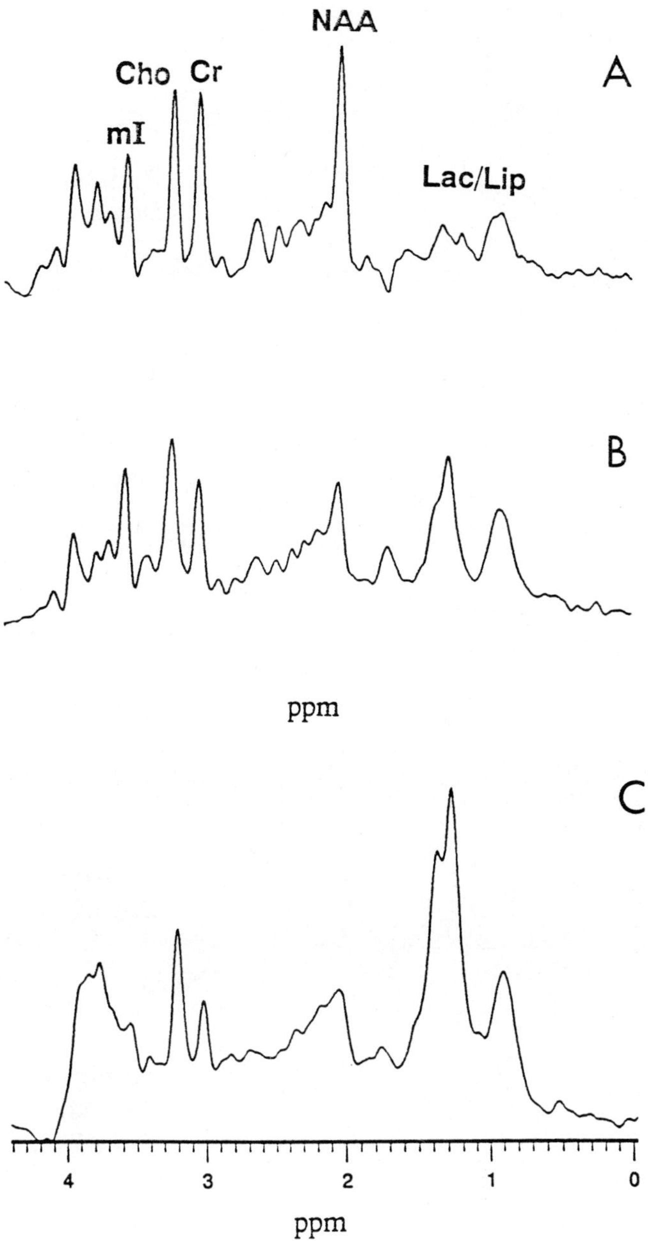

Figure 24-11

[1]H MR spectra from shaken baby syndrome. The spectrum from infant A at 7 days after-trauma is normal-appearing (good outcome). The spectra from infants B and C at 5 and 7 days after-trauma, respectively, show major abnormalities (poor outcome). Greatly reduced NAA, lower Cr, and the appearance of peaks in the Lac and lipid regions in infant B and almost absent NAA, low Cr and ml, and dominant peaks in the Lac and lipid regions in infant C.

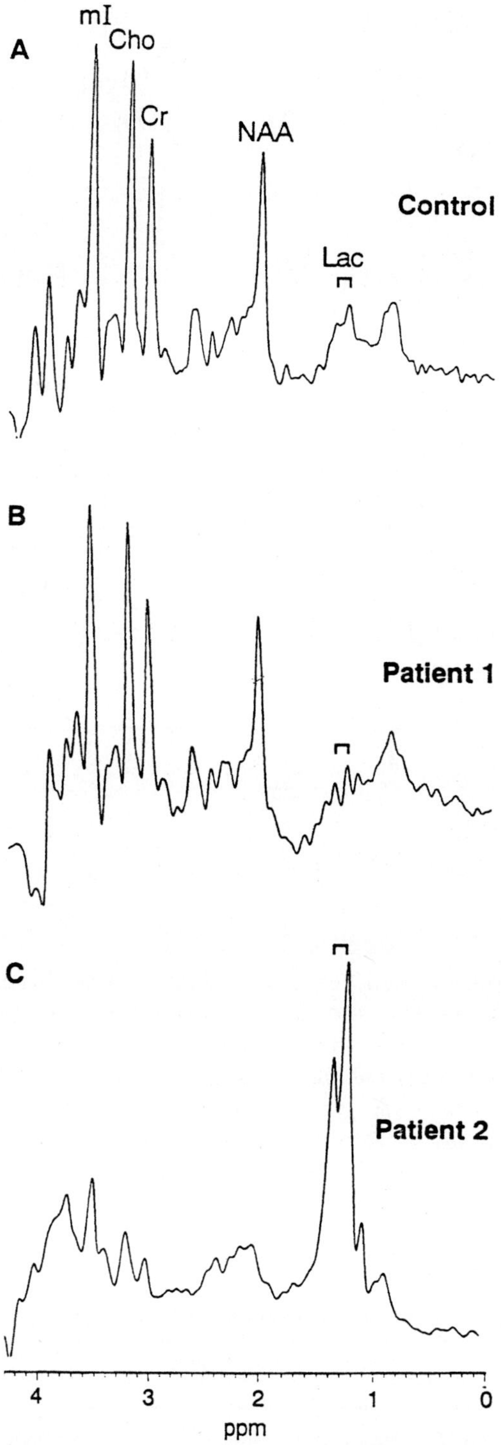

Figure 24-12

Good and bad outcomes after hypoxic encephalopathy. Localized, short echo time ^{1}H MR spectra of the gray matter in a control subject **(A)**, *patient 1* **(B)**, *and patient 2* **(C)**. *The metabolite resonances of the NAA, Cr, Cho, ml, and Lac (Lac) are indicated. In spectra* **A** *and* **B** *a possible trace of Lac is detectable, but they are otherwise identical. Since patient 1 presented as Apgar 0–0–2 after birth, hypoxic encephalopathy was prevented by the standard resuscitation measures that were applied. This contrasts with severe abnormalities in patient C. In spectrum* **C**, *major abnormalities are lack of NAA, excess Lac, excess "ml" at 3.58 ppm, and the "unknown" doublet resonance at 1.15 ppm (see also Fig. 24-44). (Modified from Ref. 147.)*

Changes in MRS appear to be irreversible and to correlate with the clinical outcome. Paradoxic recovery of cerebral metabolites after severe hypoxic encephalopathy might be best explained by cortical atrophy (Figs. 24-15 and 24-16). Despite the obvious lack of NAA at delivery, the spectrum acquired several weeks later shows NAA and an almost normal spectrum. How-

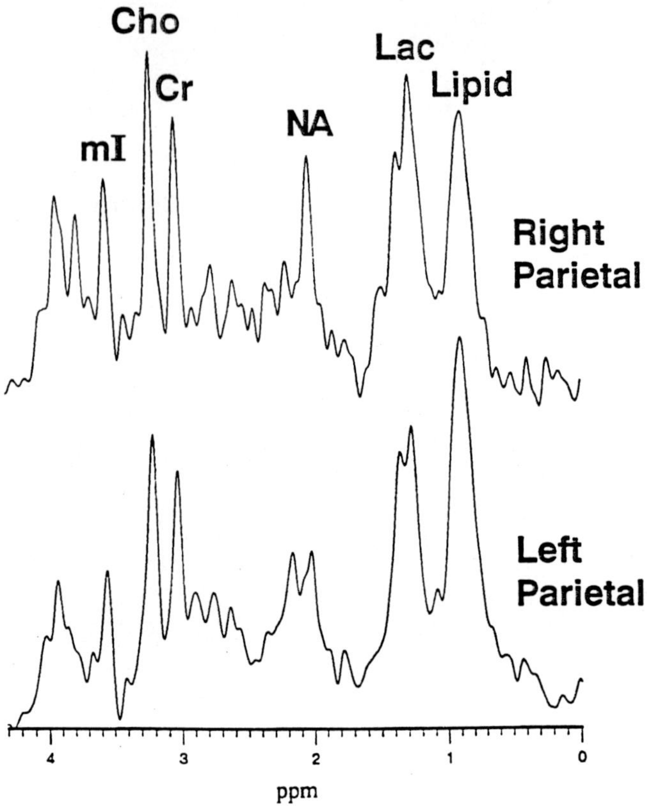

Figure 24-13
Newborn hypoxic encephalopathy.

ever, the marked ventricular dilatation on MRI (Fig. 24-16B) confirms the fact that this is most probably the result of consolidation of surviving neurons within a smaller volume of brain. Delayed neuronal development with NAA synthesis is a more speculative but very possible alternative explanation for the recovery of MRS appearances in a very premature baby.

Table 24-4
Principal neurochemical changes in stroke

	Hypoxia	*Ischemia*	*Hemorrhage*
Instant	pH ↓ lact ↑ PCr ↓ ATP ↓		?
Early	NAA ↓ Lac ≠ or normal (determines outcome)	NAA ↓ lact ↑ (lipid?) Reversible?	Poor spectral quality
Late	NAA ↓↓ lact ≠≠ Cr ↓ lipid ↑	Lac ↓	Diffuse axonal injury ± Lac ± lipid common
Chronic	NAA ↓ Cho ≠ mI ↑ lipid ↑↑	Lac	? Elevated Cho

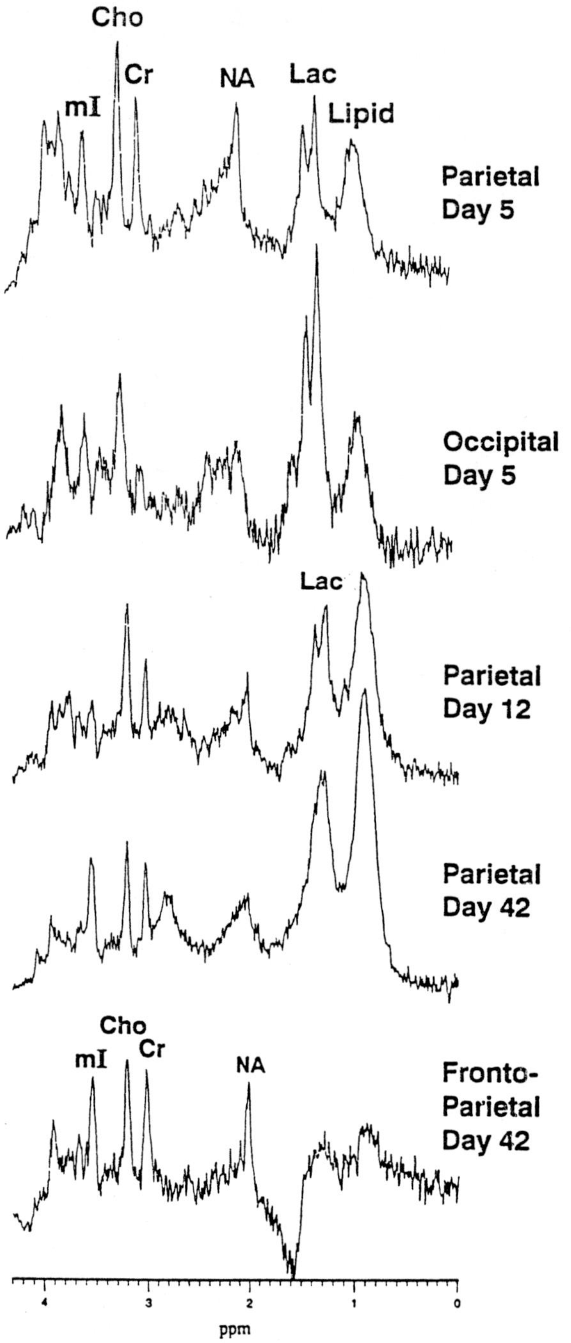

Figure 24-14
Anatomic heterogeneity of hypoxic damage and the progression of the biochemical damage over time.

Predictive Value of MRS in Neonatal Cerebral Hemorrhage

Finding hemorrhage in one location should lead to MRS examination of the contralateral hemisphere or another apparently innocent region to look for evidence of hypoxic encephalopathy. This is widespread, according to the studies of Volpe and reports from positron emission tomography (PET). MRS from the region of hemorrhage usually is not interpretable because of broad me-

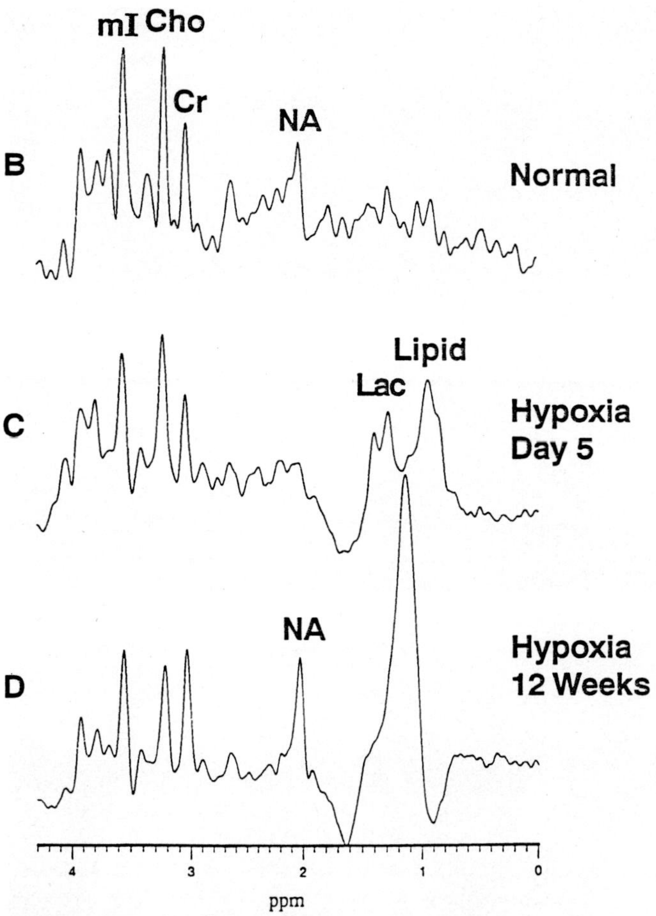

Figure 24-15

Hypoxic encephalopathy in a premature infant. ^{1}H MR spectra illustrating the paradoxic recovery of cerebral metabolites after severe hypoxic encephalopathy (see Fig. 24-16 for images) in an infant at 31 weeks gestational age (control, 34–35 weeks).

tabolite resonances (see "Appearance of Spontaneous Hemorrhage," below, and Table 24-4). However, hemorrhage also demonstrates severe hypoxic damage in apparently normal areas of the brain on MRI. MRS probably has an important contribution to make in defining the severity of hypoxic damage to surrounding brain and dating the hypoxic insult. This should be differentiated from the task of dating the hemorrhage, for which MRI is well suited.

MRS IN CHILDREN

The Similarity of MRS in Children and Adults

While undoubtedly we eventually will recognize special features, at present ^{1}H MRS in children appears to be representative of the changes seen in adults with the same pathology and for that reason is dealt with under the appropriate disease headings. Published case reports on Reye syndrome,[3,61] hypernatremia,[58] head injury,[12] and diabetes mellitus[62] illustrate this general point. MS in children 7 to 16 years old has very similar appearance on ^{1}H MRS to that in adults[63] (see the section on multiple sclerosis, below).

Seizure and Epilepsy

This common presenting symptom has so many different etiologies that it is not surprising that systematic studies with MRS are lacking. Nevertheless, we can point to several specific spectra (Figs. 24-7 and 24-8) associated with inborn errors that present as seizures and to a considerable body of work in older children with temporal lobe epilepsy. Using either symmetrically placed pairs of voxels or entire data sets of CSI, most authors can point to a significant reduction in NAA/Cr in one temporal lobe compared with the other. Even blinded studies appear to select the affected lobe with clinically useful reproducibility and precision. With this high incidence of MRS abnormalities and the prevalence of seizures in the presentation of pediatric disorders, infants and children with seizures deserve MRS as a screening procedure. A more detailed consideration of the place of MRS in epilepsy diagnosis and management is presented in the sections on MRS of epilepsy, epilepsy in children, and epilepsy in adults, below.

MRS IN ADULTS

A list of adult pathologies documented by MRS includes brain tumor, stroke, MS, hypoxia, intracranial hemorrhage, trauma, coma, metabolic disorders, hepatic encephalopathy, dementias, diabetes mellitus, focal epilepsy, and near drowning.

Focal Lesions

Cerebral Neoplasms

MRI has proved to be a boon to neuroradiologists who examine the brain for evidence of neoplasms, and in the purely diagnostic sense, there are few remaining questions MRI cannot answer. Nonenhancing lesions still present diagnostic problems, as does the differentiation between the acute edematous lesion of MS and glioma. Peritumoral edema is poorly understood on the basis of MRI alone, and since the extent of tumors visualized by computed tomography (CT) and MRI can be very different, the surgeon or radiotherapist may not have concise advice about an optimum biopsy site or the extent of desired therapy. Finally, the most often asked question concerns the appearance of recurrent tumor after radiation therapy, that is, the distinction between tumor and radiation necrosis.

MRS has addressed some of these questions and achieved a measure of success. Recent and thorough

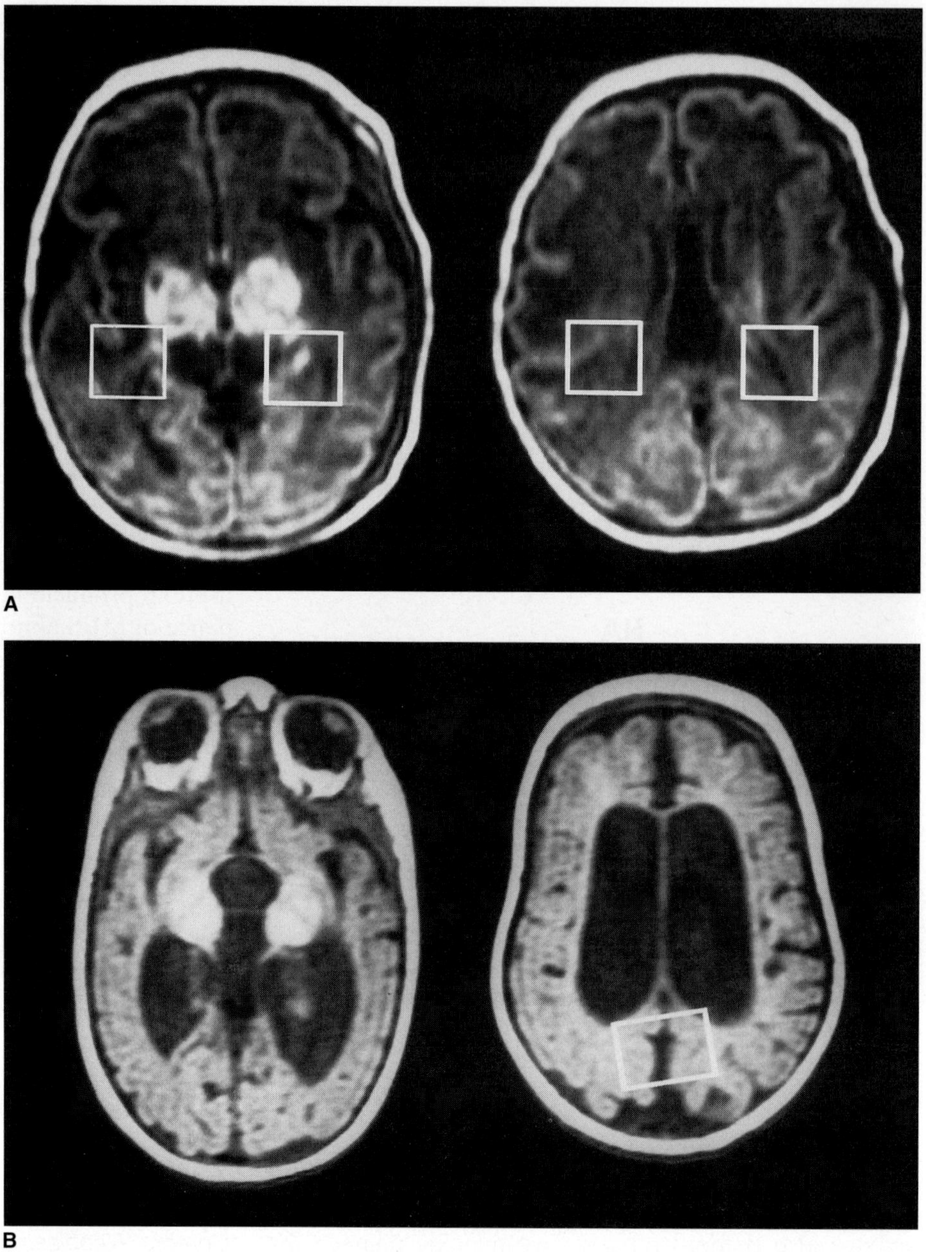

Figure 24-16
Images of patient with severe hypoxic encephalopathy at **(A)** *day 5 and* **(B)** *12 weeks of age.*

reviews are available.[64–67] Specifically, CSI performed in several different ways and in several centers readily documents the heterogeneity of brain tumors and the great regional differences in individual subjects[33,67–74] (Fig. 24-17). The loss of spectral resolution and quantitative information is compensated for by the metabolic heterogeneity now detectable in human brain tumors with three-dimensional high-spatial-resolution (0.2 to 0.4 mL) ^{1}H CSI.[75]

Diagnostic differences between solid tumor, necrosis, and viable brain tissue can be shown in single-voxel ^{1}H MRS. The areas in which MRS has special advantages include (1) the attempt to provide a better differential diagnosis than is achievable with MRI alone, (2) definition of tumor grade, aggressivity, and relevant biochemistry, in particular the importance of measuring tumor Lac and Cho, and (3) the monitoring of a successful tumor response before its regression during nonsurgical treatments and, conversely, the early definition of tumor recurrence. In all these clinical endeavors, short TE single-voxel ^{1}H MRS has clear advantages over MRI and CSI.

Basic Neurochemistry of Tumors

There are five biochemical defects common to the majority of brain tumors as measured by MRS (Fig. 24-18): NAA is decreased, Lac is increased, lipid is increased (see inset in Fig. 24-18), total Cr is decreased (as is PCr determined alone), and Cho is increased.[76] This increase

Hypoxia, Stroke and Cerebral Ischemia

Pure Hypoxia

"Pure hypoxia" is defined by interruption of oxygen supply. Near drowning is a good model for pure hypoxia and has been studied extensively.[90] ^{1}H MRS has been demonstrated to be a very useful clinical tool for predicting outcome (Fig. 24-22). The salient features are as follows:

1. ^{1}H MRS performed in occipital cortex is predictive somewhat earlier than is MRS performed in cortical white matter.
2. Five major consequences of hypoxia contribute to the sensitivity of ^{1}H MRS: loss of NAA, loss of Cr, appearance of Lac, increase in Glx, and a relative increase of Cho (while a useful indicator, this is now recognized as being due solely to the decrease in Cr noted above).
3. Poor outcome is defined as early as 48 h after resuscitation. By day 3 and day 4, changes in ^{1}H MRS have progressed to the point where a good outcome and a poor outcome can be distinguished with 100 percent accuracy.
4. The NAA/Cr ratio alone or a combination of the several MRS changes into an index rather than visual inspection of spectra is recommended if this degree of clinical precision is to be attained.

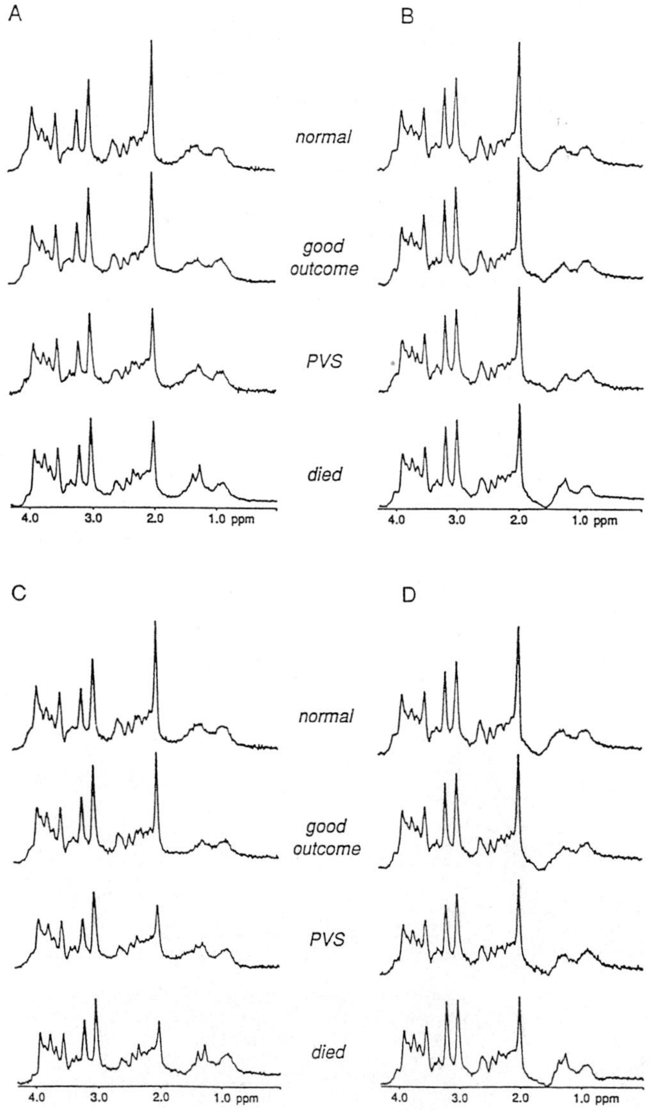

Figure 24-22
*Average ^{1}H-MR spectra in victims of near drowning (ND) grouped according to eventual outcome and time after submersion (**A** and **B** at 1–2 days, **C** and **D** at 3–4 days after ND). Spectra in **A** and **C** originated from the gray matter location; those on the right (**B** and **D**), from the white matter VOI. In all panels the largest deviations from normal occur in the spectra from ND victims who did not recover fully. There is no clear distinction between patients who died and those who developed a persistent vegetative state (PVS).*

Stroke and Cerebral Ischemia

In general, it can be stated with confidence that MRS is more sensitive than MRI in detecting hypoxic damage (caused by vascular or other disease) and is diagnostic at a much earlier stage in the disease. It is now obvious that the major changes in stroke management will demand ever-earlier emergency imaging techniques. The exquisite sensitivity of diffusion-weighted MRI to developing cerebral edema gives a warning as early as 2 to 4 h after vascular occlusion, but MRS is affected within seconds and would certainly give positive results at the earliest moment that a clinician condoned the risk of moving the patient to the MRS suite. Indeed, several studies in the past 8 years confirm in humans what was well established in experimental animals: A characteristic metabolite profile occurs in stroke. MRS of stroke has been reviewed extensively by Howe and associates.[91]

Stroke is a complex disorder with three major pathogenetic components: (1) hypoxia, (2) ischemia, and (3) hemorrhage. Each has a characteristic pathologic biochemistry. Next, the type of pathologic injury has its own impact on the biochemical evolution of the "stroke." This component is reflected in the complex events that characterize MRS changes observed in stroke over time. Finally, and probably of the greatest clinical significance, graded injuries will be apparent depending on the distance from the nearest fully "oxygenated" location. This is the concept of watershed injuries in global ischemia and of the "penumbra" of salvageable brain tissue as distance from the stroke center increases.[92] The nature, chronology, and severity of biochemical insults that can be anticipated both early and later after a major stroke are detailed in Table 24-4.

CSI of Stroke

Single-voxel MRS has been used to define all the biochemical changes in stroke: loss of NAA and Cr and accumulation of Lac and Cho. The all-important features, including the extent and severity of ischemia, and the peripheral penumbra can best be defined by CSI[72,93] (Fig. 24-23). Figure 24-23 demonstrates the presence of both lipid and Lac in typical single-voxel ^{1}H spectrum of stroke[94] by means of an editing technique.

Clinical Implications

Welch[95] emphasized the need for early assessment of stroke to determine salvageable volumes within a 6-h "therapeutic window." Very few MRS studies have actually been performed within this interval; several (including the one illustrated in Fig. 24-23) are achieved within 24 h. This may be called "acute," and the value of MRS lies in the diagnosis of ischemic damage. Late changes, including further loss of NAA, accumulation of Lac and lipid,[94] and the very late "reappearance" of Lac, that were first noted by Petroff and associates[96] also may be of clinical interest if methods for dealing with the secondary repair after stroke become available.[97]

Newer results from Graham and colleagues[98] summarize their experience in 32 patients examined at approximately day 5. Lac intensity in the "worst" CSI voxel was correlated with (1) lesion size, (2) single photon

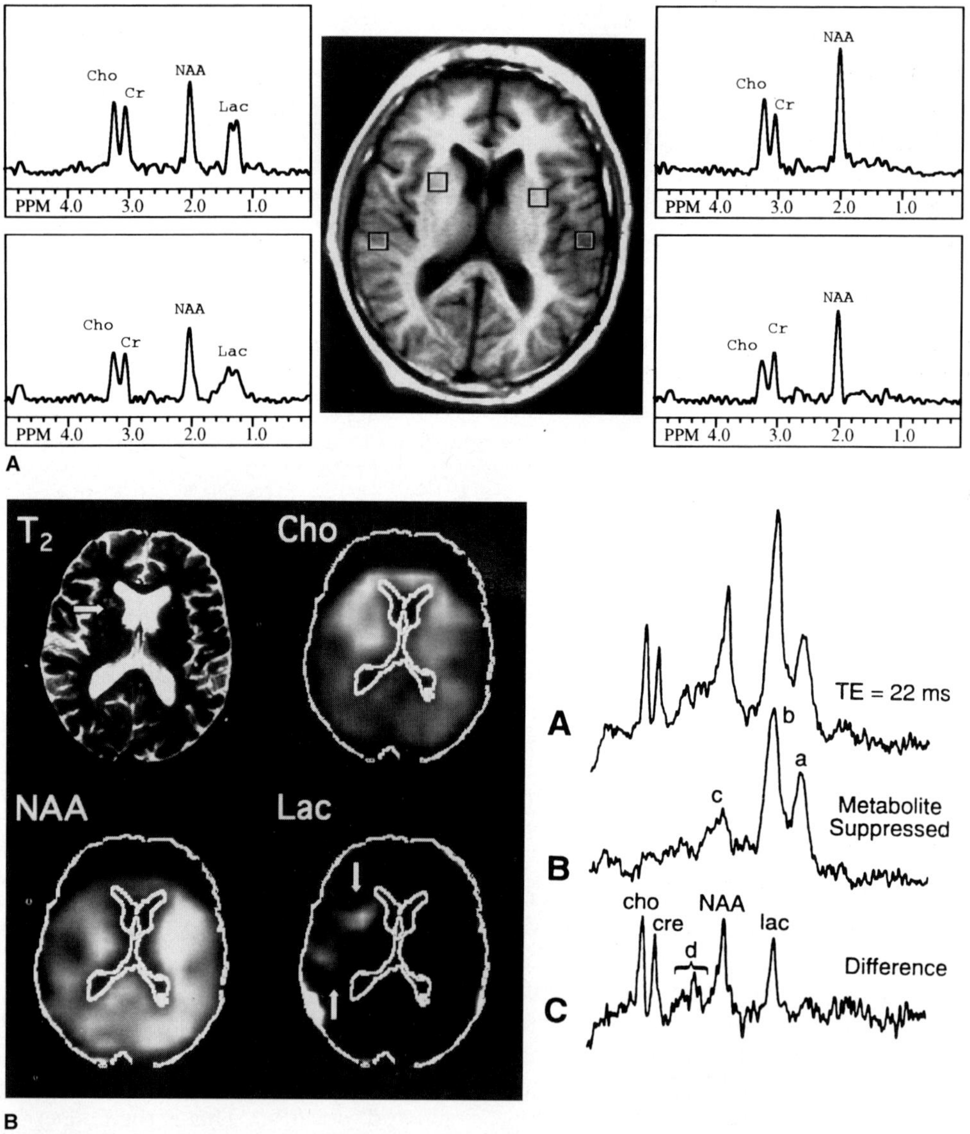

Figure 24-23

Heterogeneity of metabolism is readily identified, with the potential advantage of identifying salvageable neuronal tissue in the stroke "penumbra." Spectra obtained 23 days after a subcortical stroke. (From Dr. Peter Barker, with permission.) Inset: Definition of lipid and Lac in an infarct single-voxel difference technique based on the ability of an inversion recovery (IR) pulse to remove low-molecular-weight metabolites from the spectrum. (Courtesy of Dr. J. W. Prichard.)

emission computed tomography (SPECT) score; (3) Toronto stroke scale, and (4) "outcome" index. NAA, by contrast, correlated with 4 but not with 1 through 3. Lipid and Cho or Cr changes were not considered. Barker and coworkers[99] concurred with others that these additional biochemical markers convey clinical information and possibly have prognostic value.

In recent years, diffusion-weighted, perfusion, and mean-transit time (MTT) imaging have emerged as a vital aspect of interventional therapy planning in patients with stroke. The result is that patients with stroke enter MRI suites with 3 h of onset. While the ultimate role of MRS is therefore still unclear, to present observers it is apparent that Welch[95] is correct—the earlier MRS is performed, the more likely we are to see potentially salvageable tissues conserved by therapy. Conversely, new precision in prognosis after stroke—a notoriously difficult area of medical management—can already be offered by MRS performed as early as 5 days and as late as several weeks after a stroke.

All of the above data provide strong evidence that MRS is beneficial in stroke patients.

Neuropsychiatric Systemic Lupus Erythematosus

Systemic lupus erythematosus (SLE) is a complex disorder with overlapping pathologic processes, including inflammation, cytotoxic and vasogenic edema, stroke, demyelination, hemorrhage, and reversible ischemia. The degree to which a particular process may affect an individual patient is highly variable, resulting in a wide array of potential spectroscopic patterns. Those findings include the following:

1. Decreased NAA. This is the most common finding, occurs both in lesions and normal-appearing tissues, and appears most closely associated with previously active major neuropsychiatric systemic lupus erythematosus (NPSLE) and the presence of cerebral atrophy.
2. Increased Cho. This occurs in both lesions and normal-appearing tissues and is most closely associated with SLE patients with stroke and antiphospholipid antibody syndrome.
3. Increased T_2 of gray matter as measured by relaxometry. Increased T_2 of gray matter represents diffuse cerebral edema and is most common in patients with acute major NPSLE episodes (generalized seizures, psychosis, delirium, coma) but not stroke, suggesting a diffuse neurocytotoxic process (antineuronal antibodies?).
4. With short echo times MRS, increased resonances in the 1.3-ppm region relative to normal controls are most closely associated with active NPSLE, major or minor. These resonances do not appear to be lactate.[100–102]

White Matter Diseases

Aging Brain

The checkered history of deep white matter changes on MRI—they have been considered in turn MS, deep white matter infarcts (DWMIs), and signs of normal aging—is somewhat more clear since the advent of MRS. Even quite sizable DWMI areas in the centrum ovale have normal metabolite ratios on long echo time MRS. No evidence of Lac or an elevated Cho/Cr ratio in DWMIs has been obtained. This eliminates any suggestion that these brain regions are actually ischemic. However, the fact remains that 84 percent of patients with cerebrovascular risk factors have DWMIs compared with only 10 percent of controls. MRS shows very definite but small changes in the "normal" ^{1}H MRS profile of the aging brain. NAA/Cr and [NAA] fall in (occipital) gray matter. Cho/Cr is higher on average than it is in younger normals, while mI/Cr is somewhat lower. None of these changes exceed 10 percent (Table 24-5).

Multiple Sclerosis

The pattern of distribution rather than the specific appearance defines MS, and so MRI is greatly superior to MRS in diagnosing MS. However, despite useful studies with Gd enhancement, dating of MS plaques and in particular correlating acute activity in the plaque with neurologic activity in the patient have been only partially successful. This task becomes increasingly urgent as effective therapies are introduced in clinical trials. When the plaque is large enough to be analyzed by a single MRS voxel, the following changes are characteristic:[91] Low NAA/Cr is universally recorded, Cho/Cr is generally elevated,[103] and mI/Cr is increased in short echo time spectra.[63,104,105]

Progression of MS is more clearly documented by a reduction in NAA/Cr than by MRI.[103,106] Activity in the MS plaque is also well defined by MRS. Surveys in

Table 24-5
Normal aging

Age range	*N*	*NAA/Cr*	*Cho/Cr*	*mI/Cr*
Gray matter				
16–25	10	1.41 ± .08	0.56 ± .05	0.60 ± .04
26–37	10	1.36 ± .08	0.61 ± .08	0.60 ± .04
40–78	12	1.26 ± .09	0.60 ± .05	0.59 ± .06
White matter				
16–25	10	1.54 ± .09	0.77 ± .05	0.59 ± .05
26–37	10	1.49 ± .07	0.78 ± .06	0.60 ± .04
40–78	12	1.41 ± .12	0.82 ± .08	0.63 ± .05

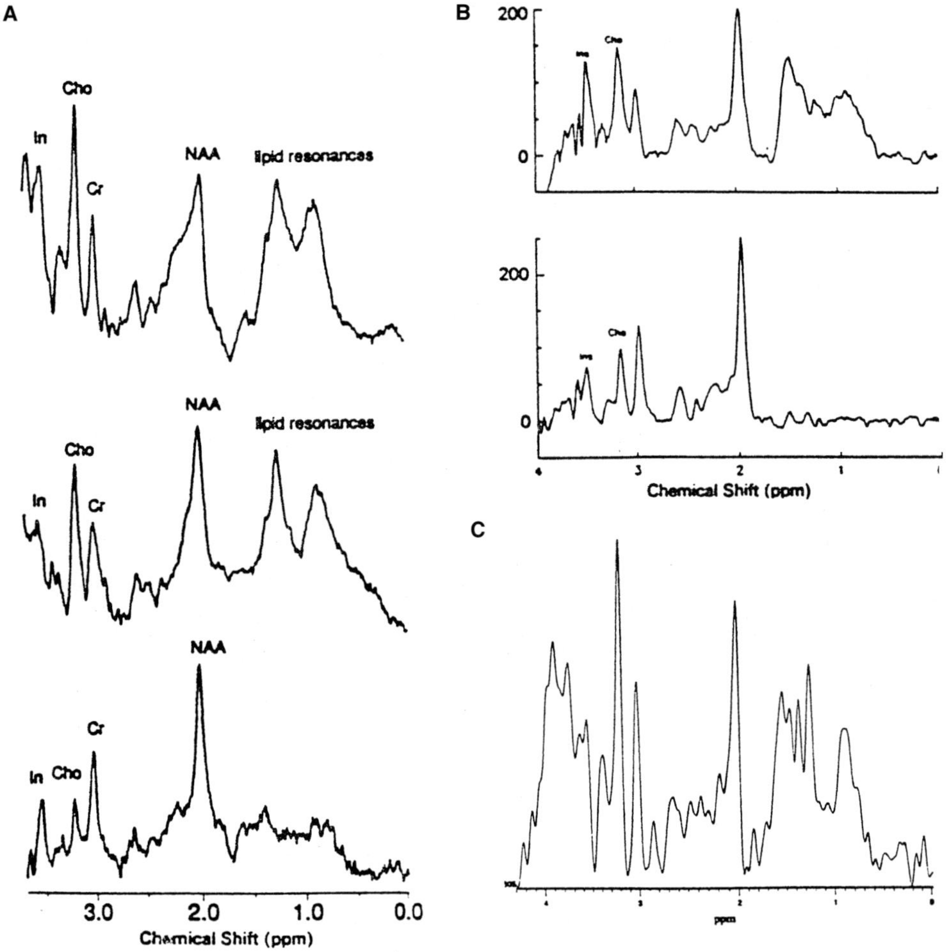

Figure 24-24
Active MS plaque. Comparable MRS appearances reported from London **(A)**, *Edmonton* **(B)**, *and Pasadena* **(C)** *in large enhancing lesions. Spectrum* **C** *is quantitative, with numbers indicating percentage of control for NAA (66 percent), Cr (50 percent), and Cho (170 percent), with lipid, Lac, and possibly alanine present.*

Canada[105] and the United Kingdom[107] indicate that large, extremely active acute MS lesions have a characteristic ^{1}H MR spectrum (Fig. 24-24). Lipid, Lac, a high Cho/Cr ratio, and elevated mI have been interpreted as evidence of myelin breakdown and acute activity in seven of eight cases[105] and 10 of 24 lesions.[107] In some instances the reversal of these changes has been reported, and there are indications that this is accompanied by regression of the acute neurologic symptoms.[108] In single-voxel MRS studies of brain regions containing chronic MS plaques, increased mI/Cr may be the only residual change (unpublished work). It seems very probable, therefore, that the addition of MRS to routine MRI in patients with established MS will improve "activity" assessment. This could translate into an improved quality of clinical trials of newer therapeutic agents, that is, patient management.

Leukodystrophies

Most MRS studies of leukodystrophies have been concerned with the childhood forms (see the section on leukodystrophies on page 737). A group of leukodystrophy patients are asymptomatic until they at some stage as adults are affected by a milder form of the disease; others never have symptoms. MRS may become an excellent tool for screening and monitoring these adult patients.

Leukoencephalitides

Diseases that clearly involve an infectious agent, such as herpes encephalitis (Fig. 24-25) and Rasmussen disease, not surprisingly result in major abnormalities of the MR spectrum. The specificity of these changes to one disease has not been established, and although the neurochemical disturbance is striking in newborns, children, and adults, it is not known whether any or all of these changes are reversible. Hence, the possible role of MRS in prognosis remains to be explored.

The anatomic extent of the disease, however, might be determined with MRS, since the focal form of Rasmussen disease, for example, appears to be accompanied by normal MRS in brain areas that are normal on MRI, with grossly abnormal spectra within the focal lesion or lesions.

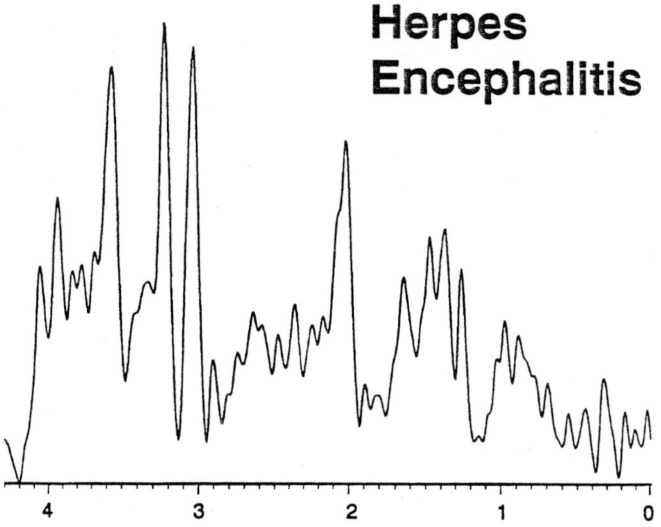

Figure 24-25

Herpes encephalitis. PROBE spectrum from parietal cortex. Low signal-to-noise ratio implies loss of brain "mass." Cho, ml, and Lac are increased relative to Cr, while NAA is reduced.

HIV and AIDS

The case of HIV is instructive and may apply to other inflammatory diseases of the brain. Several authorities report a steady decline in the NAA/Cr ratio in patients who are HIV-positive but do not yet have proven AIDS. More striking is the reporting of positive MRS findings in patients with HIV serology but normal MRI at the time of the MRS examination.[109–118] While we accept that better sequences, more careful reading, or more rigorous evaluations of immunologic status could explain such a discrepancy, the most likely answer is that MRS, by detecting the unsuspected underlying neurochemical changes of HIV infection, gives an early warning of MRI changes to come. The therapeutic consequences of this conclusion are striking, particularly in such a generally pessimistic disease. If treatment of HIV can prevent neurologic deterioration,[117] MRS will become an indispensable tool in this area. Indeed, Vion-Dury and associates[119] reported such an event, with clear evidence of MRS improvement after the treatment of HIV-positive patients.

Other infections of the CNS might behave similarly, but we do not have the results of clinical studies at hand. If herpes encephalitis can be defined before there are overt changes on MRI, it is hoped that the outcomes of treatment will be improved significantly by performing and interpreting ^{1}H MRS.

Several studies define abnormal MRS in association with abnormalities of MRI in encephalitis, HIV, and AIDS-related masses. There is persuasive evidence that MRS changes precede those in MRI, so that a serious debate surrounds the question of what to do when a patient manifests such MRS changes, in particular, reduced NAA and increased Cho.

Several neurologic complications of AIDS are recognized, and MRI is the method of choice for their detection and differentiation. In cases where focal lesions still are difficult to diagnose yet the therapeutic options demand an accurate answer, studies with MRS are very useful. Figure 24-26 shows such a study, with the authors concluding that MRS could displace unpopular and hazardous brain biopsy in this clinical arena.[120] The noninvasive, quick, and accurate differentiation of brain masses in AIDS is of great clinical benefit because (1) medicines used to treat toxoplasmosis are relatively helpful but have side effects and (2) nontoxoplasmosis infections and tumors can grow rapidly in AIDS patients, while treatment usually is attempted by starting to treat the mass as if it were toxoplasmosis.

Degenerative Diseases

Parkinson Disease

Parkinson disease is an affliction of the dopa and dopamine system, particularly in the basal ganglia. It is perhaps not surprising, therefore, that despite a carefully conducted multicenter trial, no reproducible abnormalities have been defined on ^{1}H MRS at long echo times. Treated versus untreated Parkinson disease may result in some differences in the spectra acquired from the basal ganglia, but one must be cautious because of the virtually diagnostic excess of iron in that region and the resulting susceptibility changes in Parkinson disease, as shown on MRI.

Alzheimer Disease

CT and MRI performed in a routine way make little direct contribution to the diagnosis of dementia or Alzheimer disease (AD) in particular. Their role is to eliminate other, usually space-occupying disorders or normal-pressure hydrocephalus. With special measurements, temporal lobe atrophy can become a rather specific and sensitive tool for the diagnosis of late Alzheimer disease. MRS, by contrast, is showing genuine promise of defining dementia (from the reduction in NAA/Cr and [NAA]). In more than one series the addition of even nonquantitative MRS to MRI improved the precision of Alzheimer diagnosis.[121] Elevation of Cho/Cr (although predicted by postmortem studies) is neither reproducible nor specific to Alzheimer disease, since Cho/Cr increases with age (see the section on aging brain, above) and in several other conditions, including stroke and possibly multi-infarct dementia. More specificity and a possible alternative view of pathogenesis are accorded by the measurement of mI/Cr in short echo time MRS. mI/Cr and [mI] are increased (Fig. 24-27). Although other dementias share the feature of low NAA/Cr, increased mI/Cr distinguishes AD patients from normal elderly persons and

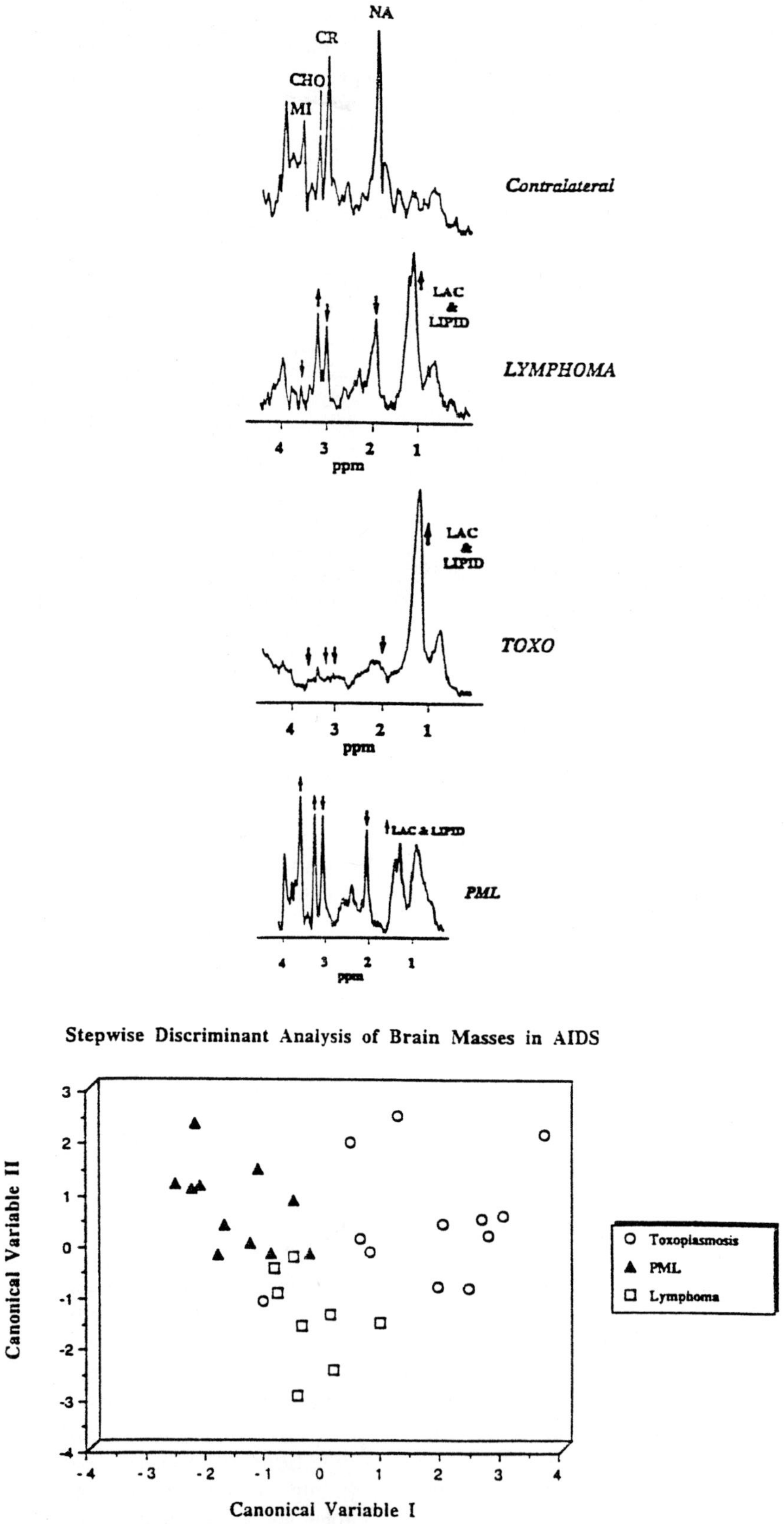

Figure 24-26
^{1}H MRS readily distinguishes the differing metabolite profiles of commonly occurring AIDS brain masses. The canonical variables I and II are weighted sums of Cho, Cr, mI, and Lac. (Courtesy of Drs. B. L. Miller, L. Chang, T. Ernst, and colleagues.)

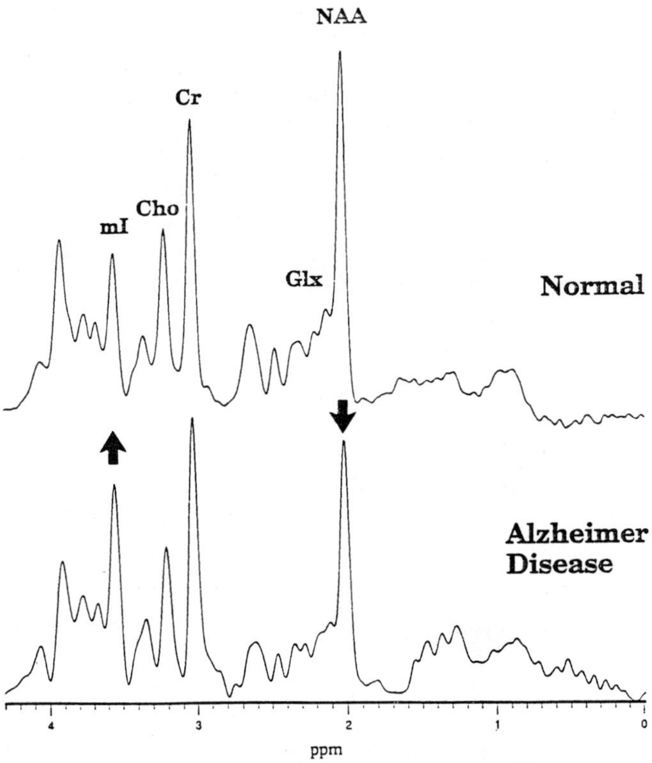

Figure 24-27
^1H MR spectra from the occipital cortex (gray matter) of a patient with probable Alzheimer disease compared with a normal elderly subject. Peaks are scaled to Cr and provide a measure of the concentrations of individual metabolites.

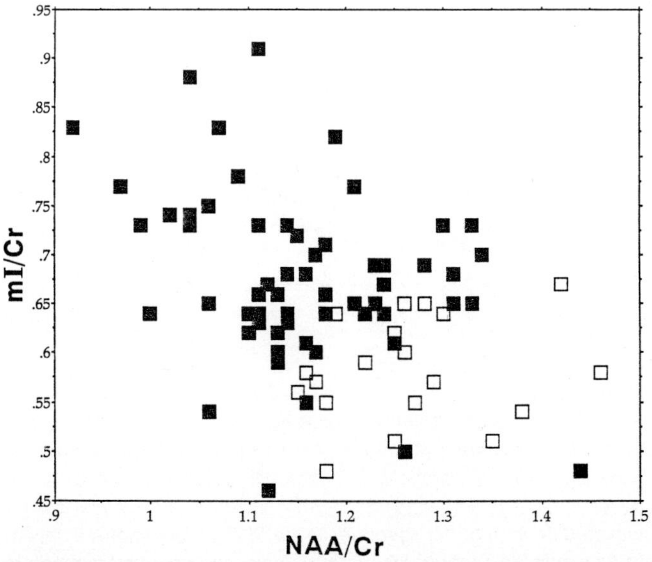

Figure 24-28
Distribution of mI/Cr and NAA/Cr in patients with clinically verified probable Alzheimer disease (■) compared with normal elderly subject (□).

patients with other dementias (Figs. 24-28 and 24-29).

Dementia in Down syndrome, which is pathogenetically similar to AD, is also marked by increased mI/Cr (Fig. 24-30). It is therefore possible that both in ruling out AD in the elderly and in making an early diagnosis of dementia in Down syndrome, MRS is superior to imaging with SPECT or MRI. At present, the clinical diagnosis of AD has a sensitivity between 80 and 90 percent. Based on the same clinical criteria (i.e., assuming this flawed gold standard = 100 percent), MRS can be equally precise in distinguishing AD from normal with a specificity of 95 percent. AD and other proven dementias are distinguished with a specificity of 64 percent, but AD is excluded with 80 percent efficiency by the MRS examination.[122]

Pick Disease

In life, the definition of Pick disease and its distinction from AD rest on the peculiarly "frontal lobe" clinical

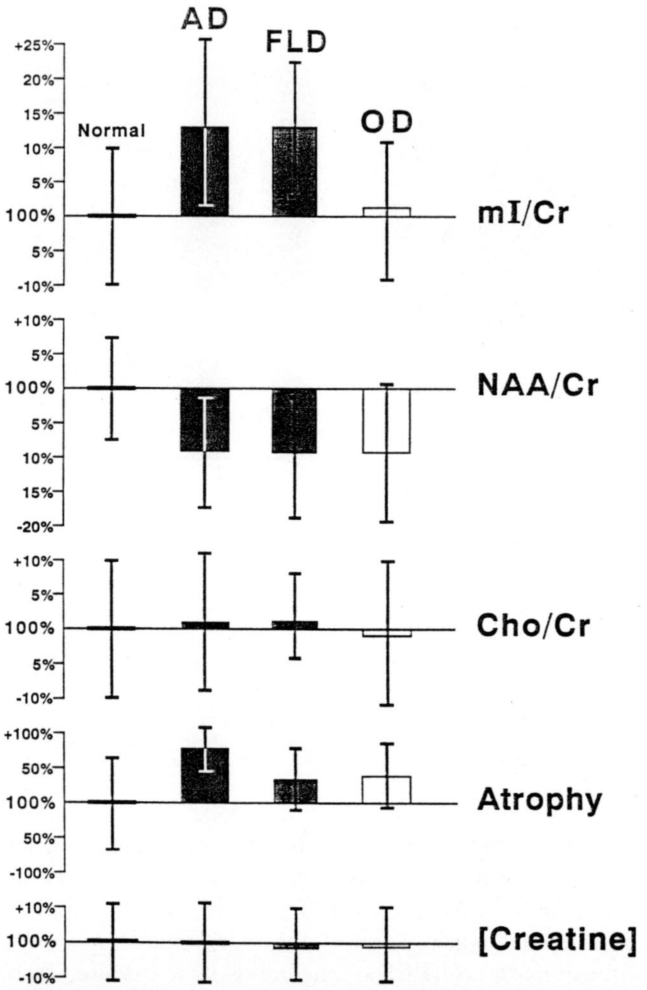

Figure 24-29
MRS and CSF volumes (atrophy index) in the differentiation of Alzheimer disease from other clinical dementias (OD). Note the marked overlap between FLD (frontal lobe dementia) and AD.

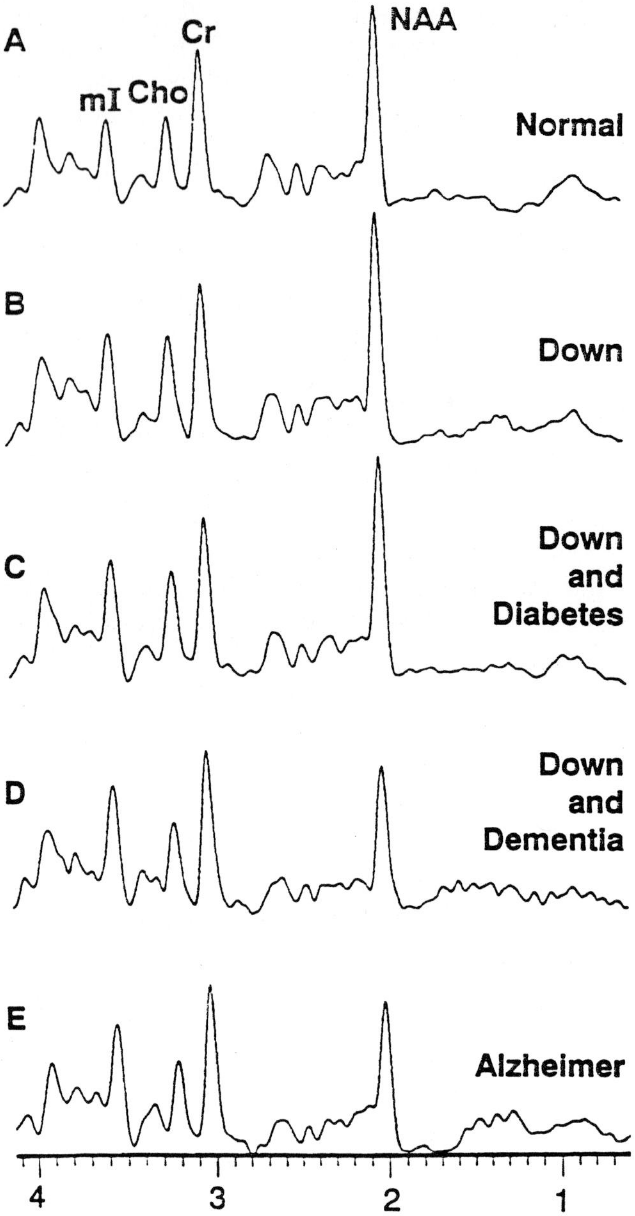

Figure 24-30
Dementia of Down syndrome. The marked similarity of this MRS to that of AD is noted, as is the presumably much earlier onset of one of the two biochemical changes, the increase in mI/Cr.

symptoms and the obvious frontal lobe atrophy on CT or MRI. Neuropathologically, Pick disease and AD are quite distinct from each other. However, in a limited series, MRS was not successful in distinguishing frontal lobe dementias (FLDs), including Pick disease, from AD when the single voxel was acquired from the occipital region (Fig. 24-29). FLDs were distinguished from AD with relative ease[123] by measuring a midfrontal region (Fig. 24-31).

Huntington Disease

Controversy surrounds an early report of lactate in the ^{1}H MRS spectrum of Huntington disease[124] and, therefore, the use of ^{1}H MRS in therapy monitoring.[125] At present, diagnostic use appears to be limited. This disease correctly belongs in the metabolic category (see "Systemic and Metabolic Disease" below) if MRS has been successful in demonstrating excess Lac in these patients.[124] Furthermore, this disease offers one of the

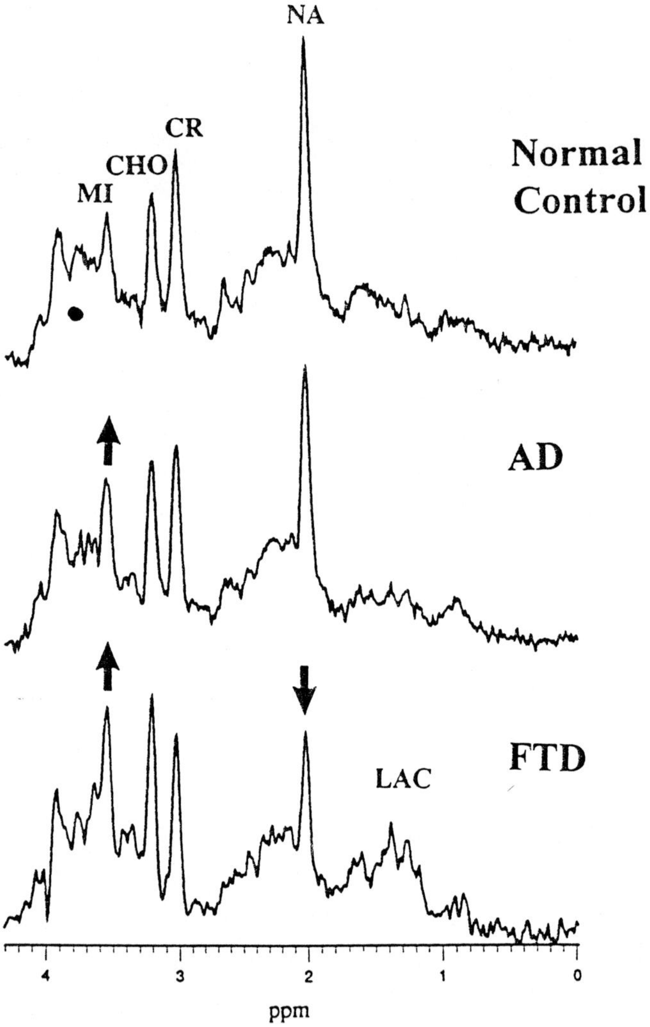

Figure 24-31
Frontal lobe spectra from a normal control, an AD patient, and a frontal lobe dementia (FLD) patient. The three spectra are scaled; peak areas reflect metabolite concentrations. While the frontal spectra of the AD patient and the normal are very similar (except for elevated mI in AD), the spectrum of the FLD patient shows a severe reduction in NAA (about 30 percent), indicating neuronal damage or loss, and a significant increase in mI (about 25 percent). The third very interersting abnormality in the FLD spectrum is the presence of the Lac doublet confirmed at long TE (270). (Reproduced with permission from Ref. 123.)

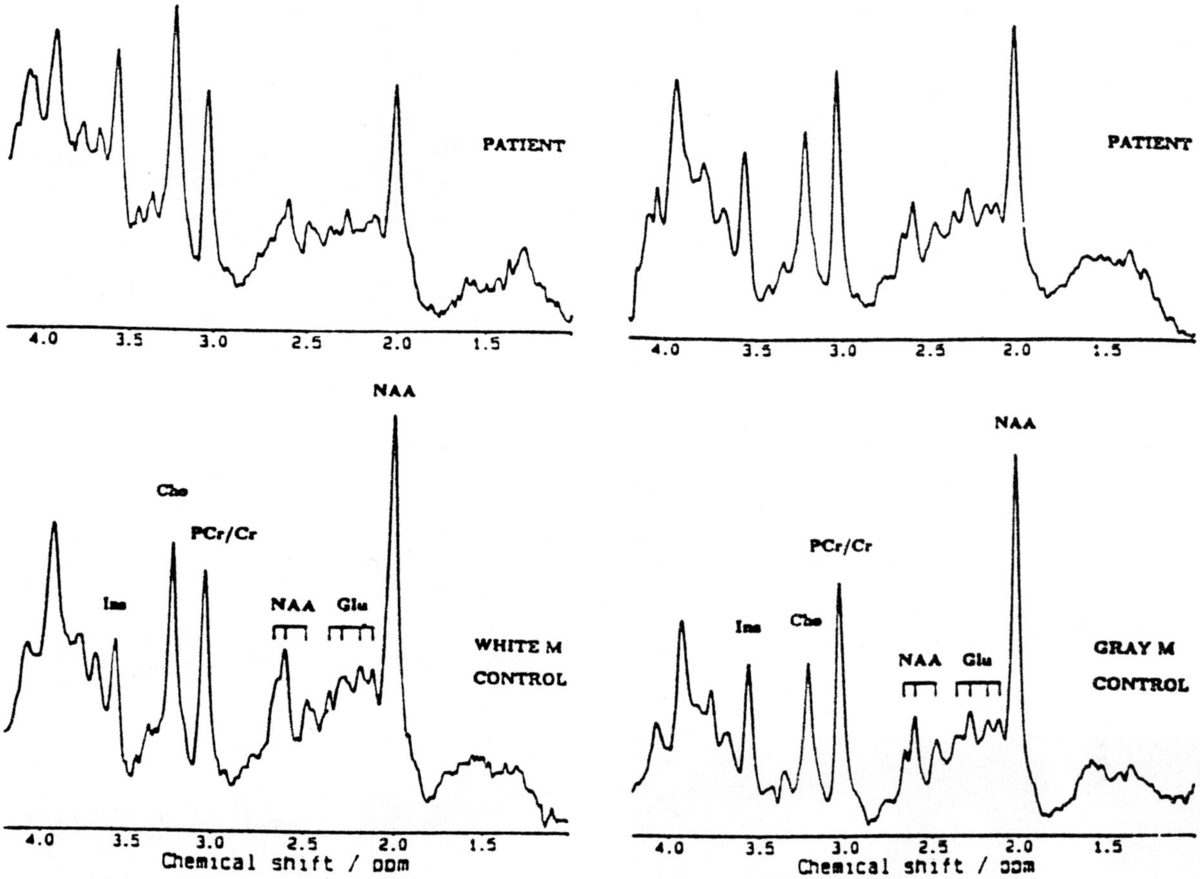

Figure 24-32

Creutzfeldt-Jakob disease (JCD) MRS at 2 tesla. Note the excellent definition of glutamate resonances at higher field. The principal change is in white matter (contrast AD), with reduction of NAA/Cr and an apparent increase in both mI/Cr and Cho/Cr. The latter is also a distinction from AD.

relatively few instances in which MRS has both guided the choice of treatment (coenzyme Q) and monitored its successful implementation.[125]

Creutzfeldt-Jakob Disease

This rare disorder gives few if any clues on MRI. MRS, by contrast, was markedly abnormal in the single case report from Bruhn and associates[126] (Fig. 24-32) and was readily distinguished from AD in that study.

Systemic and Metabolic Disease

Clinical Impact of MRS on Metabolic Disease

This area has been remarkably successful for MRI. Many reports of pattern recognition in inborn errors of metabolism serve to make MRI a necessary factor in the diagnosis.[43] However, a neuroradiologist's contact with metabolic diseases in adults is extremely limited. Central pontine myelinolysis, Leigh disease, Wilson disease, and Hallervorden-Spatz disease were the four diseases discussed in that report. In adult metabolic brain disease, the impact of MRS is now considerably greater than that of MRI.

Hepatic Encephalopathy

A triad of changes—loss of mI, increased GIx, and reduced Cho—characterizes patients with chronic hepatic encephalopathy (HE) and, more usefully, defines subclinical HE. Except in hyponatremia and central pontine myelinolysis (Fig. 24-33), the disappearance of mI is seen only in HE. Transjugular intrahepatic portal systemic shunt (TIPS) patients develop these characteristic metabolite changes as evidence of HE after shunting. Transplant patients undergo complete reversal of these biochemical abnormalities within weeks of successful transplantation. Acute fulminant HE and the rare Reye syndrome show exaggerated MRS changes even when MRI is normal.

HE is an excellent example of a metabolic encephalopathy[127] with identifiable neurotoxins originating in a systemic disease. In animal studies, several distinct neurotoxins were identified. The earliest of these was ammonia;[128,129] which normally is fully removed from

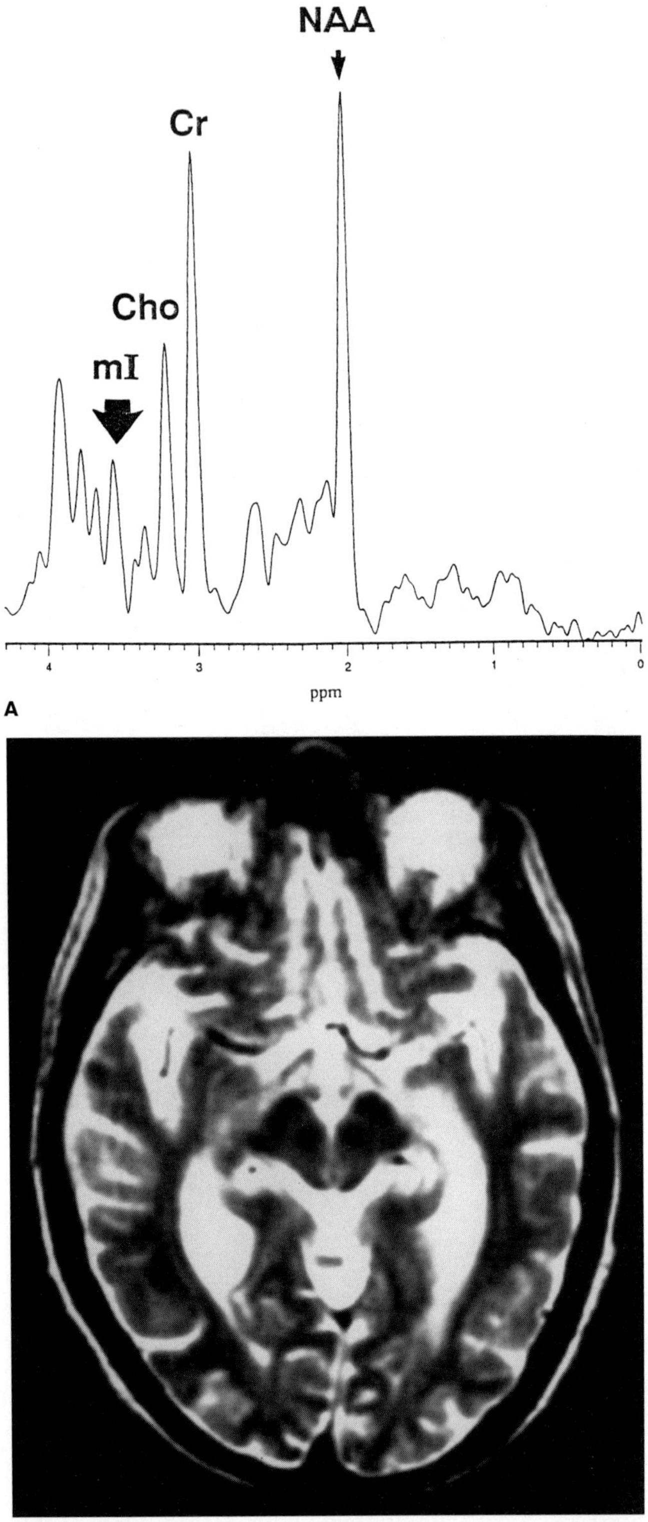

Figure 24-33
The occipital gray matter spectrum **(A)** *from a patient (F 72) examined to rule out AD. NAA is about 10 percent low; mI is not increased but is reduced about 40 percent. The MRS therefore is not consistent with AD. The very low mI was in this case explained by hyponatremia; the sodium level was 127, a conclusion supported by MRI* **(B)** *that is consistent with pontine myelinolysis.*

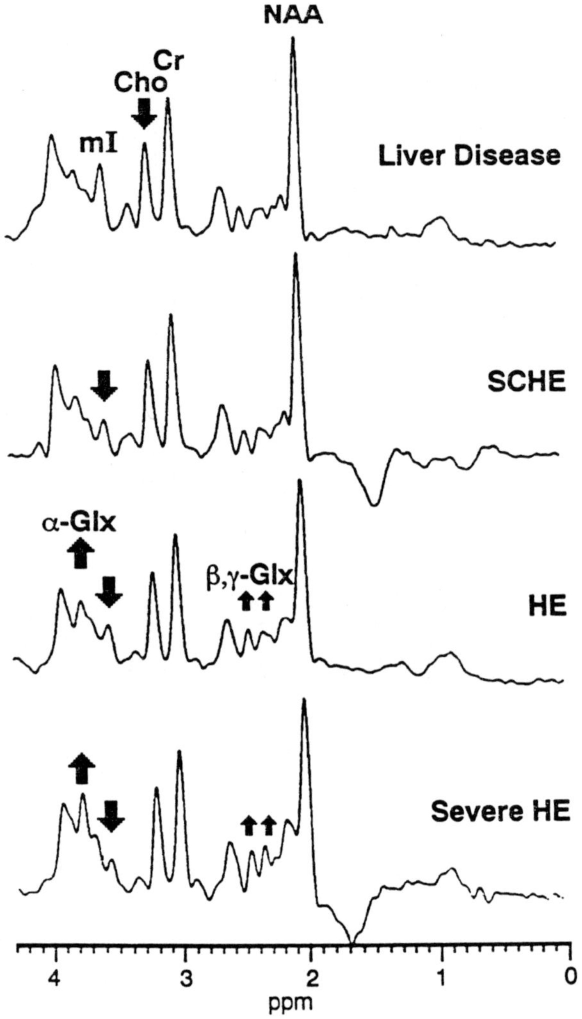

Figure 24-34
Development of hepatic encephalopathy in human subjects (1.5 tesla spectra). A series of spectra of parietal cortex (white matter) acquired under similar conditions (GE Signa 1.5 tesla, STEAM localization TR 1.5 s, Te 30 ms, NEX 128) from different patients. A normal spectrum for comparison is shown in Fig. 24-4. Liver disease (top) is a relatively normal spectrum with a slight decrease in Cho. In subclinical hepatic encephalopathy (SCHE) there is a definite decrease in mI with a minor increase in the glutamine regions (Glx). There is a very significant increase in the Glx regions in HE (grade 1), and mI is further depleted. The spectrum of grade 3 HE shows more severe changes in the biochemical markers of this disease, most notably glutamine.

portal blood by hepatic urea synthesis.[130,131] The combination of the loss of biosynthetic liver function and the diversion of nondetoxified blood to the brain by so-called portal systemic shunts (PSS) accounts for the frequently demonstrated excess of cerebral and CSF glutamine:[132]

$$NH_4^+ + \text{glutamate} \underset{\text{glutaminase}}{\overset{\text{GS}}{\longleftrightarrow}} \text{glutamine}$$

The enzyme glutamine synthetase (GS) that is responsible for this reaction is located exclusively in astrocytes.[133] The resynthesis of glutamate and GABA from glutamine (both vital neurotransmitter amino acids) occurs principally in neurons.[134]

Lest it be thought that ammonia "toxicity" accounts for all the clinical syndromes covered by the term HE, the reader is referred to Butterworth and Layrargues[135] for an extensive review of several other well-documented alternatives.

Studies using STEAM localized short echo-time ^{1}H MRS defined the changes in 10 patients with clinically confirmed chronic HE. The average increase in cerebral glutamine was estimated as more than 50 percent, Cho decreased 14 percent, and mI decreased 45 percent[5] (Fig. 24-34), so that cerebral osmolyte concentration may remain constant.[136] Very similar findings were reported at 2 tesla by Bruhn and colleagues[6,10] and at 1.5 T by McConnell and coworkers[137] using PRESS at short or long echo times.

An early study that used long echo time PRESS-localized ^{1}H MRS failed to identify depletion of mI but was the first to clearly show Cho depletion in human brain.[11]

Subclinical Hepatic Encephalopathy

As was indicated above, HE is a group of diseases presumed to have an identical etiology but presenting a great variety of distinct clinical pictures. Underlying all of them is believed to be the entity of "subclinical HE" (SCHE), although it is by no means clear that the HE and coma of fulminant (very acute) liver failure go through a truly "subclinical" phase.

^{1}H MRS accurately reflects the entity of SCHE[138,139] and in preliminary studies also appears to mirror the progressive and increasingly severe syndromes of overt HE defined by Parsons-Smith as grades 1 through 4 (Fig. 24-34). Elevation of glutamine is rather more obvious at 2 tesla (Fig. 24-35) but presents little difficulty at 1.5 tesla (or even at 0.5 T; see Fig. 24-8M).

Figure 24-34 should not be taken as proof, however, that in an individual patient this orderly progression of neurochemical dysfunction occurs. Longitudinal studies have not been performed in sufficient numbers to be certain of this. Nevertheless, it is tempting to suggest, as that figure appears to indicate, that in a brain exposed to liver "toxins," Cho depletion (possibly glycerophosphorylcholine) precedes the loss of mI and sI, with later

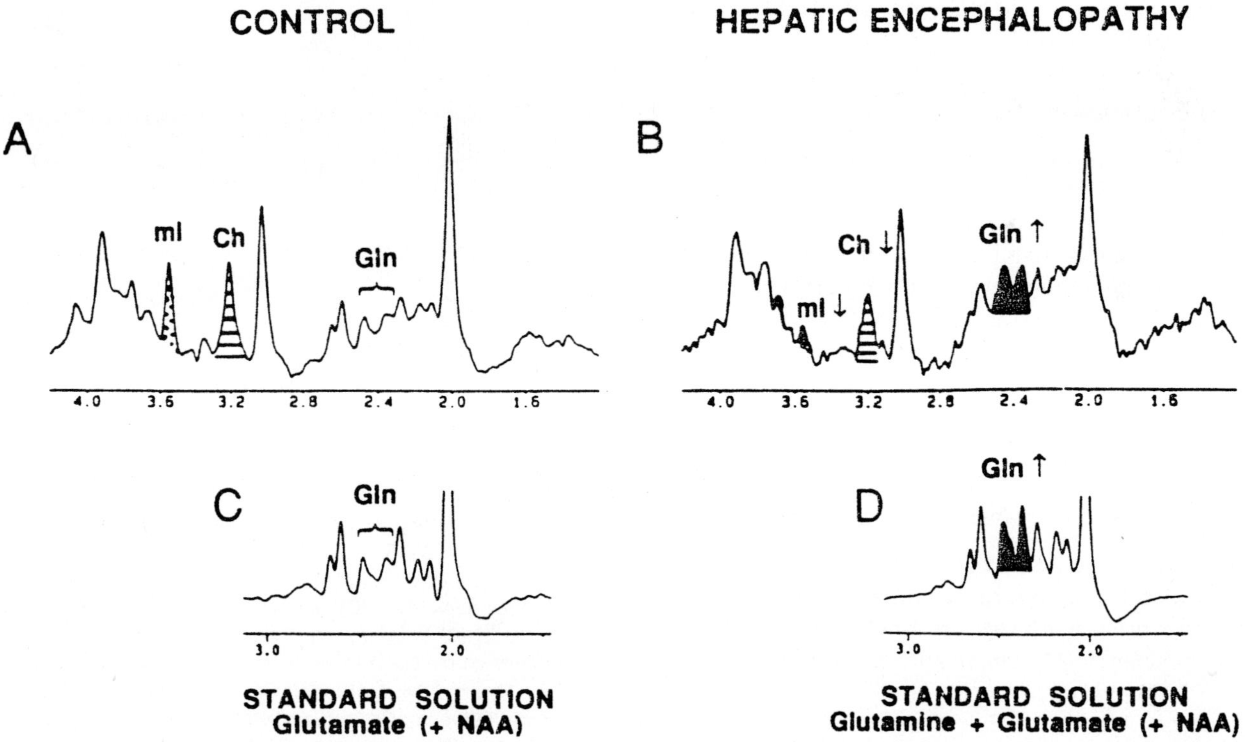

Figure 24-35

Identification of glutamine in the ^{1}H spectra at 2.0 tesla. A 51-year-old patient with HE caused by a surgical portacaval shunt is compared with a normal control. Spectra were obtained from an occipital gray matter location and show the expected changes of HE: increased glutamine and decreased Cho/Cr and mI/Cr. With the improved resolution at 2 tesla, separate analysis of glutamine and glutamate is possible. Inset shows spectra from model solutions: **(A)** *5 mM glutamate plus 5 mM NAA;* **(B)** *5 mM glutamine + 5 mM glutamate + 5 mM NAA, indicating that in this patient the increase in glutamine occurs without obvious depletion of cerebral glutamate. Spectra were acquired on a Siemens 2.0 tesla clinical spectrometer, with STEAM localization; TR 3 s, TE 20 ms. (Modified from Ref. 6. Reproduced with permission from J. Frahm, T. Michaelis, and colleagues.)*

accumulation of glutamine. If this sequence is correct, perhaps "sensitization" of the brain results from mI or Cho depletion or both. In keeping with the theory of many year's standing, increasing cerebral glutamine underlies the neurologic syndromes of grades 1 through 4 severe, overt chronic HE as well as, perhaps, the syndrome of acute fulminant HE and coma. Figure 24-36 shows the similar but more severe neurochemical changes of Reye syndrome, giving an effective indication of what may be seen in acute HE. Unfortunately, published spectra from patients with fulminant HE are limited and difficult to interpret.[140]

Transjugular Intrahepatic Portal Systemic Shunt

A human "experiment" that goes some way toward verifying this sequence is the interventional procedure known as TIPS, which is used as a lifesaving procedure in cirrhosis-induced hematemesis. Not surprisingly, TIPS induces clinical HE in up to 90 percent of survivors.[138,141] ^{1}H MRS performed both before and after TIPS in 10 patients showed a universal increase in mean intracerebral glutamine after the procedure. More important, in a small number of individuals in whom mI was normal before TIPS (these patients often show SCHE), a progressive reduction in mI/Cr and the development of subclinical and clinical HE followed the introduction of the shunt (Fig. 24-37).

Liver Transplantation

Yet another common human "experiment," that of orthotopic liver transplantation, allows the reverse process to be demonstrated unequivocally, establishing a firm, although circumstantial, link between mI depletion and the syndromes of subclinical and overt HE (Fig. 24-38). Glx and Cho also recovered. Indeed, an overshoot of cerebral Cho is consistently observed, perhaps linking the earlier Cho depletion with deficient hepatic biosynthesis of a relevant precursor of glycerophosphoryl choline.

Ornithine Transcarbamylase Deficiency

A description of MRS in HE would be incomplete without consideration of a rare but informative inborn error of hepatic urea synthesis, ornithine transcarbamylase (OTC) deficiency. The single known biochemical consequence is hyperammonemia. Gadian and colleagues[42] demonstrated the inevitable elevation of cerebral glutamine in two of these patients (Fig. 24-8), while Ross and associates[2] showed the extraordinary parallel with HE in terms of depletion of cerebral mI.

Wilson Disease

Wilson disease, which is caused by excess copper deposition, is believed to result in an encephalopathy analogous to HE. However, the ^{1}H MRS findings are, not surprisingly, rather different, lacking either mI depletion or glutamine accumulation (unpublished study from this laboratory).

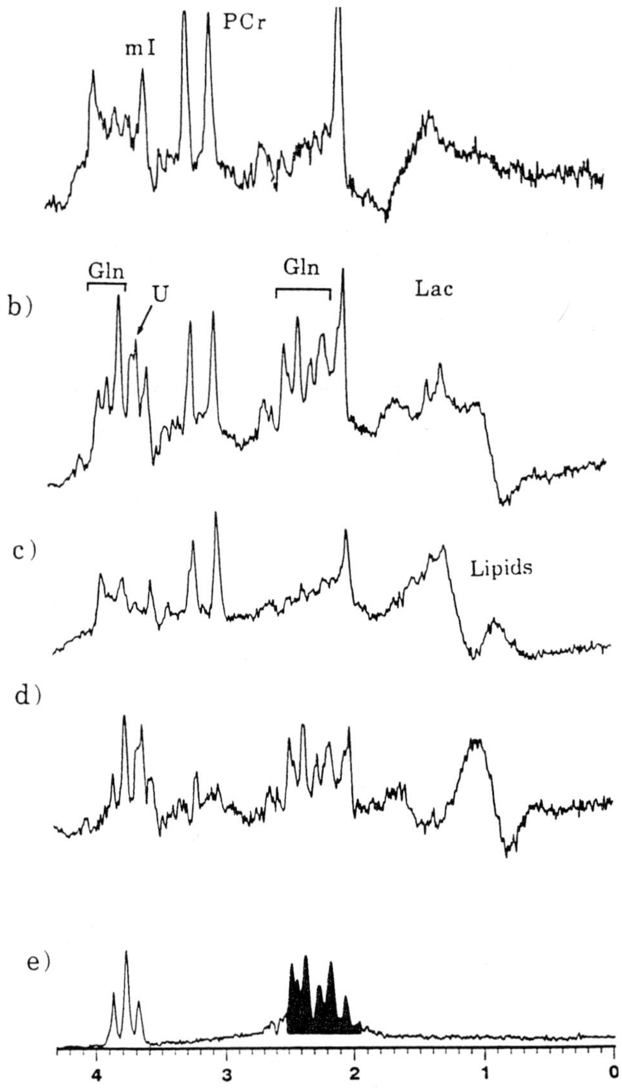

Figure 24-36
^{1}H MRS in acute hepatic encephalopathy resulting from Reye syndrome. In vivo *^{1}H MRS spectra acquired from a parietal white matter region in infant brain from* **(A)** *10-month-old normal,* **(B)** *patient on day 2 after admission,* **(C)** *patient on day 8 after admission,* **(D)** *difference* **(B–C)** *between day 2 and day 8 in patient,* **(E)** *solution with 15 mM glutamine. All spectra are scaled. Spectral assignments: Lac, 1.33 ppm; NAA, 2.02 ppm; Gln = glutamine, 2.10–2.50 ppm and 3.65–3.90 ppm; Cr (including PCr), 3.03 ppm; Cho, 3.23 ppm; mI, 3.56 ppm. U = unassigned (3.62 ppm). Notable abnormalities concern a huge accumulation of cerebral glutamine, reduced Cho, and later reduced mI, all of which reflect liver failure. In addition, there is a decrease in NAA and [Cr] and the appearance of the unassigned peak. Reye syndrome, a toxic-viral disease associated with aspirin intake, is known to produce severe neuronal damage and therefore may not completely correspond to the picture of acute liver failure. An occipital gray matter region gave almost identical results. (Reproduced with permission from Ref. 61.)*

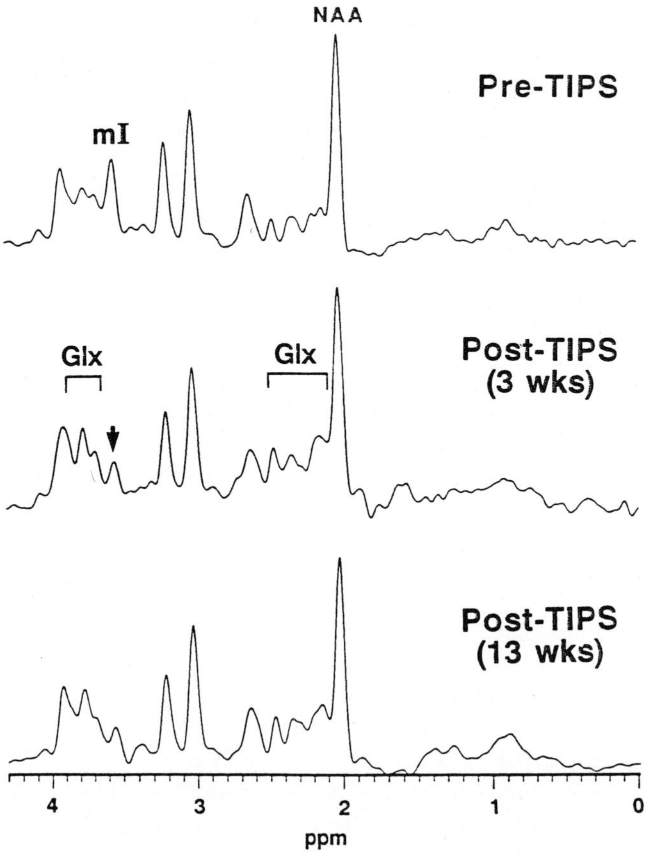

Figure 24-37
Effect of TIPS on the ¹H MR spectrum. Spectra are from a 30-year-old female 5 days after a hematemesis resulting from esophageal varices and chronic alcoholic liver disease. Spectra acquired from a parietal white matter location (GE signa 1.5 tesla, vol. 12.5 mL, STEAM TR 1.5 s, TE 30 ms, NEX 128) before TIPS procedure shows no abnormalities aside from a small but significant reduction in Cho/Cr attributable to liver disease (top). Three weeks after TIPS, changes are seen in the Glx and ml regions and there is a further reduction in Cho/Cr (middle). The bottom spectrum shows the progression of changes seen 13 weeks after TIPS. Glx is markedly increased, and ml is significantly reduced.[141]

Myelopathy and Paraplegia

An unusual form of chronic HE presents with myelopathy and paraplegia. Although neurologic considerations would suggest cord involvement, the ¹H MRS findings in the parietal cortex are typical of other patients with the more classical clinical presentation (see Fig. 4 in Ross and associates[2]).

Other Systemic Encephalopathies

Diabetes Mellitus

Like HE, diabetic encephalopathy is common and obviously "metabolic" in origin. Three principal syndromes are recognized: diabetic ketoacidosis (Fig. 24-39), lactacidosis, and nonketotic hyperosmolar coma.

Elevated cerebral glucose,[142] a significant excess of mI, a reversible accumulation of Cho, and the presence of ketone bodies have been detected in various patients with varying severity of diabetic encephalopathy.[62]

The most surprising finding of ¹H MRS, which requires further study, is the identification of acetone, rather than the more widely anticipated β-hydroxybutyrate and acetoacetate, as the ketone of human diabetic ketoacidotic encephalopathy[62] (Fig. 24-39).

Long-term neurologic and cerebral complications of diabetes contribute to the greatly increased mortality. The biochemical basis of these conditions may lie in the changes in Cho, NAA, mI, ketones, and glucose, now recognized by MRS, that are present in acutely and chronically diabetic brains.

The Hyperosmolar State: Identification of Idiogenic Organic Osmolytes by ¹H MRS

Lien and coworkers first used ¹H MRS to investigate a "new" family of cerebral metabolites that are collectively known as organic osmolytes because of their putative role in the maintenance of cerebral osmotic

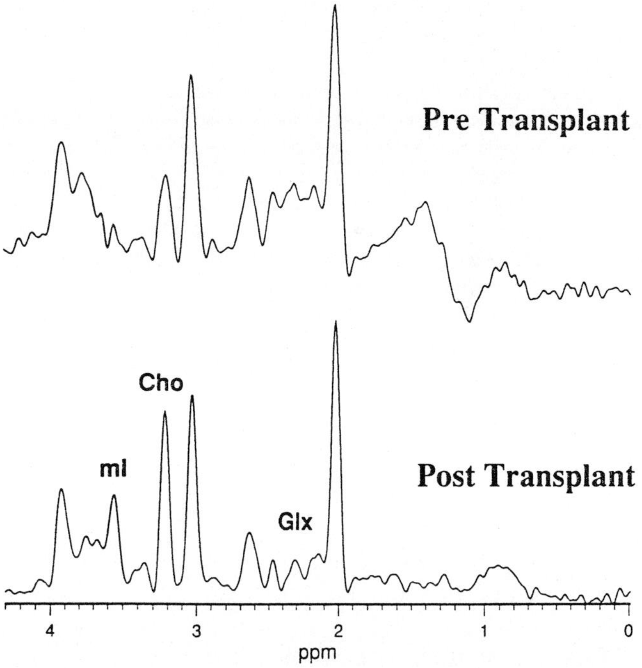

Figure 24-38
Restoration of biochemical abnormalities after a liver transplant. The patient is a 30-year-old male with acute-on-chronic hepatic encephalopathy secondary to hepatitis who subsequently was successfully treated by liver transplantation. Spectra were acquired 6 months apart from the same parietal white matter location (15.0 mL STEAM TR 1.5 s, TR 30 ms, NEX 128) and scaled to the same Cr intensity for comparison. The obvious abnormalities before liver transplantation are increased α, β, and γ glutamine and reduced Cho/Cr and ml/Cr (upper spectrum). These were completely reversed 3 months after transplantation, and Cho/Cr exceeded normal (lower spectrum).

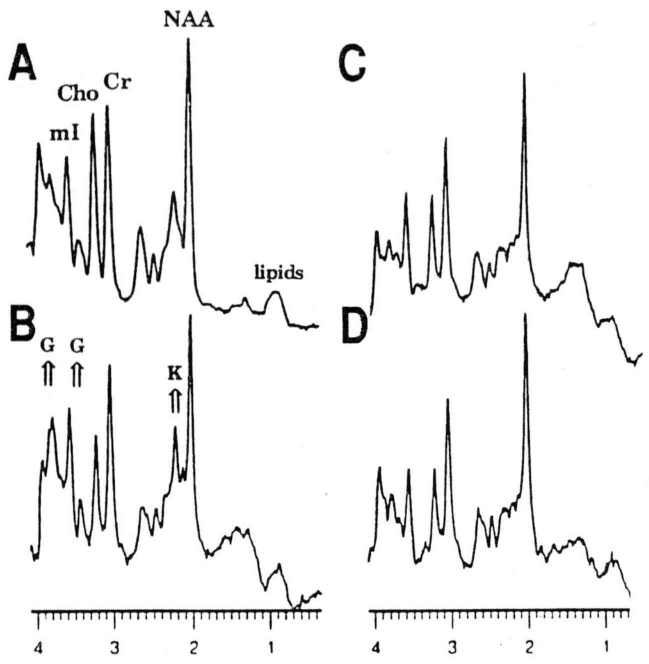

Figure 24-39

Diabetic ketoacidosis (DKA): cerebral ^1H Spectra during two episodes and recovery. **(A)** *Episode 1, acquired 3 days after admission to the hospital, at a time when the patient had supposedly totally recovered and was ready to be discharged. A peak characteristic for the presence of ketone (K) bodies was noted at 2.22 ppm, obtained from an 18-cm³ volume in the left parietal lobe. The patient relapsed into DKA 2 days later.* **(B)** *Episode 2, acquired 5 months later from an occipital gray matter location (10.3 cm³) during a second episode of DKA. In addition to the ketone peak, peaks for glucose (G) were seen.* **(C)** *Recovery 6 days after episode 2 (from the same occipital location), when no more ketone bodies were detected in the urine.* **(D)** *Occipital cortex of an age- and sex-matched healthy subject. Acquisition conditions: GE Signa 1.5 tesla, 4X software; STEAM TR 1.5 s, TE 30 ms, NEX 128. More detailed analysis of peak K indicates that the resonance frequency is that of acetone rather than acetoacetate, the ketone body more commonly identified in the blood and urine of diabetics in coma. (Reproduced by permission of the Radiological Society of North America from R. Kreis and B.D. Ross,* Radiology *184:123, 1992.)*

equilibrium.[143] These molecules were first thoroughly researched in the papilla of the kidney with the help of in vitro MRI.[144]

First in sporadic cases of diabetic hyperosmolar coma[62] and a patient after a closed head injury[44] and then, most convincingly, in a single infant with holoprosencephaly and deficient thirst mechanisms, these concepts were confirmed as contributing to human encephalopathy by the use of ^{1}H MRS (Fig. 24-40). *Myo*-inositol was 3 times the normal value, and other resonances, which also were markedly affected, returned toward normal after treatment. Difference spectroscopy is particularly helpful in identifying these changes.[145,146]

Hyponatremia

The neurologic syndromes associated with hyponatremia are postulated to be determined by the state of intracellular cerebral osmolytes. Previously inaccessible, these metabolites now can be quantitated by ^{1}H MRS. An in vivo quantitative assay of osmolytes was performed in 12 chronic hyponatremic patients (mean serum sodium, 120 meq/L) and 10 normal controls. Short echo time ^{1}H MRS of occipital gray and parietal white matter locations revealed a dramatic reduction in the concentrations of several metabolites (Fig. 24-41). In gray matter mI was most profoundly reduced at 49 percent of control value. Cho was reduced 36 percent; Cr 19 percent, and NAA 11 percent from the levels in controls. Similar changes were found in white matter. Recovery of osmolyte concentrations was demonstrated in four patients studied 8 to 14 weeks later. These results are consistent with a reversible osmolyte reduction under hypo-osmolar stress in the intact human brain and offer novel suggestions for the treatment and monitoring of this common clinical event. Pontine myelinolysis associated with hyponatremia may be found to occur more frequently than anticipated if MRS is employed to detect cerebral mI depletion (Fig. 24-33).

Diffuse metabolic changes in brain biochemistry result from complex interactions of disordered biochemistry in many other organs and tissues. Hepatic encephalopathies, diabetic coma and hyperosmolar states, and hypoxic encephalopathy are examples of conditions in which accurate application of quantitative MRS sheds new light. The diagnostic utility of MRS in metabolic encephalopathies will increase as new therapeutic options are developed.

Detection of Xenobiotics in Brain

Relatively few drugs accumulate in the millimolar range in brain because of the effectiveness of the blood-brain barrier. Three exceptions that are readily demonstrable in ^{1}H spectra are mannitol (Fig. 24-42), ethanol (Fig. 24-43), and the ubiquitous drug solvent propylene glycol (PG, 1,2 propanediol) (Fig. 24-44). These findings can, however, be of the utmost clinical importance in diagnosis, determining, for example, that a prospective liver transplant recipient is still drinking or that a pediatric lactic acidosis may be drug-related.[147]

CLINICAL DECISION MAKING WITH ^{1}H MRS

MRS Referral Guidelines

A brief justification for MRS on a case-by-case basis simplifies the task of referring physicians and (neuro)radiologists while providing a basis for claims for reimbursement of the cost of the examination by national

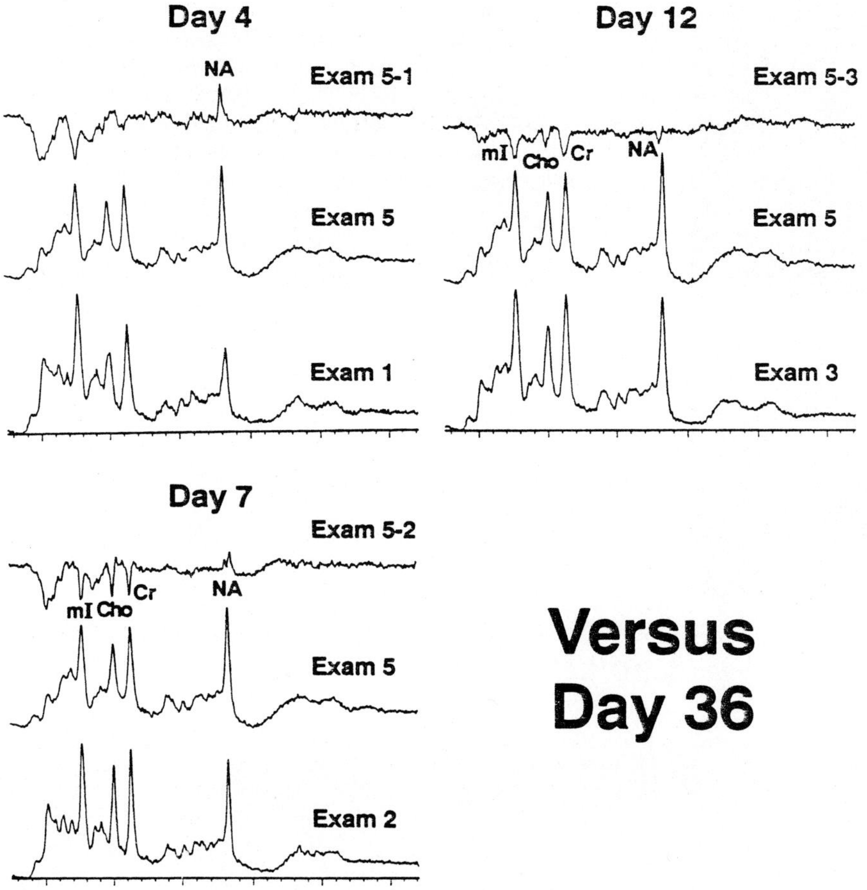

Figure 24-40

Time course of changes in principal cerebral organic osmolytes during correction of severe dehydration. A series of spectra were obtained from the same (occipital gray matter) brain location in a 14-month-old child recovering from severe dehydration and hypernatremia (plasma sodium 195 meq/L; normal range, 135–142) using identical acquisition conditions. Spectra were processed and scaled identically to permit subtraction of sequential spectra (difference spectroscopy). The day of examination refers to the interval since admission to the hospital. Examinations are numbered sequentially, from the first (Exam 1) to the last (Exam 5) on day 36. Compared with a relevant normal, the principal abnormality appears to be a reversal of the intensities of NAA (reduced) and mI (increased), so that mI dominates the spectrum. These changes slowly reversed and became nearly normal on day 36. The resultant difference spectra more clearly identify the progressively falling concentrations of several metabolites, with a possible elevation in the resonance peak assigned to the neuronal marker NAA. Quantitative MRS defines the principal abnormality as a threefold increase in the concentration of the cerebral osmolyte [mI].

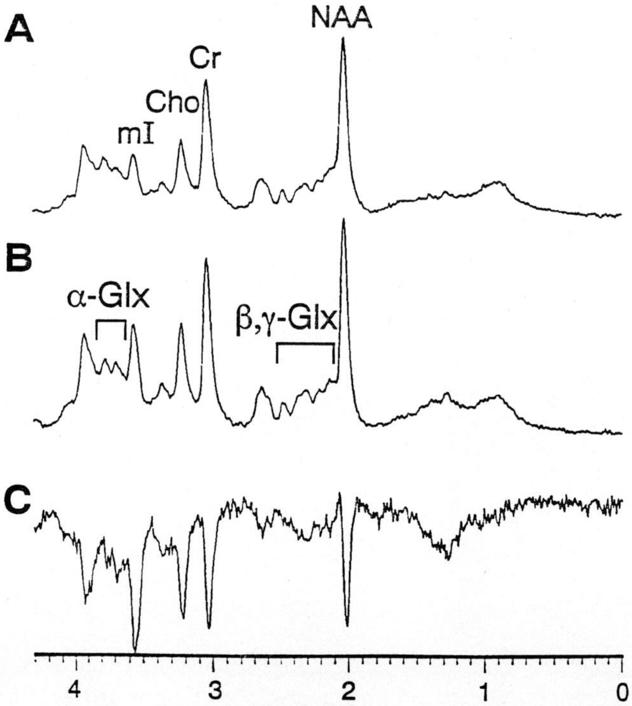

Figure 24-41

Summed and difference spectra of gray matter in hyponatremia. Individual spectra were processed on an absolute scale (see the methods section). Spectra of 11 hyponatremic patients **(A)** *and 10 controls* **(B)** *were summed and then subtracted (patients minus controls) to yield the difference spectrum* **(C)**, *which is enlarged threefold. The negative peaks of the four major metabolites represent a decline in concentration. The fifth peak at 3.95 ppm represents the methylene protons of Cr and is proportional to the methyl Cr peak at 3.05 ppm. (Courtesy of J. Videen, T. Michaelis, P. Pinto, and B. Ross,* J Clin Invest, *in press, with permission.)*

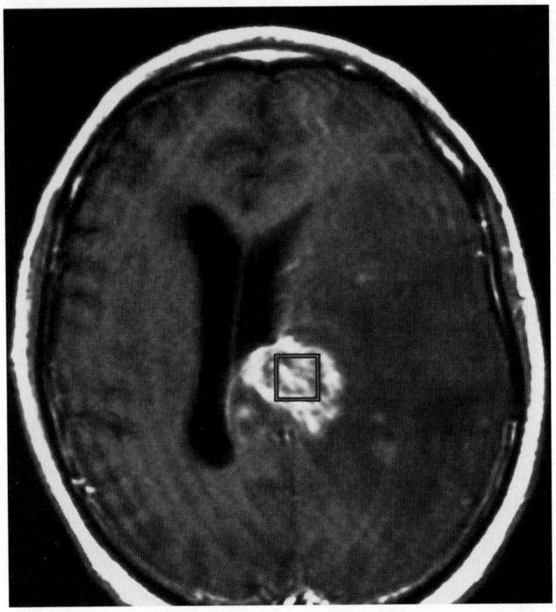

A

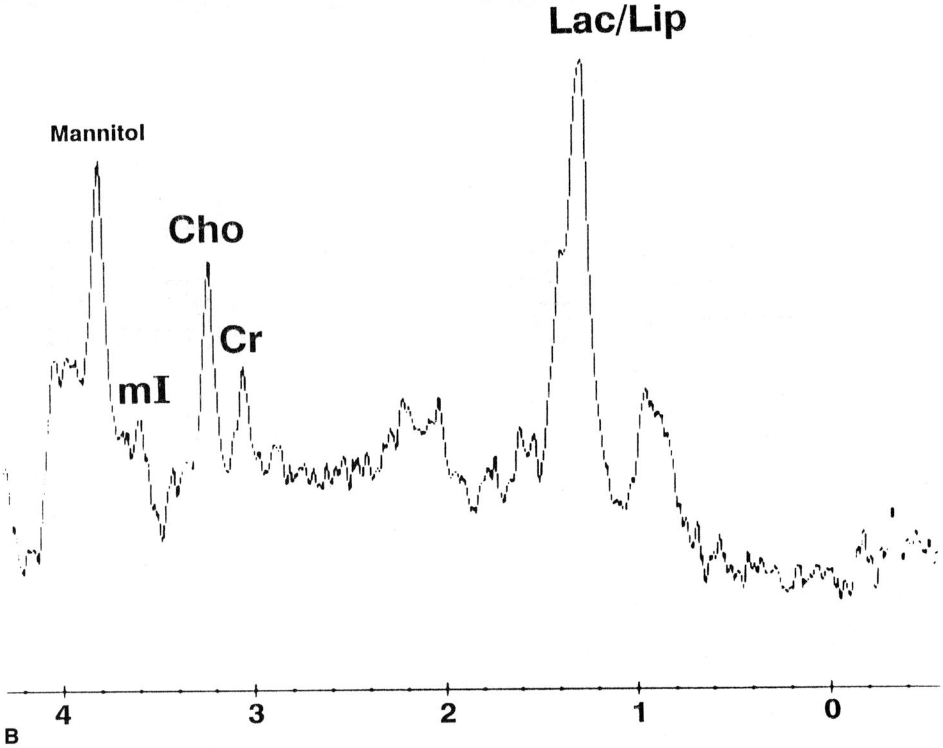

B

Figure 24-42
(A) *Axial MRI of a patient with glioma, indicating gadolinium enhancement. The volume from which the PROBE spectrum was derived is indicated by the box.* **(B)** *Automated (7 min) ^{1}H MRS PROBE spectrum from the tumor. The identities of metabolites are obtained from chemical shift (ppm) and by comparison with normal brain and model solutions.*

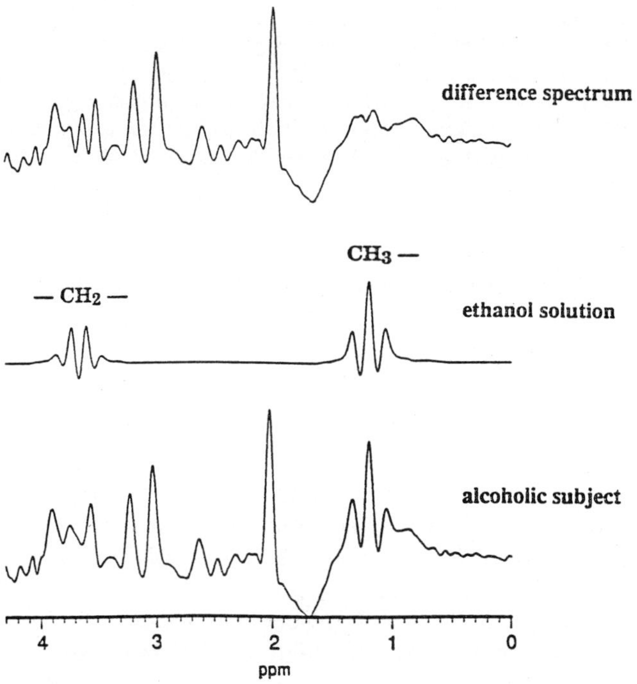

Figure 24-43

Difference spectroscopy to identify intracerebral ethanol in a patient with liver disease. ¹H MR spectrum from parietal cortex in a 30-year-old female patient with proven alcoholic liver disease shows no chronic hepatic encephalopathy (CHE) but demonstrates an additional triplet (lower spectrum). The central spectrum was recorded from an aqueous solution of ethanol. It features a triplet similar to that seen in the patient and a quartet that is not apparent in the patient's spectrum. The chemical shift scale was determined with other solutions spectra containing known internal standards. The difference spectrum (upper) shows coincidence of the resonances at 1.0–1.35 ppm seen in the patient with the triplet of ethanol, whereas negative peaks between 3.5 and 3.8 ppm indicate the absence of the expected quartet resonances.

(Medicare, Medi-Cal) or private insurers. Table 24-2 lists differential diagnostic uses of MRS, and Table 24-6 lists syndromes and clinical presentations that are frequently investigated by MRS.

Following is a summary of MRS referral guidelines for a selection of these indications. The obvious standard contraindications for a patient to be in an MRI scanner are not mentioned for each case.

Dementia

Indications: Any patient with memory deficit, progressive cognitive difficulty, prolonged depression, "pseudodementia," agitation, and/or confusion. Certain patients with unresolved cognitive change in the presence of hypertension, transient ischemic attack (TIA), or stroke. Normal CT, MRI, PET, and SPECT are not contraindications to ¹H MRS.

Contraindications: Frank psychiatric disease such as schizophrenia, focal lesions; extradural hemorrhage, and coexistent systemic diseases with neurologic consequences (diabetes mellitus, uremia, cirrhosis, hyponatremia) may complicate the interpretation of MRS.

Major Findings on ¹H MRS: Decreased NAA/Cr (and absolute [NAA]). Increased mI/Cr (and absolute [mI]). Note: the first without the second is diagnosed as another dementia (not AD). Together they are diagnosed as AD.

Confounding Entities: Stroke or copious DWMIs may increase Cho/Cr. Systemic diseases with increased cerebral mI/Cr include uremia and diabetes.

Sensitivity of MRS: Versus normal, 83 percent; versus other dementia, 82 percent.

Specificity of MRS: Versus normal, 95 percent; versus other dementia, 64 percent.

Value of MRS (PROBE) (rating): Secondary and screening.

Other Useful Investigations: Many, but less sensitive and less specific.

Key figures in the sections above: Figures 24-27 to 24-30.

Key References: 14, 15, 122, 123, 148.

Hepatic Encephalopathy

Indications: MRS should be considered as a screening examination in patients with abnormal liver function plus any abnormal neurology, dementia, liver transplant candidates, alcoholics; postoperative monitoring of TIPS candidates, and acute liver failure. Normal CT, MRI, PET, and SPECT are not contraindications to ¹H MRS.

Table 24-6
Syndromes and clinical presentations investigated with MRS

Patients with the listed syndromes and clinical presentations are obvious candidates for MRS. MRS indications, contraindications, major findings, confounding entities, sensitivity, specificity, and key references are summarized in the section "MRS Referral Guidelines" for the syndromes typed in boldface.

Elderly	confusion, depression, **dementia,** hydrocephalus, **stroke,** TIA, **tumor, trauma,** metabolic (renal diabetes)
Adult	**stroke, tumor, encephalopathy, liver disease,** liver transplant, **trauma,** hydrocephalus, MS **AIDS (mass), HIV-positive,** metabolic disease
Children	**abnormal development** (inborn error), white matter disease, hydrocephalus, **trauma,** infection, cardiac transplant, **epilepsy, hypoxia** (arrest), **near-drowning,** diabetes, hyponatremia or hypernatremia
Newborn	**hypoxic** ischemic (stroke), ECMO

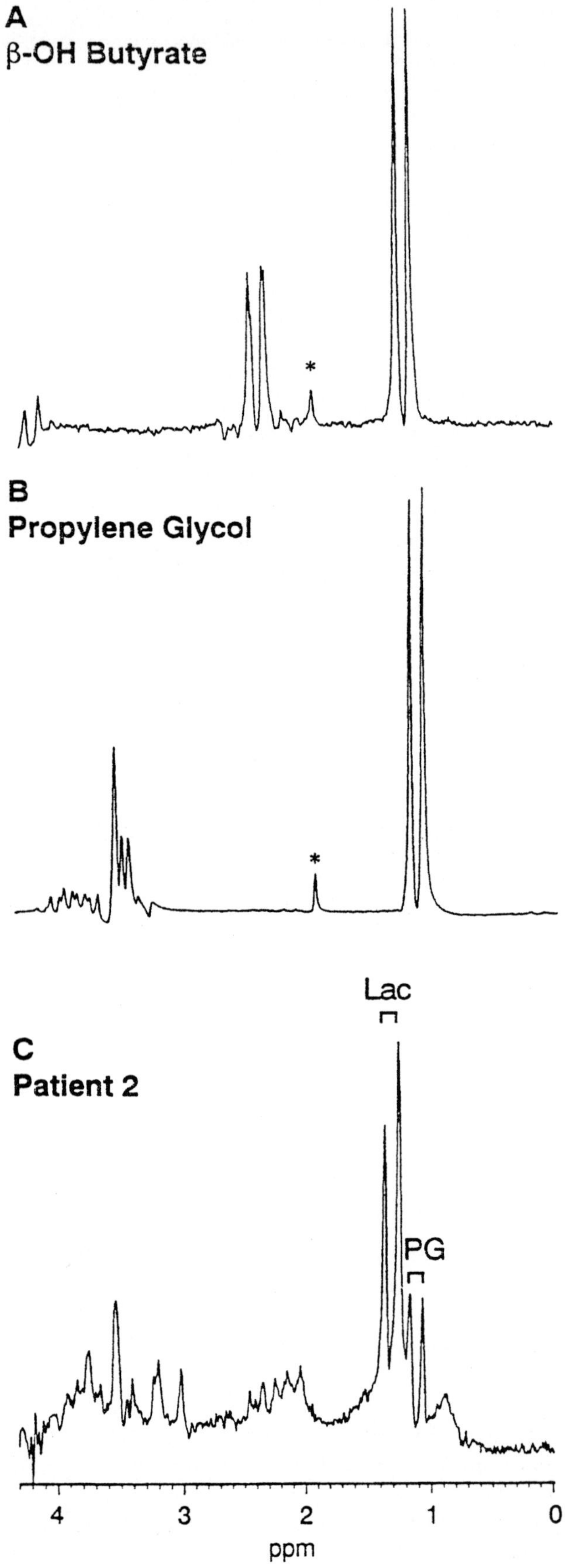

Figure 24-44
Propylene glycol (1,2 propanediol). Propanediol is clearly identified as the source of the resonances in the infant brain **(C)** *at 1.14 ppm and 3.52 ppm. Lac is possibly that of D-lactate, a toxic metabolite of DL propylene glycol. Propylene glycol is a commonly used solvent for pediatric drugs. (From T. Michaelis, K. Cooper, R. Kreis, and B. Ross, with permission.)*

Contraindications: None.

Major Findings on ^{1}H *MRS:* A triad of changes (loss of mI, increased GIx, and reduced Cho) characterizes patients with chronic HE and, more usefully, defines subclinical HE. Patients with TIPS develop these characteristic metabolite changes as evidence of HE after shunting. Transplant recipients undergo complete reversal of these biochemical abnormalities within weeks after successful transplantation. Exaggerated MRS changes are seen in patients with acute fulminant HE and the rare Reye syndrome even when the MRI results are normal:

1. Decreased NAA/Cr
2. Increased α- and β,γ-GIx
3. Decreased mI/Cr and [mI] (mI almost absent)

Confounding Entities: Hyponatremia, even 2 weeks after normalizing plasma sodium.

Sensitivity of MRS: Close to 100 percent for subclinical HE and twice as sensitive as clinical testing for overt HE.

Specificity of MRS: Almost 100 percent together with clinical history and serum sodium or osmolality. More specific than "bright" basal ganglia on T_2 MRI.

Value of MRS (PROBE) (rating): Principal and secondary.

Other Useful Investigations: Electroencephalography (EEG), number connection test, abdominal ultrasound (shunt), blood ammonia, CSF glutamine (now obsolete).

Key figures in the sections above: Figures 24-34 to 24-38.

Key References: 3–5, 8, 138, 141, 147, 149, 150.

Hypoxic Encephalopathy and Stroke

Indications: Cardiac arrest, unidentified coma, asphyxia, near drowning, stroke, TIA, congestive cardiac failure (CCF), respiratory failure, and trauma. Normal EEG, CT, MRI, PET, and SPECT are not contraindications to ^{1}H MRS.

Contraindications: None (however, technical problems arising from susceptibility to hemorrhage may arise).

Major Findings on ^{1}*H MRS:* Because simple biochemical reactions underlie the universal ^{1}H MRS response to hypoxia; (1) Lac (and Glx) accumulates when O_2 is insufficient, (2) neurons bear the main impact and probably cannot recover; NAA is lost in proportion, and (3) PCr (which constitutes 50 percent of the Cr peak) needs ATP and hence O_2 and so falls markedly after hypoxia:

1. Increased lipid and overlying Lac doublet peak (at 1.3 ppm)
2. Decreased NAA
3. Increased α- and β,γ-Glx
4. Decreased [Cr]

Confounding Entities: Mitochondrial disease, lactacidosis of any cause, inability to distinguish a persistent vegetative state (PVS) from lethal injury. The Cho/Cr ratio appears to be increased because [Cr] is decreased.

Sensitivity of MRS: Appears to be highly sensitive to a severe global hypoxic insult.

Specificity of MRS: Some overlap with posttraumatic spectrum. Best indicator of prognosis after near drowning; lack of detailed analysis of other PVS.

Value of MRS (PROBE) (rating): Screening or secondary.

Other Useful Investigations: EEG.

Key figures in the sections above: Figures 24-12 to 24-16, 24-22, 24-44.

Key References: 1, 90, 151.

Abnormal Development

Indications: Any anatomic or metabolic disorder in the neonatal or pediatric period. Normal ultrasound (US), CT, MRI, PET, and SPECT are not contraindications to ^{1}H MRS.

Contraindications: None.

Major Findings on ^{1}*H MRS:* Common but nonspecific findings are low NAA; and excess lactate. Unique metabolite profiles are to be expected in several relatively common disorders. An abundance of rare specific findings includes phenylalanine (phenylketonuria), glycine (nonketotic hyperglycemia), elevated NAA (Canavan disease), and absent Cr (Frahm-Hanefeld syndrome).

Confounding Entities: Gestational age, drugs, parenteral feeding solutions, and xenobiotics that appear in ^{1}H spectrum, including propanediol, mannitol, ethanol, and glucose.

Sensitivity of MRS: Unknown. Leukodystrophies are unique; ^{1}H MRS appears to be more sensitive than MRI.

Specificity of MRS: High specificity for single-enzyme (gene) defects.

Value of MRS (PROBE) (rating): Screening.

Other Useful Investigations: Many.

Key figures in the sections above: Figures 24-7 to 24-11.

Key Reference: 43.

Neonatal Hypoxia

Indications: Normal US, CT, MRI, PET, and SPECT are not contraindications to ^{1}H MRS.

Contraindications: None.

Major Findings on ^{1}*H MRS:* The distinction between severe hypoxic encephalopathy with a very poor prognosis and that with a prognosis of full recovery is made on the basis of excess lactate; decreased NAA, and loss of Cr. Several grades of severity can be distinguished between these extremes.

Confounding Entities: Gestational age, drugs, parenteral feeding solutions, and xenobiotics that appear in ^{1}H spectrum, including propanediol, mannitol, ethanol, and glucose.

Sensitivity of MRS: Much higher than that of US or CT.

Specificity of MRS: Not proven; overlaps with shaken baby syndrome and inborn errors.

Value of MRS (PROBE) (rating): Primary or secondary.

Other Useful Investigations: US, CT, MRI.

Key figures in the sections above: Figures 24-12 to 24-16, 24-22, 24-44.

Key References: 16, 90, 147, 151.

Epilepsy in Children

Indications: Past cerebral insult, metabolic disorders, temporal lobe focus, prelude to diet therapy.

Contraindications: None.

Major findings on ^{1}*H MRS:* Reduced NAA and elevated mI (nonspecific).

Epilepsy in Adults

Indications: Currently only during presurgical workup and possibly posttrauma.

Contraindications: None.

Major findings on ^{1}*H MRS:* Reduced ipsilateral NAA/Cr.

Cerebral Tumor

Indications: Differential diagnosis of any focal or space-occupying lesions, presurgical planning, post-radiation ("normal brain"), and recurrence (?).

Contraindications: Postsurgical clips.

Major Findings on ^{1}*H MRS:* A copious literature[32–34] explains the features of primary and secondary brain tumors. Key issues that are be addressed here concern tumor versus stroke, tumor recurrence versus radiation necrosis, edema versus tumor, and benign versus malignant. Research reports answer most of these questions, but individual experience is required in using MRS for these purposes in clinical practice:

1. Low or absent NAA
2. Lowered Cr
3. Elevated Cho
4. Lac present or absent
5. Notable excess lipid

Confounding Entities: Heterogeneity, drugs, mannitol.

Sensitivity of MRS: Very high.

Specificity of MRS: Variable owing to overlap with focal lesions.

Value of MRS (PROBE) (rating): High.

Other Useful Investigations: CSI for biopsy guidance.

Key figures in the sections above: Figures 24-18 and 24-19.

Key References: 64–67.

Closed Head Trauma (Pediatric Head Injury, Shaken Baby Syndrome)

Indications: Closed head injury, trauma, coma, seizures, mental retardation, motor disorders post-trauma, suspicion of neuronal damage. Normal US, CT, MRI, PET, and SPECT are not contraindications to ^{1}H MRS.

Contraindications: None (however, technical problems arising from susceptibility to hemorrhage may arise).

Major Findings on ^{1}*H MRS:* (1) Low NAA/Cr and/or low [NAA], (2) high Cho/Cr and/or high [Cho], (3) low [Cr], (4) hyperosmolar pattern: increased [mI], [Cho], and [Cr] in white matter, (5) SIADH (hypo-osmolar pattern of decreased [mI], [Cho], and [Cr]), (6) accumulation of Lac and lipid.

Low [NAA] and low [Cr] generally are consistent with a neurologic deficit and, in combination with an accumulation of Lac and lipid, hypoxic damage and a poor outcome are indicated. High [Cho] is viewed as a sign of axonal shear injury. The hyperosmolar state (increased mI, Cho, and Cr in white matter) persists long after the injury but is generally a sign of a moderate to good outcome. The mechanisms of the hyperosmolar pattern are not known.

Confounding Entities: Hypoxia.

Sensitivity of MRS: MRS appears to be highly sensitive to different patterns of disease in the heterogeneous disease closed head trauma.

Specificity of MRS: Some overlap with hypoxic encephalopathy. Good indicator of outcome.

Value of MRS (PROBE) (rating): Secondary; higher in prolonged posttraumatic coma.

Other Useful Investigations: Many.

Key figures in the sections above: Figures 24-11, 24-20, 24-21

Key References: 12, 44, 81.

HIV CNS Lesions and AIDS Dementia

Indications: Any HIV patient with changes in neurologic function or altered mental status, such as memory deficits, progressive cognitive difficulty, seizures, headaches, visual difficulty, and weakness. Normal CT, MRI, PET, and SPECT are not contraindications to ^{1}H MRS to evaluate AIDS dementia or HIV encephalopathy. Gadolinium injection for T1 enhancement of lesions is not contraindicated for CNS lesion studies. Sedation may be required for patients with progressive disease status. Focal lesions smaller than 10 by 10 by 10 mm are difficult to evaluate. MRI-MRS studies are recommended before stereotactic biopsy procedures.

Contraindications: Patients unable to tolerate an MRI scan for standard reasons (claustrophobia, metalic implants, pacemakers, etc.).

Acquisition: STEAM 30/2000[120], voxel sampling of the CNS lesion (T2 hyperintense area or Gd enhancing region) with minimal outervoxel contamination, plus contralateral control voxel or unaffected region. MRS acquisitions add about 15 min to a routine MRI examination.

Major Findings on ^{1}*H MRS:* See Ref. 120.

Toxoplasmosis: Decreased mI, Cho, Cr, and NAA with a 15- to 20-fold increase in lactate and lipids near 1.3 ppm; there is a predominant lipid resonance near 0.9 ppm as well.

CNS Lymphoma: Increased Cho, lactate, and lipids, but on the same order of magnitude; decreased mI and NAA and Cr.

Progressive Multifocal Leukoencephalopathy (PML): increased mI and Cho and decreased Cr and NAA. Lactate and lipids are observed, but at lower concentrations than in toxoplasmosis or lymphoma.

Cryptococcoma: Decreased mI, Cho, Cr, and NAA and increased lipids.

Confounding Entities: Drugs and systemic disorders.

Diagnostic Accuracy: Wilk lambda statistics overall diagnostic accuracy 94 percent: 100 percent toxo, 75 percent CNS lymphoma, 83 percent PML.

Value of MRS (PROBE) (rating): High.

Key figures in the sections above: Figure 24-26.

Key References: 110, 118, 120.

THE FUTURE OF NEUROSPECTROSCOPY

Neurospectroscopy has a bright clinical future if a few critical issues are addressed by its proponents, including technology, teaching, therapy, and time sharing.

Technical Limitations of Neurospectroscopy

There are several well-recognized shortcomings of modern methods of MRS when applied in the clinical arena.

Outside the brain, progress has been slow. Spinal cord and nerve monitoring are in their infancy. Muscle function, however, is one of the oldest and most successful applications of clinical MRS and can be integrated into neurologic and neuroradiologic practice through automation of ^{31}P MRS.

Inside the brain, there are too many "no-go areas." Most neurologists would instinctively reject the "global" approach to neurodiagnosis, in which large volumes of white or gray matter in seemingly unspecialized areas of the brain are used to define neuropathologies that for generations have been attributed with pinpoint accuracy to specific nuclei or tracts in the brain. However, this is the preferred method for neurospectroscopy, simply because very small structures (the nucleus accumbens, for example, and the lateral geniculate body) or histologically discrete regions such as the medial hippocampal gyrus are currently excessively difficult to examine with MRS. Even more frustrating to neurologists has been the reluctance (understandable to neurospectroscopists) to examine any infratentorial structures.

The cures for these shortcomings are not difficult but involve technical developments and a high degree of technical skill. The accelerated development of new methods while the existing armamentarium is used for diagnosis must be seen as a responsibility of everyone in neurospectroscopy.

Is there regional variation in neuropathology? It is obvious that as therapeutic options in neurology expand, the all-or-none approach that epitomizes single-voxel MRS (is it normal or abnormal?) must give way to a graded approach. If it is abnormal, how much of the brain is affected? Can I salvage neighboring brain structures by means of timely interventions? Metabolite imaging plays a role, and improved methods will be needed to speed such acquisitions. Improved radiofrequency head coils will be vital in the effort to examine specialized brain regions.

Translating STEAM into PRESS

During the preparation of this chapter, it became apparent that two technologies are competing as the gold standard. First, short TE PRESS is threatening to take over almost entirely from STEAM as the method of choice for single-voxel ^{1}H MRS. The second is short echo time CSI, the multivoxel counterpart of MRS, which radiologists have long preferred for its more objective sampling of brain regions and—the true competitive advantage—an escape from spectra to metabolic imaging. It is too early to predict the final clinical armamentarium of MRS.

QUICK REFERENCE TO ABBREVIATIONS

Clinical/Anatomic

AD	Alzheimer disease
DM	diabetes mellitus
HE	hepatic encephalopathy
ICH	intracranial hemorrhage
MS	multiple sclerosis
ND	near drowning
NPH	normal-pressure hydrocephalus
TIA	transient ischemic attack
TIPS	transjugular intrahepatic systemic shunt
GM	occipital cortex gray matter
WM	parietal cortex white matter
DWMI	deep white matter infarct
PML	progressive multifocal leukoencephalopathy

Metabolites/Biochemistry

Cr	total creatine (not creatinine) plus phosphocreatine (PCr)
Cho	total choline
Glx	glutamine (Gln) plus glutamate (Glu), α-Glx, β, γ-Glx
Lac	lactate
Lip	lipid

mI	*myo*-inositol
NAA	*N*-acetylaspartate (putative neuronal marker)
Ala	alanine
sI	*scyllo*-inositol
[NAA]	absolute concentration of NAA; similarly for the other metabolites
NAA/Cr	NAA to Cr ratio; similarly for the other metabolites
PCr	phosphocreatine

Methodologic

^{1}H	proton, hydrogen nucleus
MR	magnetic resonance
MRS	magnetic resonance spectroscopy
NMR	nuclear magnetic resonance
PROBE	proton brain examination
TE	echo time
TR	repetition time
STEAM	*st*imulated *e*cho *a*cquisition *m*ode (localization method)
PRESS	*p*oint *res*olved *s*pectroscopy (double spin echo localization method)
MRSI	magnetic resonance spectroscopic imaging
CSI	chemical shift imaging (same as MRSI)
VOI	volume of interest
Gd	gadolinium
US	ultrasound

REFERENCES

1. Kreis R, Ernst T, Arcinue E, et al: Proton MRS in children resuscitated after near-drowning: A possible prognostic indicator? *Proceedings of the 11th Society of Magnetic Resonance in Medicine,* Berlin, 1992, p 237.
2. Ross BD, Kreis R, Ernst T: Clinical tools for the 90's: Magnetic resonance spectroscopy and metabolite imaging. *Eur J Radiol* 14:128–140, 1992.
3. Kreis R, Farrow NA, Ross BD: Diagnosis of hepatic encephalopathy by proton magnetic resonance spectroscopy. *Lancet* 336:635–636, 1990.
4. Kreis R, Farrow NA, Ross BD: Localized ^{1}H NMR spectroscopy in patients with chronic hepatic encephalopathy: Analysis of changes in cerebral glutamine, choline and inositols. *NMR Biomed* 4:109–1116, 1991.
5. Kreis R, Ross BD, Farrow NA, Ackerman Z: Metabolic disorders of the brain in chronic hepatic encephalopathy detected with ^{1}H MRS. *Radiology* 182:19–27, 1992.
6. Bruhn H, Merboldt K-D, Michaelis T, et al: Proton MRS of metabolic disturbances in the brain of patients with liver cirrhosis and subclinical hepatic encephalopathy [abstract]. *Soc Magn Reson Med* 10:400, 1991.
7. Luyten PR, den Hollander JA, Boveé WMMJ, et al: ^{31}P and ^{1}H NMR spectroscopy of the human brain in chronic hepatic encephalopathy. *Proceedings of the 8th Society of Magnetic Resonance in Medicine,* Amsterdam, 1989, vol 1, p 375.
8. Ross BD, Farrow NA, Kanamori K, et al: Magnetic resonance techniques in hepatic encephalopathy (HE), in Bengtsson F (ed): *Progress in Hepatic Encephalopathy and Metabolic Nitrogen Exchange.* Boca Raton, Fla., CRC Press, 1991, pp 75–81.
9. Ernst T, Kreis R, Ross BD: Absolute quantitation of water and metabolites in the human brain: I. Compartments and water. *J Magn Reson* 102(1):1–8, 1993.
10. Bruhn H, Frahm J, Michaelis T, et al: Metabolic disturbances of the brain in patients with liver cirrhosis detected by proton magnetic resonance spectroscopy [abstract]. *Hepatology* 14(4):121, 1991.
11. Chamuleau RAFM, Bosman DK, Bovee WMMJ, et al: What the clinician can learn from MR glutamine/glutamate assays. *NMR Biomed* 4:103–108, 1991.
12. Ernst T, Ross BD, Shonk T, et al: Quantitative proton MRS for prognosis after closed head injury. *Proceedings of the 12th Society of Magnetic Resonance in Medicine,* New York, 1993, vol 1, p 323.
13. Meyerhoff DJ, MacKay S, Grossman N, et al: Effects of normal aging and Alzheimer's disease on cerebral ^{1}H metabolites. *Proceedings of the 11th Society of Magnetic Resonance in Medicine,* Berlin, 1992, vol 1, p 1931.
14. Miller BL, Moats R, Shonk T, et al: Alzheimer disease: Depiction of increased cerebral *myo*-inositol with proton MR spectroscopy. *Radiology* 187:433–437, 1993.
15. Moats RA, Ernst T, Shonk TK, Ross BD: Abnormal cerebral metabolite concentrations in patients with probable Alzheimer disease. *Magn Reson Med* 32:110–115, 1994.
16. Ross BD, Ernst T, Kreis R: Proton magnetic resonance spectroscopy in hypoxic ischemic disorders, in Bax M, Faerber EN (eds): *MRI of the Central Nervous System in Infants and Children.* London, MacKeith Press, 1995, pp 279–328.
17. Cady EB, Dawson MJ, Hope PL, et al: Non-invasive investigation of cerebral metabolism in newborn infants by phosphorus nuclear magnetic resonance spectroscopy. *Lancet* 1:1059–1062, 1983.
18. Hamilton PA, Hope PL, Cady EB, et al: Impaired energy metabolism in brains of newborn infants with increased cerebral echodensities. *Lancet* 1242–1246, 1986.
19. Huppi PS, Posse S, Lazeyras F, et al: Brain development in preterm and term babies studied with ^{1}H magnetic resonance spectroscopy using short-echo time STEAM technique. *Proceedings of the 10th Annual Meeting of the Society of Magnetic Resonance in Medicine,* San Francisco, 1991, vol 1, p 377.
20. Peden CJ, Cowan FM, Bryant DJ, et al: Proton MR spectroscopy of the brain in infants. *J Comput Assist Tomogr* 14(6):886–894, 1990.
21. Kreis R, Ernst T, Arcinue E, et al: *Myo*-inositol in short TE 1H-MRS: A new indicator of neonatal brain development and pathology. *Proceedings of the 10th Society of Magnetic Resonance in Medicine,* San Francisco, 1991, p 1007.
22. Groenendaal F, Veenhoven RH, van der Grond J, et al: Cerebral lactate and N-acetyl-aspartate/choline ratios in asphyxiated full-term neonates demonstrated *in vivo* using proton magnetic resonance spectroscopy. *Pediatr Res* 35:148–151, 1994.
23. Meyerhoff DJ, MacKay S, Bachman L, et al: Reduced

neuronal marker (N-acetylaspartate) in HIV infection. *Proceedings of the 11th Annual Meeting of the Society of Magnetic Resonance in Medicine,* Berlin, 1992, vol 1, p 1939.
24. Vion-Dury J, Nicoli F, Confort-Gouny S, et al: Assessment of AIDS dementia complex by localized brain proton MRS. *Proceedings of the European Society for Magnetic Resonance in Medicine and Biology,* Vienna, Austria, 1994, p 454.
25. Peters AR, de Jonge W, den Boer JA, et al: A longitudinal study of multiple sclerosis patients by FLAIR and 2D spectroscopic imaging. *Proceedings of the 12th Society of Magnetic Resonance in Medicine,* New York, 1993, vol 3, p 1550.
26. Doyle T, Narayana P, Jackson E, Wolinsky J: Longitudinal, short echo time proton spectroscopic imaging of MS. *Proceedings of the 12th Society of Magnetic Resonance in Medicine,* New York, 1993, vol 3, p 1551.
27. Pan JW, Hetherington HP, Mason GF, et al: Evaluation of multiple sclerosis by high field spectroscopic imaging. *Proceedings of the 12th Society of Magnetic Resonance in Medicine,* New York, 1993, vol 3, p 1552.
28. Arnold DL, Matthews PM, Francis G, Antel J: Proton magnetic resonance spectroscopy of human brain *in vivo* in the evaluation of multiple sclerosis: Assessment of the load of the disease. *Magn Reson Med* 14(1):154–159, 1990.
29. Hino A, Imahori Y, Tenjin H, et al: Metabolic and hemodynamic aspects of peritumoral low-density areas in human brain tumor. *Neurosurgery* 26(4):615–621, 1990.
30. Gill SS, Thomas DGT, Van Bruggen N, et al: Proton MR spectroscopy of intracranial tumors: *In vivo* and *in vitro* studies. *J Comput Assist Tomogr* 14:497–504, 1990.
31. Kreis R, Freeman DM, Ross BD, et al: Monitoring adoptive immunotherapy (IT) in patients with malignant glioma. *Proceedings of the Society of Magnetic Resonance in Medicine,* New York, 1990, p 1219.
32. Naruse S, Horikawa Y, Tanaka C, et al: Evaluation of the effects of photoradiation therapy on brain tumors with *in vivo* P-31 MR spectroscopy. *Radiology* 160:827–830, 1986.
33. Calabrese G, Falini A, Santino P, et al: Clinical H-1 magnetic resonance spectroscopy in brain tumors. *Proceedings of the 12th Society of Magnetic Resonance in Medicine,* New York, 1993, vol 3, p 1526.
34. Bruhn H, Michaelis T, Merboldt KD, et al: On the interpretation of proton NMR spectra from brain tumours *in vivo* and *in vitro. NMR Biomed* 5:253–258, 1992.
35. Ernst T, Hennig J, Ott D, Friedburg H: The importance of the voxel size in clinical ^{1}H spectroscopy of the human brain. *NMR Biomed* 2:216–224, 1989.
36. Berkelbach van der Sprenkel JW, Luyten PR, van Rijen PC, et al: Cerebral lactate detected by regional proton magnetic resonance spectroscopy in a patient with cerebral infarction. *Stroke* 19:1556–1560, 1988.
37. Bruhn H, Frahm J, Gyngell ML, et al: Cerebral metabolism in man after acute stroke: New observations using localized proton NMR spectroscopy. *Magn Reson Med* 9:126–131, 1989.
38. Luyten PR, Marien AJH, den Hollander JA: Acquisition and quantitation in proton spectroscopy. *NMR Biomed* 4(2):64–69, 1991.
39. Breiter SN, Soher BJ, Lesser RP, Barker PB: Proton spectroscopic imaging and MRI of epilepsy. *Proceedings of the 12th Society of Magnetic Resonance in Medicine,* New York, 1993, vol 3, p 1546.
40. Cendes F, Andermann F, Preul MC, Arnold DL: Lateralization of temporal lobe epilepsy based on regional metabolic abnormalities in proton magnetic resonance spectroscopic images. *Ann Neurol* 35:211–216, 1994.
41. Bruhn H, Kruse B, Korenke GC, et al: Proton NMR spectroscopy of cerebral metabolic alterations in infantile peroxisomal disorders. *J Comput Assist Tomogr* 16: 335, 1992.
42. Gadian DG, Connelly A, Cross JH, et al: ^{1}H spectroscopy in two children with ornithine transcarbamylase deficiency. *Proceedings of the 10th Annual Meeting of the Society of Magnetic Resonance in Medicine,* San Francisco, 1991, vol 1, p 193.
43. van der Knaap MS, Ross BD, Valk J: Inborn errors of metabolism, in Kucharcyzk J, Barkovich AJ, Moseley M (eds): *Magnetic Resonance Neuroimaging.* Boca Raton, Fla., CRC Press, 1993, chap 6.
44. Kreis R, Ernst T, Ross BD: Absolute quantitation of water and metabolites in the human brain: II. Metabolite concentrations. *J Magn Reson* 102(1):9–19, 1993.
45. Michaelis T, Merboldt K-D, Bruhn H, et al: Absolute concentrations of metabolites in the adult human brain in vivo: Quantification of localized proton MR spectra. *Radiology* 187:219–227, 1993.
46. Kreis R, Ernst T, Ross BD: Development of the human brain: *In vivo* quantification of metabolite and water content with proton magnetic resonance spectroscopy. *Magn Reson Med* 30:1–14, 1993.
47. Heerschap A, van den Berg P: Proton MR spectroscopy of the human fetus *in utero. Proceedings of the 12th Society of Magnetic Resonance in Medicine,* New York, 1993, vol 1, p 318.
48. Boesch C, Gruetter R, Martin E, et al: Variations in the *in vivo* ^{31}P MR spectra of the developing human brain during postnatal life. *Radiology* 172:197–199, 1989.
49. Michaelis T, Helms G, Merboldt KD, et al: First observation of *scyllo*-inositol in proton NMR spectra of human brain *in vitro* and *in vivo. Proceedings of the 11th Society of Magnetic Resonance in Medicine,* Berlin, 1992, vol 1, p 541.
50. Grodd W, Kragelah-Mann I, Klose U, Sauter R: Metabolic and destructive brain disorders in children: Findings with localized proton MR spectroscopy. *Radiology* 181: 173, 1991.
51. Heindel W, Kugel H, Roth B, Benz-Bohm G: Proton magnetic resonance spectroscopy reflects metabolic decompensation in maple syrup urine disease. *Pediatr Radiol* 25:296–299, 1995.
52. Zimmerman RA, Wang Z: Proton spectroscopy of the pediatric brain. *Riv Neuroradiol* 5(1):5, 1992.
53. Kugel H, Heindel W, Roth B: Localized 1H MR in the pediatric brain: A useful tool for the evaluation of metabolic diseases? *Proceedings of the 11th Society of Magnetic Resonance in Medicine,* Berlin, 1992, vol 2, p 2012.
54. Rajanayagam A, Grad J, Krivit W, et al: H-1 MR spectroscopy study of childhood adrenoleukodystrophy. *AJR* 17:1013, 1996.
55. Hanefeld F, Holzbach U, Kruse B, et al: Diffuse white

matter disease in three children: An encephalophathy with unique features on magnetic resonance imaging and proton magnetic resonance spectroscopy. *Neuropediatrics* 24(5):244–248, 1993.
56. Schiffman R, Moller JR, Trapp BD, et al: Childhood ataxia with diffuse central nervous system hypomyelination. *Ann Neurol* 35:331–340, 1994.
57. van der Knaap MS, Gabreels FJM, Barth PG, Valk J: Disease of vanishing white matter. *Neuropediatrics* 26:338, 1995.
58. Lee JH, Arcinue E, Ross BD: Organic osmolytes in the brain of an infant with hypernatremia. *N Engl J Med* 331(7):439–442, 1994.
59. Bluml S, McComb JG, Ross BD: Differentiation between cortical atrophy and hydrocephalus using ^{1}H MRS. *Magn Reson Med* 37:395–403, 1997.
60. Haseler LJ, Arcinue E, Danielsen ER, et al: Evidence from proton magnetic resonance for a metabolic cascade of neuronal injury in traumatic brain injury. *Pediatrics* 99(1):4–14, 1997.
61. Ernst T, Ross BD, Flores R: Cerebral MRS in infant with suspected Reye's syndrome [letter]. *Lancet* 340:486, 1992.
62. Kreis R, Ross BD: Cerebral metabolic disturbances in patients with subacute and chronic diabetes mellitus by proton magnetic resonance spectroscopy. *Radiology* 184:123–130, 1992.
63. Bruhn H, Frahm J, Merboldt KD, et al: Multiple sclerosis in children: Cerebral metabolic alterations monitored by localized proton magnetic resonance spectroscopy *in vivo*. *Ann Neurol* 32:140–150, 1992.
64. Negendank WG, Brown TR, Evelhoch JL, et al: Proceedings of a National Cancer Institute workshop: MR spectroscopy and tumor cell biology. *Radiology* 185:875–883, 1992.
65. Negendank W: Studies of human tumors by MRS: A review. *NMR Biomed* 5:303–324, 1992.
66. Negendank W, Zimmerman R, Gotsis E, et al: A cooperative group study of 1H MRS of primary brain tumors. *Proceedings of the 12th Society of Magnetic Resonance in Medicine,* New York, 1993, vol 3, p 1521.
67. Grad J, Stillman AE, Hall WA, et al: Serial study of brain tumors by MRS following radiation therapy. *Proceedings of the 12th Society of Magnetic Resonance in Medicine,* New York, 1993, vol 3, p 1522.
68. Bruhn H, Frahm J, Gyngell ML, et al: Non-invasive differentiation of tumors with use of localized H-1 MR spectroscopy *in vivo*. Initial experience in patients with cerebral tumors. *Radiology* 172:541–548, 1989.
69. Luyten PR, Marien AJH, Heindel W, et al: Metabolic imaging of patients with intracranial tumors: H-1 MR spectroscopic imaging and PET. *Radiology* 176:791–799, 1990.
70. Frahm J, Bruhn H, Hanicke W, et al: Localized proton NMR spectroscopy of brain tumors using short-echo time STEAM sequences. *J Comput Assis Tomogr* 15(6):915–922, 1991.
71. Segebarth CM, Baleriaux DF, Luyten PR, den Hollander JA: Detection of metabolic heterogeneity of human intracranial tumors *in vivo* by ^{1}H NMR spectroscopic imaging. *Magn Reson Med* 13:62–76, 1990.
72. Kugel H, Heindel W, Lanfermann H, Lackner K: 1H NMR spectroscopic imaging—differentiation of human brain tumors and infarcts. *Proceedings of the 12th Society of Magnetic Resonance in Medicine,* New York, 1993, vol 3, p 1525.
73. Ott D, Hennig J, Ernst T: Human brain tumors: Assessment with *in vivo* proton MR spectroscopy. *Radiology* 186:745–752, 1993.
74. de Certaines JD, Larsen VA, Podo F, et al: *In vivo* ^{31}P of experimental tumors. *NMR Biomed* 6:345–365, 1993.
75. Vigneron DB, Wald LL, Day M, et al: Detection of metabolic heterogeneity in human brain tumors by 3-dimensional high spatial resolution (0.2-0.4 cc) ^{1}H MR spectroscopic imaging. *Proceedings of the 2d Society of Magnetic Resonance,* San Francisco, 1994, vol 2, p 1170.
76. Taylor JS, Ogg RJ, Reddick WE, et al: Quantitative MRI and MRS: The St. Jude Childrens's Research Hospital experience. *Neuropediatrics* 26:339, 1995.
77. Ross BD, Narasimhan PT, Tropp J, Derby K: Amplification or obfuscation: Is localization improving our clinical understanding of phosphorus metabolism? *NMR Biomed* 2(5):340–345, 1989.
78. Negendank W, Sauter R, Brown T, et al: Intratumoral lipids and lactate in ^{1}H MRS *in vivo* in astrocytic tumors. *Proceedings of the 2d Society of Magnetic Resonance,* San Francisco, 1994, p 1296.
79. Kuesel AC, Donnelly SM, Halliday W, et al: Mobile lipids and metabolic heterogeneity of brain tumours as detectable by *ex vivo* ^{1}H MR spectroscopy. *NMR Biomed* 7:172–180, 1994.
80. Videen JS, Michaelis T, Pinto P, Ross BD: Human cerebral osmolytes during chronic hyponatremia: A proton magnetic resonance spectroscopy study. *J Clin Invest* 95:788–793, 1995.
81. Ross BD, Ernst T, Haseler LJ, et al: ^{1}H MRS in acute traumatic brain injury. *JMRI* 8:829–840, 1998.
82. Matthews PM, Andermann F, Arnold DL: A proton magnetic resonance spectroscopy study of focal epilepsy in humans. *Neurology* 40:985–989, 1990.
83. Cendes F, Andermann F, Preul MC, Arnold DL: Proton MR spectroscopic imaging in the investigation of temporal lobe epilepsy. *Proceeding of the 12th Society of Magnetic Resonance in Medicine,* New York, 1993, vol 1, p 431.
84. Constantinidis I, Epstein CM, Peterman S, et al: Can 1H MR spectroscopic imaging lateralize temporal lobe seizure foci? *Proceedings of the 12th Society of Magnetic Resonance in Medicine,* New York, 1993, vol 1, p 429.
85. Gadian DG, Connelly A, Cross JH, et al: Relationship of cognitive dysfunction to 1H MRS assessment of temporal lobe pathology. *Proceedings of the 12th Society of Magnetic Resonance in Medicine,* New York, 1993, vol 1, p 430.
86. Hugg JW, Laxer KD, Matson GB, et al: Neuron loss localizes human temporal lobe epilepsy by *in vivo* proton magnetic resonance spectroscopic imaging. *Ann Neurol* 34:788–794, 1993.
87. Ng TC, Comair Y, Xue M, et al: Proton chemical shift imaging for the presurgical localization of temporal lobe epilepsy. *Proceedings of the 12th Society of Magnetic Resonance in Medicine,* New York, 1993, vol 1, p 428.
88. Breiter SN, Arroyo S, Mathews VP, et al: Proton MR spectroscopy in patients with seizure disorders. *AJNR* 15:373–384, 1994.

89. Gadian DG, Cross JH, Gordon I, et al: ^{1}H MRS and interictal SPECT in children with intractable temporal lobe epilepsy. *Proceedings of the 2d Society of Magnetic Resonance,* San Francisco, 1994, vol 1, p 344.
90. Kreis R, Arcinue E, Ernst T, et al: Hypoxic encephalopathy after near-drowning studied by quantitative ^{1}H-magnetic resonance spectroscopy. *J Clin Invest* 97(5):1–13, 1990.
91. Howe FA, Maxwell RJ, Saunders DE, et al: Proton spectroscopy *in vivo. Magn Reson Q* 9:31–59, 1993.
92. Truwit C, Kucharczyk J: Reversible cerebral ischemia. *Neuroimaging Clin North Am* 2(3):577, 1992.
93. van der Grond J, Balm R, Eikelboom BC, Mali WPTM: ^{1}H MRSI of the hypoperfused brain. *Proceedings of the 2d Society of Magnetic Resonance,* San Francisco, 1994, vol 2, p 611.
94. Graham GD, Rothman DL, Hwang J-H, et al: Spectroscopic assessment of alterations in lipids and small molecule metabolites in human brain after stroke. *Proceedings of the 2d Society of Magnetic Resonance,* San Francisco, 1994, vol 1, p 187.
95. Welch KMA. The imperatives of magnetic resonance for the acute stroke clinician (Plenary Lecture). *Proceedings of the 11th Society of Magnetic Resonance in Medicine,* Berlin, 1992, vol 1, p 901.
96. Petroff OAC, Graham GD, Blamire AM, et al: ^{1}H spectroscopic imaging of stroke in man: Histopathology correlates of spectral changes. *Proceedings of the 10th Society of Magnetic Resonance in Medicine,* San Francisco, 1991, vol 1, p 227.
97. Graham GD, Blamire AM, Rothman DL, et al.: Early temporal variation of cerebral metabolites after human stroke monitored by *in vivo* proton magnetic resonance spectroscopy. *Proceedings of the 11th Society of Magnetic Resonance in Medicine,* Berlin, 1992, vol 1, p 642.
98. Graham GD, Kalvach P, Blamire AM, et al: Clinical correlates of proton magnetic resonance spectroscopy findings after acute cerebral infarction. *Stroke* 26:225–229, 1995.
99. Barker PB, Gillard JH, van Zijl PCM, et al: Proton magnetic resonance spectroscopic imaging in acute stroke: Identification of the ischemic penumbra. *Proceedings of the 2d Society of Magnetic Resonance,* San Francisco, 1994; vol 1, p 186.
100. Sibbitt WL: Personal communication, 1996.
101. Sibbitt WLJ, Sibbitt RR, Griffey RH, et al: Magnetic resonance and computed tomographic imaging of acute neuropsychiatric disease in systemic lupus erythematosus. *Ann Rheum Dis* 48:1014–1022, 1989.
102. Sibbitt WL, Haseler LJ, Griffey RH, et al: Analysis of cerebral structural changes in systemic lupus erythematosus by MR proton spectroscopy. *AJNR* 15:923–928, 1994.
103. Larsson HBW, Christiansen P, Jensen M, et al: Localized *in vivo* proton spectroscopy in the brain of patients with multiple sclerosis. *Magn Reson Med* 22:23–31, 1991.
104. Moats RA, Watson L, Shonk T, et al: Added value of automated clinical MRS of the brain. *J Comput Assist Tomogr* 19(3):480–491, 1995.
105. Koopmans RA, Li DKB, Zhu G, et al: Magnetic resonance spectroscopy of multiple sclerosis: In-vivo detection of myelin breakdown products. *Lancet* 341:631–32, 1993.
106. Arnold DL, Riess GT, Matthews PM, et al: Use of proton magnetic resonance spectroscopy for monitoring disease progression in multiple sclerosis. *Ann Neurol* 36:76–82, 1994.
107. Davie CA, Barker GJ, Tofts PS, et al: Detection of myelin breakdown products by proton magnetic resonance spectroscopy. *Lancet* 341:630–631, 1993.
108. Arnold DL, Matthews PM, Francis GS, et al: Proton magnetic resonance spectroscopic imaging for metabolic characterization of demyelinating plaques. *Ann Neurol* 31:235–241, 1992.
109. Menon DK, Baudouin CJ, Tomlinson D, Hoyle C: Proton MR spectroscopy and imaging of the brain in AIDS: Evidence of neuronal loss in regions that appear normal with imaging. *J Comput Assist Tomogr* 14(6):882–885, 1990.
110. Jarvik JG, Lenkinski RE, Grossman RI, et al: Proton MR spectroscopy of HIV-infected patients: Characterization of abnormalities with imaging and clinical correlation. *Radiology* 186:739–744, 1993.
111. Tracey I, Guimares AR, Carr CA, et al: The AIDS dementia complex: Localized 1H MRS on human brain detects abnormal brain metabolism following HIV infection. *Proceedings of the 2d Society of Magnetic Resonance,* San Francisco, 1994; vol 1, p 584.
112. Vion-Dury J, Confort-Gouny S, Nicoli F, et al: Localized brain proton MRS might identify different metabolic profiles in AIDS-related encephalopathies. *Proceedings of the 2d Society of Magnetic Resonance,* San Francisco, 1994; vol 1, p 585.
113. Lu D, Pavlakis S, Frank Y, et al: Localized proton MR spectroscopy of the basal ganglia in normal children and children with AIDS. *Proceedings of the 2d Society of Magnetic Resonance,* San Francisco, 1994, vol 1, p 583.
114. Wilkinson ID, Chinn RJS, Paley M, et al: Serial proton spectroscopy of brain parenchyma in HIV infection. *Proceedings of the 2d Society of Magnetic Resonance,* San Francisco, 1994, vol 1, p 582.
115. Cousins JP, Tomalski W, Peters T, Wagle WA: NAA/choline and NAA/Cr as markers of metabolic changes in HIV + patients. *Proceedings of the 2d Society of Magnetic Resonance,* San Francisco, 1994, vol 1, p 581.
116. Meyerhoff DJ, Poole N, Weiner MW, Fein G: Are proton metabolites affected in brain areas of heaviest HIV load? *Proceedings of the 2d Society of Magnetic Resonance,* San Francisco, 1994, vol 1, p 580.
117. Hall-Craggs MA, Williams I, Wilkinson ID, et al: Proton spectroscopy in a cross-section of HIV positive asymptomatic patients receiving immediate compared with deferred zidovudine. *Proceedings of the 2d Society of Magnetic Resonance,* San Francisco, 1994, vol 1, p 303.
118. Chong WK, Sweeney B, Wilkinson ID, et al: Proton spectroscopy of the brain in HIV infection: Correlation with clinical immunologic and MR imaging findings. *Radiology* 188:119–124, 1993.
119. Vion-Dury J, Nicoli F, Salvan AM, et al: Reversal of brain metabolic alterations with zidovudine detected by proton localised magnetic resonance spectroscopy. *Lancet* 345:60–61, 1995.
120. Chang L, Miller BL, McBride D, et al: Brain lesions in patients with AIDS: H-1 MR spectroscopy. *Radiology* 197:525–531, 1995.

121. Carr CA, Guimaraes AR, Growdon JH, Gonzalez RG: Combining proton MRS and MRI morphometry increases accuracy in the diagnosis of Alzheimer's disease. *Proceedings of the 12th Society of Magnetic Resonance in Medicine,* New York, 1993, vol 1, p 233.
122. Shonk TK, Moats RA, Gifford P, et al: Probable Alzheimer disease: Diagnosis with proton MR spectroscopy. *Radiology* 195:65–72, 1995.
123. Chang L, Ernst T, Miller B, Melchor R: Proton MRS in Alzheimer disease and frontotemporal lobe dementia. *Proceedings of the 3d Society of Magnetic Resonance,* Nice, 1995, p 387.
124. Jenkins BG, Koroshetz WJ, Beal MF, Rosen BR: Evidence for impairment of energy metabolism *in vivo* in Huntington's disease using localized ^{1}H NMR spectroscopy. *Neurology* 43:2689–2695, 1993.
125. Jenkins BG, Koroshetz WJ, Chen YI, et al: Lowering cerebral lactate levels in Huntington's disease by energy repletion: Assessment using MRS. *Proceedings of the 2d Society of Magnetic Resonance,* San Francisco, 1994, vol 1, p 576.
126. Bruhn H, Weber T, Thorwirth V, Frahm J: *In vivo* monitoring of neuronal loss in Creutzfeldt-Jakob disease by proton magnetic resonance spectroscopy. *Lancet* 337: 1610, 1991.
127. Sherlock S, Summerskill WHJ, White LP, Phear EA: Portal-systemic encephalopathy: Neurological complications of liver disease. *Lancet* 2:453–457, 1954.
128. Bessman S, Bessman A: The cerebral and peripheral uptake of ammonia in liver disease with an hypothesis for the mechanism of hepatic coma. *J Clin Invest* 34(4): 622–628, 1955.
129. Bessman S, Pal N: The Krebs cycle depletion theory of hepatic coma, in Grisolia S, Baguena R, Mayor F (eds): *The Urea Cycle.* Chichester, U.K.: Wiley, 1976, pp 83–89.
130. Krebs HA, Henseleit K: Untersuchungen uber die Harnstoffbildung im Tierkorper. *Hoppe-Seyler's Z Physiol Chem* 210:33–66, 1932.
131. Geissler A, Kanamori K, Ross BD: Real time study of the urea cycle using ^{15}N NMR in the isolated perfused rat liver. *Biochem J* 287(3):813–820, 1992.
132. Hourani B, Hamlin E, Reynolds T: Cerebrospinal fluid glutamine as a measure of hepatic encephalopathy. *Arch Intern Med* 127:1033–1036, 1971.
133. Norenberg MD, Martinez-Hernandez A: Fine structural localization of glutamine synthetase in astrocytes of rat brain. *Brain Res* 161:303–310, 1979.
134. Reubi J-C, van den Berg C, Cuenod M: Glutamine as precursor for the GABA and glutamate transmitter pools. *Neurosci Lett* 10:171–174, 1978.
135. Butterworth RF, Layrargues GP: *Hepatic Encephalopathy: Pathophysiology and Treatment.* Clifton, N.J., Humana Press, 1989.
136. Danielsen ER, Ernst T, Geissler A, et al: Is hepatic encephalopathy a disturbance of cerebral osmolytes? *Proceedings of the 3d Society of Magnetic Resonance,* Nice, 1995, vol 3, p 1839.
137. McConnell JR, Ong CS, Chu WK, et al: ^{1}H MRS of the brain in patients with liver failure. *Proceedings of the 11th Annual Meeting of the Society of Magnetic Resonance in Medicine,* Berlin, 1992, p 1957.
138. Ross BD, Shonk T, Moats RA, et al: Proton MRS for the diagnosis of sub-clinical hepatic encephalopathy. *Proceedings of the 12th Society of Magnetic Resonance in Medicine,* New York, 1993, vol 1, p 131.
139. Ross BD, Jacobson S, Villamil FG, et al: Cerebral *myo*-inositol depletion defines sub-clinical hepatic encephalopathy. *Hepatology* 18(4):105A, 1993.
140. Gupta RK, Saraswat VA, Poptani H, et al: Magnetic resonance imaging and localized *in vivo* proton spectroscopy in patients with fulminant hepatic failure. *Am J Gastroenterol* 88:670–674, 1993.
141. Shonk T, Moats R, Lee JH, et al: Increased incidence of sub-clinical hepatic encephalopathy associated with TIPS procedure. *Gastroenterology* 104(4):A–449, 1993.
142. Bruhn H, Michaelis T, Merboldt K-D, et al: Monitoring cerebral glucose in diabetics by proton MRS. *Lancet* 337:745–746, 1991.
143. Lien Y-HH, Shapiro JI, Chan L: Effects of hypernatremia on organic brain osmoles. *J Clin Invest* 85:1427–1435, 1990.
144. Wong GG. Studies with *in vivo* NMR. D.Phil Thesis, 1981, University of Oxford, UK.
145. Lee JH, Ernst T, Ross BD: Phosphocreatine imaging of the brain: Improved interpretation through quantitative ^{1}H MRS. *Proceedings of the 12th Society of Magnetic Resonance in Medicine,* New York, 1993, vol 3, p 1535.
146. Lee JH, Ross BD: Quantitation of idiogenic osmoles in human brain. *Proceedings of the 12th Society of Magnetic Resonance in Medicine,* New York, 1993, vol 3, p 1553.
147. Danielsen ER, Ross B: *Magnetic Resonance spectroscopy in Neurological Diagnosis.* New York, Marcel Dekker, 1999.
148. Moats RA, Shonk T: Evaluation of an automated MRS examination: Application in Alzheimer disease. *AJNR* 16:1779–1782, 1995.
149. Ross BD, Jacobson S, Villamil F, et al: Subclinical hepatic encephalopathy: Proton MR spectroscopic abnormalities. *Radiology* 193:457–463, 1994.
150. Ross BD, Kreis R, Geissler A, et al: Clinical experience with proton magnetic resonance spectroscopy in chronic (and sub-clinical) hepatic encephalopathy, in Capocaccia L, Merli M, Riggio O (eds): *Advances in Hepatic Encephalopathy and Metabolic Nitrogen Exchange.* Boca Raton, Fla., CRC Press, 1995, pp 349–356.
151. Kreis R, Arcinue E, Ernst T, et al: Secondary hypoxic encephalopathy after near-drowning studied by quantitative ^{1}H MRS: Metabolic changes and their prognostic value. *Proceedings of the 3d Society of Magnetic Resonance,* Nice, 1995, vol 1, p 380.

CHAPTER 25

INTERVENTIONAL NEUROIMAGING

Camilo R. Gomez
Marco A. Zenteno

Interventional neuroimaging includes those therapeutic techniques that require some imaging modality for their application. Practically speaking, and from the perspective of this chapter, the term is most commonly applied to the use of catheters, guidewires, and balloons to treat vascular lesions of the nervous system. In this context, it has become synonymous with such terms as *interventional neuroradiology,*[1–4] *interventional neurology,*[5,6] and *endovascular neurosurgery,*[7,8] since it now involves specialists whose primary training is not only in radiology but also in neurosurgery and neurology. Thus, the discipline may best be referred to as *neuroendovascular therapy,* and the following is a review of the most salient features of this field, with an emphasis on the application of the various techniques to the practice of neurology. Table 25-1 lists the principal procedures discussed here. Due to space limitations, the list is not all-inclusive, but the procedures reviewed here are the most important due to their frequency and level of development.

BASIC PRINCIPLES OF ENDOVASCULAR THERAPY

In general, the performance of the techniques discussed below involves the introduction of coaxial systems of catheters, microcatheters, balloons, and other devices into the cerebral blood vessels. Most commonly, the vasculature is first accessed via the femoral artery or veins, where catheterization is most comfortable, convenient, and practical for both the operator and the patient. A vascular sheath (6 to 9F in diameter) is usually introduced into the femoral vessels and left in place, ensuring repeated access by means of various types of catheters throughout the procedure. Typically, a conventional diagnostic cerebral catheter is used to engage the carotid or vertebral arteries. Once in place, this catheter allows the acquisition of scout images used to plan the procedure to be carried out.

The next step is the substitution of the diagnostic catheter for a wider-lumen guide catheter (6 to 9F in diameter). The final position of the tip of the guide catheter, as well as its size, depend upon the procedure to be performed and the target vessel. For example, the larger guide catheters are reserved for procedures in which the final localization is a vessel of large caliber (e.g., the common carotid artery or the subclavian arteries). Through this guide catheter, smaller (i.e., micro-) catheters and balloons can be introduced and navigated under fluoroscopic guidance to the target point of the procedure. This navigational process can be carried out using either a flow-directed or a wire-guided technique. The choice of which method to use is largely dependent on the disease process being treated, but also on the preferences of the operator and the availability of materials.

Flow-directed techniques depend on the utilization of extremely flexible microcatheters (e.g., Magic, from Balt, Montmercy, FR; Regatta, from Cordis Inc., Miami Lakes, FL; and Ultralite, from Medtronic MIS, Sunnyvale, CA) with tips that respond to the flow within the vessels. Once engaged in the distal intracranial arteries, a flow-directed microcatheter can be repositioned by rapid small injections of saline solution. The injections cause the catheter to recoil and thus re-engage adjacent vessels. The most frequent utilization of flow-directed microcatheters is in the treatment of arteriovenous malformations (AVMs), where the augmented flow through the anomaly preferentially affects the microcatheter.

Wire-guided microcatheters navigate by taking advantage of the geometric architecture of the vasculature. These catheters are also of small caliber, and constructed so the tip is significantly floppier than the proximal shaft (e.g., Tracker, from Target Therapeutics, Inc., Fremont, CA; Microferret, from Cook Cardiology, Inc., Bloomington, IN; and Rapid Transit, from Cordis Endovascular, Inc., Miami Lakes, FL). They are fitted with microguidewires (0.010 to 0.018 in wide) with very atraumatic tips that can be shaped by hand, allowing their navigation even through tortuous vascular structures (e.g., Taper, from Target Therapeutics, Inc., Fremont, CA; Trascend, from Meditech, Inc., Natick, MA; and Silk, from USCI, Billerica, MA).

The development of skills related to the tasks described constitutes the core of the technical aspect of training in neuroendovascular therapy. Each of these tasks must be separately mastered and concurrently applied, for it is likely that a combination of several of them will be required during any one interventional procedure. In addition to those procedures described

Table 25-1
Principal Neuroendovascular Procedures

Clinical condition	*Endovascular technique*
Vasospasm	Intra-arterial vasodilating drugs
	Angioplasty
Aneurysms	Coiling
	Therapeutic balloon occlusion
Stenotic arterial lesions	Balloon angioplasty
	Stenting
Acute ischemic stroke*	Intra-arterial thrombolysis
	Angioplasty
	Stenting
	Intra-arterial neuroprotection
	Retrograde brain perfusion
Arteriovenous malformations	Embolization
Dural and carotid-cavernous fistulas	Embolization

*Neuroendovascular rescue.

below, other, more specific tasks are required during the performance of the procedures.

ENDOVASCULAR TREATMENT OF CEREBRAL VASOSPASM

Aneurysmal vasospasm is a rather critical condition with a potentially malignant course. It accounts for a very large percentage of deaths of victims of ruptured aneurysms.[9–13] In addition, general conventional therapeutic strategies are effective only to a point, requiring the clinician to be prepared to intervene in order to save the patient's life or prevent disabling ischemic damage.[14–20]

The neuroendovascular approach to the patient with vasospasm involves either the administration of vasoactive drugs intra-arterially or the performance of angioplasty. From the pharmacologic point of view, the first and most common agent utilized in this context has been papaverine.[15,17,21,22] Although intra-arterial papaverine is certainly capable of reversing cerebral vasospasm, the main criticism of the administration of its use has been the fact that its effect is temporary, requiring the procedure to be repeated within the 24 to 48 h that follow.[15,17,21,22] On the other hand, this technique requires less sophisticated equipment and only elementary neurointerventional skills. A microcatheter is placed within the vessel affected by spasm, and approximately 200 to 300 mg of papaverine is administered by continuous infusion over 30 min. Every vessel considered for treatment is subjected to the same intervention. In most cases, it is possible to use transcranial Doppler (TCD) to follow the effectiveness of therapy and the need for reintervention.[12,23–33] Lately, we, as well as others (O. Solis and J. Wilder, personal communication), have begun using this approach to deliver other pharmacologic agents that we consider more effective. For example, in Mexico, a parenteral preparation of nimodipine is useful in this circumstance, not only because of its vasodilating property, but also because of its potential cerebral protective effect. In the United States, we have used its counterpart, nicardipine, with similar success. However, it is likely that earlier generations of calcium channel blockers are also effective. One of us (CRG) is particularly inclined to use a combination of nitroglycerin (200 to 1000 μg) followed by verapamil (500 to 1000 μg). These two drugs seem to have a synergistic effect, which lasts considerably longer than that of papaverine. In fact, it is our view that, even if angioplasty is the primary intervention, the intra-arterial administration of these medications facilitates and complements the utilization of balloon angioplasty.

The usefulness of balloon angioplasty for the treatment of aneurysmal vasospasm was first reported in 1989.[34,35] Since then, numerous reports have been added to the literature, and its application has steadily grown. The results have been somewhat variable, but, in those patients in whom conventional medical therapy has not been sufficient to prevent the development of ischemic symptoms, angioplasty has proven in many instances to be lifesaving.[34–38] Over the last few years, further development of more compliant balloons of various materials and with various inflation characteristics has resulted in easier endovascular treatment of vasospasm. However, it has been our experience that it is possible and also as effective to use moderately compliant coronary balloons to treat vasospasm endovascularly (Fig. 25-1).

An important issue is the timing of the procedure. In the majority of medical centers where endovascular treatment of vasospasm is carried out, protocols involve the utilization of "triple H" (i.e., hypertension, hypervolemia, and hemodilution) therapy as a prerequisite for deciding when to intervene. The potential danger of this approach is that the procedure may be delayed beyond the point at which it can benefit the patient. In fact, there is a current trend to treat patients endovascularly as early as possible, avoiding unnecessary delays that may prove clinically devastating.[34–38]

ENDOVASCULAR THERAPY OF CEREBRAL ANEURYSMS

Historical Perspective

The endovascular approach of managing cerebral aneurysms is relatively recent. In the 1970s, the use of detachable balloons to obliterate aneurysms began as a therapeutic alternative in very selected cases of aneurysms not suitable for surgical management.[39] These types of balloons also allowed, in some cases, complete occlusion of the vascular structures that support giant or fusiform aneurysms, a technique that continues to be valuable for the endovascular approach in extreme cases.[39–41] The latter technique makes it mandatory that the operator

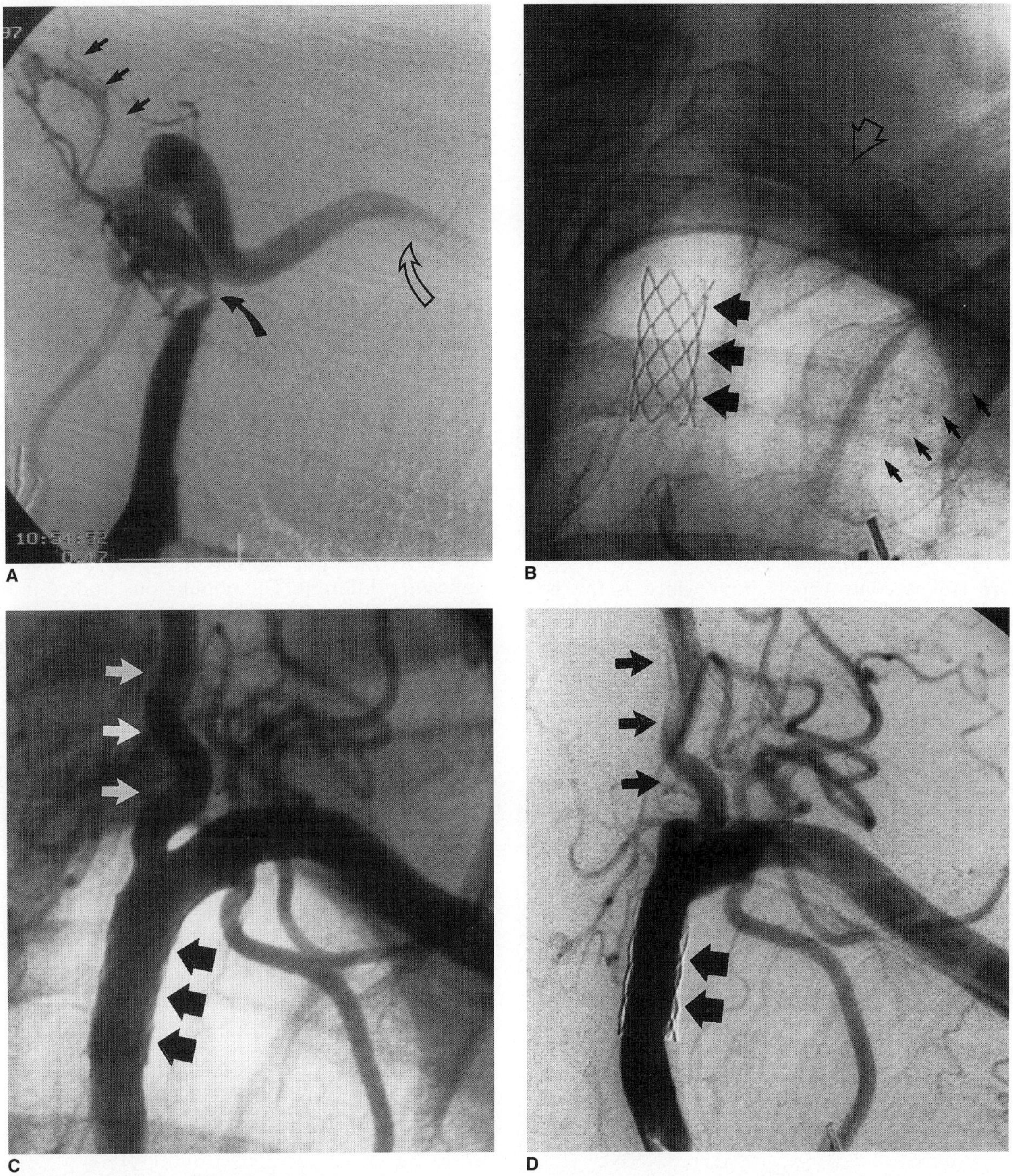

Figure 25-3

Angioplasty and stenting of subclavian artery stenosis and subclavian steal. **(A)** *Severe stenosis of the left subclavian artery is noted (curved black arrow), with poor distal run-off (open curved arrow). The vertebral artery is not visualized prior to treatment (small black arrows), since the stenosis is proximal to its origin.* **(B)** *The lesion was predilated using a peripheral balloon, and a biliary balloon expandable stent was deployed across the lesion (thick black arrows). Landmarks used during the procedure include the first rib (open straight arrow) and the clavicle (small black arrows).* **(C)** *The postoperative images show excellent results, with correction of the stenosis (thick black arrows) and restitution of antegrade flow to the vertebral artery (white arrows).* **(D)** *The six-month follow-up angiogram shows perfect placement of the stent (thick black arrows) and competent vertebral artery flow (small black arrows).*

Extracranial Carotid Artery

Treatment of the extracranial common carotid artery is perhaps the most controversial topic in neuroendovascular therapy today. The last decade has brought definitive proof of the benefit of carotid endarterectomy (CEA) for the treatment of symptomatic carotid atherosclerosis[60] and, to a lesser degree, of asymptomatic patients.[61] Therefore, the introduction of carotid artery stenting (CAS) as an alternative mode of therapy has met with considerable resistance from the surgical community.[62] However, at the time of this writing it is uncertain whether either of these methods is better for treating type A lesions of the common carotid bifurcation in low-surgical-risk patients. Already, CAS appears to be more advantageous in (1) patients whose stenotic lesion is relatively inaccessible, including proximal common carotid lesions (described earlier) and distal internal carotid pathology; (2) patients with nonatherosclerotic pathology (e.g., dissection, postradiation angiitis, or fibromuscular dysplasia),[63–68] and (3) patients with higher than average risk for CEA.

There still is controversy about which is the best method of performing CAS. The most widely used technique does not involve any specific steps for protection against distal embolism.[63,69] Essentially, it is analogous to that used in the coronary and peripheral circulations (Fig. 25-4). On the other hand, a technique introduced and championed by Theron et al involves the use of a distally placed protection balloon designed to catch and help remove any embolic material.[70–72] Although the concept of protection at first seems attractive, we think the current method is rather clumsy and we have found it to be relatively unnecessary.

An international registry of CAS has allowed compilation of the available experience in the most active centers around the world. An update of the results was recently presented at the International Congress of Endovascular Interventions.[73] At present, this registry manages data from 24 institutions in the United States and Europe, including ours (University of Alabama at Birmingham). A total of 2048 vessels has been treated using CAS over a period of approximately 6 years. The overall statistics include a mortality rate of 1.37 percent and stroke rate of 4.4 percent, which seem very competitive with those of CEA. In addition, it is important to point to two major differences between the data from the CAS registry and that from the available CEA literature. First, the populations of patients treated are significantly different. The populations studied in the major CEA trials included relatively healthy, low-risk surgical patients, as evidenced by the low proportion of severe coronary insufficiency, cardiac arrhythmias, and systemic pathologic conditions (patients with cancer, organ failure, or other degenerative conditions were

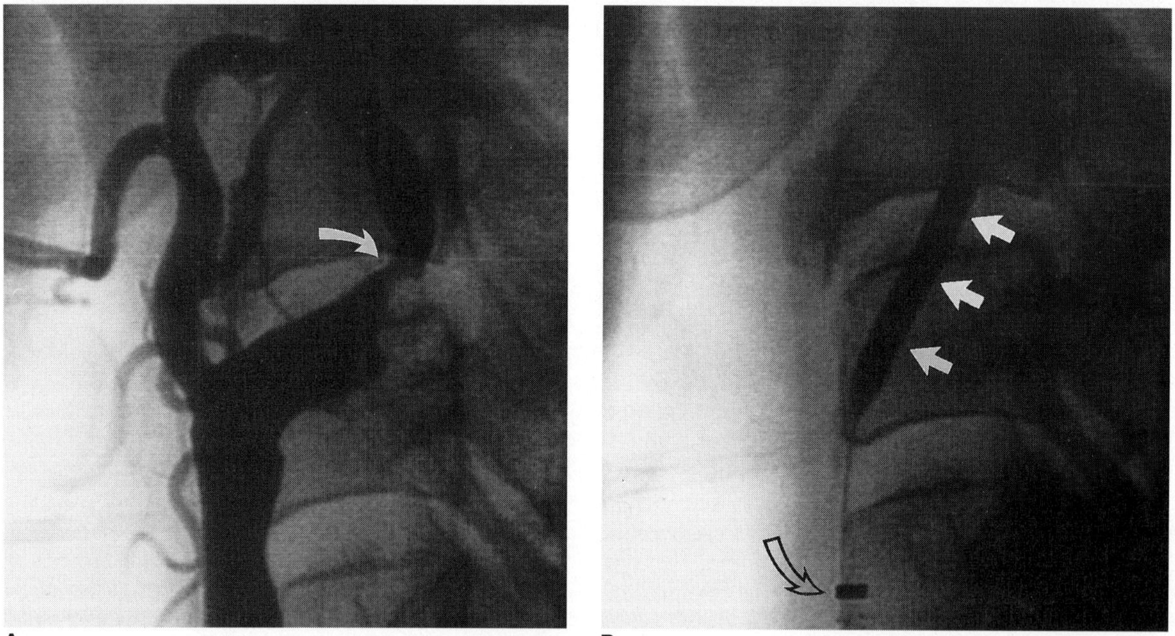

A B

Figure 25-4

Angioplasty and stenting of the extracranial internal carotid artery. **(A)** *A stenotic plaque with an irregular surface is seen in a lateral angiographic view (curved arrow).* **(B)** *The lesion is predilated with a compliant coronary balloon (white arrows).* **(C)** *Following predilation, note the degree of recoil and remaining narrowing caused by the plaque (large white arrow). Also, a small dissection is seen within the plaque (small arrow).* **(D)** *Then, a self-expandable stent is deployed across the lesion.* **(E)** *Postdilation using a noncompliant peripheral balloon is performed (black curved arrow) while the support wire is maintained across the lesion site (curved white arrows).* **(F)** *The final image shows an excellent result, with correction of the stenosis (white arrow).*

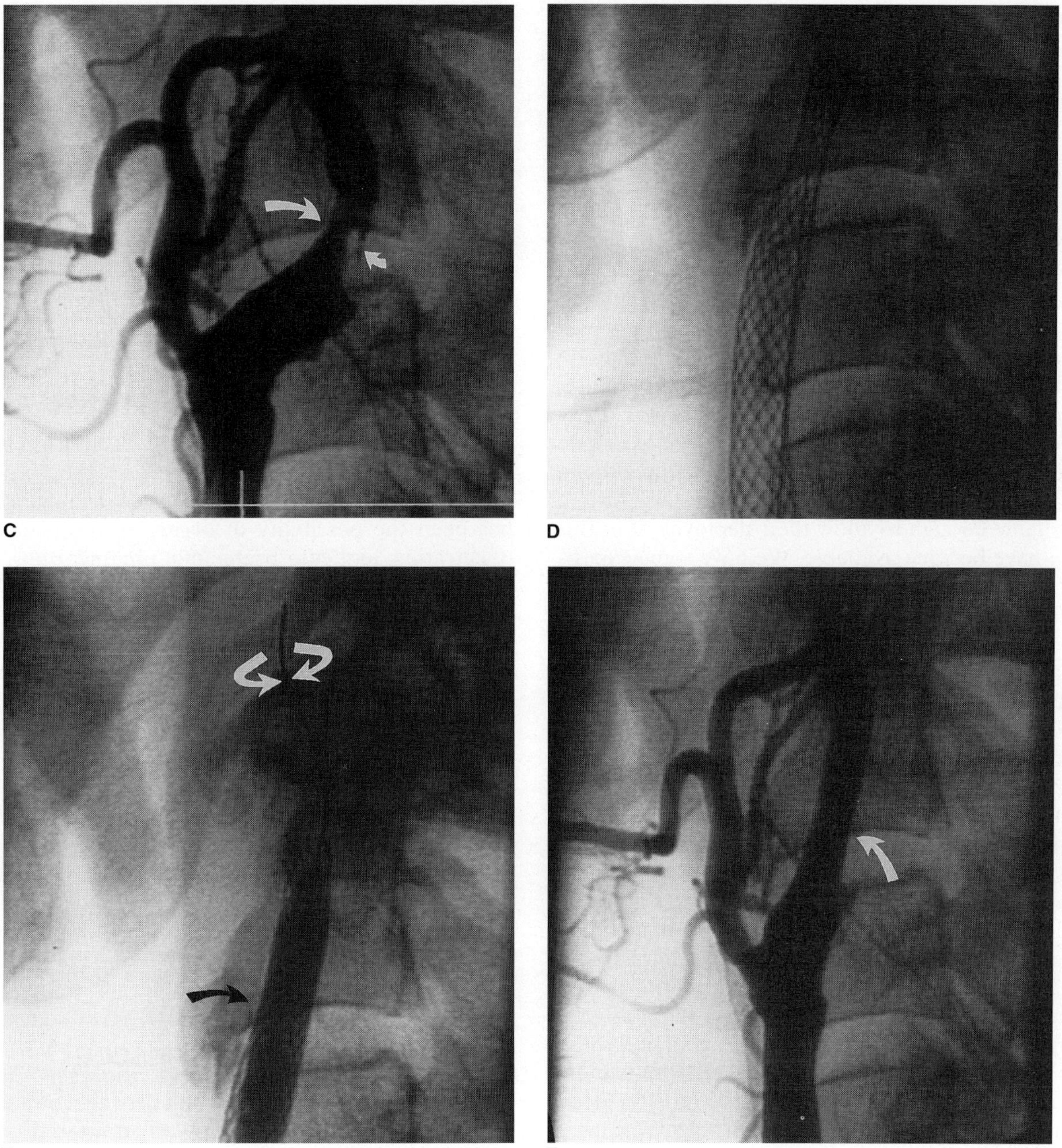

Figure 25-4 *(continued)*

excluded). The second factor is that the patients included in the CAS registry have undergone rigorous evaluations by independent neurologists prior to and following the procedure. This has allowed the diagnosis of minor events that otherwise might have been overlooked. Despite these differences, it is clear that CAS offers an exciting alternative to CEA and that further randomized prospective studies are likely to show exactly what its role and applications will be. In regard to the effectiveness of CAS, the currently available follow-up data from the CAS registry show a stroke occurrence of 3 percent over a follow-up of 24 to 36 months and a restenosis (i.e., greater than 50 percent stenosis of the treated vessel) rate of 4.5 percent over the same period. These results are also quite competitive, when one considers that the stroke rate in the surgical arm of the North American symptomatic carotid endarterectomy trial (NASCET) was 14 percent over 3 years and that of the asymptomatic carotid artery study (ACAS) was 10 percent over 5 years.[60,61] The future of CAS awaits the results of randomized prospective studies, which should probably be undertaken once the following criteria are met: (1) the procedure of CAS should be standardized; (2) there should be enough experienced endovascular therapists to carry out the study, and (3) the endovascular therapists should agree that the technology of stents has evolved to the point of using devices ideally suited to the carotid artery.

Intracranial Carotid Artery

Once the internal carotid artery penetrates the skull, issues related to its endovascular therapy change to some extent. For example, its petrous segment constitutes the only arterial structure surrounded by a continuous solid bony canal. This creates a situation in which the transmural forces to be considered during balloon angioplasty and stenting are singular. In our experience, the incidence of dissection of the petrous carotid artery following balloon angioplasty is so high that it has made us reluctant to treat these vessels without stenting them. Yet, it has not been until recently that stents flexible and pushable enough to allow their deployment in this location have become available. We have some experience placing second-generation flexible coronary stents (e.g., GRII, from Cook Cardiology, Inc., Bloomington, IN; Multilink, from Advanced Cardiovascular Systems, Inc., Santa Clara, CA; and Microstent II, from Advanced Vascular Engineering) in the petrous and precavernous internal carotid artery (Fig. 25-5). The results have been encouraging, but we anxiously await further developments of the stent technology that will allow easier treatment of this vascular segment.

The next segments of the internal carotid artery correspond to the cavernous portion, the siphon, and the clinoid portion. In these locations the vessel is surrounded by a venous sinus and then the subarachnoid space, each producing different sets of transmural forces during balloon inflation. It is relatively easy to perform balloon angioplasty of lesions located in these arterial segments (Fig. 25-6). However, in our experience, these lesions have a higher incidence of recoil following simple balloon angioplasty, and thus there is a greater need for stenting in these situations. The problem, again, is the lack of stents whose characteristics would permit us to consistently treat these lesions. This is another area in which the development of new, more flexible stents will be welcome.

Vertebral Arteries

The endovascular management of lesions in the vertebral arteries varies depending on which segment of the vessel is being considered. Stenoses of the V1 to V2 segments can be easily treated with balloon angioplasty and stenting (Fig. 25-7). We have found the latter to be indispensable, particularly in ostial lesions, which have a tendency for great recoil. In general, we have been using biliary balloon-expandable stents (e.g., Palmaz, from Cordis Endovascular, Inc. Miami Lakes, FL) to treat V1 lesions and flexible coronary stents (e.g., Flexstent or GRII, from Cook Cardiology, Inc., Bloomington, IN; Multilink, from Advanced Cardiovascular Systems, Inc., Santa Clara, CA; and Microstent II, from Advanced Vascular Engineering, Inc., Santa Rosa, CA) to treat V2 lesions.

The treatment of lesions in the V3 and V4 segments is somewhat different. The distance to navigate is longer and often tortuous, making the tracking of any of the available stents very difficult. However, balloon angioplasty is possible using coronary balloons (e.g., Predator XL, from Cordis Endovascular, Inc., Miami Lakes, FL), and stenting is not a distal reality.

Middle Cerebral and Basilar Arteries

There has been a certain reluctance to perform balloon angioplasty in patients with atherosclerotic lesions of the middle cerebral or basilar arteries. The main reason has been the possibility of occluding the ostia of the penetrating lenticulostriate and pontine branches of these arteries by causing a "toothpaste" effect when inflating the balloon. Another problem is the practical difficulty of stenting these lesions if a dissection were to occur, primarily because of the lack of suitable intracranial stents. Nevertheless, there are scattered reports of successful treatment of these lesions in selected patients, and at least three cases of successful deployment of coronary stents in the basilar artery have been reported. We have reserved this type of treatment for patients with recurrent symptoms referable to the lesion despite optimal medical treatment or for patients who are poor candidates for chronic anticoagulation. In such patients, the results can be quite good despite the lack of optimal stents (Fig. 25-8).

NEUROENDOVASCULAR RESCUE

Neuroendovascular rescue includes all intra-arterial procedures used to restore flow to an arterial territory following acute occlusion with ongoing ischemia. The original technique to which this concept refers is intra-arterial thrombolysis.[74–76] This procedure was first introduced in the early 1980s as a means of delivering "clot-busting" drugs to the site of thromboembolic occlusion. The results have been promising, particularly in specific populations, such as patients with occlusion of the basilar, internal carotid, or middle cerebral arteries. The recent approval of tissue plasminogen activator (tPA) for the intravenous treatment of patients with acute brain ischemia of less than 3 h of evolution has forced clinicians to take a critical look at who are the best candidates for intra-arterial thrombolysis. It must be remembered that, when intravenous thrombolytics were originally tested using angiographic control, the recanalization rates of large vessels were very poor, in the range of 10 to 30 percent.[77] This underscores the impor-

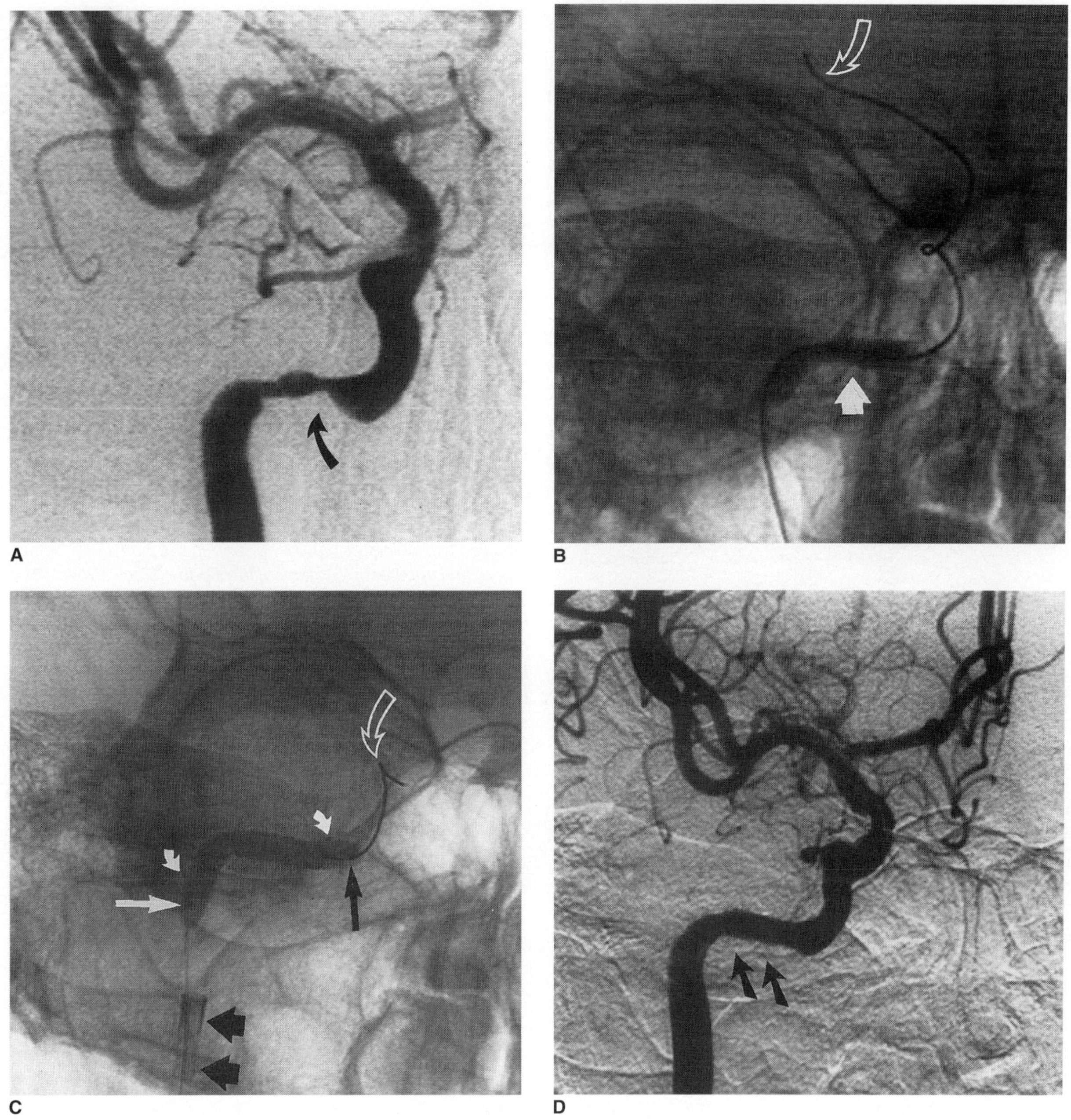

Figure 25-5

Angioplasty and stenting of the petrous portion of the internal carotid artery. **(A)** *A symptomatic stenotic lesion is displayed in the anteroposterior angiographic image (curved arrow).* **(B)** *The lesion is crossed with a floppy coronary balloon and predilated (thick white arrow). Note the microwire anchored in the distal middle cerebral artery (open arrow).* **(C)** *GRII stent is deployed across the lesion using the balloon (straight arrows) and the stent markers (small curved white arrows) to position it. The microwire is in the distal carotid (open arrow), and the guide catheter is close to the base of the skull (thick black arrows).* **(D)** *The final image shows correction of the stenosis (black arrows).*

tance of considering clot burden and the need to tailor the delivery of thrombolytic agents to the specific clinical and cerebrovascular situation. In general, the potential advantages of intra-arterial delivery of thrombolytic agents over the intravenous method include better management of clot burden, better dosing of the drug, and the opportunity to use additional revascularization procedures.

The technique involves the use of microcatheters that allow delivery of the thrombolytic agent directly into the blood clot (Fig. 25-9). In general, it has been our practice to first cross the point of occlusion using a floppy-tipped microwire (e.g., Trascend, from Meditech, Inc., Watertown, MA) and then with the microcatheter. Once the tip of the microcatheter is located distal to the point of occlusion, we obtain supraselective angio-

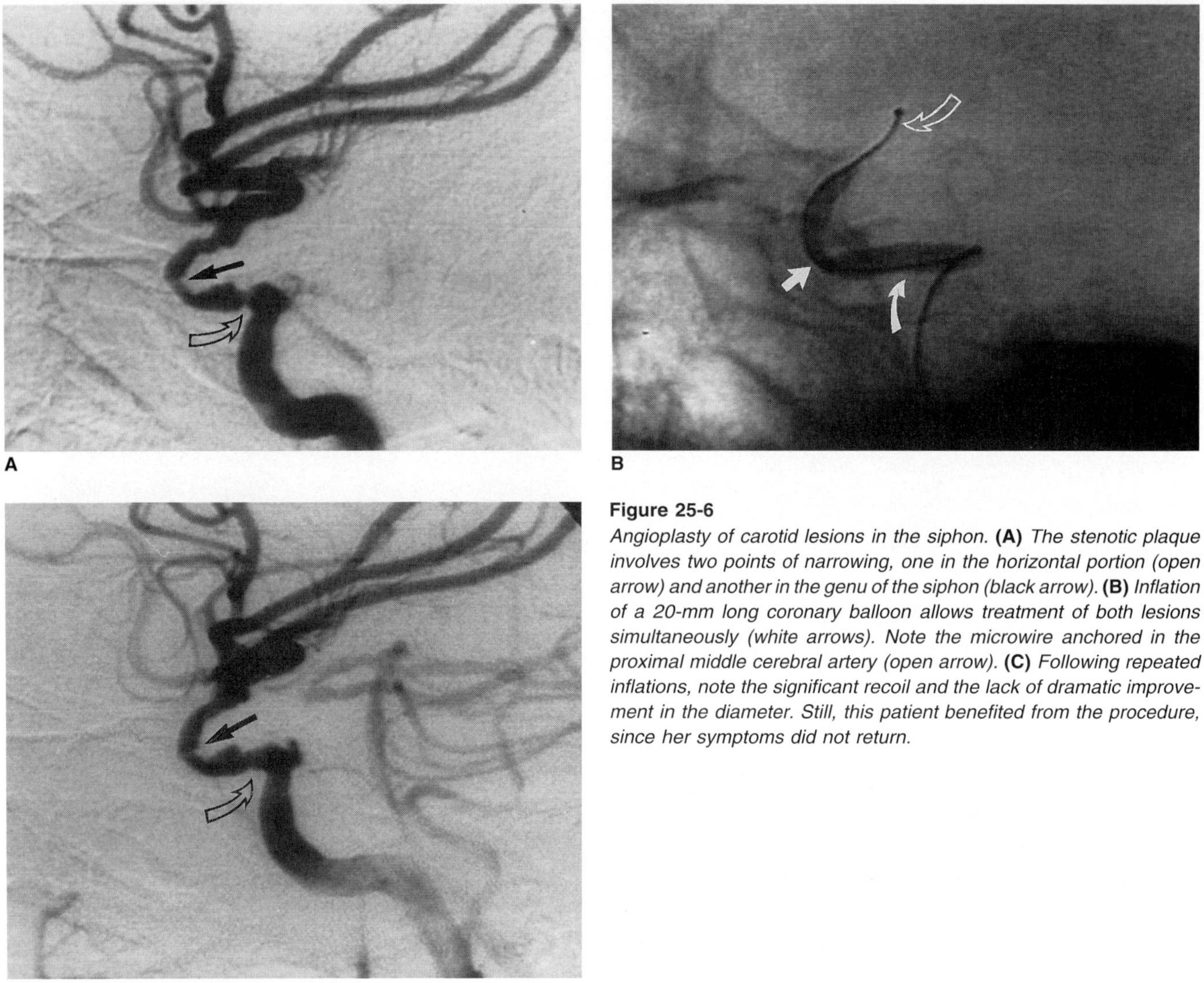

A B C

Figure 25-6
Angioplasty of carotid lesions in the siphon. **(A)** *The stenotic plaque involves two points of narrowing, one in the horizontal portion (open arrow) and another in the genu of the siphon (black arrow).* **(B)** *Inflation of a 20-mm long coronary balloon allows treatment of both lesions simultaneously (white arrows). Note the microwire anchored in the proximal middle cerebral artery (open arrow).* **(C)** *Following repeated inflations, note the significant recoil and the lack of dramatic improvement in the diameter. Still, this patient benefited from the procedure, since her symptoms did not return.*

graphic images and then inject a combination of nitroglycerin and verapamil as vasodilators (and possibly as neuroprotective agents). By vasodilating the distal arterioles, resistance to flow is theoretically reduced, and this may be of benefit in restoring flow. Next, the microcatheter tip is pulled back gently, until its tip is within the actual clot, and urokinase (Abbokinase, from Abbot Laboratories, Inc., Abbot Park, IL) is injected at a rate of 250,000 to 500,000 U over 20 min. The results are often both angiographically and clinically dramatic, although the potential for hemorrhagic complications, particularly in the territory of the lenticulostriate arteries, increases significantly as the time elapsed before treatment is prolonged over 3 h. Recently, a new kind of thrombolytic agent (pro-urokinase, Prolyse, from Abbot Laboratories, Inc., Abbot Park, IL) has been tried in a randomized, prospective, placebo-controlled fashion and has been found to be effective in a significant proportion of patients. Finally, it must be understood that the use of anticoagulants (i.e., heparin) following thrombolysis may carry an increased risk of hemorrhagic complications. It has been our practice to delay anticoagulation following treatment with thrombolytics for a few hours, until the coagulation parameters return to normal, and then to restart the heparin using a protocol that excludes the administration of bolus doses.

It is our opinion that neuroendovascular rescue therapy must not consist only of intra-arterial thrombolytics because, regardless of how they are used, thrombolytics carry the risk of cerebral or systemic hemorrhagic complications. Furthermore, there are patients whose clinical condition prevents them from being candidates for treatment with thrombolytic agents—for example, those who present beyond 6 h after onset, those who are anticoagulated with warfarin at the time of the stroke, or those who have recently undergone major surgical procedures. In these patients, other techniques must be

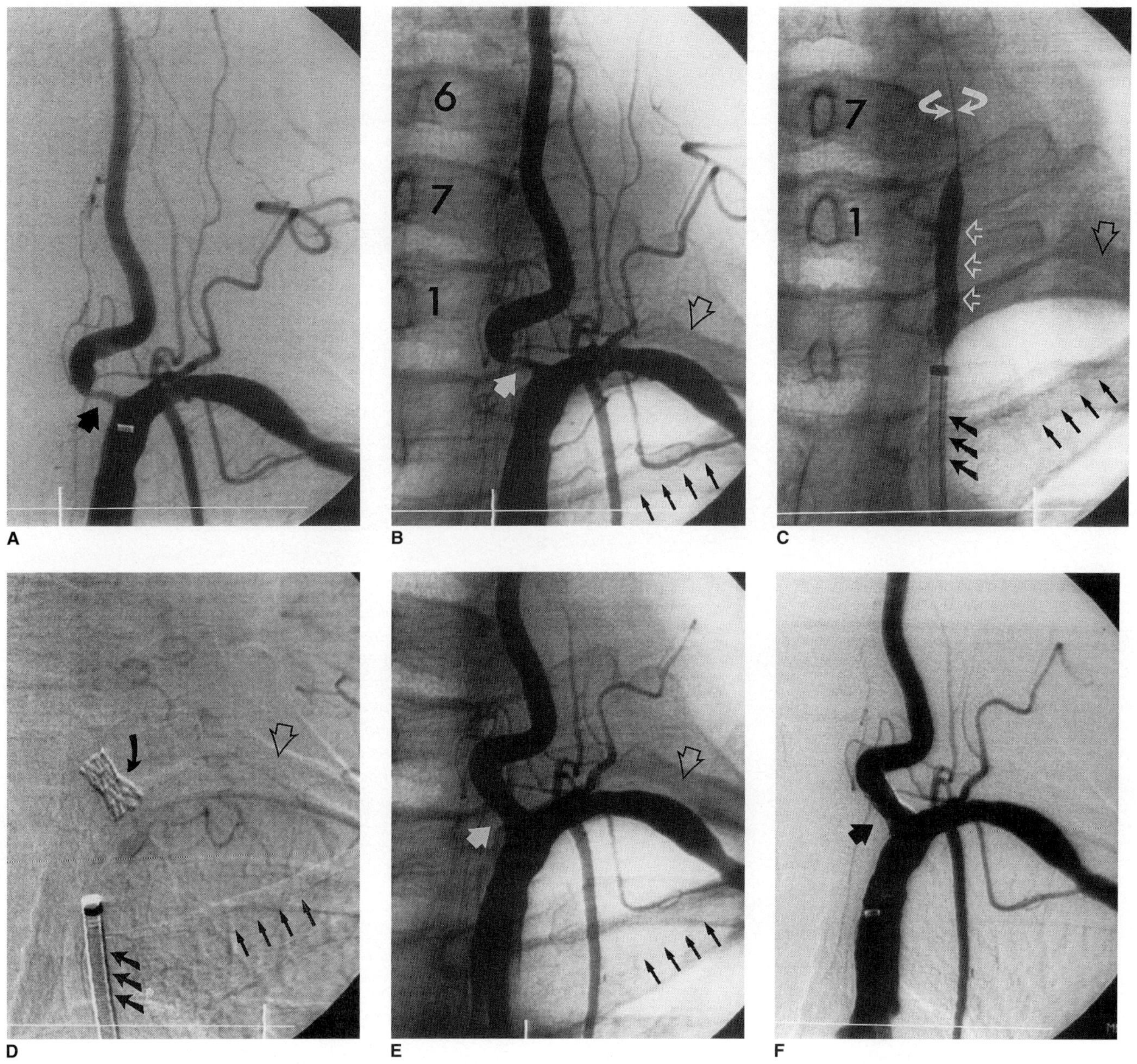

Figure 25-7

Ostial vertebral lesion treated by balloon angioplasty and stenting. **(A)** *A symptomatic ostial left vertebral artery lesion (black arrow) is displayed with full subtraction.* **(B)** *Partial subtraction allows visualization of the lesion (white arrow) and of various landmarks used during the procedure. The first rib (open arrow), the clavicle (straight black arrows), and the sixth (6) and seventh (7) cervical vertebrae as well as the first thoracic (1) vertebra are marked.* **(C)** *Predilation is performed with a coronary balloon (open straight white arrows), having the guide catheter (slanted black arrows) close to the origin of the vertebral artery. The landmarks are similar to those in the previous image, and the microguidewire (curved white arrows) is anchored in the distal vertebral artery.* **(D)** *Subtraction view of the deployed stent (curved black arrow) in relation to the previous landmarks.* **(E and F)** *Final images with partial and full subtraction, showing the results of the procedure, with correction of the stenosis (solid thick arrows).*

considered in order to restore flow to territories supplied by occluded large arteries. We and others have successfully used mechanical clot disruption and angioplasty (with or without stenting) for the treatment of acute brain ischemia (Fig. 25-10). This approach is practical, since it allows clinicians to limit the amount of thrombolytic agent used as well as to treat patients who are not candidates for thrombolysis. It has also been our experience that flow restoration, even if partial [e.g., changing the vascular occlusion from thrombolysis in myocardial infarction (TIMI) 0 flow to TIMI 2], is often accompanied by clinical improvement.

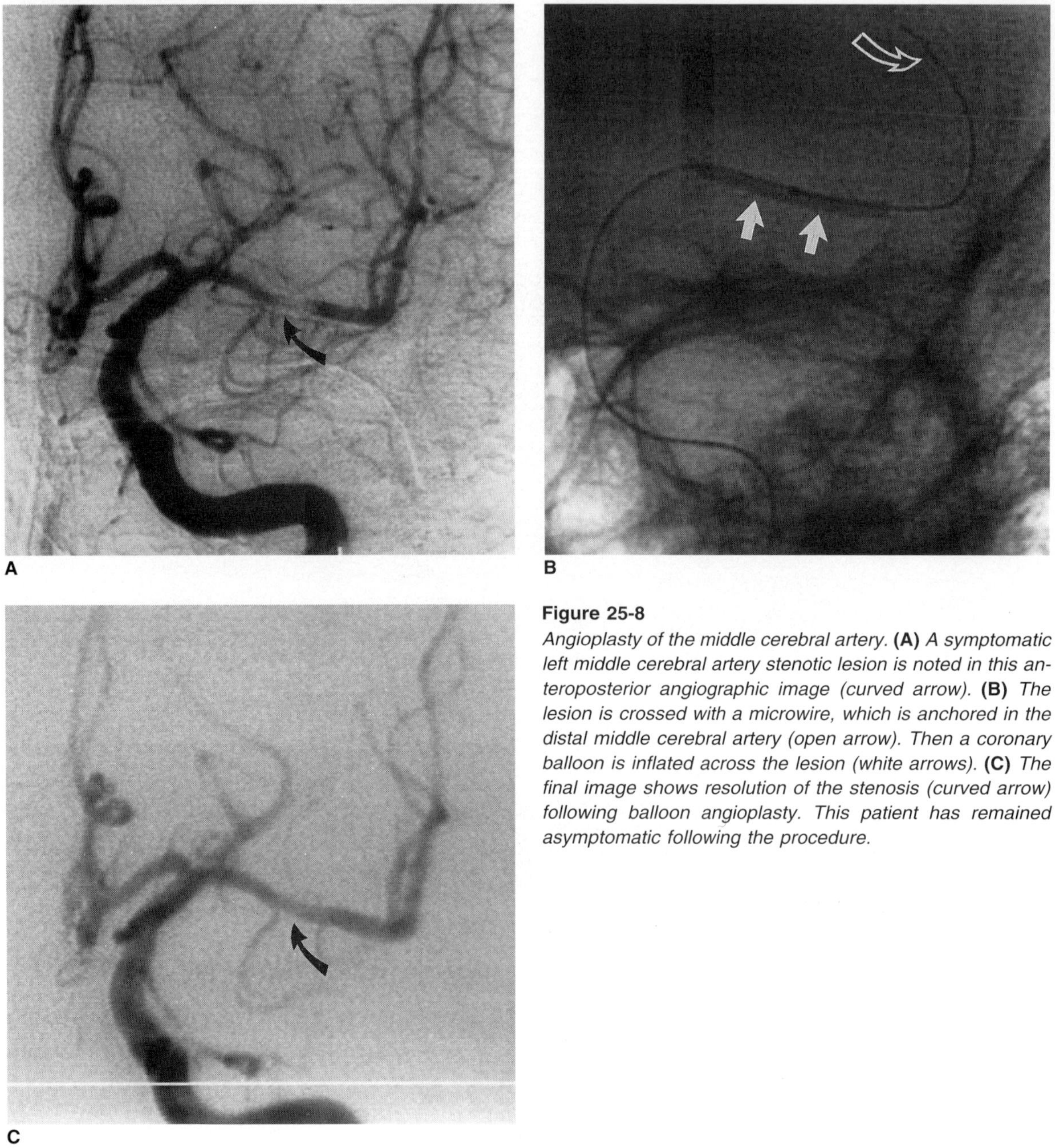

Figure 25-8
Angioplasty of the middle cerebral artery. **(A)** *A symptomatic left middle cerebral artery stenotic lesion is noted in this anteroposterior angiographic image (curved arrow).* **(B)** *The lesion is crossed with a microwire, which is anchored in the distal middle cerebral artery (open arrow). Then a coronary balloon is inflated across the lesion (white arrows).* **(C)** *The final image shows resolution of the stenosis (curved arrow) following balloon angioplasty. This patient has remained asymptomatic following the procedure.*

The explosion of new endovascular technology has also spread to devices designed to open occluded vessels or to improve flow in the ischemic area. Ultrasonic endovascular ablators, venturi-driven aspiration catheters, optico-acoustic disruptors, clot-retrieving microwires, and even lasers are currently being tested, and it is likely that they will become available for specific clinical situations. Retrograde cerebral venous perfusion is perhaps the most radical of all of the various techniques for neuroendovascular rescue. The introduction of balloon catheters into the lateral sinuses and their utilization for the retrograde delivery of oxygenated blood via femoral artery pump bypass is currently under investigation in patients with acute cerebral ischemia. Preliminary results suggest that this technique, may be of temporizing value, if nothing else, allowing time for the implementation of more definitive flow-restoring strategies.

ENDOVASCULAR THERAPY OF ARTERIOVENOUS MALFORMATIONS

Arteriovenous malformations are the most common form of congenital vascular anomalies of the central nervous system encountered in clinical practice. They are localized in the brain, the dura, or both. They can be supra- or infratentorial in location, and their vascular supply may be single or multiple. They can be associated

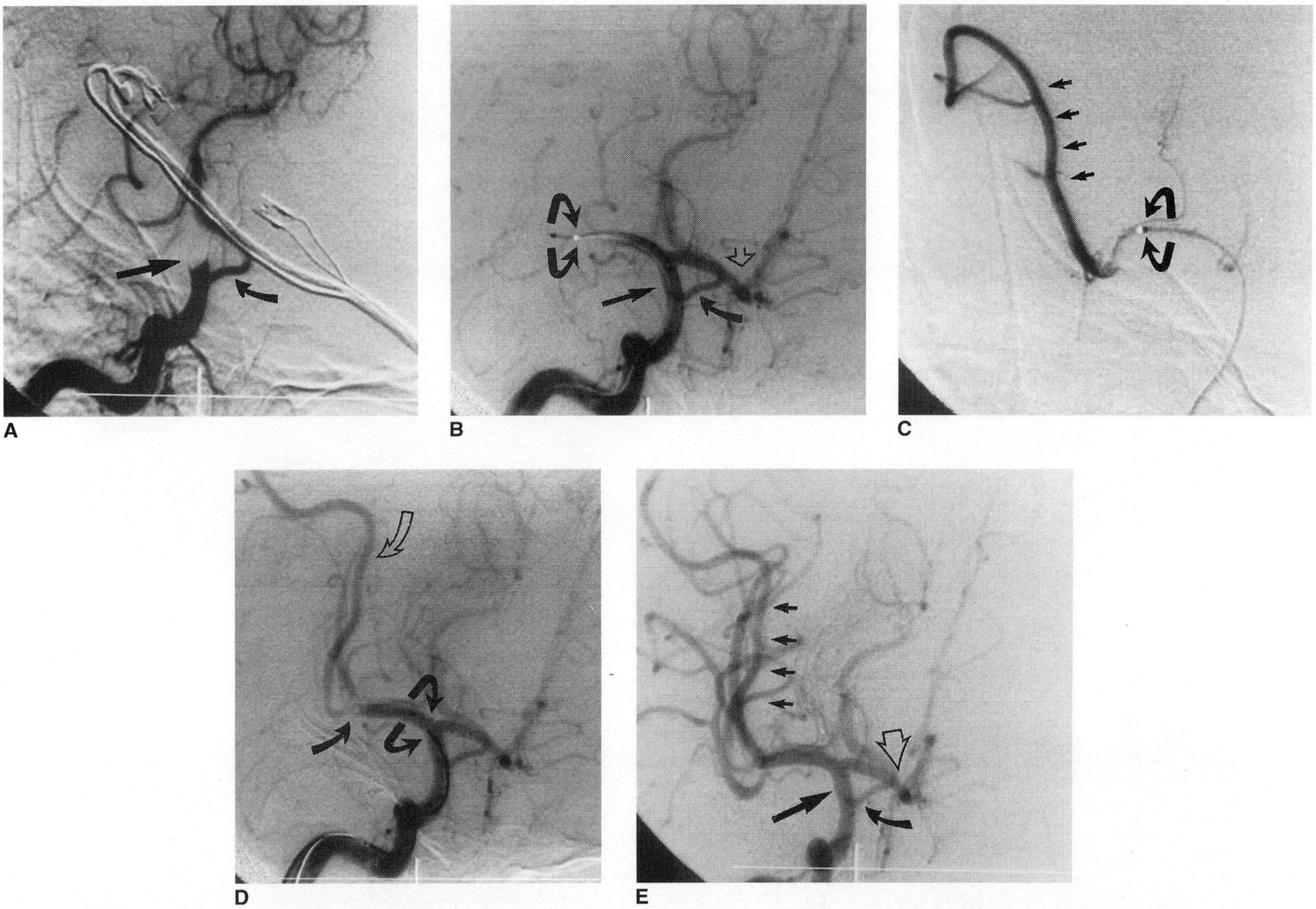

Figure 25-9

Intra-arterial thrombolysis of an occluded terminal internal carotid artery. **(A)** *The first image shows occlusion of the terminal internal carotid artery (straight arrow). The posterior cerebral artery is filling via the posterior communicating artery (curved arrow).* **(B)** *Injection of urokinase into the occluding clot results in recanalization of the distal internal carotid (straight arrow), with visualization of a normal anterior cerebral artery (open arrow) and proximal middle cerebral artery. The microcatheter (curved arrows) is advanced into the clot to continue the infusion of urokinase.* **(C)** *Prior to the infusion of additional urokinase, injection through the microcatheter (curved arrows) confirms distal middle cerebral artery flow (straight arrows). At this point nitroglycerin and verapamil are injected via the microcatheter.* **(D)** *Further microcatheter (curved arrows) infusion of urokinase results in progressive recanalization of the middle cerebral artery (open curved arrow). There is still a partial clot in its bifurcation (curved black arrow).* **(E)** *The final image displays good results, with recanalization of all branches of the internal carotid artery.*

with saccular aneurysms in 6 to 9 percent of the cases. From the clinical point of view, patients with AVM may present with one of many protean manifestations, including intracerebral hemorrhages, seizures, headaches, progressive neurologic deficit, and even mental deterioration (i.e., progressive hyperdynamic vascular dementia). In addition, the hemodynamic changes associated with AVMs, such as arterial steal, venous hypertension, and the pressure breakthrough phenomenon, are all capable of inducing neurologic symptoms.

Preinterventional Evaluation

The choice of therapy for AVM depends on the clinical presentation, the size, and the localization of the lesion. Modern neuroimaging modalities can provide both anatomic and functional information necessary for the selection of treatment strategies. Both computed tomography (CT) and magnetic resonance imaging (MRI) provide anatomic information about the size and localization of the nidus, as well as the status of the brain tissue that surrounds the AVM. From this perspective, magnetic resonance angiography (MRA) appears to be useful in the evaluation of the number and size of the feeding and draining vessels, as well as the architecture of the nidus. Finally, the incorporation of TCD into the diagnostic equipment available allows noninvasive follow-up of patients with AVM and their response to treatment.[78–82]

Conventional digital angiography remains the gold standard for the anatomic evaluation of AVMs. However, current diagnostic technology also allows the ac-

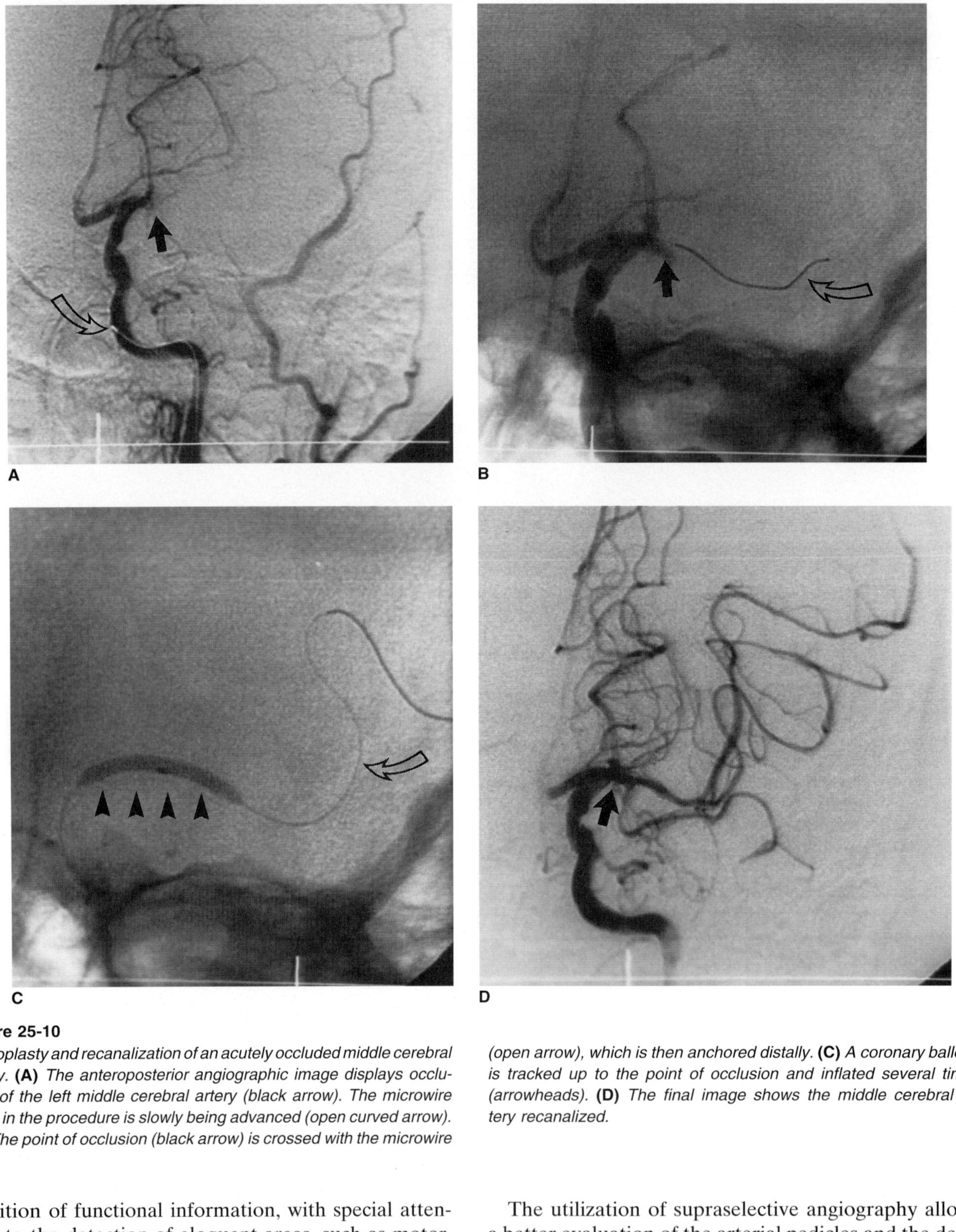

Figure 25-10

Angioplasty and recanalization of an acutely occluded middle cerebral artery. **(A)** *The anteroposterior angiographic image displays occlusion of the left middle cerebral artery (black arrow). The microwire used in the procedure is slowly being advanced (open curved arrow).* **(B)** *The point of occlusion (black arrow) is crossed with the microwire (open arrow), which is then anchored distally.* **(C)** *A coronary balloon is tracked up to the point of occlusion and inflated several times (arrowheads).* **(D)** *The final image shows the middle cerebral artery recanalized.*

quisition of functional information, with special attention to the detection of eloquent areas, such as motor, sensory, language, and visual cortexes. The most important technologic advances in this area include MRI,[83] somatosensory evoked potentials (SSEP), high-resolution electroencephalography, positron-emission tomography (PET), and the use of supraselective amytal and pressure measurement tests (e.g., the Tlalpan test).[84,85]

The utilization of supraselective angiography allows a better evaluation of the arterial pedicles and the demonstration of associated lesions, such an intracranial aneurysms (12 percent).[86] Also, angiography allows a better evaluation of the AVM nidus, and this allows for the determination of various arteriovenous circuits and their classification into plexiform (compact nidus), mixed (coexistence of a nidus and a fistula), and fistulous (true fistulas).[87] Recently, other classifications have been introduced, allowing for a more detailed analysis, including the identification of arteriovenous, arteriolovenous, and arteriolo-venular-venous circuits, favoring a more precise therapeutic approach.[88] Classifications such as that of Houdart and the hydraulic evaluation are changing current treatment schemes through a better selection of emboligenic agents.

Technical Considerations

Endovascular therapy for AVMs is considered a minimally invasive technique, with in-patient stays of less than 72 h in patients whose procedure is uncomplicated. The majority of the endovascular therapeutic approaches to AVMs are carried out within the confines of the neuroangiography or neurocatheterization suite, with the patient under conscious sedation and systemic heparinization. In general, access is obtained via the femoral arteries and, in exceptional cases (e.g., pediatric patients), under general anesthesia. The anticoagulation produced for the procedure is reversed at the end of the intervention by means of the administration of protamine at a dose of 10 mg for each 1000 U of heparin still active in the patient.

At present, catheterization and embolization of the AVM feeders is easily accomplished due to the availability of newer generations of microcatheters that can be navigated to locations very close to the AVM nidus (Fig. 25-11). In general, flow-directed microcatheters are the most commonly utilized, since they do not require microguidewires, thus reducing the morbidity related to vascular perforation. Embolization of an arterial pedicle and of an AVM nidus is generally preceded by a superselective amytal test. This test has allowed the identification of cerebral areas that, although usually not considered essential, have a certain degree of eloquence. Furthermore, the use of this test in concert with neuropsychologic testing and intrapedicular pressure measurements (i.e., the Tlalpan test) has resulted in an effective screening method for the assessment of the impact of AVM embolization.

The materials currently utilized for the embolization of AVMs include particles of polyvynilic alcohol foam (i.e., Ivalon, Unipoint Laboratories, High Point, NC), liquid agents (e.g., alcohol, *N*-butyl-cyano-acrylate), balloons, and detachable coils, among others.[89–91] In order to minimize the possibility of recanalization of the AVM, it is essential to deposit the embolic material within the nidus. In fact, occlusion of the arterial feeders without obliteration of the nidus may complicate the final extraction of the AVM due to the subsequent development of collaterals from the leptomeningeal, transmedullary, and transdural vessels. The treatment of large or giant AVMs requires a sequential obliteration or reduction of the malformation through multiple sessions of endovascular therapy. The recommended interval between embolization sessions varies between 3 and 5 days, while the interval between embolization and surgical extirpation is 7 to 10 days. This period allows hydraulic stabilization of the AVM and reduction of the edema that often follows aggressive reduction of giant AVMs by endovascular means. Finally, emergency surgical intervention is recommended whenever the endovascular procedure involves partial or total embolization of the principal drainage of the malformation, since such a situation may precipitate hemorrhagic complications, either immediately or within 72 h.

Goals of Embolization

Endovascular therapy of AVMs can be carried out as the sole method of treatment or in combination with microsurgery or radiosurgery. The elimination of deep feeding arteries, either anterior or posterior, greatly facilitates the approach to cortical malformations with subcortical or ventricular extension. The most important specific goals of endovascular therapy include (1) presurgical embolization of giant cortical AVMs, (2) preradiosurgical embolization of deep or cortical nonsurgical AVMs, (3) palliative embolization of large AVMs with progressive neurologic deficits, (4) palliative embolization of large cortical AVMs with intractable seizures, (5) palliative embolization of deep AVMs that present with progressive neurologic deficits or with hemorrhage, and (6) curative embolization of small AVMs, as a single-modality treatment.

Morbidity and Mortality Rates

The morbidity related to the endovascular treatment of cerebral AVMs is related to either ischemic or hemorrhagic complications that can occur during or immediately after the procedure. The ischemic complications have been dramatically reduced with the advances in supraselective catheterization, the new generations of microcatheters, and the utilization of supraselective amytal testing prior to embolization. The most important causes of hemorrhagic complications include arterial perforation, rupture of an intranidal aneurysm, and venous occlusion in partially embolized AVMs. In the initial series published in the literature, the mortality rate for endovascular therapy of AVMs was approximately 3.9 percent. However, the technical advances noted earlier have resulted in a reduction of the mortality rate to approximately 0.9 percent, while the surgical mortality rate approximates 1.52 percent.

DURAL ARTERIOVENOUS FISTULAS

Dural arteriovenous fistulas are abnormal communications between arterial and venous structures within the

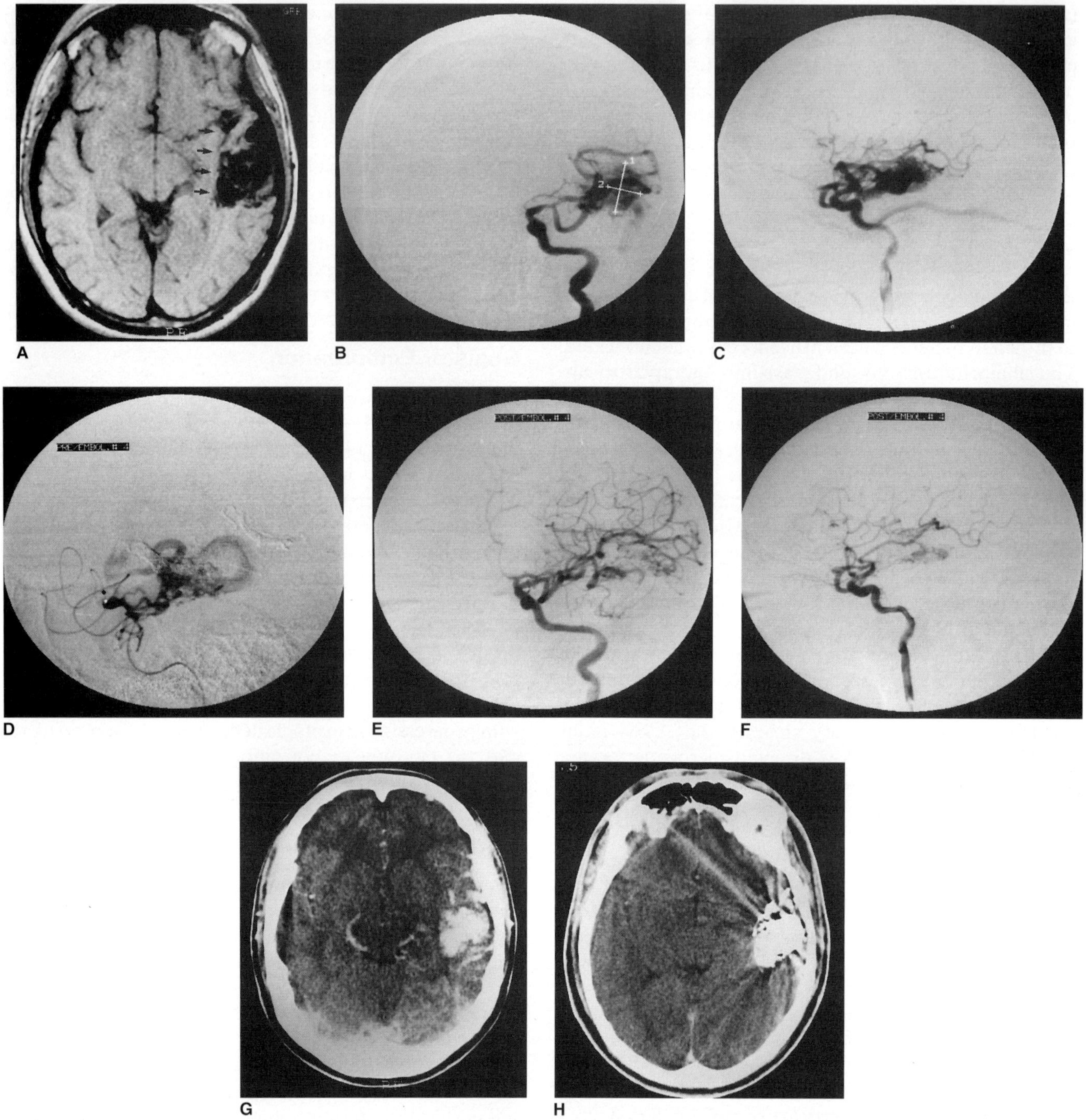

Figure 25-11

Endovascular therapy of an arteriovenous malformation. **(A)** *T1-weighted MRI demonstrates a left temporal AVM (Spetzler-Martin grade III). Pretreatment* **(B)** *anteroposterior and* **(C)** *lateral angiographic views disclose a parenchymal AVM fed by left middle cerebral artery branches. Note the absence of the left anterior cerebral artery due to steal.* **(D)** *Supraselective catheterization of the anterior temporal branch following embolization of the middle and posterior temporal branches. Postembolization control* **(E)** *oblique and* **(F)** *views show 90 percent reduction of the AVM.* **(G)** *Enhanced pre-embolization CT scan shows the AVM.* **(H)** *Unenhanced axial CT scan shows casting of the nidus with embolizing material.*

dura mater, with drainage into the dural sinuses, dural veins, or adjacent cortical veins. They are most frequently acquired and present most commonly in adults. Dural fistulas may be localized anywhere in the dura, but they are most common within the transverse and sigmoid sinuses, the cavernous sinuses, the superior sagittal sinuses, the anterior fossa dura (e.g., ethmoidal fistula), the superior petrosal sinus, and the tentorium. Much less frequent are fistulas that involve the inferior petrosal sinus and the marginal sinus.

The blood supply to the dura mater is complex, with intra- and extracranial contributions that must be studied separately. The intracranial irrigation originates from the meningeal branches of the intracavernous portion of the internal carotid artery (i.e., the meningohypopheseal and the inferolateral trunks); from the ethmoidal and anterior meningeal branches of the ophthalmic artery; and from the anterior and posterior meningeal branches of the vertebral arteries. The extracranial supply, on the other hand, originates from meningeal branches of the external carotid artery (i.e., dural branches of the ascending pharyngeal, occipital, middle meningeal, and internal maxillary arteries), as well as from the transosseous branches of the superficial temporal and posterior auricular arteries.

The clinical presentation of dural fistulas depends on their localization, arteriovenous short-circuits of high or low velocity, the presence of dural sinus thrombosis, and the recruitment of cortical veins. The latter may lead to the production of varices or to intracranial hemorrhages. When the fistula presents with minor symptoms (e.g., bruits or headaches) or when the angiogram demonstrates a low-flow fistula without cortical vein recruitment, conservative treatment by means of external compression is a reasonable therapeutic strategy.

The endovascular techniques available for the management of these lesions include transarterial and transvenous approaches and a combination of both. Deployment of embolic material on the venous side of the fistula, with preservation of the feeding artery, is the basic treatment. The embolizing agents available are similar to those used for AVMs. They include particles of Ivalon and Gelfoam, Upjohn Co., Kalamazoo, MI, which do not appear to have a permanent effect, liquid embolic materials (e.g., alcohol or acrylates), detachable balloons, and coils. The combination of current endovascular techniques results in a 95 percent rate of obliteration of dural fistulas of high flow located at the skull base, regardless of congenital or traumatic origin.

Transarterial Endovascular Treatment

From the perspective of patients who require endovascular therapy, the transarterial approach was considered the method of choice until the introduction of transvenous techniques. These involve first completing a comprehensive digital cerebral angiogram, followed by superselective injection of the dural feeding arteries, such as the middle meningeal, ascending pharyngeal, occipital, or internal maxillary arteries. Functional testing with amytal or lidocaine may precede the actual embolization, thus reducing the risk of cranial nerve paralysis. The main objective of transarterial embolization is to diminish the short-circuit, causing secondary thrombosis, or to facilitate subsequent surgical or transvenous approaches. The anatomic success of this approach is limited because it is difficult to deposit the embolic material exactly at the site of the fistula. Furthermore, proximal occlusion of the arterial feeders results in a rapid and generous development of dural collaterals, both ipsilateral and contralateral, with reactivation of the short-circuit with a more complex angioarchitectonic pattern.

The morbidity associated with this technique is rather low when it is performed by an expert. The risks of the procedure include injury to the cervical arterial structures, cerebral ischemia, and cranial nerve paralysis. The latter is related to ischemia of the nerve secondary to occlusion of meningeal branches that supply the cranial nerves as they enter or exit the skull. For example, paralysis of cranial nerves IX, X, and XI is usually due to embolization of a neuromeningeal branch of the ascending pharyngeal artery, while paralysis of the VII nerve is secondary to embolization of the superior tympanic branches of the middle meningeal artery or the stylomastoid branch of the occipital artery.

Transvenous Endovascular Approach

Transvenous embolization of dural fistulas has been popularized by Urtasun et al.[92] The intracranial navigation through the dural sinuses using the jugular, femoral, or surgical approaches is safe and allows placement of a catheter, microcatheter, and embolic material at the site of the fistula without the need for transarterial navigation. For example, embolization of the transverse sinus is possible by means of an ipsilateral transvenous approach even if the sinus is partially occluded. Also, contralateral transjugular-transocular navigation may be used to treat a transverse sigmoid sinus fistula with complete thrombosis. Cavernous fistulas may be easily embolized through catheterization of the inferior petrosal sinus or, alternatively, via the superior or inferior ophthalmic veins in the absence of posterior drainage.

Surgical Management of Dural Fistulas

The surgical treatment of dural fistulas is used as a last resort when endovascular techniques have failed to completely occlude a fistula that shows cortical venous drainage and venous hypertension. Surgery is in fact very useful in the management of fistulas that involve the superior petrosal sinus or the tentorium, and it is the treatment of choice for ethmoid sinus fistulas. Preembolization has reduced dramatically the rates of surgical morbidity and mortality of these lesions, particularly as related to uncontrolled blood loss.

Carotid-Cavernous Fistulas

For traumatic carotid cavernous fistulas, the classic technique of transarterial navigation and embolization by means of detachable balloons, as described by Serbinenko and Debrun, continues to be a very effective therapeutic approach with a high-rate of obliteration and low rates of morbidity and mortality.[92–94] However, similar results may be obtained using detachable coils delivered by transarterial or transvenous means.

CONCLUSIONS

The field of neuroendovascular therapy is rapidly growing. New technology and operators' expertise are developing at a pace that will make this discipline progressively more available and successful. Practitioners in multiple specialties can share in the growth of this field through collaboration, cross-fertilization, and mutual support. It is important that training programs expose resident physicians to these techniques and the impact that they can have in the management of neurovascular patients. Such an approach will ensure access to neuroendovascular therapy for a larger segment of the population.

REFERENCES

1. Khayata M, Aymard A, Guichard JP, et al: Interventional neuroradiology. *Curr Opin Radiol* 4:71–78, 1992.
2. Pelz DM: Interventional neuroradiology (review). *Baillieres Clin Neurol* 4:297–315, 1995.
3. Setton A, Berenstein A: Interventional neuroradiology (review). *Curr Opin Neurol Neurosurg* 5:870–880, 1992.
4. Vinuela F, Dion J, Lylyk P, et al: Update on interventional neuroradiology (review). *AJR* 153:23–33, 1989.
5. Kori SH: Interventional neurology: A subspecialty whose time has come (see comments; review). *Neurology* 43: 2395–2399, 1993.
6. Gomez CR: Interventional neurology (letter; comment). *Neurology* 45:850, 1995.
7. Hopkins LN, Strother CM: Neuroendovascular training. *Neurosurg Clin North Am* 5:565–567, 1994.
8. Guterman LR, Standard SC, Ahuja A, et al: Vascular and endovascular neurosurgery (review). *Curr Opin Neurol* 6:854–859, 1993.
9. Grosset DG, Straiton J, du Trevou M, et al: Prediction of symptomatic vasospasm after subarachnoid hemorrhage by rapidly increasing transcranial Doppler velocity and cerebral blood flow changes. *Stroke* 23:674–679.
10. Grosset DG, Straiton J, McDonald I, et al: Angiographic and Doppler diagnosis of cerebral artery vasospasm following subarachnoid haemorrhage. *Br J Neurosurg* 7:291–298, 1993.
11. Jakobsen M, Enevoldsen E, Dalager T: Spasm index in subarachnoid haemorrhage: Consequences of vasospasm upon cerebral blood flow and oxygen extraction. *Acta Neurol Scand* 82:311–320, 1990.
12. Lindegaard KF, Nornes H, Bakke SJ, et al: Cerebral vasospasm after subarachnoid haemorrhage investigated by means of transcranial Doppler ultrasound. *Acta Neurochir Suppl* 42:81–84, 1988.
13. Schaller C, Raueiser B, Rohde V, et al: Cerebral vasospasm after subarachnoid haemorrhage of unknown aetiology: A clinical and transcranial Doppler study. *Acta Neurochir* 138:560–568, 1996.
14. Zabramski JM, Spetzler RF, Lee KS, et al: Phase I trial of tissue plasminogen activator for the prevention of vasospasm in patients with aneurysmal subarachnoid hemorrhage. *J Neurosurg* 75:189–196, 1991.
15. Yoshimura S, Tsukahara T, Hashimoto N, et al: Intraarterial infusion of papaverine combined with intravenous administration of high-dose nicardipine for cerebral vasospasm. *Acta Neurochir* 135:186–190, 1995.
16. Vardiman AB, Kopitnik TA, Purdy PD, et al: Treatment of traumatic arterial vasospasm with intraarterial papaverine infusion. *AJNR* 16:319–321.
17. Eckard DA, Purdy PD, Girson MS, et al: Intraarterial papaverine for relief of catheter-induced intracranial vasospasm. *AJR* 158:883–884, 1992.
18. Konishi Y, Maemura E, Sato E, et al: A therapy against vasospasm after subarachnoidal haemorrhage: Clinical experience of balloon angioplasty. *Neurol Res* 12:103–105, 1990.
19. Le Roux PD, Newell DW, Eskridge J, et al: Severe symptomatic vasospasm: The role of immediate postoperative angioplasty. *J Neurosurg* 80:224–229, 1994.
20. Mizoi K, Yoshimoto T, Takahashi A, et al: Prospective study on the prevention of cerebral vasospasm by intrathecal fibrinolytic therapy with tissue-type plasminogen activator. *J Neurosurg* 78:430–437, 1993.
21. Fujiwara N, Honjo Y, Ohkawa M, et al: Intraarterial infusion of papaverine in experimental cerebral vasospasm (see comments). *AJNR* 18:255–262, 1997.
22. Kaku Y, Yonekawa Y, Tsukahara T, et al: Superselective intra-arterial infusion of papaverine for the treatment of cerebral vasospasm after subarachnoid hemorrhage. *J Neurosurg* 77:842–847.
23. Lennihan L, Petty GW, Fink ME, et al: Transcranial Doppler detection of anterior cerebral artery vasospasm. *J Neurol Neurosurg Psychiatry* 56:906–909, 1993.
24. Meixensberger J, Hamelbeck B, Dings J, et al: Critical increase of blood flow velocities after subarachnoid haemorrhage: Vasospasm versus hyperaemia. *Zentralbl Neurochir* 57:70–75, 1996.
25. Muttaqin Z, Arita K, Uozumi T, et al: Vasospasm after traumatic subarachnoid haemorrhage: Transcranial Doppler evaluation, case report. *Neurosurg Rev* 14:321–325, 1991.
26. Newell DW, Winn HR: Transcranial Doppler in cerebral vasospasm (Review). *Neurosurg Clin North Am* 1:319–328, 1990.

D

I

ISBN 0-07-134615-5

90000

9 780071 346153